Breastfeeding and Human Lactation

BREASTFEEDING AND HUMAN LACTATION

LACTATION

THIRD EDITION

Jan Riordan, EdD, RN, IBCLC, FAAN
Professor
School of Nursing
Wichita State University
Wichita, Kansas
Lactation Consultant
Via Christi Regional Medical Center
St. Joseph Campus
Wichita, Kansas

JONES AND BARTLETT PUBLISHERS
Sudbury, Massachusetts
BOSTON   TORONTO   LONDON   SINGAPORE

World Headquarters

Jones and Bartlett Publishers
40 Tall Pine Drive
Sudbury, MA 01776
978-443-5000
info@jbpub.com
www.jbpub.com

Jones and Bartlett Publishers Canada
2406 Nikanna Road
Mississauga, ON L5C 2W6
CANADA

Jones and Bartlett Publishers
International
Barb House, Barb Mews
London W6 7PA
UK

Library of Congress Cataloging-in-Publication Data

Breastfeeding and human lactation / [edited by] Jan Riordan.– 3rd ed.
    p. ; cm.
Includes bibliographical references and index.
  ISBN 0-7637-4585-5 (hardcover)
 1. Breast feeding. 2. Lactation.
 [DNLM: 1. Breast Feeding. 2. Infant Nutrition. 3. Lactation. 4.
Milk, Human. WS 125 B8293 2004] I. Riordan, Jan.
  RJ216.B775 2004
  649'.33–dc22   2003022400

Chief Executive Officer: Clayton Jones
Chief Operating Officer: Don W. Jones, Jr.
President of Jones and Bartlett Higher Education and Professional Publishing: Robert W. Holland, Jr.
V.P., Design and Production: Anne Spencer
V.P., Manufacturing and Inventory Control: Therese Bräuer
V.P. of Sales and Marketing: William Kane
Acquisitions Editor: Penny M. Glynn
Production Manager: Amy Rose

Editorial Assistant: Amy Sibley
Associate Production Editor: Jenny L. McIsaac
Director of Marketing: Alisha Weisman
Marketing Manager: Edward McKenna
Manufacturing Buyer: Amy Bacus
Cover Design: Anne Spencer
Composition: Modern Graphics Incorporated
Printing and Binding: Malloy Inc.
Cover Printing: Malloy Inc.

Printed in the United States of America
08 07 06 05   10 9 8 7 6 5 4 3 2

*This book is dedicated to breastfeeding women
and their babies around the globe.*

TABLE OF CONTENTS

SECTION 1

HISTORICAL AND WORK PERSPECTIVES

SECTION 2

ANATOMICAL AND BIOLOGICAL IMPERATIVES

SECTION 3

PRENATAL, PERINATAL, AND POSTNATAL PERIODS

CHAPTER 9

Breast-Related Problems   247

CHAPTER 10

Low Intake in the Breastfed Infant: Maternal and Infant Considerations   277

CHAPTER 11

Jaundice and the Breastfed Baby   311

CHAPTER 12

Breast Pumps and Other Technologies   323

CHAPTER 13

Breastfeeding the Preterm Infant 367

SECTION 4

BEYOND POSTPARTUM

CHAPTER 20

Infant Assessment 591

CHAPTER 21

Fertility, Sexuality, and Contraception During Lactation 621

SECTION 5

SOCIOCULTURAL AND RESEARCH ISSUES

CHAPTER 22

Research, Theory, and Lactation 655

I have worked in the field of lactation since the early 1960s, first as a La Leche Leader and later as a lactation consultant when it became a professional practice discipline in 1985. As I look back over those years I am struck both by how different things are now and by how much things have stayed the same. Although the breastfeeding initiation rate in the United States has risen to almost 70 percent—a vast improvement from 20 percent in the 1960s!—it still takes time and patience to help a new breastfeeding mother get her baby onto the breast.

New knowledge has changed the field. Research studies now verify that breastfed children are more intelligent and that not breastfeeding costs the U.S. health care system billions of dollars annually. Because of the new awareness of the importance of breastfeeding, the number and influence of lactation consultants has expanded. The International Board of Lactation Consultants has certified more than 10,000 health care workers in 36 countries. Most hospitals, large and small, offer lactation services of some type and employ lactation consultants. Lest anyone question the powerful, positive influence of interventions by health care workers on breastfeeding, they only need to review the table of intervention studies in Chapter 2. At the same time, lest we follow that conflicted path that led to the medicalization of childbirth, we must listen to voices that warn of the danger of lactation consultants medicalizing infant feeding.

Other changes affect lactation practice. The insurance industry now drives the health care system, reversing the reward system in favor of short hospital stays, which are now two days or less in the U.S. for vaginal births. While these short stays mean that breastfeeding mothers and babies return home less likely to be exposed to hospital infections and to supplementary feedings, this brief time allows almost no opportunity to ensure that the baby is breastfeeding effectively. Mothers still needing care themselves return home to assume full-time childcare before they feel physically able to do so. Follow-up care of a new family at home should be universal, yet many mothers of preterm and "near-term" breastfed infants who are developmentally immature leave the hospital without any plan for assistance.

This text brings together in a single volume the latest clinical techniques and research findings that direct evidence-based clinical practice. I have been fortunate in being able to enlist a dozen breastfeeding experts recognized around the world to help with the writing of this extensive volume. Dr. Kathleen Auerbach, the much-missed former co-author of this book, remains as co-author of two chapters.

Over 1,000 research studies support the clinical recommendations in this book. The Internet and MEDLINE made the literature searches so much easier for this edition—a sea of change from writing the first two editions. The Internet also made possible quick correspondence with colleagues and chapter authors as this book progressed. Addresses of helpful resources on the Internet have been added to each chapter.

Like the earlier editions, the third edition of this text has a clear clinical focus. A new chapter on infant assessment reflects current expectations that the health care worker working with the breastfeeding dyad can perform a total assessment of the baby. Nearly every chapter contains a clinical implications section. Important concepts discussed in chapters are summarized at the end of each chapter—a new feature that will make studying easier. Throughout the book are new references deemed by the authors to be the most important from the vastly expanded research and clinical literature. Some older references that introduced new ideas that are now accepted common knowledge have been regretfully removed to make room for new research. The glossary of key terms relating to lactation has been expanded in this edition.

Section 1 contrasts the past and present. Chapter 1 presents the history of breastfeeding by placing lactation and breastfeeding in its historical context. Chapter 2 fast-forwards to the work of the present-day health care worker who specializes in lactation and breastfeeding, and it addresses the reality of work-related issues of lactation consulting.

Section 2 focuses on basic anatomic and biologic imperatives of lactation. Clinical application of techniques must be based on a clear understanding of the relationships between form, function, and biological constructs. Thus this section, too, provides the background upon which to understand other aspects of lactation and breastfeeding behavior.

Section 3 is the clinical "heart" of the book that describes the basics of *what* to do, *when* to do it, and *how* to do it when one assists the lactating mother. Section 3 thus concerns itself with the perinatal period in the birth setting and concerns during the postpartum period following the family's return home—notably breast problems, neonatal jaundice, and infant weight gain. This section also addresses special needs of preterm babies and their mothers, and it critically evaluates breastfeeding devices and recommends how and when they are most appropriately used. It concludes with a review of the development and current activities of human milk banking.

The first part of *Section 4* focuses on the mother: maternal nutrition, the mother's health, and returning to work. The topics then turn to the infant and child's health and special health needs. The techniques of infant assessment are explained and demonstrated with photographs in a new chapter. The section ends with a discussion of maternal sexuality and fertility.

Section 5 begins with a careful look at research—how it is conducted, why ongoing research is needed, and how research findings can be applied in clinical settings. The principles of education, the cornerstone of clinical practice, are explored next. The book concludes with the socio-cultural context of the breastfeeding family and explores the different ways in which the breastfeeding family functions within that context.

To avoid linguistic confusion, the book uses the following conventions. The word *nursing* (in italics) in the text refers to the profession. Nursing, meaning breastfeeding, is always shown in ordinary Roman type. The masculine pronoun has been used to denote the infant or child throughout the text as a matter of convenience to distinguish the child from the breastfeeding mother. Nurses, lactation consultants, and other health care workers are referred to by feminine pronouns, although we recognize here that males serve in all health care professions.

ACKNOWLEDGEMENTS

I gratefully acknowledge the contributions to this book made by the following individuals:

Judy Angeron BA, RN, IBCLC, Coordinator, Lactation Services, Via Christi Regional Medical Center, Wichita, Kansas

Kathleen G. Auerbach PhD, IBCLC, Ferndale, Washington

Suzanne Bentley MSN, CNM, IBCLC, Clinical Nurse Specialist, University of Kansas, Clinical Instructor, University of Kansas, School of Nursing, Kansas City, Kansas

Belinda Childs MN, ARNP, CDE, Clinic/Research Coordinator, Mid-America Diabetes Associates, Wichita, Kansas

Mary Margaret Coates MS, IBCLC, TechEdit, Wheat Ridge, Colorado

Amy Ellington RN, BSN, Lactation Consultant, Via Christi Regional Medical Center, Wichita, Kansas

Barbara Gabbert-Bacon, La Leche League, Wichita, Kansas

Lenore Goldfarb, B.Comm, B.Sc, IBCLC, Herzl Family Practice Centre, Sir Mortimer B. Davis-Jewish General Hospital, Montreal, Quebec, Canada

Robert T. Hall MD, Professor, Children's Mercy Hospital and Clinics, Kansas City, Missouri

Eileen Hawkins MSN, ARNP, Wichita State University, School of Nursing, Wichita, Kansas

Kerstin Hedberg-Nyqvist PhD, RN, IBCLC, Assistant Professor in Pediatric Nursing, Department of Women's and Children's Health, Uppsala University,Uppsala, Sweden

Heather Hull MSN, PNP, Instructor, Wichita State University, Wichita, Kansas

Voni Miller RN, IBCLC, Lactation Consultant, Phoenix Children's Hospital, Phoenix, Arizona

Gerald Nelson MD, The University of Kansas School of Medicine, Wichita, Kansas

Amal Omer-Salim, MSc, Nutritionist, International Maternal and Child Health, Department of Women's and Children's Health, Uppsala University, Uppsala, Sweden

Virginia Phillips, IBCLC, Brisbane, Queensland, Australia

Christina M Smillie MD, FAAP, IBCLC, Breastfeeding Resources, Stratford, Connecticut

I am especially grateful to La Leche League International for providing the foundation for my breastfeeding education and to those institutions which encouraged and supported me in writing the book: the School of Nursing, Wichita State University, and Via Christi Regional Medical Center, both of Wichita, Kansas.

Finally, thanks to my family: Hugh, Michael, Neil and Shirley, Brian, Quinn and Rika Riordan, Teresa Riordan and Richard Chenoweth, Renee and Don Olmstead and our 11 (breastfed) grandchildren.

CHAPTER AUTHORS

Kathleen G. Auerbach, PhD, IBCLC
Ferndale, Washington

Lois D. W. Arnold, PhD (C.), MPH, IBCLC
National Commission on Donor Milk Banking
East Sandwich, Massachusetts

Debi Leslie Bocar, PhD, RN, IBCLC
Perinatal Educator, Mercy Health Center
Director, Lactation Consultant Services
Oklahoma City, Oklahoma

Yvonne Bronner, ScD, RD, LD
Professor and Director, Public Health Program
Morgan State University
Baltimore, Maryland

Mary Margaret Coates, MS, IBCLC
TechEdit
Wheat Ridge, Colorado

Lawrence M. Gartner, MD
Professor Emeritus
Departments of Pediatrics and Obstetrics/
Gynecology
The University of Chicago
Chicago, Illinois

Kathy Gill-Hopple, MSN, RN
Instructor
Wichita State University, School of Nursing
Wichita, Kansas

Thomas W. Hale, PhD, RPH
Professor of Pediatrics
Texas Tech University, School of Medicine
Amarillo, Texas

Marguerite Herschel, MD
Associate Professor of Pediatrics
Medical Director, General Care Nursery
The University of Chicago
Chicago, Illinois

Roberta J. Hewat, PhD, RN, IBCLC
Associate Professor
University of British Columbia,
School of Nursing,
Vancouver, British Columbia, Canada

Kay Hoover, MEd, IBCLC
Philadelphia Department of Public Health
Philadelphia, Pennsylvania

Nancy Hurst, RN, MSN, IBCLC
Director, Lactation Program and Mother's Own
Milk Bank
Texas Children's Hospital
Assistant Professor of Pediatrics
Baylor College of Medicine
Houston, Texas

Kathy I. Kennedy, MA, Dr.PH
Director, Regional Institute for Health and Envi-
ronmental Leadership,
University of Denver Associate Clinical Professor
of Preventive Medicine,
University of Colorado Health Sciences
Denver, Colorado

Mary Koehn, PhD, RN, MSN
Assistant Professor
Wichita State University, School of Nursing
Wichita, Kansas

Paula Meier, DNSc, RN, FAAN
NICU Lactation Program Director, Department of
Maternal-Child Nursing,
Associate Director for Clinical Research,
Section of Neonatology,
Rush-Presbyterian-St Luke's Medical Center
Chicago, Illinois

Sallie Page-Goertz, MN, CPNP, IBCLC
Assistant Clinical Professor,
KU Children's Center/Kansas University School
of Medicine
Overland Park, Kansas

Nancy Powers, MD
Medical Director, Lactation Services
Pediatrix Medical Group
Wesley Medical Center
Wichita, Kansas

Wailaiporn Rojjanasrirat, PhD, MSN
Research Assistant Professor
University of Kansas, School of Nursing
Kansas City, Kansas

Linda J. Smith, BSE, FACCE, IBCLC
Bright Future Lactation Resource Centre Ltd.
Dayton, Ohio

Marsha Walker, RN, IBCLC
Lactation Associates
Executive Director, National Alliance for Breast-
feeding Advocacy
Research, Education, and Legal Branch
Weston, Massachusetts

Karen Wambach, PhD, RN, IBCLC
Assistant Professor
University of Kansas, School of Nursing
Kansas City, Kansas

HISTORICAL AND WORK PERSPECTIVES

Just as the breastfeeding course flows and ebbs in a woman's life, so breastfeeding has experienced flows and ebbs through the centuries. It takes a village to return to breastfeeding, and community-based programs that promote breastfeeding are successfully and steadily increasing the rate of breastfeeding around the world.

As more mothers choose to breastfeed, the need for specialized help increases also. The visibility and acceptance of lactation consulting as an allied health profession offers opportunities for practice in hospitals, the community, and in private practice. Randomized clinical trials consistently demonstrate that lactation consultant services lengthen a mother's breastfeeding course and save money through healthier mothers and babies.

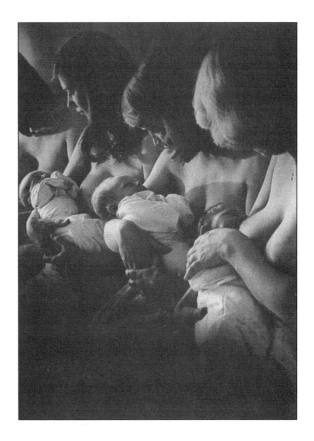

Tides in Breastfeeding Practice

Mary Margaret Coates and Jan Riordan

Throughout the world today, an infant is apt to receive less breastmilk than at any time in the past. Until the 1940s, the prevalence of breastfeeding was high in nearly all societies. Although the feeding of manufactured milks and baby milks had begun before the turn of the century in parts of Europe and North America, the practice spread slowly during the next decades. It was still generally limited to segments of population elites, and it involved only a small percentage of the world's people. During the post–World War II era, however, the way in which most mothers in industrialized regions fed their infants began to change, and the export of these new practices to developing nations was underway.

Evidence About Breastfeeding Practices

How do we know what we "know" about the prevalence of breastfeeding? (The word *prevalence* is used here to mean the combined effect of breastfeeding initiation rates and breastfeeding continuance rates.) Before attempting to trace trends in infant feeding practices, let us consider the nature of the evidence.

Large-Scale Surveys

National surveys that produce the kind of representative data that allow statistical evaluation have been available only since 1955. These surveys consist primarily of national fertility or natality surveys and of marketing surveys conducted by manufacturers of artificial baby milk. For most, exclusive breastfeeding is not a separate statistic. However, the percentage of exclusive breastmilk feedings at hospital discharge can be found in state birth certificate databases (Feldman-Winter et al., 2002). A brief description of national surveys conducted in the United States follows (Grummer-Strawn & Li, 2000):

- *National Health Interview Survey:* A personal interview is conducted in 43,000 households. Questions about incidence and duration of breastfeeding are asked.

- *National Health and Nutrition Examination Survey (NHANES):* Breastfeeding data are periodically collected from personal interviews in the home.

- *National Survey of Family Growth (NSFG):* Personal interviews are conducted every 6 years. Standard questions on incidence, duration, and exclusivity are included.

- *Pediatric Nutrition Surveillance System (PedNSS):* Statistics of breastfeeding incidence and duration in low-income populations are collected in public health clinics and reported annually. National, state, county, and clinic data are analyzed.

- *WIC Participant Characteristics Study:* Data on breastfeeding are collected each even-numbered year by the Department of Agriculture.

- *Ross Laboratories Mothers Survey:* Questionnaires are mailed to new mothers whose names are obtained from a national sample of hospitals and physicians. For marketing purposes, data on type of milk fed is collected for up to 12 months for a given cohort. Data are published on an ad hoc basis. The survey currently functions as a baseline and monitoring data source for breastfeeding goals in *Healthy People 2010.*

- *Mead-Johnson Longitudinal Study of Infant Feeding Practices:* For marketing purposes, a panel of infants is followed for 12 months. Data is collected on incidence of, duration of, and changes in breastfeeding frequencies.

Outside the United States, representative data for countries in Latin America, Asia, Africa, and the Middle East are derived from three sources. World Fertility Surveys are sponsored by the Office of Population within the United States Agency for International Development (USAID), the United Nations Fund for Population Activities, and the United Kingdom Office of Development Assistance (Lightbourne, Singh, & Green, 1982). The World Health Organization began ongoing surveys on infant feeding in the mid-1970s. Its Global Data Bank on Breast-Feeding pools information garnered from well-designed nutrition and breastfeeding surveys around the world; on the basis of these data, breastfeeding practices are periodically summarized. The most recent summary appeared in 2000 (WHO, 2000). Finally, demographic and health surveys were initiated in 1984; these ongoing surveys are sponsored jointly by USAID and governments of host countries in which the surveys are made.

Other Evidence

Until the last several decades, breastfeeding was the unremarkable norm. Thus what we "know" about breastfeeding from much earlier times often must be inferred from evidence of other methods of feeding infants. Most historical material available in English-language literature derives from a rather limited geographic area: Western Europe, Asia Minor, the Middle East, and North Africa. Written materials, which include verses, legal statutes, religious tracts, personal correspondence, inscriptions, and medical literature, extend back to before 2000 BC.

Some of the earliest existing medical literature deals at least in passing with infant feeding. An Egyptian medical encyclopedia, the *Papyrus Ebers* (c. 1500 BC), contains recommendations for increasing a mother's milk supply (Fildes, 1986). The first writings to discuss infant feeding in detail are those of the physician Soranus, who practiced in Rome around AD 100; his views were widely repeated by other writers until the mid-1700s. It is not immediately apparent to what degree these early exhortations either reflected or influenced actual practices. Many writings before AD 1800 deal primarily with wet nurses or how to hand-feed infants.

Archeological evidence provides some information about infant feeding prior to 2000 BC. Some of the earliest artifacts are Middle Eastern pottery figurines that depict lactating goddesses, such as Ishtar of Babylon and Isis of Egypt. The abundance of this evidence suggests that lactation was held in high regard (Fildes, 1986). Such artifacts first appear in sites about 3000 BC, when pottery making first became widespread in that region. Information about infant feeding may also be derived from paintings, inscriptions, and infant feeding implements.

Modern ethnography has a place of special importance. By documenting the infant feeding practices of present-day nontechnological hunter-gatherer, herding, and farming societies, ethnographers expand our knowledge of the range of normal breastfeeding practices. At the same time, they provide a richer appreciation of cultural practices that enhance the prevalence of breastfeeding. Such studies are also our best window into breastfeeding practices that may be the biological norm for *Homo sapiens sapiens.*

In summary, the historical aspect of this chapter deals with limited data from a limited social stratum in a limited geographic region. However, the common threads of these data provide a useful context within which we may better understand modern breastfeeding practices, especially in Western cultures.

The Biological Norm in Infant Feeding

Early Human Evolution

The class Mammalia is characterized principally by the presence of breasts (mammae), which secrete and release a fluid that for a time is the sole nourishment of the young. This manner of sustaining newborns is extremely ancient; it dates back to the late Mesozoic era, some 100 million years ago. (See Figure 1–1.) Hominid precursors first appeared about 4 million years ago; the genus *Homo* has existed for about 2 million years. The currently dominant human species, *Homo sapiens sapiens*, has existed for perhaps 40,000 years. Information about breastfeeding practices among our earliest ancestors is uncertain, although other information about Paleolithic societies that existed 10,000 or more years ago sheds light on this subject.

Early Breastfeeding Practices

Diets reconstructed by archeological methods reveal that the Late Paleolithic era, roughly 40,000 to 10,000 years ago, was populated by pre-agricultural peoples who ate a wide variety of fruits, nuts, vegetables, meat (commonly small game), fish, and shellfish. This diet closely resembles that of twentieth-century hunter-gatherer societies. Therefore, the infant-feeding practices of societies today may reflect breastfeeding practices of much earlier (prehistoric) times. Consider the breastfeeding practices of the iKung of the Kalahari Desert in southern Africa (Konner & Worthman, 1980) as well as hunter-gatherer societies of Papua New Guinea and elsewhere (Short, 1984). Among these people, breastfeeding of young infants is frequent (averaging four feeds per hour) and short (about 2 minutes per feed). It is equally distributed over a 24-hour period and continues, tapering off gradually, for two to six years. These breastfeeding patterns are considered a direct inheritance of practices that prevailed at the end of a long, and dietetically stable, evolutionary period that ended about 10,000 BC. This assumption is supported by observations of the human's closest primate relative, the chimpanzee, which secretes a milk quite similar to that of humans, suckles several times per hour, and sleeps with and nurses its young at night (Short, 1984).

The Replacement of Maternal Breastfeeding

Wet-Nursing

Wet-nursing may not have been the earliest alternative to maternal breastfeeding, but it was the only one likely to enable the infant to survive. Wet-nursing is common, although not universal, in traditional societies of today and (by inference) among ancient human societies. An already-lactating woman may have been the most obvious choice for a wet nurse, but women who stimulate lactation without a recent pregnancy have been described in many traditional societies (Slome, 1976; Wieschhoff, 1940).

Wet-nursing for hire is mentioned in some of the oldest surviving texts, which implies that the practice was well established even in ancient times. The Babylonian Code of Hammurabi (c. 1700 BC) forbade a wet nurse to substitute a new infant for one who had died. The Old Testament Book of Exodus (c. 1250 BC) records the hiring of a wet nurse

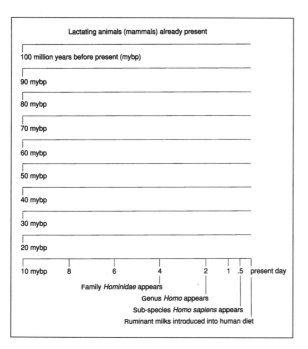

FIGURE 1–1. The antiquity of lactation. The bottom line shows the approximate times of first appearance of lactating precursors of modern humans and of regular use of nonhuman animal milk by humans.

for the foundling Moses; the fact that the "wet nurse" was Moses's own mother is incidental. The epic poems of Homer, written down around 900 BC, contain references to wet nurses. A treatise on pediatric care in India, written during the second century AD, contains instructions on how to qualify a wet nurse when the mother could not provide milk. The Koran, written about AD 500, also permits parents to "give your children out to nurse."

Although the history of wet-nursing has continued virtually unbroken from the earliest times to the present, the popularity of the practice among the elite classes who used it most has waxed and waned. In England during the 1600s and 1700s and elsewhere in Europe, the middle classes began to employ wet nurses. The use of less attentive nurses and the sending of infants greater distances from home diminished maternal supervision of either nurse or infant. Often infants were not seen by their parents from the time they were given to the nurse until they were returned home after weaning (providing they lived). However, by the latter part of the 1700s wet nursing was on the decline in North America and England (except in foundling hospitals), owing to increased public concern regarding the moral character of wet nurses and the quality of the care they provided. In France, government officials and physicians led a campaign against wet nursing. Some women recalling this period of history proudly reported that they nursed their babies themselves (Yalom, 1997). Throughout this long period, wet nurses were used sometimes because of maternal debility but more often because of the social expectations of the class of women who could afford to hire a wet nurse in order to free them for obligations incumbent upon highborn ladies. Thus the use of wet nurses by social elites foreshadows the demographic pattern later seen in the use of manufactured baby milks.

Hand-Fed Foods

The Agricultural Revolution.

The idea that animal milks are suitable foods for human infants is reflected in such myths as that of Romulus and Remus, the mythical founders of Rome, who are usually depicted as being suckled by a wolf. Surprisingly, the currently most popular hand-fed infant foods—animal milks and cereals—did not become part of the human diet until well along in human history. Cereal grains first appeared only about 10,000 years ago, and animal milks somewhat later (McCracken, 1971). The widespread adoption of these foods was made possible by the development of agriculture and (later) animal husbandry. Perhaps because of the availability of new weaning foods, periods of lactation that normally lasted three to six years were shortened to about two years in farming and herding societies (Schaefer, 1986).

Gruels.

In much of the world, the soft foods added most commonly to the infant diet have been gruels containing a liquid, a cereal, and other substances that added variety or nutritional value. The cereal might be rice, wheat, or corn. It might be boiled and mashed; ground and boiled; or, as in the case of bread crumbs, ground, baked, crushed, and heated. The liquid might be animal milk, meat broth, or water. Eggs or butter might also be added. If grains are not commonly eaten, similar soft foods for infants are based on starchy plants such as taro, cassava, or plantain.

Animal Milks.

Animal milks are a relatively recent addition to the human diet; this is implied genetically, because children beyond weaning age commonly do not produce lactase, an enzyme needed to digest the milk sugar lactose. In cultures that traditionally do not use animal milks, such as those in Mexico or Bangladesh or Thailand, some children may be lactose-intolerant before 1 year of age; in those cultures that use animal milks abundantly, the onset of lactose intolerance occurs considerably later—after age 10—in Finland (Simoons, 1980). Adult lactose tolerance is common only in cultures in which animal milks have traditionally been an important part of the diet, such as those of northern Europe and western Asia (McCracken, 1971).

Feeding Vessels.

The earliest "vessel" used to hand-feed an infant was undoubtedly the human hand, and the foods so fed were probably soft or mashed, rather than liquid. The earliest crafted vessels for feeding liquids were probably animal horns pierced by holes in the tips; such horns continued to be used into the 1900s in parts of Europe. The oldest pottery vessel thought to have been used for infant feeding, a small spouted bowl found in an infant's grave in France, is dated c. 2000–1500 bc (Lacaille, 1950). Small spouted or football-shaped bowls have been found in infant burial sites in Germany (c. 900 bc) and in the Sudan in North Africa (c. 400 bc) (Lacaille, 1950). These utensils suggest that hand-feeding of infants has been attempted for more than three millennia. (See Figure 1–2.)

Timing of the Introduction of Hand-Feeding

What archeological evidence cannot tell us is why or how much these infants were hand-fed. Neonates may temporarily be offered certain foods as prelacteal feeds; young infants may be offered occasional tastes of other foods, and they will be offered increasing amounts of soft foods as they make the transition to the adult diet (mixed feeds). Finally, infants may be reared from birth on other foods (artificial feeding).

Prelacteal Feeds. Many of the world's infants, even those who later will be fully breastfed, receive other foods as newborns. Of 120 traditional societies (and, by inference, in many ancient preliterate societies) whose neonatal feeding practices have been described, 50 delay the initial breastfeeding more than two days, and some 50 more delay it one to two days. The stated reason is to avoid the feeding of colostrum, which is described as being dirty, contaminated, bad, bitter, constipating, insufficient, or stale (Morse, Jehle, & Gamble, 1990).

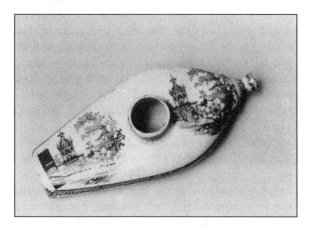

FIGURE 1–2. An English Staffordshire Spode nursing bottle, c. 1825. (Courtesy V. H. Brackett.)

Early medical writers in the eastern Mediterranean region (Greece, Rome, Asia Minor, and Arabia) and later in Europe—from Soranus through those of the 1600s—also discouraged the use of colostrum for feeding. These writers recommended avoiding breastfeeding for periods as short as one day (Avicenna, c. AD 1000) to as long as three weeks (Soranus, c. AD 100). Commonly, to promote the passage of meconium, the newborn was first given a "cleansing" food such as honey, sweet oils (such as almond), or sweetened water or wine.

In Europe, the fear of feeding an infant colostrum may have contributed to the undermining of maternal breastfeeding, at least among the upper classes, and spread wet-nursing (Deruisseau, 1940). A similar charge has been leveled at the prelacteal bottle feeds commonly given in Western (or Western-style) hospital nurseries; many studies show that early bottle-feeds undermine breastfeeding and increase the mother's use of manufactured baby milk. One can only wonder if Western hospital practices, which include delayed first breastfeeding and prelacteal feeds of water or artificial baby milk, are technological vestiges of this widespread traditional "taboo."

Not all published work supports the idea that prelacteal feeds and a delay in initiating breastfeeding reduce the likelihood of continued lactation (see Chapter 24). Some authors believe that ensuing breastfeeding is associated with the maternal perception that prelacteal feeds are appropriate. They hold that a particular set of culturally approved maternal behaviors follows the commencement of breastfeeding: nearly constant contact with or proximity to the infant; breastfeeding ad lib day and night; and no further use of feeding bottles (Nga & Weissner, 1986; Woolridge, Greasley, & Silpisornkosol, 1985).

Mixed Feeds. On the basis of current practices of many traditional societies, early mixed feedings may be the most common infant-feeding regimen (Dimond & Ashworth, 1987; Kusin, Kardjati, & van Steenbergen 1985; Latham et al., 1986).

Mixed feeding is widely practiced, even during the time when breastmilk forms the foundation of the infant diet. In many regions, such as Africa and Latin America, breastfeeding continues into the second or third year of life. In non-Western cultures, hand-fed foods include tea infusions, mashed fruits, and a variety of starchy gruels or pastes. Where the use of a particular food dominates a culture (e.g., rice in many parts of Asia), that food is usually the principal family food fed to an infant (Jelliffe, 1962). In some (mostly non-Western) cultures, such foods are offered to weaning infants in such a way that they supplement, rather than replace, breastmilk (Greiner, 1996; Whitehead, 1985) and thus do not appreciably hasten complete cessation of breast-feeding. The use of feeding bottles, however, can shorten the weaning interval, the period between full sustenance by breastmilk and full sustenance by family foods (Winikoff & Laukaran, 1989).

Hand-Feeding from Birth.   In a few regions of northern Europe (e.g., Switzerland, Finland, and Iceland) a cool, dry climate and a tradition of dairy farming permitted the survival of at least some in-fants who were fed cow milk nearly from birth. From at least the 1400s in Switzerland and Finland, breastfeeding was actively discouraged (Fildes, 1986). However, even in climatically optimal areas, hand-feeding was hazardous. In Iceland infants were hand-fed during the 1600s and 1700 despite disastrous results; married women bore as many as 30 infants because so few survived (Hastrup, 1992). In France, some foundlings and infants with syphilis were fed directly from goats; this practice was first described in writings in the 1500s, and it persisted until the early 1800s (Wickes, 1953a). Of necessity, foundling hospitals of the 1700s and 1800s in Europe and the United States hand-fed in-fants but with appalling mortality rates: up to 100 percent died. (See Figure 1–3.) However, by the mid-1900s in industrialized countries, hand-feeding from birth had become the norm and hand-fed in-fants survived and grew. Why did that happen?

Technological Innovations in Infant Feeding

The Social Context

During the late 1800s and the early 1900s, high in-fant mortality, even among infants cared for at home, was a major public concern. Physicians and parents recognized that poorly nourished children were more susceptible to illness. Between 1910 and

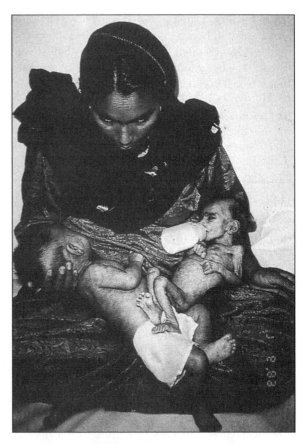

FIGURE 1–3. UNICEF photograph of thriving breast-fed twin and his dying bottle-fed sister. (Courtesy of Children's Hospital, Islamabad, Pakistan.)

1915 the newly created United States Children's Bu-reau sponsored several studies of infant mortality in major cities. Each study showed that babies fed ar-tificial milks (i.e., anything other than mother's milk) were three to five times as likely to die as those who were breastfed. The studies also docu-mented that both the rate of breastfeeding and the rate of infant mortality were linked: each increased steadily as family income decreased. In summariz-ing these results Williamson (1915) commented that "the disadvantages of a low income were sufficient to offset the greater prevalence of breast feeding among the babies of the poorer families." During this same period, a similar observation was made in England, where high infant mortality prevailed among poor, working-class mothers, 80 percent of whom breastfed their infants (Levenstein, 1983).

As women's aspirations for community service and commercial involvement were rising, Victorian beliefs about modesty discouraged breastfeeding in public. Advertising, which promoted bodily cleanliness, may have led to associating breastmilk with body fluids that were unclean or noxious, a notion that persists to this day, at least in North America (Morse, 1989). Advances in the prevention of disease, largely through public health measures related to sanitation, extended an expanding faith in "modern science" in general to "modern medicine" in particular. Women's magazines developed a wide audience of readers interested in female accomplishments outside the home, in modern attitudes, and in technological innovations; these same magazines reinforced concerns about infant health. An 1880 issue of the *Ladies' Home Journal* contained this statement (Apple, 1986):

If fed from your breast, be sure that the quantity and quality supply his demands. If you are weak or worn out, your milk cannot contain the nourishment a babe needs.

The Technological Context

Between about 1860 and 1910, scientific advances and technological innovations created many new options in infant feeding that appeared to enhance infant survival. The upright feeding bottle and rubber nipple, each of which could be cleaned thoroughly, made artificial feeding easier and safer. New foods to be used with this equipment appeared. Large-scale dairy farming produced abundant supplies of cow milk, which was marketed first as canned evaporated milk and later in condensed (i.e., highly sweetened to retard spoilage) or dried forms.

This technological ferment, fueled both by the need for improved infant health care and by a popular belief in the ability of science and technology to provide answers, attracted analytical chemists. Around 1850 chemists had begun to turn their attention to food products. Early investigations (now viewed as rudimentary) into the composition of human and cow milk convinced them that "the combined efforts of the cow and the ingenuity of man" could construct a food the equal of human

milk (Gerrard, 1974). Patented foods, such as Liebig's Food and Nestle's Milk Food, were first marketed in Europe and the United States in the 1860s. The Nestle's product was a mixture of flour, cow milk, and sugar that was to be dissolved in milk or water before feeding. Milk modifiers, such as Mellin's Food, and milk foods, such as Horlick's Malted Milk, were popular in the United States by the 1880s.

Extravagant claims for these foods (Liebig's Food was called "the most perfect substitute for mother's milk") were combined with artful advertising that played on fears for the health of the infant and faith in modern science (Apple, 1986). (See Figure 1–4.) A hundred years later we see these advertising themes played again and again.

In the 1890s, physician Thomas Rotch developed a complex system of modifying cow milk so that it more closely resembled human milk. Rotch observed that the composition of human milk varies, as do digestive capacities in infants. He devised mathematical formulas to denote the proportions of fat, sugar, and protein in cow milk that some infants required at a particular age (Rotch, 1907). The result was an exceedingly complex system of feeding that required constant intervention by the physician, who often changed the "formula" weekly. Supervising infant feeding then became a principal focus of the newly emerging specialty of pediatrics.

Commercial advertising promoted the use of manufactured infant milks to both mothers and physicians. The basic themes—a mother's concern for her infant's health, the perfection of the manufactured product, and the difficulty of breastfeeding—have persisted over the years (Apple, 1986).

The Role of the Medical Community

Regulation of Childbirth. During the early part of this century, childbirth moved from home or midwife-attended births largely to hospitals, where a birthing woman was separated from her family and attended by hospital staff. During the middle part of this century, hospital routines and the use of general anesthesia during labor and delivery separated mother and infant much of the time in the early postpartum period. Bottle-feedings by nursery

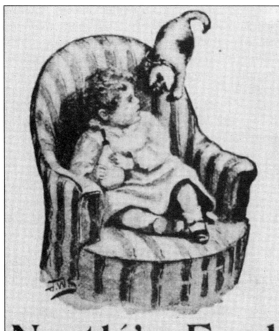

Nestlé's Food

Nestlé's Food is a complete and entire diet for babies. Over all the world Nestlé's Food has been recognized for more than thirty years as possessing great value as a protection against Cholera Infantum and all other forms of Summer Complaint.

Nestlé's Food is safe. It requires only the addition of water to prepare it for use. The great danger always attendant on the use of cow's milk is thus avoided.

Consult your doctor about Nestlé's Food, and send to us for a large sample can and our book, "The Baby," both of which will be sent free on application.

THOMAS LEEMING & CO.
73 Warren Street, New York

FIGURE 1–4. An advertisement for artificial infant milk that appeared in the *Ladies' Home Journal* in 1895.

staff became increasingly common. Normal postpartum hospital stays in the United States lengthened; during the 1930s and 1940s, they were sometimes as long as two weeks. This period, intended to permit the mother to recuperate from (an often highly medicated) childbirth, resulted as well in a return home with an impaired breastmilk supply and a baby who was accustomed to bottle-feeding. Bain (1948) notes that babies who were older than eight days at discharge were less apt to be breastfed than were younger ones.

Regulation of Breastfeeding. Underlying many changes in the feeding of infants was a "regulatory" frame of mind, the seeds of which had been sown in Europe as early as the 1500s. The advent of book printing about this time permitted a much wider dissemination of works on infant care. Their authors shared a concern for the high incidence of gastrointestinal illness in infants and for high infant-mortality rates. For reasons not at all clear today, overfeeding was deemed a central factor in both. Writers concerned with child care responded by advocating the regulation of feeding in order to prevent presumed overfeeding.

Writing in the mid-1600s, Ettmuller (1703; cited in Wickes, 1953a) was not the first to recommend infrequent feedings:

Nothing is more apt to disorder the child than suckling it too often, since large quantities of milk stagnating in the stomach, must needs corrupt . . . especially if fresh milk be pour'd in before the preceding be digested.

Some 250 years later in 1900, Pierre Budin (1907; cited in Wickes, 1953b), a French obstetrician famous for his early interest in premature infants and for his advocacy of breastfeeding, was nonetheless typical of many others in recommending small feedings: "It is better at first to give too little than too much, (for an underfed infant failed to gain weight but it was free from digestive troubles)."

Even medical writers who strongly recommended breastfeeding also recommended highly regulated times for feedings—a fixed number of feedings at fixed times. William Cadogan (1749; cited in Kessen, 1965), whose firm endorsement of breastfeeding and largely sound advice prompted many privileged English women to breastfeed, advocated only four feeds per day at equal intervals, and no night feeds! A prototype mothercraft manual by Hugh Smith (1774; cited in Fildes, 1986) contains excellent advice: to feed colostrum and to allow the newborn to suckle frequently to stimulate lactation. (See Figure 1–5.) However, it then instructs mothers to limit feeds, (beginning at 1

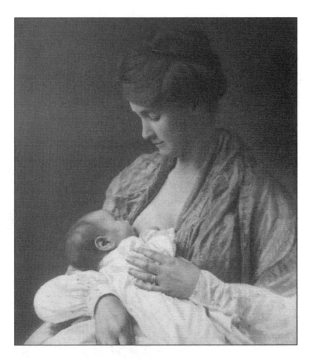

FIGURE 1–5. A mother nursing her infant about 1900s. (With permission from M. M. Coates.)

month), to five per day timed at 7 and 10 A.M. and 1, 6, and 11 P.M. About 50 years later, after recommending ad lib feeds for the first 10 days, Thomas Bull (1849; cited in Wickes, 1953a) instructed mothers to feed for the rest of the first month at regular 4-hour intervals day and night, because he also believed that irregular feeding harmed the infant. After 1 month the night feed was to be eliminated.

These influential publications began the process of removing the management of infant feeding from the mother (or from the realm of women in general) and placing it in the hands of (usually male) "authorities." Cadogan (1749; cited in Kessen, 1965) commended this change that put "men of sense rather than foolish unlearned women" in charge, and Rotch a century and a half later (1907) deplored that "mothers and nurses . . . dominated the physicians." Even as late as the 1950s US physicians ordered that newborns be given nothing by mouth for the first 24 hours after birth. In Australia, midwifery texts of the 1940s recommended that the baby not go to the breast until 12 hours after birth (Thorley, 2001). Now (2004) we are anxious if a baby has not latched on to the breast by 12 hours after birth!

Social censure and in some places statutory laws have dictated not only when breastfeeding should take place but also *where.* American women have only just recently gained the legal right to breastfeed in public places. Seventeen states have passed laws that prevent women who breastfeed in public from being charged with indecent exposure, and a 1999 federal law makes breastfeeding legal on all federal property (Tiedje et al., 2002).

Regulation and Industrialization. This "regulatory" frame of mind fit nicely with the needs of the growing industrial sector of the economy, which relied on efficiency and schedules governed by the clock. Societal perceptions of infants' innate characteristics and needs were interpreted in this light (Millard, 1990). Early in the twentieth century, infants were seen as needing order imposed onto their characters from the outside (Rossiter, 1908):

An infant two days old may be forming either a good or a bad habit. A child that is taken up whenever it cries is trained into a bad habit; the same principle is true in reference to nursing a baby to stop its crying. Both these habits cultivate self-indulgence and a lack of self-control.

"Good" mothering thus drifted toward meeting the letter of schedules often imposed by the medical profession rather than meeting the mutual needs of mother and infant as expressed by and interpreted within the dyad.

Although rigid, externally imposed schedules diminished after the 1960s, it is still assumed in most literature that lactation functions better when mother and baby develop feeding routines. The lack of some routine is usually perceived as abnormal by both mother and physician (Millard, 1990). Unfortunately, certain attitudes required of most employees, such as an awareness of time and responsiveness within a hierarchical authority structure, are those least apt to enable a mother or a pediatrician to accommodate the normal irregularities of early breastfeeding.

Regulation of Contraception. During the late 1950s and early 1960s, the widespread acceptance of oral contraceptives may have also reinforced the decline in breastfeeding (Meyer, 1968). Contraceptives containing estrogen and progestin reduce breastmilk volume and thus contribute to lactation insufficiency, early supplementation, and early weaning from the breast. Moreover, women who planned to use combined estrogen and progestin oral contraceptives were discouraged from breastfeeding in order to avoid passing those hormones to the infant. During this period, several million women per year in the United States alone were thereby removed from the pool of potential breastfeeders. Currently marketed low-progestin contraceptives pose fewer hazards to the maternal milk supply and the baby, and often they are routinely recommended to mothers nursing young infants (Kelsey, 1996).

Accommodation Between Physicians, Other Health Professionals, and Infant Milk Manufacturers.

The relationship between physicians and other health professionals, on the one hand, and infant food manufacturers on the other has in general promoted mothers' dependency on either the manufacturer or the physician for information on infant feeding. In the late 1800s as proprietary infant foods were being developed, manufacturers advertised to both groups. By the 1920s, some preparations were advertised to mothers but could be purchased only by prescription or used only after consulting a physician: the package contained no instructions for use. By 1932 the American Medical Association essentially required baby milk manufacturers to advertise only to the medical profession (Greer & Apple, 1991). The mutual economic benefits of this policy were clearly spelled out in many advertisements placed by formula manufacturers such as Mead Johnson (1930) in medical journals:

When mothers in America feed their babies by lay advice, the control of your pediatric cases passes out of your hands, Doctor. Our interest in this important phase of medical economics springs, not from any motives of altruism, philanthropy or paternalism, but rather from a spirit of enlightened self-interest and co-operation because (our) infant diet materials are advertised only to you, never to the public.

For several decades this unwritten agreement has extended also to medical education. Formula companies spend about $10,000 per medical student during a student's medical education (Walker, 2001). Many nursing and dietetic professional organizations also accept money from formula companies to fund continuing education, grants, and other projects.

Despite several early studies that showed breastfed infants to be healthier than bottle-fed ones (Grulee, Sanford & Herron, 1934; Howarth, 1905; Woodbury, 1922), for years many physicians advised mothers that there was little advantage to breastfeeding. This persistent view was expressed up through the 1960s. For instance, Aitken and Hytten (1960) reported that "with modern standards of hygiene artificial feeding on simple mixtures of cow's milk, water and sugar is a satisfactory substitute for breast feeding."

The Prevalence of Breastfeeding

United States, England, and Europe

The Recent Past.   The net result of these shifts in technology and attitudes has been a rapid decline in the prevalence of breastfeeding in Western nations since the 1940s. In the United States, the proportion of newborns receiving any breastmilk at 1 week postpartum declined steadily to a low of 25 percent in 1970 (Martinez & Krieger, 1985). The proportion of newborns exclusively breastfed at hospital discharge was even lower: it declined from 38 percent in 1946 (Bain, 1948) to 21 percent in 1956 and only 18 percent by 1966 (Meyer, 1968). The period of most dramatic decline of breastfeeding coincided with economic factors in the United States that encouraged major migrations from rural to urban areas. For example, between 1945 and 1970 approximately five million African-Americans moved from the rural South to the urban North. The association between internal migration from rural to urban areas and a decline in breastfeeding also has been noted in developing countries. Breastfeeding rates reversed in the 1970s and rose gradually until the mid-1980s, when 52 percent of women initiated exclusive breastfeeding in hospitals and 17 percent persisted in exclusive breastfeeding at 6 months postpartum. Breastfeeding prevalence then dipped for a few years but has slowly risen since the early 1990s; breastfeeding rates recorded in 2001 were the highest ever (see below; Ryan, Wenjun, & Acosta, 2002).

Current Breastfeeding Practices. Breastfeeding rates are slowly rising. Almost 70 percent of hospital-born infants received any breastmilk in the hospital; of those, 31.4 percent were still receiving any breastmilk by six months of age. (See Figures 1–6 and 1–7.) Only about half of breastfeeding mothers are exclusively breastfeeding at the time of hospital discharge (Feldman-Winter et al., 2002).

In 2000, over 80 percent of mothers living in the Rocky Mountain and Pacific Northwest regions reported breastfeeding their infants in the hospital. The highest rates of breastfeeding at 6 and 12 months occurred among mothers who are white or of Hispanic origin, over age 35, college educated, living in the western United States, and not en-

rolled in the Women, Infants, and Children (WIC) program.

Developing Regions

The Role of Colonial Empires. Declines in the prevalence of breastfeeding were noted in non-Western regions somewhat later than in the West. Between World Wars I and II, British, French, and German colonial empires controlled fully one fourth of the inhabited globe and one fourth of the world's population. These empires served as vehicles for the expansion of markets for artificial baby milks.

Colonial ruling elites who followed the practices of their social class in their country of origin (which moreover placed social distance between the elites and the nationals of the country in which they resided) were much more likely to feed their infants artificial milks than to breastfeed. That most of these infants survived is due in large part to the higher levels of sanitation and medical care that their position in life afforded them. To some degree,

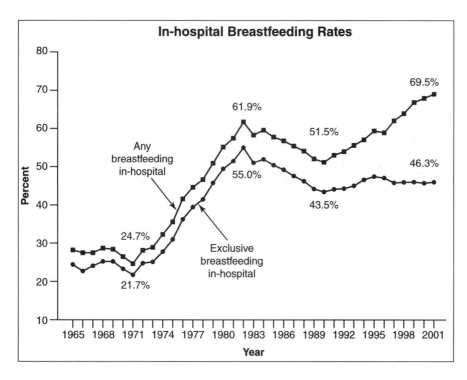

FIGURE 1–6.
In-hospital breastfeeding and exclusive breastfeeding rates, 1965–2001.
(With permission from American Academy of Pediatrics.)

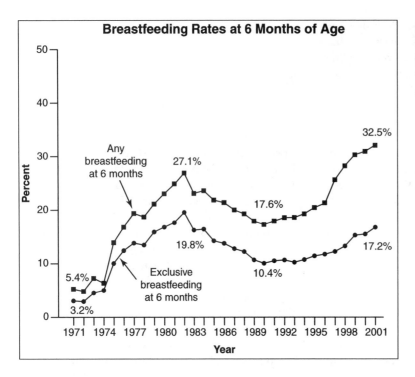

FIGURE 1–7.
Breastfeeding and exclusive breast-feeding rates at 6 months of age, 1971–2001. (With permission from American Academy of Pediatrics.)

these colonial elites served as unwitting role models for indigenous peoples.

Concern for the health of indigenous peoples led many health-care workers to transmit Western attitudes toward infant feeding to the populations they served by example, by direct recommendations, and by the training provided to indigenous health-care providers. Westerners have traditionally assumed that foods good for them must be good for all people and have passed these prejudices on to foreign nationals trained in Western schools (McCracken, 1971). Perhaps because Western medical personnel were successful at treating many other health problems, local populations were prepared to accept attitudes that encouraged the use of artificial baby milks. Health-care personnel in hospitals helped to introduce the use of manufactured baby milks and contributed to undermining breastfeeding (Winikoff & Laukaran, 1989).

Colonial transportation and communication networks and health clinics and hospitals aided the advertisement and sale of artificial baby milks to this huge population. The decline in breastfeeding accelerated after World War II, in part because of greater contact between Western health-care personnel and populations in developing countries,

and in part because relief projects shipped to war-torn countries the surplus of skim milk, produced in abundance by the large dairy industry in the United States. Between 1976 and 1977, 42 transnational companies manufactured, distributed, and marketed infant milk products in four countries surveyed: Ethiopia, Nigeria, India, and the Philippines (WHO, 1981).

Infant Feeding and Infant Mortality. The relation between infant feeding and infant mortality is complex. Infant mortality has tended to be highest among populations in which breastfeeding was most common: the poor. Rural mothers in Ethiopia and Zaire reported that at least 30 percent of their infants died, although 97 percent of mothers were breastfeeding at 18 months postpartum, as were 80 percent of a similar group of mothers in rural Zaire (WHO, 1981). The same relationship held in the United States during the early 1900s.

Although widespread artificial feeding has been associated with poorer infant survival, both in Western nations early in this century and in developing nations in the mid-1900s, the reverse is not always the case. The advent of primary health care for a large portion of a population may explain decreases in infant mortality in the face of declines in breastfeeding. In Nicaragua, the proportion of infants breastfed at 6 months declined 25 percentage points (from 58 to 33 percent) between 1977 and 1988. During this same period, infant mortality declined from about 10 percent to about 6.5 percent (Sandiford et al., 1991). It seems clear that the pervasive problems of poverty, in both Western and non-Western locales, were at the root of the appalling infant mortality in impoverished populations.

Current Breastfeeding Practices. During the 1970s, when breastfeeding rates were generally increasing in Western nations, they continued to decline in the more populous developing regions. Despite overall improvement in worldwide breastfeeding patterns made during the 1990s, fewer than half of all infants are exclusively breastfed for up to 4 months. During the 1990s, rates increased from 48 to 52 percent in the developing world (based on 37 countries). Although global levels of continued breastfeeding are relatively high at 1 year of age (79 percent), only around half of infants are still breastfeeding at age 2. Thus current breastfeeding patterns are still far from the recommended levels. Canada, with a 73 percent breastfeeding initiation rate, lags behind many other industrialized nations (Sheehan et al., 2001). East Asian and Pacific infants are most likely to be exclusively breastfed (57 percent) and have the longest median duration of breastfeeding.

African investigators report a relatively low rate of exclusive breastfeeding, about 33 percent, but a relatively long median duration (21 months). Generalizing breastfeeding rates reported in Europe (a rate of 16 percent and median duration of 11 months) is difficult because only four of 50 countries, representing perhaps 20 percent of all European infants, provided WHO with survey results. On the whole, the foregoing figures are estimated to represent almost 60 percent of the world's infants. However, it is surmised that infants in countries that did not provide WHO with information regarding breastfeeding practices are even less likely to be exclusively breastfed and are breastfed for even shorter periods.

Although breastfeeding, and particularly exclusive breastfeeding, continued to decline during the 1990s in some countries (Kenya, Jordan, Pakistan, Turkey), in other regions exclusive breastfeeding increased at rates *per year* of about 1 percent (Asia exclusive of China) to nearly 13 percent (Latin America and the Caribbean) (UNICEF, 2001).

Characteristics of Breastfeeding Women in Developing Regions. Generalizations about demographic characteristics most likely to predict who will breastfeed have many exceptions. In general, rural women are more likely to begin breastfeeding and to breastfeed longer than urban women; poorer mothers are more likely to breastfeed than more affluent ones. The urban poor, often recent immigrants from more rural areas, are the mothers among whom breastfeeding rates are declining most rapidly. However, in Kenya and Trinidad/Tobago, increases in median duration during the 1980s occurred in a broad range of socioeconomic and educational levels. During this same period in the Dominican Republic, the median duration of breastfeeding rose among urban mothers and among employed mothers, although the overall median duration dropped 15 percent.

The Cost of Not Breastfeeding

To see a world in a grain of sand
And a heaven in a wild flower,
Hold infinity in the palm of your hand
And eternity in an hour.

—William Blake, "Auguries of Innocence," c. 1803

Although isolated voices championed breastfeeding throughout its years of steady decline, not until the 1970s did the trend toward artificial feeding reverse (see again Figure 1-6). What prompted this change? The reasons are not clear but seem to reflect a widespread desire by many to include simpler, more natural practices in their lives. Basic, clinical, and demographic research increasingly demonstrated the benefits of breastmilk and breastfeeding to the infant and of lactation and breastfeeding to the mother. Later still, it has come to be recognized that there is a cost to not breastfeeding.

Health Risks of Using Manufactured Infant Milks

Risks to the Infant.   It has been recognized since the advent of manufactured infant milks that infants fed these products suffer more illness (Howarth, 1905; Woodbury, 1922; Grulee, Sanford, & Herron, 1934; Cunningham, Jelliffe, & Jelliffe, 1991). Artificially fed infants are denied the benefits of autoimmunization, whereby the breast produces antibodies to organisms to which the infant has been exposed. This observation is confirmed by more recent studies that are discussed in later chapters. At the time of the earlier studies, the immunological role of breastmilk was unclear; most deleterious effects of manufactured milks were attributed to contamination. In more recent decades, it has become established that artificial baby milk increases the risk of ill health by many pathways (Walker, 1993). Not only can these foods be (or easily become) contaminated, but they lack the immunological and other health-promoting factors present in human milk. In addition, they contain nutrients that are foreign to humans or are mixed in nonphysiologic proportions. Furthermore, the act of bottle-feeding differs from that of breastfeeding in ways that may contribute to cardiopulmonary problems in some infants. The effects of artificial feeding may extend well beyond infancy.

Risks to the Mother.   Artificial feeding is also detrimental to maternal health. In the absence of lactational amenorrhea, additional pregnancies may ensue that adversely affect the mother's health. As discussed in Chapter 16, mothers who artificially feed their infants are more likely than breastfeeding mothers to later develop health problems such as osteoporosis, premenopausal breast cancer, and ovarian cancer. Bottle-feeding mothers who have diabetes will not enjoy the same amelioration of symptoms that may be experienced by breastfeeding mothers who have diabetes (Butte et al., 1987).

Economic Costs of Using Manufactured Infant Milks

The presence or absence of breastfeeding affects the economics of the family, the community, and the nation. Some of these effects are more pronounced in less developed regions, but to a degree they also affect all segments of populations in technologically advanced regions.

Costs to the Family.   Although lactation imposes some demands on the mother's body stores, these demands are moderated by gastric changes that allow women to metabolize foods more efficiently while lactating (Illingworth, 1986; Uvnas-Moberg et al., 1987) and by the water-conserving effect of prolactin (Dearlove & Dearlove, 1981). Moreover, the contraceptive effect of full, unrestricted breastfeeding reduces a woman's physical and economic costs of childbearing (Jackson, 1988; Kennedy et al., 1989).

The direct monetary costs of rearing a breastfeeding infant are markedly lower than those of rearing one who is artificially fed. Approximately 150 cans of ready-to-feed manufactured baby milk are used during the first six months of full artificial feeding. In industrial nations, the cost of manufactured baby milk may exceed the cost of additional food for the lactating mother by two or three times (Jarosz, 1993). The cost of infant formula for 1 month in the midwestern United States is about $80. If the baby needs a special formula because of allergies or other problems, the monthly cost to families can be as high as $300 to $400. In developing nations, the ratio is many times higher. In regions where one third to one half of those in large urban areas live in poverty, the cost of manufactured milks required to provide adequate nutrition (and implements with which to feed them) is a significant portion of the family income (Serva, Karim, & Ebrahim, 1986). Other members of the family may eat more poorly because the baby is artificially fed.

An equally important consideration is the reduced need for medical care by breastfed infants (particularly those who are exclusively breastfed). The frequency and severity of illnesses in a young infant is often inversely related to the proportion of the diet that comes from breastmilk (Chen, Yu, & Li, 1988). More breastfeeding increases infant intake of high quality protein and a variety of other needed nutrients, and it decreases infant exposure to potential pathogens in other foodstuffs (Habicht, DaVanzo, & Butz, 1988). Several studies confirm that the annual cost of not breastfeeding to the

Table 1–1

THE COSTS OF NOT BREASTFEEDING REPORTED BY VARIOUS RESEARCHERS

Costs of Not Breastfeeding	Study	Sample	Additional Costs
Total Cost per Year			
Over $3 billion annually	Weimer, 2001	United States and Britain general population	Otitis media, $365 million Gastroenteritis, $10 million Necrotizing entercolitis, $3 billion
Over $1 billion annually	Riordan, 1997	United States general population	Gastroenteritis, $291.3 million Respiratory syncytial virus, $225 million; Insulin-dependent diabetes, $10 to $125 million; Otitis media, $660 million
AU$11.5 million annually	WABA, 1998	South Australia	Health care costs for infants (if exclusive breastfeeding increased from 60 to 80 percent)
Cost per First 12 Months per Family			
$478 first 12 months per family	Montgomery & Splett, 1997	Colorado WIC	Food vouchers for breastfeeding mothers vs. medical costs for gastroenteritis and otitis media in formula-fed infants
$331 to $475 per infant first 12 months	Ball & Wright, 1999	Arizona HMO; Scotland general population	Office visits, drug prescriptions, hospitalizations of breastfed vs. nonbreastfed infants
Extra $200 first 12 months for medical costs	Hoey & Ware, 1997	North Carolina HMO	Office visits, drug prescriptions, hospitalizations of breastfed vs. nonbreastfed infants
Cost per First 6 Months per Family			
$450–$800 first 6 months per family in WIC	Tuttle & Dewey, 1996	California WIC	Medicaid expenditures for additional health care in first 6 months vs. food vouchers and administrative costs
Excess Cost of Formula During First Two Months			
Extra $45 to $70 for first 62 days for each neonate	Jarosz, 1993	Hawaii	Cost of extra maternal food vs. cost of formula

health care system is in the billions of dollars (see Table 1–1). Weimer (2001) calculated that a minimum of $3.6 billion would be saved if breastfeeding were increased from current levels to those recommended by the US Surgeon General (75 percent initiation and 50 percent continuation at 6 months). This figure is likely an underestimation of the total savings because it represents cost savings from the treatment of only a few types of childhood illnesses.

The United States Breastfeeding Committee (2002) estimated the nonmedical costs of artificial feeding as follows:

• Families spend $2 billion per year on formula.

- The WIC spends $578 million per year in federal funds to buy formula.

- Every 10 percent increase in breastfeeding rates among WIC recipients would save WIC $750,000 per year.

- If a parent misses 2 hours of work for the excess illness attributable to formula feeding, greater than 2000 hours—the equivalent of 1 year of employment—are lost per 1000 never-breastfed infants.

- The United States uses 110 billion BTUs of energy ($2 million) each year for processing, packaging, and transporting formula.

Because full breastfeeding, which includes frequent feeds throughout a 24-hour period, tends to delay resumption of ovulation (Lewis et al., 1991), spacing between births tends to increase. Births spaced less than two years apart may increase the mortality risk of both the older and the younger infant (Retherford et al., 1989). Especially in families living at subsistence level, the older a child is when he or she is displaced from the breast and the fewer the number of children in a family, the more likely each child is to be healthy. In malnourished communities, breastfeeding may substantially increase child survival up to three years of age (Briend, Wojtyniak, Rowland, 1988).

Thus the breastfed infant stands a significantly greater likelihood of surviving. The mother's physical and emotional investment in pregnancy and lactation and the familial investment in time and money are repaid by the survival of a child; they are lost to the family when that child dies.

Cost to the Community and State. Community or national units that provide health care must respond to the local epidemiology of infant illness, in which feeding may play a major role. Morbidity is more prevalent in artificially fed infants (Jason, Nieburg, & Marks, 1984; Kovar et al., 1984) regardless of location. The increase of the infant population, resulting from the loss of the contraceptive effect of breastfeeding, also serves to increase the need for pediatric health care.

The debate on the economic value of breastfeeding has focused on health costs, but estimates of the value of the time and energy women expend on breastfeeding are not discussed. The value of time spent breastfeeding is neglected (along with all the other unwaged caring work women do, including caring for children who fall ill as a result of not breastfeeding).

Another little-discussed aspect of the replacement of breastfeeding by use of manufactured products is that certain sectors of an economy can become economically dependent on the payrolls met and taxes paid by infant milk manufacturers, especially if capital funds are obtained from outside the country. Once they become a financial presence in a country, those manufacturers may be politically and economically difficult to dislodge, despite increases in health costs elsewhere in the economy. In the United States, infant formula is a $3.1 billion per year industry that generates a large payroll in the community and tax revenues to governmental entities.

Nonetheless, manufactured milk products widely used for infant feeding are subsidized by the diversion of resources (land, dairy cattle, and people to manage both)—and by manufacturing capacity pulled from other possible uses.

When one considers that more than 20 million babies are born annually in Africa alone, it becomes apparent that providing adequate volumes of manufactured milks represents a staggering burden and a largely unnecessary diversion of human and monetary resources from other more beneficial programs. At a time when environmental issues have become paramount, these unnecessary uses of power and raw material, not to mention the disposal of discarded packaging, is an increasing concern.

The Promotion of Breastfeeding

The many ways of encouraging mothers to breastfeed their own infants—breastfeeding promotion—may be considered to lie on a continuum. At one end, in societies where breastfeeding is the cultural norm, "promotion" consists of assuming that mother and infant will breastfeed. This assumption is combined with social arrangements, such as special foods for the mother or lightened duties, especially within the first few weeks after birth, to ensure that breastfeeding becomes well established. At the other end, in societies in which artificial feeding is the norm, promotion often consists of encouragement to breastfeed, sometimes offered by government officials and often by healthcare professionals or members of elite population groups, without at the same time removing cultural barriers to breastfeeding.

Breastfeeding Promotion in the United States

Healthy People Statements. In 1978, the US Public Health Service defined national health objectives with a report, *Healthy People* (USDHHS, 1979). One objective stated that 75 percent of women should breastfeed at hospital discharge and 35 percent at 6 months, as opposed to the actual 1978 figures of 45 percent and 21 percent. Although year 2000 goals were not met, even higher percentages were set as goals for the year 2010. *Healthy People 2010* (USDHHS, 2000) calls for an increase in the rate of newborn breastfeeding to 75 percent, at age 6 months to 50 percent, and at age 1 year to 25 percent (see Table 1–2).

In 2000, the US Department of Human Services Office on Women's Health developed a *Blueprint for Action on Breastfeeding*, a policy-setting document issued by the federal government to affirm breastfeeding. However, although the *Blueprint* supports the Baby-Friendly Hospital Initiative (BFHI), it does not endorse that program nor does it make specific recommendations for legislation that would support breastfeeding.

The WIC Program. Although other government agencies in the United States also work to improve infant nutrition, the Special Supplemental Nutrition Program for Women, Infants, and Children—the WIC program—probably directly affects the greatest number of people. Established in 1972, this program provides free nutrition counseling and food supplements, including manufactured baby milk, to low-income mothers and their infants. Clients come from the population segment in the United States least likely to breastfeed (MacGowan et al., 1991).

The WIC program follows in the footsteps of infant welfare programs of the 1890s and at the turn of the century in France, England, and the United States that operated centers where infants could be weighed and examined weekly. These centers also provided cow milk ("fresh and clean" in some cases, sterilized in others) to nonbreastfeeding mothers in an effort to reduce infant illness and death caused by the use of contaminated milks. By 1903, such milk dispensaries were already being accused of discouraging breastfeeding because they seemed to endorse the use of other infant milks (Wickes, 1953b). Even today, government-sponsored distribution of free milk (as has occurred in Nicaragua since 1970) has been considered one reason for the decline of breastfeeding (Sandiford et al., 1991). The WIC Program is still the largest purchaser of formula sold in the United States, with a

Table 1–2

BREASTFEEDING RATES (PERCENTAGES) AND US *HEALTHY PEOPLE 2010* BREASTFEEDING OBJECTIVES FOR THE NATION

	1998 Actual	2000 Actual	2010 Goal
Initiate breastfeeding within the early postpartum period	64	68	75
Breastfeeding at 6 months after birth	29	31	50
Breastfeeding at 12 months of age	16	18	25

Source: Available at http://www.ross.com/aboutross/Survey.pdf. Accessed March 17, 2002.

budget in 2000 of about $4 billion, up from $3.7 billion in 1997.

In the late 1980s, the promotion of breastfeeding became an important goal within WIC. The Child Nutrition and WIC Reauthorization Act of 1989 required that a certain proportion of its budget was to be spent on the promotion and support of breastfeeding and that each state health department would establish a breastfeeding promotion coordinator. Today breastfeeding women have a higher priority for enrollment in WIC programs than do nonbreastfeeding mothers: they are provided more, and increasingly varied, foods, and their benefits persist longer—one year, as opposed to 6 months for nonbreastfeeders.

Despite these efforts, the increases in breastfeeding rates of WIC enrollees have been minimal. WIC infants initiate breastfeeding at a much lower rate than non-WIC infants (56 percent vs. 77 percent) and continue breastfeeding at 6 months at an even lower rate compared with non-WIC infants (20 percent vs. 40 percent). Tuttle (2000) notes that although these increases may provide some cause for optimism, the results "beg the question of how the rates of breastfeeding initiation and duration might have been different if formula were not being dispensed from the same agency providing the education and support." Women enrolled in WIC who worked full-time had the lowest breastfeeding rate even though they initiated breastfeeding at the same rate as other enrollees.

US Breastfeeding Committee.   In 1998, supported by the Maternal and Child Health Bureau, a national breastfeeding conference was convened to form a breastfeeding committee as had been recommended by the Innocenti Declaration on 1990. The United States Breastfeeding Committee (USBC) was established, composed of representatives from government and nongovernment organizations and health professional associations. The committee's goals have been to expand awareness of the value of breastfeeding and to recommend policies to government and corporate organization that increase breastfeeding prevalence (USBC, 2001).

Legislation.   Legislation intended to increase the prevalence of breastfeeding may mandate actions that encourage breastfeeding or discourage feeding of artificial baby milk (or use of wet nurses) or both. One of the earliest examples was set in around 350 BC by Lycurgus, the king of Sparta: he required not only that mothers nurse their own infants, but that nursing mothers be shown kindness and respect (Hymanson, 1934).

During the past decade, breastfeeding legislation on the state level has chipped away at the US bottle-feeding culture in an attempt to encourage a breastfeeding culture. *The Breastfeeding Promotion Act*, introduced into Congress in 2001 to protecting women from being discriminated against in the workplace for pumping milk or breastfeeding, is an example. State laws in 27 states have been enacted to protect a woman's right to breastfeeding her child in public and private locations. Several states have passed laws that excuse breastfeeding women from jury duty (Humenick & Gwayi-Chore, 2001; Walker, 2001).

Statements by Health Organizations.   In 1997 the American Academy of Pediatrics Work Group on Breastfeeding issued a policy statement endorsing breastfeeding (AAP, 1997). The statement received considerable attention from the press, accelerating nationwide interest in breastfeeding. Other professional organizations have published similar public endorsements of breastfeeding: the American College of Obstetricians and Gynecologists (2000; rev. 2002), the American Dietetic Association (1997), the American College of Nurse-Midwives (1992), the American Academy of Family Physicians (2001), the Association of Women's Health, Obstetric and Neonatal Nurses (1999), and the National Association of Pediatric Nurse Practitioners (2003).

International Breastfeeding Promotion

The International Code of Marketing of Breast-Milk Substitutes.   In the 1970s, the deleterious effects of manufactured baby milks on infant health and survival became better appreciated, and the role of advertising in spreading the use of these milks became increasingly suspect. In 1981 WHO, by a vote of 118 to 1 (the United States was the dissenting country), approved the International Code of Marketing of Breast-Milk Substitutes. The code provides a model of marketing practices that permits the availability of manufactured baby milk but

BOX 1–1

WHO/UNICEF Code for Marketing Breast-Milk Substitutes

- No advertising of these products to the public.
- No free samples to mothers.
- No promotion of products in health-care facilities.
- No company mothercraft nurses to advise mothers.
- No gifts or personal samples to health workers.
- No words or pictures idealizing artificial feeding, including pictures of infants, on the products.
- Information to health workers should be scientific and factual.

- All information on artificial feeding, including the labels, should explain the benefits of breastfeeding, and the costs and hazards associated with artificial feeding.
- Unsuitable products, such as condensed milk, should not be promoted for babies.
- All products should be of a high quality and take into account the climatic and storage conditions of the country where they are used.

Source: From WHO (1981).

---

forbids its advertisement or free distribution directly to consumers. (See Box 1–1.)

The code also seeks to balance the information provided by infant milk manufacturers, in both written "educational" material and in the text or pictures on containers of the product (Armstrong, 1988; IBFAN/IOCU, 1985). In 1996, the World Health Assembly passed six resolutions that further clarify the intent of the International Code. Of these six, one reaffirms the use of local family foods to complement the diet of breastfeeding infants beyond about 6 months of age. Another reaffirms the need to end the free or low-cost (subsidized) distribution of artificial baby milk to newly parturient women in the hospital. Two other resolutions proscribe receipt of funds from manufacturers or distributors of artificial baby milk or feeding supplies to be used for professional training in infant and child health, or for financial support of any organization that monitors compliance with the International Code (UNICEF, 1996).

An individual country may adopt the International Code in the manner that best fits the needs of that country. In some, no action has been taken,

and formula manufacturers are bound only by voluntary adherence to the industry-written "codes of ethics" that lack sanctions for noncompliance. A few other countries have adopted and do enforce various aspects of the code.

The International Code focuses attention on ways in which the infant formula industry influences both consumers and professionals to support the use of their products. Direct advertising to consumers may be the most obvious ploy, but what Jelliffe and Jelliffe (1978) called "manipulation by assistance" is also effective. For example, formula manufacturers not only provide free formula to hospital nurseries but also assist in the design of those nurseries (to separate mothers and infants), donate equipment and supplies to hospitals and individual physicians (bottles of formula and sterile water, for example), and support conferences (including some dealing with breastfeeding). They even entertain hospital staff at company-sponsored events; hospital staff in one US city was taken on an outing to the dog races. These "gifts" are treated by the companies as marketing expenses. Lactation consultants should be watchful in order to avoid succumbing to such "manipulation by assistance" provided by manufacturers of artificial baby milk and of other feeding products banned by the International Code.

As individuals and institutions become financially dependent on such gifts and enmeshed in social relationships with company salespeople, they are more likely to tacitly endorse, or even recommend, artificial baby milks. By highlighting such practices as marketing ploys, the code may make health-care professionals more aware of the intent behind them, and thus perhaps more resistant to their allure.

Innocenti Declaration. In 1990, the World Health Organization and the United Nations Inter-national Children's Emergency Fund (UNICEF) were instrumental in the development of the Innocenti Declaration, which restated the importance of breastfeeding for maternal and child health. It set forth four goals to be met by 1995: (1) the establishment of national breastfeeding coordinators and a national breastfeeding committee, (2) the practice of Ten Steps to Successful Breastfeeding by maternity services (see Box 1–2), (3) the implementation of the WHO International Code, and (4) enactment of enforceable laws for protecting the breastfeeding rights of employed women (UNICEF, 1990).

Some 140 countries now have national breastfeeding committees, and about 185 offer maternity leaves of at least 12 weeks, usually only to those formally employed (UNICEF, 1996). Not all countries

---

BOX 1–2

Ten Steps to Successful Breastfeeding

Every facility providing maternity services and care for newborn infants should

1. Have a written breastfeeding policy that is routinely communicated to all health-care staff.

2. Train all health-care staff in skills necessary to implement this policy.

3. Inform all pregnant women about the benefits and management of breast-feeding.

4. Help mothers initiate breastfeeding within 30 minutes after birth.

5. Show mothers how to breastfeed, and how to maintain lactation even if they should be separated from their infants.

6. Give newborn infants no food or drink other than breast milk, unless medically indicated.

7. Practice rooming-in—allow mothers and infants to remain together 24 hours a day.

8. Encourage breastfeeding on demand.

9. Give no artificial teats or pacifiers (also called *dummies* or *soothers*) to breastfeeding infants.

10. Foster the establishment of breast-feeding support groups and refer mothers to them on discharge from the hospital or clinic.

Source: From WHO (1989).

Note: These steps and the complete elimination of free and low-cost supplies of breastmilk substitution, bottles, and teats from health care facilities form the basis for the Baby-Friendly Hospital Initiative.

have achieved the Innocenti goals; for example, in Italy, the country that hosted the Innocenti conference, the government has made little progress toward fulfilling its goals as a signatory of the declaration (Chapin, 2001). The World Alliance for Breastfeeding Action (WABA) is a multinational coalition of individuals and private organizations involved in research and promotion of breastfeeding. It works to ensure that the goals of the Innocenti Declaration are met, and it annually supports activities presented during World Breastfeeding Week—an opportunity for people worldwide to celebrate and support breastfeeding.

Baby-Friendly Hospital Initiative. The Baby-Friendly Hospital Initiative (BFHI) was launched by the World Health Organization and UNICEF in 1991 to encourage specific hospital practices in all countries that promote exclusive breastfeeding. In order to be designated "baby-friendly," a hospital must demonstrate to an external review board that it practices each of the ten steps to successful breastfeeding outlined in the Innocenti Declaration. With the principal exception of the Scandinavian countries, industrialized nations have moved more slowly than developing nations, primarily because it is difficult to meet the requirement that hospitals should accept no free formula. Breastfeeding advocates in the industrialized world labor against three impediments: an artificial milk industry that is powerful enough, both financially and politically, to avoid regulation; a pervasive bottle-feeding culture that does not consider breastfeeding important to child or maternal health; and the lack of much precedence for government-mandated health programs. As a result, all industrialized nations together can claim only a small percentage of all baby-friendly hospitals. The United States has only 33 hospitals (of 16,000 worldwide) designated as having achieved baby-friendly status.

Several studies have examined the degree to which the "Ten Steps" are being implemented and their effect on hospital practices and breastfeeding outcomes (DiGirolamo, Grummer-Strawn, & Fein, 2001; Dodgson et al., 1999; Hannon et al., 1999; Merewood & Philipp, 2001; Wright, Rice, & Wells, 1996). Without exception, these studies show improved breastfeeding outcomes. A high proportion of mothers delivering in a hospital or birthing center certified as baby-friendly choose to breastfeed because of the consistent support they receive from the staff and from their birth experience in a breastfeeding-friendly environment. Table 1–3 lists organizations that promote breastfeeding.

Private Support Movements

During the 1970s, the trend to artificial feeding reversed. (See Figure 1–6.) The reasons are not clear but seem to have been part of a widespread desire of many to include simpler, more natural practices in their lives. In the 1950s and 1960s, voluntary groups that offer information and support to women interested in breastfeeding, such as La Leche League International (LLLI) in the United States, Nursing Mothers' Association of Australia, and Ammenhjelpen of Sweden, had been formed. Such groups assist individual women and have focused national attention on the benefits of breastfeeding. La Leche League is officially recognized as a nongovernmental organization qualified to consult on breastfeeding to organizations such as the United Nations and the United States Agency for International Development. In 2001, LLLI had over 7000 accredited leaders and some 3000 groups around the world. It offers information in 32 languages (LLLI, 2002) and provides $33 million per year in in-kind services. Members of groups such as these, by their demonstration that even "modern" mothers can breastfeed, and by their requests to medical personnel for information about medical practices that support breastfeeding, have been a major force behind the dissemination of technical information concerning lactation, human milk, and breastfeeding.

To better reach low-income women, who are not commonly La Leche League members, LLLI has trained more than 3000 peer counselors—low-income women who have breastfed and have completed a training program. Offering breastfeeding advice and support in clinics that serve low-income populations, such counselors can be very effective (see Chapter 23).

Table 1–3

ORGANIZATIONS AND EVENTS THAT PROMOTE BREASTFEEDING

Year	Organization	Event/Policy
1978	World Health Organization (WHO)	International Conference on Primary Care
1979	US Department of Health and Human Services (USDHHS)	*Healthy People: The Surgeon General's Report on Health Promotion and Disease Prevention* www.surgeongeneral.gov/library/reports.htm
1980	USDHHS	*Promoting Health and Preventing Disease: Objectives for a Nation* www.surgeongeneral.gov/library/reports.htm
1981	WHO	The International Code of Marketing Breast-Milk Substitutes www.waba.org.br/folders94.htm
1990	USDHHS	*Healthy People 2000: National Health Promotion and Disease Prevention* www.cdc.gov.nchs/about/otheract/hp000/hp2000.htm
1990	UNICEF	Innocenti Declaration: On the protection, promotion and support of breastfeeding. www.unicef.org/crc/crc.htm
1991	WHO	Baby-Friendly Hospital Initiative www.uniceforg/programme/nutrition/infantfe/tensteps.htm
1995	World Alliance for Breastfeeding Action	Platform for Action www.waba.org.br
1997	American Academy of Pediatrics	Guidelines and Recommendations for Breastfeeding www.aap.org/policy/re9729.html
1998	United States Breastfeeding Committee	US National Breastfeeding Policy Conference United States Breastfeeding Committee, 2001
1999	US Congress	The Right to Breastfeed Act passed to ensure a woman's right to breastfeed on federal property www.lalecheleague.org/LawBills.html
2000	American Academy of Nursing	Expert Panel on Breastfeeding
2001	USDHHS	Breastfeeding Blueprint www.4woman.gov/breastfeeding/blueprint.htm

Source: From: Humenick & Gwayi-Chore (2001).

S u m m a r y

Humans evolved within the mammalian lineage, which has provided a species-specific milk for the nourishment and protection of the young of each species. For millennia, the staple of the human infant's diet has been human milk obtained directly from the human breast, commonly in situations where no other food was suitable. Within the last century or so, as breastfeeding became associated with more restrictive aspects of women's lives, as breastmilk was thought by some to be inferior to increasingly available manufactured infant milks, and as use of manufactured milks became a hallmark of privileged segments of society, large portions of both lay and health-care populations came to believe that there was little reason to persist in traditional breastfeeding practices.

Since the early 1990s, however, it has become increasingly clear that breastfeeding confers health and psychological advantages on the breastfeeding infant and also benefits the child and adult into which that infant will grow. Breastfeeding enhances aspects of maternal health as well. Breastfeeding is economically frugal and ecologically sound. Breastfeeding is important. Most mothers and health-care providers now recognize these benefits.

The promotion efforts outlined in this chapter are needed because, to some degree in most countries (and particularly those in the industrialized world), the most important requirements are missing: acceptance by society at large of the need for a mother and child to be together, and the right of the breastfeeding dyad to participate in social, civic, and commercial activities outside the home. For many women, the ultimate barrier to breastfeeding is not sore nipples, night-time nursing, or employment outside the home. It is the disapproval they encounter for "wasting" their education and career skills by staying home with their breastfeeding infants, or for being considered disruptive or even ob-

scene for taking their breastfeeding infant with them to work or to worship, or perhaps to a city council or parent-teacher meeting, or simply to a restaurant or to a park. A goal for women should be to empower all mothers so that they are able to attend to all of their duties, maternal as well as civic, religious, and professional.

Those who breastfeed or who promote the reestablishment of breastfeeding as the norm in infant feeding do so not because there are no alternatives but because the alternatives are inferior. Unfortunately, the belief that breastfeeding is the optimal way to nourish an infant may not be enough to empower a woman to breastfeed. Knowledge of beneficial breastfeeding practices and society's acceptance of those practices are also required. Currently, the prevalence of breastfeeding reflects the importance that society places on it, as measured by the degree to which breastfeeding mothers and infants are accepted in the life of the community at large. Returning breastfeeding wisdom to the public domain and reintegrating breastfeeding into the social fabric so that women who wish to breastfeed may do so without hindrance is the challenge that awaits.

Key Concepts

- The class Mammalia is characterized by breasts (mammae), which secrete and release a fluid that for a time is the sole nourishment of the young; breastfeeding dates back some 100 million years.

- Before about 1900, information about breastfeeding incidence, prevalence, and practices came from indirect sources; since the mid-twentieth century, national surveys and World Health Organization data have been available.

- Among modern hunter-gatherers, whose breastfeeding practices may be very ancient, breastfeeds tend to be frequent (average 4/hour), short (about 2 minutes), equally distributed throughout a 24-hour day, and persist for 2 to 6 years.

- Before about 1900, wet-nursing was the only alternative to breastfeeding that was likely to allow the infant to survive.

- The currently typical hand-fed infant foods did not become part of the human diet until late in human history; cereal grains were domesticated only about 10,000 years ago and animal milks about 5000 years ago.

- In the decades around 1900, high infant mortality was a major public concern, standards of modesty strictly limited breastfeeding outside the home, and advances in science and technology led to the creation of dry or tinned artificial infant foods.

- In the 1890s, physician Thomas Rotch developed a complex system of progressive modifications of cow milk to make it more digestible by infants of various ages; this system required constant intervention by the physician, who might change an infant's "formula" weekly.

- Beginning in the 1700s, mothercraft manuals began to shift the management of infant feeding from the mother (or women in general) to (usually male) "authorities," and by the early part of the twentieth century, "good mothering" drifted toward meeting feeding and infant-care schedules imposed by authorities.

- In the United States, the proportion of newborns receiving any breastfeeding declined steadily after 1940 to a low of 25 percent in 1970; the trend then reversed and despite a dip in the late 1980s, has risen steadily since then.

- In 2000, more than 80 percent of mothers in the Mountain and Pacific Northwest breastfed their infants in the hospital.

- After World War II, the United States and Western Europe exported hand-feeding practices to countries that they colonized or otherwise influenced.

- Infants fed manufactured infant milks suffer more illness because such milks lack the nutritive qualities and immunologic factors of breastmilk; mothers who use manufactured infant milks are more susceptible to osteoporosis, premenopausal breast cancer, and ovarian cancer.

- Infants who are fed manufactured infant milks are more costly to raise, in part because of the considerable cost of the formula and in part because they suffer more, and more severe, illness as compared with breastfed infants.

- The diversion of land, power, and raw material to the manufacture of artificial infant milks, and the disposal of discarded packaging, is an increasing ecological concern.

- Voluntary groups dedicated to promoting breastfeeding, such as La Leche League International in the United States, Nursing Mothers' Association of Australia, and Ammenhjelpen in Sweden, began in the 1960s and 1970s and paved the way for governmental efforts.

- In the United States, national breastfeeding goals were first stated in 1979 in *Healthy People: The Surgeon General's Report on Health Promotion and Disease Prevention.*

- During the 1980s, the promotion of breastfeeding in the United States became an important goal within the Women, Infants, and Children (WIC) Program; however, increases in breastfeeding rates of WIC enrollees, who typically come from population segments least likely to breastfeed, have come slowly.

- The International Code of Marketing of Breast-Milk Substitutes was approved in 1981 by the World Health Organization; it permits manufactured infant milks to be available but forbids their advertisement or free distribution directly to consumers.

- The Innocenti Declaration was approved in 1990 by the World Health Organization and the United Nations International Children's Emergency Fund; it encourages specific hospital perinatal practices that promote exclusive breastfeeding.—

Internet Resources

Baby-Friendly Hospital Initiative:
www.uniceforg/programme/nutrition/infantfe/tensteps.htm
www.babyfriendlyusa.org

Blueprint for Action on Breastfeeding, Department of Health and Human Services:
www.woman.gov/breastfeeding

Breastfeeding rate in the United States:
www.ross.com/aboutross/Survey.pdf

Information on breastfeeding in 44 developing countries:
www.childinfo.org/eddb/brfeed/probl3/htm

UNICEF Breastfeeding and Complementary Feeding:
www.childinfo.org/eddb/brfeed/test/database.htm

US Breastfeeding Committee:
www.usbreastfeeding.org

US Congressional legislative action on breastfeeding:
http://thomas.loc.gov

World Alliance for Breastfeeding Action (WABA):
www.waba.org.br

References

Aitken FC, Hytten FE. Infant feeding: comparison of breast and artificial feeding. *Nutr Abstr Rev* 30:341–71, 1960.

American Academy of Family Physicians. AAFP Policy and position statement on breastfeeding. Available at: www.aafp.org/x633.xml; 2001. Accessed May 2003.

American Academy of Pediatrics Work Group on Breast-feeding. Breastfeeding and the use of human milk. *Pediatrics* 100:1035–39, 1997. *Guidelines and Recommendations for Breastfeeding.* Available at: www.aap.org/policy/re9729.html.

American College of Nurse-Midwives. *Position Statement on Breastfeeding.* Washington: ACNM, July 1992.

American College of Obstetricians and Gynecologists. Breastfeeding: maternal and infant aspects. *ACOG Educational Bulletin* 258, July 2000. Available at: www.acog.org/from_homepublications/press_releases/nr07-0100.htm. Accessed July 2002.

American Dietetic Association. Position of the American Dietetic Association: promotion of breast-feeding. *ADA Reports* 97(6): 662–66, 1997. Available at: www.eatright.org/adar1_101801.html.

Apple RD. "Advertised by our loving friends": the infant formula industry and the creation of new pharmaceutical markets, 1870–1910. *J Hist Med Allied Sci* 41:3–23, 1986.

Armstrong H. The International Code of Marketing of Breast-Milk Substitutes (Part 2) *J Hum Lact* 4:194–99, 1988.

Association of Women's Health, Obstetric and Neonatal Nurses (AWHONN). AWHONN position statement. *NAACOG Newsletter* 19, 1992.

Bain K. The incidence of breast feeding in hospitals in the United States. *Pediatrics* 2:313–20, 1948.

Ball TM, Wright AL. Health care costs of formula-feeding in the first year of life. *Pediatrics* 103:870–76, 1999.

Briend A, Wojtyniak B, Rowland MGM. Breast feeding, nutritional state, and child survival in rural Bangladesh. *Br Med J* 296:879–82, 1988.

Butte NF et al. Milk composition of insulin-dependent diabetic women. *J Pediatr Gastroenterol Nutr* 6:936–41, 1987.

Chapin EM. The state of the Innocenti Declaration targets in Italy. *J Hum Lact* 17:202, 5, 2001.

Chen Y, Yu S, Li W. Artificial feeding and hospitalization in the first 18 months of life. *Pediatrics* 81:58–62, 1988.

Cunningham AS, Jelliffe DB, Jelliffe EFP. Breast-feeding and health in the 1980s: a global epidemiologic review. *J Pediatr* 118:659–66, 1991.

Dearlove JC, Dearlove BM. Prolactin fluid balance and lactation. *Br J Obstet Gynaecol* 88:652–54, 1981.

Deruisseau LG. Infant hygiene in the older medical literature. *Ciba Symposia* 2:530–60, 1940.

DiGirolamo AM, Grummer-Strawn LM, and Fein S. Maternity care practices: Implications for breastfeeding. *Birth* 28(2):94–100, 2001.

Dimond HJ, Ashworth A. Infant feeding practices in Kenya, Mexico and Malaysia: the rarity of the exclusively breast-fed infant. *Hum Nutr Appl Nutr* 41A:51–64, 1987.

Dodgson JE et al. Adherence to the Ten Steps of the Baby-Friendly Hospital Initiatives in a Minnesota hospital. *Birth* 26:239–47, 1999.

Feldman-Winter L et al. Breastfeeding initiation rates derived from electronic certificate data in New Jersey. *J Hum Lact* 18:373–77, 2002.

Fildes VA. *Breasts, bottles, and babies: a history of infant feeding.* Edinburgh: Edinburgh University Press, 1986.

Gerrard JW. Breast-feeding: second thoughts. *Pediatrics* 54:757–64, 1974.

Greer FR, Apple RD. Physicians, formula companies, and advertising: a historical perspective. *Am J Dis Child* 145:282–86, 1991.

Greiner T. The concept of weaning: definitions and their implications. *J Hum Lact* 12:123–28, 1996.

Grulee CG, Sanford HN, Herron PH. Breast and artificial feeding: influence on morbidity and mortality of twenty thousand infants. *JAMA* 103:735–39, 1934.

Grummer-Strawn LM, Li R. U.S. national surveillance of breastfeeding behavior. *J Hum Lact* 16:283–90, 2000.

Habicht J-P, DaVanzo J, Butz WP. Mother's milk and sewage: their interactive effect on infant mortality. *Pediatrics* 88:456–61, 1988.

Hannon PR et al. A multidisciplinary approach to promoting a Baby Friendly environment at an urban university medical center. *J Hum Lact* 15:289–96, 1999.

Hastrup K. A question of reason: breastfeeding patterns in seventeenth and eighteenth-century Iceland. In: Maher V, ed. *The anthropology of breast-feeding—natural law or social construct.* Oxford: Berg Publishers, 1992:91–108.

Hoey C, Ware J. Economic advantages of breastfeeding in an HMO setting: a pilot study. *Am J Managed Care* 3:861–65, 1997.

Howarth WJ. The influence of feeding on the mortality of infants. *Lancet* 2 (July 22):210–13, 1905.

Humenick SS, Gwayi-Chore MO. Leader or left behind: national and international policies related to breastfeeding. *JOGNN* 30:529–40, 2001.

Hymanson A. A short review of the history of infant feeding. *Arch Pediatr* 51:1–10, 1934.

Illingworth PJ. Diminution in energy expenditure during lactation. *Br Med J* 292:437–41, 1986.

International Baby Food Action Network/International Organization of Consumers Unions (IBFAN/IOCU). *Protecting infant health: a health worker's guide to the International Code of Marketing of Breast-milk Substitutes.* Penang, Malasia: IBFAN/IOCU, 1985.

Jackson RI. Ecological breastfeeding and child spacing. *Clin Pediatr* 27:373–77, 1988.

Jarosz LA. Breast-feeding versus formula: cost comparison. *Hawaii Med J* 52:14–16 passim, 1993.

Jason JM, Nieburg P, Marks JS. Mortality and disease associated with infant-feeding practices in developing countries. *Pediatrics* 74:702–27, 1984.

Jelliffe DB. Culture, social change and infant feeding: current trends in tropical regions. *Am J Clin Nutr* 10:19–45, 1962.

Jelliffe DB, Jelliffe EFP. *Human milk in the modern world.* Oxford: Oxford University, 1978.

Kelsey JJ. Hormonal contraception and lactation. *J Hum Lact* 12:315–18, 1996.

Kennedy K et al. Consensus statement on the use of breast-feeding as a family planning method. *Contraception* 39:447–96, 1989.

Kessen W. *The child.* New York: Wiley, 1965.

Konner M, Worthman C. Nursing frequency, gonadal function, and birth spacing among Kung hunter-gatherers. *Science* 207:788–91, 1980.

Kovar MG et al. Review of the epidemiologic evidence for an association between infant feeding and infant health. *Pediatrics* 74:615–38, 1984.

Kusin JA, Kardjati S, van Steenbergen W. Traditional infant feeding practices: right or wrong? *Soc Sci Med* 21:283–86, 1985.

Lacaille AD. Infant feeding-bottles in prehistoric times. *Proc R Soc Med* 43:565–68, 1950.

La Leche League International (LLLI). Available at: www.lalecheleague.org, Statistics, 2002.

Latham MC et al. Infant feeding in urban Kenya: a pattern of early triple nipple feeding. *J Trop Pediatr* 32:276–80, 1986.

Levenstein H. "Best for babies" or "Preventable infanticide"? The controversy over artificial feeding of infants in America, 1880–1920. *J Am Hist* 70:75–94, 1983.

Lewis PR et al. The resumption of ovulation and menstruation in a well-nourished population of women breastfeeding for an extended period of time. *Fertil Steril* 55:529–36, 1991.

Lightbourne R, Singh S, Green CP. The World Fertility Survey: charting global childbearing. *Popul Bull* 37:7–55, 1982.

MacGowan RJ et al. Breast-feeding among women attending Women, Infants, and Children clinics in Georgia, 1987. *Pediatrics* 87:361–66, 1991.

Martinez GA, Krieger FW. 1984 Milk-feeding patterns in the United States. *Pediatrics* 76:1004–8, 1985.

McCracken RD. Lactase deficiency: an example of dietary evolution. *Curr Anthrop* 12:479–517, 1971.

Mead Johnson [advertisement]. *JAMA* 95:22, 1930.

Merewood A, Philipp B. Implementing change: becoming Baby-Friendly in an inner city hospital. *Birth* 28:36–40, 2001.

Meyer HF. Breastfeeding in the United States: report of a 1966 national survey with comparable 1946 and 1956 data. *Clin Pediatr* 7:708–15, 1968.

Millard AV. The place of the clock in pediatric advice: rationales, cultural themes, and impediments to breastfeeding. *Soc Sci Med* 31:211–21, 1990.

Montgomery D, Splett P. Economic benefit of breastfeeding infants enrolled in WIC. *J Am Dietetic Assoc* 97:379–85, 1997.

Morse JM. "Euch, those are for your husband!" Examination of cultural values and assumptions associated with breast-feeding. *Health Care Women Int* 11:223–32, 1989.

Morse JM, Jehle C, Gamble D. Initiating breastfeeding: a world survey of the timing of postpartum breastfeeding. *Int J Nurs Stud* 27:303–13, 1990.

National Association of Pediatric Nurse Practitioners (NAPNAP). *Position Paper on Breastfeeding.* Available at: www.napnap.org/practice/position/breastfeeding. Accessed May 2003.

Nestlé's Food [advertisement]. *The Ladies' Home Journal* 9:26, 1892.

Nga NT, Weissner P. Breast-feeding and young child nutrition in Uong Bi, Quang Ninh Province, Vietnam. *J Trop Pediatr* 32:137–39, 1986.

Retherford RD et al. To what extent does breastfeeding explain birth-interval effects on early childhood mortality? *Demography* 26:439–50, 1989.

Riordan J. Cost of not breastfeeding: a commentary. *J Hum Lact* 13:93–97, 1997.

Ross Products Division. *Mothers' Survey.* Columbus, OH: Abbott Laboratories, 2000.

Rossiter FM. The practical guide to health, a popular treatise on anatomy, physiology, and hygiene, with a scientific description of diseases, their causes and treatment, designed for nurses and home use. Pacific Press Publishing, 1908. (Reprinted in part in *J Hum Lact* 7:89–91, 1991.)

Rotch TM. An historical sketch of the development of percentage feeding. *NY Med J* 85:532–37, 1907.

Ryan AS, Wenjun Z, Acosta A. Breastfeeding continues to increase into the new millennium. *Pediatrics* 110:1103–1109, 2002.

Sandiford P et al. Why do child mortality rates fall? An analysis of the Nicaraguan experience. *Am J Public Health* 81:30–37, 1991.

Schaefer O. The impact of culture on breastfeeding patterns. *J Perinatol* 6:62–65, 1986.

Serva V, Karim H, Ebrahim GJ. Breast-feeding and the urban poor in developing countries. *J Trop Pediatr* 32:127–29, 1986.

Sheehan D et al. The Ontario mother and infant survey: breastfeeding outcomes. *J Hum Lact* 17(3):211–19, 2001.

Short RV. Breast feeding. *Sci Am* 250:35–41, 1984.

Simoons FJ. Age of onset of lactose malabsorption. *Pediatrics* 66:646–48, 1980.

Slome C. Nonpuerperal lactation in grandmothers. *J Pediatr* 49:550–52, 1976.

Thorley V. Initiating breastfeeding in postwar Queensland. *Breastfeeding Review* 9(3):21–26, 2001.

Tiedje LB et al. An ecological approach to breastfeeding. *MCN: Am J Matern Child Nurs* 27:154–61, 2002.

Tuttle CR. An open letter to the WIC program: the time has come to commit to breastfeeding. *J Hum Lact* 16:99–103, 2000.

Tuttle CR, Dewey, KG. Potential cost savings for Medi-Cal, AFDC, food stamps, and WIC programs associated with increasing breastfeeding among low-income Hmong women in California. *J Am Diet Assoc* 96:885–90, 1996.

United Nations Children's Emergency Fund (UNICEF). *Innocenti Declaration on the Protection, Promotion and Support of Breastfeeding, Florence, Italy, August 1990.* New York: UNICEF, Nutrition Cluster (H-8F), 1990.

———. *Breastfeeding/Baby-Friendly Hospital Initiative, Update on progress, 1996.* BFHI, Nutrition Section, New York:

UNICEF, November 1996.

———. *State of the world's children: trends in exclusive breastfeeding of children aged 0–3 months in the developing world, 2001.* Available at: www.unicef.org/. Accessed November 4, 2003.

United States Breastfeeding Committee (USBC). *Breastfeeding in the United States: a national agenda.* Rockville MD: USDHHS, Health Resources and Services Administration, Maternal and Child Bureau, 2001.

———. *Economic benefits of breastfeeding* (issue paper). Raleigh, NC: United States Breastfeeding Committee, 2002.

United States Department of Health and Human Services (USDHHS). *Healthy people: The Surgeon General's report on health promotion and disease prevention.* Washington: Government Printing Office, 1979. Available at: www.surgeongeneral.gov/ library/reports.htm. Accessed June 2002.

———. *Healthy people 2010*, vol. 11. Washington: Government Printing Office, 2000. Available at: www.cdc.gov. nchs/about/otheract/hp000/hp2000.htm. Accessed June 2002.

Uvnas-Moberg K et al. Release of GI hormones in mother and infant by sensory stimulation. *Acta Paediatr Scand* 76:851–60, 1987.

Walker M. A fresh look at the risks of artificial infant feeding. *J Hum Lact* 9:97–107, 1993.

———. *Selling out mothers and babies: marketing of breast milk substitutes.* Weston, MA: National Alliance for Breastfeeding Action, 2001.

Weimer JP. *The economic benefits of breastfeeding: a review and analysis.* Food and Rural Economics Division, Economic Research Service, U.S. Department of Agriculture, Food Assistance and Nutrition Research report No. 13, March 2001.

Whitehead RG. The human weaning process. *Pediatrics* 75(suppl 1):189–93, 1985.

Wickes IG. A history of infant feeding: III. Eighteenth and nineteenth century writers. *Arch Dis Child* 28:332–40, 1953a.

———. A history of infant feeding: V. Nineteenth century concluded and twentieth century. *Arch Dis Child* 28:495–502, 1953b.

Wieschhoff HA. Artificial stimulation of lactation in primitive cultures. *Bull Hist Med* 8:1403–15, 1940.

Williamson MA. *Infant mortality: Montclair, NJ. A study of infant mortality in a suburban community.* Washington: US Department of Labor, Children's Bureau, 1915.

Winikoff B, Laukaran VH. Breast feeding and bottle feeding controversies in the developing world: evidence from a study in four countries. *Soc Sci Med* 29:859–68, 1989.

Woodbury RM. The relation between breast and artificial feeding and infant mortality. *Am J Hyg* 2:668–87, 1922.

Woolridge MW, Greasley V, Silpisornkosol S. The initiation of lactation: the effect of early versus delayed contact for suckling on milk intake in the first week postpartum. A study in Chiang Mai, northern Thailand. *Early Hum Dev* 12:269–78, 1985.

World Alliance for Breastfeeding Action (WABA). *Platform for action, 1995.* Available at: www.waba.org.br. Accessed June 2003.

———. *Action Folder '98: breastfeeding—the best investment. 1998.* Available at: www.waba.org.br/folder98.htm. Accessed November 4, 2003.

World Health Organization (WHO). *Declaration of Alma-Ata.* Report of the International Conference on Primary Health Care, jointly supported by the World Health Organization and United Nations Children's Fund. Health for All series 1. Geneva: WHO, 1978.

———. *Contemporary patterns of breast-feeding.* Geneva: WHO, 1981.

———. *International code of marketing breast-milk substitutes.* Geneva: WHO, 1981.

———. *Protecting, promoting and supporting breastfeeding: the special role of maternity services.* A joint WHO/UNICEF statement, Geneva: WHO, 1989.

———. *Baby-Friendly Hospital Initiative* (A joint WHO/ UNICEF statement). Launched at the International Paediatric Association Meeting in Ankara, Turkey, 1991.

———. *WHO Global Data Bank on Breast-Feeding.* Geneva: Nutrition Unit of the World Health Organization, 2000.

Wright A, Rice S, Wells S. Changing hospital practices to increase the duration of breastfeeding. *Pediatrics* 97:669–75, 1996.

Yalom M. *A history of the breast.* New York: Ballantine Books, 1997.

Work Strategies and the Lactation Consultant

Jan Riordan

A lactation consultant (LC) is a specialist trained to focus on the needs and concerns of the breastfeeding mother-baby pair and to prevent, recognize, and solve breastfeeding difficulties. LC services do not replace those of other health-care workers; instead, the LC is an extender of maternal-child services. Lactation consultants work with the public in many settings: hospitals, clinics, private medical practices, community health departments, home health agencies, and private practices. Almost all LCs are women; many have educational and clinical backgrounds in the health professions. The majority of LCs are also registered nurses.

Lactation consulting is a rapidly growing new health-care specialty. Prior to recognition of the LC as a paid specialist in 1985, individuals serving breastfeeding women did so as volunteers or as unrecognized practitioners. The lack of standardization of skills and minimal competencies led to formal development of the specialty practice. This occurred in part through a certification examination, and through the establishment of the International Lactation Consultant Association (ILCA), which publishes the *Journal of Human Lactation* and documents relating to lactation consultant education and practice. La Leche League International and the Australian Breastfeeding Association (for-merly Nursing Mother's Association of Australia) also publish professional materials that teach and support the LC. This chapter traces the historical roots of lactation consultants and discusses work-related issues.

History

In a cultural setting in which nearly all mothers breastfed, help with breastfeeding was available through the shared knowledge of other family members, neighbors, and friends. As childbirth came to be managed by health professionals in hospital settings, however, knowledge of lactation, which a mother formerly shared with her daughters or a sister with her younger siblings, was set aside.

Thus, during the 1960s (at the nadir of breastfeeding) in the United States and shortly thereafter in other countries (such as Australia and Scandinavia), volunteer breastfeeding support groups became a major source of assistance and information about how to breastfeed (Phillips, 1990). As the numbers of breastfeeding mothers increased, health-care providers at first denounced these groups; later they came to appreciate them for the important role they played in helping mothers and in forcing the medical profession to consider lactation an integral part of prenatal and postpartum care.

As these volunteers relearned the art of breastfeeding, they also sought more knowledge of the science of lactation. La Leche League responded by providing research information to their group leaders, who serve as mother-to-mother helpers, and by publishing a quarterly newsletter, *Breastfeeding Abstracts*, which focuses exclusively on the scientific literature. Through La Leche League's professional liaison department, key individuals seek to cultivate and maintain communication links to health providers in local communities.

Out of this context, some experienced breastfeeding support group members began to look beyond what they could accomplish as volunteers. Many of these women sought to apply in a paid work setting what they had learned from many years of helping breastfeeding mothers. In 1982 La Leche League formed the Lactation Consultant Department. From this beginning grew the notion of the need for a new health-care worker and in 1985 an independent certification board, the International Board of Lactation Consultant Examiners, was formed.

Do Lactation Consultants Make a Difference?

In this day of cost containment in health care, administrators want to know if lactation consultants are effective. Do interventions by LCs and other health-care providers make a difference in outcomes of breastfeeding? Table 2–1 presents randomized controlled trials, the highest level and most rigorous type of research study, of breastfeeding interventions worldwide. Most of the studies show that the interventions have a positive effect on breastfeeding. Note from the table that even if the results do not reach significance, any intervention (even a booklet given to the mother) results in higher rates of breastfeeding than no intervention. These results hold constant regardless of where the studies were done.

If the data from the randomized controlled trials in the table were translated to health-care costs saved by breastfeeding, it would show that LC services save the health care system enormous amounts of money through reduction in illness of both baby and mother. Studies that show peer counselor interventions are also effective (see Chapter 25). Clearly lactation services improve the health of our nation, but we have yet to document the extent of this effect in terms of money savings.

Certification

In 1981, experienced La Leche League leaders JoAnne Scott and Linda Smith were asked to develop a certification and training program for lactation consultants. This need derived from (1) an awareness that many health-care providers discredited the accomplishments of the volunteer because she was unpaid, and (2) a need to establish minimum standards for individuals who were already providing LC services for a fee. A certification program was viewed as a way to recognize the important role of the volunteer and to provide a credential that identified competence.

Scott and Smith assembled a small group of breastfeeding experts who had come to the field of lactation through voluntary service, mostly through La Leche League. In 1984, these individuals gathered and concluded that legitimacy of the field would be heightened if minimal standards of knowledge and skills were recognized through a certification examination. Subsequently, they developed the IBLCE Examination based on a three-dimensional content outline or test blueprint and derived from practice analysis.

The first examination was administered in July 1985 under the International Board of Lactation Consultant Examiners (IBLCE). Since 1985, a certification examination has been given annually. To date, more than 10,000 candidates have been certified, the majority of whom live in the United States and Canada. In 2003, IBLCE administered its 19th annual examination to 2094 candidates in 130 locations across 37 counties and territories. The test has been administered in English, Dutch, French, German, Italian, Korean, and Spanish. The largest numbers of candidates have been in Australia, Canada, and the United States. Since the number of candidates from Australia and Canada peaked in 1996 and 1997, the largest candidate growth has

Table 2–1

RANDOMIZED CONTROLLED TRIALS ON THE EFFECT OF LACTATION CONSULTANT AND HEALTH PROVIDER INTERVENTION ON BREASTFEEDING OUTCOMES

Author	Intervention Description	Outcome: Intervention vs. Control
Albernaz et al., 2003 (Brazil)	Lactation support visit in the hospital and 7 visits at home	Twice as likely to be still BF at 4 mo as control group
Susin et al., 1999 (Brazil)	Video, explanatory leaflet, discussion and 4 home visits; N=400	6.5 times higher exclusive BF at end of 3 mo than control
Jakobsen et al., 1999 (Guinea Bissau)	Individual session at first prenatal visit and until 9 mo; N=1154	Any BF at 13 wk 29% vs. 18% .003* Full BF at 4 mo 31% vs. 25%*
Froozani et al., 1999 (Iran)	Hospital session, individual counseling in clinic or at home until 4 mo; N=134	Exclusive BF at 4 mo 54% vs. 6%*
Bolam et al., 1998 (Nepal)	Individual session (20 min); N=540 Intervention 1: at birth and at 3 mo Intervention 2: at birth Intervention 3: at 3 mo	Exclusive BF 33% vs. 28%** 24% vs. 28%** 29% vs. 28%**
Pugh and Milligan, 1998 (United States)	2 home visits with help in home tasks at day 3–4. Phone call	Any BF at 6 mo 50% vs. 27%*
Curro et al., 1997 (Italy)	Booklet: instruction for breastfeeding given during first pediatric visit	Full BF at 6 mo 48% vs. 44%** Any BF at 6 mo 59% vs. 52%**
Duffy, 1997 (Australia)	Group session 3 times: 2 hr + 25 min video	Any BF at 6 wk 91% vs. 29%*
Gagnon et al., 1997 (Canada)	Home visits, early postpartum discharge, phone calls until d 10 postpartum; N = 201	Any BF at 1 mo 55% vs. 39%*
Brent et al., 1995 (United States)	Daily round at hospital 1 phone call, prenatal and postnatal one-on-one consult until 1 yr; N=115	Any BF at 2 mo 37% vs. 9%*
Barros et al., 1994 (Brazil)	Home visits at d 5, 10, 20; N= 900	Any BF at 2 mo 73% vs. 62%
Hauch and Dimmock, 1994 (Australia)	33–page breastfeeding booklet sent home shortly after discharge; N=150	Any BF at 6 mo 59% vs. 56%** Any BF at 12 mo 16% vs. 22%**
Rossiter, 1994 (Australia)	Group session 3 times: 2 hr + 25 min video (after 12th week); N=194	Any BF at 4 wk 50% vs. 26%*

Table 2–1 (cont.)

Chen, 1993 (Taiwan)	Intervention 1: home visits, wk 1, 2, 4, 8 Intervention 2: phone calls, wk 1, 2, 4, 8; N=180	Any BF duration wk mean Home visit: 4.07 Phone call: 3.62 Control: 3.35
Serafino-Cross and Donovan, 1992 (United States)	5–8 home visits during 2 mo + counselor's phone number available; N=52	Any BF at 2 mo 62% vs. 35%**
Neyzi et al., 1991 (Turkey)	Hospital group session + 10 min video, 1 home visit at 5–7 d + booklet; N=941	Any BF at 4 mo 95% vs. 81%** Exclusive BF at 2 mo 4% vs. 2%**
Hill, 1987 (United States)	Group session 1 time: 40 min lecture, 5-10 min questions + pamphlets; N=64	Any BF at 6 wk 39% vs. 30%**
Frank et al., 1987 (United States)	Intervention 1: bedside session in hospital; phone calls until 3 mo + research discharge pack; N=343 Intervention 2: research discharge pack	Exclusive BF at 3 mo 20% vs. 6%* Any BF at 4 mo 71% vs. 54%* Exclusive BF at 2 mo 15% vs. 6%** Any BF at 4 mo 56% vs. 54%**
Lynch et al., 1986 (Canada)	1 home visit within 5 days of post-discharge + phone calls until 6 mo; N=270	Any BF at 1, 3, 6, 9 mo**
Bloom et al., 1982 (Canada)	Phone calls at d 10, 17, 21 + referral to nurse	Any BF at 6 mo 89% vs. 77%*

Significant.
**Not significant.*
Source: Adapted from de Oliveira (2001).

been in other countries in Asia, Europe, and South America (Gross, 2003).

The percentage of candidates who passed the examination has ranged from 83.7 (1997) to 94.6 (1985) (Table 2–2). Periodic recertification as an LC is required through the acquisition of continuing education credits and by reexamination. This dual-recertification option increases the likelihood that the LC will remain current. Guidelines for becoming certified by IBLCE are found in Appendix C.

IBLCE maintains a current registry of certified lactation consultants on its Web site, and at least one state (Louisiana) has a listing of registered LCs who are certified by the International Board of Certified Lactation Consultants. Employers and regulators can thus confirm that an individual is currently certified. The National Certification Corporation for Neonatal and Obstetric Nurses also offers a subspecialty exam in breastfeeding for RNs. It is considered a first step to becoming certified by IBLCE. For more information on lactation consultant certification, go to the International Board of Lactation Consultant Examiners Web site at www.iblce.org.

Certification, a process by which an individual demonstrates clinical competence in a specialty, is

Table 2–2

IBLCE EXAMINATION SUMMARY DATA, 1985–2003

Year of Examination	Number of Candidates	Mean Score	Pass-Fail Score	Pass Rate (%)
1985	259	72.8	61.8	94.6
1986	222	72.6	62.9	93.2
1987	281	72.5	63.8	90.7
1988	281	74.0	64.6	91.1
1989	306	76.1	67.5	92.5
1990	428	72.1	64.6	89.3
1991	683	72.9	63.6	91.1
1992	834	71.9	64.0	88.0
1993	1,171	76.4	64.0	93.3
1994	1,198	73.4	63.8	87.3
1995	1,556	73.8	61.8	94.1
1996	1,764	74.8	63.0	92.0
1997	1,670	71.8	64.0	83.7
1998	1,812	74.7	64.7	88.8
1999	1,757	75.0	66.8	83.8
2000	1,862	72.7	60.9	87.8
2001	2,070	76.7	66.7	88.6
2002	2,536	75.4	65.0	90.4
2003	2,094	78.4	67.0	93.3

Source: From International Board of Lactation Consultant Examiners (IBLCE).

a valued and popular credential, especially in the United States. More than 40 specialty certifications exist in the field of nursing alone, despite the fact that certification is a voluntary credential.

In a study of nurses in the United States and Canada who earned certification in a specialty area (Cary, 2000; Raudonis & Anderson, 2002), the nurses reported that they felt more confident and experienced fewer errors in patient care since they had become certified. The authors concluded that certified health professionals appear to be more motivated to achieve high levels of performance and professionalism; thus certification may be a marker for excellence in practice and improved health care. Clearly, certified health professionals believe there is value in holding certification (Simpson & Creehan, 2001).

Getting a Job as a Lactation Consultant

Most lactation consultants are health professionals, usually nurses, who start their career in a job where they work with breastfeeding dyads. They learn about breastfeeding "on the job" and by personal experience rather than as part of their formal education. Others begin by affiliation with La Leche League and take the necessary courses and gain clinical experience to become certified. Applying for an LC position takes planning to be successful.

Interviewing for a Job

Insider information tells you that a position for a lactation consultant is available and you want to apply. Here are some steps to follow to prepare for the interview:

- Research the position. What are the expected skills and experiences needed? Does your background match these skills and experiences? Some state laws limit clinical service to licensed medical or nursing staff, often for legal reasons. A common requirement for a hospital-based job as a lactation consultant is experience working with new mothers and babies, and certification by the IBLCE.

- Research the organization. Is it a clinic, medical office, small or large hospital? If it is a hospital, how many deliveries does it have each year? What is its competition? If it does not provide lactation services and a competing hospital does, develop this lack as major selling point for your services.

- Identify your strengths and weaknesses. Be ready to highlight skills, experience, personal qualities, and accomplishments you would bring to the health-care agency.

- Keep in mind that first impressions count. Your appearance tells the interviewer quite a bit about your character. You want the interviewer to see you as a professional in every way including personal hygiene and wardrobe. An expensive outfit is not necessary but your clothing should fit well and be clean and pressed. A business suit with a knee-length skirt is always appropriate.

- Know what salary to expect before you begin to interview. LCs employed by a hospital or birth center are usually paid on the same scale as staff nurses. Wages will differ according to the region you live in; however, US hospital staff nurses receive an average hourly rate of about $24. Average annual nursing income is listed in Table 2–3. Note that nurses working in a physician's medical office receive the lowest pay.

Table 2–3

AVERAGE ANNUAL INCOME OF US NURSES

Setting	Average Annual Income ($)
Hospital	69,710
Community/home health	58,720
Outpatient services/clinic	56,880

Source: Derived from Steltzer et al. (2003).

- Follow the general rule that if an employer does not bring up the subject of salary, don't ask about it until you have a job offer. Until you have that offer, salary doesn't matter. Once you have the offer, you can negotiate from a position of greater power.

- Evaluate the benefits being offered. Insurance (disability, life, and medical) and a 401(k) or 401(b) retirement plan with matches from your employer must be kept in mind. These extras can make a difference in the total compensation package. Although malpractice is rare with breastfeeding situations, it is not rare in obstetrics and the LC might become involved in a legal case. Generally, LCs working in a hospital or community health agency will not need malpractice insurance.

Hafner-Eaton (2000) reported a wide range in hourly wages in her survey of 169 LCs (Table 2–4). She found that nurse practitioners or certified nurse midwives who are also lactation consultants make the highest annual salary ($61,000).

Gaining Clinical Experience

IBLCE certification requires a considerable number of clinical hours of direct care of the breastfeeding dyad: from 900 clinical hours if one has a doctorate in medicine to 4000 for those without a college degree.

Table 2–4

AVERAGE WAGE AND CONSULT TIME OF LACTATION CONSULTANTS

Practice Setting	Hourly Wage ($)	Initial Consult ($)	Length of Consult (min)
Private	55	79	95
Clinic	43	69	64
Hospital	28	62	74

Source: Hafner-Eaton (2000).

A health-care professional who needs clinical hours to qualify as an applicant to take the LC certification examination should seek out a job where she will work with breastfeeding mothers to accumulate clinical hours. Working on a mother-baby unit is an example.

The individual who is still in a school to become a health-care professional can investigate the possibility of taking a supervised clinical practicum as a part of a degree. For each hour spent in a clinical practicum, a student can reduce the number of hours needed to take the exam by 5 to 1, up to 500 hours. For example, a 40-hour practicum counts as 200 hours toward the number of hours of breastfeeding experience needed.

Opportunities for clinical experience working with breastfeeding dyads is an issue when the individual who wishes to become an LC does not have access to clinical learning. Not everyone who desires to work as a lactation consultant wishes to become a nurse or other type of health professional. There are other ways to acquire practical experience working with breastfeeding dyads:

- Seek out a formal clinical teaching program in lactation management. The few available programs are of high quality but you may have to travel to another part of the state (or country) in order to do the clinical practice. Sometimes a clinical arrangement can be made in your own area. For example, some students have completed their clinical requirements by working with a local pediatrician (Smillie, 2000).

- Join La Leche League and become an LLL Leader. The IBLCE will give credit for each year of active practice as a leader. Because the women attending LLL meetings are either pregnant or have breastfed for a long time, it will give you an opportunity to observe the needs and concerns of mothers just learning about breastfeeding and those who have extensive experience.

- Become a WIC peer counselor. As a peer counselor IBLCE will grant 500 practice hours for each year that you are active in the field.

- Work in a medical office as a breastfeeding specialist teaching breastfeeding classes and counseling mothers.

- Contract with an IBLCE certified health professional to observe and assist in a clinical setting. Sometimes called "shadowing," observing a qualified practitioner at work can take place in a clinical agency such as a hospital, in a community health clinic, or in a medical office (see Box 2–1). Permission for such an experience will need to be obtained from both the LC and the supervisor or director of the clinical agency.

- "Round out" your experience by visiting different work settings. For example, if your experience has been in a hospital, visit a WIC clinic to learn about the issues associated with breastfeeding older children or make arrangements to observe a breastfeeding mother in her home environment. Conversely, if your work setting has been a medical office or WIC clinic, go to a hospital setting.

- Keep track of and document the hours spent working with breastfeeding mothers either as paid staff or in a volunteer capacity. Accurate records of contact hours are necessary in order to apply to take the certification examination.

LC Education

Most lactation consultants have another health-care degree in areas such as nursing, medicine, dietetics, or physical therapy, and they obtain certification as

Shadowing Guidelines

- Seek permission from the preceptor and the client being observed. The facility or LC may welcome you, but the mother may feel uncomfortable. Obey protocols such as wearing scrubs.
- As an observer, introduce yourself and speak only when appropriate.
- Take copious notes on what you've observed.
- Arrange with the preceptor to spend time after the observation period to discuss the cases and ask questions.
- Always thank the client being observed for her willingness to allow you into her "space."
- Do not observe on a day when you have a cold, sore throat, diarrhea, or allergies.
- Thank the preceptor in person and again with a note. Let her know how she has facilitated your education. Stress the positive things you experienced and saw.
- If there were problems during the observation, discuss these with your faculty or mentor.

Source: From Smith (2002).

an LC as a second credential. Being a health professional who is also a lactation consultant will offer you greater job security. In addition, this also means you will have already taken many of the courses that are required to be eligible to take the IBLCE certification examination.

As the number of lactation consultants working in health care increases, so does the availability of educational courses on lactation. Since the role of the LC has only recently been developed, the history of formal lactation education in the United States is short (Table 2–5).

Although lactation certification by IBLCE is considered the "gold standard," other certifications have sprung up, including certification as a "lactation counselor" and as a "lactation educator." These programs are geared toward people, such as WIC personnel, who do not wish to become lactation consultants but want to be more knowledgeable about breastfeeding.

Wilson-Clay (2000) believes that LCs have an identity crisis partly due to inconsistent professional education. Claiming that a common education creates a sense of shared values, tradition, and practice, she calls for a comprehensive course of study on lactation followed by examination and certification to guarantee consumers that someone with the LC title will be competent. In response to a call for educational standards, ILCA has moved toward planning a formal accreditation of educational programs that meet criteria for preparing lactation consultants.

Lactation Programs

A New York state law mandated in 1984 that any institution providing care for new mothers and babies had to have at least one person on staff who was designated to serve as a resource for other staff members and to provide breastfeeding assistance to patients. This landmark event helped launch the subsequent growth of the lactation consultant as a clinical specialty.

The 1990s could be characterized as the decade for the emergence of breastfeeding programs and clinics. Only a small number of hospitals in the United States had a lactation program in the early 1990s. But within the past decade lactation programs have proliferated rapidly and most hospitals and birth centers now have lactation services staffed by certified LCs, who have thus grown in numbers and visibility. Although lactation expertise has long been integrated into midwifery practice in countries where midwives predominate, LCs are becoming more common, especially in Australia, Canada, and Europe (Figure 2–1).

Table 2–5

HISTORY OF LACTATION EDUCATIONAL PROGRAMS

Program Start Date	Description
Late 1950s and 1960s	• La Leche League International in Chicago develops first educational programs for mothers and professionals worldwide.
1970s	• Wellstart Program in San Diego provides lactation training for professionals from teaching hospitals in developing nations (sponsored by USAID).
	• Lactation Institute and Breastfeeding Clinic in Los Angeles starts in 1979.
	• LLLI starts annual Physician Seminar in 1975.
1980s	• LLLI initiates lactation consultant continuing education programs.
	• Lactation counselor certification programs offered.
	• IBLCE forms and develops LC certification.
	• ILCA forms and provides continuing education courses for lactation consultant credit.
	• First European seminar held in 1987 in Switzerland by VELB, European Lactation Associates.
1990s	• Education programs specifically for LC training continue to grow.
	• Wichita State University offers first graduate course on lactation entirely on the Internet.
2000–present	• Degree program as lactation specialist is offered at Union College.
	• Lactation education programs continue to proliferate worldwide.

Opportunities for paid positions have increased to the point that hospitals now advertise for lactation consultants. Medical centers tend to hire registered nurses into lactation consultant positions because of state practice regulations concerning direct care of patients and because nurses can work in other units of the hospital if the maternity area census is low.

A lactation program may take many guises and offer a variety of services (Box 2–2). A breast pump rental depot, because it is so likely to generate revenue, may serve as a first kind of service for breastfeeding women (Rago, 1987). A lactation service may be part of a community health program already in place but funded for a breastfeeding clinic or promotion program (Dublin, 1989). Such programs often require that the LC become cognizant of both the political and social climates, not only of the particular agency for whom she works but also of the larger community that it serves. For example, in a community in which health-care workers are already well versed in assisting breastfeeding mothers and babies, a lactation clinic may simply be part of an environment supportive of lactation. In another community, in which breastfeeding is not seen as part of regular health care, establishing such a clinic may represent a threatening but potentially exciting departure from previous care patterns.

A lactation program may also develop out of a patient education program that began with childbirth preparation and other classes designed to meet the many needs of pregnant and postpartum women and their families. For clientele who have already developed rapport with the patient educator, additional classes may be provided, including prenatal breastfeeding classes, and follow-up services after the baby is born.

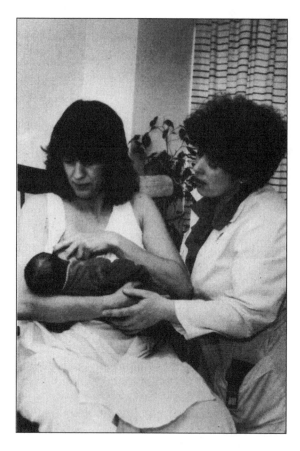

FIGURE 2–1. Early assistance promotes maternal confidence.

Other programs may have begun in neonatal intensive care units and later expanded to the rest of the hospital, or they may be the outcome of patient surveys that indicate the need for lactation services. Still others may have developed from a hospital needing to "keep up with the medical Joneses"—i.e., when a competing hospital provides and then publicizes its lactation consultant services, other hospitals compete by providing similar services, such as the lactation clinic seen in Figure 2–2.

How those services are structured varies by the institution. In some programs, the LC sees all new mothers who indicate that they plan to breastfeed. In other cases, she sees all new mothers, identifying her clients when they tell her how they are feeding or planning to feed their babies. A few LCs counsel both breastfeeding and bottle-feeding mothers. Other institutions restrict the LC's contact only to those breastfeeding mothers for whom the referring physician has asked for a consultation and follow-up care. Most of the time hospital-based LCs work on the birthing unit and/or postpartum area but they also assist breastfeeding mothers who are hospitalized in other areas. Thus their rounds take them to the surgical and medical units and to intensive care. Women in the hospital for premature labor can also be seen by the LC.

BOX 2–2

Hospital-Based Lactation Programs and Services

- Daily one-on-one mother-baby rounds. Every breastfeeding mother seen by LC without referral or breastfeeding mothers seen only with referral
- Telephone hotline or "warmline"; post-discharge telephone calls
- Prenatal classes on breastfeeding
- Home postpartum visits and assistance with breastfeeding
- Pump rental and sales
- Postpartum breastfeeding consults for

problems by appointment or "open clinic" hours
- Continuing education for staff, area seminars, preceptorships, and breastfeeding classes
- Research on lactation and breastfeeding issues (most often at a tertiary-care medical center)
- Evaluation of lactation products, devices, and services

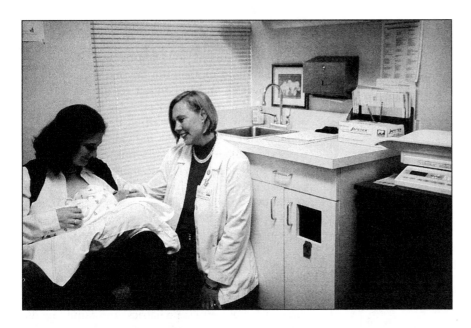

FIGURE 2–2.
A hospital-based lactation clinic (With permission, Pardee Hinson)

Workload Issues

Whatever system is used, it is wise to estimate the anticipated workload prior to the start of the lactation service. Most hospital-based programs have been in existence six or seven years and employ two to four LCs who mostly work part-time. Thus one must measure full-time equivalent hours (FTEs) in order to determine the completeness of coverage. For example, in some hospitals, three part-time LCs share seven days per week coverage. The actual number of work hours should be based upon the number of births in the institution and the percentage of mothers who are breastfeeding. Daily rounds on breastfeeding women may be feasible in a hospital in which the LC sees fewer than 10 patients per day; it may not be feasible if more than 10 breastfeeding mothers are housed in the maternity unit on a given day—unless there is more than one LC in the service or staff members providing other care are trained to provide optimal lactation-related care as well, thus reserving the LC for mothers and babies needing additional help and as a resource for the staff.

Thus, in a hospital with 200 births per month with an 80 percent breastfeeding rate, the LC will see about six to eight patients on weekdays (and fewer on the weekend). A hospital with 3000 deliveries each year should have a minimum of three full-time LC positions or six part-time positions (Box 2–3). This staffing produces a bare minimum coverage that usually results in understaffing and/or part-time coverage. The service—to be effective—should be available seven days a week, on all shifts.

Lactation consultant Pardee Hinson reported 2.6 FTEs LC positions (about 90 hours) for a hospital with 1600 deliveries (Hinson, 2000). These lactation consultants used to see each breastfeeding mother every day but now, in order to be able to keep up with the demand for their services, they see each breastfeeding mother once and see her again only if there is a referral. In an effort to meet patient needs, it is not uncommon for LCs to volunteer additional time for which they are unpaid. Heinig (1998) addressed this issue as "closet consulting," warning that when the caseload is invisible to the employer, the LC's professional time is undervalued and may result in further limits on LC time.

Developing a Lactation Program

In proposing a lactation program, it is essential to realize that such a service will overlap with the interests of several ongoing departments or programs. As a result, it is both politic and appropriate to involve all such departments in the early stages of the proposal process. Touching base with hospital decision-makers and developing a working relationship with them is critical. Without it, any hope

BOX 2–3

Sample Time Expended to Provide LC Services in a Hospital

Assume one to three visits per mother per day (to coincide with recommended frequency of offering the breast in an eight- to nine-hour period).

Time per visit: 20 minutes – average length of first visit;

+ 15 minutes × 2 (average length of each of the next two visits)

× 10 breastfeeding mothers in the mother-baby unit

= 8.3 hours of work for the LC

This does not take into account other time factors for the LC: time spent charting, having lunch, meeting with colleagues, planning, outpatient visits and prenatal education classes, participating in staff in-services, and the like. Hospital-based lactation consultant jobs are often strenuous and exhausting. Many LCs are on their feet for most of the 8 (or 10 or 12!) hours of their shift and have little opportunity to sit down. Time to chart, eat lunch, or drink a cup of coffee is precious and short.

of establishing and maintaining a program is seriously undermined, and the likelihood of the program becoming and remaining an integral part of the institution remains low. The hospital-based LC often creates her own position when hospital administrative personnel respond to patient demands for lactation services. Most LCs working in hospitals develop a plan for providing lactation services and then present a proposal to administration for approval.

No new program will be implemented without someone in power pushing it, especially in a downsizing environment. A sponsor with "clout" is needed to lend momentum beyond the actions of the innovators and to commit resources from the institutional budget. This person can be a high-level administrator, a chief of staff, or department chair. Kantor (1983) calls this individual the "prime mover" or an "idea sponsor": "prime movers push in part by repetition by mentioning the new idea or practice on every possible occasion in every speech and at every meeting."

Department heads particularly critical to securing support for the new program include the director of maternity nursing (who may oversee labor and delivery, postpartum and nursery units, and sometimes the intensive care nursery); the director of the pediatric unit; and the chairman or medical director for obstetrics, pediatrics, and family medicine. If the institution has a midwifery service, the support of its director should also be sought. Usually, department heads meet as a committee to review requests and attempt to solve problems. These committees should be approached when proposing a new lactation service. One option is a lactation service that contracts with the hospital for services. Using the contract services, the hospital saves money because it does not pay for benefits for the lactation consultants who see its patients (Ferrarello, 2001).

If the institution has an employee health service or a women's health clinic, their supervisors should be informed of the proposal and asked for their support. Written proposals or documents that highlight how the new program will assist and support the services that are already being provided helps build their acceptance. For example, the head of employee health may be particularly interested in learning that the lactation program will include services to employees, such as a special place where employees returning to work after the birth of a baby can hand express or pump their breasts or nurse their babies during work hours (Dodgson & Duckett, 1997). The women's health service may want to know how to refer clients to the lactation service and how they can take advantage of the resources of such a service.

Experienced LCs who have started a lactation service point out the importance of not taking for granted that everyone knows about the service and what it offers. Being as visible as possible around the hospital helps to get the word out. The LC is a member of the staff and thus able to attend staff meetings for the departments (nursing service, family practice, pediatrics, obstetrics) in which the lactation service will have the greatest effect. In all cases, each contact and presentation must focus on the ways in which the department and institution will benefit from the service. Although improved patient care is an obvious item to mention, most hospital administrators hope that any new service will generate income.

Hospital administrators choose new programs from dozens of possibilities for hospital investment (for example, another magnetic resonance imager versus a new diabetes center). Administration looks at two "bottom-line" factors—revenue and marketing potential—of proposed services before selecting which to offer. In deciding on any new health program, money speaks loudest.

Lactation services are usually provided in a single area that serves as the home base for telephone follow-up and inpatient services, as well as record keeping and as a site for professional resources. LCs can also see mothers who return for outpatient care in this area. In addition to outpatient services, some hospitals offer free postpartum home visits as a part of the insurance coverage for the delivery. This "perk" differs according to the insurance company with which the hospital contracts for deliveries. Income generated from inpatient care is managed through the regular accounting or finance office and submitted for insurance coverage, as occurs for other hospital-based charges.

Although lactation services will generate minimal revenue compared to high-tech medical equipment, they are an effective marketing tool for the hospital. Women make most of the decisions about health-care services for family members. Health strategists claim that if the mother uses a certain hospital for her baby's birth and she liked the service she received there, she will probably use that same hospital again for the family's future health-care needs. In the United States and many other developed countries, the women most likely to breastfeed are educated and in middle-to-higher income brackets; thus, a lactation service increases the hospital's visibility and credibility with young,

educated families who have a high earning potential later on. The income-generating nature of patient care makes such a service attractive, particularly in settings in which several local hospitals are competing for the same patient dollars. The new trend in hospitals is product-line management, an approach that markets a product-line of services: lactation services are a "product" that medical centers can offer to their "customers."

Just as the lack of physicians' support can prevent a program from being added to the array of services already offered, physician support can pave the way for the addition of a lactation program. Such support is most likely to be obtained if the key physicians—often chiefs of service or department heads—see that a lactation program will meet needs that they feel are important. In some cases, the need for such a service is championed by a female physician who has personal breastfeeding experience.

Physicians are still influential figures in the hospital although their power has diminished since managed care; therefore, maintaining positive relations with physicians is critical. Even with managed care, the physician as "gatekeeper" plays a major role in the fiscal health of a hospital. If the physician's patients do not want to go to a particular hospital because it lacks certain amenities—such as a lactation service—the birthing service administrator, with the backing of physicians, may create such a program rather than lose patients to a competing institution. Supportive physicians are more likely to be mothers who breastfed, fathers of breastfed children, those building a new practice, and those from countries where breastfeeding is the norm.

Changing well-established routines is a major source of conflict between other health-care workers and the lactation service personnel, even when the change is supported by research. Because few people like to do things differently and most health professionals tend to provide service as they were taught in medical or nursing school, recommendations from the LC can cause resentment and irritation among the nursing and medical staff.

When any change in protocols or routines, however small, is contemplated, the wise LC will enlist the assistance of those most likely to be affected by the change. Such planning can go a long way toward defusing potential antagonism and reducing resistance to change. Nearly always, this means consulting with the physicians who write orders and the nurses who are expected to carry them out. Even something so apparently insignificant as the removal of supplemental water bottles from the cribs of neonates will require meetings and discussions, often with a committee mandated to initiate the change.

In addition, in-service programs are needed to explain the change. A team approach is more likely to accomplish a change, and compliance is more likely. After change is instituted, additional in-servicing is often necessary—to ensure that all staff members are following the new protocol and to iron out any difficulties that may arise as the new protocol is put into effect.

Marketing

Marketing—a discipline used by business to convert people's needs into profitable company opportunities—is still poorly understood and appreciated by health workers; either they need to learn marketing techniques themselves or to seek assistance from marketing experts. Nurse/entrepreneurs can seek help from small-business centers at universities that help small-business people at no cost, attend marketing classes, and read books on marketing.

The following are basic marketing techniques that LCs may find useful:

- Collect data such as the number and percentage of women giving birth who breastfeed, and survey women who have used lactation services.

- Analyze strengths and weaknesses of competitors and focus on service needs not currently being met.

- Establish a small niche within the health-care market that is ignored by large health-care providers—for example, a postdischarge visit for a back-to-work consult.

- Promote the practice by advertising and public relations: brochures, newsletters, letterhead stationery, business cards, fact sheets, and radio and TV interviews all help to inform clients and other health workers about LC services (Gardner & Weinrauch, 1988).

The Unique Characteristics of Counseling Breastfeeding Women

There are unique aspects of working with breastfeeding women that differ from other aspects of health care.

- Breastfeeding is an emotion-laden subject that may be viewed as an integral part of human sexuality, not just an infant feeding method. It touches deep-seated feelings that people have about themselves and their bodies that reach back to childhood. This emotional content makes breastfeeding counseling, like sex counseling or childbirth education, unusually sensitive. Health-care workers assisting breastfeeding families must be especially intuitive, caring listeners and advisors.

- Working with new mothers and babies is a popular and thus, competitive, activity. Not only are newborns adorable, but the mothers and fathers are (generally) healthy and happy. By working on the hospital maternity unit or in a birth center, the nurse gets to play a paid, starring, ongoing role in the usually joyous family dramas of birthing and early breastfeeding. As a result, nurses compete to work there, and the mother-baby unit tends to have a low rate of staff turnover. This situation is especially true for nurses who work in lactation services.

- Breastfeeding counseling is almost exclusively provided by women who must daily interact and work with other women: mothers and other female health workers. Women interact in the workplace differently than men do. Awareness and understanding of the typical ways that women interact with women and compete with each other gives the nurse or LC who comes onto the unit or into the community agency as a "new kid on the block" an advantage (Gilligan, 1982). Table 2–6 summarizes how women tend to work together and how they *need* to work together.

Three characteristics—the emotional quality of breastfeeding, the popularity of caring for babies, and the dysfunctional, covert games that women bring to the work environment—set the stage for potential difficulties between the LC and the nurse, the nurse and the breastfeeding mother, the volunteer counselor and the LC, and the female physician and the LC.

Although workplace standards of behavior tend to follow men's rules, it does not negate feminine elements. Feminine, nurturing qualities help us in working with breastfeeding families. Our best qualities have to do with becoming attached and developing close relationships and friendships with others. These attributes are critical for all healthcare workers, including LCs, if they are to empathize with breastfeeding mothers. However, when women personalize the business or professional setting, it is counterproductive to their professional or business goals.

Survival in the workplace requires that we learn to operate within two concurrent cultures: the culture of nurturing and caring and the culture of the profession's business, which is about accomplishing tasks efficiently. Virginia Woolf noted that the values of women differ from the values of men; yet, she added, "it is the masculine values that prevail" (Woolf, 1929). Women succeed in the workplace when they use their womanly strengths of compassion and intuitiveness in their work, while playing by men's rules.

Roles and Responsibilities

The LC is responsible to the mothers she sees to provide up-to-date and accurate information and

---

Table 2–6

CORRECTING NEGATIVE FEMALE WORKPLACE BEHAVIORS

What Women Tend to Do	What Women Need to Learn to Do
Women tend to express anger covertly behind their co-workers' backs rather than openly and confrontationally. Girls learn that they should be "nice" to everyone, not fight, and especially not hit anyone. These concepts are called Mommy's Rules (Davidson-Crews, 1989), and they are deeply embedded female behaviors, especially in white, middle-class, American women.	Be overt, not covert. If there's a problem, confront, forget, and move on.
Women try to avoid being criticized; they often take it personally. Women are socialized to derive their self-worth from external, rather than internal, sources; therefore, they tend to react excessively to others' opinions, whether positive or negative. Women are more likely to hold grudges for long periods.	Communicate. Do not make scenes or public outbursts.
Women are less likely than men to have used the give-and-take team concept of "you help me and I'll help you and we'll both get ahead." Women operate on a higher utopian level: what is right and just is more important than any other consideration. Women act as police officers of one another, making sure that what their coworkers do is right and correct and "trashing" them to keep them in their place.	Be friendly, but do not strive to be close friends.
Women tend to become over friendly, one-to-one. Women who work together and become fast friends tell each other their deepest secrets, which are sometimes used against them when the friendship dissolves. Women give away power by giving away too much of themselves. Women are more likely to work for social rewards; men work for money.	Accept and love yourself. Accept (and appreciate) that some people are not your friends, now or ever.

appropriate assistance. In a medical center setting, however, such service will be molded by the other services also provided there. Table 2–7 lists the six competency areas or functions required by an LC practice.

Although there are no studies on the time allocation of various role components, LCs report that the majority of their time is spent in direct care of clients. The role of the LC closely parallels that of the clinical nurse specialist insofar as it requires in-depth clinical knowledge and expertise in a particular area. Gibbins et al. (2000) describe a model of the Nurse Practitioner (NP) or Clinical Nurse Specialist (CNS) in the role as a lactation consultant in a breastfeeding clinic. This advanced practice role encompasses the dimensions of the advanced practice model: research, leadership, education, and clinical practice. Like the clinical specialist, the LC does the following:

- Gives direct care
- Teaches
- Consults
- Conducts or assists in conducting research

Giving breastfeeding mothers consistent breast-feeding information is vital. The patient takes for granted that the person to whom she spoke knows exactly what should be done. If confusion or controversy is found among the staff, we cannot expect the patient to become knowledgeable and comfortable with learning mother-infant tasks. Staff in-ser-

vices on breastfeeding increase the likelihood that the staff will provide consistent information.

Although providing in-service education is an important, perhaps even essential, role of the lactation consultant, one can (like the proverbial horse brought to a watering hole) offer but not impel other health-care workers to drink from the pool of knowledge. Other nursing staff may have fallen into the habit of expecting the LC to take care of all breastfeeding issues. If an LC is not available on all shifts or all days, this person cannot possibly always take care of things. Rather than expecting the LC to do it all, it is more effective for her to teach the staff, so that all health-care workers are operating from the same frame of reference in how they assist breastfeeding mothers and when they will intervene to resolve a difficulty (Shrago, 1995).

Another function of the LC, whether she is located in a hospital or has a private practice, is to evaluate services and products related to lactation. Evaluating new products and then publishing the results is a professional responsibility. Seeking feedback from patients helps ensure that quality service is being provided (Turner, 1996).

Stages of Role Development

Roles of health professionals have been extensively studied and shown to progress through stages of development. For example, Benner (1984) used the Dreyfus and Dreyfus (1980) model of skill acquisition to describe the progression of skills and competencies of nurses in the clinical setting. This model, a structure for the metamorphosis that occurs as nurses persevere in their practice, can also apply to lactation consultants. According to Benner (1984), there are five stages of role acquisition:

- *Novice:* Develops technical skills; has narrow scope of practice; needs a mentor.
- *Advanced beginner:* Enhances clinical competencies; develops diagnostic reasoning and clinical decision-making skills; begins to incorporate research findings into practice.
- *Competent:* Expands scope of practice; becomes competent in diagnostic reasoning and clinical skills; senses nuances; develops organizational skills.

Table 2–7

REQUIRED COMPETENCIES FOR LACTATION PRACTICE

1. Breastfeeding education and advocacy
2. Clinical management of breastfeeding
3. Technical knowledge
4. Special knowledge and assistance
5. Professional responsibilities and activities
6. Business practices/legal considerations

- *Proficient:* Achieves highest level of clinical expertise; conducts or directs research projects; acts as change agent; uses holistic approach; interprets nuances.
- *Expert:* Global scope of practice; consults widely; empowers patients and families; serves as mentor.

Benner derived these insights from the stories nurses told about their practice and applied them into a logical, orderly progression of skill development. Joel (1997, p. 7) paints a vivid picture of the journey from novice to expert:

At first we see situations as tidbits of equal significance; later we move to the idea of a highly complex integrated whole where some pieces are just more important to solving the problem. And, finally the nurse becomes as one with the clinical situation. Rather than looking from the outside in, at the zenith of your practice, you are indivisible from the puzzle you are challenged to solve. You move right to the heart of the matter without responding to distraction.

Using Benner's model from novice to expert as discussed earlier, LCs—such as experienced clinical nurse specialist—will spend more time as consultant and in scholarly work as they gain experience in the field (Auerbach, Riordan, Gross, 2000). Because the role of the lactation consultant is relatively new, other health providers may be unclear about what to expect of this new health-care worker. To clarify areas of expertise that can be expected of such an individual, the International Lactation Consultant Association has developed a set of recommendations and related competencies for LC practice (see Appendix A).

Lactation Consultants in the Community Setting

Because of the heightened awareness of the importance of breastfeeding, community health workers are becoming educated about breastfeeding; some of them go on to certify as an LC. The 1989 WIC Reauthorization Act that mandated a breastfeeding coordinator in each state accelerated community health workers' interest in breastfeeding. Most of these coordinators are registered dietitians or registered nurses. Home health nurses are another group of community-based health workers who frequently care for breastfeeding families.

Community-based health care is different from hospital-based care in that the health-care provider works with the mother over the long term—throughout her pregnancy, childbirth, and postpartum course; thus they have an advantage over those working in the hospital in that they see the mother and her family in a total environment. Someone once described this as seeing a whole movie, whereas in the hospital one sees only one frame. Being in the family home gives a much wider perspective on the mother's needs that are not otherwise apparent. For example, I visited a breastfeeding mother in her home along with a student nurse as a clinical experience. The client was a 15-year old new mother who recently arrived from Mexico and had no family members here. She was having trouble putting the baby to breast because of extreme engorgement. After we pumped and got the baby on the breast, I suggested that we freeze the milk, since I thought she probably had not thought of this, given her youth and inexperience. She motioned me to her refrigerator and opened the freezer section, which held many bottles of breastmilk that she had expressed and saved. Clearly, this young woman had much more knowledge about lactation than I could have surmised by seeing her one time in the hospital before she was discharged.

Moreover community-based services are organized around a system of interdisciplinary community services and resources. Many times the community heath nurse works with mothers who are poor and receive welfare assistance, where breastfeeding problems are but a minor star in a firmament of despairing circumstances.

Medical Office

Physicians, especially pediatricians, realize the value of having staff who are knowledgeable about breastfeeding and can quickly and effectively work with breastfeeding women in their practice; thus lactation consultants are employed in the medical office. Their responsibilities include answering phone calls from breastfeeding women, making home visits, and working with the physician during postpartum visits to the medical office and making hospital rounds. The physician office usually pays the lactation consultant a salary; however, advanced practice nurses such as pediatric nurse practitioners may do their own billing.

Lactation Consultants and Volunteer Counselors

The client is apt to obtain more complete services when lactation consultants maintain a congenial, reciprocal relationship with volunteer counselors as well as other health-care professionals in their community.

The volunteer counselor and the lactation consultant provide similar services. They most often differ about where such service is provided, the nature of clinical assistance, and the degree of follow-up care. For example, volunteer counselors are an excellent source of preventive health-care information pertaining to breastfeeding and lactation. They also spend more time giving long-term assistance than the LC, particularly if the latter sees clients in a clinic or hospital setting. It is not uncommon for a mother to continue to receive assistance and caring concern from a volunteer counselor through the entire lactation course; only rarely will an LC meet with a client regularly through that entire period. Instead, she is more apt to have sporadic contact, initiated by the client when a specific question or concern arises. The LC is more apt to assist a mother when specific clinical skills are needed to assess or to resolve a problem.

Volunteer breastfeeding helpers and LCs can assist one another (Thorley, 2000). The volunteer may have seen a certain mother in her own home and thus may be able to alert the LC working in a hospital, doctor's office, or clinic to elements about the mother's home life that may bear on her lactation course. The LC may serve as a referral source for persons with complex problems. When the LC works in a medical center where ongoing research is part of her role, she helps generate new knowledge. Both the volunteer and the paid LC can review materials written for clients. The volunteer may be sensitive to ongoing issues that crop up after the mother has left the hospital or does not choose to mention to her health-care providers.

The LC may be aware of aspects of the health-care system that influence breastfeeding.

Networking

Networking is an established mechanism used by members of groups to exchange information, to assist others, and to get help in solving problems (Harter et al., 1987). Most people think first of networking with physicians and others from whom referrals are sought and reports sent (Williams, 1995). However, LCs also network with other lactation consultants and with volunteer breastfeeding counselors—a "good ole girl" network (see Figure 2–3). Generally, these contacts are with LCs who work in a similar setting such as a hospital or in a private practice or with LCs who belong to city- or countywide task forces or other groups of like-minded individuals.

Networking serves several purposes. It offers LCs an opportunity to learn from one another. When a difficult case arises, they feel more comfortable if they can use the phone to work through the situation with another lactation consultant. Additional assessment of the problem and how to begin moving toward a solution might offer new insights or

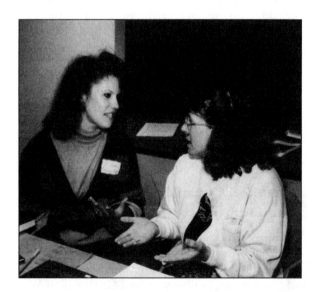

FIGURE 2–3. Making their "net" work for them, two LCs share experiences. (Courtesy of Via Christi Medical Center, Wichita, Kansas.)

creative alternatives to the plan of action already considered. Networking also identifies job possibilities, colleagues who will cover for one another, and referrals for clients needing equipment or specialized help. Networks may also be used to change systems and improve methods of providing care.

Opportunities to communicate with others also abound on the Internet. Foremost among these offerings is LACTNET, a worldwide breastfeeding listserv. Other networks have started, including one for Spanish-speaking individuals, and one exclusively set up for and run by private practice LCs. The benefits of electronic contact include ease of communication with persons for whom telephone contact would be too expensive and postal contact would be too slow. In addition, being able to vent and obtain sympathetic electronic "clucks" within minutes or hours or to seek assistance for a troubling case supports the private LC in a way that can be duplicated only by the existence of as many knowledgeable professionals in the local area. It is the rare setting in which so many colleagues would be gathered in a single place. Electronic networking is here to stay.

In addition to email discussion groups, numerous Web sites also provide information on items of interest to LCs. Exploring the Internet can take hours of time, and new links are created daily. La Leche League International, the Australian Breastfeeding Association, and the International Lactation Consultant Association all have Web sites that describe their purpose, services, and coming events. The ability to access such disparate resources as the National Library of Medicine, Web sites created by proprietary companies, and professional organizations means that LCs can now quite easily electronically "reach out and touch someone," or something, at any time of the day or night, by means of the computer.

Reporting and Charting

It is the responsibility of the LC, regardless of where she practices, to chart each contact with her clients and to provide complete reports to referring physicians and other health-care providers (Williams, 1995). Almost all record keeping involves using a computer. Computer skills are a necessity for health-care workers. As with other health

providers, computers can be used to generate records, reports, and charts that do the following:

- Provide other health workers with valuable information.
- Reflect quality of care delivered (quality assurance, continuous quality improvement).
- Highlight sometimes subtle observations or findings.
- Validate health services for insurance companies to determine reimbursement payment.
- Provide data that can be used for research.
- Serve as evidence in a legal dispute.

In the hospital, the mother's and infant's charts are clinical records that contain information about the hospital stay and all contacts with everyone involved in their care. Because the mother and infant usually have separate charts, it is sometimes necessary to "double chart." At the same time, care plans tend to be geared to the mother, because it is she who is taught and the baby who is the recipient of her learning.

Health professionals are rapidly adopting small hand-held computers known as personal digital assistants (PDAs) to document their interventions by entering coding and pinpointing diagnosis, among other things. Software for items such as coding and medications can be downloaded from the Internet for a trial period and then purchased if one desires.

The most commonly used methods of charting are narrative charting and problem-oriented charting. Flow sheets and standard care plans that are individualized are becoming more popular. They reduce paperwork and save time (and money).

Narrative Charting. Narrative documentation uses a diary or story format to document client-care events. A simple paragraph describes the client's status and the care that was given. Narrative notes, sometimes called *progress notes*, are used less now, with the advent of flow sheets and clinical care plans, which capture the routine aspects of care. Narrative notes (Box 2–4) can be easily combined with flow sheets or any other client record.

Problem-Oriented Charting. Charting based on a problem uses a structured problem list and logical

BOX 2–4

An Example of a Narrative Note

Date	Time	Progress note
05–22–03	0800	Infant alert. Rooting and suckling movements noted. Infant latched on breast and suckled effectively until asleep. Breastfeeding assessment score 9/10.
05–22–03	1500	Discussed basic breastfeeding information including normal infant elimination patterns to watch for after discharge. Mother given written materials on sore nipples, engorgement, use of breast pump, and breastmilk storage.
05–23–03	1100	Explained that a follow-up call will be made 2 to 3 days after discharge. Mother will have the option of a home visit.

format for each entry in the medical record. The format used in problem-oriented charting is called the SOAP or SOAPIE method. Each letter stands for a different phase of the nursing process: subjective data, objective data, assessment and nursing diagnosis, plan, interventions, and evaluation of care (see Box 2–5).

In private practice the completeness of reports also assists the referring health-care worker to understand the "how" as well as the "why" of an LC's practice and methods. Reporting provides a database for all types of information (e.g., an increase in the number of referrals from a particular physician's practice). Early referrals may be for one or two common problems, whereas tracking over a time period may show that later referrals are for a wider variety of problems.

Clinical Care Plans

A clinical care plan provides basic information about client assessment, diagnosis, and planned interventions. It also offers a guide for care, establishes a continuity of care, and represents a means of communication among all caregivers. There are two types of care plans: individual and standard. Individual care plans are developed "from scratch" for each client based on her specific needs. A standard care plan is a preprinted plan of care for a group of patients within the same diagnosis. Because each standard care plan must be tailored according to the needs of a particular client, they are designed to include space for adding information.

The Joint Commission on Accreditation of Healthcare Organizations (JCAHO) requires a care plan for each patient in the hospital as a necessity for accreditation; however, the plan of care can be computer generated, preprinted, or appear in progress notes or standards of care (American Nurses Association, 1991). Care plans are legal requirements of practice and may also serve as protocols or standards of care.

Traditionally, individual care plans are divided into columns. Column headings change over the years to reflect new ideas in nursing, and some column labels are preferred over others. In this book, for instance, the clinical care plans include *assessment/interventions/rationale*. Other commonly used labels are *problem, evaluation, nursing diagnosis, patient outcomes, nursing action,* or simply *intervention-*

BOX 2–5

Problem-Oriented Medical Records

S = *Subjective data.* What the mother herself tells you. *Example:* "My nipples feel sore." *Note:* If the charting relates to only the infant, there will be no subjective data.

O = *Objective data.* Concrete data you can observe. *Examples:* Infant position at breast, temperature, and infant weight.

A = *Assessment and nursing diagnosis.* An assessment of physical and psychosocial factors based upon subjective and objective data; what you think is going on. *Examples:* Infant poorly positioned on the breast; breastfeeding at margin of nipple; ineffective breastfeeding; Latch score = 3 (1 low; 10 high).

P = *Plan.* Organized plan for care. Based upon the assessment, what you plan to do about the problem to help the breastfeeding mother and baby. *Exam-* *ple:* Will reposition infant on breast at next feeding.

I = *Interventions.* What you've done to/for the problem or what you plan to do. Includes teaching, referrals, finding the right pump. *Example:* Infant repositioned on mother's breast so that infant is grasping adequate breast tissue during suckling.

E = *Evaluation.* Review of outcomes. What happened? Was it effective? *Examples:* Infant appears to be suckling effectively at the breast. Infant breastfed four times during shift, three times following repositioning. Infant had bowel movement during feeding—appears well hydrated. In some cases in which a nursing care plan with diagnoses is used, evaluation may reflect only the presenting problem. Outcomes are then charted in the flow sheet.

evaluation. A Nursing Diagnosis and Nursing Care Plan from County of Orange (1999) is seen in Box 2–6. The critical care path or clinical path is a commonly used type of care plan in hospitals. These paths, abbreviated care plans that focus on the client's length of stay in the hospital, integrate infant feeding into the overall care plan.

Legal and Ethical Considerations

Whenever an LC offers advice or touches a mother or baby, she is risking a potential legal action. The action that is most likely to be brought includes battery (when a client does not consent to being touched by another person), breach of warranty (meaning that a service promised verbally or in writing is not provided), or the infliction of emotional distress (usually through a reckless, intentional, or negligent act that harms the patient) (Bornmann, 1986). People usually sue health-care workers not because of their clinical actions but because they are angry with them or for some other reason. Therefore, the most effective protection against such actions is establishing a mutually respectful relationship and rapport. The LC's pattern of practice should include the following:

- Obtain permission—at least verbal, but preferably written—before touching the client or her infant. In different cultures, how one touches a baby may be important. For example, in some cultures, use of the left hand to do a digital

BOX 2-6

Clinical Care Plan

COUNTY OF ORANGE • HEALTH CARE AGENCY • FIELD NURSING
NURSING INTERVENTIONS • NURSING CARE PLAN

Client's Name:_____ Client's Number:_____

Lactation Counseling — 5244

DEFINITION: Use of an interactive helping process to assist in maintenance of successful breastfeeding.

ACTIVITIES:	DATE:					
Determine knowledge base about breastfeeding						
Educate parent(s) about infant feeding for informed decision-making						
Provide information about advantages and disadvantages of breastfeeding						
Correct misconceptions, misinformation, and inaccuracies about breastfeeding						
Determine mother's desire and motivation to breastfeed						
Provide support of mother's decisions						
Give parent(s) recommended education material, as needed						
Inform parent(s) about appropriate classes or groups for breastfeeding (e.g., La Leche League)						
Evaluate mother's understanding of infant's feeding cues (e.g., rooting, sucking, and alertness)						
Determine frequency of feedings in relationship to baby's needs						
Monitor maternal skill with latching infant to the nipple						
Evaluate newborn suck/swallow pattern						
Demonstrate suck training, as appropriate						
Teach mother about:						
• Relaxation techniques, including breast massage						
• Ways of increasing rest, including delegation of household tasks and ways of requesting help						
• Record keeping of length and frequency of nursing sessions						
• Infant stool and urination patterns						
• Adequacy of breast emptying with feeding						
• Quality and use of breastfeeding aids						
• Appropriateness of breast pump use						
• Formula information for temporary low supply problems						
• Skin integrity of nipples						
• Nipple care						
• Relieving breast congestion						
• Applying warm compresses						
• Signs of problems to report to health care practitioner						
• How to relactate						
• Continuing lactation upon return to work or school						
• Signs of readiness to wean						
• Options for weaning						
• Alternative methods of feeding						
• Contraception						

(With permission, Parris KM., 1999).

assessment of the baby's mouth is a highly offensive action and would be deeply resented by the mother. One way to avoid inadvertently offending a client is to ask if the baby may be touched—and to explain how the baby will be touched before doing so.

• Avoid causing the mother, the baby, or any other member of the client's family emotional distress as a result of words said, reports written, or other actions that reflect the LC's relationship with the mother and baby.

- Maintain confidentiality about the mother, baby, and family. To fail to do so is an invasion of privacy, a tort (wrongful act) that involves confidential information that is revealed without permission to someone not entitled to know it.

A clearly written, detailed record of the health provider's actions, initial recommendations, and follow-up assistance (by phone and in person) is one of the most effective ways of avoiding legal action. Referrals increase following a well-written, complete report that is sent in a timely and professional manner. Client records are considered business records of the agency and are admissible as such under legal (court) rules of evidence. Records will often prevent cases from going to court; lawsuits often are won and lost based on what is in the record. Although testimony is another form of evidence, the written health chart is viewed as more accurate and reliable.

The LC who works in a doctor's office, clinic, or hospital is very apt to be part of the staff who are covered in an "umbrella" professional liability policy. The LC in private practice must determine for herself how much coverage she needs and what she can afford. Although legal action against an LC is rare, it does occur; therefore, every individual practitioner needs to consider how she will protect herself and her family against a judgment that could ruin her financially.

A Code of Ethics, established specifically for LCs, covers professional practice and conduct to safeguard interests of clients. These ethical principles seen in Appendix B of this book guide the profession and outline commitments and obligations of the LC to self, client, colleagues, society, and the profession. This code applies to all individuals who hold the credential of IBCLC. To address complaints of misconduct against an LC, the certification board has procedures for discipline. Following the complaint and information gathering, a Discipline Committee decides if the behavior in question was a serious breach of ethics (Kelley, 1999).

Reimbursement

In most countries lactation services are a part of the national health care system and reimbursement for these services is mainly through salaried positions paid for by government programs. In the United States, reimbursement for lactation services is extremely complex and depends upon the setting where the services are provided, educational qualifications of the provider, and the type of insurance involved.

LCs who work in a birthing center, hospital, or medical office are usually salaried employees reimbursed with a set hourly or weekly wage. Hospitals usually include LC services as part of the total cost of the maternity "package." The cost package is an agreement between the insurance company and the hospital to charge a certain amount of money for health-care coverage for each birth. This is known as capitation. Managed care companies compete with each other with price bids to win the health care contract, the lowest bid gaining the contract.

If postpartum home visits are part of a maternity insurance package, breastfeeding assistance is given as a part of a routine postpartum visit to the mother's home. Nurses providing these home visits are usually salaried by the home health company that employs them. Services above and beyond the packaged LC services are paid for either by a separate insurance claim or by the family themselves.

For the LC in private practice, cash payment for services rendered or for equipment is usually requested from the client at the time of the service. The client in turn seeks reimbursement from her insurance company and provides the third-party payer with the information it needs. The client may give the LC forms to complete and send to the insurer in the hope of being reimbursed. Insurance companies expect to be sent the HCFA form that can be downloaded from www.medela.com. A "Superbill" with ICD-9 codes is displayed in Box 2–7. This form, along with an instruction booklet, is available from Pat Lindsey, IBCLC, at www.patlc.com.

Insurance and Third-Party Payment

Insurance and third-party payment for lactation services is a complex issue. Third-party payment—insurance or payment by another entity besides the patient—varies according to the state (and country) where the services were given. In the United States, third-party payers can be divided into two general categories: government or public health insurance

BOX 2–7

Superbill (Lactation Visit Receipt)

Pat Lindsey, IBCLC - Lactation Services
Board Certified Lactation Consultant - Registered Lactation Consultant
TAX ID/PROVIDER # 59-3579433
3849 Oakwater Circle, Orlando, FL 32806 - Telephone 407-859-7239 - Fax 407-850-9185 - Email PatlBCLC@aol.com

"Affordable Health Care Begins with Breastfeeding"

© 2002 Pat Lindsey, IBCLC

PATIENT INFORMATION

PATIENT'S LAST NAME	FIRST	INITIAL	PT'S BIRTHDATE	PATIENT: MALE FEMALE	RELATIONSHIP TO SUBSCRIBER

ADDRESS	CITY	STATE	ZIP	REFERRING PHYSICIAN

PHONE ( )	SUBSCRIBER		INSURANCE CARRIER

ADDRESS - IF DIFFERENT	CITY	STATE	INS. ID	COVERAGE CODE	GROUP

LACTATION   ILLNESS   DATE SYMPTOMS APPEARED:
ACCIDENT   PREGNANCY
INDUSTRIAL

OTHER HEATH COVERAGE?   YES   NO   IDENTIFY:

ASSIGNMENT. I hereby assign my insurance benefits to be paid directly to the undersigned health care provider. I am financially responsible for non-covered services.

RELEASE: I authorize the undersigned health care provider to release any information acquired in the course of my examination or treatment.

SIGNED: (Insured or Authorized Person)   Date:

SIGNED: (Insured or Authorized Person)   Date:

NEW	ESTAB	OFFICE SERVICE	FEE
99203 30min	99213 15min	Hx Evaluation and Management	
99204 45min	99214 25min	Hx Evaluation and Management	
99205 60min	99215 40min	Hx Evaluation and Management	

NEW	ESTAB	HOME SERVICE	FEE
99342 30min	99348 25min	Hx Evaluation and Management	
99343 45min	99349 40min	Hx Evaluation and Management	
99344 60min	99350 60min	Hx Evaluation and Management	

NEW	ESTAB	HOSPITAL SERVICE	FEE
99221 30min	99231 15min	Hx Evaluation and Management	
99222 50min	99232 25min	Hx Evaluation and Management	
99223 70min	99233 35min	Hx Evaluation and Management	

NEW	ESTAB	TELEPHONE CONSULT	FEE
99371	99371	Brief	
99372	99372	Intermediate	
99373	99373	Lengthy/complex	

TRAVEL	# Miles @	

SUPPLIES					CPT/MOD	FEE
BREAST PUMPS						
Breast Pump Collection Kit	Single	Double	Conversion		A7002	
Pump In Style	Orginial	Traveler	Companion		E0603	
Purely Yours					E0603	
Nurse II & III	with case	w/out case			E0603	
Manual Pump					E0603	
Hand Pump	Medela	Ameda	Avent		E0602	
Other Pump					E0603	
SUPPLEMENTAL NURSING SYSTEM	Starter	Regular			A7002	
BREAST SHELLS					99070	
NIPPLE SHIELDS					99070	
BOOKS/PAMPHLETS					99071	
OTHER Feeding Supplies					99070	
Baby Weigh Scale Rental - Serial #		# days @ $			E1399	
ELECTRIC HOSPITAL GRADE PUMP RENTAL					E0604	
Equipment Serial Number						
Rented Date		Return Date				
# days @ $		# months @ $				
Delivery / Extra Cleaning Charge on Rental Pump						
TOTAL SUPPLIES AND/OR RENTAL						
SALES TAX IF NO PRESCRIPTION						

LACTATION DX ICD 9 CM CODES

CHILD

BREASTFEEDING PROBLEM
783.21   Abnormal Weight Loss
775.5   Dehydration Newborn
783.41   Failure to Gain Weight
779.3   Newborn Feeding Problem
          Breast Refusal
          Latch-on Difficulties
          Regurgitation of food
          Slow feeding
          Vomiting
          Other
783.3   Infant Feeding Problem
          Breast Refusal
          Latch-on Difficulties
          Mismanagement of feeding
          Other
783.6   Polyphagia-Overeating
783.2   Under weight

SUCKING PROBLEMS
796.1   Suck Reflex Abnormal

JAUNDICE   (V12.3)
774.39   Breastmilk Jaundice
774   Newborn - Physiologic
774.2   Newborn - Premature

ABNORMAL FUSSINESS/COLIC
777.8   Newborn - Colic
789.0   Infant - Colic
780.59   Sleep Disturbences Infant

DERMATITIS/INFECTION
691.0   Diaper Rash
693.1   Due to Food
691.8   Eczema
771.7   Thrush-Newborn
112.0   Thrush-Infant

OTHER
750.0   Ankyloglossia - Tongue Tie
530.81   GEReflux-NoInflam(V12.79)
530.11   GEReflux-Inflam(V12.79)
750.15   Macroglossia (V12.4)
750.16   Microglossia (V12.4)
520.7   Teething Syndrome

CHILD DIAGNOSIS
PRIMARY DX_____
SECONDARY DX_____
SECONDARY DX_____
SECONDARY DX_____

MOTHER

NIPPLE/AREOLA PROBLEM
676.14   Cracked/Fissured
692.9   Dermatitis Contact
676.04   Dimpled/Folded/Creviced
676.34   Flat
675.9   Infection (unspecific/Thrush)
676.04   Inverted (Retracted)
676.34   Sore Nipples
676.3   Trauma
676.3   Ulceration
676.34   Unusual Shape

BREAST PROBLEM
676.3   Breast Pain
692.9   Dermatitis Contact
676.9   Disorder of Lactation
676.8   Galactocele
757.6   Hypoplasia of Breast
611.72   Mass (es) / Lump (s)

ENGORGEMENT, BREAST
676.20   After the Perinatal Period
676.24   Perinatal, Moderate/Severe

MASTITIS
675.14   Breast Abscess
675.04   Filled Duct
675.20   Non-Purulent Infection
675.24   Plugged Duct
675.14   Purulent Infection

MILK SUPPLY
676.44   Agalactia (No Milk)
676.64   Galactorreah
676.8   Polygalactia (Over Supply)
676.54   Suppressed (Reduced)

LACTATION
676.50   Induced (Adoption) (v61.29)
676.54   Relactation

OTHER
_____
_____
_____

MOTHER DIAGNOSIS
PRIMARY DX_____
SECONDARY DX_____
SECONDARY DX_____
SECONDARY DX_____

NOTES

INSTRUCTIONS TO PATIENT FOR FILING INSURANCE CLAIMS:

COMPLETE THE PATIENT INFORMATION SECTION AT THE TOP OF THIS FORM. SIGN AND DATE. THEN MAIL THIS FORM DIRECTLY TO YOUR INSURANCE COMPANY. PLEASE ATTACH YOUR OWN INSURANCE CARRIER'S CLAIM FORM.

PLEASE REMEMBER THAT PAYMENT IS YOUR OBLIGATION. REGARDLESS OF INSURANCE OR OTHER THIRD PARTY INVOLVEMENT.

REC'D BY		
CHARGE	TODAY'S FEE	
CASH	OLD BALANCE	
CHECK	TOTAL DUE	
#	AMT. REC'D	
	NEW BALANCE	

NEXT APPOINTMENT	PROVIDER'S SIGNATURE	DATE OF SERVICE

(With permission, Pat Lindsey, 2003).

(Medicare, Medicaid) and managed care organizations (MCOs).

Medicare applies to individuals over age 65 and is not applicable for breastfeeding except that insurance companies usually follow Medicare rules for payment. Medicaid is a federal program administered by the states, and state regulations apply to mothers and children who qualify on the basis of poverty. The regulations in various states may differ in billing rules and regulations. About one third of US births are paid for under Medicaid. Medicaid reimbursement for health care is further complicated by the fact that some Medicaid recipients are also enrolled in managed care plans. The plans' policies on reimbursement differ from the state and federal rules governing reimbursement when the patient is not enrolled in managed care.

Insurance policies usually spell out by title who may be reimbursed with third-party payment. Physicians and "mid-level" providers such as nurse practitioners and certified nurse midwives are recognized by third-party payers as providers who can receive direct payment for their services.

To receive reimbursement from Medicaid, the lactation consultant must be accepted as a Medicaid provider by her state Medicaid agency in order to be admitted to the provider panel of an MCO. Generally, providers are accepted on the basis of having a medical or medically-related degree and national certification. Lactation consultants can receive direct reimbursement if they are a physician or an advanced registered nurse practitioner (NP) (including a certified nurse-midwife) who has graduated from an accredited educational program and is certified nationally in a specialty.

Physicians or nurse practitioners can apply for a provider number through the state Medicaid agency by filing a provider application. If accepted as a provider, they can bill the state Medicaid agency on a HFCA 1500 form using the patient's name and identifying information, the ICD-9 code, the Current Procedural Terminology (CPT) code, the charge, the provider's name, number, and location for services. Fees for CPT codes vary according to locations and providers. For example, in many states in order to receive third-party payment, LC services must be provided in collaboration with a physician.

As an example of a successful private medical practice, Pediatrician Tina Smillie set up her breastfeeding practice right after passing the IBLCE exam. She began by writing a series of two- or three-page letters to the HMOs in her area stating benefits of breastfeeding and emphasizing the benefits for the HMO. These letters got her into most of the HMOs as a provider and cover fees for about 95 percent of her patients. She recommends writing these letters as a first step for any physician (or nurse practitioner) going into practice (Smillie, 2000).

If the company rejects a bill, the HCFA 1500 is returned with a short explanation about why it is being rejected. Sometimes several letters back and forth are necessary before the bill will be paid. Persistence is the key, as many claims may not be paid on the first submission. Anyone in a medically-related practice quickly learns from trial and error how to best file third-party insurance claims in order to maximize the number of paid claims.

Payers may require documentation to validate that the care was given, the site of the care, and the medical necessity and appropriateness of services provided. Fees for care of breastfeeding women on Medicaid are based on number and type of services provided using the CPT, published in the ninth edition of *International Classification of Diseases* (ICD-9) (see Box 2–8) and Health Care Financing Administration's Common Procedure Coding System (HCPCS) codes (see Box 2–9).

Major barriers to third-party reimbursement for nonphysician health-care workers such as lactation consultants have been third-party payers who fear expansion of provider eligibility, state licensure laws, and opposition by the medical profession. The 1997 passage of a provision contained in the budget bill Public Law 105-33 to expand Medicare reimbursement for nurse practitioners allows for reimbursement of NP services including lactation services; however each state has the option of covering NP services. Even though the law has passed, these nonphysician providers have difficulties in getting third-party payment.

BOX 2–8

Common Lactation ICD-9 Codes/Diagnosis Codes

Code	Mother	Code	Infant
675.2	Nonpurulent mastitis	276.5	Volume depletion, dehydration, hypovolemia
675.1	Abscess of breast		
676.1	Cracked nipple	524.06	Microgenia; major anomalies of jaw size
676.3	Other and unspecified disorder of breast	783.2	Abnormal loss of weight
675.8	Other specified infection of breast and nipple	750.1	Abnormal tongue position
		774.39	Breastmilk jaundice
692	Dermatitis contact	749	Cleft palate/lip
651.04	Twin pregnancy postpartum condition or complication	750	Tongue tie
		758	Down's syndrome
676.2	Engorgement of breasts	787.2	Dysphagia
676.5	Suppressed lactation	784.41	Failure to thrive, failure to gain weight
676.0	Retracted nipple		
676.4	Failure of lactation	783.3	Feeding difficulty—infant
676.6	Galactorrhea	779.3	Feeding problems in newborn
676.8	Other disorders of lactation	771.7	Neonatal candida infection

Coding

Accurate and complete coding for services and supplies is vital to the financial success of a lactation program or service. The HCPCS is a uniform method for health providers to report professional services and supplies. Box 2–8 presents a listing of HCPCS codes for breast pumps. Keep in mind that payment coding requirements and polices vary

BOX 2–9

HCPCS Codes For Breast Pumps

HCPCS Code	Description
E0602	Breast pump, manual, any type
E0603	Breast pump, electric (AC and/or DC) any type
E0604	Breast pump, heavy duty, hospital grade, piston operated, pulsatile vacuum suction/release cycles, vacuum regulator, supplied, transformer, electric (AC and/or DC)

from payer to payer, and new codes may not be recognized by all payers (International Lactation Consultant Association, 2002). The *Reimbursement Tool Kit* available from ILCA at www.ilca.org is a valuable source of information. The *Healthcare Insurance Guide for Breastfeeding Families* can be downloaded free at the Medela Web site (www.medela.com).

Private Practice

Rising rates of breastfeeding and short hospital stays have resulted in lactation services as a private practice. Some physicians are successful in building a practice that is limited to breastfeeding families. Both professional health workers and those without a health-care background are finding they can enjoy the work they love, assisting women with breastfeeding, and still survive.

Auerbach (Riordan & Auerbach, 1999) surveyed lactation consultants in private practice in the United States and Canada to gain information about their experiences. A majority of the private practice LCs reported that they work 4 to 5 hours a day, qualifying for "part-time" status when seeking professional liability coverage, which all maintained. The number of clients seen in a given week or month varied widely, and was related to several factors, including how long the LC had been in practice, whether she limited herself to home visits (more time-consuming and thus less frequent), and whether her practice was located in a rural or more densely populated metropolitan area. LCs in practices for only two to three years reported seeing the fewest number of clients but their practices grew over time as satisfied customers made referrals to friends, neighbors, and colleagues.

Some LCs started by opening a breast pump rental depot. Others set up a private practice after receiving numerous calls from mothers who requested their help with breastfeeding. Several had been (or still were) hospital nurses who wanted to do more to help breastfeeding mothers than could be accomplished in the hospital. Still others found that a private practice in lactation consulting was an extension of their previous work as volunteer LLL leaders.

The LC's own home is the most common practice setting for non–health professional LCs. For health professionals, practice locations are a clinic, physician's office, or hospital where the LC receives referrals from the staff members of these organizations. Some residential neighborhoods have restrictive covenants that prevent home business or signage that a business is located in a home. Using a post office box for an address avoids neighborhood zoning restrictions. These details must be checked out in advance of opening such a facility. Inadequate road signs in suburban settings or in rural areas will make maps on the backs of flyers and other advertisements a necessity. In North American practices, busy periods clustered in March, April, and May, reflecting the higher birth rates during the warmer months, while slower periods tended to occur in November, December, and January.

The Business of Doing Business

One of the hardest lessons for an LC to learn is that a private practice is a business; if she has no business experience, she must learn about it (Auerbach, 1995). Advertising is essential in establishing and/or maintaining a client pool. Generally, the best advertising is word-of-mouth referral from clients who are satisfied with the LC's services. Other successful advertising includes distributing business cards, flyers, and magnets, and sending personal letters to hospital staff, local physicians (pediatricians, family physicians, obstetricians), community women's groups, childbirth educators, and La Leche League leaders. Teaching a prenatal breastfeeding class is a form of advertising. At the same time, the LC has to make it clear that she charges for later visits. Additional techniques include listings in the telephone book (white or yellow pages), newspaper articles, and press releases for new activities or special events relating to the business.

Lactation consultants disagree about whether to advertise in local newspapers or on the radio. Such visibility has the potential to attract the people merely posing as clients, is expensive, and rarely results in generating clients. The choice of words in advertisements or signs should be considered carefully. In one case, an LC posted a large sign with her name but not the word *breast* or *lactation*, to alert passersby to her business. Using family, parenting, or mother-related phrases works well in lieu of more obvious words. In other communities, inclusion of the words *breastfeeding* or *breast* may not be controversial.

More effective marketing techniques include meeting face-to-face with local physicians, their office staff, and hospital nurse managers, as well as attending professional meetings, such as hospital grand rounds and continuing education programs for nurses. Presenting a case history to hospital physicians, midwives, doulas, childbirth educators, and other health providers raises the visibility of the LC practice and generates referrals.

Incorporating the private practice should be considered only after carefully reviewing the advantages and disadvantages. The advantages are that the business is a legal entity with possible tax advantages and that the business can be sold or transferred. The disadvantages are the expenses of incorporation and that the business is regulated by state and federal controls.

Payment and Fees

Most clients pay for their visits by cash, check, or credit card at the time of service. Lactation consultants, however, harbor a strong streak of idealism and on occasion refrain from charging a client when it is clear that the client cannot pay. Others establish an informal sliding scale for people for whom a total payment at the time of service is not possible or offer a payment plan for those who cannot pay in full at the time of the visit. Only rarely are LC bills not paid. Most people prefer to pay something rather than nothing. And when clients pay even a very small amount for the care they receive, they are more inclined to follow through with the suggestions.

Another aspect of doing business is setting fees. This issue seems to generate the greatest concern when LCs first go into practice. Anxiety about how much to charge for their services may stem from having been a volunteer breastfeeding support person for many years and coming to value the helping relationships with the mothers without thinking of charging for the service. This problem is not confined to LCs. Women tend to be reluctant to charge what their services are worth. This undervaluing of skills or services is part of a woman's socialization when she is growing up. In addition, lack of familiarity with running a business results in undervaluing the service provided. Setting fees too low

degrades lactation consultant services and lowers expectations for insurance company payments.

The prospective private practice LC needs to set her fees on the basis of what other comparable professionals in her community are charging for similar services (e.g., other LCs in private practice, nurses who make home health visits, and medical office visits). Other factors to consider in setting fees are the length of visits. While well-baby visits to a physician's office may last only 15 to 20 minutes, the usual first LC visit may run 60 to 90 minutes. One lactation clinic charges $29 for 15 minutes; $46 for 30 minutes and $68 for one hour (ILCA, 2002).

If the visits take place in the mother's home, a set time for travel is included in the charge: one lactation consultant adds 1 hour to account for travel time to and from the client's home when she bills the visit. Still others charge a set fee according to the number of miles/kilometers they travel in addition to their usual visit fee. Saturday and Sunday visits are sometimes charged at double the usual rate.

Phone consultations should be considered in establishing a fee structure. Some LCs do not charge for phone consultations at all, preferring instead to limit calls to no more than 10 minutes. If more time is needed, they suggest that a visit for which they will be paid is in order. LCs bill differently for phone consultations. Some bill for a specific amount of time within a set framework, such as up to 1 hour of calls within a week after the first visit. Others bill for each call separately. Still others provide free phone consultation for minor issues.

Overhead costs such as rent, taxes, phone, computers, and traveling should be added to determine fee structure. If the annual cost of overhead is added to annual salary and divided by 52 weeks, the amount should equal weekly income (Ferrarello, 2001).

LCs in private practice are most successful when they have an ongoing, mutually respectful relationship with other health-care providers in the community who refer clients to them. A physician in private practice found the following:

Initially some physicians raised their eyebrows. They thought breastfeeding was not worthy of a physician's time. However, as I have seen more and more of their patients, and spoken on grand rounds, I have gained their respect and lots of referrals. Once they discover that there is a science behind the art, the breast is as complex and elegant as any other organ system, they are eager to learn more (Smillie, 2000, p. 51).

Relationships with physicians have established rules, one of which is that if a baby is thought to have a medical problem, before proceeding with lactation assistance, the LC refers the family to their baby's own health-care provider. The LC who is also a nurse practitioner can assess and treat a nursing mother/baby with a medical problem in collaboration with a physician according to the nursing practice laws in her state.

Essential to developing a professional reputation and high ethical standards is sending a written report to the referring physician or calling the physician after the patient has been seen. Referrals increase following a well-written, complete report sent in a timely and professional manner (Williams, 1995).

Partnerships

Partnerships differ in how they are structured. In some cases, each partner sees all clients, and income that is generated is shared equally. In other practices, each partner maintains her own client group. Having a partner to cover for you (as long as the partner is available) is the biggest advantage. Going into a partnership requires that each LC be clear about what she wants from the arrangement at the outset. Complementary ways of working are a plus; it is not necessary for each partner to be a "clone" of the other. However, when very different philosophies exist about how to provide client services, conflicts that cannot be resolved are more likely to arise. Like a marriage, a partnership has its high and low points. Sometimes, partners can simply create a whole new set of problems such as disagreements about workload, methods of practice, and income.

Private practice is clearly not for every lactation consultant. However, those who have done so and have weathered the first five years report that it can provide rewards that are rarely found in another occupation. The independence, which is most frightening to persons who are used to a guaranteed salary and set working hours, also offers an opportunity to structure one's workday in a way that may allow the LC more time with her family than is possible otherwise.

Persons already in the field are the best to ask what others entering the field should know. Linda Smith's book, *The Lactation Consultant in Private Practice: The ABCs of Getting Started* is a valuable resource for starting a private practice. Box 2–10 lists dos and don'ts suggested by LCs in practice—either when establishing a private practice or when initiating an office-, clinic-, or hospital-based LC service.

BOX 2–10

Dos and Don'ts of Lactation Consulting

DO ...

- Insist on gaining credibility for the profession by passing the IBLCE examination. Ensure that people know this is the minimum credential for any person practicing as an LC in the community.

- From the very first client, behave with the utmost professionalism.
- Charge what you are worth; do not apologize for your fees.
- Set limits immediately, so that people know the boundaries of your availability.

BOX 2–10   (cont.)

- Establish your own knowledge and skills boundaries. Do not be afraid to ask for help.
- Develop a network of LCs in the community; they can serve as a sounding board for problems and as back-up when you are not available.
- Avoid repeating problems other LCs have experienced by learning from those with more experience than you have.
- Know what you are doing if you rent or sell equipment. Learn how the equipment works, and who should and should not use it. Be aware that its availability from you may influence what you tell a client to do.
- Use a computer to maintain a database of clients and practice documents and for maintaining your business.
- Learn as much as possible about running a business. It can take years to break even.
- Get a competent business advisor for accounting, marketing, and taxes. Ensure that those advisors understand exactly what you are trying to do.
- Bill the client directly for the service. The client then files a claim to her insurance company. Use standard forms for billing and a letter that the client can use to seek insurance coverage.
- Develop a specialization within the field and make your work visible to others through good care (Brimdyr, 2002).

- Document what you have done and send the original to the primary care provider, whether or not this individual made the initial referral.
- Recognize that this business is a labor of love. Do not expect to get rich.

DON'T

- Don't get heavily involved in phone consultations, paid or unpaid, without having seen the mother and baby. An overall assessment is needed.
- Don't give away your time without reimbursement.
- Don't waste your money on a lot of expensive advertising. Advertise judiciously and be patient.
- Don't use someone else's opinion as a reason for doing something. Experiment; be creative. What works in one practice may not work in another one.
- Don't get too many partners at the beginning. Knowing how each partner works as an individual will not necessarily predict how each works as part of a group. The more partners one has the greater the number of problems that can arise.
- Never forget that a happy mother and thriving baby are your best advertisements.

Summary

The field of lactation, well into its second decade, is widely accepted as a health-care specialty. Most hospitals now offer lactation services and employ nurse lactation consultants; women physicians are starting up breastfeeding specialty private practices. And no wonder: of the 4 million women who give birth each year in the United States, ap-

proximately 65 percent or 2.5 million start off breastfeeding. The opportunity to work with healthy families and adorable babies—and to enhance early parenting and child health—has made it a popular, satisfying field. Although growth is welcomed, rapid growth causes growing pains. Some health professionals feel threatened by the emergence of new practitioners who expect to share their turf.

The experiences of the lactation consultant in this decade are similar to those of the childbirth educator in the 1960s and 1970s. At that time, it was the childbirth educator who was the innovator and change agent who flew against the prevailing wind and traditional practices in birthing. These two disciplines share more than a common history: both empower mothers and act as change agents for women and for families during an age when technology and defensive medicine rule medical practice.

Those working with breastfeeding families cannot expect to become wealthy. However, they reap the reward of personal fulfillment as they assist other women in becoming empowered by their own breastfeeding experiences. This outcome has no price.

Key Concepts

- A lactation consultant (LC) is a specialist trained to focus on the needs and concerns of the breastfeeding mother-baby pair in hospitals, clinics, private medical practice, community health departments, home health agencies, and private practices. LCs usually have educational and clinical backgrounds in the health professions.

- Randomized clinical trials consistently show that interventions by health-care workers have a positive effect on breastfeeding. Translated to health-care costs, these studies would show that LC services save the health-care system enormous amounts of money through reduction in illness of both baby and mother.

- The number of candidates taking the international IBLCE certification examination for lactation consultants has grown steadily since its inception in 1985. Most candidates have been from Australia, Canada, and the United States. Passing rates usually range from 85 to 95 percent. Periodic recertification is required.

- Salaries for working as a lactation consultant for a clinical agency are similar to those paid to hospital nurses; working in a medical office pays the least. The fee charged for consultation with a mother ranges from about 70 to 95 dollars.

- Opportunities to gain clinical experience working with breastfeeding dyads can be obtained through La Leche League, finding a preceptor arrangement with an experienced nurse or physician, serving as a WIC peer counselor, and teaching prenatal classes.

- Certification by the IBLCE is the "gold standard" for working as a lactation consultant; other "short course" certifications with titles have caused confusion to the public and to employers.

- Most hospitals now have lactation services. These services usually include mother-baby rounds; telephone hotline and postdischarge telephone calls; prenatal classes on breastfeeding; pump rental or sales; postpartum breastfeeding consults; and continuing education for staff.

- A hospital with 3000 births per year should have at least three full-time LC positions that can be split into six part-time positions. The usual time per visit with mothers when doing daily rounds is 15 to 20 minutes. The majority of LC work time is spent in direct care of clients.

- A "prime mover" (i.e., a nursing director, administrator, or physician) who has institutional power is needed in order to develop a lactation program as well as to obtain the wide support of those who have influence in deciding budget allocations.

- The role of the LC is based on an advanced practice model. Roles develop sequentially according to experience as follows: novice, advanced beginner, competent, proficient, and expert.

- A major responsibility of the LC is documentation, through reports and charting. Narrative and problem-oriented charting and clinical care plans are popular methods to organize and chart clinical care. Computer skills are mandatory for getting and keeping a job.

Internet Resources

Breastfeeding photos and images: www.jump.net/~bwc/index.html

Breastfeeding Support Consultants Center for Lactation Education; lactation courses, study modules, products, certification requirements: www.bsccenter.org

Health Share Lactation Services, Inc.; setting up lactation services: www.hsls.com

International Board for Lactation Consultant Examiners; provides numerous documents for lactation consultants, including registry of certified lactation consultants and how to become certified: www.iblce.org

International Lactation Consultant Association (ILCA) conferences, courses, professional practice documents, reimbursement Tool Kit: www.ilca.org

Jones and Bartlett Publishing Company; books on breastfeeding include *The Lactation in Private Practice* by Linda Smith: www.jbpub.com

La Leche League International; publications, seminars, answers to breastfeeding questions: www.lalecheleague.org

Medela Healthcare Insurance Reimbursement Guide:www.medela.com/NewFiles/reburstmt_pro.html

Pat Lindsey, IBCLC Lactation Services; instruction booklet for ICD-9 codes, lactation visit receipt and other documents to help LCs receive reimbursement: www.PATLC.com

References

Albernaz E et al. Lactation counseling increases breastfeeding duration but not breast milk intake as measured by isotopic methods. *J Nutr* 133:205–10, 2003.

American Nurses Association (ANA). Has JCAHO eliminated care plans? *Am Nurse* June 1991:6.

Auerbach KG. Record-keeping: making the business end of doing business work for you. *J Hum Lact* 11:220–21, 1995.

Auerbach KG, Riordan J, Gross A. The lactation consultant: an increasingly visible health care role. *Mother Baby Jr* 5(1):41–46, 2000.

Barros FC et al. A randomized intervention trial to increase breast-feeding prevalence in southern Brazil [in Portuguese]. *Rev Saude Publ* 28:177–83, 1994.

Benner P. *From novice to expert: excellence and power in clinical nursing practice.* Menlo Park, CA: Addison-Wesley, 1984.

Bloom I et al. Factors affecting the continuance of breastfeeding. *Acta Paediatr Scand* 300(suppl):9–14, 1982.

Bolam A et al. The effects of postnatal health education for mothers on infant care and family planning practices in Nepal: a randomized controlled trial. *Br Med J* 316:805–11, 1998.

Bornmann PG. *Legal considerations and the lactation consultant—USA* (Unit 3), Lactation Consultant Series. Garden City Park, NY: Avery Publishing, 1986.

Brent NB et al. Breast-feeding in a low-income population: program to increase incidence and duration. *Arch Pediatr Adolesc Med* 149:798–803, 1995.

Brimdyr K. Lactation management: a community of practice. In: Cadwell K, ed. *Reclaiming breastfeeding for the United States.* Sudbury, MA: Jones and Bartlett, 2002:51–63.

Cary AH. *International survey of certified nurses in the U.S. and Canada.* Washington: Nursing Credentialing Center, 2000.

Chen C-H. Effects of home visits and telephone contacts on breastfeeding compliance in Taiwan. *Maternal Child Nurs J* 21:82–90, 1993.

Curro V et al. Randomised controlled trial assessing the effectiveness of a booklet on the duration of breast feeding. *Arch Dis Child* 76:500–4, 1997.

de Oliveira MI. Extending breastfeeding duration through primary care: a systematic review of prenatal and postnatal intervention. *J Hum Lact* 17:326–43, 2001.

Dodgson JE, Duckett L. Breastfeeding in the workplace: building a support program for nursing mothers. *AAOHN J* 45:290–98, 1997.

Dreyfus SE, Dreyfus HO. *A five-stage model of the mental activities involved in directed skill acquisition* (USAF Contract No. F49620-79-C-0063) Berkeley, CA: University of California, 1980.

Dublin P. Options for lactation consultants: the public health arena, *J Hum Lact* 5:19–20, 1989.

Duffy EP, Percival P, Kershaw E. Positive effects of an antenatal group teaching session on postnatal nipple pain, nipple trauma and breastfeeding rates. *Midwifery* 13:189–96, 1997.

Ferrarello DP. The entrepreneurial LC: the mission and the math. Presented at: Annual meeting and conference of the ILCA; Acapulco, Mexico, July 2001.

Frank DA et al. Commercial discharge packs and breastfeeding counseling effects on infant-feeding practices in a randomized trail. *Pediatrics* 80:845–54, 1987.

Froozani MD et al. Effect of breastfeeding education on the

feeding pattern and health of infants in their first 4 months in the Islamic Republic of Iran. *Bull WHO* 77:381–85, 1999.

Gagnon AF et al. A randomized trial of a program of early postpartum discharge with nurse visitation. *Am J Obstet Gynecol* 176:205–11, 1997.

Gardner KL, Weinrauch D. Marketing strategies for nurse entrepreneurs. *Nurse Pract* 13:46–49, 1988.

Gibbins S et al. The role of the clinical nurse specialist/neonatal nurse practitioner in a breastfeeding clinic: a model of advanced practice. *Clinical Nurse Specialist* 14:56–59, 2000.

Gilligan C. *In a different voice.* Cambridge, MA: Harvard University Press, 1982.

Gross LJ. Statistical report of the 2002 IBCLE examination. Available at: www.iblce.org. Accessed July 20, 2003.

Hafner-Eaton C. Lactation consultant reimbursement, consultation, charges/fees, and hours worked: beginning the resource-based relative value scale (RBRVS) method of reimbursement. Presented at: Annual meeting of the International Lactation Consultant Association; Boca Raton, FL, July 2000.

Harter C et al. Networking to implement effective health care. *MCN* 14:387–92, 1987.

Hauch YL, Dimmock JE. Evaluation of an information booklet on breastfeeding duration: a clinical trial. *J Adv Nurs* 20:836–43, 1994.

Heinig MJ. Closet consulting and other enabling behaviors. *J Hum Lact* 14:181–182, 1998.

Hill PD. Effects of education on breastfeeding success. *Maternal Child Nurs J* 16:145–56, 1987.

Hinson P. The business of clinical practice. In: Auerbach KG, ed. *Current issues in clinical lactation 2000.* Sudbury, MA: Jones and Bartlett, 2000:43–47.

International Lactation Consultant Association (ILCA). *Recommendations and competencies for lactation consultant practice.* Raleigh NC: ILCA, 2003.

———. *Reimbursement tool kit.* Raleigh, NC: ILCA, 2002.

Jakobsen MS et al. Promoting breastfeeding through health education at the time of immunizations: a randomized trial from Guinea Bissau. *Acta Paediatr* 88:741–47, 1999.

Joel LA. An epiphany in retrospect [editorial]. *Amer J Nurs* 97(11):7, 1997.

Kantor MB. *The change masters: innovation for productivity in the American corporation.* New York: Simon and Schuster, 1983:409.

Kelley KJ. The IBLCE discipline process. *J Hum Lact* 15:61–62, 1999.

Lynch SA et al. Evaluating effect of a breastfeeding consultant on the duration of breastfeeding. *Can J Public Health* 77:190–95, 1986.

Neyzi O et al. An educational intervention on promotion of breastfeeding. *Paediatr Perinat Epidemio* 5:286–98, 1991.

Parris KM. Integrating nursing diagnosis, interventions, and outcomes in public health nursing practice. *Nurs Diag* 10:49–56, 1999.

Pugh LC, Milligan RA. Nursing intervention to increase the duration of breastfeeding. *Appl Nurs Res* 11:190–94, 1998.

Phillips V. The Nursing Mother's Association of Australia as a self-help organization. In: Katz AH and Bender EL, eds. *Helping one another: self-help groups in a changing world.* Oakland, CA: Third Party Publishing, 1990.

Raudonis BM, Anderson CM. A theoretical framework for specialty certification in nursing practice. *Nursing Outlook* 50:247–52, 2002.

Rago JL. Breast pump rental depot: a way to bridge the gap. *J Hum Lact* 3:156–57, 1987.

Riordan J, Auerbach K. Breastfeeding and human lactation, second edition. Sudbury, MA: Jones and Bartlett, 1999.

Rossiter JC. The effect of a culture-specific education program to promote breastfeeding among Vietnamese women in Sydney. *Int J Nurs Stud* 31:369–79, 1994.

Serafino-Cross P, Donovan PR. Effectiveness of professional breastfeeding home-support. *J Nutr Educ* 24:117–22, 1992.

Shrago LC. Fostering collegial relationships among lactation consultants [editorial]. *J Hum Lact* 11:1–2, 1995.

Simpson KC, Creehan, PA. *AWHONN Perinatal Nursing.* 2nd ed. Philadelphia, PA: Lippincott, 2001.

Smillie C. A specialty practice in breastfeeding. In: Auerbach KG, ed. *Current issues in clinical lactation 2000.* Sudbury, MA: Jones and Bartlett, 2000:49–54.

Smith L. Shadowing Guidelines. Personal communication. January 2002.

Steltzer TM, Woods A, Gasda KA. Salary survey 2003. *Nurs Manage* 34:28–32, 2003.

Susin L et al. Does parental breastfeeding knowledge increase breastfeeding rates? *Birth* 26:149–56, 1999.

Thorley V. Complementary and competing roles of volunteers and professionals in the breastfeeding field. *Int Self Help Self Care* 1(2):171–79, 2000.

Turner MR. Twenty questions for the consumer: a quality assurance tool for the lactation consultant. *J Hum Lact* 12:50–52, 1996.

Williams EL. Increasing your credibility with physicians: strategies for lactation consultants [editorial]. *J Hum Lact* 11:3–4, 1995.

Wilson-Clay B. Lactation consultants: are we a profession yet? In: Auerbach K, ed. *Clinical Issues in Clinical Lactation.* Sudbury, MA: Jones and Bartlett, 2000:57–72.

Woolf V. *A room of one's own.* New York: Harcourt, Brace and World, 1929.

SECTION 2

ANATOMICAL AND BIOLOGICAL IMPERATIVES

After pregnancy, the mother continues to nourish her child through breastmilk—energy now synthesized and stored in the breast. Breastmilk, a living fluid that benefits infants, mothers, and society, changes throughout lactation to meet the infant's nutriment needs. No human-made substitute nourishes the infant as well.

What drugs and viral infections pose a risk to the breastfeeding baby? Most drugs are compatible with breastfeeding, as this chapter shows. Viruses and bacteria stimulate antibodies in the mother's body, which, except for HIV, protect the vulnerable infant through mother's milk. Scientists are attempting to catch the elusive thread that unravels the tragedy of AIDS and the mystery of the HIV virus within breastmilk cells.

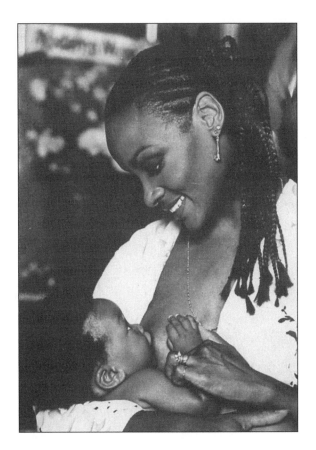

Anatomy and Physiology of Lactation

Jan Riordan

It is essential that health-care providers understand the anatomy of the human female breast and the physiological mechanisms of milk production. It is equally necessary to recognize the unique anatomy of the infant's oral structures and the physiological mechanisms of suckling. This chapter is divided into two parts: the first focuses on the mother, the second on the infant. In lactation, as in all human biological systems, there is a working relationship between anatomy (form) and physiology (function). Although function changes as form changes, the functional capacity of the human breast is not wholly dictated by form. Breast size, for instance, is a poor predictor of lactational capability. It is the infant's appetite that determines milk yield, rather than the mother's capacity to produce milk. Throughout this book, the developmental cycle of the mammary gland has four phases: mammogenesis, lactogenesis (stages I and II), galactopoiesis, and involution (Table 3–1).

Mammogenesis

The mammary system is unlike other organ systems. From birth through puberty, pregnancy, and lactation, no other human organ displays such dramatic changes in size, shape, and function as does the breast. The Latin term for breasts, *mammae*, developed from the infant's cry, "mamma," in seeking the breast. In some cultures, female breasts serve more than one function: they attract the sexual attentions of the male adult and then give nourishment and nurturing to the suckling infant. The first part of this chapter, which focuses on the mother, describes breast development from embryo to adulthood, breast anatomy, changes during pregnancy and lactation, and hormones that influence the course of lactogenesis.

Breast development begins early, by the fourth week of gestation when two parallel primitive milk streaks develop from axilla to groin on the trunk of the embryo. These streaks become the mammary ridge or milk line by the fifth week of embryonic life. This ridge or line is actually a thickening of epithelial cells in a localized ventrolateral area on the embryo (the "milk hill" stage) that continues through weeks 7 and 8 and is accompanied by inward growth into the chest wall. Between 12 and 16 weeks' gestation, these specialized cells differentiate further into the smooth muscle of the nipple and areola. Also during this period, epithelial cells continue to develop into mammary buds and then, in a treelike pattern, proliferate to form epithelial branches that eventually become alveoli (Dawson, 1934; Vorherr, 1974).

Table 3–1

STAGES OF LACTATION

Mammogenesis	• Mammary (breast) growth; increased size and weight of breast
	• Proliferation of ducts and glandular system under estrogen and progesterone
Lactogenesis, stage I (mid-pregnancy to day 2 postpartum)	• Initiation of milk synthesis from mid-pregnancy to late pregnancy
	• Differentiation of alveolar cells from secretory cells
	• Prolactin stimulates mammary secretory epithelial cells to produce milk
Lactogenesis, stage II (day 3 to day 8)	• Closure of tight junctions in alveolar cell (Figure 3–6)
	• Triggered by rapid drop in mother's progesterone levels
	• Onset of copious secretion of milk
	• Fullness and warmth in breasts
	• Switch from endocrine to autocrine control
Galactopoiesis (day 9 to beginning of involution)	• Maintenance of established secretion
	• Control by autocrine system (supply–demand)
	• Breast size decreases between 6 and 9 months postpartum
Involution (average 40 days after last breastfeeding)	• Additions of regular supplementation
	• Decreased milk secretion from build-up of inhibiting peptides
	• High sodium levels

Placental sex hormones enter fetal circulation and stimulate formation of channels (canalization) of the branched epithelial tissue. This process continues until the fetus is 32 weeks old. From 32 to 40 weeks' gestation, lobular-alveolar structures containing colostrum develop. During this time, the fetal mammary gland mass increases four times over its original mass, and the nipple and areola develop further and become pigmented. After birth, the neonate's mammary tissue may secrete colostral milk (so-called witch's milk).

Mammary gland development during childhood is limited to general growth. However, at puberty, estrogen and a pituitary factor, probably growth hormone, become the major influence on breast growth in a girl when, at 10 to 12 years of age, primary and secondary ducts grow and divide and form club-shaped terminal end buds that are associated with beginning function of the hypothalamus-pituitary-ovarian axis. The buds develop into new branches and small ductules of areolar buds, which later become the acini or alveoli in the ma-

ture female breast. During each menstrual cycle, proliferation and active growth of duct tissue occurs during the follicular and ovulatory phases, reaching a maximum in the late luteal phase and then regressing. During each ovulatory cycle, peaks of ovarian steroids, primarily progesterone, foster further mammary development that never regresses to its former state of the preceding cycle. Trauma, incisions, or radiation therapy to the breast bud in the prepubertal era can trigger maldevelopment with hypoplasia of the vestigal breast that has future consequences for lactation. For example, radiation during childhood can be associated with an inadequate breastmilk supply as an adult.

Complete development of mammary function occurs only in pregnancy when the breasts increase in size and the nipple pigment darkens. Except for the uterus, no other organ changes so dramatically as the breast does during pregnancy and lactation. New budding of structures continues until about age 35. In addition to progesterone, prolactin or human placental lactogen is thought to be necessary for the final stages of mammary growth and differentiation (Neville, 2001).

Breast Structure

The basic units of the mature glandular tissue are the *alveoli*, which are composed of secretory acinar units in which the ductules terminate. Each cluster of secretory cells of an alveolus is surrounded by *myoepithelial cells*, a contractile unit responsible for ejecting milk into the *ductules*. Each ductule then merges, without communicating with its neighbors, into a larger duct (Figure 3–1). An ultrasound image of a lactating breast is shown in Figure 3–2, where ducts filled with milk can be clearly seen. Each breast has nine to ten duct openings, sometimes called nipple "pores." The ducts are lined with stratified squamous epithelium near the nipple, by columnar epithelium at more distal areas and highly vascular connective tissue.

The alveolus or milk-secreting unit is a single layer of epithelial cells with surrounding supporting structures: myoepithelial cells, contractile cells for milk ejection, and connective tissue. Milk is continuously secreted into the alveolar lumina where it is stored until the letdown reflex triggers the myoepithelial cells to contract and eject the milk. (Neville, 2001).

Mammary ducts do not widen into *sinuses* located behind the nipple and the areola as previously thought. Figure 3–3, which shows contrast opacification of a single lactiferous duct, confirms that the duct does not widen before it branches in mammary ducts. In each breast, there are 15 to 20 subdivided *lobes*.

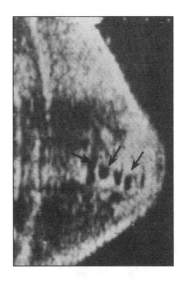

FIGURE 3–2. Ultrasound image showing milk-filled ducts. Mother lactating 10 months. (From Division of Ultrasound, Dept. of Radiology and Dept. of Pathology. *Atlas of breast ultrasound.* **Philadelphia: Thomas Jefferson University Medical College and Hospital, 1980:121.)**

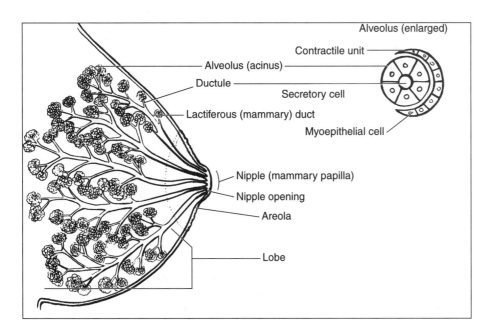

FIGURE 3–1. Schematic diagram of breast.

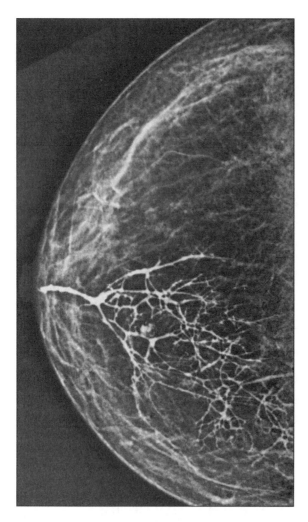

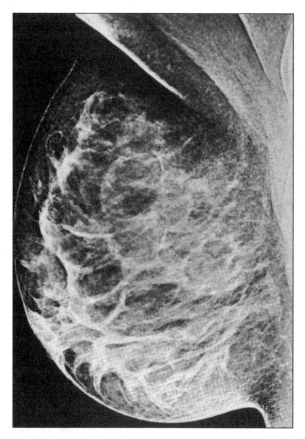

FIGURE 3–4. Curvilinear densities represent Cooper's ligaments. (From Kopans DB. *Breast imaging*. Philadelphia: Lippincott, 1989:20.)

FIGURE 3–3. Contrast opacification of a single lactiferous duct demonstrates a branching network that defines a single lobe of the breast. (From Kopans DB. *Breast imaging*. Philadelphia: Lippincott, 1989:20.)

Between and around the uneven edges of the lobes is a thick layer of fat. As seen in Figure 3–4, running vertically through the breast and attaching the deep layer of the subcutaneous tissue to the dermis of the skin are the *suspensory ligaments* or *Cooper's ligaments*. The breast's structure is mainly the result of fibrous tissues that surround and course through it. Glandular tissue that extends toward the axilla partly under the lateral border of the pectoralis ma-

jora is known as the *axillary tail* (Figure 3–5). Each breast of an adult woman weighs, on average, 150 to 200 gm and doubles in weight to 400 to 500 gm (about 1 pound) during lactation. Between 6 and 9 months after the beginning of lactation, breast size decreases slightly. Whether this results from mobilization of breast fatty tissue or greater breast tissue efficiency in making milk, milk production remains constant (Hartmann, Sherriff, & Kent, 1995).

The breast is highly vascularized. Blood is supplied to the breast through the internal mammary (60 percent) and lateral thoracic (30 percent) arteries. The lymph vessels of the breast are numerous and, for the most part, join the lymph nodes of the axilla. The majority of lymph vessels

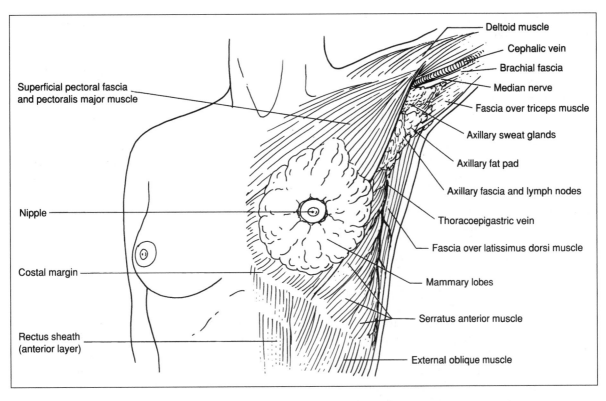

Deltoid muscle

Cephalic vein

Brachial fascia

Median nerve

Fascia over triceps muscle

Axillary sweat glands

Axillary fat pad

Axillary fascia and lymph nodes

Thoracoepigastric vein

Fascia over latissimus dorsi muscle

Mammary lobes

Serratus anterior muscle

External oblique muscle

Superficial pectoral fascia and pectoralis major muscle

Nipple

Costal margin

Rectus sheath (anterior layer)

FIGURE 3–5. Anterior pectoral dissection. The diagram shows the lobular nature of the mammary gland extending toward the axilla and its location anterior to the pectoralis major muscle. Includes the superficial axillary lymph and sweat glands. (Adapted from Clemente CD. *Anatomy: a regional atlas of the human body.* **Philadelphia: Lea & Febiger, 1978.)**

follow the lactiferous ducts and thus converge toward the nipple, where they join a plexus situated beneath the areola (subareolar plexus).

The nerve supply of the breast is derived from the intercostal nerves of the fourth, fifth, and sixth intercostal spaces. The fourth intercostal nerve penetrates the posterior aspect of the breast (left breast at 4 o'clock, right breast 8 o'clock) and supplies the greatest amount of sensation to the nipple and to the areola. The breast has uneven patterns of sensation: the areola is the most sensitive part of the breast, the skin adjacent to the areola is less sensitive, and the nipple itself is the least sensitive. Women with larger breasts report less sensation than women with smaller breasts. Of women with small- or moderate-sized breasts, those who have never been pregnant report greater sensation in their nipples and areolae. Midway to the nipple and areola, the fourth intercostal nerve

becomes more superficial. As it reaches the areola, it divides into five branches: one central, two upper, and two lower. The lowermost branch consistently pierces the areola at 5 o'clock on the left side and 7 o'clock on the right side. Any trauma to this nerve will cause some loss of sensation in the breast (Courtiss & Goldwyn, 1976). If the lowermost nerve branch is severed, the mother loses sensation to the nipple and areola (Farina, Newby, & Alani, 1980).

The covering smooth skin is modified at the center of each breast to form a *mammary papilla* or nipple into which the ducts open. Some of these ducts join so that 5 to 10 openings appear on the nipple surface. The nipple projects as a small cylindrical body with pigmented wrinkled skin slightly below the center of each breast at about the level of the fourth intercostal space. Surrounding the nipple is the *areola*. Within the areola lie the glands of

Montgomery—or Montgomery's "tubercles" as they are commonly called—accompanying sebaceous glands, and a few scattered sweat glands (Smith, 1982). Long a focus of anatomic debate, the tubercles are true mammary glands whose ducts and secretory parenchyma are the same as those of the mammary glands that open at the tip of the nipples. As such, they are an integral part of the mammary structure and total breast tissue (Montagna & MacPherson, 1974). It is widely held that these glands provide nipple lubrication and antisepsis but no evidence of this function exists. From an evolutionary standpoint, it is of interest that the rhesus monkey does not have tubercles of Montgomery (MacPherson & Montagna, 1974).

The nipple and areola contain erectile smooth muscles. Hair follicles surround the nipple and areola but are not within the nipple/areola proper; most women have at least some nipple hair. In a lactating mother, the average diameter of the areola is 6.4 cm, and the average diameter of the erectile portion of the nipple is 1.6 cm and the length is 0.7 cm (Ziemer, 1993). Contraction of bundles of smooth muscles beneath the nipple and areola cause the nipple to be firm and protruding. These structures are seen in Color Plates 1–3.

Variations

From woman to woman, breasts vary in color, size, shape, and placement on the chest wall. Lobular size varies within a single breast, from one breast to another, and from woman to woman. Moreover, breast asymmetry is common; the left breast is often larger than the right. Areola and nipple color vary according to complexion: pink in blonds, browner in brunettes and black in dark-skinned women. *Supernumerary breasts (polymastia)* and/or an *accessory nipple* may occur at any point along the milk line from the axilla to the groin. They occur in about 1 to 2 percent of the population and may be associated with renal or other organ-system anomalies (Berman & Davis, 1994). Polymastia occurs in different forms: breast tissue with a nipple but lacking an areola; breast with a nipple and areola; or breast tissue only. Only rarely does a true or complete accessory mammary gland develop (Grossl, 2000). The most common areas in which an accessory breast might develop are in the axilla and on the thorax (Color Plate 21).

Lack of full protraction of the nipple on the common pinch test (see Figure 3–11, later in this chapter) is fairly common in primigravid women. Poor nipple protractibility in women during their first pregnancy has been reported to range from 10 to 35 percent (Alexander et al., 1992; Blaikeley et al., 1953; Hytten & Baird, 1958; Waller, 1946). Protractility of the nipple gradually improves during pregnancy and, by puerperium, most women have good nipple protraction. Generally, nipple protraction continues to improve with each subsequent pregnancy and lactation experience. The relationship between protractility and subsequent breastfeeding difficulty is minimal. Because the infant makes a teat not from the nipple alone but from the surrounding breast tissue, the actual shape of the nipple may be a secondary consideration.

Nipple inversion is found in about 3 percent of women and is usually bilateral (87 percent) (Park, Yoon, & Kim, 1999). Of the total number of inverted nipples, 96 percent are umbilicated and only 4 percent are invaginated ("true" inversion). Although true inversion is uncommon, its treatment can be difficult. If the inversion is on one breast only, the mother can breastfeed from a single breast and use a silicone breast shield on the other breast. Placing a silicone breast shield over the inverted nipple allows the infant to grasp on to the breast and suckle effectively. When the inversion is bilateral, feedings at the breast may have to be supplemented. The mother's first breastfeeding experience may be more difficult than subsequent ones—frequent suckling by the infant helps to evert the previously inverted tissue.

Pregnancy

During pregnancy, the breasts grow larger, the skin appears thinner, and the veins become more prominent. The diameter of the areola increases from about 34 mm in early pregnancy to 50 mm postpartum (Hytten, 1954), although there is a wide range of areolar width in any population. As the nipples become more erect, pigmentation of the areola increases and the glands of Montgomery enlarge.

Serum hormones stimulate breast growth during pregnancy: nipple growth is related to serum prolactin levels; areolar growth is related to serum placental lactogen (Cregan & Hartmann, 1999). Estrogen and progesterone also exert their specific effect on the breast during pregnancy; the ductal system proliferates and differentiates under the influence of estrogen, whereas progesterone promotes an increase in size of the lobes, lobules, and alveoli. Adrenocorticotropic hormone (ACTH) and growth hormone combine synergistically with prolactin and progesterone to promote mammary growth.

Breast growth during pregnancy varies among women. In a study of eight pregnant women, most had a gradual increase in breast growth throughout their pregnancy; however one mother had a spurt of breast growth between 10 and 15 weeks and afterward very little growth; another had little or no breast growth (Cregan & Hartmann, 1999).

Lactogenesis

The transition from pregnancy to lactation is called *lactogenesis*. The first half of pregnancy is characterized by growth and proliferation of the ductal tree and further formation of lobules. During the second half of pregnancy, secretory activity accelerates and the acini or alveoli become distended by accumulating colostrum (Russo & Russo, 1987). After 16 weeks of pregnancy, lactation occurs even if the pregnancy does not progress. An accessory breast may also swell. Just before and during childbirth, a new wave of mitotic activity increases the total DNA of the mammary gland (Salazar & Tobon, 1974; Vorrher, 1974).

The capacity of the mammary gland to secrete milk from mid-pregnancy to late pregnancy is called *lactogenesis, stage I* (or *lactogenesis I*) (see again Table 3–1). During lactogenesis I, breast size increases as epithelial cells of the alveoli differentiate into secretory cells for milk production. Fat droplets accumulate in these cells and plasma concentration of lactose and α-lactalbumin increase. The milk droplets move through the cell membrane and into the ductules (see Figure 3–6). The onset of copious milk secretion after birth is *lactogenesis, stage II* (days 2 or 3 to 8 postpartum). During lactogenesis II, milk volume increases rapidly from 36 to 96 hours postpartum and then abruptly levels off.

Lactogenesis II is triggered by a rapid drop of serum progesterone (and possibly estrogen) after the delivery of the placenta. It is also accompanied by a significant fall in breastmilk levels of sodium, chloride, and protein and a rise in lactose and milk lipids. These changes in cellular metabolism are a result of closure of junction complexes between alveolar cells. Before lactogenesis (first 3 to 4 days), there are large gaps between the alveolar cells. During full lactation, the passage of substances between alveolar cells is stopped by a gasketlike structure called the *tight junction*, which joins the epithelial

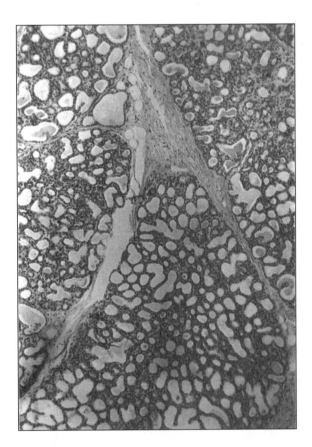

FIGURE 3–6. Milk is secreted from the alveolar cells, where small droplets form and migrate through the cell membrane and into the alveolar ductules. Photomicrograph. (With permission, Victor B. Eichler, PhD.)

cells tightly to one another (Figure 3–7). The closure of these tight junctions precedes the onset of copious milk secretion. (Neville, 2001).

As lactation begins, these hormonal changes are essential:

- Drop in progesterone levels.
- Release of prolactin from the anterior pituitary, which stimulates lactogenesis and initiates milk secretion.
- Removal of breastmilk by the infant or pump.
- Release of oxytocin from the posterior pituitary (at least by day 3).

Delay in Lactogenesis

Not all women experience the coming in of the milk on the third or fourth day postpartum. A delay or diminishment in lactogenesis, common in cer-

tain situations (as listed in Table 3–2), invites us to gain a better understanding of the specific biochemical or hormonal nature of lactogenesis that may lead to a delay in lactogenesis. We do know that high breastmilk sodium levels on or before the third day after birth are significant for impending breastfeeding problems and for lactation involution (Morton, 1994; Humenick et al., 1998). Although the reasons for lactogenesis delay are not always clear, it does appear that lactogenesis is susceptible to outside influence and is thus fragile.

Hormonal Influences

Lactogenesis II is triggered following the expulsion of the placenta by a fall in progesterone levels and the continued presence of prolactin. A great deal of information about these hormonal functions during lactation is now known through radioimmunoassay

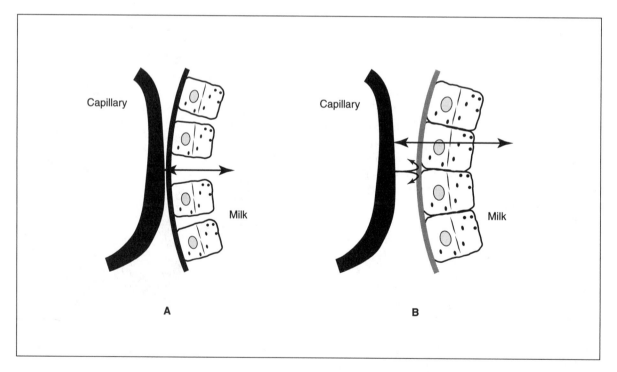

FIGURE 3–7. (A) Gaps between alveolar cells before lactogenesis. **(B)** Intracellular gaps close tightly to one another following lactogenesis (With permission, Hale T. *Medications and mother's milk,* 9th ed. 2000:6.)

Table 3-2

MATERNAL CONDITIONS THAT CAN DELAY OR IMPAIR LACTOGENESIS

Cesarean birth	Sozmen, 1992
Diabetes, type I	Neubauer et al., 1993
Labor analgesia	Hildebrandt, 1999
Obesity	Rasmussen et al., 2001
Polycystic ovary syndrome	Marasco et al., 2000
Theca lutein cysts	Hoover et al., 2002
Placental retention	Neifert, 1981
Stress	Chen, 1999 Grajeda & Perez-Escamilla, 2002

studies. A programmed transformation of the mammary epithelium mediated by a cascade of hormonal changes leads to a rapid synthesis of breastmilk by day 4 following birth. The postpartum period is characterized hormonally by a drop in progesterone and elevated levels of prolactin, which act synergistically with cortisol, thyroid-stimulating hormone, prolactin-inhibiting factor, and oxytocin to establish and maintain lactation. If the delicate interplay of these hormones are disturbed—for example, by high testosterone levels in the woman with theca lutein cysts (Hoover, Barbalinardo, & Pia Platia, 2002) or polycystic ovary syndrome (Marasco, Marmet, & Shell, 2000), lactogenesis is delayed and possibly suppressed (see Chapter 16).

Progesterone

Progesterone is required to maintain pregnancy and remains high throughout pregnancy. Lactation during pregnancy is inhibited by high levels of progesterone, which interfere with prolactin action at the alveolar cell receptor level. The inhibiting influence of progesterone is so powerful that lactation is delayed if placental fragments are retained after birth (Neifert et al., 1981). Following birth, progesterone decreases about tenfold during the first four days. This rapid fall of progesterone in the presence of maintained prolactin levels triggers lactogenesis. Once lactation is initiated, the principal hormone in maintaining milk biosynthesis is prolactin.

Prolactin

Prolactin is essential for both initiating and maintaining milk production. Though oxytocin appears to be keyed more closely to milk ejection, milk is not made if there is an absence of prolactin. During pregnancy, prolactin, which is secreted by the anterior pituitary gland, has an important role in increasing breast mass and cell differentiation. A group of peptides, including angiotensin II, gonadotropin-releasing hormone (GnRH), and vasopressin, stimulate the release of prolactin. The mammary ducts and alveoli mature and proliferate as prolactin levels steadily rise from the normal nonpregnancy level of 10 to 20 ng/ml to a peak of 200 to 400 ng/ml at term (Tyson et al., 1972).

As progesterone and estrogen levels abruptly drop after a woman gives birth, the anterior pituitary gland, no longer inhibited by these two hormones, releases pustile prolactin 7 to 20 times in 24 hours and greater amounts during sleep; thus, for accurate measurement of prolactin, samples should be taken in close intervals around the clock (Madden et al., 1978). Episodic peaks are superimposed on a stable ongoing level of secretion. Because human placental lactogen (HPL) competes with prolactin for breast receptors, the decline of HPL after delivery of the placenta also promotes prolactin action. Figure 3–8 describes the rise and fall of hormones during pregnancy and lactation.

Following lactogenesis II, when milk secretion shifts from endocrine to autocrine control, prolactin secretion continues to be controlled by the hypothalamus. This control is largely inhibitory; that is, whenever the pathway between the hypothalamus and the pituitary is disrupted, prolactin levels rise. During galactopoiesis, the hypothalamus is dependent upon removal of milk in order for lactation to continue. When the nipple is stimulated and milk is removed from the breast, the hypothalamus inhibits the release of dopamine, a prolactin inhibiting fac-

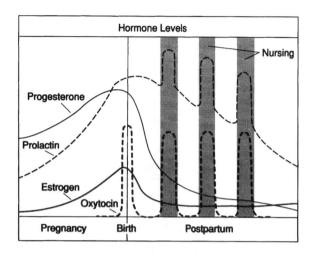

FIGURE 3–8. Hormone levels during pregnancy and lactation. (Adapted from Love S. *Dr. Susan Love's breast book*. Boston: Addison-Wesley, 1990:34.)

tor; this drop in dopamine stimulates the release of prolactin and causes milk production (Chao, 1987).

Plasma prolactin levels increase the most in the immediate postpartum period but rise and fall in proportion to the frequency, intensity, and duration of nipple stimulation. Prolactin concentration in blood doubles in response to suckling and peaks approximately 45 minutes after the beginning of a breastfeeding session (Noel, Suh, & Frantz, 1974). If lidocaine is applied to the nipples to deaden sensation, prolactin does not increase (Neville, 2001).

During the first week after birth, prolactin levels in breastfeeding women fall about 50 percent. If a mother does not breastfeed, prolactin levels usually reach nonpregnant levels by 7 days postpartum (Tyson et al., 1972).

During lactation, maternal prolactin levels are described as follows:

- They follow a circadian rhythm; levels during the night (sleep) are higher than during the day.
- They decline slowly over the course of lactation (Battin et al., 1985; Cox, Owens, & Hartmann, 1996) but remain elevated for as long as the mother breastfeeds, even if she breastfeeds for years (Stallings et al., 1996).
- They rise with suckling: the more feedings, the higher the level of serum prolactin. More than eight breastfeedings per 24 hours prevents de-

cline of the concentration of prolactin before the next breastfeeding (Cox, Owens, & Hartmann, 1996; Tay, 1996).

- They are not necessarily related to milk yield especially after lactation becomes established (Hill, Chatterton, & Aldag, 1999; Ueda et al., 1994), although feeding two babies simultaneously doubles prolactin surge (Tyson et al., 1972).
- They delay the return of ovulation by inhibiting ovarian response to follicle-stimulating hormone and is higher in amenorrheic than in cycling women during the first year postpartum (Battin et al., 1985; Stallings et al., 1996).
- They are not related to the degree of postpartum breast engorgement (West, 1979).
- They drop with cigarette smoking (Baron et al., 1986) and rise with beer drinking (Mennella & Beauchamp, 1993).
- They rise with anxiety and psychological stress (Hill, Chatterton, & Aldag, 1999) even though feeding at the breast and let-down are calming (because of oxytocin release).

Normal prolactin levels in nonpregnant or nonlactating women are 20 ng/ml or less. In lactating women, mean baseline prolactin levels are 90 ng/ml at 10 days postpartum; afterward, these levels slowly decline but remained elevated at 180 days postpartum (44.3 ng/ml). Women who remain amenorrheic have higher (about 110.0 ng/ml) baseline prolactin levels as compared to women (about 70.1 ng/ml) who menstruate prior to 180 days (Battin et al., 1985). An overview of prolactin serum levels during pregnancy and breastfeeding is shown in Figure 3–9.

Prolactin also is present in breastmilk. The release of prolactin into intraalveolar secretions of the breast plays a role in establishing and maintaining lactation. Milk prolactin concentration is lower than its concentration in blood plasma and is highest in early transitional milk (about 43 ng/ml) and the foremilk rather than the hindmilk (Cox, Owens, & Hartmann, 1996). This early transmission of prolactin in the aqueous foremilk is thought to have an effect on intestinal fluid and electrolyte exchange in the newborn (Yuen, 1988). Milk prolactin levels are about the same between left and right breasts and

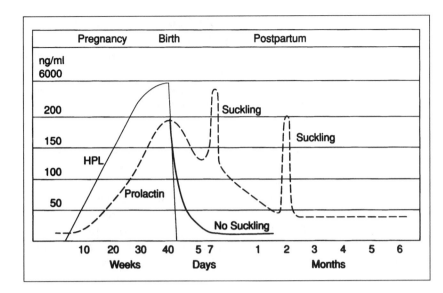

FIGURE 3–9.
Fluctuation of human placental lactogen and prolactin serum levels in pregnancy and lactation. (From Battin DA et al. Effect of suckling on serum prolactin, luteinizing hormone, follicle-stimulating hormone, and estradiol during prolonged lactation. *Obstet Gynecol* 65:785–8, 1985; Tyson JE et al. *Am J Obstet Gynecol* 113:14–20, 1972; Speroff L, Glass RH, Kase NG. *Clinical gynecology, endocrinology and infertility,* 4th ed. Baltimore: Williams & Wilkins, 1989:283.

are highest in the morning (Cregan, Mitoulas, & Hartmann, 2002). Breastmilk prolactin steadily declines but remains detectable in mature milk (about 11 ng/ml) until weaning up to 40 weeks postpartum (Yuen, 1988).

The Prolactin Receptor Theory. De Carvalho et al. (1983) postulated that frequent feeding in early lactation stimulates a faster increase in milk output because suckling stimulates the development of receptors to prolactin in the mammary gland. According to this approach, the number of these receptors per cell increases in early lactation and remains constant thereafter (Hinds & Tyndale-Biscoe, 1982; Sernia & Tyndale-Biscoe, 1979).

Some understanding of the impact of early breastfeeding on prolactin-receptors is provided by Zuppa et al. (1988). In this study, although serum prolactin levels were slightly lower in multiparous mothers as compared with primiparous mothers in the first 4 postpartum days, the volume of milk obtained by the infants of the multiparous mothers was significantly higher. They concluded that multiparous women had a greater number of mammary gland receptors for prolactin. The implication here is that the controlling factor in breastmilk output is the number of prolactin receptors rather than the amount of prolactin in serum. More receptors may result in more than adequate milk production, even in the presence of lower prolactin levels. This finding helps to ex-

plain why infants of multiparous mothers begin gaining weight somewhat faster than do those of primiparous mothers.

Cortisol

Cortisol, a main glucocorticoid, acts synergistically on the mammary system in the presence of prolactin (Neville & Berga, 1983). The final differentiation of the alveolar epithelial cell in a mature milk cell takes place because prolactin is present, but only after prior exposure to cortisol and insulin. Glucocorticoids are hormones secreted by the adrenal glands and help to regulate water transport across the cell membranes during lactation. A high cortisol level is associated with a delay in lactogenesis (Chen, 1998).

Thyroid-Stimulating Hormone

The thyroid hormone (TSH) promotes mammary growth and lactation through a permissive rather than a regulatory role. Dawood et al. (1981) established a marked and significant increase in plasma thyroid-stimulating hormone level on the third to fifth postpartum days.

Prolactin-Inhibiting Factor

Prolactin-inhibiting factor (PIF) is a hypothalamic substance, either dopamine itself or mediated by dopamine. It stimulates dopamine releases and thus inhibits prolactin secretions (dopamine agonist). Bromocriptine, a drug that suppresses lactation, is an example of a dopamine agonist. Dopamine antagonists have the opposite effect. Nipple stimulation and milk removal suppresses PIF and dopamine, causing prolactin levels to rise and the breast to produce milk. Drugs, such as metoclopramide, phenothiazines, and reserpine derivatives, increase breastmilk production because they inhibit PIF (Bohnet & Kato, 1985).

Oxytocin

In response to suckling, the posterior pituitary hormone oxytocin causes the *milk-ejection reflex* (MER) or *letdown*, a contraction of the myoepithelial cells surrounding the alveoli necessary for the removal of milk from the breast. Oxytocin is released in pulsatile waves and is carried though the bloodstream to the breast where it interacts with receptors on myoepithelial cells, causing contraction and forcing milk from the alveoli into the ducts where it becomes available to the newborn through the nipple openings. Most women feel pressure and a tingling, warm sensation during milk ejection. After lactation becomes established, women will experience multiple milk ejections during a feed.

Oxytocin plays a major role in the continuance of lactation. During suckling or breast stimulation, oxytocin is released in discrete pulses. Blood levels rise within 1 minute of remaining elevated during stimulation, and they return to baseline levels within 6 minutes after cessation of nipple stimulation. This rise and fall of oxytocin levels continues at each feeding throughout the lactation course, even when the mother breastfeeds for an extended period (Leake et al., 1983). The posterior pituitary contains a surprisingly large store of oxytocin (3000–9000 mU) when compared with the amount required to elicit the ejection reflex (50–100 mU) (Lincoln & Paisley, 1982).

Oxytocin has another important function—to contract the mother's uterus. Uterine contractions help to control postpartum bleeding and to aid in uterine involution. The uterus not only contracts during breastfeeding but continues to contract rhythmically for as long as 20 minutes after the feeding. These cramps may be painful during the first few days postpartum. After involution is complete,

however, these rhythmical pulsations may be a source of pleasure to the mother. Oxytocin also has peripheral effects, notably dilation of peripheral vascular beds and increased blood flow without increased systemic arterial pressure. As a result, breastfeeding is accompanied by increased skin temperature not unlike that of a menopausal hot flash (Marshall, Cumming, & Fitzsimmons, 1992). New mothers often report an increase in thirst while breastfeeding, which appears to be closely related to the increase in plasma oxytocin (James et al., 1995). Women who have had emergency cesarean births (Nissen et al., 1996) or are under stress (Ueda et al., 1994) have significantly less oxytocin pulses during breastfeeding. Breast massage raises the maternal plasma oxytocin level (Yokoyama et al., 1994).

Through oxytocin mediation, these afferent pathways become so well established that letdown can occur even when the mother merely thinks of her baby. There are many anecdotal reports of spontaneous lactation in mothers who have weaned. Milk synthesis is a complex interplay of the hypothalamic-pituitary-gonadal axis (Figure 3–10) that is susceptible to emotional upheaval and can potentially inhibit the letdown reflex.

The calmness while breastfeeding that mothers report is partly governed by oxytocin. Oxytocin infusion in rats produces sedation, lower blood pressure, and lower levels of corticosteroids (Uvnas-Moberg, 1997). Goer and Davis (2002) make the case that breastfeeding women have a diminished response to stressors and to pain. When exposed to stress, lactating women had lower levels of ACTH, cortisol, glucose, and norepinphrine than did nonlactating women (Altemus et al., 1996).

The influence of supplemental feedings on oxytocin and prolactin peaks was measured by Johnstone and Amico (1986). These investigators found that mothers who were exclusively breastfeeding had higher oxytocin levels over time than did women who were giving their babies replacement feedings. The exclusively breastfeeding women's oxytocin levels not only remained higher but also tended to climb over time, so that their oxytocin levels were higher at 15 to 24 weeks than they were at earlier periods (2 to 4 weeks and 5 to 14 weeks). In sharp contrast, the oxytocin levels of the mothers who were supplementing were lower at all times examined, and no rise in oxytocin peaks was noted

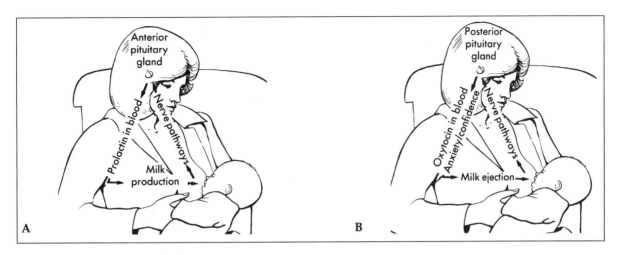

FIGURE 3–10. (A) Release and effect of prolactin on milk ejection. (B) Release and effect of oxytocin.

over time. In both groups of women, prolactin levels tended to decline over time. Among mothers who were not supplementing, however, prolactin levels were consistently higher at all times examined. These data suggest that over time prolactin levels can be expected to fall, but oxytocin levels will continue to climb. However, when a mother supplements with formula-feedings, prolactin levels decline markedly and fall even further over time, and oxytocin levels remain depressed and do not climb.

Milk Production

With closure of tight junctions in the cells of the alveoli (Figure 3–7) and through the mediation of the hypothalamus, the alveolar cells respond with milk secretion at the base of the alveolar cell, where small droplets form and migrate through the cell membrane and into the alveolar ducts for storage (see again Figure 3–6). The rate of milk synthesis after each breastfeeding episode varies, ranging from 17 ml/hr to 33 ml/hr in one study (Arthur et al., 1989). Milk synthesis is related to the degree of breast fullness. For example, a woman who did not breastfeed her baby for 6 hours will have a lower rate of milk synthesis than if she had breastfed every 90 minutes (Cregan & Hartmann, 1999).

The highly vascularized secretory cells extract water, lactose, amino acids, fats, vitamins, minerals, and numerous other substances from the mother's blood, converting them to milk for her infant. Stores of adipose tissue laid down during pregnancy are drawn upon to provide substrate for milk synthesis. When the milk "comes in" or rapidly increases in volume, creating breast fullness 3 to 4 days after birth, closure of the junctional complexes between the mammary alveolar cells prevents direct access of extracellular space to the lumen of the mammary alveoli (Neville, 2001). Thus sodium, chloride, and lactose concentrations are altered. Mothers then begin to feel a tightening in their breasts as the myoepithelial cells contract to expel the milk (Color Plate 3). This physiologic response is known as "letdown" and also as mammary-ejection reflex.

Autocrine Versus Endocrine

It is at this point that lactation shifts from *endocrine control* (hormone-driven) to *autocrine control* (milk removal-driven) (Prentice et al., 1989). It follows, then, that the amount of colostrum secreted by nonbreastfeeding women during the first few days postpartum is similar to that of breastfeeding women; however, this reverses abruptly after the first few days. Thus breastfeeding is not a major factor for the *initiation* of lactation but it is essential for the *continuation* of lactation (Kulski & Hartmann, 1981). From a clinical standpoint the onset of copious milk secretion after birth or the milk "coming in" will happen whether the baby is being put to the breast or not since it is hormonally driven.

Galactopoiesis

Galactopoiesis is the maintenance of the established milk production (Table 3–1). The breast is not a passive container of milk but an organ of active production that is infant- rather than hormone-driven. The removal of milk from the breasts facilitates continued milk production; conversely, lack of adequate milk removal or stasis tends to limit breastmilk synthesis in the breasts. It is the quantity and quality of infant suckling or milk removal that governs breastmilk synthesis. Milk production reflects the infant's appetite rather than the woman's ability to produce milk, which in fact can be severalfold higher (Daly & Hartmann, 1995). As long as milk is removed regularly from the breast, the alveolar cells will continue to secrete milk almost indefinitely.

This phenomenon, the *supply-demand response,* is a feedback control that regulates the production of milk to match the intake of the infant. A common adage that expresses this response is "The more the mother breastfeeds, the more milk there will be" (La Leche League International, 1997). Because lactation is an energy-intensive process, it makes teleological sense that there should be safeguards against wasteful overproduction as well as mechanisms for a prompt response to the infant's need.

A case of a new mother who became pregnant three months after having a pituitary resection supports the concept of autocrine control (de Coopman, 1993). After delivering a healthy infant, this mother had sufficient milk to completely sustain her baby by breastfeeding without supplementation. This unusual situation was attributable to the pituitary abscess that caused milk production to continue through her pregnancy after she weaned her first child; thus her milk yield postpartum was based on milk removal as much as on hormonal stimulation.

Galactorrhea

Galactorrhea is the spontaneous secretion of milk from the breast under nonphysiological circumstances. Small amounts of milk or serous fluid are commonly expressed for weeks, months, or years from women who have previously been pregnant or lactating. Many anecdotal reports of spontaneous lactation present an intriguing enigma. Thyrotoxicosis, certain drugs (reserpine, methyldopa, phenothiazines), and the use of intrauterine devices containing copper (Horn & Scott, 1969) can trigger abnormal milk secretion.

Surprisingly, only 30 percent of women with galactorrhea have higher-than-normal prolactin levels (Frantz, Kleinberg, & Noel, 1972); these women are otherwise healthy and have no history of menstrual irregularity or infertility. These women may be overly sensitive to normal circulating prolactin levels (Friesen & Cowden, 1989). For other women, galactorrhea is a symptom of a larger problem of hyperprolactinemia; in addition to a spontaneous milk secretion, they may also complain of amenorrhea, difficulty in becoming pregnant, and lack of libido. Any woman with persistent galactorrhea should be referred to a physician for a thorough physical examination and biochemical assessment.

Clinical Implications: Mother

Breast Assessment

Usually little attention is given to prenatal assessment of the breast and nipples because of Western cultural inhibitions about the breast and lack of recognition of its importance. As a consequence, after giving birth, mothers may experience feeding difficulties that could have been prevented. Nurses and lactation consultants practicing as primary caregivers are the ideal people to perform a prenatal breast assessment, particularly because physicians (especially males) are often reluctant to do so.

Ideal for teaching as well as for data gathering, physical assessment of the breast and nipples includes both inspection and palpation. While one is assessing the breasts, the following observations and questions are relevant.

Inspection. Size, symmetry, and shape of the breasts proper have minimal effect on lactation. The assessment provides the opportunity to reassure the woman with small breasts that she will be able to breastfeed and have a sufficient supply of milk. Asymmetry of breast size is usually normal, but *marked* asymmetry may be an indication of inadequate glandular tissue in a small minority of women (see Color Plate 27). Hypoplasia (lack of breast tissue) accompanied by a wide space between breasts (intramammary space) is another anatomical "red flag" associated with insufficient lactation (Huggins, Petok, & Mireles, 2000). When mothers with possible hypoplasia (underdeveloped breasts) are identified, their newborn baby should be monitored closely for adequate milk intake. Inadequate glandular tissue might prevent the mother from exclusively breastfeeding her baby; however, she can continue to enjoy the breastfeeding relationship if she provides the baby with additional nutrition while feeding from the breast.

For the woman with large breasts, discussing the importance of a support bra and where such a bra may be obtained is helpful. Holding and feeding her infant will not be the same for the large-breasted woman as for mothers with average-sized breasts. Instead of simply holding the breast, the mother with large breasts may need to lift her breast and to hold or push part of the breast back to permit her infant to grasp the nipple and maintain an adequate airway. During prenatal discussions, the mother may talk about some of her deeper feelings about having large breasts and her decision to breastfeed.

The skin of the breast should be inspected for any deviations. Skin turgor and elasticity can be assessed by gently pinching the skin, although the effect of elasticity on lactation is questionable: women who have been pregnant before have more elastic skin because it has been stretched from a previous pregnancy; women pregnant for the first time have firmer tissue.

A lateral incision in the vicinity of the cutaneous branch of the fourth intercostal nerve (left breast, 5 o'clock position; right breast, 7 o'clock position) made during breast augmentation or reduction surgery may mean severed innervation of the nipple and areola (Farina, Newby, & Alani, 1980). Surgery on the breast, especially if it involves an incision at the areolar margin, is likely to interfere to some degree with milk production. However, even having undergone such surgery, most mothers still can breastfeed. Breast-reduction surgery, because of the greater likelihood of the movement and replacement of nipple tissue, is more likely than augmentation surgery (Hurst, 1996) to negatively

influence later lactation performance (Neifert et al., 1990). Scar tissue from injury should be evaluated for its effect on skin elasticity and the degree to which nerve reactivity may have been affected.

Note should also be taken of any skin thickening and dimpling of the breast or nipple tissue. Although rare in a woman of childbearing age, such a change could be an early sign of a tumor a nd should be promptly referred to a physician for evaluation.

Now is the time to ask questions: "Have your breasts grown during pregnancy?" "Have you had any tenderness and soreness?" An increase in breast size, swelling, and tenderness usually indicates adequately functioning breast tissue responsive to hormonal changes.

Next, the nipple should be carefully inspected. (For the purpose of this discussion, nipple will refer to the areola as well as the nipple shaft and pores.) If the nipples appear small, explain that the size of a woman's nipples is of secondary importance to their functional ability. Likewise, any nipple structural abnormality such as inversion should be assessed only in terms of its function.

The look of the breast does not dictate its ability to function. A case in point may be women who have sustained significant scarring from burns (see Color Plate 25). Second- and third-degree burns rarely extend so deeply into the parenchyma that they destroy the glandular tissue of the breast, even when the burns have occurred in adulthood. Significant scarring of the dermis and epidermis, however, may result in (1) reduced maternal sensation when the infant suckles, (2) minimal tissue elasticity, thus requiring the mother to alter the baby's position at the breast, and (3) reduced milk ejection if a nipple has been surgically reconstructed. Nevertheless, scar tissue on the breast or nipple does not, by itself, preclude breastfeeding.

Palpation. After thorough hand washing, the nurse or lactation consultant should assess the nipple by compressing or palpating the areola between the forefinger and the thumb just behind the base of the nipple (the pinch test). This action simulates the compression that occurs when the infant is at the breast. Because of possible nipple adhesions within the underlying connective tissue, a nipple that initially appears everted may retract inwardly on stimulation. Conversely, a nipple that appears flattened or inverted may, on palpation, evert; therefore, differentiation must be made between structure and function in assessing the nipples.

The classification of nipple function in Table 3–3 is suggested as standard terminology. It must be emphasized that although many primigravidas have nipples that tend to retract during pregnancy, most evert easily by the end of pregnancy and do not interfere with breastfeeding. Thus nipple assessment should be performed periodically through the pregnancy to track changes and to inform the mother how her body is preparing to feed her baby.

Classification of Nipple Function

When the nipple is compressed using the pinch test, it responds in one of the ways identified in Figure 3–11. This response may reflect degree of function.

Flat or retracted nipples may be treatable during pregnancy. Dysfunction may be present in one nipple while the other is perfectly normal, or it may be present in both nipples. Retraction or inversion can prevent the infant from effectively milking milk ducts that lie beneath the areola. Retraction or simple inversion identified in early pregnancy, however, does not necessarily foretell later difficulty. The infant forms a teat not only from the nipple but from the surrounding breast tissue. When inversion is noted early in pregnancy, time is on the mother's side. As pregnancy progresses, hormonal changes increase the size and protractibility of the nipples. The mother also has time to use interventions that help prevent subsequent feeding problems.

Concepts to Practice

Encouraging early and frequent breastfeeding is a simple, low-cost recommendation for breastfeeding initiation. If the infant is able to suckle effectively at the breast soon after birth, there is a direct relationship between the frequency and strength of suckling and subsequent availability of breastmilk. There appears to be an early "window of opportunity" for the infant's suckling to stimulate prolactin receptors (discussed earlier in this chapter), which in turn enhances milk production. A basic knowledge of anatomy and physiology is put to valuable use when the lactation consultant or nurse translates basic concepts into easily understandable teaching materials. If a client realizes a stressful environment

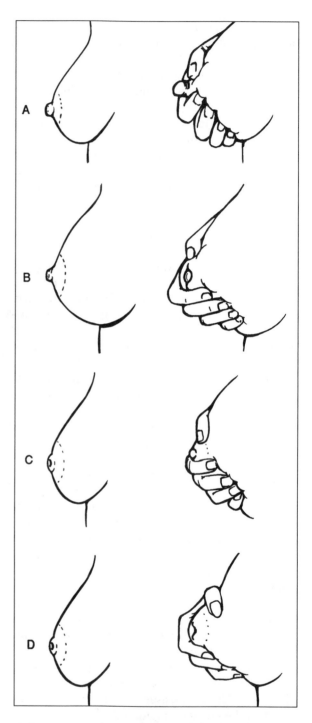

FIGURE 3–11. (A) Protracting normal nipple. (B) Moderate to severe retraction. (C) Inverted-appearing nipple, which when compressed using pinch test, will either invert farther inward or will protract forward. (D) True inversion; nipple inverts further.

Table 3–3

CLASSIFICATION OF NIPPLE FUNCTION

Protraction	Nipple moves forward; considered a normal functional response. No special interventions are needed.
Retraction	Instead of protracting, the nipple moves inward.
Minimal	An infant with a strong suck exerts sufficient pressure to pull the nipple forward. A weak or premature infant may have difficulties at first.
Moderate to severe	Nipple retracts to a level even with or behind the surrounding areola. Intervention is helpful to stretch the nipple outward and improve protractility.
Inversion	On visual inspection, all or part of the nipple is drawn inward within the folds of the areola.
Simple	The nipple moves outward to protraction with manual pressure or when cold (pseudoinversion).
Complete	The nipple does not respond to manual pressure because adhesions bind the nipple inward; very rarely there is congenital absence of the nipple.

may inhibit her milk supply, she may take action to reduce stressful situations over which she has control. If a woman understands that the reason she needs less covering when she breastfeeds is that she literally has "hot flashes" during feedings, she will take measures to "keep cool." Examples of the application of basic biologic principles of maternal lactation are legion and form the basis of many of the chapters that follow.

Newborn Oral Development

Infants perform a series of complex oral movements to obtain sufficient nutriment from their mother's breast to meet daily nutritional requirements and to support rapid growth, especially during the first few months of life. Suckling is a dynamic process, as the infant is continually adjusting to a changing anatomy. The act of suckling is far more than simply obtaining food. The infant's earliest autonomous functions are focused about his mouth and pharynx area. The infant's mouth is the cockpit of his awareness and is the principal site of interaction with his environment.

In the embryo, facial and pharyngeal regions develop from neural-crest cells at about the time of neural-tube closure. Further development is due to tissue differentiation from the endoderm, which later forms the digestive tract. During gestation, the fetus is able to swallow fluid as early as 11 weeks (Miller, 1982) and has a suckle reflex at 24 weeks (Herbst, 1981). Older studies reported that the rooting response and the link between suckling and swallowing was not established until 32 weeks (Amiel-Tison, 1967; Bu'Lock, Woolridge, & Baum, 1990) and not well coordinated until 37 weeks (Bu'Lock, Woolridge, & Baum, 1990). However, in a study of Swedish preterm infants (Nyqvist, Sjoden, & Ewald, 1999), efficient rooting, areolar grasp and latching on at the breast were observed at 28 weeks—much earlier than previously thought.

At birth, the infant's mouth is vertically short in comparison with that of the adult. There is so little room that when the newborn's mouth is closed, the tongue is in lateral contact with the gums and with the roof of the mouth. There are other proportional differences in size and shape between the infant and the adult skull (Figures 3–12 and 3–13). The infant's lower jaw (mandible) is small and somewhat receded. Whereas the adult's hard palate is deeply arched and situated on a higher plane relative to the base of the skull, the infant's is short, wide, and only slightly arched at birth. Corrugated transverse folds (rugae) on the hard palate assist the newborn in holding the breast during suckling.

Because the infant's tongue fills the small oral cavity, the extent and the direction of tongue movement is limited. Taste buds on the tongue (mostly on the tongue tip) are present at birth, but the newborn has an increased suckling response only to sweet taste. The entire surface of the tongue is within the oral cavity. The infant's lips are well adapted to effect an airtight closure around the breast. The lips are partially everted so that the oral mucosa presents slightly externally; they have tiny swellings on the inner surface (eminences of the

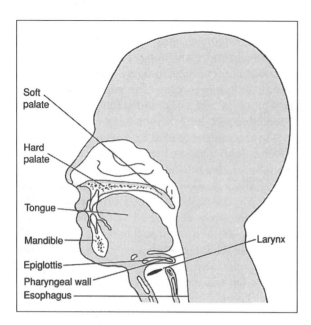

FIGURE 3–12. Midsagittal section of cranial and oral anatomy of an adult while swallowing.

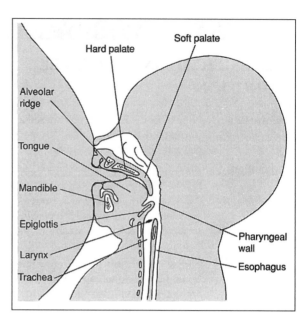

FIGURE 3–13. Midsagittal section of cranial and oral anatomy of an infant while swallowing.

pars villosa) that facilitate holding the breast and areola in place.

The largest increments in craniofacial growth occur during the first 4 years of life. During the first year after birth, the lower jaw grows downward, creating a larger intraoral space. Active breastfeeding encourages mandibular development and strengthens the jaw muscles. The tongue also gradually descends. By the fourth or fifth year of age, the tongue is attached directly to the epiglottis of the larynx. The frenulum is a fold of mucous membrane midline on the undersurface of the tongue that helps to anchor the tongue to the floor of the mouth. If the frenulum is too short to allow freedom of tongue movement or is placed too far forward to permit tongue extension upward or forward, it can interfere with an infant's ability to suckle (Notestine, 1990).

The infant's epiglottis lies just below the soft palate, unlike the adult's, as seen in Figure 3–13. This makes it possible for food to move laterally on the outside of the epiglottis and to pass directly into the esophagus. The epiglottis plays an important role by closing off the pathway to the lungs when the infant swallows. Such closure ensures that the milk will travel into the esophagus rather than into

the trachea. Relative to an adult larynx, the infant larynx is much higher in the oral cavity and occupies a larger space. It is short and funnel-shaped. As fluid passes through the mouth, the larynx elevates so that fluid can move easily into the pharynx. Because the larynx is high and elevated during swallowing, it depends much less on the action of the epiglottis and on closure of the vocal folds to protect the airway. The shape of the pharynx gradually changes as the child grows. At birth, the pharynx curves very gradually downward to join the oral cavity. This curvature would prevent articulate speech even if the necessary central nervous system linkage were present. By puberty, the posterior walls of the nasal and oral segments join almost at a right angle.

The infant has pads of fat on both cheeks to assist with suckling. Each pad is a circumscribed layer of fat enclosed within its own capsule of fibrous connective tissue. It lies between the buccinator and masseter muscles. It is thought that buccal fat pads provide stability for suckling and reduce the likelihood of collapsing of the cheeks and buccinator muscles between the gums. When babies suck their own tongues, the degree of negative pressure is such that drawing in of the cheeks occurs, creating a characteristic dimpling. Collapsing of the cheeks is more likely in a premature baby who lacks the layer of fat (including that in the cheeks) that gives full term infants their characteristic plump facial appearance.

The shape and softness of the human breast is beneficial to shaping the hard palate into a round U-shaped configuration because it broadens and flattens in response to the infant's tongue movements. Compared with the V shape associated with bottle-fed children, the broad and wide palate of a breastfed child is physiologically ideal because it aligns teeth properly and most likely reduces the incidence of malocclusions (Palmer, 1998).

Suckling

Suckling behavior develops early in gestation. Fetuses display a suckle reflex by 24 weeks gestation. By 28 weeks preterm babies can coordinate the suckle/swallow/breathe cycle at the breast and by 32 weeks can suckle in repeated bursts of more than 10 suckles and maximum suckling bursts of over 30 (Nyqvist, Sjoden, & Ewald, 1999).

The precise way in which infants use their oral and facial muscles to efficiently take in nourishment from their mothers' breasts is vital information for health professionals, because some breastfeeding infants have initial difficulty getting on the breast, and a few continue to have suckling dysfunction. In a study of spontaneous feeding behavior, infants placed in a prone position between their mothers' breasts after an unmedicated delivery began licking, suckling, and rooting movements after about 15 minutes, began hand-to-mouth movements after about 34 minutes, and spontaneously began to suckle after 55 minutes. Licking movements both preceded and followed the rooting reflex in alert infants (Widstrom et al., 1987).

Suckling might be strongest in neonates soon after delivery. When suckling ability was measured using the Neonatal Oral Motor Assessment Scale (NOMAS), an instrument to digitally assess oral motor behavior and suckling ability, younger newborns had a stronger suckle than did older newborns (MacMullen & Kulski, 2000).

The position of the neonate's tongue is critical to the feeding. After the rooting stimulus, the infant opens the mouth wide (the gape), keeping the tongue at the bottom of the mouth. This tongue position enables the infant to "catch" the mother's nipple and attach to the breast without help. It is important to note that an infant places the tongue in the palate when crying, which might be a security reflex, to prevent obstruction of the trachea during the inspiration phase. Forcing a crying baby to the breast might thus cause the infant to place the tongue in his or her palate, a defensive response that inhibits suckling and disturbs the rooting-tongue reflex system (Widstrom & Thingstrom-Paulsson, 1993).

In the literature, *sucking* and *suckling* are not distinguished, both terms being used interchangeably to refer to suckling. In this book, we too use these terms interchangeably, though some individuals feel strongly about the distinction (Montagu, 1979):

The baby is said to "suck" at its mother's nipple. The baby knows better than to do anything so foolish, for were he to "suck" the nipple all he would, for the most part, succeed in achieving would be to produce a partial vacuum in his mouth and fail to develop the ability to suckle properly. A baby sucks at the nozzle on the top of a bottle, but at the mother's breast a baby suckles.

Does the infant suckle or suck at the breast? Now that we have discovered that the mechanism by which babies extract milk from the breast differs considerably from the method that they use on a bottle teat, we urge that separate words are needed to differentiate the two acts. The word *suckle* seems ideal for breastfeeding, and it has come to be used in this sense in modern American breastfeeding literature. However, this term still retains its original meaning in the breastfeeding literature of many of the British Commonwealth countries. *The Oxford English Dictionary* (1961) defines the two words thus:

Suck: *(1) the action or an act of sucking milk from the breast; the milk or other fluid sucked at one time; (2) to apply the lips to a teat, breast, the mother, nurse, or dam, for the purpose of extracting milk from, with the mouth.*

Suckle: *(1) To give suck to; to nurse (a child) at the breast; (2) to cause to take milk from the breast or udder; to put to suck.*

Babies suckle and swallow at a frequency of about once per second or faster when breastmilk is actively flowing. This rate is similar to that of other primates. If the milk flow lessens or stops, the infant will increase this rate to about two suckles per second (Wolff, 1968). In other words, when the milk flow increases, the rate of suckling decreases. Conversely, when milk flow is low, the rate of suckling is higher. Inch and Garforth (1989) describe the suckling rhythm as follows:

When the baby first goes to the breast, short fast bursts of sucking can be observed. During this period no milk is flowing and unrelieved suction is applied to the surface of the nipple. With the letdown, milk begins to flow and fill the oral cavity and the sucking pattern changes to long, slow, continuous, suckling. Very little milk transfer is necessary to cause the shift away from short, fast, continuous suckling.

Drewett and Woolridge (1979) observed that suckling rates fluctuate at different stages of the feeding and that these rates are greater than those reported by Wolff (1968). These authors reported a rate of 72.4 sucks per minute during the first 2 minutes of feeding. This rate drops at 2 to 4 minutes to 70.8 sucks per minute, and increases again to 73.3 and 74.9 sucks per minute at 4 to 7 and 7 to 10 minutes respectively.

In addition to yielding milk and calories, suckling facilitates feelings of calm, reduces heart rate and metabolic rate, and elevates both the baby's and mother's pain threshold (Blass, 1994; Gray, 2002; Goer, 2002). Wolff (1968) originally defined two categories of suckling: nutritive (full and continuous milk flow) and nonnutritive (alternating suckling bursts and rests during minimal milk intake). Bowen-Jones, Thompson, and Drewett (1982) challenged the validity of these two categories. The latter study showed that breastfeeding babies *always* suckle in bursts, with resting periods or pauses between bursts. The term *nonnutritive suckling* is now accepted to mean either spontaneous suckling in the absence of anything being introduced into the infant's mouth (common during sleep) or suckling as prompted by something that is not a liquid nutriment (e.g., a pacifier) (McBride & Danner, 1987).

Nonnutritive suckling has important implications for infant development, especially under special circumstances such as prematurity. Nonnutritive suckling in premature infants increases peristalsis, enhances secretion of digestive fluids, and decreases crying in these infants (Measel & Anderson, 1979).

Suckling at the breast has been examined in great detail. With the advent of ultrasonography and other technologies, it is now possible to accurately quantify suckling patterns, replacing earlier descriptions that only inferred what actually occurred. When infants feed from both breasts, milk transfer from the second breast decreases by 58 percent as compared with the first breast, even though there are no significant changes in suckling pressure (Prieto et al., 1996). Detailed descriptions of infant suckling mechanics at the breast have been described by Marmet and Shell (1984), Woolridge (1986), McBride and Danner (1987), and Smith et al. (1985). The following description of functional suckling at the breast is based on the work of these investigators. Figure 3–14 illustrates the complete suck cycle:

- The nipple and its surrounding areola and underlying breast tissue are drawn deeply into the infant's mouth; the infant's lips and cheeks then form a seal. The infant's lips are flanged outward around the mother's breast and are minimally involved.

- The tip of the infant's tongue is maintained behind the lower lip and over the lower gum while the rest of the anterior tongue cups the areola of the breast.

- During the feeding, the mother's highly elastic nipple elongates (two to three times its resting length) into a teat by suction created within the baby's mouth. The nipple extends back as far as the posterior tongue junction between the hard and soft palates. At its base, the nipple is held between the upper gum and tongue that covers the lower gum. The mother's nipple and areolar tissue undergo extensive changes during feeding.

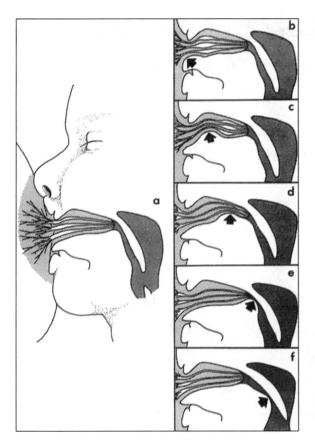

FIGURE 3–14. Complete suck cycle. Shown in median section, the baby exhibits good feeding technique: the nipple is drawn well into the mouth, extending back to the junction of the hard and soft palate.

- The jaw moves the tongue up, compressing the maternal areola against the infant's alveolar ridge.

- As the anterior portion of the tongue is raised, the posterior tongue is depressed and retracted in undulating or peristaltic motions, forming a groove that channels the milk to the back of the oral cavity where it stimulates receptors that initiate the swallowing reflex. This backward movement produces a negative pressure, similar to withdrawing a piston in an airtight syringe.

- If the volume of milk taken is sufficient to trig-

ger swallowing, the back of the tongue elevates and presses against the posterior pharyngeal wall. The soft palate rises and closes off the nasal passageways. The larynx then moves up and forward to close the trachea, propelling the milk into the esophagus. Afterward, the larynx returns to its previous position.

- The infant lowers the jaw, and a new cycle begins. A rhythm is created by this sequence of vertical jaw movements and the depression and elevation of the posterior tongue. Each suck sequence is followed by a swallow.

The differences between bottle-feeding and breastfeeding are shown in Table 3–4. Generally, breastfeeding infants suckle more times per day and maintain a higher level of oxygen pressure (tcPO$_2$) and skin temperature (Mathew, 1988; Meier & Anderson, 1987) than do bottle-feeding infants. The differences between bottle-feeding and breastfeeding premature infants are even greater (Meier & Pugh, 1985).

Breathing and Suckling

In a normal, coordinated, nutritive suckling cycle, swallowing does not inhibit respiration. Breathing appears to continue throughout the sucking cycle; however, at the onset of the swallow, as the bulk of the bolus enters the pharynx, airflow might be momentarily interrupted and then immediately restored (Ardran, Kemp, & Lind, 1958). In a perfectly coordinated cycle of suckling, swallowing, and breathing, breathing movements appear to be related in a 1:1:1 sequence. The rate of suckling is high for the first 1 or 2 minutes until the milk-ejection reflex occurs, then it slows down (Bu'Lock et al., 1990; Weber, Woolridge, & Baum, 1986; Wolff, 1968). This sequence reoccurs with each milk ejection during a feeding. As the feeding progresses, suckling bursts become shorter with more frequent pauses.

Although suckling, swallowing, and breathing are generally well coordinated during a feeding, infant cyanosis is a relatively common event, especially in neonates. The neonate almost always

Table 3–4

COMPARISONS BETWEEN BREASTFEEDING AND BOTTLE-FEEDING IN FULL-TERM INFANTS

Breastfeeding	Bottle-feeding	References

More frequent suckling/min
  Nonnutritive: 1 suckle/sec
  Nutritive: 2 suckles/sec
	Less frequent suckling/min	Drewett & Woolridge, 1979;
		Mathew, 1988; Wolff, 1968

Breathing patterns
  Shortening of expiration
  Prolonging of inspiration
	Breathing patterns
	  Prolonged expiration
	  Shortening of inspiration
		Mathew, 1988

Oxygen saturation < 90%
  2 of 10 infants
	Oxygen saturation < 90%
	  5 of 10 infants
		Mathew, 1988

Bradycardia
  0 of 10 infants
	Bradycardia
	  2 of 10 infants
		Hammerman & Kaplan, 1995;
		Mathew, 1988

Extended opening of mouth to grasp mother's nipple	Less extension to grasp rubber teat	Marmet & Shell, 1984
Infant's lips flanged outward, relaxed and resting against the breast to make a seal	Lips closer together and pursed to maintain contact with rubber teat	McBride & Danner, 1987
Extensive mandibular (jaw) action	Minimal mandibular action	Palmer, 1998
Tongue grooved around nipple; remains under nipple through out feeding. Moves in peristaltic, rolling action from front to back	Tongue upward and thrust forward against end of teat, "piston-like," to control milk flow	Marmet & Shell, 1984; Woolridge, 1986; Weber, Woodbridge, & Baum, 1986
Silent, except for soft swallow sounds, and (in older infants), cooing or "singing"	High-pitched squeak at end of intake of air prior to new suck	
Duration of feeding varies from short (few minutes) to long (30 min or longer)	Duration of feeding is usually 5 to 10 min	Ardan et al., 1958
Includes nutritive and nonnutritive suckling throughout the feeding	Involves nearly exclusively nutritive suckling	Ardran et al., 1958; Hornell et al., 1999; Woolridge, 1986

recovers spontaneously and often continues to suckle and swallow despite cyanosis. Oxygen saturation in the feeding infant normally declines. Mean levels drop from 96 percent (during feeding) to 93 percent (postfeeding) in breastfed infants and from 95 percent (during feeding) to 92 percent (postfeeding) in bottle-fed infants (Hammerman & Kaplan, 1995).

Unless hypoxic, the newborn is usually a nose breather, owing in part to the positioning of the soft palate and to the lack of space in the mouth through which air can travel in and out. Although it is true that babies have ventilatory problems when the nasal passages are occluded, an infant is capable of breathing through the mouth when necessary (Rodenstein, Perlmutter, & Stanescu, 1985).

Frequency of Feedings

How often does the exclusively breastfed infant feed? Hornell et al. (1999) recorded the daily number of feedings of 506 Swedish infants for the first 6 months. These mothers live in a country where breastfeeding is the norm. Each had previously breastfed at least one infant for at least 4 months and considered that they breastfed on demand.

During the first 6 months of life, median frequency of feeds was eight feeds per 24 hours. This is consistent with the data by Howie et al. (1981) and Quandt (1986) but different from the studies by Butte et al. (1985) and de Carvalho (1982) who noted a decline in feeding frequency during the first months. It also differs from a study of La Leche League mothers that showed an average daily number of 15 feedings (Cable & Rothenberger, 1984).

In the Hornell study, the median frequency of daytime feeds of exclusively breastfed infants was slightly below 6 during the first 26 weeks. The median number of night feeds declined from 2.2 at 2 weeks to 1.3 at 12 weeks, after which it increased up to 1.8 at 20 weeks (see Figure 3–15). The frequency and duration of daily feedings varied widely among mothers. For example, at 2 weeks, the frequency of feeds during the day ranged from 2.9 to 10.8 and night feeds from 1.0 to 5.1. Daytime suckling duration ranged from 20 minutes to over 4 hours and night-time duration from 0 to 2 hours, 8 minutes. Increased feeding frequencies or so-called appetite or "growth spurts" were not observed in this study.

The neonate's ability to suckle effectively at the breast takes time and practice. For the first few feedings, even in full-term infants, suckling is usually disorganized. Drugs given to the mother during childbirth can also inhibit early suckling. Usually, after several attempts, the infant latches onto the breast and begins to suckle vigorously and effectively. These first feedings are critical because they imprint a suckling pattern that tends to be repeated in subsequent feedings. A healthy infant unaffected by labor or birth analgesia or anesthesia should be allowed to demonstrate hunger before being offered the breast. Practicing lactation consultants are fully aware that it is difficult, if not impossible to "make" a baby breastfeed when he is in a deep

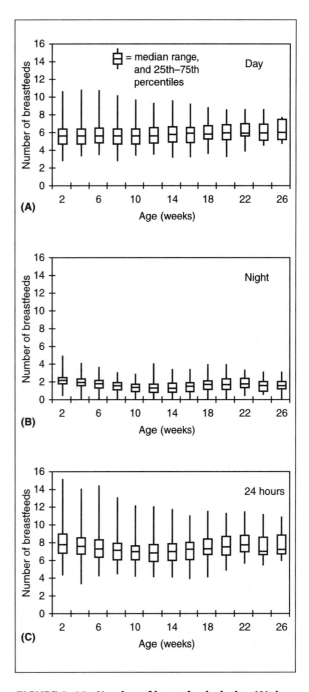

FIGURE 3–15. Number of breastfeeds during (A) daytime, (B) night-time, and (C) 24 hours at different ages. Median, 25th and 7th percentiles and range. (From Hornell A et al. Breastfeeding patterns in exclusively breastfed infants: a longitudinal prospective study in Uppsala, Sweden. *Acta Paediatr* 88, 203–11, 1999.)

sleep. Forcing the infant to the breast might abolish the rooting reflex and disturb placement of the tongue (Widstrom & Thingstrom-Paulsson, 1993).

Consistent breastfeeding assessment and identification of early problems so that they can be resolved before they worsen is essential. Several breastfeeding assessment tools have been developed over the last decade. While there is not yet general agreement on which is the most valid tool in predicting how well breastfeeding will progress, an evidence-based tool undoubtedly will be developed (Riordan & Koehn, 1997). The more popular breastfeeding assessment tools are discussed in Chapter 20. The PIBBs breastfeeding tool, developed for assessing preterm infants, can be found as an appendix to Chapter 13.

Summary

Knowledge of maternal breast anatomy and the physiology of lactation are necessary antecedents to clinical practice. The fundamental biological principles of lactation discussed in this chapter are used, although not always consciously, in almost every clinical situation in which lactation is involved. Knowledge of the structure and function of the normal breast and of infant suckling are necessary for assessment; knowing what is normal must precede recognizing the abnormal and recommending actions designed to support an optimal breastfeeding experience. Enabling the natural physiological mechanisms to function optimally is more likely to lead to an uncomplicated breastfeeding experience; interference with these mechanisms can result in difficulty with breastfeeding for mother and infant. For example, restrictive policies in breastfeeding for preterm babies are commonly based on bottle-feeding studies, not on knowledge about the early development of infants' capacity for suckling at the breast (Nyqvist, Sjoden, & Ewald, 1999).

At the same time, anatomy and physiology are the building blocks in a larger picture of the breastfeeding and lactation experience. Most women are physiologically equipped to produce sufficient milk for their infant or infants. Yet the most commonly cited problem in breastfeeding worldwide is the mother's perception that she has insufficient milk (Hill & Humenick, 1989). Social and cultural influences play a major role in the mother's perceptions of her ability to nourish her infant from her breasts. Succeeding chapters build on the anatomy and physiology of lactation and address the clinical implications as well as its social and cultural aspects.

Key Concepts

- Breastmilk removal (through feeding or pumping) in the first two days postpartum is not necessary for lactogenesis II to occur; however, milk removal must begin by day 3 after birth or the likelihood of successful establishment of lactation is decreased.

- Three factors are necessary for lactation: (1) oxytocin released from the posterior pituitary, (2) removal of breastmilk by the infant or pump, and (3) prolactin release from the anterior pituitary, which stimulates lactogenesis and initiates milk secretion.

- Lactogenesis occurs earlier if breastmilk is removed by feeding or pumping within the first 2 to 3 days after birth. Early breastfeeding or pumping is associated with higher milk volume by day 5.

- Short-term rate of milk synthesis is considerably higher when most of the available milk has been removed from the breast.

- Frequency of breastfeedings varies widely; however, exclusively breastfed term infants (living in a country where breastfeeding is the norm) feed a median of 8 times per day (6 times during the day, and twice during the night).

- Mammary ducts do not widen into sinuses behind the nipple as previously thought.

- Suspensory ligaments of the breast are called Cooper's ligaments.

- Each breast of an adult woman weighs, on average 150 to 200 gm. It doubles in weight to 400 to 500 gm (about 1 pound) during lactation.

- Nerves that supply the breast are from the intercostal nerves of the fourth, fifth, and sixth intercostal spaces. The fourth intercostal nerve, which penetrates the left breast at 4 o'clock and right breast 8 o'clock, supplies the greatest amount of sensation to the nipple and areola.

- If the lowermost nerve branch of the fourth intercostal nerve is severed, the mother loses sensation to the nipple and areola.

- Breast asymmetry is common; the left breast is often larger than the right.

- Marked asymmetry and breast hypoplasia may indicate problems with breastmilk production.

- Areola and nipple color vary according to complexion: pink in blonds, brown in brunettes, and black in dark-skinned women.

- Supernumerary breasts (polymastia) and/or an accessory nipple may occur in about 1 to 2 percent of the population at any point along the milk line from the axilla to the groin.

- Poor nipple protractility occurs in 10 to 35 percent of women during their first pregnancy.

- Nipple inversion is found in about 3 percent of women, and it is bilateral in 87 percent of these women. Only 4 percent of nipple inversion is "true" inversion.

- Prolactin influences nipple growth; areolar growth is related to serum placental lactogen; the ductal system proliferates and differentiates under the influence of estrogen; progesterone promotes enlargement of the lobes, lobules, and alveoli.

- Lactogenesis, stage I occurs mid- to late pregnancy when breast size increases as epithelial cells of the alveoli differentiate into secretory cells for milk production.

- Lactogenesis II (days 2 to 8 postpartum) is the onset of copious milk secretion after birth when milk volume increases rapidly and then abruptly levels off.

- Before lactogenesis II large gaps occur between the alveolar epithelial cells. These gaps close suddenly after 3 to 4 days via a gasketlike structure (the tight junction) and trigger the onset of copious milk secretion.

- Maternal conditions that can delay or impair lactogenesis include cesarean birth, type I diabetes, labor analgesia, obesity, polycystic ovary syndrome, placental retention, and stress.

- The developmental cycle of the mammary gland has four phases: (1) mammogenesis, (2) lactogenesis, (3) galactopoiesis, and (4) involution.

- After delivery, progesterone levels drop and prolactin levels rise; both act synergistically with cortisol, thyroid-stimulating hormone, prolactin-inhibiting factor, and oxytocin to establish and maintain lactation.

- Following lactogenesis II, milk production shifts from endocrine to autocrine control. When the nipple is stimulated and milk removed from the breast, the hypothalamus inhibits dopamine, which in turn stimulates the release of prolactin and causes milk production.

- The basic unit of the breast is the alveoli which is surrounded by a contractile unit of myoepithelial cells responsible for ejecting milk into the ductules. Each ductule merges into a larger duct. The ducts are lined with epithelium and highly vascular connective tissue.

- Milk is secreted into the alveolar lumina where it is stored until the posterior pituitary hormone oxytocin causes the milk-ejection reflex or letdown, a contraction of the myoepithelial cells surrounding the alveoli.

- Oxytocin plays a major role in lactation. Blood levels rise within 1 minute of suckling, remain elevated during the feeding, and return to baseline levels within 6 minutes.

- Oxytocin contracts the mother's uterus, which help to control postpartum bleeding and to aid in uterine involution.

- The supply-demand response is a feedback control that regulates the production of milk to match the intake of the infant.

- Galactorrhea is the spontaneous secretion of milk from the breast from unexpected or unknown circumstances.

- Before lactogenesis, lactation is driven hormonally (endocrine control); after, it is driven by suckling and milk removal (autocrine control).

- Suckling and milk removal is not a major factor for the initiation of lactation but is essential for its continuation.

- If the frenulum—a fold of mucous membrane midline on the undersurface of the baby's tongue—is too short or is too far forward, it can interfere with an infant's ability to suckle.

- The suckling reflex is present at 24 weeks gestation. By 28 weeks preterm, babies can coordinate the suckle/swallow/breathe cycle; by 32 weeks, they can suckle in repeated bursts.

- Forcing a crying baby to the breast evokes a defensive response (tongue to palate) that inhibits suckling and disturbs the rooting-tongue reflex system.

- Nutritive suckling is intake of continuous flow of liquid nutriment; nonnutritive suckling is suckling in the absence of liquid nutriment being introduced into the baby's mouth.

- Breastfeeding infants suckle more times per day and maintain a higher level of oxygen pressure ($tcPO_2$) and skin temperature compared with bottle-fed infants.

- Babies suckle and swallow at a frequency of about once per second. When milk flow increases, the rate of suckling decreases; when milk flow is low, the rate of suckling increases.

References

Alexander JM, Grant AM, Campbell MJ. Randomized controlled trial of breast shells and Hoffman's exercises for inverted and non-protractile nipples. *Br Med J* 304:1030–32, 1992.

Altemus J et al. Suppression hypothalamic-pituitary-adrenal axis responses to stress in lactating women. *J Clin Endocr Metab* 80:2954–59, 1996.

Amiel-Tison C. Neurological evaluation of the maturity of newborn infant. *Arch Dis Child* 43:89, 1967.

Ardran GM, Kemp MB, Lind J. A cineradiographic study of breast feeding. *Br J Radiol* 31:156–62, 1958.

Arthur PG et al. Measuring short-term rates of milk synthesis in breast-feeding mothers. *Q J Exp Physiol* 74:419–28, 1989.

Baron JA et al. Cigarette smoking and prolactin in women. *Br Med J* 293:482, 1986.

Battin D et al. Effect of suckling on serum prolactin, luteinizing hormone, follicle-stimulating hormone, and estradiol during prolonged lactation. *Obstet Gynecol* 65:785–88, 1985.

Berman MA, Davis GD. Lactation from axillary breast tissue in the absence of a supernummeray nipple: a case report. *J Reprod Med* 39:657–59, 1994.

Blaikeley J et al. Breastfeeding—factors affecting success. *J Obstet Gynaecol Br Emp* 60:657–69, 1953.

Blass EM. Behavioral and physiological consequences of suckling in rat and human newborns. *Acta Paediatr Suppl* 397:71–76, 1994.

Bohnet HG, Kato K. Prolactin secretion during pregnancy and puerperium: response to metoclopramide and interactions with placental hormones. *Obstet Gynecol* 65:789–92, 1985.

Bowen-Jones A, Thompson C, Drewett RF. Milk flow and sucking rates during breastfeeding. *Dev Med Child Neurol* 24:626–33, 1982.

Bu'Lock F, Woolridge MW, Baum JD. Development of coordination of sucking, swallowing and breathing: ultrasound study of term and preterm infants. *Dev Med Child Neurol* 32:669–78, 1990.

Butte NF et al. Feeding patterns of exclusively breast-fed infants during the first four months of life. *Early Hum Dev* 12:291–300, 1985.

Cable TA, Rothenberger LA. Breast-feeding behavioral patterns among La Leche League mothers: a descriptive survey. *Pediatrics* 73:830, 1984.

Chao S. The effect of lactation on ovulation and fertility. *Clin Perinatol* 14(1):39–49, 1987.

Chen DC et al. Stress during labor and delivery and early lactation performance. *Am J Clin Nutr* 68:335–44, 1998.

Courtiss EH, Goldwyn RM. Breast sensation before and after plastic surgery. *Plast Reconstr Surg* 58:1–12, 1976.

Cox DB, Owens RA, Hartmann PE. Blood and milk prolactin and the rate of milk synthesis in women. *Exp Physiol* 81:1007–20, 1996.

Cregan M, Hartmann PE. Computerized breast measurement from conception to weaning: clinical implications. *J Hum Lact* 15:89–95, 1999.

Cregan MD, Mitoulas LR, Hartmann PE. Milk prolactin, feed volume, and duration between feeds in women breastfeeding their full-term in-fants over a 24-hour period. *Exp Physiol* 87:207–14, 2002.

Daly SEJ, Hartmann PE. Infant demand and milk supply. Part 1: Infant demand and milk production in lactating women. *J Hum Lact* 11:21–23, 1995.

Dawood MY et al. Oxytocin release and plasma anterior pituitary and gonadal hormones in women during lactation. *J Clin Endocrinol Metab* 52:678–83, 1981.

Dawson EK. A histological study of the normal mamma in relation to tumour growth: 1. Early development to maturity. *Edinb Med J* 41:653–82, 1934.

de Carvalho M et al. Milk intake and frequency of feeding in breast-fed infants. *Early Hum Dev* 7:155–63, 1982.

———. Effect of frequent breast-feeding on early milk production and infant weight gain. *Pediatrics* 72:307–11, 1983.

de Coopman J. Breastfeeding after pituitary resection: support for a theory of autocrine control of milk supply? *J Hum Lact* 9:35–40, 1993.

Division of Ultrasound, Department of Radiology and Department of Pathology. *Atlas of breast ultrasound.* Philadelphia: Thomas Jefferson University Medical College and Hospital, 1980:121.

Drewett RF, Woolridge M. Sucking patterns of human babies on the breast. *Early Hum Dev* 315:315–21, 1979.

Farina MA, Newby BG, Alani HM. Innervation to the nipple-areola complex. *Plast Reconstr Surg* 66(4):497–501, 1980.

Frantz A, Kleinberg DL, Noel G. Studies on prolactin in man. *Recent Prog Horm Res* 28:527–34, 1972.

Friesen HG, Cowden EA. Lactation and galactorrhea. In: DeGroot LJ, ed. *Endocrinology in pregnancy.* Philadelphia: Saunders, 1989: 2074–86.

Goer M, Davis MW. Postpartum stress: current concepts and the possible protective role of breastfeeding. *JOGN Nursing* 31:411–17, 2002.

Grajeda R, Perez-Escamilla R. Stress during labor and delivery is associated with delayed onset of lactation among urban Guatemalan women. *J Nutr* 132:3055–60, 2002.

Gray L et al. Breastfeeding is analgesic in healthy newborns. *Pediatrics* 109:590–93, 2002.

Grossl NA. Supernumerary tissue: historical perspectives and clinical features. *South Med J* 93:29–32, 2000.

Hammerman C, Kaplan M. Oxygen saturation during and after feeding in healthy term infants. *Biol Neonate* 67:94–99, 1995.

Hartmann PE, Sherriff JL, Kent JC. Maternal nutrition and milk synthesis. *Proc Nutr Soc* 54:379–89, 1995.

Herbst JJ. Development of suck and swallowing. In: Lebenthal E, ed. *Textbook of gastroenterology and nutrition in infancy,* Vol. 1. New York: Plenum, 1981:97–107.

Hildebrandt HM. Maternal perception of lactogenesis time: a clinical report. *J Hum Lact* 15:317–23, 1999.

Hill PD, Chatterton RT, Aldag AC. Serum prolactin in breastfeeding: state of the science. *Biol Res Nurs* 1:65–75, 1999.

Hill PD, Humenick SS. Insufficient milk supply. *Image* 21:145–48, 1989.

Hinds LA, Tyndale-Biscoe CH. Prolactin in the marsupial *Macropus engenii* during the estrous cycle, pregnancy, and lactation. *Biol Reprod* 26:391–98, 1982.

Hoover K, Barbalinardo L, Pia Platia M. Delayed lactogenesis 2 secondary to gestation ovarian theca lutein cysts in two normal singleton pregnancies. *J Hum Lact* 18:264–68, 2002.

Horn HW, Scott JM. IUD insertion and galactorrhea. *Fertil Steril* 20:400–04, 1969.

Hornell A et al. Breastfeeding patterns in exclusively breast-fed infants: a longitudinal prospective study in Uppsala, Sweden. *Acta Paediatr* 88:203–11, 1999.

Howie PW et al. Effect of supplementary food on suckling patterns and ovarian activity during lactation. *Br Med J* 283:757–59, 1981.

Huggins K, Petok E, Mireles O. Markers of lactation insufficiency: a study of 34 mothers. In: Auerbach K, ed. *Current issues in clinical lactation.* Sudbury, MA: Jones and Bartlett, 2000:25–35.

Humenick SS et al. Breast-milk sodium as a predictor of breastfeeding patterns. *Can J Nurs Res* 30:67–81, 1998.

Hurst N. Lactation after augmentation mammoplasty. *Obstet Gynecol* 87:30–34, 1996.

Hytten FE. Clinical and chemical studies in lactation: IX. Breastfeeding in hospital. *Br Med J* 18:1447–52, 1954.

Hytten FE, Baird D. The development of the nipple in pregnancy. *Lancet* 1(June 7):1201–04, 1958.

Inch S, Garforth S. Establishing and maintaining breastfeeding. In: Chalmers I, Enkin M, Keirse M, eds. *Effective care in pregnancy and childbirth.* Oxford, England: Oxford University Press, 1989:1359–74.

James RJA et al. Thirst induced by a suckling episode during breast feeding and its relation with plasma vasopressin, oxytocin and osmoregulation. *Clin Endocrinol* 43:277–82, 1995.

Johnstone JM, Amico JA. A prospective longitudinal study of the release of oxytocin and prolactin in response to infant suckling in long-term lactation. *J Clin Endocrinol Metab* 62:653, 1986.

Kopans DB. *Breast imaging.* Philadelphia: Lippincott, 1989:20.

Kulski JK, Hartmann PE. Changes in human milk composition during the initiation of lactation. *Aust J Exp Biol Med Sci* 59:101–14, 1981.

La Leche League International. *The womanly art of breastfeeding,* 6th ed. Schaumberg, IL: La Leche League, 1997.

Leake R et al. Oxytocin and prolactin responses in long-term breast-feeding. *Obstet Gynecol* 62:565–68, 1983.

Lincoln DW, Paisley AC. Neuroendocrine control of milk ejection. *J Reprod Fertil* 65:571–86, 1982.

MacMullen NJ, Kulski LA. Factors related to suckling ability in healthy newborns. *JOGN Nursing* 29:390–96, 2000.

MacPherson EE, Montagna W. The mammary glands of rhesus monkeys. *J Invest Derm* 63:17–18, 1974.

Madden JD et al. Analysis of secretory patterns of prolactin and gonadotropins during twenty-four hours in a lactating woman before and after resumption of menses. *Am J Obstet Gynecol* 132:436–41, 1978.

Marasco L, Marmet C, Shell E. Polycystic ovary syndrome: A connection to insufficient milk supply? *J Hum Lact* 16:143–48, 2000.

Marmet C, Shell E. Training neonates to suck correctly. *MCN* 9:401–7, 1984.

Marshall WM, Cumming DC, Fitzsimmons GW. Hot flushes during breast feeding? *Fertil and Steril* 57:1349–50, 1992.

Mathew OP. Regulation of breathing patterns during feeding. In: Mathew OP, Sant Ambrogio G, eds. *Respiratory function of the upper airway.* New York: Marcel Dekker, 1988:535–60.

McBride MC, Danner SC. Sucking disorders in neurologically impaired infants: assessment and facilitation of breastfeeding. *Clin Perinatol* 14(1):109–30, 1987.

Measel CP, Anderson GC. Nonnutritive suckling during tube feedings: effect on clinical course in premature infants. *JOGN Nursing* 8:265–72, 1979.

Meier P, Anderson GC. Responses of small preterm infants to bottle- and breast-feeding. *MCN* 12:97–105, 1987.

Meier P, Pugh EJ. Breastfeeding behavior in small preterm infants. *MCN* 10:396–401, 1985.

Mennella JA, Beauchamp GK. Beer, breastfeeding, and folklore. *Dev Psychobiol* 26:459–66, 1993.

Miller AJ. Deglutition. *Physiol Rev* 62:129–83, 1982.

Montagna W, MacPherson EE. Some neglected aspects of the anatomy of the breasts. *J Invest Derm* 63:10–16, 1974.

Montagu A. Breastfeeding and its relation to morphological, behavioral, and psychocultural development. In: Rapheal D, ed. *Breastfeeding and food policy in a hungry world.* New York: Academic, 1979:189–93.

Morton JA. The clinical usefulness of breast milk sodium in the assessment of lactogenesis. *Pediatrics* 93:802–6, 1994.

Neifert M et al. The influence of breast surgery, breast appearance, and pregnancy-induced breast changes on lactation sufficiency as measured by infant weight gain. *Birth* 17:31–38, 1990.

Neifert MR, McDonough SL, Neville MC. Failure of lactogenesis associated with placental retention. *Am J Obstet Gynecol* 140:477–78, 1981.

Neubauer SH et al. Delayed lactogenesis in women with insulin-dependent diabetes mellitus. *Am J Clin Nutr* 58:54–60, 1993.

Neville, MC. Anatomy and physiology of lactation. In: Schanler RJ, ed. Breastfeeding 2001, Part 1: The evidence for breastfeeding. *Pediatr Clin No Amer* 48:13–34, 2001.

Neville MC, Berga SE. Cellular and molecular aspects of the hormonal control of mammary function. In: Neville MC, Neifert MR, eds. *Lactation: physiology, nutrition, and breastfeeding.* New York: Plenum, 1983:141–77.

Nissen E et al. Different patterns of oxytocin, prolactin but not cortisol release during breast-feeding in women delivered by cesarean section or by the vaginal route. *Early Hum Dev* 45:103–8, 1996.

Noel GL, Suh HK, Frantz AG. Prolactin release during nursing and breast stimulation in postpartum and nonpostpartum subjects. *J Clin Endocrinol Meta* 38:413–23, 1974.

Notestine GE. The importance of the identification of ankyloglossia (short lingual frenulum) as a cause of breastfeeding problems. *J Hum Lact* 6:113–15, 1990.

Nyqvist K, Sjöden PO, Ewald U. The development of preterm infants' breastfeeding behavior. *Early Hum Dev* 55:247–64, 1999.

Oxford English dictionary, Vol. 10. Oxford, England: Clarendon Press, 1961.

Palmer B. The influence of breastfeeding on the development of the oral cavity: a commentary. *J Hum Lact* 14:93–99, 1998.

Park HS, Yoon CH, Kim HJ. The prevalence of congenital inverted nipple. *Aesthetic Plast Surg* 23:1446, 1999.

Prentice A et al. Evidence for local feed-back control of human milk secretion. *Biochem Soc Trans* 17:489–92, 1989.

Prieto CR et al. Sucking pressure and its relationship to milk transfer during breastfeeding in humans. *J Reprod Fertil* 108:69–74, 1996.

Quandt SA. Patterns of variation in breast-feeding behaviors. *Soc Sci Med* 23:445–53, 1986.

Rasmussen KM, Hilson JA, Kjolhede CL. Obesity may impair lactogenesis 2. *J Nutr* 131:3009S–11S, 2001.

Riordan J, Koehn M. Reliability testing of three breastfeeding assessment tools. *JOGN Nursing* 26:181–87, 1997.

Rodenstein DO, Perlmutter N, Stanescu DC. Infants are not obligatory nose breathers. *Am Rev Respir Dis* 131:343–47, 1985.

Russo J, Russo IH. Development of the human mammary gland. In: Neville MD, Daniel CW, eds. *The mammary gland: development, regulation, and function.* New York: Plenum, 1987: 67–93.

Salazar H, Tobon H. Morphologic changes of the mammary gland during development, pregnancy and lactation. In: Josimovich J, ed. *Lactogenic hormones, fetal nutrition and lactation.* New York: Academic Press, 1974:1–18.

Sernia C, Tyndale-Biscoe CH. Prolactin receptors in the mammary gland, corpus luteum and other tissues of the Tammar wallaby. *Macropus engenii. J Endocrinol* 26:391–98, 1979.

Smith DM. Montgomery's areolar tubercle: a light microscopic study. *Arch Pathol Lab Med* 106:60–63, 1982.

Smith WL et al. Physiology of sucking in the normal term infant using real-time ultrasound. *Radiology* 156:379–81, 1985.

Sozmen M. Effects of early suckling of cesarean-born babies on lactation *Biol Neonate* 62:67–68, 1992.

Speroff L, Glass RH, Kase NG. *Clinical gynecology, endocrinology and infertility,* 4th ed. Baltimore: Williams and Wilkins, 1989:283.

Stallings JF et al. Prolactin response to suckling and maintenance of postpartum amenorrhea among intensively breastfeeding Nepali women. *Endocrinol Res* 22:1–28, 1996.

Tay CCK, Glasier AF, McNeil AS. Twenty-four hours patterns of prolactin secretion during lactation and the relationship to suckling and the resumption of fertility in breast-feeding women. *Hum Reprod* 11:950–55, 1996.

Tyson JE et al. Studies of prolactin in human pregnancy. *Am J Obstet Gynecol* 113:14–20, 1972.

Ueda T, Yokoyama Y, Irahara M et al. Influence of psychological stress on suckling-induced pulsa-tile oxytocin release. *Obstet Gynecol* 84:259–62, 1994.

Uvnas-Moberg K. Oxytocin linked antistress effects—the relaxation and growth response. *Acta Physiol Scand Supp* 640:38–42, 1997.

Vorherr H. Development of the female breast. In: Vorrherr H, ed. *The breast.* New York: Academic, 1974:1–18.

Waller H. The early failure of breastfeeding. *Arch Dis Child* 21:1–12, 1946.

Weber F, Woolridge MW, Baum JD. An ultrasonographic study of the organization of sucking and swallowing by newborn infants. *Dev Med Child Neurol* 28:19–24, 1986.

West CP. Hormonal profiles in lactating and non-lactating women immediately after delivery and their relationship to breast engorgement. *Am J Obstet Gynecol* 86:501–6, 1979.

Widstrom AM et al. Gastric suction in healthy newborn infants: effects on circulation and developing feeding behaviour. *Acta Paediatr Scand* 76:566–72, 1987.

Widstrom AM, Thingstrom-Paulsson J. The position of the tongue during rooting reflexes elicited in newborn infants before the first suckle. *Acta Paediatr* 82:281–83, 1993.

Wolff PH. The serial organization of sucking in the young infant. *Pediatrics* 42:943–56, 1968.

Woolridge MW. The "anatomy" of infant sucking. *Midwifery* 2:164–71, 1986.

Yokoyama Y et al. Releases of oxytocin and prolactin during breast massage and suckling in puerperal women. *Eur J Obstet Gynecol Reprod Biol* 53:17–20, 1994.

Yuen BH. Prolactin in human milk: the influence of nursing and duration of postpartum lactation. *Am J Obstet Gynecol* 158:583–86, 1988.

Ziemer M. Nipple skin changes and pain during the first week of lactation. *JOGN Nursing* 22:247–56, 1993.

Zuppa AA et al. Relationship between maternal parity, basal prolactin levels and neonatal breast milk intake. *Biol Neonate* 53:144–47, 1988.

The Biological Specificity of Breastmilk

Jan Riordan

Breastmilk is sometimes referred to as *white blood*, because it is considered similar to the placental blood of intrauterine life. Indeed, human milk is similar to unstructured living tissue, such as blood, and is capable of transporting nutrients, affecting biochemical systems, enhancing immunity, and destroying pathogens. With the use of sophisticated laboratory techniques, many scientific investigators have substantiated the life-sustaining properties of breastmilk. Organs themselves provide evidence of the profound influence of breastfeeding. For example, the thymus plays a role in the development of the immune system by providing the environment for T-cell differentiation and maturation. At age 4 months, the thymus is about twice as large in exclusively breastfed infants as in infants fed only infant formula. This difference in size continues until the child is at least 10 months old (Hasselbalch et al., 1999). Although thymus size can be influenced by many factors, it would not be unreasonable to generate a variety of hypothetical mechanisms whereby breastfeeding might influence thymic size (Prentice & Collinson, 2000).

Breastmilk, like all other animal milks, is species-specific. It has been adapted throughout human existence to meet nutritional and antiinfec- tive requirements of the human infant to ensure optimal growth, development, and survival. National and international health organizations consistently recommend that mothers breastfeed for the entire first year of life and thereafter as long as it is beneficial to the mother and infant (American Academy of Pediatrics, 1997; US Department of Health and Human Services, 2000).

Because an infant's birth weight normally requires about 4 to 6 months to double, the nutritional needs of the human baby must be substantially different from those of other mammals whose birth weight doubles much more rapidly. In addition, breastmilk enhances brain development: breastfed children may be more intelligent than children not breastfed. A meta-analysis of 11 studies in which confounding variables were adjusted showed an average 3.2 point higher cognitive development score among breastfed infants. This advantage was seen early on and continued through childhood (Anderson, Johnstone, & Remley, 1999). Chapter 18 presents a detailed discussion of this topic.

This chapter breaks down the general properties of human milk into specific components and describes for each component species-specific "biochemical messages" that contribute to the well-being of the baby and mother. The chapter also explores the concept that these "messages" can be nutritional programming, triggering an early stimulus or insult during a critical or sensitive period with long-term effects on health and disease (Nommsen-Rivers, 2003; Lucas, 1998). Knowledge of biological constructs of lactation is critical to the clinician because it forms the rationale for effective practice in the clinical setting.

Milk Synthesis and Maturational Changes

Major components of human milk (protein, fat, lactose) are synthesized and secreted by the mammary secretory epithelial cells. Cregan (1999) labeled these cells "lactocytes." During pregnancy these cells further develop under the influence of prolactin. Four of the five milk-secretion pathways necessary for milk secretion are synchronized in the alveolar cell of the mammary gland. In the fifth pathway, the passage of components is between epithelial cells, rather than through them, and is known as the paracellular pathway (Neville, 2001).

Factors that influence milk composition include stage of lactation, gestational age of the infant, stage (beginning or end) of the feeding, frequency of the baby's demand for milk, and degree of fullness or emptiness of the breasts. As discussed in Chapter 3, lactogenesis occurs in two stages. Stage I refers to the development, during late pregnancy, of the mammary gland's capacity to synthesize milk. Stage II, traditionally based on postpartum day, refers to the onset of copious milk secretion or the time at which the mother feels her milk "coming in."

Arthur, Smith, and Hartmann (1989) and Humenick (1987) have proposed two different biological markers as objective measures to define stages of breastmilk maturation. Arthur, Smith, and Hartmann hold that in the first stage of lactogenesis, average concentrations of lactose, citrate, and glucose are low. A sudden and rapid increase in concentrations of these components between 24 to 48 hours after birth heralds the transition from stage I to stage II lactogenesis. Stage II lactogenesis markers (lactose, citrate, and total nitrogen) take an additional 24 hours to attain concentration in women who have insulin-dependent diabetes

compared with women who do not (Hartmann & Cregan, 2001).

Humenick et al. (1994), on the other hand, consider the breakdown of an emulsion dependent on the ratio of sterols plus phospholipids to fat content of milk (maturation index of colostrum and milk [MICAM]) as the biological marker for breastmilk maturation (Figure 4–1). Both of these methods appear to be valid in that they were positively related to greater milk yield (Casey, Hambridge, & Neville, 1985; Saint, Smith, & Hartmann, 1984), infant weight gain, and lower transcutaneous bilimeter readings (Humenick, 1987). These studies also show that breastmilk maturation during lactogenesis proceeds more rapidly in some mothers than in others and is not consistent with the coming in of the milk. Neville (2001) believes that the terms *colostrum* and *transitional milk* used to describe breastmilk during the early postpartum do not define clear-cut changes in milk composition and are not a useful distinction. Instead, they should be viewed as part of a continuum of events where changes in breastmilk occur rapidly during the first few days after birth and are followed by slow changes. The time at which mothers report that their milk comes in is highly variable and ranges from 38 to 98 hours after birth, with an average of 50 to 59 hours (Arthur, Smith, & Hartmann, 1989; Kulski & Hartmann, 1981; Hildebrandt, 1999).

Compared with mature milk, colostrum is richer in protein and minerals and lower in carbohydrates, fat, and some vitamins. This high concentration of total protein and total ash (minerals) and whey in colostrum and early milk gradually changes to reflect the infant's needs over the first two to three weeks as lactation becomes established. The total dose of such key components as immunoglobulins, which the infant receives from breastmilk, remains relatively constant throughout lactation, regardless of the amount of breastmilk provided by the mother. This happens because concentrations decrease as total volume increases as lactation is established; and, at weaning, concentration increases as total volume decreases.

Energy, Volume, and Growth

Human milk is rich in nutrient proteins, nonprotein nitrogen compounds, lipids, oligosaccharides, vita-

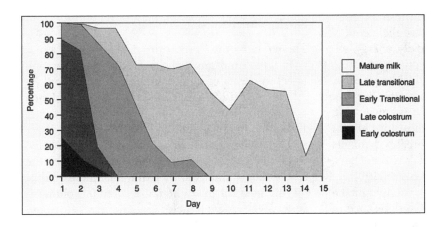

FIGURE 4–1.
Milk type by day. (From Humenick, 1987).

mins, and certain minerals. In addition, it contains hormones, enzymes, growth factors, and many types of protective agents. Human milk contains about 10 percent solids for energy and growth; the rest is water, which is vital for maintaining hydration. The pH of early colostrum is 7.45; it falls to a low of 7.0 during the second week of lactation. Thereafter, the pH of milk remains at 7.0 and then rises gradually to 7.4 by 10 months. The significance of these changes is not known (Morriss et al., 1986). Infants can digest breastmilk much more rapidly than formula. The average gastric half-emptying time for breastmilk is substantially less (48 minutes) than for infant formula (78 minutes) (Cavell, 1981).

Healthy infants, even preterm infants, who consume enough breastmilk to satisfy their energy needs receive enough fluid to satisfy their requirements even in hot and dry environments (Almroth & Bidinger, 1990; Brown et al., 1986b; Cohen et al., 2000). Exclusive and prolonged breastfeeding in healthy infants enhances infant growth during the first three months of life and growth and does not affect the normal growth pattern during the first year (Kramer et al., 2002).

Caloric Density

The caloric content or energy density of human milk is generally considered to be 65 kcal/dl, although published values differ. Garza et al. (1983) reported 57.7/dl.; Lepage et al. (1984) reported 66.6, and Lemons et al. (1982) reported 72.2. Using breastmilk as the "gold standard," the American Academy of Pediatrics (AAP, 1976) recommended a calorie content of 67 kcal/dl for commercial formulas.

Nature abhors waste and breastmilk is efficiently utilized. During their first 4 months, exclusively breastfed infants attain adequate growth with nutrient intakes substantially less than the current dietary recommendation (Butte, Smith, & Garza, 1990). Energy requirements of breastfed infants is about 20 percent below recommended levels (Butte et al., 2000; Stuff & Nichols, 1989). Caloric intake does not increase after solid foods are added to the baby's diet, strongly suggesting that the calorie value of breastmilk feeds is sufficient for the infants' needs. Kilocalories of breastmilk ingested per kilogram by exclusively breastfed babies decrease significantly during the first few months of life (Table 4–1).

Table 4–1

KILOCALORIES OF BREASTMILK INGESTED PER KILOGRAM ACCORDING TO INFANT AGE

Time Post Birth	Kcal per Kg
14 Days	128
3rd Month	70–75
5th Month	62.5

Source: From Garza, Stuff, & Butte (1986); Wood et al. (1988).

The energy intakes of breastfed and formula-fed infants differ significantly because their energy expenditure differs greatly. Total daily energy expenditure, minimal rates of energy expenditure, metabolic rates during sleep, rectal temperature, and heart rates are all lower in breastfed infants. Total body water and fat-free mass is lower, and body fat is higher in breastfed infants at 4 months of age (Butte, 1995). By 8 months, breastfed infants have consumed about 30,000 kcal less than have bottle-fed infants (Butte, Smith, & Garza, 1990).

Although this difference in energy intake should result in about a 2.7–kg mean difference of weight, such is not the case. To explain this discrepancy, Garza, Stuff, and Butte (1986) suggested that (1) differences in intake in the general population are not as great as those found in the babies studied; (2) energy expenditure differs substantially between breastfed and bottle-fed infants; or (3) composition of newly acquired tissue differs between these two groups. A possibility is that the energy density of milk taken by a 4-month-old is higher on the average than that taken by the same baby 3 months earlier. The 4-month-old baby's suckle is more active, leading to a higher fat intake that more than compensates for the volumes needed, because breastmilk is used more completely and with less waste than is artificial milk.

Milk Volume and Storage Capacity

The volume of milk must provide sufficient caloric energy to permit normal growth and development. Small amounts of colostrum—averaging about 37 ml (range, 7–123)—are yielded in the first 24 hours postpartum (Hartmann, 1987; Hartmann & Prosser, 1984); the infant ingests approximately 7 to 14 ml at each feeding (Houston, Howie, & McNeilly, 1983). This milk yield gradually increases for the first 36 hours, followed by a dramatic increase during the next 49 to 96 hours. By day 5, volume is about 500 ml/day; it increases more slowly to about 800 ml/day at month 6 of full breastfeeding, with a range between 550 and 1150 (Daly, Owens, & Hartmann, 1993; Cox et al., 1996; Cregan, Mitoulas, & Hartmann, 2002; Neville et al., 1988). These volumes are similar to others established by test-weighing the infant (using prefeeding and postfeeding infant weighings). As seen in Figure 4–2, the volume of milk taken by thriving breastfed infants varies little from 1 to 4 months. Breastmilk intake slowly declines as other foods are added to the baby's diet.

Even if a mother feels that she had insufficient milk to feed her first baby, health professionals should reassure women that it is well worth trying a second time. Multiparous mothers produce more

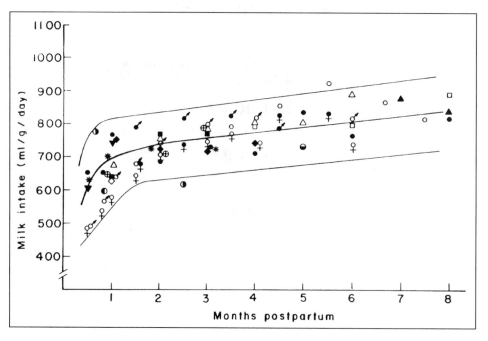

FIGURE 4–2. Milk intakes during established lactation. The lines show the smoothed mean from this study and ± 1 SD. Points are data from the literature obtained by test-weighing of fully breastfed infants. (From Neville MC et al. *Am J Clin Nutr* 48:1375–1386, 1988.)

breastmilk (about 140 ml) at 1 week than primiparous women (those giving birth for the first time) (Ingram, Woolridge, & Greenwood, 2001). Breastmilk of adolescent mothers is not different from breastmilk of adult women although adolescents breastfeed fewer times per day (Motil, Krtz, & Thotathuchery, 1997).

It is well established that breastmilk production and intake are related to infant demand. Infants have the capacity to self-regulate their own milk intake. This important concept of lactation has been extensively studied. Australian researchers measured the short-term rates of milk synthesis using a computerized system in which a camera relays video images to a computer that produces a model of the chest by active triangulation (Cregan, 1999; Daly, Owens, and Hartmann, 1993). Their findings and practical applications (Cregan & Hartmann, 1999; Daly & Hartmann, 1995a, 1995b) are summarized in Box 4–1. Breast storage capacity is important in determining how the infant's demand for milk is met by the mother. Further discussion on how these research-based principles are used in lactation practice is found in later chapters.

BOX 4–1

Application of Physiological Principles

Principle from Physiological Research	Application in Practice
The breast does balance supply to meet the infant's demand for breastmilk.	Watch the baby for hunger cues.
The breast can rapidly change its rate of milk synthesis from one feed to the next.	Encourage the mother when she thinks she has "run out of milk."
The breasts have the capacity to synthesize more milk than the infant usually requires.	As above.
Breast production varies from one breast to the other; breasts operate independently of each other.	Reassure the mother that infant preference for one breast is normal.
The larger the breasts, the greater the milk storage capacity (i.e., the difference between maximum and minimum breast volumes during a 24-hour period).	Women with large breasts have more flexibility in feeding intervals.
There is no relationship between total milk storage capacity and total 24-hour milk production.	Women with smaller breasts can produce as much milk as women with larger breasts but they must breastfeed more often.
The greater the degree of emptying at a breastfeed, the greater the rate of milk synthesis after that feed.	Advise the mother to avoid fast "switching" from one breast to another and to try to empty one breast as much as possible.
The length of time between feeds (up to 6 hours) does not appear to decrease milk synthesis.	Feeding interval can be flexible once lactation is established.

Differences in Milk Volume Between Breasts

Daly et al., (1993) were able to determine the rate of synthesis of human milk. Figure 4–3(A) shows the volume of milk produced by a small-breasted woman who had a storage capacity of 111 ml for her right breast and a capacity of 81 ml for her left breast. Thus the maximum amount of milk that this woman appeared to be able to store was about 20 percent of her infant's 24-hour milk intake. From her breast volume changes over time, it appears that her infant met its demand for milk by breastfeeding frequently. Conversely, Figure 4–3(B) displays a larger-breasted woman who produced similar volumes of milk but with larger storage capacities for her breasts (right breast, 600 ml; left breast, 180 ml), allowing her to store nearly 90 percent of her infant's 24-hour milk intake. Further, there was no relationship between total milk storage capacity and 24-hour milk production. Thus we can conclude that small breast size does not restrict a woman's ability to provide milk for her infant. On the other hand, mothers with a greater storage capacity do have more flexibility with patterns of breastfeeding.

There appear to be wide differences among women in the rate of milk synthesis, which among some women can be double or triple the rate of other women (Arthur et al., 1989; Daly et al., 1992). Milk volume between breasts also differs. Milk yield from right breasts appear to be higher than that from left breasts, clearly demonstrating that the rate of milk synthesis within one breast is independent of the rate of milk synthesis in the other breast (Cox, Owens, & Hartmann, 1996; Daly et al., 1993).

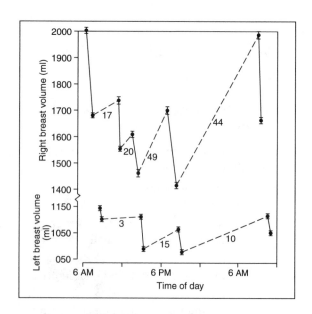

FIGURE 4–3(B). Breast-volume changes. The right and left breast volume changes of one subject over a period of 28 hours. Each point represents the mean plus or minus the standard error of the mean of replicate breast-volume measurement. Lines link prefeeding and postfeeding mean breast volumes. Dashed lines link postfeeding mean breast volume of a breastfeeding to the prefeeding mean breast volume of the next breast; their slope thus indicates rate of milk synthesis between the two breastfeedings. Rate of milk synthesis also is given by the number (in milliliters per hour) accompanying each dashed line. (From Daly SE, Owens RA, Hartman PE. The short-term synthesis and infant-regulated removal of milk in lactating women. *Exp Physiology* 78:209–220, 1993.)

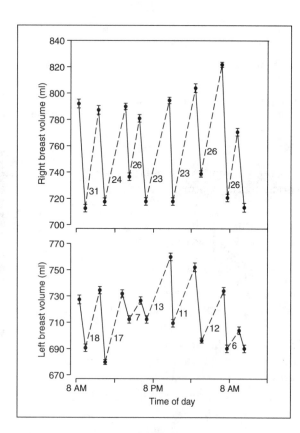

FIGURE 4–3(A). The right and left breast volume changes of one subject over a period of 24 hours.

At the same time, the amount of milk available in the breast is not necessarily an important determinant of the amount removed by the infant at feedings. Infant intake of breastmilk also varies widely. For example, at 5 months, infant intake of breastmilk can range from 200 ml/day for partial breastfeeding to 3500 ml/day if a wet nurse is used (Neville & Oliva-Rasbach, 1987). These differences appear to be culturally based. Australian women, for example, have been reported to make more breastmilk than do US women. The average daily yield of well-nourished Australian mothers during the first 6 months of lactation was found to be in excess of 1100 ml in one study (Hartmann, 1987) and to range from 535 to 1078 ml in another (Daly et al., 1993). Mothers breastfeeding twins produce in excess of 2100 ml/day in the early months. Breast volume and production decrease in extended lactation. After 6 months of lactation, breast volume, milk production, and storage capacity all decline.

Seasonal changes in breastmilk volume may be influenced by some mothers' need to work during harvest and by their reluctance to introduce supplementary food for fear of diarrheal disease (Serdula, Seward, & Marks, 1986). The nutritional status of the mother does not appear to affect milk volume unless the mother is severely malnourished (Brown et al., 1986a; Forman et al., 1990).

A healthy, breastfeeding, full-term neonate breastfeeds an average of 4.3 times during the first 24 hours (range 0–11) and 7.4 times during the next 24 hours (range 1–22) (Yamauchi & Yamanouchi, 1990), and an overall median of 8 times per day after the first several days (see Hornell's study, p. 89). Breastmilk intake shows little or no correlation with maternal factors, such as weight-for-height, weight gain, nursing frequency, maternal age, and parity (Dewey & Lönnerdal, 1983). Although birth weight is not a strong predictor of milk intake throughout lactation, infant weight at 1 month is. Thus lactation performance during the first 4 weeks postpartum is a strong predictor of milk output during the subsequent period of full lactation (Neville & Oliva-Rasbach, 1987).

Infant Growth

Normal human growth is greatest during infancy. The infant gains about 10 g/kg/day (about 5 to 7 oz/week) until about 4 weeks; then the gain drops to 1 g/kg/day (about 3 oz/week) by the end of the first year.

There are growth differences between breastfed and formula-fed infants. Infants breastfed exclusively have the same or somewhat greater weight gain in the first 3 to 4 months than do bottle-fed or mixed-fed infants (Fawzi et al., 1997; Juex et al., 1983; Motil et al., 1997). After this time, bottle-fed or mixed-fed infants clearly weigh more. The greatest differences are evident between 6 and 20 months of age, when breastfed infants are lighter than bottle-fed or mixed-fed infants (Dewey et al., 1993; Dewey et. al., 1995; Yoneyama, Nagata, & Asano, 1994). Increases in length and head circumference growth remain the same for both groups. Length is a reliable indicator for evaluating infant growth and the absence of significant difference in length between breastfed and nonbreastfed infants suggest that formula-fed infants are overfed. Small for gestational age infants who are breastfed show faster postnatal growth and are more likely to have significant catch-up growth than those who are fed a standard term infant formula (Lucas et al., 1997).

Nutritional Values

Around the world, breastmilk is remarkably stable, varying only within a relatively narrow range. Constituents of colostrum and breastmilk and their amounts are shown in Appendix 4-A of this chapter. A profile of lactose protein and lipid concentrations in human milk for the first 30 days of lactation is seen in Figure 4–4. Yet, because breastfeeding is an interactive process, the infant helps to determine composition of the feed. During weaning (involution phase), for example, the concentrations of sodium and protein in breastmilk progressively increase and the milk is saltier; in contrast, concentrations of potassium, glucose, and lactose gradually decrease (Prosser, Saint, & Hartmann, 1984).

Fat

The fat of human milk, which provides about one half of the milk's calories, is its most variable component. The total fat content of human milk ranges from 30 to 50 g/L. The energy density of preterm mother's milk is much greater than that of full-term mother's milk, owing to a 30 percent higher fat concentration (Atkinson, Anderson, & Bryan, 1980). Triglycerides, the main constituent (98–99 percent)

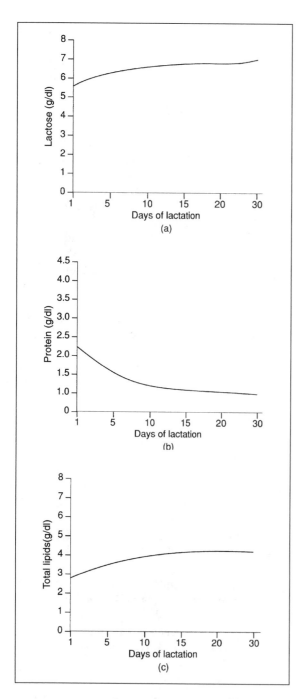

FIGURE 4–4. Lactose protein and total lipid concentration in human milk.

of milk fat, are readily broken down to free fatty acids and glycerol by the enzyme lipase, which is found not only in an infant's intestine but in the breastmilk itself.

The lipid fraction of human milk provides essential fatty acids. The main concern about fatty acid intake is its effect on brain growth. The rate of brain growth is greatest in the last trimester of pregnancy and continues throughout the first year of life. Tissues of breastfed and formula-fed infants have distinctly different plasma fatty acid compositions. Breastmilk contains a wide range of long-chain polyunsaturated fatty acids (LC-PUFAs), which represent 88 percent of milk fat and are the most variable element in milk (Jensen, 1999). Interestingly, levels of fatty acids are low in lactating women, which indicates that transfer to breastmilk is at the expense of the maternal stores (Koletzko & Rodriquez-Palmero, 1999).

LC-PUFAs include docosahexanoic acid (DHA) and arachidonic acid (AA), which are associated with higher visual acuity and cognitive ability of the child. An analysis of studies of human-milk feedings, DHA-supplemented, and unsupplemented formula documented advantages of DHA on visual acuity (SanGiovanni et al., 2000).

An essential fatty acid that enhances the developing human visual system, DHA is found in extremely high levels in the photoreceptors and the visual cortex and may ameliorate neurovisual developmental disorders such as the retinopathy of prematurity (Hylander et al., 2001). Breastfed infants accumulate DHA in the cortex, whereas formula-fed infants merely maintain the same amount of DHA present at birth. As a result, breastfed infants have higher levels of DHA than an age-matched group of formula-fed infants (Baur et al., 2000).

Until recently, commercial infant formula was fortified only with precursor essential fatty acids, α-linolenic acid, and linoleic acid. In an attempt to narrow the "nutrient gap" between formula and breastmilk, two formula companies (Mead Johnson and Ross) added DHA and AA to their infant formula after the FDA approved it as an additive in 2001. Critics charge that there is insufficient evidence that these additives are safe. DHA is extracted from fermented microalgae and AA from soil fungus. Human fatty acids are structurally different from those manufactured from plant source and interact with each other in a special matrix that cannot be duplicated.

Breastfed infants have a higher proportion of acetic acid in the short-chain fatty acid spectra than do formula-fed infants, which, along with the monoglycerides generated by milk lipases, act against envelope viruses, bacteria, and fungus (Garza et al., 1987; Siigur, Ormission, & Tamm, 1993). The paler color, softer consistency, and milder odor of breastmilk stools, as compared with formula stools, are due in part to a higher concentration of fatty acid soaps (Quinlan et al., 1995). Fatty acid composition also differs between mothers whose babies develop atopic manifestation during the first year of life and those who remain healthy. Specifically, lower levels of α-linolenic acid and *n*-3 long chain polyunsaturated fatty acid in mature milk of atopic mothers, especially in those with atopic babies, suggest that the low levels of this fatty acid could be associated with the development of atopy in the infants (Duchen, Yu, & Björkstén, 1999).

Although maternal dietary fat intake does not affect the total amount of fat in a mother's milk, the types of fat in the diet do influence the composition of fatty acids in milk. For example, black mothers in South Africa consuming a traditional maize diet have higher levels of monounsaturated fatty acid in their milk than do their urban counterparts who eat more animal fats (van der Westhuyzen, Chetty, & Atkinson, 1988). If the mother eats a high-carbohydrate, energy-replete diet, the proportion of triglycerides of medium-chain fatty acid increases (Garza et al., 1987).

The effects of breastfeeding can depend on the formerly breastfed individual's age. A prime example is cholesterol. Because cholesterol levels (10–20 mg/dl) in human milk are considerably higher than those of formulas derived from bovine milk (Wagner & Stockhausen, 1988), one would expect cholesterol levels in adulthood to be higher in breastfed individuals. The reverse, however, is true. Exposure to cholesterol in breastmilk may have long-term benefits for cardiovascular health. Coronary artery disease in persons up to 20 years of age is less frequent in individuals who were breastfed (Bergstrom et al., 1995). Serum total cholesterol and LDL levels (1) tend to be higher among breastfed infants compared to nonbreastfed infants, (2) tend not to be different by infant-feeding group during childhood, and (3) tend to be lower among adults who were breastfed rather than artificially fed as infants (Owen et al., 2002). In addition to higher cholesterol concentration, adults who were bottle-fed had higher plasma glucose concentra-

tions and impaired glucose tolerance (Ravelli et al., 2000).

Fat content of milk changes throughout a breastfeeding and, generally speaking, increases more steeply as more milk is taken. Fat content varies according to the degree to which the breast is emptied at that breastfeeding, and that fat content increases markedly after most of the milk in the breast has been taken (Daly et al., 1993). The longer the time interval between two breastfeedings, the less likely the infant is to empty the breast and, thus, the lower the fat concentration will be in the subsequent feeding. Although the work of Daly et al. (1993) indicated that the pattern of feedings dictates the infant's fat intake, this is not necessarily the case. Woolridge, Ingram, and Baum (1990) studied mothers who fed in two patterns—either feeding at one breast or at two breasts during a feeding. The infants thus fed were able to regulate their fat intake and to achieve stable fat intakes in spite of disparate patterns of feedings. His findings support flexible "baby-led" feedings.

Lactose

Lactose, a disaccharide, accounts for most of the carbohydrates in human milk, although small quantities of oligosaccharides, galactose, and fructose are also present. Although lactose concentration is relatively constant (7.0 gm/dl) in mature milk, it is affected by maternal diet.

Lactose enhances calcium absorption and metabolizes readily to galactose and glucose, which supply energy to the rapidly growing brain of the infant. Some oligosaccharides promote the growth of *Lactobacillus bifidus*, thus increasing intestinal acidity and stemming the growth of pathogens (Dai et al., 2000).

The enzyme lactase is necessary to convert lactose into simple sugars that can be easily assimilated by the infant. The enzyme is present in the infant's intestinal mucosa from birth. Congenital or primary lactase deficiency is exceedingly rare (Montgomery et al., 1991). Lactose intolerance, however, is common in many mammals as they grow older and is the result of diminishing activity of intestinal lactase after weaning. In humans, lactose intolerance is more prevalent in adults of Asian and African heritage.

Protein

Protein content of mature human milk from well-nourished mothers is about 0.8 to 0.9 gm of protein per deciliter. Some of the protein in human milk is probably not nutritionally available to the infant; it serves immunological purposes instead. The high quality of protein in human milk and its precisely balanced quantity meet the energy needs of infants (Gaull, 1985; Raiha, 1985).

Human milk contains casein and whey protein. Casein and whey levels change as lactation progresses to meet the nutritional needs of the infant. Casein is lower in early lactation, then increases rapidly. Whey proteins are at their highest in early lactation and continue to fall. These changes result in a whey/casein ratio of about 90:10 in early lactation, 60:40 in mature milk, and 50:50 in late lactation (Kunz & Lönnerdal, 1992). Whey proteins are acidified in the stomach, forming soft, flocculent curds. These quickly digest, supplying a continuous flow of nutrients to the baby. By contrast, caseins (the primary protein in untreated bovine milk) form a tough, less digestible curd that requires high expenditure of energy for an incomplete digestive process.

Whey protein is composed of five major components: (1) alpha-lactalbumin, (2) serum albumin, (3) lactoferrin, (4) immunoglobulins, and (5) lysozyme. The latter three elements play important roles in immunological defense. Lactoferrin concentration of milk is higher in iron-deficient women as compared with well-nourished mothers; therefore milk lactoferrin may also help protect the infant against iron deficiency (Raiha, 1985). A large number of other proteins (enzymes, growth modulators, and hormones) are present in low concentrations.

Nonprotein Nitrogen. Milk proteins are synthesized from amino acids derived from the bloodstream. Nonprotein nitrogen contains a number of free amino acids, including glutamic acid, glycine, alanine, valine, leucine, aspartic acid, serine, threonine, proline, and taurine. When amino acids exist singly or in free form, they are known as *free amino acids*. Of these, leucine, valine, and threonine are essential amino acids; they must be consumed in the diet because the body does not manufacture them.

The percentage of protein in human colostrum is greater than that in mature breastmilk. This high level is due to the fact that in colostrum lactose and water haven't yet flooded the system and also because of the presence of additional amino acids and antibody-rich proteins, especially secretory IgA and lactoferrin. All ten essential amino acids are present in colostrum and account for approximately 45 percent of its total nitrogen content.

Nucleotides. Nucleotides are low-molecular-weight compounds with a nitrogenous base. Necessary for energy metabolism, enzymatic reactions, and growth and maturation of the developing gastrointestinal tract, they also play several roles in immune function, including enhanced lymphocytic proliferation, stimulation of immunoglobulin production in lymphocytes, and increased natural killer-cell activity. Infant formula manufacturers seek to emulate the many nucleotides of breastmilk in their formulas (Cosgrove, 1998; Leach et al., 1995).

The importance to the baby of available nitrogen cannot be overstated. Atkinson, Anderson, and Bryan (1980) have shown that the concentration of nitrogen in the milk of women who deliver preterm infants is 20 percent greater than that in the milk of women delivering at term. The higher levels of available protein and fat in preterm mother's milk underscore the importance of using the milk of the preterm infant's mother rather than pooled milk from women in other stages of lactation (Table 4–2). Donated milk (not preterm milk), however, can be modified with components from other human milk to make a preterm human milk formula with none of the dangers of commercial bovine-based preterm formulas.

Vitamins and Micronutrients

The amounts of vitamins and micronutrients in human milk vary from one mother to another because of diet and genetic differences. However, it is generally true that human milk will satisfy the micronutrient requirements of a full-term healthy infant and thus can be taken as the primary yardstick of dietary recommendations, or reference values. Generally, as lactation progresses, the level of water-soluble vitamins in breastmilk increases, and

Table 4–2

COMPOSITION OF TERM AND PRETERM MILK DURING THE FIRST MONTH OF LACTATION

Nutrients	3–5 Days		8–11 Days		15–18 Days		26–29 Days	
	Full Term	**Preterm**	**Full Term**	**Preterm**	**Full Term**	**Preterm**	**Full Term**	**Preterm**
Energy (kcal/dl)	48	58	59	71	62	71	62	70
Lipid (gm/dl)	1.85	3.00	2.9	4.14	3.06	4.33	3.05	4.09
Protein (gm/dl)	1.87	2.10	1.7	1.86	1.52	1.71	1.29	1.41
Lactose (gm/dl)	5.14	5.04	5.98	5.55	6.00	5.63	6.51	5.97

Source: From Anderson (1985).

the level of fat-soluble vitamins declines. The levels of fat-soluble vitamins (A, D, K, E) in human milk are minimally influenced by recent maternal diet, as these vitamins can be drawn from storage in the body.

Vitamin A. Human milk is a good source of vitamin A (200 IU/dl), which is present mainly as retinol (40–53 ng/dl). Required for vision and maintenance of epithelial structures, vitamin A is at highest levels in the first week after birth and then gradually declines. Deficiency of vitamin A is a serious health problem for young children in many developing countries, leading to blindness through damage to the corneal epithelium (xerophthalmia) and to increased morbidity from infectious diseases. The prolongation of even partial breastfeeding provides an important source of vitamin A to children in developing countries (Bates & Prentice, 1994).

Vitamin D. Human milk has very little fat-soluble vitamin D and breastfed infants can develop rickets, although it is uncommon. The risk of rickets is greatest for dark-skinned children living in inner-city areas, children whose clothing deters skin exposure to the sun, and children of mothers eating vegetarian diets that exclude meat, fish, and dairy products. The child who is adequately exposed to the sun (and thus to radiation-formed precursors of vitamin D) and whose mother consumes adequate nutrients usually does not need routine vitamin D supplements (Greer & Marshall, 1989). Concentrations in human milk range between 5 IU and 20 IU per liter. Increased vitamin D intake results in increased levels in human milk (Specker et al., 1985). Vitamin D may constitute an exception to the general rule that breastmilk micronutrient levels are protected from the effect of maternal deficiency. Scattered reports of rickets led the American Academy of Pediatrics in 2003 to recommend vitamin D supplements not only for children subject to certain conditions but to all infants (Gartner & Greer, 2003).

Vitamin E. Human colostrum is particularly rich in vitamin E (tocopherol). Milk of mothers with preterm and term infants have similar levels of vitamin E (3 IU/100 kcal) and carotenoid levels, which are higher than those in bovine milk (Ostrea, 1986) or formula (Sommerburg et al., 2000). A deficiency of vitamin E in infancy can result in hemolytic anemia, especially in the premature infant. Because it is an antioxidant, vitamin E protects cell membranes in the retina and lungs against oxidant-induced injury. The requirement for vitamin E increases with intake of polyunsaturated fatty acids in breastmilk. Mothers who eat foods high in polyunsaturated fats and "fast foods" add to oxidant stress (Guthrie, Picciano, & Sheehe, 1977).

Vitamin K. Vitamin K, which is required for the synthesis of blood-clotting factors, is present in human milk in small amounts. A few days after birth, a baby normally produces vitamin K in sufficient quantities by enteric bacteria. However, neonates are susceptible to vitamin K deficiency until ingestion of copious amounts of breastmilk can promote gastrointestinal bacterial colonization, which enhances their low levels of vitamin K. Vitamin K supplements taken by the mother will increase breastmilk levels and infant plasma levels of the vitamin (Greer, 1999).

Insufficient vitamin K in neonates can lead to vitamin K–responsive hemorrhagic disease. To prevent hemorrhage and to raise prothrombin levels, 1 mg vitamin K is routinely given intramuscularly postpartum. Alternatively, a 1 mg oral dose of vitamin K administered at birth, at 1 to 2 weeks, and at 4 to 6 weeks is absorbed in the intestinal tract in amounts sufficient to prevent bleeding, and the infant is spared the pain of an injection and the risk of nerve damage always possible with any intramuscular injection. Formula-fed infants need not receive vitamin K routinely because formula (other than soy) contains vitamin K (Medves, 2002).

Water-soluble vitamins—ascorbic acid, nicotinic acid, B_{12} (thiamine), riboflavin, and B_6 (pyridoxine)—are readily influenced by the maternal diet. If maternal supplements are present, the vitamin levels in the milk increase and then plateau. Although supplementation may be beneficial for undernourished women, it is not necessary if the mother is well nourished and eating a diet that contains foods close to their natural state.

Vitamin B_{12}. Vitamin B_{12} is needed for early development of the baby's central nervous system. A mother eating a vegan diet (i.e., without meat or dairy products) may produce milk deficient in B_{12}. A deficiency of B vitamin folate during pregnancy is associated with neural tube defects. The March of Dimes' campaign to educate women on the importance of taking B_{12} folate supplements during preconception and pregnancy has reduced neural tube deformities.

Unlike other micronutrients, folate (which is bound to a folate-binding protein) remains at the same level throughout all stages of lactation. Folate supplementation of a breastfeeding mother with megaloblastic anemia results in an increase in milk folate levels even though her plasma values remain the same. Maternal stores of folate diminish slightly from 3 to 6 months to maintain milk folate levels (Mackey & Picciano, 1999).

Vitamin B_6. High pharmacological doses of vitamin B_6 have been reported to suppress prolactin and thus lactation. However, low nutritionally relevant doses have no effect on plasma prolactin or on breastmilk volume. Doses as high as 4.0 mg of vitamin B_6 taken as part of a vitamin B complex supplement are considered safe for both the lactating mother and the infant (Andon et al., 1985).

Minerals

The total mineral content in human milk is fairly constant. Excepting magnesium, minerals tend to have their highest concentration in human milk in the first few days after birth and decrease slightly in a consistent pattern throughout lactation, with little diurnal or within-feeding variation. Maternal age, parity, and diet, even when supplemented, usually have minimal influence on mineral concentrations in milk, probably because of their regulation from maternal body stores (Butte et al., 1987; Casey, Neville, & Hambridge, 1989).

Sodium. Breastmilk sodium is elevated in early colostrum but falls dramatically by the third day postpartum and declines at a slower rate for 6 months. Elevated human milk sodium levels occur during weaning, in women with mastitis, and during the first months of gestation. A high concentration of sodium has also been found in the milk of mothers whose infants develop malnutrition, dehydration, and hypernatremia. Persistent high levels may be a marker for impaired lactation (Morton, 1994).

Zinc. Zinc is actively transported into the mammary gland. Zinc levels rise to a peak on the second day postpartum and then decline for the duration of lactation (Casey, Neville, & Hambidge, 1989). Zinc is eight times as abundant in human colostrum as in mature milk. Zinc requirements are based on growth velocity; therefore, requirements are relatively high in the very young infant and decrease with increasing age of the infant (Krachler, Rossipal, & Irgolic, 1998; Krebs & Hambidge, 1986). For fully breastfed infants, a combination of high absorption and efficient conservation of intestinal endogenous zinc retain enough zinc to meet the demands of infant growth in the face of modest intake (Abrams, Wen, & Stuff, 1996; Krebs et al., 1996).

Zinc dramatically improves acrodermatitis enteropathica, a rare but serious congenital metabolic disorder that manifests itself in part in severe dermatitis (Evans & Johnson, 1980). While infants with this disorder continue to receive human milk, they have no symptoms. The high bioavailability of zinc in human milk is brought about by a low-molecular-weight zinc-binding ligand that facilitates zinc absorption. Abnormally low zinc levels in breastmilk are rare but apparently can sometimes occur in mothers of infants with low birth weight. A slowing growth rate and persistent perioral or perianal rash (with or without diarrhea) in infants fed solely breastmilk may be due to zinc depletion (Atkinson et al., 1989). These infants should continue to breastfeed but they may require zinc supplementation. Maternal diet does not affect breastmilk zinc levels. In the rare case where a woman has low concentrations of breastmilk zinc, she is likely to have delivered her infant prematurely (Lönnerdal, 2000).

Iron. Although human milk has only a small amount of iron (0.5–1.0 mg/L), breastfed babies rarely are iron deficient. They maintain their iron status at the same level as that of formula-fed infants receiving iron supplements for up to 9 months (Duncan et al., 1985; Salmenpera et al., 1986; Siimes et al., 1984). Breastfed infants are sustained by sufficient iron stores laid down in utero and by the high lactose and vitamin C levels in human milk, which facilitate iron absorption. Iron in human milk is absorbed five times as well as is a similar amount from cow's milk.

For the first few months of life, healthy, full-term infants draw on extensive iron reserves generally present at birth. Normally, an infant's hemoglobin level is high (16–22 gm/dl) at birth and decreases rapidly as physiological adjustment is made to extrauterine life. At 4 months of age, normal hemoglobin ranges between 10.2 and 15 gm/dl. Iron is well absorbed by older infants and is not affected by mineral intake from solid foods in the diet or by vegetarianism (Abrams, Wen, & Stuff, 1996; Dorea, 2000; Lönnerdal, 2000). Breastmilk iron is not affected by the mother's iron intake.

Iron supplementation is not usually needed and may in fact be detrimental to the breastfeeding baby during the first half-year after birth. Excess iron tends to saturate lactoferrin and thereby diminish its antiinfective properties. The authors of a randomized double-blind controlled trial concluded that routine iron supplementation of Swedish and Honduran breastfed infants with normal hemoglobin presented a greater risk of diarrhea (Dewey et al., 2002).

Calcium. Like iron, calcium appears in only small quantities in human milk (20–34 mg/dl). Yet babies absorb 67 percent of the calcium in human milk as compared to only 25 percent of that in cow's milk. Neonatal hypocalcemia and tetany are more commonly seen in the formula-fed infant, because cow's milk has a much higher concentration of phosphorus (calcium-phosphorus ratio of 1.2:1.0 versus 2:1 in human milk), which leads to decreased absorption and increased excretion of calcium. Calcium and phosphorus supplements are sometimes given to breastfed infants with low birth weight who should be monitored for hypercalcemia (calcium > 11 mg/dl) (Steichen, Krug-Wispe, & Tsang, 1987).

Magnesium. Magnesium is present in low levels in breastmilk and decreases in mature milk during 3 to 6 months (Picciano, 2001). Women who have been treated with magnesium sulfate for preeclampsia have high milk magnesium concentrations for the first day postpartum. After that time, levels return to normal (Lönnerdal, 2000).

Other Minerals. Copper levels are highest on the first few days postpartum, decrease for about 5 to 6 months, and then tend to remain stable. The mother's serum levels have no influence on milk concentration (Dorea, 2000). Selenium is usually higher in human milk than in formula (Kumpulain et al., 1987; Smith, Piccano, & Milner, 1982).

Minute amounts of aluminum, iodine, chromium, and fluorine are also found in breastmilk. Formula-fed infants ingest as much as 80 times more manganese than breastfed infants. Manganese enters the neonatal brain at a much higher rate than in the adult brain. Nenoates are therefore at risk of neurotoxicity from excess manganese. High manganese levels in infant formula have been identified as being possibly related to neurocognitive deficits (Tran et al., 2002). Very little is known about the mechanisms or control of the secretion of trace elements into human milk. Table 4–3 lists the major components of human milk and their functions.

Preterm Milk

The milk of a woman who delivers a preterm infant is different from that of a woman who delivers at term, probably to meet the special needs of the low birth weight neonate. Compared with term breastmilk, preterm breastmilk has higher levels of energy, lipids, protein, nitrogen, fatty acids, some vitamins, and minerals (see Table 4–2). In addition, preterm breastmilk has higher levels of immune factors, including cells, immunoglobulins, and anti-inflammatory elements than term breastmilk. In the United States, the extra health-care costs of not

---

Table 4–3

MAJOR COMPONENTS OF HUMAN MILK AND THEIR FUNCTION

Cells	Function
Phagocytes (macrophages)	Engulf and absorb pathogens; release IgA; polymorphonuclear and mononuclear.
Lymphocytes	T cells and B cells; essential for cell-mediated immunity; antiviral activity; memory T cells give long-term protection.
Anti-inflammatory Factors	
Prostaglandins PGE1, PGE2	Cytoprotective
Cytokines/chemokines	Immunodulating agents that bind to specific cellular receptors, activate the immune system, promote mammary growth, and move lymphocytes into breastmilk and across neonatal bowel wall. TGF-β is the dominating cytokine in colostrum.
Growth factors	Promote gut maturation, epithelial cell growth. EGF is a type of cytokine.
Enzymes	
Amylase	Facilitates infant digestion of polysaccharides.
Lipase	Hydrolizes fat in infant intestine; bactericidal activity.
Growth Factors/Hormones	
Human growth factors	Polypeptides that stimulate proliferation of intestinal mucosa and epithelium; strengthens mucosal barrier to antigens.
Cortisol, insulin, thyroxine cholecystokinin (CCK)	Promotes maturation of the neonates intestine and intestinal host-defense process. Thyroxin protects against hypothyroidism; CCK enhances digestion.
Prolactin	Enhances development of B and T lymphocytes.
Lipids (Fat)	Major source of calories.
Long-chain polyunsaturated fatty acids (LC-PUFA)	DHA and AA associated with higher visual acuity and cognitive ability; breastmilk content dependent on maternal diet.
Free fatty acids (FFA)	Anti-infective effects.
Triglycerides	Largest source of calories for infant; broken down to free fatty acids and glycerol by lipase; types of fat depend on maternal diet

Table 4–3 (cont.)

Lactose	Carbohydrate, major energy source; breaks down into galactose and glucose; enhances absorption of Ca, Mg, and Mn.
Oligosaccharides	Microbial and viral ligands.
Glycoconjugates	Microbial and viral ligands.
Minerals	Regulates normal body functions; minimal influence by maternal diet.
Protein	
Whey	Contains lactoferrin, lysozyme, and immunoglobulins, alpha-lactalbumin
Immunoglobulins (SIgA, IgM, IgG)	Immunity response to specific antigens in environment. SIgA pathways to mammary gland called GALT and BALT.
Lactoferrin	Antibacterial especially against *E. coli*; iron carrier.
Lysozyme	Bacteriocidal and anti-inflammatory; activity progressively increases starting 6 months after delivery.
Taurine	Abundant amino acid; associated with early brain maturation and retinal development.
Casein	Inhibits microbial adhesion to mucosal membranes.
Vitamins A, C, E	Anti-inflammatory action; scavenges oxygen radicals.
Water	Constitutes 87.5% of human milk volume; provides adequate hydration to infant.

using human milk for preterm infants is estimated to be $9889 per baby (Wight, 2001). Chapter 13 also discusses preterm breastmilk.

Anti-infective Properties

Breastmilk offers the newborn protection against disease. This benefit has been recognized for hundreds of years; however, only in the last few decades have investigators begun to identify the specific anti-infective components of human milk that make it a peerless substance for feeding the human infant. Breastmilk has been viewed from ancient times as living tissue and rightly so. This "white blood" contains enzymes, immunoglobulins, and leukocytes in abundance. These components, one frequently enhancing the efficacy of another, account for most of the unique anti-infective properties of human milk. In some cultures, fresh breastmilk is used as eyedrops to treat conjunctivitis; elsewhere, it is common practice to apply breastmilk on the skin to heal cracked nipples. Breastmilk provides several tiers of defense

against diseases of infants that include a top tier of secretory antibodies against specific pathogens, next a tier of fatty acids and lactoferrin that provide broad-spectrum protection, followed by glyco-conjugates and oligosaccharides, each protecting against one or more specific pathogens (Newberg et al., 1998).

Studies that measured the protectiveness of human milk reaffirm its significance in preventing infections (Dewey, Heinig, & Nommsen-Rivers, 1995; Frank et al., 1982; Gulick, 1986; Kovar et al., 1984; Kramer et al., 2001; Pullan et al., 1980; Rosenberg, 1989; Victora et al., 1987). The evidence is strongest for bacterial infections, gastroenteritis, and necrotizing enterocolitis but is less convincing for respiratory infections (Kramer et al., 2001).

Gastroenteritis and Diarrheal Disease

Wherever infant morbidity and mortality are high, breastfeeding conclusively helps to prevent infantile diarrhea and gastrointestinal infections (Almroth & Latham, 1982; Brown et al., 1989; Clavano, 1982; Duffy, 1986; Espinoza, 1997; Granthan-

McGregor & Back, 1972; Habicht, DaVanso, & Butz, 1988; Jason, Niebury, & Marks, 1984; Koopman et al., 1985; Kovar et al., 1984; Mitra & Rabbani, 1995; Perera et al., 1999; Ravelomanana et al., 1995; Ruuska, 1992). Breastfeeding minimizes diarrhea both by providing protective factors and by reducing exposure to other foods or water that may contain enteropathogens (Van Derslice, Popkin, & Briscoe, 1994). As antibiotic resistance becomes a global problem, discoveries about the protective effect of breastfeeding become even more important (Hakansson et al., 2000).

Protection is dose-dependent. In a review of field studies conducted to identify the effect of breastfeeding on childhood diarrhea in Bangladesh, children partially breastfed had a greater risk of diarrhea than had those who were exclusively breastfed (Glass & Stoll, 1989). Although breastmilk's protective effect is most easily demonstrated in areas of poverty and malnutrition, evidence of this protection is worldwide. In China, Chen, Yu, and Li (1988) showed that compared with breastfed infants, artificially-fed infants are more likely to be admitted to the hospital for gastroenteritis and other conditions. In the Cebu region of the Philippines, giving water, teas, and other liquids to breastfed babies doubled or tripled the likelihood of diarrhea (Popkin et al., 1990). Young Nicaraguan children who develop rotavirus infections very early are partially protected by specific IgA antibodies in their mothers' milk. Rotavirus in stool samples correlated significantly with the concentration of anti-rotavirus IgA antibodies in colostrum (Espinoza et al., 1997). Canadian infants exclusively breastfed for the first 2 months had significantly fewer episodes of diarrhea than did infants bottlefed from birth (Chandra, 1979). Breastfed children in Burma required less oral rehydration solution than did those who were not breastfed during the early acute phase of diarrhea and recovered from diarrhea more quickly (Khin-Maung et al., 1985).

A major methodological problem in breastfeeding research on disease is the dose response effect—i.e., the greater the amount of breastmik the infant receives, the greater the protection against disease; protection improves with the duration of breastfeeding. A lack of a clear consistent definition of breastfeeding is a flaw in many breastfeeding studies given the fact that there is a wide variation in feeding practices and that mothers often erroneously report supplements given to the infant (Aarts, Kylberg, Hornell et al., 2000; Zaman et al., 2002). Moreover, it is neither feasible nor ethical to randomly assign mother/infant dyads to breastfeeding or formula feeding groups.

Kramer et al. (2001) got around this problem by looking at infant outcomes of hospitals and clinics in Belarus that introduced Breastfeeding Friendly Hospital Initiatives and compared them with hospitals and clinics that continued their traditional practices. Results indicated that infants at the intervention site were more likely to breastfeed to any degree at 12 months and were more likely to be exclusively breastfeeding at 3 and 6 months. The risk of gastrointestinal infections and atopic eczema were significantly lower in the intervention group but there was not significant reduction in respiratory tract infection.

Epidemiological evidence indicates that human milk continues to confer protection even with supplementation. Partial breastfeeding is better than no breastfeeding at all. This protection is specific to pathogens in the mother's and infant's environment. Moreover, the infant receives protection against the pathogens it is most likely to encounter. Table 4–4 summarizes the ameliorating and protective effects of human milk. We assume that breastfeeding is the norm and that artificial feeding is a deviation from the norm that brings about hazards to infant health. Two infant health problems exacerbated by lack of breastfeeding—respiratory illness and otitis media—are discussed here. Others are discussed throughout this book, especially in Chapters 18 and 19.

Respiratory Illness

Studies of the protective effects of breastfeeding against respiratory tract infections are conflicting and complex because of error in parents' reports and other conditions not related to feeding. Several studies suggest that breastfeeding helps to prevent respiratory illnesses (Abdulmoneim & Al-Gamdi, 2001; Cushing et al., 1998; Lopez-Alarcon, Villalpando, & Fajardo, 1997) and others indicate little protection (Dewey, Heinig, & Nommsen-Rivers, 1995; Kramer et al., 2001). There is, however, strong evidence that breastmilk protects against res-

Table 4–4

AMELIORATION BY HUMAN MILK OF DISEASE IN INFANTS AND CHILDREN

Disease in Child	Ameliorating Properties of Human Milk
Acrodermatitis enteropathica	More efficient zinc absorption (Evans & Johnson, 1980).
Appendicitis	Anti-inflammatory properties (Pisacane et al., 1995b).
Asthma	Introduction of milk other than human milk prior to 4 months is a risk factor for asthma at age 6 years (Dell & To, 2001; Oddy, 2000). Breastfeeding provides protection against asthma in children with family history of atopy (Gdalevich et al., 2001), especially if the child is exposed to tobacco smoke (Chulada et al., 2003).
Bacterial infections, neonatal sepsis	Leukocytes, lactoferrin, immune properties (Ashraf et al., 1991; Fallot et al., 1980; Leventhal et al., 1986).
Celiac disease	Longer duration and greater exclusivity of breastfeeding associated with later diagnosis; protects against development of villous atrophy in intestinal mucosa; later introduction of gluten in breastfeeders (Ascher et al., 1997; Auricchio, 1983; Bouguerra et al., 1998; Greco et al., 1988; Ivarsson et al., 2000; Kelly et al., 1989).
Childhood cancer (lymphoma, leukemia neuroblastoma)	Modulates and strengthens defenses against carcinogenic insult by enhancing long-term development of infant immune system (Davis, 1998). Cancer cells undergo apoptosis (destruction) in human milk (Bener, Kenic, & Galadari, 2001; Daniels et al., 2002; Davis, Savitz, & Graubard, 1988; Franke, Custer, & Tanaka, 1998; Gimeno & Pacheco, 1997; Hakansson et al., 1995; Mathur et al., 1993; Shu et al., 1995; Smulevich et al., 1999; Svanborg et al., 2003; Swartzbaum et al., 1991).
Colitis	Less exposure to cow's milk proteins (Anveden-Hertzberg, 1996; Jenkins et al., 1984; Rigas et al., 1993).
Crohn's disease	Uncertain (Bergstrand & Hellers, 1983; Koletzko et al., 1989; Rigas et al., 1993).
Diabetes, type I (IDDM)	Lack of antigenic peptides helps protect against autoimmune disease. Less risk 2% to 26%. (Borch-Johnson et al., 1984; Gimeno & de Suza, 1997; Kostraba et al., 1993; Mayer et al., 1988; Perez-Bravolt et al., 1996; Verge et al., 1994; Virtanen et al., 1992; Wasmuth & Kolb, 2000 and many more articles).
Dental caries	Less occurrence of dental caries (Erickson, 1999).
Gastrointestinal infection/ diarrheal disease	Humoral and cellular anti-infectious factors (Dewey et al., 1995; Espinoza et al., 1997; Howie et al., 1990; Long et al., 1999; numerous other studies discussed throughout this book).
Gastroesophageal reflux	More rapid gastric emptying; lower esophageal pH (Heacock et al., 1992).
Hypertrophic pyloric stenosis	Uncertain; breastfeeding may prevent pyloric spasm and edema (Habbick, Kahnna, & To, 1989).
Inguinal hernia	Hormones in breastmilk might stimulate neonatal testicular function to close inguinal canal and promote descent of testes. One-fourth incidence (Pisacane et al., 1995a).
Juvenile rheumatoid arthritis	Anti-inflammatory properties protect against autoimmune disease (Mason et al., 1995).
Liver disease	Protease inhibitors (including antitrypsin) protect children with alpha-antitrypsin deficiency (Udall et al., 1985).

Table 4–4 (cont.)

Malocclusion	Physiological suckling patterns (Labbok & Hendershot, 1987).
Multiple sclerosis	Protects against autoimmune disease (Pisacane et al., 1994).
Necrotizing entercolitis	Immunological factors, macrophages, osmolarity of human milk, high levels of platelet-activating acetyl-hydrolase (Aksu et al., 1998; Lucas & Cole, 1990).
Otitis media	Antibody, T- and B-cell protection; lack of irritation from cow's milk; upright feeding position (Aniansson et al., 1994; Duncan et al., 1993; Sassen, Brand, & Grote, 1994).
Oral development	Fewer malocclusions and reduced need for orthodontic intervention because breastfed children have well-rounded, U-shaped dental arch. Fewer problems with snoring and sleep apnea in later life (Palmer, 1998).
Respiratory syncytial virus	IgA, IgG antibody transmitted to breastmilk and infant through gut-associated lymphoid tissue (GALT) or bronchus-associated lymphoid tissue (BALT). Lactadherin, a glycoprotein binds to rotavirus and inhibits activity (Bell, 1988; Duffy et al., 1986; Holberg et al., 1991; Naficy et al., 1999; Newburg et al., 1998; Rahman et al., 1987).
Lower respiratory tract disease	Meta-analysis of 33 studies on healthy infants in developed nations. Severe respiratory tract illnesses with hospitalization were tripled for infants who were not breastfed compared with those who were exclusively breastfed for 4 months (Bachrach, Schwarz, & Bachrach, 2003).
Retinopathy of prematurity	Antioxidants (inositol, Vitamin E, beta-carotene) and DHA may protect against the development of retinopathy of prematurity (Hylander et al., 2001).
Sudden infant death syndrome	Uncertain; possibly anti-infectious, antiallergic (Ford et al., 1993; Gilbert et al., 1995; Kum-Nji et al., 2001).
Urinary tract infections	Antibacterial properties (Marild et al., 1990; Pisacane et al., 1990).

piratory syncytial virus (RSV) infection (Bell et al., 1988; Downham et al., 1976; Duffy et al., 1986; Holberg et al., 1991; Naficy et al., 1999; Newburg et al., 1998; Rahman et al., 1987). Downham et al. (1976) compared 115 infants hospitalized with RSV who were younger than 12 months with 162 control infants. Only 7 percent of the hospitalized infants were breastfed, compared with 27.5 percent of the control infants, a statistically significant difference. In the case of pneumonia caused by *Streptococcus*, researchers recently discovered a novel folding variant of alpha-lactalbumin that is a naturally occurring antibacterial compound in breastmilk (Hakansson et al., 2000).

As with gastroenteritis, the preventive effect of breastmilk is global. When Chen, Yu, and Li (1988) looked for an association between type of feeding and hospitalization of infants in Shanghai,

they found that artificial feeding was associated with more frequent hospitalizations for respiratory infections during the first 18 months of life. In Brazil, babies who were not being breastfed were 17 times more likely than those being exclusively breastfed to be admitted to the hospital for pneumonia (Cesar, Victoria, & Barros, 1999). Similar protection has been established for *Haemophilus influenzae* bacteremia and meningitis (Cochi et al., 1986; Istre et al., 1985; Takala et al., 1989).

Otitis Media

Breastfeeding protects against ear infections (otitis media) for reasons that are not completely clear. However, immunological factors, the feeding position, and lack of irritation from bovine-based formula may explain it. Saarinen et al. (1982) followed healthy term infants for 3 years. Up to 6 months of age, no infant had otitis during the period of exclusive breastfeeding, whereas 10 percent of the babies who were given any cow's milk did. These significant differences persisted up to 3 years of age. Other studies (Aniansson et al., 1994; Dewey, Heinig, & Nommsen-Rivers, 1995) support an inverse relationship between ear infections and breastfeeding.

Controversies and Claims

In contrast to global evidence that breastfeeding helps to protect infants against health problems, Bauchner, Levanthal, and Shapiro (1986), and Leventhal et al. (1986) have challenged the claim that breastfeeding protects infants in developed countries, citing lack of control for potentially confounding factors, such as low birth weight, parental smoking, crowding, sanitation, and other characteristics of socioeconomic status.

Howie et al. (1990) settled this controversy by examining the effect of breastfeeding on childhood illness in Scotland in a study using an adequate sample that met the methodological criteria set by Bauchner, Levanthal, and Shapiro (1986). Howie concluded that breastfeeding during the first 13 weeks of life confers protection against gastrointestinal illness beyond the period of breastfeeding itself. A few years later, Fuchs, Victor, and Martines

(1996) questioned this long-term protection for diarrhea. They found that children who stopped breastfeeding in the previous 2 months were vulnerable to developing dehydrating diarrhea. Certain supplemental foods such as herbal teas prolonged diarrheal disease in Mexican children (Long et al., 1999).

In a prospective multicenter study on the effect of breastmilk in preventing necrotizing enterocolitis in premature infants, Lucas and Cole (1990) found that the disease was six to ten times more common in exclusively formula-fed babies than in exclusively breastmilk-fed babies. This held true even though the human milk received was often pooled, not derived from the baby's mother. These findings support the contention that breastfeeding is more than a lifestyle choice; it has profound implications for the health of the child. Parents sometimes ask how long breastmilk protective effects last. Table 4–5 presents research on the length of breastfeeding and expected protection.

Chronic Disease Protection

The protection offered by breastmilk against illness extends beyond infancy to childhood and adulthood. Breastfeeding contributes to prevention of celiac disease, diabetes, multiple sclerosis, sudden infant death syndrome, childhood cancer, and

---

Table 4–5

MINIMUM LENGTH OF BREASTFEEDING FOR PROTECTION AGAINST INFECTIOUS DISEASES

Health Problem	Minimum Length of Breastfeeding	Length of Protection	Source
Gastroenteritis/diarrheal disease	13 weeks	7 years	Howie, 1990
Otitis Media	4 months	3 years	Duncan et al., 1993
Respiratory infections	15 weeks	7 years	Wilson et al., 1998
Wheezing bronchitis	—	6–7 years	Burr et al., 1993; Porro et al., 1993;
Haemophilus influenzae, type b	—	10 years	Silfverdal et al., 1997
Hodgkin's disease	6 months	Not specified	Davis, 1998

many other health problems that are discussed throughout this book. The longer the duration of breastfeeding and the more complete exclusivity of breastmilk, the greater its protective effect.

Childhood Cancer

Does a mother's milk modulate the interaction between the developing infant immune system and infectious agents that helps protect an infant against carcinogenic insults? When Davis (1998) reviewed nine case-control studies on the association between infant feeding and childhood cancer, she confirmed that children who are never breastfed or are breastfed short-term have a higher risk of developing Hodgkin's disease than those breastfed for at least 6 months. It is possible that a type of human alpha-lactalbumin found in breastmilk lessens the risk of childhood cancer. This alpha-lactalbumin, a protein-lipid complex called HAMLET, induces apoptosis-like death in tumor cells but leaves fully differentiated cells unaffected (Hakansson et al., 1995; Svanborg et al., 2003). Other researchers contend that evidence showing that breastfeeding is protective against childhood cancer is limited and that further evidence is needed to support this conclusion (Heinig & Dewey, 1996).

Allergies and Atopic Disease

The incidence of food-induced allergic disease in children has been estimated to be between 0.3 to 7.5 percent (Metcalfe, 1984). Heredity is a significant predictor of allergic disease, even when the mother is on a milk-free diet during late pregnancy and lactation (Lovegrove, Hampton, & Morgan, 1994). Sixty percent of all those who will develop atopic eczema do so within the first year of life, and 90 percent do so within the first 5 years. Before 6 to 9 months of age, the infant intestinal mucosa is permeable to proteins; moreover, secretory IgA, which will later "paint" the mucosa and bind sensitizing proteins to itself, is not yet functioning effectively. After following 150 infants from birth to 17 years of age, Saarinen and Kajosaari (1995) concluded that breastfeeding is prophylactic against allergies—including eczema, food allergy, and respiratory allergy—throughout childhood and adolescence.

Bovine milk is the most common single allergen affecting infants. Proteins in bovine milk known to act as allergens include lactoglobulin, casein, bovine serum albumin, and lactalbumin. Modern heat treatment of formula has reduced—but certainly not eliminated—the allergic potential of these proteins. The problem is probably increased by the sizable dose of allergens in formula and by the large volume of formula ingested. At 2 to 4 months of age, for example, infants consume their body weight in milk each week. This is the equivalent of nearly 7 quarts per day for an adult—truly a macrodose!

Vomiting, diarrhea, colic, and occult bleeding are symptoms of allergy. It also affects the respiratory tract (runny nose, cough, asthma) and the skin (dermatitis, urticaria). Because the symptoms are varied and nonspecific, the diagnosis is often mistaken or missed.

At birth, the IgE system is defective in the potentially allergic infant, and problems arise if this system is activated by allergens. When the introduction of foreign proteins is delayed for 4 to 6 months, the baby's own IgA system is permitted to become more fully functional; thus allergic responses may be minimized or entirely avoided. Exclusive consumption of breastmilk facilitates the early maturation of the intestinal barrier and provides a passive barrier to potentially antigenic molecules until the baby's own natural barriers develop. The rationale for delay of solids for the first half year after birth is thus reinforced.

High levels of neonatal blood IgE are thought to predict later development of atopic symptoms. When the relationship between fecal IgE levels (a reliable indicator of serum IgE levels) was compared in infants 1 month old, formula-fed babies showed a higher incidence of high fecal IgE levels than did the breastfed infants (Furukawa et al., 1994).

A few breastfed infants develop atopic eczema. Of those who do, the culprit is often foods ingested by the mother—especially cow's milk. Cow's milk antigen can be detected in breastmilk (Axelsson et al., 1986; Cavagni et al., 1988; Odze et al., 1995; Paganelli, Cavagni, & Pallone, 1986). Early and occasional exposure to cow's milk protein sensitizes neonates so that even minute amounts of bovine milk protein in human milk may later act as booster doses that elicit allergic reactions (Host, Husby, & Osterballe, 1988). Prolonged breastfeeding exclusively or combined with infrequent exposure to small amounts of cow's milk during the first 8 weeks induces the development of IgE-mediated cow's milk allergy (Saarinen et al., 2000). By almost completely excluding milk, other dairy products, eggs, fish, beef, and peanuts throughout pregnancy and lactation, Chandra et al. (1986) documented a significant reduction in the incidence and severity of atopic eczema among breastfed infants of these mothers.

Problems in conducting research on allergies and breastfeeding are manifold. Because it is not possible to classify mothers randomly into breastfeeding and nonbreastfeeding groups, are those infants with a family history of atopic eczema more likely to be breastfed because the parents are aware that it has a protective effect? When the infant is identified as breastfed, does that mean that the baby received no other nutriments? If so, for how long was breastfeeding continued? After conducting a meta-analysis of 22 original research reports on infant feeding and atopic disease, Kramer (1988) decided that errors in research methods are conflicting and seriously flawed, which thus, precludes definitive conclusions.

Asthma

Outcomes of epidemiological and clinical studies on asthma and breastfeeding are inconsistent and the longstanding question of whether breastfeeding prevents or reduces the incidence of asthma has been controversial. To help settle the question Gdalevich, Mimouni, and Mimouni (2001) conducted a meta-analysis of research on the effect of breastfeeding on bronchial asthma. They found 41 studies that showed a protective effect, five studies that had no association, and two studies that had a positive association. Twelve of these studies were prospective and met the standards for study methodology as determined by Kramer (1988). Meta-analysis of these 12 showed that exclusive breastfeeding during the first months after birth is associated with lower asthma rates during childhood (Odds Ratio 0.70, 95% CI 0.60 to 0.81).

Finally, in regard to breastfeeding's protective effect against chronic disease, Palmer (1998) makes a convincing case that artificial feedings alter normal early oral cavity development so much that it can cause later problems such as snoring, sleep apnea, and malocclusion. For the mother herself, breastfeeding promotes health because it helps to prevent breast and ovarian cancer (see Chapter 16).

The Immune System

The body's overall immune system is known as the *systemic immune system*. Another immune system, the *secretory immune system*, invokes surfaces of the body (such as the breast) and acts locally. Lymphocytes in the secretory immune system are different from other lymphocytes. Sensitized to antigens found in the gastrointestinal or the respiratory tracts, these lymphocytes travel through mucosal lymphoid tissues (e.g., breasts, salivary glands, bronchi, intestines, and genitourinary tract) where they secrete antibodies.

Most antigens to which a mother has been exposed sensitize lymphocytes migrating to the breast. There they secrete immunoglobulins into the milk—hence, the term *secretory IgA* or *sIgA*. These components are described later in this chapter where immunoglobulins are discussed.

Active Versus Passive Immunity

Immunity occurs actively and passively. Maternal antibodies passed to the fetus through the placenta before birth present an example of passive immunity. Passive immunological protection is only temporary, as the infant's immune system has not itself responded. Breastfeeding can also confer long-term protection by stimulating an active immune response. Active immunity is a specific immunity whereby the immune system formulates a long-term memory of exposure to a certain antigen. Later exposure to the same antigen will produce an immune response. Poliovirus or rubella immunization of women or any attenuated virus immunization of the mother provides active immunity to the infant, as the virus will likely appear in her milk and thus immunize the infant. Reports indicate enhanced vaccine responses in breastfed infants compared with those not breastfeeding. After being vaccinated for measles-mumps-rubella (MMR), only breastfed children had increased production of interferon-gamma (Pabst et al., 1997). Another example of active immunity is the breastfed infant's immune response to cytomegalovirus in human milk.

Cells

Human milk contains two main types of white cells (leukocytes): phagocytes and lymphocytes (Figures 4–5 and 4–6). Although phagocytes (mostly macrophages) are most abundant (90 percent), the lymphocyte population (10 percent) provides significant protective effects to the recipient infant. The concentration of these cells and the predominant cell type vary with the duration of lactation. After birth, the number of these cells is higher than at any other time; they decline progressively thereafter.

Phagocytes.   Macrophages, a type of leukocyte, are the dominant phagocyte in human milk. They engulf and absorb pathogens. Macrophages release IgA, although they probably do not synthesize it. Macrophages are both polymorphonuclear (PMN) and mononuclear. Because PMN numbers increase dramatically during inflammation of the breast, they may function to protect the mammary tissue per se rather than to impart protection to

the newborn (Buescher & Pickering, 1986). Macrophages also produce complement, lactoferrin, and lysozyme (discussed later in this chapter). Neutrophils are yet another phagocytic leukocyte. Short-lived but effective, they are first to arrive at an inflamed site, such as that which may occur during mastitis.

Lymphocytes.   Lymphocytes are also leukocytes and include T cells, B cells, and assorted T-cell subsets. Lymphocytes compose about 4 percent of the total leukocytes in early lactation; about 83 percent of the lymphocytes are T cells that appear to transfer through human milk to infants (Wirt et al., 1992). The various ways in which lymphocytes recognize and help to destroy antigens are called *cell-mediated immunity.* Such immunity is important in the destruction of viruses because the cells within which viruses live shield them from the action of antibodies. Formula-fed and breastfed infants have different types of lymphocyte subsets (Hawkes & Gibson, 2001).

Decreasing rapidly in the first week after birth and continuing to decline steadily, T cells are a special and separate immune component that can be activated into memory T cells (Wirt et al., 1992). These memory cells are the key to active immunity. Antibodies persist for only a few weeks before breaking down; however, memory cells can live for

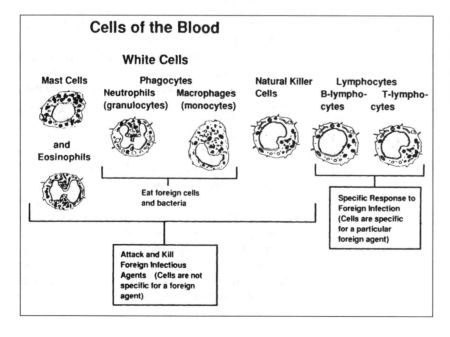

FIGURE 4–5.
White cells of the blood.
(From Fan H, Conner R, Villarreal L. *The biology of AIDS.* Boston: Jones and Bartlett, 1989: 28.)

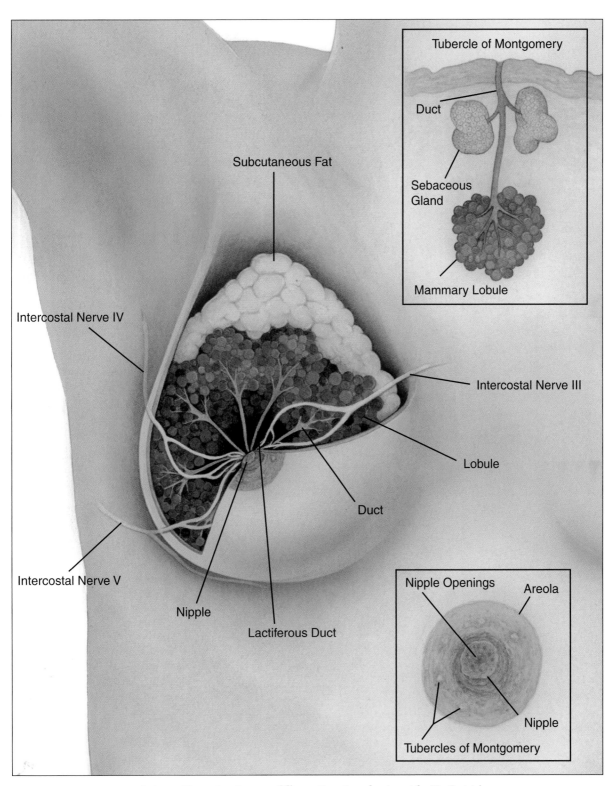

COLOR PLATE 1. Frontal view of lactating breast. *(Illustrations in color insert by Ka Botzis)*

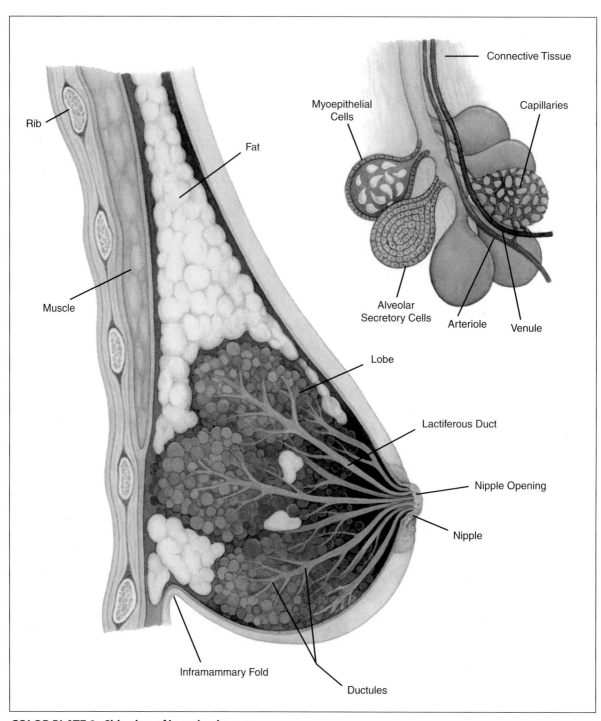

COLOR PLATE 2. Side view of lactating breast.

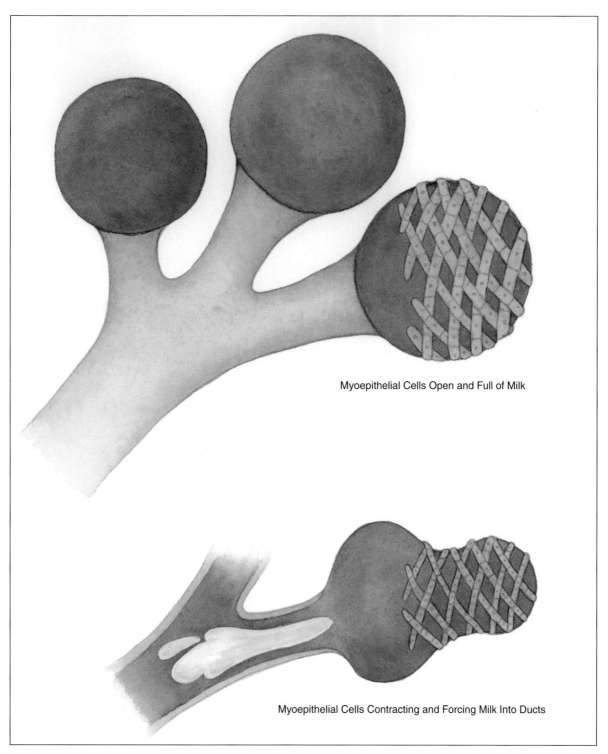

Myoepithelial Cells Open and Full of Milk

Myoepithelial Cells Contracting and Forcing Milk Into Ducts

COLOR PLATE 3. Myoepithelial cells.

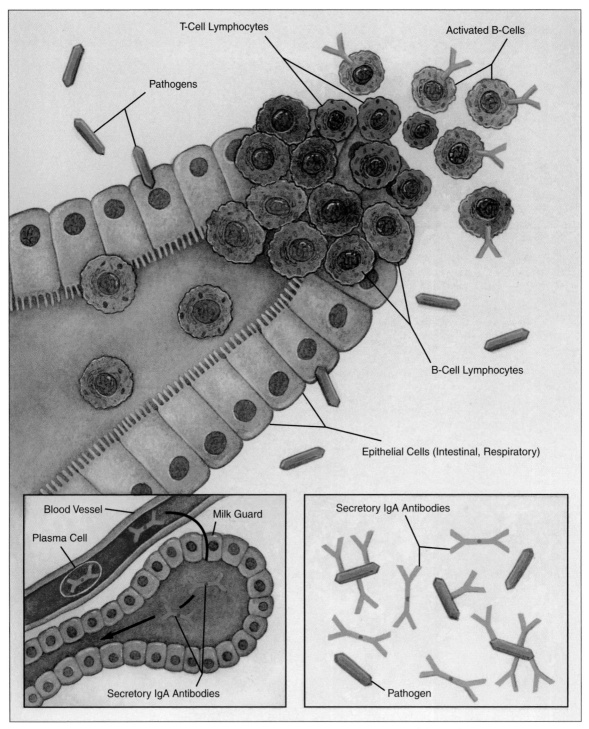

COLOR PLATE 4. BALT and GALT migration. *B cells originate in the epithelium of the mother's intestinal tract or respiratory tract. These B-cell lymphocytes are sensitized by microbial antigens from bacteria in the mother's intestines and activated by a chemical from T-cell lymphocytes. The sensitized B cells migrate to the mother's breast by a special "homing" system (GALT or BALT) described in the text. Once there, they can secrete IgA that enters into breastmilk. When the infant consumes the milk, it coats his intestinal walls, providing protection. The B-cell lymphocytes can also travel in milk to the baby and secrete IgA antibodies in the infant's own intestinal tract. Either way, the infant has secretory IgA antibodies against the specific bacteria he will most likely encounter in his environment.*

COLOR PLATE 5. Nipple bruised and cracked from poor positioning. This trauma occurred on post-partum day 1. It was corrected by lifting the baby out of the mother's lap and into her arms and turning the baby so that his entire body faced the mother.

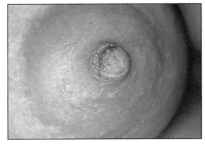

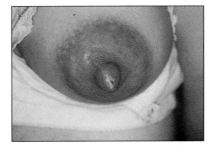

COLOR PLATE 6. Sore nipple with trauma from poor positioning. The white streak across the face of the nipple is a sign that the baby's lower jaw was too close to the tip of the nipple. Positioning the baby centrally across the mother's torso resulted in the baby driving his chin in closer to the breast rather than to the nipple. (Photo with permission from Barbara Wilson-Clay.)

COLOR PLATE 7. Nipple fissure that resulted from use of a poorly designed breast pump for three days. Even short-term use of a poorly designed pump can cause significant nipple damage. (Photo with permission of Catherine Watson Genna.)

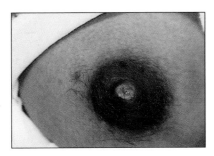

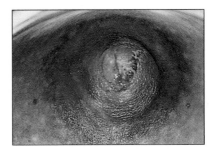

COLOR PLATE 8. Badly cracked nipple with possible bacterial infection. Such trauma can become an entry point for bacterial invasion and subsequent inflammation or infection. (Photo with permission of Kay Hoover.)

COLOR PLATE 9. Extreme engorgement. Engorgement occurred 30 to 36 hours postpartum, secondary to ineffective and infrequent breastfeeding and no expression or pumping when the infant did not obtain milk. (With permission from Chele Marmet/ Lactation Institute.)

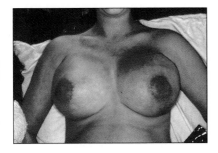

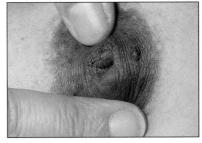

COLOR PLATE 10. Abraded folded nipple. The abrasion occurred when the nipple tissue remained wet between feedings; air-drying after each breast-feeding resolved the problem.

COLOR PLATE 11. Milk plugs at nipple pores, often characterized by acute pain. When milk is released from the duct, relief is immediate.

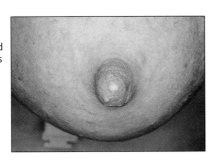

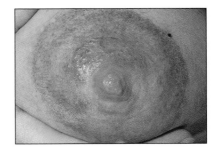

COLOR PLATE 12. *Candidiasis* **(thrush) of the breast.** This mother experienced four separate episodes in which her breasts, but not the baby's mouth, were treated. Within one week of simultaneous treatment of mother and baby, neither the baby's mouth nor the mother's breasts were infected.

COLOR PLATE 13. Breast abscess prior to excision. A breast abscess will often present with generalized redness. When the affected area is palpated, it is hot and hard to the touch. (Photo with permission from Barbara Wilson-Clay.)

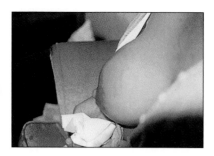

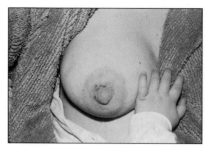

COLOR PLATE 14. Herpes on the areola. A thirteen-month-old nursing toddler contracted oral herpes by using a playmate's contaminated rattle; the mother was then infected. The breast lesion appeared soon after the baby's infection was identified. (With permission from Chele Marmet/Lactation Institute.)

COLOR PLATE 15. Psoriasis of the nipples. Although previous lesions had occurred on her breasts (but never on her nipples or areolae), this mother developed psoriasis on her nipples within a week of her baby's birth. When the baby latched on at the beginning of each breastfeeding session, she felt pain, which gradually subsided as the feeding progressed. (Photo with permission of Karen Foard.)

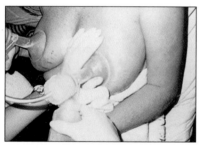

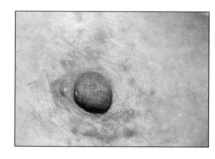

COLOR PLATE 16. Breast abscess with iodoform gauze drain in place; the safety pin is not holding the drain in place. (Photo with permission of Donna Corrieri.)

COLOR PLATE 17. Pumping the breast following abscess drainage. When a mother cannot put a baby to breast following treatment for a breast abscess, pumping may be necessary. The LC's gloved hand is placing gentle, even pressure over the area of the abscess drain to create a seal, in order to pump both breasts simultaneously and comfortably. (Photo with permission from Donna Corrieri.)

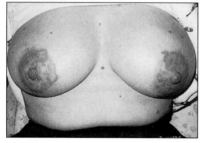

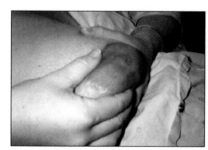

COLOR PLATE 18. Poison ivy on the areola. (Photo with permission of Kay Hoover.)

COLOR PLATE 19. Mastitis involving the lower outer quadrant of the breast. The mother was placed on intravenous antibiotics in the hospital, and lactation continued throughout the IV therapy. Her baby was housed with her during her hospitalization.

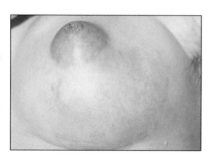

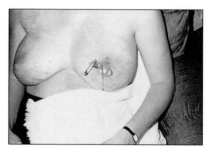

COLOR PLATE 20. This mother is displacing breast edema (different from engorgement) by applying pressure from the areola backwards toward the chest wall, rotating the fingers around the "clock" and moving back, holding the pressure until the tissue becomes soft. The procedure can take a few minutes to 30 minutes depending on the severity of the edema.

COLOR PLATE 21. Auxiliary breast and nipple tissue. A common site for additional breast or nipple tissue. In the absence of stimulation, milk production and tissue swelling ceases.

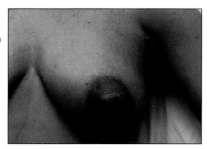

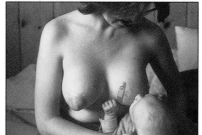

COLOR PLATE 22. Breastfeeding following biopsy for a benign tumor. The mother, with a totally breastfed infant, is shown four months post-partum. The tumor was discovered during lactation two weeks prior to biopsy. The baby is breastfeeding four hours after biopsy, the mother keeping the baby's hand away from the biopsy incision area. (With permission from Chele Marmet/ Lactation Institute.)

COLOR PLATE 23. Nipple inversion. The mother had successfully breastfed her previous baby using both breasts.

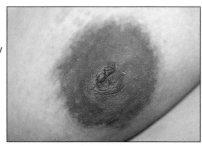

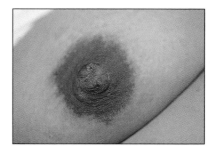

COLOR PLATE 24. Nipple eversion. Following gentle suction with a hand breast pump, the nipple completely everted.

COLOR PLATE 25. Burn scars on breast. This mother sustained third-degree burns as a child and experienced numerous subsequent reconstructive surgeries, including one to reconstruct her nipples. Although the breast tissue was difficult to compress because of extensive scar tissue, the baby was able to breastfeed.

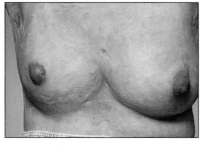

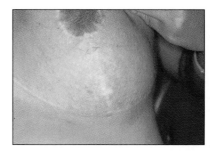

COLOR PLATE 26. Breast-reduction scars. This mother had breast surgery at age 28, two years before her first pregnancy; her bra size changed from a 32HH to a 36B prior to her first pregnancy. The nipples were not entirely detached, but both areolae were reduced in size and repositioned on the breast. Following surgery, the left breast had heightened sensation; the right nipple had no sensation at all. Some milk was obtained from each breast. (With permission from Chele Marmet/ Lactation Institute.)

COLOR PLATE 27. Significantly different breast size and shape, suggestive of primary breast insufficiency; this mother was referred for a lactation consultation for her inadequate milk supply. (Photo with permission from Kay Hoover.)

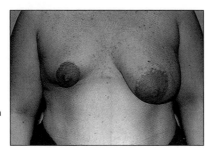

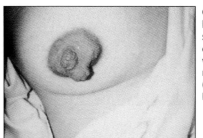

COLOR PLATE 28. Double nipple on the same breast. This mother's baby needed to gape widely enough to take both nipples into his mouth. (Photo with permission of Linda Stewart.)

COLOR PLATE 29. Oral *Candidiasis* (thrush). When first seen, the baby was fifteen days old; the gums and inner cheeks were as involved as his tongue. The mother's nipples were also inflamed. After four weeks of intermittent treatment, neither the baby's mouth nor the mother's breasts were infected. (With permission from Chele Marmet/Lactation Institute.)

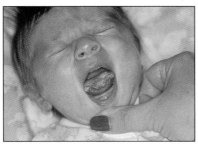

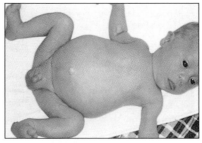

COLOR PLATE 30. Baby with Down syndrome. Note the small genitalia characteristic of a child with Down syndrome. Poor head and neck control, weak jaw and other motor abilities, and a poor suck often require special assistance while the baby is learning how to suckle the breast. (With permission from Chele Marmet/ Lactation Institute.)

COLOR PLATE 31. Baby with FTT. At birth, this baby weighed 8 lbs 12 oz. When referred to the LC at 4½ months, he still weighed only 10 lbs 11 oz. He avidly sucked his own fingers and slept for long periods; when put to breast, he was extremely lethargic. In addition, he sucked in his cheeks, generating no effective negative pressure on the breast. (Photo with permission from Jane Bradshaw.)

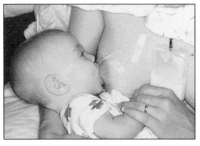

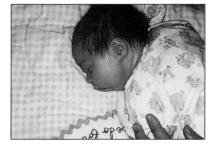

COLOR PLATE 32. Hemangioma of the infant's lip. Although it may appear to be troublesome, this condition did not cause feeding problems for the baby. (Photo with permission of Barbara Wilson-Clay.)

COLOR PLATE 33. Cleft of the soft palate. Such a cleft can occur without a cleft of the lip. (Photo with permission from Jane Bradshaw.)

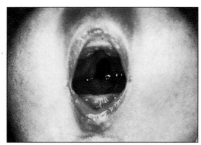

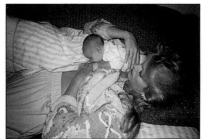

COLOR PLATE 34. Baby with Pierre Robin syndrome. This syndrome is characterized by a severely receded chin, which can often require special assistance and creative positioning to help the baby latch on. Other characteristics of this syndrome, such as cleft palate, may also render breastfeeding difficult or impossible to achieve for varying lengths of time. (Photo with permission from Jane Bradshaw.)

COLOR PLATE 35. Baby being fed by NG tube while at breast. Sometimes a baby unable to feed directly can be fed with a nasogastric tube. Doing so while holding her baby next to her breast and allowing the baby to suck on a finger or thumb can help the mother to normalize this feeding situation. (Photo with permission of Jane Bradshaw.)

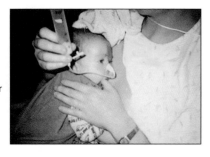

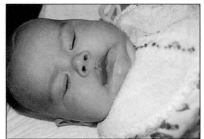

COLOR PLATE 36. Over-the-shoulder positioning of baby. This mother with extremely sore nipples was referred to a lactation consultant. The position shown here was taught as an alternative, to move the baby's mouth away from very tender areas and allow breastfeeding to continue during the healing period. The mother was placed on the LC's couch on her back, with the baby approaching the breast from over her shoulder. (Photo with permission from Jane Bradshaw.)

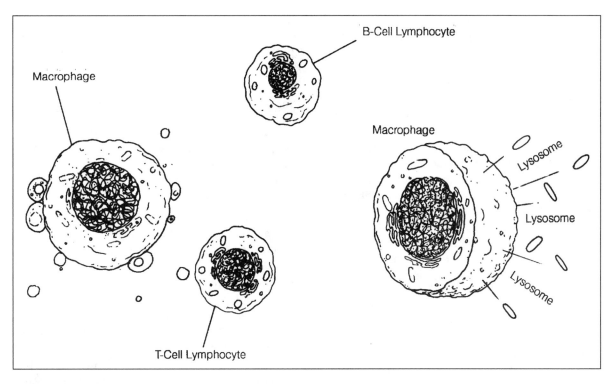

FIGURE 4–6. Microscope view of living cells in human milk. The cells of human milk consist mainly of macrophages and T-cell and B-cell lymphocytes. Macrophages secret lyzozyme, which help destroy the cell walls of bacteria (Drawing by Ka Botzis).

years, providing long-lasting protection. It is not clear whether T cells are activated in human milk or whether there is a specific homing of activated and memory T lymphocytes to the breast. B cells have functional capabilities similar to those of T cells. They mature into plasmalike cells that travel to epithelial tissues in the breast and release antibodies (Bellig, 1995; Newman, 1995) that reflect exposure to pathogens encountered in their environment. For example, milk from mothers living in Nigeria and exposed to malaria was compared with milk from a control population of mothers living in Washington, DC. The Nigerian mothers carried a high IgA level of antimalaria antibodies compared with the Washington mothers (Kassim et al., 2000).

Antibodies/Immunoglobulins

Antibodies are immunoglobulins that recognize and act on a particular antigen. Immunoglobulins are proteins produced by plasma cells in response to an immunogen. There are five types of immunoglobulins: (1) IgG, (2) IgA, (3) IgM, (4) IgE, and (5) IgD. Both IgA and IgE play a critical role in biological specificity of human milk on the recipient infant.

Secretory IgA (sIgA) is the major immunoglobulin in all human secretions. SIgA provides the initial bolus that supplements immunoglobulins transferred earlier across the placenta to the fetus. It is the immunoglobulin most frequently noted in medical literature as having immense immunological value to the neonate. SIgA, which is both synthesized and stored in the breast, reaches levels up to 5 mg/ml in colostrum; then it decreases to 1 mg/ml in mature milk. Interleukin-6 in human milk may be partly responsible for the genesis of IgA- and IgM-producing cells in the mammary gland (Rudloff et al., 1993). As the mother yields more milk, the infant receives more sIgA so that the total dose of sIgA the baby receives throughout lactation is constant or even increases (depending on the milk intake). Mothers of infants with a systemic infection and poor suckling have higher IgA levels in their breastmilk (Feist, Berger, & Speer, 2000; Groer, Humenick, & Hill, 1994).

SIgA synthesis via the secretory immune system described is an elegant lymphocyte traffic pathway called *gut-associated lymphoid tissue* (GALT) or *bronchus-associated lymphoid tissue* (BALT). This pathway leads to the development of lymphoid cells in the mammary gland, which produce IgA antibodies after exposure to specific microbial or environmental antigens on the intestinal or the respiratory mucosa (Goldman et al., 1983; Okamoto & Ogra, 1989). This migration of immunological responsiveness from both BALT and GALT to the mammary glands supports the unique concept of a common mucosal immune system (see Color Plate 4).

Because the infant's own IgA is deficient and only slowly increases during the first several months after birth, sIgA in human milk provides important passive immunological protection to the digestive tract of newborn infants. SIgA protects the newborn's entire intestinal track. It is only minimally absorbed from the intestine because it is bound to the human milk fat globule membrane, travels through the newborn's entire intestinal track, and is found unaltered in the newborn feces (Schroten et al., 1999).

A number of IgA antibodies in human milk that act upon viruses or bacteria that cause respiratory and gastrointestinal tract infections have been reported. These infecting agents include *E. coli, V. cholerae, Clostridium difficile, Salmonella, G. lamblia, E. histolytica, Campylobacter,* rotavirus, and poliovirus (Pickering & Kohl, 1986; Ruiz-Palacios et al., 1990). As stated earlier, immunizing breastfeeding women with poliovirus or rubella creates IgA antibodies in milk that specifically target these agents. IgA$_4$ may also play a role in host defense of mucosal surfaces; in some women IgA$_4$ is produced locally in the mammary gland (Keller et al., 1988). In addition to IgA, other Ig classes, including IgD, may be involved in local immunity of the breast. Several investigators (Litwin, Zehr, & Insel, 1990; Steel & Leslie, 1985) have demonstrated high levels of locally produced IgD in breast tissues and breastmilk.

As shown in Figure 4–7, clear biological rhythms of protective factors predictably rise and fall as lactation progresses. The reasons for waxing and waning of various anti-infective components are not always clear but are assumed to be adapted to the needs of the infant (see Figure 4–7 and Color Plate 4).

Nonantibody Antibacterial Protection

Nonantibody factors in human milk comprise an elegant and intricate system that protects the infant against bacterial infection. These factors include lactoferrin, the bifidus factor, lactoperoxidase, and oligosaccharides.

Lactoferrin. Lactoferrin, a potent bacteriostatic iron-binding protein, is abundant in human milk (1–6 mg/ml) but is not present in bovine milk. It is present in higher proportions relative to total protein in preterm milk (de Ferrer et al., 2000). Lactoferrin inhibits adhesion of *Escherichia coli* to cells and helps prevent diarrheal disease (de Araujo & Gugliano, 2001). In the presence of IgA antibody and bicarbonate, lactoferrin readily absorbs enteric iron and thus prevents pathogenic organisms, particularly *Escherichia coli* and *Candida albicans* (Borgnolo et al., 1996; Kirkpatrick et al., 1971), from obtaining the iron needed for survival. Because exogenous iron may well interfere with the protective effects of lactoferrin, giving iron supplements to the healthy breastfed infant must be carefully weighed. Lactoferrin also has been shown to be an essential growth factor for human B and T lymphocytes (Hashizume, Kuroda, & Murakami, 1983) and to inhibit fungal growth.

The Bifidus Factor. The intestinal flora of breastfed infants is dominated by gram-positive lactobacilli, especially *Lactobacillus bifidus.* This bifidus factor in human milk, first recognized by Gyorgy (1953), promotes the growth of these beneficial bacteria. The buffering capacities of milk (bifidus factor), together with the low protein and phosphate, contribute to the low pH (5–6) of stools. This acid environment, present even in the first days of life of the breastfeeding infant (Rubaltelli et al., 1998) discourages replication of enteropathogens such as *Shigella, Salmonella,* and some *E. coli.* This protection does not appear to be complete, however. Although breastmilk inhibits bacterial-cellular adhesion to intestinal epithelial cells, a sign of the beginning of the infectious process, it does not prevent loss of epithelial barrier (Kohler, 2002).

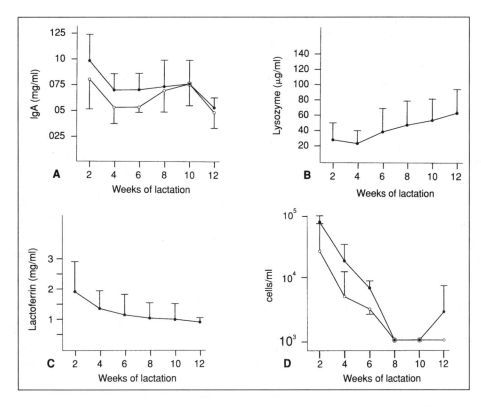

FIGURE 4–7.
A longitudinal study of selected resistance factors in human milk. (A) Total (·) and secretory (○) IgA. (B) Lysozyme. (C) Lactoferrin. (D) Macrophages-neutrophils (·--·) and lymphocytes (○–○). (Modified from Goldman AS et al. Immunological factors in human milk during the first year of lactation. *J Pediatr* 100:663, 1982.)

Whether the breastfed infants in the study were fed other liquids and foods was not addressed.

Lactoperoxidase. Although levels of the enzyme lactoperoxidase are low, substantial amounts are present in the newborn's saliva. It is thought that IgA in milk enhances the ability of lactoperoxidase to kill streptococci.

Oligosaccharides. Oligosaccharides (carbohydrates composed of a few monosaccharides) in human milk help to block antigens from attaching to the epithelium of the gastrointestinal tract. This blocking mechanism prevents the attachment of *Pneumococcus*, which is particularly adhesive (Goldman et al., 1986). There are about 130 different oligosaccharides in human milk. Breastmilk contains many times the amount of oligosaccharides that are found in bovine milk or formula. A few formula companies are adding a limited number of simple oligosccaharides to infant formula; yet the oligosaccharides found in human milk can be thought of as 130 reasons to breastfeed (McVeagh & Miller, 1997).

Cytokines and Chemokines. Cytokines and chemokines—polypeptids that bind to specific cellular receptors—are called immunomodulators in that they operate in networks and orchestrate activation of the immune system (Goldman et al., 1996) probably by moving lymphocytes into breastmilk and across the neonatal bowel wall (Michie et al., 1998). Several different cytokines and chemokines have been discovered in human milk recently and the list is growing rapidly (Garofolo & Goldman, 1998). In addition to activating the immune system to protect the infant against infection (Wallace et al., 1997), these biologically active molecules also appear to play a role in growth and differentiation of the mammary gland (Goldman et al., 1996). Much has yet to be learned about cytokines.

Anti-inflammatory and Immunomodulating Components

Many host defense agents in human milk have more than one function. Secretory IgA, lactoferrin, and lysozyme are examples. Human milk, rich in anti-inflammatory agents, supplies key protection during the vulnerable period of infancy. Major biochemical pathways of inflammations are either absent or poorly represented in breastmilk. Garofalo and Goldman (1999) have identified several anti-inflammatory factors in breastmilk, such as antioxidants (vitamins A, C, and E and enzymes), alpha$_1$-antitrypsin, cortisol, epidermal growth factor, IgA, lysozyme, prostaglandins, and cytokines. The anti-inflammatory effects of these components have not as yet been directly demonstrated in the nursing infant but they are thought to modulate cytokine responses to infection and facilitate defense mechanisms while minimizing tissue damage (Kelleher & Lönnerdal, 2001).

Goldman et al. (1996) suggest that the immunomodulating properties of human milk have a long-term influence on the development of the immune system and explain why the long-term risk for many diseases are lessened by breastfeeding. An immunomodulator changes the function of another defense agent and thus changes the quality or magnitude of the immune response. Fibronectin in human milk is an example of an immunomodulator that acts by augmenting the clearance of bacteria and intravascular debris. Interferon-alpha is not in human milk; yet breastfed infants with respiratory syncytial virus infection have higher blood levels of this element than nonbreastfed infants. Cytokines are also thought to immunomodulate the immune system. For example, Interleukin-18, which is activated by macrophages, is higher in colostrum compared with early milk and mature milk. Interleukin-10 increases the development of IgA antibody production, thus playing an important role in host defense of neonates (Takahata et al., 2001).

Bioactive Components

Hamosh (2001) designates a special group of substances in human milk as *bioactive components*. These substances promote growth and development of the newborn by special activities that continue after the infant ingests breastmilk. Many are not available to the infant in commercial infant formula. Research on bioactive components is a growing area of investigation. These bioactive components may play a significant role in child health.

Enzymes

Mammalian milk contains a large number of enzymes, some of which appear to have a beneficial effect on the development of the newborn. The enzyme content of human milk and bovine milk differ substantially (Hamosh, 1996). For example, lysozyme activity is several thousand times greater in human milk than in bovine milk. The alkaline pH of the human infant's stomach has a limited effect on the antitrypsin activity of breastmilk, thereby protecting children with alpha$_1$-antitrypsin deficiency against severe liver disease and early death (Udall et al., 1985). Most mammal milks contain many enzymes that appear to be species-specific because of their varying level of activity in different species. The enzymes discussed next serve a digestive function in the infant or may be important to neonatal development.

Lysozyme. Lysozyme, a major component of human milk whey fraction, produces both bacteriocidal and anti-inflammatory action. It acts with peroxide and ascorbate to destroy *E. coli* and some *Salmonella* strains (Pickering and Kohl, 1986). Lysozyme is much more abundant in human milk (400 ug/ml) than in bovine milk. Rather than slowly declining as lactation progresses, lysozyme activity increases progressively, beginning about 6 months after delivery (Goldman et al., 1982; Prentice et al., 1984). The lysozme differs from other protective factors in this respect because babies begin receiving solid foods around 6 months, and high levels of lysozyme may be a teleological, practical safeguard against the greater risk from pathogens and diarrheal disease at this time.

Lipase. In order for human infants to digest fat, adequate lipase activity and bile salt levels must be present. The bile salt–stimulated lipase and lipoprotein lipase present in human milk compensate for immature pancreatic function and for the absence of amylaze in neonates, especially in the premature infant. When human milk is frozen or refrigerated (Hamosh et al., 1997), lipase is not affected; however, heating severely reduces lipase activity. Several protozoa—*Giardia lamblia*, *Entamoeba histolytica*, and *Trichomonas vaginalis*—have been shown in vitro to be killed rapidly by exposure to salt-stimulated lipase, which is found only in the milk of humans and mountain gorillas (Blackberg et al., 1980).

Amylase. Amylase is necessary for the digestion of starch. Although amylase is synthesized and stored in the pancreas of the newborn, the infant is around 6 months old before amylase is released into the duodenum. Human milk contains about 10 to 60 times as much alpha-amylase as does normal human serum, thus providing an alternate source of this starch-digestive substance. No alpha-amylase is present in bovine, goat, or swine milk, suggesting that this enzyme appeared late in the evolutionary continuum. Breastfed infants have fewer problems digesting solid foods than do formula-fed infants, even if these foods are introduced early, because of the alpha-amylase provided by breastmilk. Amylase is stable when refrigerated (95–100 percent activity after 24 hours storage at 15–25° C) (Hamosh et al., 1997).

Growth Factors and Hormones

Human milk contains growth-promoting components also known as *growth modulators.* As with the anti-infective properties of breastmilk, these substances are more pronounced in colostrum than in mature milk. Neither their biological significance nor their method of action is yet clear. Many questions remain: Do growth factors influence growth and repair of mammary tissue or promote growth and repair of cells within the intestines of the neonate? Are these factors absorbed from the neonatal gastrointestinal tract or do they enter the circulation of the neonate and exert an effect on enteric or target organs? Or is it some combination of these possible actions that occurs? (Morriss et al., 1986). Different growth factors may have overlapping functions, both stimulating cell growth and indirectly affecting the infant's defense mechanisms against disease.

Epidermal Growth Factor. Epidermal growth factor (EGF), a type of cytokine, is a major growth-promoting agent in breastmilk which stimulates proliferation of intestinal mucosa and epithelium and strengthens the mucosal barrier to antigens (Carpenter, 1980; Petschow et al., 1993). A polypeptide that contains 53 amino acids, EGF is highest in human milk after delivery and decreases rapidly thereafter (Matsuoka & Idota, 1995). There is no diurnal variation or variation between preterm and term milk. EGF is also present in plasma, saliva, and amniotic fluid, but human milk contains a higher concentration. EGF may also be involved in the development of low-density lipoprotein receptors and in cholesterol metabolism.

Human Growth Factors I, II, and III. Three polypeptides—called *human milk growth factors* (HMGF) I, II, and III—have been isolated (Shing & Klagsburn, 1984). HMGF III stimulates DNA synthesis and cellular proliferation, suggesting that it is an epidermal growth factor. In vivo studies (Heird, Schward, & Hansen, 1984; Widdowson, Colombo, & Artavanis, 1976) on growth factors in animal milk have shown striking increases in the mass of intestinal mucosa. Growth factors in human milk influence the growth of target tissues in the breastfed infant by provoking an endogenous hormonal response that is different from that provoked by formula—a possible stimulus of nutritional programming.

Insulinlike Growth Factor. An insulinlike growth factor (IGF-I) in human milk is thought to have a growth-promoting role. The concentration of this factor in colostrum is about 30 times that in human serum, significantly higher than cow's milk, and very low to almost absent in formula (Shehadeh et al., 2001). These high levels (4.1 nmol/L) decrease rapidly (to 1.3 nmol/L) as colostrum alters to transitional milk (Read et al., 1984) but do not decline further. In fact, Corps et al. (1988) found that the concentration of an insulinlike growth factor in human milk increased (2.5 nmol/L) by the sixth week postpartum.

Thyroxine and Thyrotropin-Releasing Hormone. Thyroxine is present in human milk in small quantities but is not found in commercial formulas. The concentration in colostrum is low, increases by the first week postpartum, and gradually declines thereafter. It has been suggested that thyroxine may stimulate the maturation of the infant's intestine (Morriss, 1985).

Although the thyroxine level is significantly higher in breastfed children than in formula-fed children at 1 and 2 months of age (Rovet, 1990), it is unclear whether breastfeeding protects breastfed infants against clinical evidence of congenital hypothyroidism (Latarte et al., 1980; Rovet, 1990). Some infants receive sufficient thyroxine in their mother's milk to compensate for hypothyroidism; thus the symptoms may be masked for several months. Although this does not appear to be true for all infants, the results of thyroid studies after the first week of life should be interpreted with caution in breastfed infants and should include measurements of both thyroxine and thyroid-stimulating hormone (TSH) concentrations.

Cortisol. Cortisol is present in relatively high concentrations in colostrum, declines rapidly by the second day, and remains low thereafter. Its role in infant physiology is not clear. Three theories have been presented concerning the function of cortisol in infants. The first is that it may control the transport of fluids and salts in infants' gastrointestinal tract (Kulski & Hartmann, 1981). Another theory is that it may play a role in the growth of an infant's pancreas (Morisset & Jolicoeur, 1980). Or cortisol may serve as a hormone released during chronic stress. Mothers' higher level of satisfaction with breastfeeding is associated with lower levels of cortisol in her milk. The amount of cortisol in milk is inversely related to sIgA, suggesting that cortisol may suppress the function of immunoglobulin-producing cells in milk (Groer, Humenick, & Hill, 1994).

Cholecystokinin. Cholecystokinin (CCK) is a gastrointestinal hormone that enhances digestion, sedation, and a feeling of satiation and well-being. During suckling, vagal stimulation causes CCK release in both mother and infant, producing a sleepy feeling. The infant's CCK level peaks twice after suckling. The first peak occurs immediately after the feeding. It peaks again 30 to 60 minutes later. The first CCK rise is probably induced by suckling; the second by the presence of milk in the gastrointestinal tract (Marchini & Linden, 1992; Uvnas-Moberg, Marchini, & Windberg, 1993).

Beta-Endorphins. Beta-endorphins are higher in the colostrum of women who delivered (1) prematurely, (2) vaginally and, (3) without epidural analgesia. It is hypothesized that elevated beta-endorphin concentrations in colostrum may contribute to post-natal fetal adaptation to overcoming birth stress of natural labor and delivery, and at the same time contribute to the postnatal development of several related biological functions of the growing newborn (Zanardo et al., 2001).

Prostaglandins. Prostaglandins, a special group of lipids, are present in most mammal cells and tissues and affect almost every biological system. Formed by numerous body tissues, prostaglandins affect many physiological functions, including local circulation, gastric and mucous secretion, electrolyte balance, zinc absorption, and the release of brush border enzymes. The protective activity of milk lipids is thought to be due to the presence of prostaglandins PGE_2 and PGF_{2a} present both in colostrum and in mature milk. Concentrations there are about 100 times as great as their levels in adult plasma (Lucas & Mitchell, 1980). PGE_2 particularly is thought to exert a cytoprotective action (protection against inflammation and necrosis) on the gastric mucosa by promoting the accumulation of phospholipids in the neonatal stomach (Reid, Smith, & Friedman, 1980). The full extent of the beneficial effects of prostaglandins in human milk awaits future scientific investigation.

Taurine

Taurine, absent in bovine milk, is the second most abundant amino acid in human milk (Raiha, 1985). This unusual amino acid, which may function as a neurotransmitter, plays an important role in early brain maturation (Gaull, 1985). Before 1983, taurine was thought to act only in the conjugation of bile acids. Infants who do not receive taurine in their diet conjugate bile acids with glycine, which less effectively assists in absorbing dietary fats. Although deleterious effects of low taurine levels are not known in humans, deficiencies have caused retinal problems in cats and monkeys (Jensen et al., 1988). Taurine was added to most commercial formulas when formula-fed infants were found to have plasma taurine levels only half as high as those of breastfed infants.

Implications for Clinical Practice

Human milk is a species-specific fluid of diverse composition that includes both nutrient and non-nutrient substances, all of which protect the infant. Although the significance to young infants of these components is well-known, the influence of their nutritional programming on the subsequent health of infants is a relatively new field.

A thorough understanding of the biological components of human and bovine milks and of manufactured formulas is essential for the health-care specialist who is providing lactation assistance. When prenatal discussion with the parents and pre-natal classes include information about the im-munological protection available from breastmilk but absent from formula, parents can then make an informed choice of infant feeding method.

This chapter objectively describes human milk components—but what about mothers' views of their breastmilk? Bottorff and Morse (1990) re-vealed that mothers clearly recognize the difference between colostrum and mature breastmilk. Because of the relative thickness of colostrum, some mothers believe it is the "strongest" milk, significant for its "rich" supply of antibodies rather than for its nutri-tional properties. Breastmilk was frequently de-scribed by using fat-related terms (e.g., lean, creamy, rich) and evaluated by drawing compar-isons to cow's milk and infant formula, as if some similarities should exist between the two.

Knowledge of lactation physiology and breast-milk components provides us direction for lactation practice and advice to mothers. For example, the high fat (and thus calories) in hindmilk—the milk that appears when the breast is nearly empty—imply caution in routinely recommending "switch" nursing (repeatedly switching feedings from breast to breast during a breastfeeding) (Woolridge & Fisher, 1988). On the other hand, infants whose re-quirements may fluctuate with time are amazingly adept at self-regulating their nutrient intake (Wool-ridge, Ingram, & Baum, 1990). Thus we can encour-age women to be flexible about breastfeedings and to be led by infants' cues that tell mothers when to continue and when to stop a feeding.

Given the differences between the growth pat-terns of breastfed infants and infants fed human-milk substitutes, practitioners need to evaluate infant growth using standardized growth charts based on breastfed infants. Otherwise, breastfeed-ing mothers might be told that their babies are gain-ing too slowly and that their milk production must

be insufficient, when their babies are healthy in all respects. (See Chapter 10 on slow weight gain for a more detailed discussion of this issue.)

The drop of infant CCK levels 10 minutes after a feeding implies a "window" within which the in-fant can be awakened to feed from the second breast or to reattach to the first side for additional fat-rich milk. Waiting 30 minutes after the feeding before laying the baby down takes advantage of the second CCK peak to help the infant to stay asleep.

The studies cited here support giving fresh, rather than heat-treated or frozen, human milk whenever possible. Some living cells are killed by both of these treatments. Also, due to the action of the bile salt–stimulated lipase, fat in fresh human milk is absorbed more completely than that in pas-teurized milk. Mixing mother's milk with formula is acceptable. It is particularly important for prema-ture infants, who lack digestive enzymes, and mix-ing fresh human milk with formula improves fat absorption. Ideally, preterm infants will be receiv-ing high volumes of their own mother's milk or mother's milk enriched with human milk compo-nents, both of which sustain excellent growth with-out the risks of bovine milk.

During the assessment phase of working with a breastfeeding family, the practitioner needs to ask if there is a family history of allergies. If so, the mother should be encouraged to breastfeed for a minimum of 12 months and to delay feeding the in-fant solid foods until the baby shows signs of readi-ness. Because of the risk of sensitization to allergenic proteins, particularly in babies who have a family history of allergies, even occasional for-mula supplements can trigger an allergic reaction and should be avoided as long as possible. In addi-tion to preventing allergies, infant malabsorption problems, such as celiac disease, are lessened when the baby is breastfed and solid foods are delayed. Solid foods are usually started around 6 months of age as a baby's intestinal enzymes mature and be-come increasingly capable of digesting complex proteins and starches. After 6 months, babies can eat whatever they like and in any order they want.

In the maternal diet, dairy products are par-ticularly potential allergens to the breastfeeding baby. If the mother notices that a particular food seems to cause an allergic response in her infant, she needs to consider eliminating it from her diet.

A case report (Wilson, Self, & Hamburger, 1990) describes rectal bleeding in a four-day-old infant who was exclusively breastfed: Her mother was drinking four to five glasses of cow's milk per day. Although this case is extreme and rare, it demonstrates the potential for problems when a breast-feeding mother drinks large quantities of cow's milk. Discussion of diet and appropriate substitution should be part of the care provided the mother by the health-care worker offering lactation consultation and support.

Summary

The nutritional components of human milk, combined with its immune and antiallergic properties, make it the ideal foundation for optimal infant health. Immunological and allergy protection are obvious, but it is more difficult to substantiate the protection by breastfeeding against inflammatory and immunologically determined disorders that emerge later in life. There appears to be a threshold level for passive immunity conferred by breastmilk that is related to the amount of breastmilk a baby receives—i.e., a dose response effect where exclusively breastfed infants benefit far more than infants who receive minimum amounts of breastmilk (Raisler, 1999).

Allowed to breastfeed at will in response to their own needs, infants generally obtain milk in amounts that satisfy their energy needs and maintain normal growth. Practical experience clearly supports the benefits of breastfeeding. In recent years, scientific data from all parts of the world confirm what the practitioner has long observed. It is ironic that many of the complex properties of human milk described in this chapter have been identified through research funded by formula companies, which stand to make large sums of money if they can develop products for which they can claim a close resemblance to human milk.

With the advent of managed care that rewards prevention of health problems and avoidance of using health services, health-care corporations look for cost-effective ways to keep their insured clients healthy. Studies discussed in Chapter 1 show additional billions of dollars in health-care costs for not breastfeeding

Human milk has a remarkable fitness in terms of the demands and needs of the infant. The configuration of elements in breastmilk are nutritional programming with a reciprocal fitness between the mother and the infant. In special cases, such as the accelerated energy needs of the premature infant, this adaptability is seen in the greater availability of energy in preterm milk. Human milk is a carrier of important physiological messages to the recipient infant.

Key Concepts

- Human milk—the gold standard for infant nutriment—has between 57 to 65 kcal per deciliter.

- Breastfed infants ingest less volume than formula-fed infants because human milk is more energy efficient.

- Babies do not usually remove all the milk available in the breast during a single feeding.

- Small amounts of colostrum are produced in the first day or two after delivery followed by rapid increases to about 500 ml at five days postpartum.

- Milk storage capacity differs among women. Women with larger breasts have a greater milk storage capacity and may breastfeed less often; women with small breasts may need to breastfeed more often; otherwise breast size does not affect the ability to breastfeed.

- Milk synthesis and volume differs between breasts.

- The nutritional status of a lactating mother has a minimal effect on milk volume unless she is malnourished.

- Multiparous women produce more breastmilk than primiparous women; mothers produce significantly more breastmilk with their second baby.

- Breastfed infants grow at about the same rate as those not breastfed for the first 3 to 4 months.

- Fat in human milk varies according to the degree to which the breast is emptied; high volume is associated with low milk fat content; accordingly, fat content progressively increases during a single feeding.

- Breastfeeding should be early and frequent; the longer the interval between feedings, the lower the fat content.

- The type of fat the mother eats affects the type of fatty acids present in her milk.

- Primary or congenital lactose deficiency or intolerance in infants is rare or nonexistent.

- Lactose in human milk supplies quick energy to the infant's rapidly growing brain.

- Human milk contains two main proteins: casein and whey. Casein is tough and less digestible curd; whey is soft and flocculent, and it digests rapidly.

- The amount of protein in colostrum is greater than that in mature milk because of the immune factors (IgA, lactoferrin) present in colostrum.

- Preterm mother's milk contains high levels of protein and fat compared with nonpreterm milk; thus using the milk of the preterm infant's mother is preferred.

- Generally speaking, human milk contains sufficient amounts of vitamins and minerals to meet the needs of full-term infants. Exceptions are premature infants and vitamin D supplementation for dark-skinned babies living in northern climates.

- Mineral content in human milk is fairly constant, tending to be highest right after birth and decreasing slightly throughout lactation.

- Healthy infants who consume enough breastmilk to satisfy their energy needs receive enough fluid to satisfy their requirements even in hot and dry environments.

- In the first 1 to 2 days after birth, the infant ingests small amounts, approximately 7 to 14 ml of colostrum at each feeding. Milk yield gradually increases for the first 36 hours, then rapidly increases. By day 5, volume is about 500 ml/day and 800 ml/day (range 550 and 1150) during months 1 and 6 of full breastfeeding.

- Immunity occurs actively and passively. Colostrum is densely packed with antibodies and immunoglobulins.

- Human milk contain two types of white cells: phagocytes and lymphocytes. Phagocytes (1) engulf and absorb pathogens and (2) release IgA. Lymphocytes (83 percent are T cells) protect an infant by destroying cell walls of viruses in a process called cell-mediated immunity.

- Antibodies are immunoglobulins that act against specific antigens or pathogens. Secretory IgA is the major immunoglobulin. Total sIgA remains relatively constant throughout lactation.

- SIgA passes from the mother's mucosa (intestinal, respiratory) to the mammary gland/breastmilk through lymphocyte traffic pathways (GALT and BALT).

- Immunity has a dose-response effect—i.e., the more breastmilk the infant ingests, the greater the immunity.

Internet Resources

CDC growth charts based on both breastfed and formula-fed infants: www.cdc.gov/growthcharts/

References

Aarts E, Kylberg A, Hornell A et al. How exclusive is breast-feeding? A comparison data since birth with current status data. *Int J Epidemiol* 29:1041–46, 2000.

Abrams SA, Wen H, Stuff JE. Absorption of calcium, zinc, and iron from breast milk by five to seven-month-old infants. *Pediatr Res* 39:384–90, 1996.

Abdulmoneim I, Al-Gamdi SA. Relationship between breastfeeding duration and acute respiratory infections in infant. *Saudi Med J* 22:347–50, 2001.

Adebonojo FO. Artificial vs. breast-feeding: relation to infant health in a middle class American community. *Clin Pediatr* 11:25–29, 1972.

Aksu M, Kultursay N, Ozkayin N, et al. Platelet-activating factor levels in term and pre-term milk. *Biol Neonate* 74:289–83, 1998.

Almroth S, Bidinger PD. No need for water supplementation for exclusively breast-fed infants under hot and arid conditions. *Trans Roy Soc Trop Med Hyg* 84:602–4, 1990.

Almroth SG, Latham MC. Breast feeding practices in rural Jamaica. *J Trop Pediatr* 28:103–9, 1982.

American Academy of Pediatrics, Committee on Nutrition. Commentary on breastfeeding and infant formulas, including standards for formulas. *Pediatrics* 57:278–85, 1976.

American Academy of Pediatrics, Work Group on Breastfeeding. Breastfeeding and the use of human milk. *Pediatrics* 100:1034–39, 1997.

Anderson CH. Human milk feeding. *Pediatr Clin No Amer* 32:335–52, 1985.

Anderson JW, Johnstone BM, Remley DT. Breastfeeding and cognitive development: a meta-analysis. *Am J Clin Nutr* 70:25–35, 1999.

Andon MB et al. Nutritionally relevant supplementation of vitamin B6 in lactating women: effect on plasma prolactin. *Pediatrics* 76:769–73, 1985.

Aniansson G et al. A prospective cohort study on breastfeeding and otitis media in Swedish infants. *Pediatr Infect Dis J* 13:183–88, 1994.

Anveden-Hertzberg L. Proctocolitis in exclusively breast-fed infants. *Eur J Pediatr* 155:464–67, 1996.

Arthur PG et al. Measuring short-term rates of milk synthesis in breast-feeding mothers. *Q J Exp Physiology* 47:419–28, 1989.

Arthur PG, Smith M, Hartmann PE. Milk lactose, citrate, and glucose as markers of lactogenesis in normal and diabetic women. *J Pediatr Gastroenterol Nutr* 9:488–96, 1989.

Ascher H et al. Influence of infant feeding and gluten intake on celiac disease. *Arch Dis Child* 76:113, 1997.

Ashraf RN et al. Breast feeding and protection against neonatal sepsis in a high risk population. *Arch Dis Child* 66:488–90, 1991.

Atkinson SA, Anderson G, Bryan MH. Human milk: comparison of the nitrogen composition of milk from mothers of premature infants. *Am J Clin Nutr* 33:811–15, 1980.

Atkinson SA et al. Abnormal zinc content in human milk: risk for development of nutritional zinc deficiency in infants. *Am J Dis Child* 143:608–11, 1989.

Auricchio S et al. Does breast feeding protect against the development of clinical symptoms of celiac disease in children? *J Pediatr Gastroenterol Nutr* 2:428–33, 1983.

Axelsson I et al. Bovine beta-lactoglobulin in the human milk. *Acta Pediatr Scand* 75:702, 1986.

Bachrach VR, Schwarz E, Bachrach LR. Breastfeeding and the risk of hospitalization for respiratory disease in infancy: a meta-analysis. *Arch Pediatr Adolesc Med* 157:237–43, 2003.

Bates CJ, Prentice A. Breast milk as a source of vitamins, essential minerals and trace elements. *Pharmacol Ther* 62:193–220, 1994.

Bauchner J, Levanthal JM, Shapiro ED. Studies of breastfeeding and infections: how good is the evidence? *JAMA* 256:887–92, 1986.

Baur LA et al. Relationships between the fatty acid composition of muscle and erythrocyte membrane phospholipid in young children and the effect of type of infant feeding. *Lipids* 35:77–82, 2000.

Bell LM et al. Rotavirus serotype-specific neutralizing activity in human milk. *Am J Dis Child* 142:275–78, 1988.

Bellig LL. Immunization and the prevention of childhood diseases. *J Obstet Gynecol Neonatal Nurs* 24:469–77, 1995.

Bener A, Kenic S, Galadari S. Longer breast-feeding and protection against childhood leukaemia and lymphomas. *European J Cancer* 37:234–38, 2001.

Bergstrand O, Hellers G. Breast-feeding during infancy in patients who develop Crohn's disease. *Scand J Gastroenterol* 18:903–6, 1983.

Bergstrom O et al. Serum lipid values in adolescents are related to family history, infant feeding, and physical growth. *Atherosclerosis* 17:1–13, 1995.

Blackberg LD et al. The bile salt stimulated lipase in human milk is an evolutionary newcomer derived from a non-milk protein. *FEBS Lett* 112:51, 1980.

Borch-Johnson K et al. Relation between breast-feeding and incidence rates of insulin-dependent diabetes mellitus. *Lancet* 2:1083–86, 1984.

Borgnolo G et al. A case-control study of Salmonella gastrointestinal infection in Italian children. *Acta Paediatr* 85:804–8, 1996.

Bottorff JL, Morse JM. Mother's perceptions of breast milk. *JOGN Nursing* 19:518–27, 1990.

Bouguerra F et al. Effect of breastfeeding relative to the age at onset of celiac disease. *Arch Pediatr* 5:621, 1998.

Brown KH et al. Lactational capacity of marginally nourished mothers: relationships between maternal nutritional status and quantity and proximate composition of milk. *Pediatrics* 78:909–19, 1986a.

Brown KH et al. Milk consumption and hydration status of exclusively breast-fed infants in a warm climate. *J Pediatr* 108:677–80, 1986b.

Brown KH et al. Infant-feeding practices and their relationship with diarrheal and other diseases in Huascar (Lima), Peru. *Pediatrics* 83:31–40, 1989.

Buescher ES, Pickering LK. Polymorphonuclear leukocytes in human colostrum and milk. In: Howell RR, Morriss

FH, Pickering LK, eds. *Human milk in infant nutrition and health.* Springfield, IL: Thomas, 1986:160–73.

Burr ML et al. Infant feeding, wheezing, and allergy: a prospective study. *Arch Dis Child* 68:724–28, 1993.

Butte NF, Smith EO, Garza C. Energy utilization of breast-fed and formula-fed infants. *Am J Clin Nutr* 51:350–58, 1990.

Butte NF et al. Macro- and trace-mineral intakes of exclusively breast-fed infants. *Am J Clin Nutr* 45:42–47, 1987.

Butte NF et al. Influence of early feeding mode on body composition of infants. *Biol Neonate* 67:414–24, 1995.

Butte NF et al. Energy requirements derived from total energy expenditure and energy deposition during the first 2 years of life. *Am J Clin Nutr* 72:1558–69, 2000.

Carpenter G. Epidermal growth factor is a major growth-promoting agent in human milk. *Science* 210:198–199, 1980.

Casey CE, Hambridge KM, Neville MC. Studies in human lactation: zinc, copper, manganese and chromium in human milk in the first month of lactation. *Am J Clin Nutr* 41:1193–200, 1985.

Casey CE, Neville MC, Hambridge KM. Studies in human lactation: secretion of zinc, copper, and manganese in human milk. *Am J Clin Nutr* 49:773–85, 1989.

Cavagni G et al. Passage of food antigens into circulation of breast-fed infants with atopic dermatitis. *Ann Allergy* 61:361–65, 1988.

Cavell B. Gastric emptying in infants fed human or infant formula. *Acta Paediatr Scand* 70:639–41, 1981.

Cesar JA, Victoria CG, Barros FC. Impact of breastfeeding on admission for pneumonia during postneonatal period in Brazil: Nested case-control study. *Br Med J* 318:1316–20, 1999.

Chandra RK. Prospective studies of the effect of breast-feeding on incidence of infection and allergy. *Acta Paediatr Scand* 68:691–94, 1979.

Chandra RK et al. Influence of maternal food antigen avoidance during pregnancy and lactation on incidence of atopic eczema in infants. *Clin Allergy* 16:563–69, 1986.

Chen Y, Yu S, Li W. Artificial feeding and hospitalization in the first 18 months of life. *Pediatrics* 81:58–62, 1988.

Chulada PC et al. Breast-feeding and the prevalence of asthma and wheeze in children: analyses from the third national health and nutrition examination survey, 1988-1994. *J Allergy Clin Immunol* 111:328–36, 2003.

Clavano NR. Mode of feeding and its effect on infant mortality and morbidity. *J Trop Pediatr* 28:287–93, 1982.

Cochi SL et al. Primary invasive *Haemophilus influenzae* type b disease: a population-based assessment of risk factors. *J Pediatr* 108:87–96, 1986.

Cohen RJ et al. Exclusively breastfed, low birthweight term infants do not need supplemental water. *Acta Paediatr* 89:550-52, 2000.

Corps AN et al. The insulin-like growth factor I content in human milk increases between early and full lactation. *J Clin Endocrinol Metab* 67(1):25–29, 1988.

Cosgrove M. Perinatal and infant nutrition: nucleotides. *Nutrition* 14:748, 1998.

Cox DB, Owens RA, Hartmann PE. Blood and milk prolactin and the rate of milk synthesis in women. *Exp Physiol* 81:1007–20, 1996.

Cregan M, Hartmann PE. Computerized breast measurement from conception to weaning: clinical implications. *J Hum Lact* 15:89–95, 1999.

Cregan MD, Mitoulas LR, Hartmann PE. Milk prolactin, feed volume, and duration between feeds in women breastfeeding their full-term infants over a 24-hour period. *Exp Physiol* 87:207–14, 2002.

Cushing AH et al. Breastfeeding reduces the risk of respiratory illness in infants. *Am J Epidemiol* 147:863–70, 1998.

Dai D et al. Role of oligosaccharides and glycoconjugates in intestinal host defense. *J Pediatr Gastroenterol Nutr* 30 (suppl):23, 2000.

Daly SE, Hartmann PE. Infant demand and milk supply. Part 1: Infant demand and milk production in lactating women. *J Hum Lact* 11:21–26, 1995a.

———. Infant demand and milk supply. Part 2: The short-term control of milk synthesis in lactating women. *J Hum Lact* 11: 27–36, 1995b.

Daly SE, Owens RA, Hartmann PE. The short-term synthesis and infant-regulated removal of milk in lactating women. *Exp Physiol* 78:209–20, 1993.

Daly SE et al. The determination of short-term breast volume changes and the rate of synthesis of human milk using computerized breast measurement. *Exp Physiol* 77:79–87, 1992.

Daly SE et al. Degree of breast emptying explains changes in the fat content, but not fatty acid composition of human milk. *Exp Physiol* 78:741–55, 1993.

Daniels JL et al. Breast-feeding and neuroblastoma, USA and Canada. *Cancer Causes Control* 13:401–5, 2002.

Davis MK. Review of the evidence for an association between infant feeding and childhood cancer. *Int J Cancer* S11:29–33, 1998.

Davis MK, Savitz DA, Graubard B. Infant feeding and childhood cancer. *Lancet* 2(8607):365–68, 1988.

de Araujo AN, Giagliano LG. Lactoferrin and free secretory component of human milk inhibits the adhesion of enteropathic *Escherichia coli* to HeLa cells. *BMC Microbiology* 1:25, 2001.

de Ferrer PA et al. Lactoferrin levels in term and preterm milk. *J Amer College Nutr* 19:370–73, 2000.

Dell S, To T. Breastfeeding and asthma in young children: findings from a population-based study. *Arch Pediatr Adolesc Med* 155:1261–65, 2001.

Dewey KG, Heinig J, Nommsen-Rivers LA. Differences in morbidity between breast-fed and formula-fed infants. *J Pediatr* 126(5):697–702, 1995.

Dewey KG, Lönnerdal B. Milk and nutrient intake of breast-fed infants from 1 to 6 months: relation to growth and fatness. *J Pediatr Gastroenterol Nutr* 2:497–506, 1983.

Dewey KG et al. Breast-fed infants are leaner than formula-fed infants at 1 year of age: the DARLING study. *Am J Clin Nutr* 57:140–45, 1993.

Dewey KG et al. Growth of breast-fed infants deviates from current reference data: a pooled analysis of US, Canadian, and European data sets. *Pediatrics* 96:495–503, 1995.

Dewey KG et al. Iron supplementation affects growth and morbidity of breast-fed infants: results of a randomized trial in Sweden and Honduras. *J Nutr* 132:3249–55, 2002.

Dorea JG. Iron and copper in human milk. *Nutrition* 16:209–20, 2000.

Downham MA et al. Breast-feeding protects against respiratory syncytial virus infection. *Br Med J* 2:274–76, 1976.

Duchen K, Yu G, Björkstén B. Polyunsaturated fatty acids in breast milk in relation to atopy in the mother and her child. *Int Arch Allergy Immunol* 118:321–23, 1999.

Duffy LC et al. The effects of infant feeding on rotavirus-induced gastroenteritis: a prospective study. *Am J Public Health* 76:259–63, 1986.

Duncan B et al. Iron and the exclusively breast-fed infant from birth to six months. *J Pediatr Gastroenterol Nutr* 4:412–25, 1985.

Duncan J et al. Exclusive breast-feeding for at least 4 months protects against otitis media. *Pediatrics* 91:867–72, 1993.

Erickson PR, Mazhari E. Investigation of the role of human breast milk in caries development. *Pediatr Dent* 21:86–90, 1999.

Espinoza E et al. Rotavirus infections in young Nicaraguan children. *Pediatr Infect Dis* 16: 564–71, 1997.

Evans GS, Johnson PE. Characterization and quantitation of a zinc-binding ligand and human milk. *Pediatr Res* 14:876–80, 1980.

Fallot MB et al. Breast-feeding reduces incidence of hospital admissions for infections in infants. *Pediatrics* 65:1121–24, 1980.

Fan H, Conner R, Villareal L. *The biology of AIDS*. Boston: Jones and Bartlett, 1989:28.

Fawzi WW et al. Maternal anthropometry and infant feeding practices in Israel in relation to growth in infancy: the North African Infant Feeding Study. *Am J Clin Nutr* 65:1731–37, 1997.

Feist N, Berger D, Speer CP. Anti-endotoxin antibodies in human milk: correlation with infection of the newborn. *Acta Paediatr* 89:1087–92, 2000.

Ford RPK et al. Breastfeeding and the risk of sudden infant death syndrome. *Int J Epidemiol* 22:885–90, 1993.

Forman MR et al. Undernutrition among Bedouin Arab infants: the Bedouin Infant Feeding Study. *Am J Clin Nutr* 51:339–43, 1990.

Frank AL et al. Breast-feeding and respiratory virus infection. *Pediatrics* 70:239–45, 1982.

Franke AA, Custer LJ, Tanaka Y. Isoflavones in human breast milk and other biological fluids. *Am J Clin Nutr* 68(suppl):1466S–73S, 1998.

Fuchs SC, Victor CG, Martines J. Case-control study of risk of dehydrating diarrhoea in infants in vulnerable period after full weaning. *BMJ* 313:391–94, 1996.

Furukawa SK et al. Fecal IgE in infants at 1 month of age as indicator of atopic disease. *Allergy* 49:791–94, 1994.

Garofalo RP, Goldman AS. Cytokines, chemokines, and colong-stimulating factors in human milk. *Biol Neonate* 74:134–42, 1998.

Garofalo RP, Goldman AS. Expression of functional immunomodulating and anti-inflammatory factors in human milk. *Clin Perinatol* 26:361, 1999.

Gartner LM, Greer FR. Prevention of rickets and vitamin D deficiency: new guidelines for vitamin D intake. *Pediatrics* 111(Part 1):908–10, 2003.

Garza C, Stuff J, Butte N. Growth of the breast-fed infant. In: Goldman AS, Atkinson SA, Hanson LA, eds. *Human lactation: the effects of human milk on the recipient infant*. New York: Plenum, 1986:109–21.

Garza C et al. Changes in the nutrient composition of human milk during gradual weaning. *Am J Clin Nutr* 37:61–65, 1983.

Garza C et al. Special properties of human milk. *Clin Perinatol* 14:11–31, 1987.

Gaull GE. Significance of growth modulators in human milk. *Pediatrics* 75(suppl):142–45, 1985.

Gdalevich M, Mimouni D, Mimouni M. Breast-feeding and the risk of bronchial asthma in childhood: a systematic review with meta-analysis of prospective studies. *J Pediatr* 139:261–66, 2001.

Gilbert RE et al. Bottle-feeding and the sudden infant death syndrome. *BMJ* 310:88–90, 1995.

Gimeno, SGA, de Suza JMP. IDDM and milk consumption. *Diabetes Care* 20:1256–60, 1997.

Glass RI, Stoll BJ. The protective effect of human milk against diarrhea: a review of studies from Bangladesh. *Acta Paediatr Scand* 351(suppl):131–36, 1989.

Goldman AS et al. Immunologic factors in human milk during the first year of lactation. *J Pediatr* 100:563–67, 1982.

Goldman AS et al. Immunologic components in human milk during gradual weaning. *Acta Paediatr Scand* 72:133–34, 1983.

Goldman AS et al. Anti-inflammatory properties of human milk. *Acta Paediatr Scand* 75:689–95, 1986.

Goldman AS et al. Cytokines in human milk: properties and potential effects upon the mammary gland and the neonate. *J. Mammary Gland Biol and Neoplasia* 1:251–58, 1996.

Grantham-McGregor SM, Back EH. Breast feeding in Kingston, Jamaica, *Arch Dis Child* 45:404–9, 1972.

Greco L et al. Case control study on nutritional risk factors in celiac disease. *J Pediar Gastroenterol Nutr* 7:395–99, 1983.

Greer FR. Vitamin K status of lactating mothers and their infants. *Acta Paediatr* 88(suppl):95, 1999.

Greer FR Marshall S. Bone mineral content, serum vitamin D metabolite concentrations and ultraviolet B light exposure in infants fed human milk with and without vitamin D2 supplements. *J Pediatr* 114:204–12, 1989.

Groer MW, Humenick S, Hill P. Characterizations and psychoneuroimmunolgic implications of secretory immunoglobulin A and cortisol in preterm and term breast milk. *J Perinat Neonatal Nurse* 7(4):42–51, 1994.

Gulick EE. The effect of breast-feeding on toddler health. *Pediatr Nurs* 12:51–54, 1986.

Guthrie HA, Picciano MF, Sheehe D. Fatty acid patterns of human milk. *J Pediatr* 90:39–41, 1977.

Gyorgy P. A hitherto unrecognized biochemical difference between human milk and cow's milk. *Pediatrics* 11:98–104, 1953.

Habbick BF, Kahnna C, To T. Infantile hypertropic pyloric stenosis: a study of feeding practices and other possible causes. *Can Med Assoc J* 140:401–4, 1989.

Habicht JP, DaVanso J, Butz WP. Mother's milk and sewage: their interactive effects on infant mortality. *Pediatrics* 81:456–60, 1988.

Hakansson A, Svensson M, Mossberg A-K et al. A folding variant of α-lactalbumin with bactericidal activity against *Streptococcus pneumoniae*. *Molec Microbiol* 35(3):589–600, 2000.

Hakansson A et al. Apoptosis induced by a human protein. *Proc Natl Acad Sci* 92:8064, 1995.

Hamosh M. Human milk. Digestion in the neonate. *Clin Perinatol* 23:191, 1996.

Hamosh M. Boactive factors in human milk. In: Schanler, RJ *The evidence for breastfeeding*. ed. Breastfeeding 2001, Part I. *Ped Clin N Amer* 48:69–86, 2001.

Hamosh M et al. Digestive enzymes in human milk: stability at suboptimal storage temperatures. *J Pediatr Gastroenterol Nutr* 24:38–43, 1997.

Hartmann PE. Lactation and reproduction in Western Australian women. *J Reprod Med* 32:543–57, 1987.

Hartmann PE, Cregan M. Lactogenesis and the effects of insulin-dependent diabetes mellitus and prematurity. *J Nutrition* 131:3016S–20S, 2001.

Hartmann PE, Prosser CG. Physiological basis of longitudinal changes in human milk yield and composition. *Fed Proc* 43:2448–53, 1984.

Hashizume S, Kuroda K, Murakami H. Identification of lactoferrin as an essential growth factor for human lymphocytic cell lines in serum-free medium. *Biochem Biophys Acta* 763:377, 1983.

Hasselbalch H et al. Breastfeeding influences thymic size in late infancy. *Eur J Pediatr* 158:964–67, 1999.

Hawkes JS, Gibson RA. Lymphocyte subpopulations in breast-fed and formula-fed infants at six months of age. *Adv Exp Med Biol* 501:497–504, 2001.

Heacock H et al. Influence of breast versus formula milk on physiological gastroesophageal reflux in healthy, newborn infants. *J Pediatr Gastroenterol* 14:41–46, 1992.

Heinig J, Dewey KG. Health advantages of breast feeding for infants: a critical review. *Nutr Res Rev* 9:89–110, 1996.

Heird WC, Schward SM, Hansen IH. Colostrum-induced enteric mucosal growth in beagle puppies. *Pediatr Res* 18:512, 1984.

Hildebrandt HM. Maternal perception of lactogenesis time: A clinical report. *J Hum Lact* 15(4):317–23, 1999.

Holberg CJ et al. Risk factors for respiratory syncytial virus-associated lower respiratory illnesses in the first year of life. *Am J Epidemiol* 133:1135–51, 1991.

Host A, Husby S, Osterballe O. A prospective study of cow's milk allergy in exclusively breast-fed infants. *Acta Paediatr Scand* 77:663–70, 1988.

Houston MJ, Howie PW, McNeilly AS. Factors affecting the duration of breast feeding: 1. Measurement of breast milk intake in the first week of life. *Early Hum Dev* 8:49–54, 1983.

Howie PW et al. Protective effect of breast feeding against infection. *Br Med J* 300:11–16, 1990.

Humenick SS. The clinical significance of breastmilk maturation rates. *Birth* 14(4):174–79, 1987.

Humenick SS et al. The maturation index of colostrum and milk (MICAM): a measurement of breast milk maturation. *J Nurs Measurement* 2:16–86, 1994.

Hylander MA et al. Association of human milk feedings with a reduction in retinopathy of prematurity among very low birth weight infants. *Jr Perinatology* 21:356–62, 2001.

Ingram JC, Woolridge MS, Greenwood RJ. Breastfeeding: It is worth trying with the second baby. *Lancet* 358:986-87, 2001.

Istre GR et al. Risk factors for primary *Haemophilus influenzae* disease: increased risk from day care attendance and school-aged household members. *J Pediatr* 106:190–95, 1985.

Ivarsson A et al. Epidemic of celiac disease in Swedish children. *Acta Pediatr* 89:165, 2000.

Jason JM, Niebury P, Marks JS. Mortality and infectious disease associated with infant-feeding practices in developing countries. *Pediatrics* 74(suppl):702–27, 1984.

Jenkins HR et al. Food allergy: the major cause of infantile colitis. *Arch Dis Child* 59:326–29, 1984.

Jensen RG. Lipids in human milk. *Lipids* 34:1243, 1999.

Jensen RG et al. Human milk as a carrier of messages to the nursing infant. *Nutr Today* 23:20–25, 1988.

Juex G et al. Growth pattern of selected urban Chilean infants during exclusive breast feeding. *Am J Clin Nutr* 38:462–68, 1983.

Kassim OO et al. Inhibitory factors in breast milk, maternal and infant sera against in vitro growth of *Plasmodium falciparum* malaria parasite. *J Trop Pediatr* 46:92–96, 2000.

Kelleher SL, Lönnerdal B. Immunological activities associated with milk. *Adv Nutr Res* 10:39–65, 2001.

Keller MA et al. IgAG₄ in human colostrum and human milk: continued local production or selective transport form serum. *Acta Paediatr Scand* 77:24–29, 1988.

Kelly DW et al. Rise and fall of coeliac disease 1960–1985. *Arch Dis Child* 64:1157–60, 1989.

Khin-Maung-U J et al. Effect of clinical outcome of breast-feeding during acute diarrhea. *Br Med J* 290:587–89, 1985.

Kirkpatrick CH et al. Inhibition of growth of *Candida albicans* by iron-unsaturated lactoferrin: relation to host defense mechanisms in chronic mucocutaneous candidiasis. *J Infect Dis* 124:539, 1971.

Kohler H et al. Antibacterial characteristics in the feces of breast-fed and formula-fed infants during the first year of life. *J Pediatr Gastroenterol Nutr* 34:188–93, 2002.

Koletzko B, Rodriquez-Palmero M. Polyunsaturated fatty acids in human milk and their role in early human development. *J Mammary Gland Biol Neoplasia* 4:269, 1999.

Koletzko S et al. Role of infant feeding practices in development of Crohn's disease in childhood. *Br Med J* 298:1617–18, 1989.

Koopman JS et al. Infant formulas and gastrointestinal illness. *Am J Public Health* 75:477–80, 1985.

Kostraba JN et al. Early exposure to cow's milk and solid foods in infancy, genetic predisposition and risk of IDDM. *Diabetes* 42:288–95, 1993.

Kovar MG et al. Review of the epidemiologic evidence for an association between infant feeding and infant health. *Pediatrics* 74(suppl):615–38, 1984.

Krachler M, Rossipal SE, Irgolic KJ. Changes in the concentrations of trace elements in human milk during lactation. *J Trace Elements Biol* 12:159–76, 1998.

Kramer MS. Infant feeding, infection, and public health. *Pediatrics* 81:164–66, 1988.

Kramer MS et al. Promotion of breastfeeding intervention trial (PROBIT): A randomized trial in the Republic of Belarus. *JAMA* 285:413–20, 2001.

Kramer MS et al. Breastfeeding and infant growth: biology or bias? *Pediatrics* 110:343–47, 2002.

Krebs NF, Hambidge KM. Zinc requirements and zinc intakes of breast-fed infants. *Am J Clin Nutr* 43:288–92, 1986.

Krebs NF et al. Zinc homeostasis in breast-fed infant. *Pediatr Res* 39:661–65, 1996.

Kulski JK, Hartmann PE. Changes in the concentration of cortisol in milk during different stages of human lactation. *Aust J Exp Biol Med Sci* 59:769, 1981.

Kum-Nji et al. Reducing the incidence of Sudden Infant Death Syndrome in the delta region of Mississippi: a three-pronged approach. *South Med J* 94:704–10, 2001.

Kumpulainen J et al. Formula feeding results in lower selenium status than breast-feeding or selenium-supplemented formula feeding: a longitudinal study. *Am J Clin Nutr* 45:49–53, 1987.

Kunz C, Lönnerdal B. Re-evaluation of the whey protein/casein ratio of human milk. *Acta Paediatr* 81:107–12, 1992.

Labbok M, Hendershot GE. Does breast-feeding protect against malocclusion? An analysis of the 1981 Child Health Supplement to the National Health Interview survey. *Am J Priv Med* 3:227–32, 1987.

Latarte J et al. Lack of protective effect of breast-feeding in congenital hypothyroidism: report of 12 cases. *Pediatrics* 65:703–5, 1980.

Leach JL et al. Total potentially available nucleotides of human milk by stage of lactation. *Am J Clin Nutr* 61:1224–30, 1995.

Lemons JA et al. Differences in the composition of preterm and term human milk during early lactation. *Pediatr Res* 16:113–17, 1982.

Lepage G et al. The composition of preterm milk in relation to the degree of prematurity. *Am J Clin Nutr* 40:1042–49, 1984.

Leventhal JM et al. Does breastfeeding protect against infection in infants less than 3 months of age? *Pediatrics* 78:896–903, 1986.

Litwin SD, Zehr BD, Insel RA. Selective concentration of IgD class-specific antibodies in human milk. *Clin Exp Immunol* 80:262–67, 1990.

Long K et al. The impact of infant feeding patterns on infection and diarrheal disease due to *Enterotoxigenic Escherichia coli. Salud Publica Mex* 41:263–70, 1999.

Lönnerdal B. Regulation of mineral and trace elements in human milk: exogenous and endogenous factors, *Nutr Review* 58:223–29, 2000.

Lopez-Alarcon M, Villalpando S, Fajardo A. Breast-feeding lowers the frequency and duration of acute respiratory infection and diarrhea in infants under six months of age. *J Nutr* 127:436–43, 1997.

Lovegrove JA, Hampton SM, Morgan JB. The immunological and long-term atopic outcome of infants born to women following a milk-free diet during late pregnancy and lactation: a pilot study. *Br J Nutr* 71:223–38, 1994.

Lucas A. Programming by early nutrition: an experimental approach. *J Nutr* 128:401S–406S, 1998.

Lucas A, Cole TJ. Breast milk and neonatal necrotizing enterocolitis. *Lancet* 336:1519–23, 1990.

Lucas A, Mitchell MD. Prostaglandins in human milk. *Arch Dis Child* 55:950, 1980.

Lucas A et al. Breastfeeding and catch-up growth in infants born small for gestational age. *Acta Paediatr* 86:564–69, 1997.

Mackey AD, Picciano MF. Maternal folate status during extended lactation and the effect of supplemental folic acid. *Am J Clin Nutr* 69:285, 1999.

Marchini G, Linden A. Cholecystokinin, a satiety signal in newborn infants? *J Dev Physiol* 17:215–19, 1992.

Marild S et al. Breastfeeding and urinary tract infection [letter]. *Lancet* 336(8720):942, 1990.

Mason T et al. Breast feeding and the development of juvenile rheumatoid arthritis. *J Rheumatol* 22:1166–70, 1995.

Mathur GP et al. Breastfeeding and childhood cancer. *Indian Pediatr* 30:651–57, 1993.

Matsuoka Y, Idota T. The concentration of epidermal growth factor in Japanese mother's milk. *J Nutr Sci Vitaminol* 41:24–51, 1995.

Mayer EJ et al. Reduced risk of IDDM among breast-fed children. *Diabetes* 37:1625–32, 1988.

McVeagh P, Miller JB. Human milk oligosaccharides: only the breast. *J Paediatr Child Health* 33:281–86, 1997.

Medves JM. Three infant care interventions: reconsidering the evidence. *JOGNN* 31:563–69, 2002.

Metcalfe DD. Food hypersensitivity. *J Allergy Clin Immunol* 73:749–62, 1984.

Michie et al. Physiological secretion of chemokines in human breast milk. *Eur Cytokine Netw* 9:123–29, 1998.

Mitra AK, Rabbani F. The importance of breastfeeding in minimizing mortality and morbidity from diarrhoeal diseases: the Bangladesh perspective. *J Diarrhoeal Dis Res* 13(1):1–7, 1995.

Montgomery RK et al. Lactose intolerance and the genetic regulation of intestinal lactose-phlorizin hydrolase. *Federation of American Societies for Experimental Biology J* 5:2824–32, 1991.

Morriss FH. Method for investigating the presence and physiologic role of growth factors in milk. In: Jensen RG, Neville MC, eds. *Human lactation: milk components and methodologies.* New York: Plenum, 1985:193–200.

Morriss FH et al. Relationship of human milk pH during course of lactation to concentrations of citrate and fatty acids. *Pediatrics* 78:458–64, 1986.

Morrisset J, Jolicoeur L. Effect of hydrocortisone on pancreatic growth in rats. *Am J Physiol* 239:295, 1980.

Morton JA. The clinical usefulness of breast milk sodium in the assessment of lactogenesis. *Pediatrics* 93:802–6, 1994.

Motil, KJ, Krtz B, Thotathuchery M. Lactation performance of adolescent mothers show preliminary differences from that of adult women. *J Adolescent Med* 20:442–49, 1997.

Motil KJ et al. Human milk protein does not limit growth of breast-fed infants. *J Pediatr Gastroenterol Nutr* 24:10–17, 1997.

Naficy AB et al. Epidemiology of rotavirus diarrhea in Egyptian children and implications for disease control. *Am J Epidemiol* 150:770–77, 1999.

Neville MC. Lactogenesis. In: Schanler RJ, ed. Breastfeeding 2001, Part I. *The evidence for breastfeeding. Ped Clin N Amer* 48 69–86, 2001.

Neville MC, Oliva-Rasbach J. Is maternal milk production limiting for infant growth during the first year of life in breast-fed infants? In: Goldman AS, Atkinson SA, Hanson LA, eds. *Human lactation. Vol. 3. The effects of human milk on the recipient infant.* New York: Plenum, 1987: 123–33.

Neville MC et al. Studies in human lactation: milk volumes in lactating women during the onset of lactation and full lactation. *Am J Clin Nutr* 48:1375–86, 1988.

Newburg DS et al. Role of human-milk lactadherin in protection against symptomatic rotavirus infection. *Lancet* 351:1160, 1998.

Newman J. How breast milk protects newborns. *Scientific American.* December 1995:76–79.

Nommsen L. The long-term effects of early nutrition: the role of breastfeeding on cholesterol levels. *J Hum Lact* 19:103–4, 2003.

Oddy WH. Breastfeeding and asthma in children: findings from a West Australian study. *Breastfeeding Rev* 8(1):5–11, 2000.

Odze RD et al. Allergic colitis in infants. *J Pediatr* 126:163–70, 1995.

Okamoto Y, Ogra P. Antiviral factors in human milk: implications in respiratory syncytial virus infection. *Acta Paediatr Scand* 351(suppl):137–43, 1989.

Ostrea EM et al. Influence of breast-feeding on the restoration of the low serum concentration of vitamin E and beta-carotene in the newborn infant. *Am J Obstet Gyncecol* 154:1014–17, 1986.

Owen CD et al. Infant feeding and blood cholesterol: a study in adolescents and a systematic review. *Pediatrics* 110:597–608, 2002.

Pabst HE et al. Differential modulation of the immune response to breast- or formula-feeding of infants. *Acta Paediatr* 86:1291-97, 1997.

Paganelli R, Cavagni G, Pallone F. The role of antigenic absorption and circulating immune complexes in food allergy. *Ann Allergy* 57:330–36, 1986.

Palmer B. The influence of breastfeeding on the development of the oral cavity: a commentary. *J Hum Lact* 14:93–99, 1998.

Perera BJ et al. The impact of breastfeeding practices on respiratory and diarrhoeal disease in infants: a study from Sri Lanka. *J Trop Pediatr* 45(2):115–18, 1999.

Perez-Bravolt F et al. Genetic predisposition and environmental factors leading to the development of insulin-dependent diabetes mellitus in Chilean children. *J Mol Med* 74:105–9, 1996.

Petschow B et al. Influence of orally administered epidermal growth factor on normal and damaged intestinal mucosa in rats. *J Pediatr Gastroenterol Nutr* 17:49–57, 1993.

Picciano MF. Nutrient composition of human milk. In: Schanler RJ, ed. Breastfeeding 2001, Part I. *The evidence for breastfeeding. Ped Clin N Amer* 48:69–86, 2001.

Pickering LK, Kohl S. Human milk humoral immunity and infant defense mechanisms. In: Howell RR, Morriss FH, Pickering LK, eds. *Human milk in infant nutrition and health.* Springfield, IL: Thomas, 1986:123–40.

Pisacane A et al. Breast feeding and urinary tract infection. *Lancet* 336:50, 1990.

Pisacane A et al. Breast feeding and multiple sclerosis. *Br Med J* 308:1411–12, 1994.

Pisacane A et al. Breast-feeding and inguinal hernia. *J Pediatr* 127:109–11, 1995a.

Pisacane A et al. Breast feeding and acute appendicitis. *BMJ* 310:836–37, 1995b.

Popkin BM et al. Breast-feeding and diarrheal morbidity. *Pediatrics* 86:874–82, 1990.

Porro E et al. Early wheezing and breast feeding. *Asthma* 30:23–28, 1993.

Prentice AM, Collinson AC. Does breastfeeding increase thymus size? *Acta Paediatr* 89:8–10, 2000.

Prentice AM et al. Breast-milk antimicrobial factors of rural Gambian mothers. *Acta Paediatr Scand* 73:796–812, 1984.

Prosser CG, Saint L, Hartmann PE. Mammary gland function during gradual weaning and early gestation in women. *Aust J Exp Biol Med Sci* 62:215–28, 1984.

Pullan CR et al. Breast-feeding and respiratory syncytial virus infection. *Br Med J* 281(6247):1034–36, 1980.

Quinlan PT et al. The relationship between stool hardness and stool composition in breast- and formula-fed infants. *J Pediatr Gastroenterol Nutr* 20:81–90, 1995.

Rahman MM et al. Local production of rotavirus specific IgA in breast tissue and transfer to neonates. *Arch Dis Child* 62:401–5, 1987.

Raiha NCR. Nutritional proteins in milk and the protein requirement of normal infants. *Pediatrics* 75(suppl):136–41, 1985.

Raisler J, Alexander C, Campo P. Breastfeeding and infant illness: a dose-response relationship? *Am J Public Health* 89(1):25–30, 1999.

Ravelli A et al. Infant feeding and adult glucose tolerance, lipid profile, blood pressure, and obesity. *Arch Dis Child* 82:248–52, 2000.

Ravelomanana N et al. Risk factors for fatal diarrhoea among dehydrated malnourished children in a Madagascar hospital. *Eur J Clin Nutr* 49:91–97, 1995.

Read L et al. Changes in the growth-promoting activity of human milk during lactation. *Pediatr Res* 18:133–38, 1984.

Reid B, Smith H, Friedman Z. Prostaglandins in human milk. *Pediatrics* 66:870–72, 1980.

Rigas A et al. Breast-feeding and maternal smoking in the etiology of Crohn's disease and ulcerative colitis in childhood. *Ann Epidemiol* 3:387–92, 1993.

Rosenberg M. Breast-feeding and infant mortality in Norway 1860–1930. *J Biosoc Sci* 21:335–48, 1989.

Rovet JF. Does breast-feeding protect the hypothyroid infant whose condition is diagnosed by newborn screening? *Am J Dis Child* 144:319–23, 1990.

Rubaltelli FR et al. Intestinal flora in breast- and bottle-fed infants. *J Perinat Med* 26:186–91, 1998.

Rudloff EH et al. Interleukin-6 in human milk. *J Reprod Immunol* 23:13–20, 1993.

Ruiz-Palacios GM et al. Protection of breast-fed infants against *Campylobacter diarrhea* by antibodies in human milk. *J Pediatr* 116:707–13, 1990.

Ruuska R. Occurrence of acute diarrhea in atopic and nonatopic infant: the role of prolonged breast-feeding. *J Pediatr Gastroenterol Nutr* 14:27–33, 1992.

Saarinen KM et al. Breast-feeding and the development of cow's milk protein allergy. *Adv Exp Med Biol* 478:121–30, 2000.

Saarinen UM, Kajosaari M. Breastfeeding as prophylaxis against atopic disease: prospective follow-up study until 17 years old. *Lancet* 346:1065–69, 1995.

Saarinen UM et al. Prolonged breast feeding as prophylaxis for recurrent otitis media. *Acta Paediatr Scand* 71:567–71, 1982.

Saint L, Smith M, Hartmann PE. The yield and nutrient content of colostrum and milk of women giving birth to 1 month postpartum. *Br J Nutr* 52:87–95, 1984.

Salmenpera L et al. Folate nutrition is optimal in exclusively breast-fed infants but inadequate in some of their mothers and in formula-fed infants. *J Pediatr Gastroenterol Nutr* 5:283–89, 1986.

SanGiovanni JP et al. Meta-analysis of dietary essential acuity in healthy preterm infants. *Pediatrics* 105:1292–98, 2000.

Sassen ML, Brand R, Grote JJ. Breast-feeding and acute otitis media. *Amer J Otolaryngol* 15:351–57, 1994.

Schroten H et al. Secretory immunoglobulin A is a component of the human milk fat globule membrane. *Pediatr Res* 45:82–86, 1999.

Serdula MK, Seward J, Marks JS. Seasonal differences in breast-feeding in rural Egypt. *Am J Clin Nutr* 44:405–9, 1986.

Shehadeh N et al. Importance of insulin content in infant diet: suggestion for a new infant formula. *Acta Paediatr* 90:93–95, 2001.

Shing YW, Klagsburn M. Human and bovine milk contain different sets of growth factors. *Endocrinology* 115:273, 1984.

Shu XO et al. Infant breastfeeding and the risk of childhood lymphoma and leukaemia. *Int J Epidemiol* 24:27–34, 1995.

Siigur U, Ormission A, Tamm A. Faecal short-chain fatty acids in breast-fed and bottle-fed infants. *Acta Paediatr* 82:536–38, 1993.

Siimes MA et al. Exclusive breast-feeding for nine months: risk of iron deficiency. *J Pediatr* 104:196–99, 1984.

Silfverdal SA et al. Protective effect of breastfeeding on invasive *Haemophilus influenzae* infection: a case-control study in Swedish preschool children. *Int Epidemiol* 26:443–50, 1997.

Smith AM, Picciano MF, Milner JA. Selenium intakes and status of human milk and formula fed infants. *Am J Clin Nutr* 35:521, 1982.

Smulevich et al. Parental occupation and other factors and cancer risk in children: 1. Study methodology and non-occupational factors. *Int J Cancer* 83:712, 1999.

Sommerburg O et al. Carotenoid supply in breast-fed and formula-fed neonates. *Eur J Pediatr* 159:86–90, 2000.

Specker BL et al. Sunshine exposure and serum 25-hydroxyvitamin D concentrations in exclusively breast-fed infant. *J Pediatr* 107:372–76, 1985.

Steichen JJ, Krug-Wispe SK, Tsang RC. Breastfeeding the low birth weight preterm infant. *Clin Perinatol* 14:131–71, 1987.

Steel MG, Leslie GA. Immunoglobulin D in rat serum, saliva and milk. *Immunology* 55:571–77, 1985.

Stuff JE, Nichols GL. Nutrient intake and growth performance of older infants fed human milk. *J Pediatr* 115:959–68, 1989.

Swartzbaum JA et al. An exploratory study of environmental and medical factors potentially related to childhood cancer. *Med Pediatr Oncol* 19:115–21, 1991.

Svanborg C et al. HAMLET fills tumor cells by an apoptosis-like mechanism—cellular, molecular, and therapeutic aspects. *Adv Cancer Res* 8:1–29, 2003.

Takahata Y et al. Interleukin-18 in human milk. *Pediatr Res* 50:268–72, 2001.

Takala AK et al. Risk factors of invasive *Haemophilus influenzae* type b disease among children in Finland. *J Pediatr* 115:694–701, 1989.

Tran TT et al. Effects of neonatal dietary manganese exposure on brain dopamine levels and neurocognitive functions. *Neurotoxicology* 145:1–7, 2002.

Udall JN et al. Liver disease in a1-antitrypsin deficiency. *JAMA* 253:2679–82, 1985.

US Department of Health and Human Services. *Healthy people 2010*. Washington, DC, 2000.

Uvnas-Moberg K, Marchini G, Windberg J. Plasma cholecystokinin concentrations after breastfeeding in healthy 4 day old infants. *Arch Dis Child* 68:46–48, 1993.

Van Derslice J, Popkin B, Briscoe J. Drinking-water quality, sanitation, and breast-feeding: their interactive effects on infant health. *Bull WHO* 72(4):589–601, 1994.

van der Westhuyzen, Chetty M, Atkinson PM. Fatty acid composition of human milk from South African black mother consuming a traditional maize diet. *Eur J Clin Nutr* 42:213–20, 1988.

Verge CF et al. Environmental factors in childhood IDDM: a population-based case-control study. *Diabetes Care* 17:1381, 1994.

Victora CG et al. Evidence for protection by breastfeeding against infant deaths from infectious diseases in Brazil. *Lancet* 2(8554):319–21, 1987.

Virtanen SM, Rasanen L, Aro A et al. childhood diabetes in Finland Study Group: feeding in infancy and the risk of type 1 diabetes mellitus in Finnish children. *Diabet Med* 9:815, 1992.

Wagner V, Stockhausen JG. The effect of feeding human milk and adapted milk formulae on serum lipid and lipoprotein levels in young infants. *Eur J Pediatr* 147:292–95, 1988.

Wallace JM et al. Cytokines in human milk. *Br J Biomed Sci* 54:85–87, 1997.

Wasmuth HE, Kolb H. Cow's milk and immune-mediated diabetes. *Proc Nutr Sco* 59:573–79, 2000.

Widdowson EM, Colombo VE, Artavanis CA. Changes in the organs of pigs in response to feeding for the first 24 hours after birth: II. The digestive tract. *Biol Neonate* 28:272, 1976.

Wight NE. Donor human milk for preterm infants. *J. Perinatol* 21:249–54, 2001.

Wilson AC et al. Relation of infant diet to childhood health: seven year follow-up of cohort of children in Dundee infant feeding study. *BMJ* 316(7124):21–25, 1998.

Wilson JV, Self TW, Hamburger R. Severe cow's milk induced colitis in an exclusively breast-fed neonate. *Clin Pediatr* 29:77–80, 1990.

Wirt DP et al. Activated and memory T lymphocytes in human milk. *Cytometry* 13:282–90, 1992.

Wood CS et al. Exclusively breast-fed infants: growth and caloric intake. *Pediatr Nurs* 14(2):117–24, 1988.

Woolridge MW, Fisher C. Colic, "overfeeding," and symptoms of lactose malabsorption in the breast-fed baby: a possible artifact of feed management? *Lancet* 2:382–84, 1988.

Woolridge MW, Ingram JC, Baum JD. Do changes in pattern of breast usage alter the baby's nutrient intake? *Lancet* 336:395–97, 1990.

Yamauchi Y, Yamanouchi I. Breast-feeding frequency during the first 24 hours after birth in full-term neonates. *Pediatrics* 86:171–75, 1990.

Yoneyama K, Nagata H, Asano H. Growth of Japanese breast-fed and bottle-fed infants from birth to 20 months. *Ann Hum Biol* 21:597–608, 1994.

Zaman K et al. Children's fluid intake during diarrhoea: a comparison of questionnaire responses with data from observations. *Acta Paediatr* 91:376–82, 2002.

Zanardo V et al. Beta endorphin concentrations in human milk. *J Pediatr Gastroenterol Nutr* 33:160–64, 2001.

Appendix 4–A

COMPOSITION OF HUMAN COLOSTRUM AND MATURE BREASTMILK

Constituent (per 100 mL)	Colostrum 1–5 days	Mature Milk > 30 days	Constituent (per 100 mL)	Colostrum 1–5 days	Mature Milk > 30 days
Energy, kcal	58	70	**Vitamins (Water Soluble)**		
Lactose, g	5.3	7.3	Thiamine, µg	15	16
Total nitrogen, mg	360	171	Riboflavin, µg	25	35
Protein nitrogen, mg	313	129	Niacin, µg	75	200
Nonprotein nitrogen, mg	47	42	Folic acid, µg	—	5.2
Total protein, g	2.3	0.9	Vitamin B_6, µg	12	28
Casein, mg	140	187	Vitamin B_{12}, ng	200	26
α-lactalbumin, mg	218	161	Vitamin C, mg	4.4	4.0
Lactoferrin, mg	330	167	**Minerals and Trace Elements**		
IgA, mg	364	142	Calcium, mg	23	28
Urea, mg	10	30	Sodium, mg	48	15
Creatine, mg	—	3.3	Potassium, mg	74	58
Total fat, g	2.9	4.2	Iron, µg	45	40
Cholesterol, mg	27	16	Zinc, µg	540	166
Vitamins (Fat Soluble)					
Vitamin A, µg	89	47			
Beta-carotene, µg	112	23			
Vitamin D, µg	—	0.04			
Vitamin E, µg	1280	315			
Vitamin K, µg	0.2	0.21			

Source: From Casey CE, Hambridge KM. Nutritional aspects of human lactation. In: Neville MC, Neifert MR, eds. *Lactation: physiology, nutrition and breastfeeding.* New York: Plenum 1983:203–4.

DRUG THERAPY AND BREASTFEEDING

Thomas W. Hale

The nutritional and immunologic benefits of human milk are now well known and many national and international health organizations strongly recommend the breastfeeding of infants (Work Group on Breastfeeding, 1997). Key benefits to the infant include perfect nutrition, enhanced neurocognitive development, stronger immune function, and significant reductions in various syndromes such as upper respiratory infections, otitis media, sudden infant death syndrome, and necrotizing enterocolitis (Cochi et al., 1986a, 1986b; Ford et al., 1993; Goldman, 1993; Goldman et al., 1994; Pisacane et al., 1992).

Although recent studies have suggested that the number of women who choose to breastfeed their infant is rising, the number of women who discontinue breastfeeding in order to take a medication is simply too high. Surveys in Western countries indicate that 90–99 percent of women who breastfeed will receive a medication during the first week postpartum (Bennett, 1996). Another study of Scandinavian women suggests that medication use is a major reason for mothers to discontinue breastfeeding, and that 17–25 percent of breastfeeding women had taken a medication during the prior 2 weeks (Matheson, Kristensen, & Lunde, 1990). The most frequently used drugs included analgesics, hypnotics, and methylergometrine (Matheson, 1985).

Without exception almost all breastfeeding mothers will take a medication, so it is not at all surprising that one of the most common questions asked of health-care professionals concerns drugs and breastfeeding. Far too often clinicians recommend discontinuing breastfeeding while a mother is using a medication simply because they do not know if it is safe. Unfortunately, discontinuing breastfeeding is often the wrong decision and most mothers could easily continue to breastfeed their infants and take the medication without risk to the infant. However, the risk of taking a medication is not always clear. New medications are introduced into this field almost daily, and it is therefore difficult to cull the safe from the hazardous among these newer products.

We do know that certain pharmacokinetic parameters can be used to help distinguish between safe and unsafe medications. Certainly the most useful data available would be a study reporting the amount of drug that enters milk, but with new medications this is seldom available. Therefore the health-care practitioner must use available tools to evaluate the overall risk to the infant.

The following review is designed to aid readers in their evaluation of medications in breastfeeding mothers and to distinguish between hazardous and safe medications and to provide some techniques that consultants can use to evaluate the mother's situation and determine the true risk to the infant from the medication. Lactation risk categories (see Box 5–1), a tool for determining possible risks associated with taking a medication while breastfeeding is used throughout this chapter.

The Alveolar Subunit

The parenchyma of the breast consists of approximately 10 to 15 ductal regions, which ultimately drain toward the nipple (Figure 5–1). As the ducts course through the mammary fat and as progestins,

estrogens, and placental lactogen rise during pregnancy, the terminal duct lobular units undergo a dynamic change such that each lobular unit ultimately resembles a large bunch of grapes (Neville & Morton, 2001). The alveolar subunit is lined with a specialized epithelial cell called the *lactocyte*. The entire alveolar subunit is thoroughly perfused with capillaries and lymphatics and is innervated with small nerves. Closely juxtaposed with the basal membrane of the alveolus are numerous capillaries that are the primary source of immunoglobulins, fats, and many other components (including drugs) needed for the production of human milk. During pregnancy, the size and number of alveolar complexes increase significantly, due to the high level of maternal estrogen, progesterone, placental lactogen, prolactin, and oxytocin, all of which act

---

BOX 5–1

Lactation Risk Category Descriptions

- **L1 Safest:** Drug that has been taken by a large number of breastfeeding mothers without any observed increase in adverse effects in the infant. Controlled studies in breastfeeding women fail to demonstrate a risk to the infant and the possibility of harm to the breastfeeding infant is remote; or the product is not orally bioavailable in an infant.

- **L2 Safer:** Drug that has been studied in a limited number of breastfeeding woman without an increase in adverse effects in the infant. And/or, the evidence of a demonstrated risk that is likely to follow use of this medication in a breastfeeding woman is remote.

- **L3 Moderately Safe:** There are no controlled studies in breastfeeding women; however, the risk of untoward effects to a breastfed infant is possible; or, controlled studies show only minimal nonthreatening adverse effects. Drugs should be given only if the potential benefit justifies the potential risk to the infant.

- **L4 Possibly Hazardous:** There is positive evidence of risk to the breastfed infant or to breastmilk production but the benefits from use in breastfeeding mothers may be acceptable despite the risk to the infant (e.g., if the drug is needed in a life-threatening situation or for a serious disease for which safer drugs cannot be used or are ineffective).

- **L5 Contraindicated:** Studies in breastfeeding mothers have demonstrated that there is significant and documented risk to the infant based on human experience; or, it is a medication that has a high risk of causing significant damage to an infant. The risk of using the drug in breastfeeding women clearly outweighs any possible benefit from breastfeeding. The drug is contraindicated in women who are breastfeeding an infant.

Source: Adapted from Hale (2002).

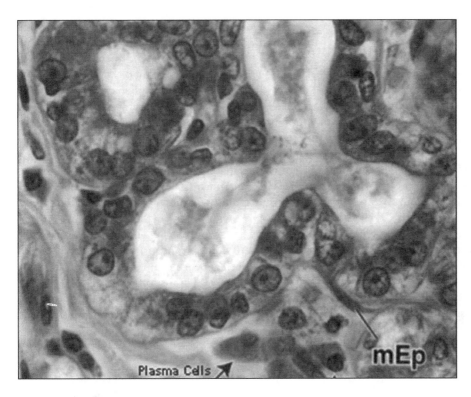

FIGURE 5–1.
Structure of the alveolar subunit with blood supply and other structures. (Reproduced with permission from Ross M, Gordon K, Pawlina W. *Histology: a text and atlas.* **Philadelphia: Lippincott, Williams & Wilkins, 2002.)**

directly on the mammary gland to bring about developmental changes (Neville, McFadden, & Forsyth, 2002). At this stage, the high levels of progestins largely suppress the lactocyte. But with delivery of the placenta, progestins and estrogens rapidly disappear from the plasma of the mother and the lactocyte begins a rapid change from a quiescent state to a fully active secretory state (lactogenesis).

During the early stages of lactation (the colostral phase) when the lactocytes are small in size and the intercellular spaces are large, maternal substances including drugs, lymphocytes, immunoglobulins, proteins, and other plasma substances can easily transfer into human milk via these large intercellular gaps. But with the drop in progestins, the lactocytes grow in size and subsequently narrow the intercellular gaps, eventually closing most of them.

As can be seen from the transition from colostrum to mature milk, these changes in milk occur due to the rapid growth of the lactocytes ending in closure of the tight junctions between the cells. At 36 hours following delivery, a major change in the components of milk begins to occur and is complete by 5 days postpartum. With closure of the intercellular spaces, the transfer of maternal medications and other maternal proteins into the mother's milk is greatly reduced.

Drug Transfer into Human Milk

Drugs transfer into human milk largely as a function of their physicochemical characteristics, which include molecular weight, lipophilicity, protein binding, and pKa (Atkinson & Begg, 1990). Maternal factors include the plasma level of the medication, with higher transfer occurring when levels peak in the maternal plasma compartment (C_{max}). Of these many factors, the most influential are as follows:

- Maternal plasma concentration of the drug, with most transfer at C_{max}.
- Molecular weight of the medication, with higher transfer at lower molecular weights.
- Protein binding of the medication, with higher transfer of unbound drugs.
- Fat content of the milk, with higher transfer of lipid soluble drugs.

Passive Diffusion of Drugs into Milk

The transfer of drugs into human milk is usually facilitated by passive diffusion down a concentration gradient formed by the nonionized, free drug on each side of the semipermeable membrane (Miller, Banerjee, & Stowe, 1967). Normally drugs transfer from areas of high concentration to areas of low concentration (passive diffusion). As described above, the overall rate and degree of transfer may be initially affected by the stage of alveolar development and the junctional condition of the lactocytes (Figure 5–2).

In the first 2 to 3 days, the alveolar epithelial structure of the breast is quite open and porous, thus permitting easy transfer of maternal proteins, lipids, immunoglobulins, and medications into the milk compartment. Often drug levels in milk reach equilibrium with the plasma compartment (M/P ratio =1). As the lactocyte begins to swell, the inter-

cellular junctions close. This subsequently leads to dramatically lower levels of drugs in the milk compartment after the first week postpartum. Although it is true that the transfer of medications or any substance into milk may be higher during the initial stages of early lactation, fortunately the absolute amount of colostrum delivered is often quite low (50–60 mL/day on days 1 and 2), which means that the clinical dose of medication delivered to the infant during this time is actually very low.

Milk and maternal plasma should be viewed as distinct and separate compartments. For most drugs, their transfer in and out of the milk compartment is accomplished by passive diffusion. While some active transport systems exist for iodides, as well as for immunoglobulins and electrolytes, facilitated transport systems are rather limited. Transport systems for medications may be indicated by drugs that have high milk/plasma ratios, although many drugs are ion-trapped in milk

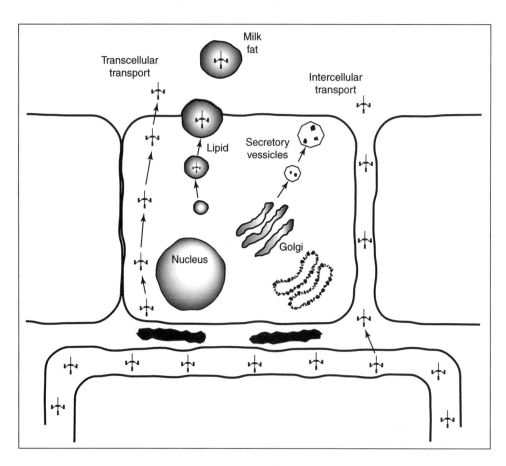

FIGURE 5–2. Compartment representation of drug transfer from plasma to the milk compartment.

due to the lower pH of milk and higher pKa of the medication (see below). Regardless, in the case of higher milk/plasma ratios, it is apparent that either the drug is ion-trapped in the milk or that it is pumped into the milk at higher levels (e.g., iodides).

Drugs enter the milk compartment and in almost all instances exit as well, largely as a function of equilibrium forces. The retrograde diffusion of drugs from the milk back into the plasma is well documented and is probably controlled by the same kinetic factors as entry (Schadewinkel-Scherkl et al., 1993). As the maternal plasma level of medication increases, so does the transfer into milk. As the mother metabolizes or eliminates the medication and her plasma levels drop, most drugs diffuse out of the milk compartment and back into the maternal plasma compartment to be eliminated by the mother (Figure 5–3). Following this reasoning, it is obvious that the diffusional forces that push medications into milk are highest at C_{max} (peak) in the mother and lowest during the trough period when the medication is being eliminated by the mother. Thus with shorter half-life medications, higher exposure to medications can be reduced by avoiding breastfeeding when the maternal plasma levels are highest and instead breastfeeding when the maternal levels are much lower. While this works for some drugs, it simply will not work for medications with long half-

lives, as the time period between C_{max} and trough is prolonged.

Ion Trapping

Because the pH of milk is slightly more acidic than plasma (milk pH = 7.2; plasma pH = 7.4), certain weak bases (pKa > 8) may become more polarized and therefore fail to diffuse backward into the plasma once in milk. Thus they are "trapped" in milk (ion trapping) and may produce higher milk/plasma ratios (Rasmussen, 1971). Ion trapping probably occurs with medications such as the barbiturates, ranitidine, and many others. Conversely, a weak acid is often trapped in the plasma compartment, where it is more polar and enters milk relatively poorly due to its polar state and its inability to transfer through the lactocyte bilayer lipid membrane.

Molecular Weight

With closure of the intercellular gaps, most medications must transfer via the "transcellular" pathway. To do so they must enter the basal membrane of the lactocyte, diffuse gently through the cell, and exit via the luminal surface. The lower the molecular weight of the medication and the more lipid soluble, the greater the diffusion across these bilayer lipid membranes. Although medications with lower molecular weights can easily transfer this way, it be-

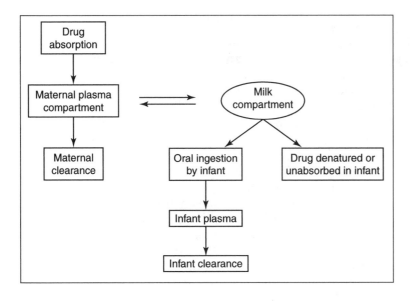

FIGURE 5–3.
Transport of drugs and other substances through the alveolar epithelial cell.

comes increasingly difficult for those with molecular weights exceeding 500 to 800 daltons to diffuse through these bilayer membranes and to enter breastmilk. Thus medications whose molecular weights exceed 1000 daltons seldom enter the milk compartment in clinically relevant amounts. Medications such as heparin, insulin, interferon (Kumar et al., 2000), and other large molecular weight drugs simply do not pass into milk in clinically relevant amounts. A medication such as lithium, with no protein binding and low molecular weight, transfers into milk readily (Sykes, Quarrie, & Alexander, 1976). Many of the psychotropic drugs such as the amphetamines are low in molecular weight and highly lipid soluble, which accounts for their rapid entry into the central nervous system as well as their higher milk/plasma ratios in human milk.

Lipophilicity

Although plasma contains lipid, it is relatively low compared to the 5–15 percent triglyceride found in human milk. As such, some medications that are lipid soluble may immerse themselves in the lipid fraction of milk and become concentrated therein. We actually know very little about the diffusion into and out of the lipid fraction of milk, but it is known that by selectively extracting the lipid fraction in milk, certain drugs are found there in higher concentrations. Some medications, during their transfer through the lactocyte, dissolve themselves in the lipid droplets and are subsequently dumped into the alveolar lumen. Others may actually transfer completely through the cell and subsequently transfer into the lipid droplets. For highly lipid-soluble drugs such as many neuroleptic drugs (diazepam, chlorpromazine, etc.), a vast majority of the drug is found in the lipid fraction (Syversen & Ratkje, 1985). While scientifically interesting, the clinical use of this information is relatively small. The most important feature of lipophilicity is that the more lipid soluble the medication, the more likely it will transfer into human milk. A more practical feature of this is that most Central Nervous System (CNS) active drugs are both low in molecular weight and very lipid soluble, two kinetic parameters that permit them to transfer through the blood-brain barrier as well as into human milk. Hence, greater concern for the infant should be taken with CNS active drugs.

Milk/Plasma Ratio

The ratio of the concentration of drug in the milk to that in the plasma is known as the milk/plasma ratio (M/P). The M/P ratio is quite useful in determining the relative transfer of medication into milk, but there are significant difficulties in accurately measuring it. Because of differences in the rate of drug transfer, the plasma and milk concentrations of medications do not always follow one another and the time at which the samples are drawn becomes incredibly important. The M/P ratio may be 1.14 at zero time and 0.31 at 3 hours following administration (Hale et al., 2002). As a result, the M/P ratio actually reflects the differential rate of entry of drug into plasma and milk, and it will often change from hour to hour (Sykes, Quarrie, & Alexander, 1976). Most importantly, the M/P ratio is of limited clinical use in assessing the likelihood that a clinically relevant dose will be transferred to the infant during breastfeeding. Even with those drugs that have high M/P ratios (e.g., ranitidine, cimetidine), the absolute dose transferred to the infant is subclinical. Ultimately, it is the concentration of drug in the milk and the volume of milk ingested that determine the clinical dose transferred to the infant. For this reason, low M/P ratios suggest that very little drug enters milk. Conversely, high M/P ratios may or may not indicate high levels in milk, because it ultimately depends on the maternal plasma level of medication.

Maternal Plasma Levels

Ultimately one of the most important kinetic factors determining drug transfer to the infant is the maternal plasma level of the drug. Plasma concentrations of drugs vary according to the dose administered, the half-life of the medication, the volume of distribution, the oral bioavailability, and its protein binding. Drugs vary enormously in potency, some requiring only microgram doses, whereas others required huge doses (grams). Because of the enormous difference in potency, plasma levels of various drugs can vary from nanograms per mL to milligrams per mL. In general, as the molar concentrations of a drug in solution increases, the equilibrium gradient also increases to force the drug into other compartments. Thus the more drug present, the higher the forces pushing it into the milk compartment. For this reason alone, the degree and rate of transfer of a drug into milk generally correlates with the plasma concentration curve. As the concentration in the plasma peaks (C_{max}), it is quite common that milk levels will then peak as well. Although this is certainly not always true—for example, as happens with metformin (Hale et al., 2002)—the majority of drugs exhibit this feature. Thus it is important to understand that if a drug is not absorbed in the mother or if it is rapidly depleted from her plasma compartment to other compartments (rapid redistribution), the transfer to her milk compartment will be quite low. Drugs with brief half-lives will be eliminated so quickly that they seldom pose a major risk to the infant, unless the infant is feeding at C_{max}.

Bioavailability

The bioavailability of a medication generally refers to the amount of drug that reaches the systemic circulation after administration. Depending on the route of administration (oral, IV, IM, SC, topical), medications must ultimately pass into the systemic circulation prior to reaching their intended site of action or the milk compartment. Fortunately, many medications are unstable in the gastric milieu, or are incompletely absorbed by infants. Most topical medications are poorly absorbed transcutaneously, so they seldom attain significant plasma levels. If administered orally, the liver often sequesters or metabolizes many medications, preventing their entry into the plasma compartment. Thus the poor bioavailability of many products reduces the exposure level in breastfed infants. Because infants receive drugs via the mother's milk, oral bioavailability is of major importance in evaluating potential risks to the infant. The absolute dose of a medication received via milk must by design be decreased by the percentage of oral bioavailability. Obviously, poorly bioavailable drugs are ideal for breastfeeding mothers, as their absorption in the infant is likely to be poor. Box 5–2 provides examples of medications that are virtually unabsorbed orally and are unlikely to cause problems in an infant. In some instances, however, the active medication may be concentrated in the GI tract of the infant and cause problems. Diarrhea and thrush are a common complication following the use of various antibiotics.

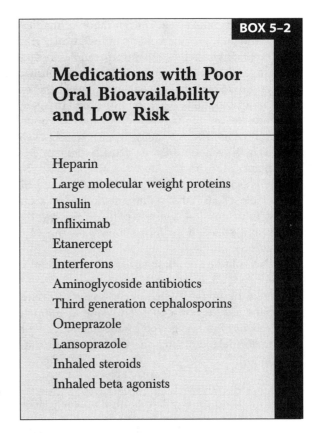

BOX 5–2

Medications with Poor Oral Bioavailability and Low Risk

Heparin
Large molecular weight proteins
Insulin
Infliximab
Etanercept
Interferons
Aminoglycoside antibiotics
Third generation cephalosporins
Omeprazole
Lansoprazole
Inhaled steroids
Inhaled beta agonists

Drug Metabolites

Ordinarily the primary function of drug metabolism is to make a drug more soluble so that it will be excreted by the renal system. However, there are situations in which the parent drug (prodrug) is actually metabolized to an active drug. This is true of valacyclovir, codeine, hydroxyzine, fluoxetine, and many others. In certain drugs—e.g., norfluoxetine, (from Prozac), normeperidine (from Demerol), cetirizine (from Atarax, hydroxyzine)—some of these metabolites actually have much longer half-lives than the parent drug. In these cases, both the metabolite and parent drug must be evaluated for levels in milk and for side effects. In the case of meperidine, it is the metabolite (normeperidine) that is believed to account for some of the toxicities of this drug.

Calculating Infant Exposure

Perhaps the most important clinical parameter is to calculate the actual dose received by the infant

(D_{inf}). To do so, the actual concentration of medication in the milk and the volume of milk transferred must be known. While this information is not always available, many drugs do have published studies providing the C_{max} concentrations or the average concentrations (C_{av}) for the drug. In many previous studies, the C_{max} was the most commonly reported value. Unfortunately, this frequently overestimates the amount of drug actually delivered to the infant. More recent studies now calculate the area under the curve (AUC) value for the medication (Hale et al., 2002). This methodology accurately estimates the average daily intake by the infant and is much more accurate than the C_{max} estimates.

The volume of milk ingested is highly variable and depends on the age of the infant, and the extent to which the infant is exclusively breastfed. Many clinicians use the 150 cc/kg/day value to estimate the amount of milk ingested by the infant. The following formula estimates the clinical dose to the infant:

$$D_{inf} = \frac{\text{Drug concentration in milk}}{\text{(at } C_{max}, \text{ or } C_{av}) \text{ X Volume of milk ingested}}$$

Ultimately, the simplest method for determining the safety of the medication is to relate the weight-normalized dose to that used during therapy in infants where specific data are available. For instance, if the normal dose the mother would receive of a drug is 10 mg/kg/day, and the infant is receiving 1 mg/kg/day via milk, then you can estimate that the relative infant dose (RID) is 10 percent of the maternal dose. Thus, the most useful and accurate measure of exposure is to calculate the relative infant dose (RID):

$$\frac{\text{Relative infant}}{\text{dose}} = \frac{D_{inf} \text{ (mg/kg/day)}}{\text{Maternal dose (mg/kg/day)}}$$

Generally expressed as a percentage of the mother's dose, this value provides a standardized method of relating the infant's dose to the maternal dose. In full-term infants, Bennett (1996) recommends that a relative infant dose of >10 percent should be the theoretical "level of concern" for most medications. Nevertheless, the 10 percent level of concern is relative and each situation should be individually evaluated according to the overall toxicity of the medication. In premature infants, this level of concern may have to be lowered appropriately, depending on the medication. In this regard, it should always be remembered that many neonates may have been exposed in utero to drugs taken by their mothers and that such exposure may be an order of magnitude greater than that received via breastmilk. This is the reason that infants exposed in utero to methadone go through significant withdrawal upon delivery even with breastfeeding.

Unique Infant Factors

A major function of all clinicians is to evaluate the relative risk of a medication to the infant. All infants should be categorized as low, moderate, or high risk for the medication of interest. Infants at low risk are generally older infants (6 to 18 months), who can metabolize and handle drugs relatively efficiently. Moderate-risk infants are those less than 6 months old, who suffer from various metabolic problems such as complications of delivery, apnea, GI anomalies, or other metabolic problems. High-risk infants would include premature infants, neonates, unstable infants, or infants with poor renal output.

Pediatric patients are often referred to as "therapeutic orphans" due to the lack of pharmacodynamic studies in neonates and infants. Less than 1 percent of all therapeutic agents have recommended dosing guidelines for the newborn or premature infant. Early postpartum, a state of relative achlorhydria, exists the first week and the pH continues to decrease slowly toward adult values in the next two years. Weak acids (phenobarbital) may have reduced absorption and weak bases may have enhanced absorption due to the higher pH of the infant's stomach. Since the infant's exposure is via the oral route, the oral bioavailability of the medication is of paramount importance. Drugs with high first-pass clearance (morphine) are rapidly cleared from the portal circulation by the liver, even in infants. Drugs with poor stability in the gut (aminoglycosides, insulin, heparin) are rapidly degraded in the stomach or intestine. Poor biliary function subsequently leads to poor lipid absorption and relative steatorrhea in newborn or premature infants. Thus lipid soluble drugs presented in milk would have poorer bioavailability. Gastric emptying time is prolonged in premature infants and in some cases may alter the absorption kinetics altogether. Values for total body water are higher in neonates than in adults. Protein binding is decreased and the oxidative and conjugative capacity of the liver is greatly reduced in neonates (Besunder, Reed, & Blumer, 1988). Interestingly, while the metabolic capacity of the liver is reduced at first, it rapidly increases and actually supersedes adult capacity in subsequent months (Morselli, Franco-Morselli, & Bossi, 1980). Ultimately, the evaluation of the safety of drugs in breastmilk depends on three major factors: (1) the amount of medication presented in milk, (2) the oral bioavailability of the medication, and (3) the ability of the infant to clear the medication. Table 5–1 provides a list of medications of particular risk to newborn or premature infants. While the amount present in milk has been published for many drugs and their bioavailability is reasonably well known in adults, the ability of the infant to clear the medication is highly variable and requires evaluation by the clinician. Begg (2000) has estimated infant clearance to be 5, 10, 33, 50, 66, and 100 percent of adult maternal levels at 24–28, 28–34, 34–40, 40–44, 44–68, and more than 68 weeks post conceptual age, respectively.

Table 5–1

DRUGS TO AVOID IN BREASTFEEDING MOTHERS OF PREMATURE OR NEWBORN INFANTS

Drug	Possible Side Effect
Acebutolol	Has potential to cause hypotension in infant (Boutroy et al., 1986).
ACE inhibitors	May cause neonatal hypotension; wait several weeks postpartum (Hale & Berens, 2003).
Alcohol	May reduce milk production significantly (Mennella & Beauchamp, 1991).
Amphetamines	Potentially high milk levels reported; may cause stimulation of infant (Steiner et al., 1984).
Anticancer agents	Cytotoxicity, immune suppression reported (Hale & Berens, 2003).
Caffeine	Milk levels small, but neonatal half-life long; symptoms include jitteriness, stimulation (Stavchansky et al., 1988; Nehlig & Debry, 1994).
Cocaine	Potential high milk levels, intoxication, and stimulation of infant reported (Chasnoff, Lewis, & Squires, 1987).
Demerol	Neonatal sedation reported; neurobehavioral delay in neonates (Wittels, Scott, & Sinatra, 1990).
Dostinex	Reduces milk supply by inhibiting prolactin (Caballero-Gordo et al., 1991).
Ergotamine	Reduces milk supply by inhibiting prolactin (White & White, 1980).
Estrogens	May reduce milk supply (Booker & Pahl, 1967; Booker, Pahl, & Forbes, 1970; Gambrell, 1970).
Fluoxetine	Tremulousness, colic, crying, hypotonia reported (Lester et al., 1993).
Iodine	High levels in milk reported; may inhibit thyroid function in neonate (Postellon & Aronow, 1982).
Lithium	Levels high in milk, risk high to infant unless monitored closely (Llewellyn, Stowe, & Strader, 1998).
Marijuana	May suppress prolactin and/or milk supply; infant will be drug-screen positive for long periods (Hale & Berens, 2003; Perez-Reyes & Wall, 1982).
Parlodel	Reduces milk supply by inhibiting prolactin (Spalding, 1991; Canales et al., 1981).
Progestins	Early postnatal use may reduce milk supply (Hale, 2002).
Pseudoephedrine	May inhibit milk supply (Aljazaf et al., 2003).
Sulfonamides	Displaced bilirubin from binding site; hyperbilirubinemia possible; do not use in G6PD deficiency (Hale & Ilett, 2002).

Maternal Factors

The plasma compartment is the only source of medication for the milk compartment. If drugs are not absorbed by the mother and do not produce significant plasma levels, then they are of no risk to the infant. Medications that are not orally bioavailable in the mother (for example, oral vancomycin, magnesium hydroxide, magnesium sulfate, and many others) do not attain significant plasma levels and are therefore not hazardous to a breastfed infant. This also includes most, but not all, topical preparations. Many topical steroids, antibiotics, and retinoids used over minimal surface areas are not well absorbed transcutaneously and are virtually undetectable in the plasma compartment. One-time injections of local anesthetics such as those used for dental procedures provide so little drug that plasma levels are minuscule. Hence, the acute use of many medications is not usually problematic as the overall dose transferred to the infant is low over time.

The amount of milk the mother produces is very important as well. Milk production the first or second day postpartum is so low that the overall dose of medication transferred is usually insignificant. Also, mothers who are 1 to 2 years postpartum generally have a significantly reduced milk supply, their infants are much older, and thus the clinical dose transferred is reduced as well. Therefore the risk of a medication in a mother with an 18-month-old infant is relatively small.

Minimizing the Risk

The observation of certain procedures may profoundly reduce exposure to medications and risk in the infant:

- Avoid feeding the infant or pumping breastmilk at C_{max}. Because milk levels are invariably a function of maternal plasma levels, collecting/breastfeeding at the peak (C_{max}) will always produce higher drug levels in milk. While useful for shorter half-life medications, avoiding breastfeeding at C_{max} is of questionable use with long half-life medications.

- Temporarily withhold breastfeeding for brief exposures. If the mother can store sufficient milk for a brief exposure to medication, then the risk to the infant is eliminated. Milk produced during the exposure can be pumped and discarded.

- Choose medications that produce minimal levels in milk. For example, the antidepressants sertraline (Zoloft) or paroxetine (Paxil) produce milk levels far less than fluoxetine (Prozac) (Bennett, 1996; Kristensen et al., 1998; Kristensen et al., 1999; Wisner, Perel, & Blumer, 1998).

- Choose medications that are commonly used in pediatric patients and are considered safe.

- Choose medications such as warfarin with high protein binding because tissue and milk levels will be lower.

- Choose medications such as domperidone with poor blood/brain penetration as they usually produce lower milk levels.

- Choose medications such as heparin with higher molecular weights as this factor greatly reduces transfer into milk.

Effect of Medications on Milk Production

Drugs That May Inhibit Milk Production

Some medications are well known to affect the rate of milk production. Because infant weight gain and development are directly associated with milk production, even modest changes in milk supply can produce major growth complications for the infant. Drugs that may potentially inhibit milk production include ergot alkaloids—bromocriptine, cabergoline (Dostinex, ergotamine)—estrogens (Treffers, 1999; Sweezy, 1992), progestogens, pseudoephedrine (Aljazaf et al., 2003), and to a minor degree alcohol (Mennella & Beauchamp, 1991). Table 5–2 presents a list of drugs generally contraindicated in breastfeeding mothers.

Estrogens have a long but poorly documented history of suppressing milk (Booker & Pahl, 1967; Booker, Pahl, & Forbes, 1970; Gambrell, 1970). While they may have no effect whatsoever in some mothers, others may be exceedingly sensitive to them. The onset may be rapid or slow, and the change in milk production may not be readily no-

Table 5–2

Drugs Generally Contraindicated in Breastfeeding Mothers

Drug	Possible Side Effect in Infant/Mother
Amiodarone	High risk of accumulation due to long half-life and high volume of distribution; cardiovascular risks are high; thyroid suppression risk is high (Brackbill, Kane, & Manniello, 1974a; Chatterton, 1978).
Antineoplastic agents	Some antineoplastic agents may be used following pumping and discarding of milk; others may not.
Chloramphenicol	Blood dyscrasias, aplastic anemia, etc. Possible in mother but not reported as a result of breastfeeding (Kuhnert et al., 1979b).
Doxepin	Dangerous sedation and respiratory arrest reported.
Ergotamine, Cabergoline, ergot alkaloids	Ergotism poisoning (vomiting and diarrhea) reported; may inhibit prolactin secretion; reduces milk production; Cabergoline in particular is a potent inhibitor of milk production.
Iodides	Iodides concentrate in milk; thyroid suppression has been noted; Betadine douches should be avoided.
Methotrexate and immunosuppressants	Potential for a range of symptoms associated with suppression of the immune system; cyclosporine appears to be low risk (Kuhnert et al., 1979a, 1980); methotrexate may concentrate in neonatal GI cells.
Lithium	RID high (18–23%); high potential for toxicity; monitor plasma levels and thyroid function routinely.
Radiopharmaceuticals	Brief to full interruption of breastfeeding recommended.
Ribavirin	No reported milk levels, but following chronic use may lead to hemolytic anemia; caution recommended.
Tetracycline (chronic)	Brief use ok (< 3 weeks); chronic use not recommended.
Pseudoephedrine	May reduce milk supply; caution recommended.

Source: Adapted from Hale and Ilett (2002).

ticed by many mothers. Regardless, all mothers who take estrogen-containing birth control preparations should be forewarned of the possible effect on milk production. When necessary, low-dose progestogen-only oral contraceptives should be used, although even these can suppress milk production in some mothers if used too early postpartum. The most sensitive time for suppression is early postpartum before the mothers' milk supply is established. Waiting as long as possible (weeks to months) prior to use is recommended. All mothers should be warned that in some cases reduced milk supply may result and they should be observant for such changes.

Some members of the ergot family are well known to suppress prolactin levels. Bromocriptine has been used in the past to reduce engorgement and inhibit milk production, although it was associated with numerous cases of cardiac dysrhythmias, stroke, intracranial bleeding, cerebral edema, convulsions, and myocardial infarction (Dutt, Wong, & Spurway, 1998; Iffy et al., 1998; Pop et al., 1998; Webster, 1996). A newer analog, cabergoline, has proved much safer and is now recommended for both hyperprolactinemia and inhibition of lactation (Ferrari, Piscitelli, & Crosignani, 1995; Webster et al., 1992). Doses of 1 mg administered early postpartum will completely inhibit lactation. For established lactation, 0.25 mg twice daily for 2 days has been found to completely inhibit lactation (Anonymous, 1991; Caballero-Gordo et al., 1991).

There are recent suggestions that the nasal decongestant pseudoephedrine may suppress milk production (Aljazaf et al., 2003a). Studies are still under way, but mothers should be cautious using pseudoephedrine, particularly during late-stage lactation (> 8 months), or if they have a poor milk supply. Box 5–3 provides a list of drugs that are known to affect milk production negatively.

Drugs That May Stimulate Milk Production

The pituitary hormone prolactin is one of the major determinants of milk production. It is well known that while prolactin levels must be elevated for milk production to occur, higher levels of prolactin do no necessarily increase production (Chatterton et al., 2000). Hence, prolactin levels and milk production are not necessarily related. Initially antenatal prolactin levels are quite high and then over the next 6 months drop significantly almost to normal ranges even though milk production levels are virtually unchanged.

In some mothers, particularly those with premature infants, prolactin levels may not be sufficient to support adequate lactation. In these patients,

medications that inhibit dopamine receptors in the hypothalamus (metoclopramide, domperidone) may or may not stimulate milk production. Dopamine antagonists such as domperidone, metoclopramide, risperidone, or the phenothiazine neuroleptics are all well known to stimulate milk production in some patients. The two most commonly used dopamine antagonists are metoclopramide (Reglan)(Budd et al., 1993; Ehrenkranz & Ackerman, 1986; Kaupila, Kivinen, & Ylikorkala, 1981; Kauppila et al., 1983) and domperidone (Motilium)(Hofmeyr & Van Iddekinge, 1983; Hofmeyr, Van Iddekinge, & Blott, 1985; Petraglia et al., 1985). Metoclopramide is the most frequently used agent, and in some cases, profoundly stimulates milk production as much as 100 percent. Unfortunately, it may induce significant depression if therapy is continued for more than 1 month. The prolactin-stimulating effect of metoclopramide is dose-related, with doses of 10 to 15 mg TID required for efficacy. The amount transferred into milk is small, ranging from 28 to 157 µg/L in the early puerperium (Kauppila, Kivinen, & Ylikorkala, 1981), which is far less than the clinical dose administered directly to infants (800 µg/kg/d). The most significant side effect of metoclopramide is extra-pyramidal jerks, gastric cramping, and in some cases major depression.

Domperidone is another dopamine antagonist that stimulates prolactin levels. It is apparently much safer since it does not penetrate the blood-brain barrier and thus causes no CNS side effects. However, it is unfortunately not available in the United States except through compounding pharmacies. A recent study of domperidone suggests a mean milk volume increase of 44.5 percent over 7 days. Milk levels of domperidone were only 1.2 ng/mL (da Silva, Knoppert, & Angelini, 2001). These agents apparently do not always stimulate milk production in patients with prolactin levels already above normal, or in those patients with inadequate breast tissue. But in many mothers of premature infants, they may be quite efficacious. Because the milk supply is dependent on elevated prolactin levels, a precipitous withdrawal of these agents may result in a significant loss of milk supply. A slow withdrawal is generally recommended over several weeks to a month to prevent loss of milk supply.

The dopamine antagonists are often used inappropriately to stimulate milk production in mothers

---

BOX 5–3

Drugs That May Reduce Milk Production

- Progestins
- Estrogens
- Ethanol
- Bromocriptine
- Ergotamine
- Cabergoline
- Pseudoephedrine

with moderate to low milk production. In these cases, breastfeeding more often, pumping, and reduced intervals between breastfeeding may work much better. In cases where the maternal prolactin levels are probably already elevated, dopamine agonists often fail to work at all.

Herbs

The stimulation of milk production by the use of herbals is extraordinarily common therapy today. However, good supporting data suggesting that these agents stimulate milk production is minimal to nil. Fenugreek is the most commonly used herbal for this purpose. In a recent abstract of 10 women who ingested three capsules three times daily, the average milk production during the week increased significantly from 207 mL/day (range 57–1057 mL) to 464 mL/day (range 63–1140 mL) (Swafford & Berens, 2000). No untoward effects were reported; however, this was not a blinded or controlled study.

Review of Selected Drug Classes

Analgesics

Analgesics are the most commonly used medications in breastfeeding mothers. While the nonsteroidal anti-inflammatory agents (NSAIDS) are most frequently used, opioids such as morphine, codeine, and hydrocodone are most commonly given during the early postpartum period for pain relief. Selected analgesics are reviewed in Table 5–3.

NSAIDS. Of the NSAID family, ibuprofen and ketorolac are perhaps ideal agents with low relative infant doses (< 0.6 percent). Not only is ibuprofen cleared for use in infants, its milk levels are generally subclinical. Naproxen is suitable for short-term use (a few days), but bleeding, hemorrhage, and acute anemia have been reported in a 7-day-old infant (Figalgo, 1989). Recent data from unpublished research on newer COX2 inhibitors

---

Table 5–3

RELATIVE INFANT DOSE AND CLINICAL SIGNIFICANCE OF SELECTED ANALGESICS

Drug	Relative Infant Dose	Clinical Significance	Lactation Risk Category
Fentanyl	< 3	Milk levels low; no untoward effects rom exposure to milk.	L2
Indomethacin	0.4	Milk levels low; plasma levels low to undetectable in infants; caution with chronic administration.	L3
Ketorolac	0.16–0.4	Milk levels are very low; no untoward effects reported.	L2
Meperidine; pethidine	1	Neurobehavioral delay, sedation noted from long half-life metabolite; avoid.	L2 L3 postpartum
Methadone	2.6, 5.6, 2.4, 1.0	Milk levels low; approved for use in breastfeeding mothers; will not prevent neonatal abstinence syndrome.	L3
Morphine	5.8	Oral bioavailability poor; milk levels generally low; considered safe; observe for sedation.	L3
Naproxen	3.0	Long half-life; may accumulate in infant; bleeding, diarrhea reported in one infant; short-term use acceptable; avoid chronic use.	L3 L4 (chronic)

Source: Adapted from Hale and Ilett (2002).

such as celecoxib and valdecoxib suggest that milk levels are quite low, much less than 200 µg/L and even lower with valdecoxib. These agents may yet prove to be useful and suitable alternatives to the older NSAIDs.

Aspirin, due to its causal association with Reye's syndrome, is not generally recommended in breastfeeding mothers. However, the amount of aspirin in milk is quite low and it could be used in low maternal doses (82 mg/d) to inhibit platelet function, but this involves some risk to the infant. The relative infant dose is reported to be about 2.4 percent of the maternal dose (Bailey et al., 1982).

Methadone. Methadone is widely used in the treatment of opiate addiction and is commonly used in pregnant patients. Methadone levels in milk are dependent on the dose, but generally range from 2.8 to 5 percent of the maternal dose (Begg et al., 2001; Wojnar-Horton et al., 1997). Because of these low levels in milk, neonatal abstinence syndrome may occur in a high percentage of breastfed newborns whose mothers take methadone during pregnancy (Ostrea et al., 1976; Strauss et al., 1974). In a recent study by McCarthy (2000), methadone concentrations in milk ranged from 27 to 260 µg/L in patients receiving 25 to 180 mg/d. Assuming milk intake of 475 mL/d, the average infant would receive only 50 µg/d or 0.97 percent of the maternal dose in these studies.

Morphine and Congeners. The data on morphine are unfortunately somewhat varied. Older studies suggested the amount of morphine in milk was minimal to undetectable. In a study of epidural morphine, the concentration in milk following two 4 mg epidural doses was only 82 µg/L (Wittels, Scott, & Sinatra, 1990) Other studies (Robieux et al., 1990) suggest higher levels (10-100 µg/L). Combined with its poor oral bioavailability (< 25 percent), and minimal milk levels, morphine does not appear to be significantly hazardous to most breastfeeding infants so long as the maternal doses are low to moderate, and the infant is stable.

Codeine and hydrocodone are without doubt the most commonly used opiate analgesics in breastfeeding mothers. Although some cases of neonatal sedation and apnea have been reported with codeine, the majority of infants are unaffected by these agents. While the studies on these drugs are poor, they suggest that after 48 hours of exposure to 12 doses of 60 mg codeine, the estimated dose of codeine in 2000 ml of milk was only 0.7 mg or 0.1 percent of the maternal dose. Bennett (1996) suggests the relative infant dose is 1.4 percent. Few problems have been reported although infant sedation can occur. Codeine and hydrocodone are considered safe when used in moderate to low doses in most patients. No data are available for hydrocodone.

Meperidine. The use of meperidine in the perinatal period is increasingly controversial. Although the use of meperidine in obstetrics is common, it is gaining disfavor as more and more sedation is reported in newborn infants. Meperidine administered to mothers has been found to produce neonatal respiratory depression, decreased Apgar scores, lower oxygen saturation, respiratory acidosis, and abnormal neurobehavioral scores.(Brackbill, Kane, & Manniello, 1974a, 1974b; Hodgkinson et al., 1978, 1979). Meperidine is metabolized to normeperidine, which is both active and has a half-life of approximately 62 to 73 hours in newborns. Because of this prolonged half-life, neonatal depression after exposure to meperidine may be profound and prolonged (Brackbill, Kane, & Manniello, 1974a). Small but significant amounts of meperidine and normeperidine are secreted into human milk (Quinn et al., 1986), and have been found to produce changes in neurocognitive function in some infants (Wittels, Scott, & Sinatra, 1990).

Fentanyl. The transfer of fentanyl into human milk is low. In women receiving doses varying from 50 to 400 µg intravenously during labor, the amount found in milk was exceedingly low (< 0.05 µg/L), generally below the limit of detection (Leuschen, Wolf, & Rayburn, 1990).

Antibiotics

Aside from analgesics, the most commonly used class of medications in breastfeeding mothers is antibiotics. Virtually all of the penicillins and cephalosporins have been studied and are known to produce only trace levels in milk (Blanco et al., 1983; Kafetzis, Lazarides, & Siafas, 1980; Kafetzis, Siafas, & Georgakopoulos, Matsuda, 1984; Shyu et al., 1992; Yoshioka et al., 1979; Bourget, Quinquis-Desmaris, & Fernandez, 1993). Some changes in intestinal flora are to be expected (Table 5–4).

Table 5–4

RELATIVE INFANT DOSE AND CLINICAL SIGNIFICANCE OF ANTIBIOTICS

Drug	Relative Infant Dose (%)	Clinical Significance	Lactation Risk Category
Acyclovir	1.1, 1.5	Infant dose low; safe.	L2
Amoxicillin	1.3	Observe for change in intestinal flora; compatible.	L1
Ampicillin	0.24	Observe for change in intestinal flora; compatible.	L1
Azithromycin	5.8	Observe for change in intestinal flora; compatible.	L2
Cefazolin	0.8	Observe for change in intestinal flora; compatible.	L1
Cefepime	0.3	Observe for change in intestinal flora; compatible.	L2
Cefoperazone	0.9	Observe for change in intestinal flora; compatible.	L2
Cefotaxime	0.3	Observe for change in intestinal flora; compatible.	L2
Cefoxitin	0.2	Observe for change in intestinal flora; compatible.	L1
Cefprozil	0.3	Observe for change in intestinal flora; compatible.	L1
Ceftazidime	0.9	Observe for change in intestinal flora; compatible.	L1
Ceftriaxone	0.9	Observe for change in intestinal flora; compatible.	L2
Cephalexin	0.5	Observe for change in intestinal flora; compatible.	L1
Ciprofloxacin	2.6, 2.0	Recently approved by AAP; one case of pseudomembranous colitis reported; observe for changes in gut flora.	L4
Clindamycin (oral)	1.6	Observe for changes in intestinal flora; pseudomembranous colitis reported in one infant; probably safe.	L3
Cloxacillin	0.8	Observe for change in intestinal flora; compatible.	L2
Dicloxacillin	1.2	Observe for change in intestinal flora; compatible.	L1
Doxycycline	4	Infant dose low; bioavailability poor; safe for acute use; do not use chronically.	L3 L4 chronic
Erythromycin	1.4	Observe for change in intestinal flora; compatible; hypertonic pyloric stenosis reported in one case.	L1
Fluconazole	12.6	Safe; no untoward effects have been reported.	L2
Gentamicin	2.1	Observe for change in intestinal flora; compatible.	L2
Isoniazid	13.5	Caution; monitoring of infant for liver toxicity and neuritis recommended.	L3
Metronidazole	13, 9.9, 12.6, 29	Milk levels moderately high, but significantly less than pediatric therapeutic dose (15mg/kg/d); with high doses, discontinue breastfeeding for 12–24 hr after dose.	L2
Nitrofurantoin	0.7	Safe; no untoward effects reported; caution for infants with G6PD	L2
Ofloxacin	3.2	Probably safe but observe for changes in intestinal flora.	L3
Rifampicin	11	Probably safe; minimal data available.	L2

Table 5–4 (cont.)			
Streptomycin	0.6	Observe for change in intestinal flora; compatible.	L3
Tetracycline	1.35	Short-term use safe; bioavailability in milk is low to nil; caution with long-term use.	L2
Vancomycin	6.6	Safe; oral bioavailability low to nil; observe for changes in intestinal flora.	L1

Source: Adapted from Hale and Ilett (2002).

The transfer of the older tetracyclines into human milk is very low. Furthermore, when mixed with calcium salts, the bioavailability of these tetracyclines is significantly reduced and it is unlikely that the infant would absorb the minuscule levels present in milk. However, doxycycline absorption is largely delayed, not blocked. Short-term administration of these compounds for up to 3 weeks is permissible. Long-term use such as treatment for acne, is not recommended in breastfeeding mothers due to the possibility of dental staining in the infant and reduced growth rate in the epiphyseal growth plates.

The fluoroquinolones are somewhat controversial. Although the dose received via milk is far too low to induce arthropathy, pseudomembranous colitis has been reported, although this can occur with any antibiotic (Harmon, Burkhart, & Applebaum, 1992). Ciprofloxacin concentrations in human milk vary over a wide range (Cover & Mueller, 1990; Gardner, Gabbe, & Harter, 1992; Giamarellou, Kolokythas, & Petrikkos, 1989). Studies of the new fluoroquinolones suggest that ofloxacin concentrations in milk are probably lowest. Ciprofloxacin has recently been approved for use in breastfeeding mothers by the Academy of Pediatrics (Anonymous, 2001).

Metronidazole is a commonly used antimicrobial in pediatric patients. Older studies in rodents suggesting that metronidazole may be mutagenic have never been duplicated in humans. Following an oral dose of 400 mg three times daily, the maximum concentration in milk averaged 15.5 mg/L (Passmore et al., 1988).

Relative infant doses reported are moderate approximating 9–13 percent of the maternal dose. Thus far no untoward effects have been reported in a breastfed infant. High maternal doses (PO) such as 2 g for treatment of trichomoniasis may potentially produce high milk levels. In these patients a brief interruption of breastfeeding is recommended for 12 to 24 hours.

Following the use of intravenous metronidazole, milk levels have not been reported. However, with a short withholding period of a few hours (2–3 hr) to avoid the peak, maternal plasma levels rapidly fall to levels similar to those following oral administration. Intravaginal and topical applications do not produce significant plasma levels and do not require changes in breastfeeding recommendations.

Erythromycin and azithromycin levels in milk are quite low. Following a dose of 2 g erythromycin daily, milk levels varied from 1.6 to 3.2 mg/L of milk (Knowles, 1972). However, recent data suggests that erythromycin when given to breastfeeding mothers early postpartum (1–2 weeks) may increase the risk of pyloric stenosis (Sorensen et al., 2003). Azithromycin transfer to milk is minimal and produces a clinical dose of approximately 0.4 mg/kg/day (Kelsey et al., 1994).

Sulfonamides displace bilirubin from its albumin-binding site, and therefore they should not be used in newborns. However, they can be used later. Sulfisoxazole milk levels are low and only 1 percent of the maternal dose is transferred to the infant (Kauffman, O'Brien, & Gilford, 1980). The transfer of trimethoprim, which is commonly used in sulfonamide products, is minimal.

The use of antifungals in breastfeeding mothers is popular due to suggestions of topical and intraductal candidiasis. Without doubt, traumatized nipples are sometimes colonized with *C. albicans*. Virtually all infants have oral thrush at one time or another. Thus far, no data are available that support the growth of *C. albicans* in ductal tissue, particularly in immunocompetent mothers.

Topical antifungals such as nystatin or miconazole are often used to treat topical candidiasis. Although there is some controversy about the migration of *C. albicans* deep into ductal tissues of the breast, some patients respond quite well to several weeks of oral antifungals such as fluconazole. The transfer of fluconazole has been studied and is reported to be < 12 percent of the maternal dose. This is still considerably less than the clinical dose commonly used in neonates. While there is some risk of elevated liver enzymes, none have been reported following exposure to fluconazole in breastmilk.

Acyclovir is a potent antiviral commonly used for herpes infections. Levels in milk are quite low and the oral bioavailability in an infant is low as well. Following doses as high as 4 g/day, breastmilk concentrations ranged from 4.2 to 5.8 mg/L or about 1.3 percent of the maternal dose (Taddio, Klein, & Koren, 1994). Because the oral bioavailability is poor (< 15 percent), the clinical dose to the infant via milk is small.

Antihypertensives

Antihypertensives are commonly used early postpartum, and longer in breastfeeding mothers, but as a family they require a higher degree of caution. Several beta blockers (atenolol, acebutolol) have been reported to produce dangerous cyanosis, bradycardia, and hypotension in some breastfed infants (Boutroy et al., 1986). Infants should be closely monitored for these symptoms following therapy. Certain beta blockers are safer than others and the careful selection of an appropriate medication is highly recommended.

Early postpartum, some infants have difficulty controlling their blood pressure. Angiotensin converting enzyme inhibitors (ACEi), due to their potency, are significantly dangerous early postpartum, particularly in infants who are borderline hypotensive. ACE inhibitors should not be used in breastfeeding mothers until their infants can maintain adequate control of their blood pressure. It is therefore recommended that the ACEi family be avoided for at least several weeks postpartum in breastfeeding mothers. Afterward, captopril and enalapril are preferred due to lower milk levels.

Of the calcium channel blockers, nifedipine has been studied and its concentration in milk is quite low. It has also been used extensively to control blood pressure in hypertensive breastfeeding patients and to treat Raynaud's phenomenon of the nipple. While the amount in milk varies depending on study, the clinical dose received by the infant is generally less than 8 µg/kg/day (Penny & Lewis, 1989). Two other studies of verapamil transfer into milk have reported relative infant doses of 0.1 to 1 percent (Andersen, 1983; Anderson et al., 1987).

Other antihypertensives such as hydralazine and methyldopa are commonly used in pregnant patients. Studies suggest that their breastmilk levels are quite low and do not produce clinical changes in breastfed infants (Jones & Cummings, 1978; Liedholm et al., 1982; White et al., 1985).

Psychotherapeutic Agents

Sedatives and Hypnotics. The most commonly used sedative medications are benzodiazepines. Most benzodiazepine anxiolytics have been thoroughly studied in breastfeeding mothers. Levels of diazepam (Wesson et al., 1985), lorazepam (Whitelaw, Cummings, & McFadyen, 1981; Summerfield & Nielsen, 1985), and midazolam (Matheson, Lunde, & Bredisen, 1990b) have been reported and are quite low (Table 5–5). However, some in this family have rather prolonged half-lives and some medication does transfer to the infant as is evidenced by minor withdrawal symptoms.

The intermittent use of diazepam, midazolam, or lorazepam has not been associated with significant sedation in breastfed infants. In a prospective study of 42 women ingesting sedatives while breastfeeding, there were only three reports of slight sedation in their infants (Ito, Blajchman, & Stephenson, 1993). Lorazepam has a shorter half-life than diazepam (12 hr). When administered as premedication in 3.5 mg oral doses, milk concentrations were only 8–9 µg/L, which is far too low to be clinically relevant (Summerfield & Nielsen, 1985). Other studies suggest high levels (23–82 µg/L), but were not reported to produce neurobehavioral effects in breastfed infants (McBride et al., 1979).

In a mother who received alprazolam 0.5 mg 2 to 3 times daily (PO) during pregnancy, a neonatal withdrawal syndrome was reported in the breastfed

Table 5–5

RELATIVE INFANT DOSE AND CLINICAL SIGNIFICANCE OF PSYCHOTROPIC DRUGS

Drug	Maternal Dose	Relative Infant Dose (%)	Clinical Significance	Lactation Risk Category
Citalopram	20–60 mg/d	3.7	Infant levels extremely low; somnolence reported; most studies show no untoward effects.	L3
Diazepam	30 mg/d 30 mg/d	3.0 2.7	Sedation minimal; acute or occasional use acceptable; avoid prolonged exposure.	L3 L4 chronic
Fluoxetine	20–80 mg/d (0.51 mg/kg/d) 7–65 mg/d (0.17–0.85 mg/kg/d)	3.4 4.4	Fluoxetine and norfluoxetine found in 55–77% of infants; not recommended in preterm or very young neonates, or in high maternal doses.	L2 in older infants L3 in neonates
Fluvoxamine	200 mg/d (2.86 mg/kg/d) 100 mg/d	0.5 0.52	No adverse effects in 2 infants; probably safe.	L2
Haloperidol	10 mg/d 29 mg/d	2.4 0.2	Infant dose minimal; no untoward effects noted; caution recommended.	L2
Lithium	15 mmol/d	56	Severe sedation in some infants; monitoring of milk and/or infant serum concentrations mandatory; plasma levels in infants vary from 30–40% of maternal levels 2 weeks postpartum.	L4
Lorazepam	5 mg/d 3.5 mg/d	2.5 2.8	Infant dose low; no untoward effects noted in breastfeeding infants; observe for sedation.	L3
Midazolam	15	0.6	Milk levels are low; no sedation noted in infants; use caution but probably safe.	L3
Olanzapine	15 mg/d	1.05	No adverse effects noted but data are preliminary; probably safe.	L3
Paroxetine	20–30 mg/d 10–50 mg/d	1.4 1.7–2.3	Minimally detected in several infants; no adverse effects; safe.	L2
Risperidone	6 mg/d	0.84	Single case; no infant data; use caution.	L3
Sertraline	50 mg/d 25–200 mg/d	0.9 0.3–1.9	Milk levels low; levels in some infants extremely low; no adverse effects; preferred; safe.	L2
Temazepam	10–20 mg/d	No data	Milk concentrations in 9 mothers were extremely low; depending on dose, should be relatively safe.	L3

Table 5–5 (cont.)				
Venlafaxine	150–450 mg/d (6.1 mg/kg/d)	3.5	No adverse effects reported; use cautiously.	L3
	225–300 mg/d (2.9 mg/kg/d)	3.2		

Source: Adapted from Hale and Ilett (2002).

infant the first week postpartum (Anderson & McGuire, 1989). Such data suggest that the amount of alprazolam in breastmilk is insufficient to prevent a withdrawal syndrome following prenatal exposure. Furthermore, in another case of infant exposure solely via breastmilk, the mother took alprazolam (dosage unspecified) for 9 months while breastfeeding and withdrew herself from the medication over a 3-week period (Anderson & McGuire, 1989). The mother reported withdrawal symptoms in the infant, including irritability, crying, and sleep disturbances. Thus short-term use of certain benzodiazepines (i.e., diazepam, midazolam, or lorazepam) for 1 or 2 weeks is unlikely to produce problems, but long-term daily exposure could be problematic.

The use of phenothiazine sedatives such as Phenergan or Thorazine may increase sleep apnea (Kahn, Hasaerts, & Blum, 1985) and the risk of SIDS (Cantu, 1989), and should probably be avoided in breastfeeding mothers if possible. The transfer of phenobarbital is moderate, averaging 2.74 mg/L following a dose of 30 mg four times daily (Nau et al., 1982). Maternal and infant plasma levels should be monitored occasionally and kept in the normal range to prevent high levels in the infant. Phenobarbital is not usually a major problem in neonates or premature infants, as the bioavailability of phenobarbital in premature infants is generally considered poor, but caution is recommended.

Antidepressants. The incidence of postpartum depression has either risen markedly or is being reported more often. At present, about 10–15 percent of postpartum women report clinical depression, although approximately 80 percent experience postpartum blues (O'Hara et al., 1990). In the past, the use of antidepressants in breastfeeding mothers has been discouraged. However, recent information

suggests that depression itself has major negative implications for infants and that it may interfere with optimal parenting producing significant neurobehavioral delay in infants (Lee & Gotlib, 1991; Sinclair & Murray, 1998; Zekoski, O'Hara, & Wills, 1987). Many women presenting with depressive symptoms may not require pharmacotherapy. Early postpartum, sleep deprivation, and stress are clearly normal, and general support may be all that is required. But in some patients with severe depression, therapy is clearly indicated. For these reasons, it is important that major depression in breastfeeding women be closely monitored and if necessary, treated.

In past years, the older tricyclic antidepressants were the mainstay of depressive therapy. While they have been thoroughly studied in breastfeeding mothers and are generally considered safe, poor patient compliance and a high side effect profile generally preclude their use. Weight gain, sedation, and anticholinergic symptoms such as dry mouth, blurred vision, and constipation are major drawbacks to their use as antidepressants.

With the introduction of the selective serotonin reuptake inhibitors (SSRIs), the use of antidepressants has increased enormously. In general, the SSRIs are well tolerated and highly effective, and there are an increasing number of studies showing they are relatively safe in breastfeeding mothers. Clinical studies of sertraline (Zoloft) and paroxetine (Paxil) clearly suggest that transfer of these agents into milk is quite minimal and virtually no side effects have been reported in numerous breastfed infants (Altshuler et al., 1995; Kristensen et al., 1998; Stowe et al., 1997; Stowe et al., 2000). At least three cases of colic, prolonged crying, vomiting, tremulousness, and other symptoms have been reported following the use of fluoxetine (Prozac) in breastfeeding women, although these numbers are probably quite small compared to the thousands of infants who have breastfed without side effects. Recent data suggest that fluoxetine may reduce weight gain in breastfed infants (Chambers et al., 1999) and may reduce growth and development in adolescents (Weintrob et al., 2002). Therefore, fluoxetine should be viewed as a less preferred SSRI for breastfeeding mothers.

The mixed serotonin and norepinephrine reuptake inhibitor venlafaxine has now been studied in nine breastfeeding women (Ilett, Kristensen, & Hackett, 2002; Ilett et al., 1998). In the nine infants, the relative infant dose for venlafaxine averaged 3.5 percent and for its active metabolite (o-desmethylvenlafaxine), 6.8 percent. Moreover, no adverse effects were noted in their infants despite milk concentrations of up to 8.2 mg/kg/d.

Citalopram is a new SSRI antidepressant similar in effect to Prozac and Zoloft although more selective for the receptor site. In an excellent study of seven women receiving an average of 0.41 mg/kg/d citalopram, the average peak level (C_{max}) of citalopram was 154 µg/L and 50 µg/L for demethylcitalopram (Rampono et al., 2000). However, average milk concentrations (AUC) were lower and averaged 97 µg/L for citalopram and 36 µg/L for demethylcitalopram during the dosing interval. Low concentrations of citalopram (around 2 to 2.3 µg/L) were detected in only three of the seven infant's plasma. No adverse effects were found in any of the infants. The authors estimate the daily intake to be approximately 3.7 percent of the maternal dose.

We have limited data on bupropion (Wellbutrin, Zyban), but milk levels have been reported to be low (Briggs, Samson, & Ambrose, 1993). However the author has received three case reports suggesting that bupropion may reduce milk supply. Close monitoring of infant weight gain and the mother's milk supply is suggested.

Neonatal withdrawal symptoms characterized by poor adaptation, jitteriness, irritability, and poor gaze control after gestational exposure to selective SSRIs has been reported for fluoxetine (Chambers et al., 1996; Spencer & Escondido, 1993), sertraline, and paroxetine (Stiskal et al., 2001). However, long-term changes in psychomotor or neurodevelopment have not been noted (Nulman et al., 1997).

Antimanic Preparations. The treatment of bipolar syndrome in breastfeeding mothers is somewhat controversial. Lithium, valproate, and carbamazepine have relatively well-established efficacy in acute mania. However, due to the significant toxicity of lithium, some caution is recommended. Lithium is both small in molecular weight and unbound in the plasma compartment. As such, it produces relatively high levels in human milk and some reported toxicity (Llewellyn et al., 1998; Sykes, Quarrie, & Alexander, 1976; Tunnessen & Hertz, 1972). Recent data suggest that lithium plasma levels in breastfed infants are moderate, approximately 30–40 percent of the maternal level (Fries, 1970; Sykes, Quarrie, & Alexander, 1976; Tunnessen & Hertz, 1972). However, lithium plasma levels can change dramatically with state of hydration, particularly in the infant with dehydration, and careful monitoring of plasma lithium levels in mother and infant is strongly recommended. Because lithium affects thyroid function, thyroid panels should be routinely ordered as well.

Newer studies of valproic acid suggest that this medication is quite efficacious in treating acute mania. More rapid in onset, two placebo-controlled studies have reported clinically significant superiority of divalproex over placebo (Bowden et al., 1994; Pope et al., 1991). The transfer of valproic acid into milk is generally considered quite low. In a study of six women receiving 9.5 to 31 mg/kg/d valproic acid, milk levels averaged 1.4 mg/L while maternal serum levels averaged 45.1 mg/L (Nau et al., 1981). The average milk/serum ratio was 0.027. Most authors agree that the amount of valproic acid transferring to the infant via milk is low. Breastfeeding would appear safe. However, the infant should be closely monitored for liver and platelet changes. Thus in breastfeeding mothers with mania, valproic acid may be effective and safer than lithium.

Antipsychotics. The published literature on the transfer of antipsychotics into milk is limited. However, older data seem to suggest that the phenothiazines and thioxanthenes transfer into milk in rather limited amounts.(Blacker, 1962; Wiles, Orr, & Kolakowska, 1978). Moderate sedation has been reported in some infants (Wiles, Orr, & Kolakowska, 1978) and the use of phenothiazines has been reported to produce significant increases in sleep apnea in neonates (Kahn, Hasaerts, & Blum, 1985). An increased risk of sudden infant death syndrome has also been suggested (Kahn, Hasaerts, & Blum, 1985; Pollard & Rylance, 1994). For these reasons, the older phenothiazines and thiozanthines should probably be avoided in breastfeeding women.

The transfer of haloperidol into milk is limited and no sedation has been reported (Stewart, Karas, & Springer, 1980; Whalley, Blain, & Prime, 1981). However, the newer atypical antipsychotics may be the best choice of therapy. Risperidone levels are reportedly quite low with an estimated relative infant dose of 4.3 percent (Hill et al., 2000). Levels of olanzapine have just been published. In a study of five lactating women, the median relative infant dose was 1.6 percent of the maternal dose. No effects were noted in any of the infants. It is not known if this would be detrimental to an infant, but these levels are quite low (Croke, Buist, & Hackett, 2002).

Corticosteroids

Corticosteroids in general do not apparently transfer well into human milk. Following moderately high doses of prednisone (80 mg), the clinical dose transferred via milk is only 10 µg/kg, which is approximately 10 percent of the endogenous production (Ost et al., 1985). Prednisone and prednisolone transfer into milk has been found to be limited, even with larger doses (Berlin, 1979). Even following chronic doses of methylprednisolone (6–8 mg/d), no untoward side effects were noted in the infants (Coulam, Moyer, & Jiang, 1982).

The use of high-potency inhaled steroids in asthmatics should pose no problem whatsoever primarily because plasma levels are exceedingly low. In the case of high intravenous doses, such as those given with multiple sclerosis or acute immune reactions, plasma levels of these steroids fall rapidly due to redistribution. A brief interruption of a few hours should suffice to limit exposure in the milk (Hale & Ilett, 2002).

With most lower-potency topical steroids, the transcutaneous absorption is generally minimal. However, following the use of high-potency topical steroids over a large body surface, significant plasma levels are measurable. In these instances, a risk versus benefit assessment may be required concerning breastfeeding, particularly because these agents are extremely potent.

Thyroid and Antithyroid Medications

The primary objective of treating patients with thyroid supplements is to increase their plasma thyroxine levels into the euthyroid range. Hence it should be obvious that once accomplished that supplementation with thyroxine is no different than breastfeeding in a normal euthyroid mother. Regardless, the amount of thyroxine transferred into human milk is invariably low (Mizuta et al., 1983; Oberkotter, 1983). There are no contraindications to breastfeeding and using thyroid supplements as long as normal thyroxine levels in the maternal plasma are maintained.

In hyperthyroid states both propylthiouracil (PTU) and methimazole have been thoroughly studied. PTU levels in milk are at least ten times lower than the maternal plasma level. Following a dose of 400 mg, the average amount of PTU transferred over 4 hours was only 99 ug (Kampmann, Johansen, & Hansen, 1980). Using radio labeled PTU, only 0.08 percent of the maternal dose transferred into milk over 24 hours (Low, Lang, & Alexander, 1979). Thus far no changes in the infants thyroid function have been reported.

Carbimazole is metabolized to the active metabolite, methimazole. Levels depend on maternal dose but appear too low to produce clinical effect. In one study of a patient receiving 2.5 mg methimazole every 12 hours, the dose to the infant was calculated at 16 to 39 µg/d (Tegler & Lindstrom, 1980). This was equivalent to 7–16 percent of the maternal dose. In a study of 35 lactating women receiving 5 to 20 mg/day of methimazole, no changes in the infant thyroid function were noted in any infant, even in those mothers at higher doses (Azizi, 1996).

Furthermore, in a study of 11 women who were treated with the methimazole derivative carbimazole (5 to 15 mg daily, equal to 3.3 to 10 mg methimazole), all 11 infants had normal thyroid function following maternal treatments (Lamberg et al., 1984). In a large study of over 139 thyrotoxic lactating mothers and their infants, even at methimazole doses of 20 mg/day, no changes in infant TSH, T4, or T3 were noted in over 12 months of study (Azizi et al., 2000).

Drugs of Abuse

The risk versus benefit determination in women with a history of drug abuse and who want to breastfeed is enormously difficult. Each health-care provider must evaluate the relative risk that the mother will return to the use of these various medications. While with some of these drugs the overall risk of the medication may be lower, some drugs of abuse could be horribly detrimental to breastfeeding infants, and the risk assessment is thus extremely important. Mothers who appear unlikely to adhere to a drug-free existence should probably be advised to feed formula.

Because most drugs of abuse are psychotropics, they pass readily into the brain and in some instances, the breast milk compartment as well. The most dangerous compounds are the hallucinogens, such as LSD and phencyclidine. Mothers who are drug-screen positive for these substances should be strongly warned that these agents are the most dangerous of this group and pose significant hazard to their infants. Amphetamines and methylphenidate do pass into milk but the levels may not be high enough to pose a major hazard to most infants, although this is as yet unclear. Milk/plasma ratios with the amphetamines range from 3 to 7 (Steiner et al., 1984). Interestingly, cocaine levels in milk have never been reported. Cocaine undoubtedly enters milk avidly but as yet we do not have explicit data. However, we do know that cocaine can induce excitement in a breastfed infant when ingested by the mother (Chasnoff, Lewis, & Squires, 1987).

The effect of marijuana in breastfeeding mothers is unclear. Thus far, neurobehavioral effects on the infants have not been reported even in heavy users (Perez-Reyes & Wall, 1982; Tennes et al., 1985). Marijuana passes rapidly out of the plasma compartment and enters adipose tissue. Because of this rapid redistribution, milk levels are apparently low. However, infants will continue to be drug-screen positive for long periods (perhaps weeks).

Ingestion of heroin in breastfeeding mothers has not been well studied. Heroin is almost instantly deacetylated to its metabolite, morphine. While morphine is considered a good choice analgesic for breastfed infants, the major problem with heroin ingestion is the enormous dose sometimes used by addicts. Hence, levels of the metabolite (morphine) in milk could be potentially quite large and therefore hazardous to the infant.

Mothers should be advised that all of these psychotropic medications readily enter milk, and that their infants may be at high risk of sedation, apnea, or death if the dose is high enough. Furthermore, all mothers should be advised that regardless of the clinical effect on the infant, their infants will be drug-screen positive for many days, perhaps weeks, following their use. Suggested pumping and discarding periods are suggested in Table 5–6.

Table 5–6

SUGGESTED DURATION FOR INTERRUPTED BREASTFEEDING FOLLOWING USE OF DRUGS OF ABUSE

Drug	Interrupt Feeding
Amphetamines, Ecstasy, MDMA	24–36 hours
Barbiturates	48 hours
Cocaine, crack	24 hours
Ethanol	1 hour per drink, or until sober
Heroin, morphine	24 hours
LSD	48 hours
Marijuana	24 hours
Phencyclidine, PCP	1–2 weeks

Source: Adapted from Hale and Ilett (2002).

Radioisotopes

The use and transfer of radio-labeled substances is of major importance to breastfeeding mothers. Commonly used as diagnostic tools, the majority of these radioactive compounds have rather brief half-lives and do not pose a major problem for breastfeeding mothers. They can simply pump and discard their milk for 12 to 24 hours and continue to breastfeed. However, with the use of I-131, Gallium-67, or Thallium-201, longer pumping periods may be necessary and may preclude breastfeeding altogether.

The most comprehensive source of information is published by the Nuclear Regulatory Commission (NRC) (Table 5–7) and is both accurate and thorough. Mothers who are required to take these medications are urged to follow these guidelines. The most dangerous radioisotope is Iodine-131. It is concentrated in human milk (by a factor of approximately 23), and may potentially destroy the infant's thyroid or could ultimately increase the risk of thyroid carcinoma in the infant exposed to this isotope via milk. The NRC recommends discontinuing breastfeeding altogether. Women who require high doses of I-131 should probably discontinue breastfeeding for several weeks prior to use to avoid high exposure to their breasts.

Radiocontrast Agents

Radiocontrast agents, or radiopaque agents, are used to enhance visualization of various tissue compartments. Two types are used: one group contains high concentrations of iodine; the other group contains the gadolinium ion. The iodinated groups are used for CAT scans while the gadolinium products are used for magnetic resonance imaging (MRI) scans.

In general, we recommend against the use of iodine-containing products in breastfeeding mothers. But in the case of the radiocontrast agents, the iodine molecule is covalently bound to the structure and is not generally released. Thus following the use of radiocontrast agents, the amount of free iodine is minimal and they are not considered a risk to breastfed infants. In addition, the plasma half-life of these agents is quite short, less than 1 hour for most, and the oral bioavailability is virtually nil. Therefore the absorption of clinically relevant amounts by breastfeeding infants is low. Table 5–8 provides the radiocontrast agents and their reported milk concentrations. While most of the package inserts on these products suggest a 24-hour pumping and discarding of milk, this is obviously not necessary.

In MRI scans, gadolinium-containing compounds are used. Milk levels of gadopentetate are reported to be very low (Rofsky, Weinreb, & Litt, 1993). Only 0.23 percent of the maternal dose was excreted over 24 hours of exposure. Furthermore, the oral bioavailability of the gadolinium products is about 0.8 percent.

Table 5–7

NUCLEAR REGULATORY GUIDELINES ON RADIOISOTOPES AND BREASTFEEDING

Radiopharmaceutical	Activity Above Which Instructions Are Required		Examples of Recommended Duration of Interruption of Breastfeeding*
	Mbq	*mCi*	
I-131 NaI	0.01	0.0004	Complete cessation (for this infant or child)
I-123 NaI	20	0.5	
I-123 OIH	100	4	

Table 5–7 (cont.)

Radiopharmaceutical	Activity Above Which Instructions Are Required		Examples of Recommended Duration of Interruption of Breastfeeding*
	Mbq	*mCi*	
I-123 mIBG	70	2	24 hr for 370 MBq (10 mCi) 12 hr for 150 MBq (4 mCi)
I-125 OIH	3	0.08	
I-131 OIH	10	0.30	
Tc-99m DTPA	1000	30	
Tc-99m MAA	50	1.3	12.6 hr for 150 Mbq (4 mCi)
Tc-99m Pertechnetate	100	3	24 hr for 1,100 Mbq (30 mCi) 12 hr for 440 Mbq (12 mCi)
Tc-99m HAM	400	10	
Tc-99m MIBI	Tc-99m DISIDA	1000	
Tc-99m MDP	Tc-99m Glucoheptonate	1000	
Tc-99m PYP	900	25	
Tc-99m red blood cell in vivo labeling	400	10	6 hr for 740 Mbq (20 mCi)
Tc-99m red blood cell in vitro labeling	1000	30	
Tc-99m sulfur colloid	300	7	6 hr for 440 Mbq (12 mCi)
Tc-99m DTPA aerosol	1000	30	
Tc-99m MAG3	1000	30	
Tc-99m white blood cells	100	4	24 hr for 1,100 Mbq (5 mCi) 12 hr for 440 Mbq (2 mCi)
Ga-67 citrate	1	0.04	1 month for 150 Mbq (4 mCi) 2 weeks for 50 Mbq (1.3 mCi) 1 week for 7 Mbq (0.2 mCi)
In-111 white blood cells	10	0.2	1 week for 20 Mbq (0.5 mCi)
T1-201 chloride	40	1	2 weeks for 110 Mbq (3 mCi)

*The duration of interruption of breastfeeding is selected to reduce the maximum dose to a newborn infant to less than 1 millisievert (0.1 rem), although the regulatory limit is 5 millisieverts (0.5 rem). The actual doses that would be received by most infants would be far below 1 millisievert (0.1 rem). Of course, the physician may use discretion in the recommendation, increasing or decreasing the duration of the interruption.

Notes: Activities are rounded to one significant figure, except when it was considered appropriate to use two significant figures. Details of the calculations are shown in NUREG-1492, Regulatory Analysis on Criteria for the Release of Patients Administered Radioactive Material (Ref.2).

If there is no recommendation in Column 3 of this table, the maximum activity normally administered is below the activities that require instructions on interruption or discontinuation of breastfeeding.

Source: Adapted from US Nuclear Regulatory Commission. *Nuclear Regulatory Commission Guideline 8.39.* Washington, DC, April 1997.

Table 5–8

RADIOCONTRAST AGENTS AND THEIR REPORTED MILK CONCENTRATIONS

Drug	Dose	Milk (C_{max})	Clinical Significance	Bioavailability	Lactation Risk Category
Gadopentetate	6.5 g	3.09 µmol/L	Only 0.023% of maternal dose; total dose = 0.013 µmol/24 hr; safe.	0.8%	L2
Iohexol	0.755 g/kg	35 mg/L	Mean milk level was only 11.4 mg/L; virtually unabsorbed; safe.	< 0.1%	L2
Iopanoic Acid	2.77 g	20.8 mg/19–29 hr	Only 0.08% of maternal dose; virtually unabsorbed; safe.	Nil	L2
Metrizamide	5.06 g	32.9 mg/L	Only 0.02% of maternal dose recovered over 44.3 hr; poor oral absorption; safe.	0.4%	L2
Metrizoate	580 mg	14 mg/L	Mean milk level 11.4 mg/24 hr; only 0.3% of maternal dose; safe.	Nil	L2

Source: Adapted from Hale and Ilett (2002).

S u m m a r y

Breastfeeding provides enormous medical and physical benefits to the infant and is strongly supported by numerous national academies and health-care organizations. Too often, and largely out of ignorance, mothers are advised to discontinue breastfeeding so that they can be treated with a medication. In the vast majority of these situations, the medication is quite safe for the infant or it is not even transferred into milk, but the infant ultimately suffers due to the lack of breastmilk.

It is true that all medications transfer into human milk. However, the vast majority do so in levels that are incredibly low and subclinical and pose no real risk for most infants. Nevertheless, all infants should be evaluated for risk prior to being exposed to medications used by their mothers, and those infants deemed at high risk should only be exposed to medications that carry a minimal risk associated with their use.

By understanding the various mechanisms of transfer and those medications that pose the most risk, the clinician can usually develop strategies that can provide the safe use of medications in mothers who breastfeed their infants. Such strategies involve using a safer medication or breastfeeding when the medication is low in the maternal plasma supply, or as a last resort, pumping and discarding the milk while the mother is treated.

There are always alternative medications that may be more suited for a breastfeeding mother and these should always be part of the overall evaluation of treatment. Following a few rules, the clinician can almost always find some suitable medication with low risk and allow the mother to be treated, and to continue breastfeeding the infant.

Ultimately, it is the clinician's role to take the time to do these simple evaluations and choose the appropriate therapy in order to avoid the unnecessary discontinuation of breastfeeding.

Key Concepts

- Avoid using medications when not absolutely necessary. This includes most herbal drugs.
- Choose drugs with shorter half-lives over those with longer half-lives.
- Choose drugs with less toxicity and those commonly used in infants.
- Choose drugs with poorer bioavailability to reduce oral absorption in infants.
- Choose drugs for which we have published milk studies.
- Advise the mother to feed the infant and then to take her medication to avoid breastfeeding when it peaks in the maternal plasma.
- Evaluate the infant's medications.
- Evaluate the age, stability, and condition of the infant in order to determine if the infant can handle exposure to the medication.

- Evaluate preterm or unstable neonates with special care; they may be more susceptible to adverse effects of medications because their clearance mechanisms have not matured.
- Understand that it is likely that drugs that enter the CNS will also enter breastmilk. An increased level of concern is recommended.
- Always advise the mother to watch for changes in milk production with various drugs. Mothers forewarned are more observant of subtle changes.
- Make a risk versus benefit assessment prior to the use of any drug, even though most drugs can be safely used in breastfeeding mothers.
- Keep in mind that only a very few medications are unsafe under any circumstances.

Internet Resources

Information on drugs and breastfeeding: www.neonatal.ama.ttuhs.edu/lact/

List of drugs and other chemicals that transfer into human milk, issued by: www.aap.org

References

Aljazaf K et al. Pseudoephedrine: effects on milk production in women and estimation of infant exposure via breastmilk. *Br J Clin Pharmacol* 56:18–24, 2003.

Altshuler LL et al. Breastfeeding and sertraline: a 24-hour analysis. *J Clin Psychiatry* 56:243–45, 1995.

Andersen HJ. Excretion of verapamil in human milk. *Eur J Clin Pharmacol* 25:279–80, 1983.

Anderson P et al. Verapamil and norverapamil in plasma and breast milk during breast feeding. *Eur J Clin Pharmacol* 31:625–27, 1987.

Anderson PO, McGuire GG. Neonatal alprazolam withdrawal—possible effects of breast feeding. *DICP* 23:614, 1989.

Anonymous. Single dose cabergoline versus bromocriptine in inhibition of puerperal lactation: randomized, double blind, multicentre study. European Multicentre Study Group for Cabergoline in Lactation Inhibition [see comments]. *BMJ* 302:1367–71, 1991.

Anonymous. Transfer of drugs and other chemicals into human milk. *Pediatrics* 108:776–89, 2001.

Atkinson HC, Begg EJ. Prediction of drug distribution into human milk from physicochemical characteristics. *Clin Pharmacokinet* 18:151–67, 1990.

Azizi F. Effect of methimazole treatment of maternal thyrotoxicosis on thyroid function in breast-feeding infants. *J Pediatr* 128:855–58, 1996.

Azizi F et al. Thyroid function and intellectual development of infants nursed by mothers taking methimazole. *J Clin Endocrinol Metab* 85:3233–38, 2000.

Bailey DN et al. A study of salicylate and caffeine excretion in the breast milk of two nursing mothers. *J Anal Toxicol* 6:64–8, 1982.

Begg EJ. *Clinical pharmacology essentials. The principle behind the prescribing process.* Auckland, New Zealand: Adis International, 2000.

Begg EJ et al. Distribution of R- and S-methadone into human milk during multiple, medium to high oral doseing. *Br J Clin Pharmacol* 6:681–85, 2001.

Bennett PN. Use of the monographs on drugs. In: Bennett PN, ed. *Drugs and human lactation.* Amsterdam: Elsevier, 1996:67–74.

Berlin CM. Excretion of prednisone and prednisolone in human milk. *The Pharmacologist* 21:264, 1979.

Besunder JB, Reed MD, Blumer JL. Principles of drug biodisposition in the neonate. A critical evaluation of the pharmacokinetic-pharmacodynamic interface (Part II). [Review; 390 refs]. *Clin Pharmacokinet* 14:261–86, 1988.

Blacker KH. Mothers milk and chlorpromazine. *Am J Psychiat* 114:178–79, 1962.

Blanco JD, Jorgensen JH, Castaneda YS, Crawford SA. Ceftazidime levels in human breast milk. *Antimicrob Agents Chemother* 23:479–80, 1983.

Booker DE, Pahl IR. Control of postpartum breast engorgement with oral contraceptives. *Am J Obstet Gynecol* 98:1099–101, 1967.

Booker DE, Pahl IR, Forbes DA. Control of postpartum breast engorgement with oral contraceptives. II. *Am J Obstet Gynecol* 108:240–42, 1970.

Bourget P, Quinquis-Desmaris V, Fernandez H. Ceftriaxone distribution and protein binding between maternal blood and milk postpartum. *Ann Pharmacother* 27:294–97, 1993.

Boutroy MJ et al. To nurse when receiving acebutolol: is it dangerous for the neonate? *Eur J Clin Pharmacol* 30:737–39, 1986.

Bowden CL et al. Efficacy of divalproex vs. lithium and placebo in the treatment of mania. The Depakote Mania Study Group. *JAMA* 271:918–24, 1994.

Brackbill Y, Kane J, Manniello RL. Obstetric meperidine usage and assessment of neonatal status. *Anesthesiology* 40:116–20, 1974a.

Brackbill Y et al. Obstetric premedication and infant outcome. *Am J Obstet Gynecol* 118:377–84, 1974b.

Briggs GG, Samson JH, Ambrose PJ. Excretion of bupropion in breast milk. *Annals Pharmacother* 27:431–33, 1993.

Budd SC et al. Improved lactation with metoclopramide. A case report. *Clin Pediatr (Phila)* 32:53–57, 1993.

Caballero-Gordo A et al. Oral cabergoline. Single-dose inhibition of puerperal lactation. *J Reprod Med* 36:717–21, 1991.

Canales ES, Garcia IC, Ruiz JE, Zarate A. Bromocriptine as prophylactic therapy in prolactinoma during pregnancy. *Fertil Steril* 36:524–6, 1981.

Cantu TG. Phenothiazines and sudden infant death syndrome. *DICP* 23:795–96, 1989.

Chambers CD et al. Birth outcomes in pregnant women taking fluoxetine [see comments]. *NEJM* 335:1010–15, 1996.

Chambers CD et al. Weight gain in infants breastfed by mothers who take fluoxetine. *Pediatrics* 104:e61, 1999.

Chasnoff IJ, Lewis DE, Squires L. Cocaine intoxication in a breast-fed infant. *Pediatrics* 80:836–38, 1987.

Chatterton RT Jr. Mammary gland: development and secretion. *Obstet Gynecol Annu* 7:303–24, 1978.

Chatterton RT Jr. et al. Relation of plasma oxytocin and prolactin concentrations to milk production in mothers of preterm infants: influence of stress. *J Clin Endocrinol Metab* 85:3661–68, 2000.

Cochi SL et al. Primary invasive *Haemophilus influenzae* type b disease: a population-based assessment of risk factors. *J Pediatr* 108:887–96, 1986a.

———. Primary invasive *Haemophilus influenzae* type b disease: a population-based assessment of risk factors. *J Pediatr* 108:887–96, 1986b.

Coulam CB, Moyer TP, Jiang NS. Breast-feeding after renal transplantation. *Transplant Proc* 14:605–9, 1982.

Cover DL, Mueller BA. Ciprofloxacin penetration into human breast milk: a case report [see comments]. *DICP* 24:703–4, 1990.

Croke S, Buist A, Hackett LP. Olanzapine excretion in human breast milk: estimation of infant exposure. *Int J Neuropsychopharmacol* 5:243–47, 2002.

da Silva OP, Knoppert DC, Angelini MM. Effect of domperidone on milk production in mothers of premature newborns: a randomized, double-blind, placebo-controlled trial. *CMAJ* 164:17–21, 2001.

Dutt S, Wong F, Spurway JH. Fatal myocardial infarction associated with bromocriptine for postpartum lactation suppression. *Aust N Z J Obstet Gynaecol* 38:116–17, 1998.

Ehrenkranz RA, Ackerman BA. Metoclopramide effect on faltering milk production by mothers of premature infants. *Pediatrics* 78:614–20, 1986.

Ferrari C, Piscitelli G, Crosignani PG. Cabergoline: a new drug for the treatment of hyperprolactinaemia. *Hum Reprod* 10:1647–52, 1995.

Figalgo I. Anemia aguda, rectaorragia y hematuria asociadas a la ingestion de naproxen. *Anales Espanoles de Pediatrica* 30:317–19, 1989.

Ford RP et al. Breastfeeding and the risk of sudden infant death syndrome. *Int J Epidemiol* 22:885–90, 1993.

Fries H. Lithium in pregnancy. *Lancet* 1:1233, 1970.

Gambrell RDJ. Immediate postpartum oral contraception. *Obstet Gynecol* 36:101–6, 1970.

Gardner DK, Gabbe SG, Harter C. Simultaneous concentrations of ciprofloxacin in breast milk and in serum in mother and breast-fed infant. *Clin Pharm* 11:352–54, 1992.

Giamarellou H, Kolokythas E, Petrikkos G. Pharmacokinetics of three newer quinolones in pregnant and lactating women. *Am J Med* 87:49S–51S, 1989.

Goldman AS. The immune system of human milk: antimicrobial, antiinflammatory and immunomodulating properties. *Pediatr Infect Dis J* 12:664–71, 1993.

Goldman AS et al. Immunologic protection of the premature newborn by human milk. *Semin Perinatol* 18:495–501, 1994.

Hale TW. *Medications and mothers' milk*. Amarillo, TX: Pharmasoft, 2002.

Hale TW, Berens PD. *Clinical therapy in breastfeeding patients*. Amarillo, TX: Pharmasoft Publishing LP, 2003.

Hale TW, Ilett KF. *Drug therapy and breastfeeding. From theory to clinical practice*. London: Parthenon Press, 2002.

Hale TW, Shum S, Grossberg M. Fluoxetine toxicity in a breastfed infant. *Clin Pediatr (Phila)* 40:681–84, 2001.

Hale TW et al. Transfer of metformin into human milk. *Diabetologia* 45:1509–14, 2002.

Harmon T, Burkhart G, Applebaum H. Perforated pseudomembranous colitis in the breast-fed infant. *J Pediatr Surg* 27:744–46, 1992.

Hill RC et al. Risperidone distribution and excretion into human milk: case report and estimated infant exposure during breast-feeding [letter]. *J Clin Psychopharmacol* 20:285–86, 2000.

Hodgkinson R, Huff RW, Hayashi RH, Husain FJ. Double-blind comparison of maternal analgesia and neonatal neurobehaviour following intravenous butorphanol and meperidine. *J Int Med Res* 7:224–30, 1979.

Hodgkinson R et al. Neonatal neurobehavior in the first 48 hours of life: effect of the administration of meperidine with and without naloxone in the mother. *Pediatrics* 62:294–98, 1978.

Hofmeyr GJ, Van Iddekinge B. Domperidone and lactation [letter]. *Lancet* 1:647, 1983.

Hofmeyr GJ, Van Iddekinge B, Blott JA. Domperidone: secretion in breast milk and effect on puerperal prolactin levels. *Br J Obstet Gynaecol* 92:141–44, 1985.

Iffy L et al. Severe cardiac dysrhythmia in patients using bromocriptine postpartum. *Am J Ther* 5:111–15, 1998.

Ilett KF, Kristensen JH, Hackett LP. Distribution of venlafaxine and its O-desmethyl metabolite in human milk and their effects in breastfed infants. *Br J Clin Pharmacol* 53:17–22, 2002.

Ilett KF et al. Distribution and excretion of venlafaxine and O-desmethylvenlafaxine in human milk. *Br J Clin Pharmacol* 45:459–62, 1998.

Ito S, Blajchman A, Stephenson M. Prospective follow-up of adverse reactions in breastfed infants exposed to maternal medication. *Am J Obstet Gynecol* 168:1393–99, 1993.

Kafetzis DA, Lazarides CV, Siafas CA. Transfer of cefotaxime in human milk and from mother to foetus. *J Antimicrob Chemother* 6 (suppl A):135–41, 1980.

Kafetzis DA, Siafas CA, Georgakopoulos PA, Papadatos CJ. Passage of cephalosporins and amoxicillin into the breast milk. *Acta Paediatr Scand* 70:285–88, 1981.

Kahn A, Hasaerts D, Blum D. Phenothiazine-induced sleep apneas in normal infants. *Pediatrics* 75:844–47, 1985.

Kampmann JP, Johansen K, Hansen JM. Propylthiouracil in human milk. Revision of a dogma. *Lancet* 1:736–37, 1980.

Kauffman RE, O'Brien C, Gilford P. Sulfisoxazole secretion into human milk. *J Pediatr* 97:839–41, 1980.

Kauppila A, Arvela P, Koivisto M, Kivinen S, Ylikorkala O, Pelkonen O. Metoclopramide and breast feeding: transfer into milk and the newborn. *Eur J Clin Pharmacol* 25:819–23, 1983.

Kauppila A, Kivinen S, Ylikorkala O. A dose response relation between improved lactation and metoclopramide. *Lancet* 1:1175–77, 1981.

Kelsey JJ et al. Presence of azithromycin breast milk concentrations: a case report. *Am J Obstet Gynecol* 170:1375–76, 1994.

Knowles JA. Drugs in milk. *Pediatr Currents* 21:28–32, 1972.

Kristensen JH et al. Distribution and excretion of sertraline and N-desmethylsertraline in human milk. *Br J Clin Pharmacol* 45:453–57, 1998.

Kristensen JH et al. Distribution and excretion of fluoxetine and norfluoxetine in human milk. *Br J Clin Pharmacol* 48:521–27, 1999.

Kuhnert BR et al. Meperidine and normeperidine levels following meperidine administration during labor. II. Fetus and neonate. *Am J Obstet Gynecol* 133:909–14, 1979a.

Kuhnert BR et al. Meperidine and normeperidine levels following meperidine administration during labor. I. Mother. *Am J Obstet Gynecol* 133:904–8, 1979b.

Kuhnert BR et al. Meperidine disposition in mother, neonate, and nonpregnant females. *Clin Pharmacol Ther* 27:486–91, 1980.

Kumar AR, Hale TW, Mock RE. Transfer of interferon alfa into human breast milk. *J Hum Lact* 16:226–28, 2000.

Lamberg BA et al. Antithyroid treatment of maternal hyperthyroidism during lactation. *Clin Endocrinol (Oxf)* 21:81–87, 1984.

Lee CM, Gotlib IH. Adjustment of children of depressed mothers: a 10-month follow-up. *J Abnorm Psychol* 100:473–77, 1991.

Lester BM et al. Possible association between fluoxetine hydrochloride and colic in an infant. *J Am Acad Child Adolesc Psychiatry* 32:1253–55, 1993.

Leuschen MP, Wolf LJ, Rayburn WF. Fentanyl excretion in breast milk [letter]. *Clin Pharm* 9:336–37, 1990.

Liedholm H et al. Transplacental passage and breast milk concentrations of hydralazine. *Eur J Clin Pharmacol* 21:417–19, 1982.

Llewellyn A, Stowe ZN, Strader JRJ. The use of lithium and management of women with bipolar disorder during pregnancy and lactation [review; 67 refs]. *J Clin Psychiat* 59 (suppl 6):57–64; discussion 65:57–64, 1998.

Low LC, Lang J, Alexander WD. Excretion of carbimazole and propylthiouracil in breast milk [letter]. *Lancet* 2:1011, 1979.

Matheson I. Drugs taken by mothers in the puerperium. *Br Med J (Clin Res Ed)* 290:1588–89, 1985.

Matheson I, Kristensen K, Lunde PK. Drug utilization in breast-feeding women. A survey in Oslo. *Eur J Clin Pharmacol* 38:453–59, 1990.

Matheson I, Lunde PK, Bredesen JE. Midazolam and nitrazepam in the maternity ward: milk concentrations and clinical effects. *Br J Clin Pharmacol* 30:787–93, 1990.

Matsuda S. Transfer of antibiotics into maternal milk. *Biol Res Pregnancy Perinatol* 5:57–60, 1984.

McBride RJ et al. A study of the plasma concentrations of lorazepam in mother and neonate. *Br J Anaesth* 51:971–78, 1979.

McCarthy JJ, Posey BL. Methadone levels in human milk. *J Hum Lact* 16:115–20, 2000.

Mennella JA, Beauchamp GK. The transfer of alcohol to human milk. Effects on flavor and the infant's behavior. *N Eng J Med* 325:918–85, 1991.

Miller GE, Banerjee NC, Stowe CM Jr. Diffusion of certain weak organic acids and bases across the bovine mammary gland membrane after systemic administration. *J Pharmacol Exp Ther* 157:245–53, 1967.

Mizuta H et al. Thyroid hormones in human milk and their influence on thyroid function of breast-fed babies. *Pediatr Res* 17:468–71, 1983.

Morselli PL, Franco-Morselli R, Bossi L. Clinical pharmacokinetics in newborns and infants: age-related differences and therapeutic implications. *Clin Pharmacokinet* 5: 485–527, 1980.

Nau H et al. Valproic acid and its metabolites: placental transfer, neonatal pharmacokinetics, transfer via mother's milk and clinical status in neonates of epileptic mothers. *J Pharmacol Exp Ther* 219:768–77, 1981.

Nau H et al. Anticonvulsants during pregnancy and lactation: transplacental, maternal and neonatal pharmacokinetics. *Clin Pharmacokinet* 7:508–43, 1982.

Nehlig A, Debry G. Consequences on the newborn of chronic maternal consumption of coffee during gestation and lactation: a review. *J Am Coll Nutr* 13:6–21, 1994.

Neville MC, McFadden TB, Forsyth I. Hormonal regulation of mammary differentiation and milk secretion. *J Mammary Gland Biol Neoplasia* 7:49–66, 2002.

Neville MC, Morton J. Physiology and endocrine changes underlying human lactogenesis II. *J Nutr* 131: 3005S–3008S, 2001.

Nulman I et al. Neurodevelopment of children exposed in utero to antidepressant drugs. *N Engl J Med* 336:258–62, 1997.

O'Hara MW et al. Controlled prospective study of postpartum mood disorders: comparison of childbearing and nonchildbearing women. *J Abnorm Psychol* 99:3–15, 1990.

Oberkotter LV. Thyroid function and human breast milk [letter]. *Am J Dis Child* 137:1131, 1983.

Ost L et al. Prednisolone excretion in human milk. *J Pediatr* 106:1008–11, 1985.

Ostrea EM, Chavez CJ, Strauss ME. A study of factors that influence the severity of neonatal narcotic withdrawal. *J Pediat* 88:642–45, 1976.

Passmore CM et al. Metronidazole excretion in human milk and its effect on the suckling neonate. *Br J Clin Pharmacol* 26:45–51, 1988.

Penny WJ, Lewis MJ. Nifedipine is excreted in human milk. *Eur J Clin Pharmacol* 36:427–28, 1989.

Perez-Reyes M, Wall ME. Presence of delta9-tetrahydrocannabinol in human milk [letter]. *N Engl J Med* 307:819–20, 1982.

Petraglia F et al. Domperidone in defective and insufficient lactation. *Eur J Obstet Gynecol Reprod Biol* 19:281–87, 1985.

Pisacane A et al. Breast-feeding and urinary tract infection. *J Pediatr* 120:87–89, 1992.

Pollard AJ, Rylance G. Inappropriate prescribing of promethazine in infants [letter]. *Arch Dis Child* 70:357, 1994.

Pop C et al. Postpartum myocardial infarction induced by Parlodel. *Arch Mal Coeur Vaiss* 91:1171–74, 1998.

Pope HG Jr. et al. Valproate in the treatment of acute mania: a placebo-controlled study. *Arch Gen Psychiatry* 48:62–68, 1991.

Postellon DC, Aronow R. Iodine in mother's milk. *JAMA* 247:463, 1982.

Quinn PG et al. Measurement of meperidine and normeperidine in human breast milk by selected ion monitoring. *Biomed Environ Mass Spectrom* 13:133–35, 1986.

Rampono J et al. Citalopram and demethylcitalopram in human milk; distribution, excretion and effects in breast fed infants. *Br J Clin Pharmacol* 50:263–68, 2000.

Rasmussen F. *Excretion of drugs by milk.* New York: Springer-Verlag, 1971.

Robieux I et al. Morphine excretion in breast milk and resultant exposure of a nursing infant. *J Toxicol Clin Toxicol* 28:365–70, 1990.

Rofsky NM, Weinreb JC, Litt AW. Quantitative analysis of gadopentetate dimeglumine excreted in breast milk. *J Magn Reson Imaging* 3:131–32, 1993.

Ross M, Gordon K, Paulina W. *Histology: a text and atlas.* Lippincott, Williams & Wilkins, 2002.

Schadewinkel-Scherkl AM et al. Active transport of benzylpenicillin across the blood-milk barrier. *Pharmacol Toxicol* 73:14–19, 1993.

Shyu WC et al. Excretion of cefprozil into human breast milk. *Antimicrob Agents Chemother* 36:938–41, 1992.

Sinclair D, Murray L. Effects of postnatal depression on children's adjustment to school. Teacher's reports. *Br J Psychiatry* 172:58–63, 1998.

Sorensen HT et al. Risk of infantile hypertrophic pyloric stenosis after maternal postnatal use of macrolides. *Scan J Infect Dis* 35:104–6, 2003.

Spalding G. Bromocriptine (Parlodel) for suppression of lactation. *Aust NZ J Obstet Gynecol* 31:344–45, 1991.

Spencer MJ, Escondido CA. Fluoxetine hydrochloride (Prozac) toxicity in a neonate. *Pediatrics* 92:721–22, 1993.

Stavchansky S, Combs A, Sagraves R, Delgado M, Joshi A. Pharmacokinetics of caffeine in breast milk and plasma after single oral administration of caffeine to lactating mothers. *Biopharm Drug Dispos* 9:285–99, 1988.

Steiner E et al. Amphetamine secretion in breast milk. *Eur J Clin Pharmacol* 27:123–24, 1984.

Stewart RB, Karas B, Springer PK. Haloperidol excretion in human milk. *Am J Psychiat* 137:849–50, 1980.

Stiskal JA et al. Neonatal paroxetine withdrawal syndrome. *Arch Dis Child Fetal Neonatal Ed* 84:F134–35, 2001.

Stowe ZN et al. Sertraline and desmethylsertraline in human breast milk and nursing infants [see comments]. *Am J Psychiatry* 154:1255–60, 1997.

Stowe ZN et al. Paroxetine in human breast milk and nursing infants. *Am J Psychiatry* 157:185–89, 2000.

Strauss ME et al. Methadone maintenance during pregnancy: pregnancy, birth, and neonate characteristics. *Am J Obstet Gynecol* 120:895–900, 1974.

Summerfield RJ, Nielsen MS. Excretion of lorazepam into breast milk [letter]. *Br J Anaesth* 57:1042–43, 1985.

Swafford S and Berens P. Effect of fenugreek on breast milk production [Annual meeting abstracts Sept 11–13, 2000.] *BM News and Views* 6(3), 2000.

Sweezy SR. Contraception for the postpartum woman. *NAACOG Clin Issu Perinat Womens Health Nurs* 3:209–26, 1992.

Sykes PA, Quarrie J, Alexander FW. Lithium carbonate and breast-feeding. *Br Med J* 2:1299, 1976.

Syversen GB, Ratkje SK. Drug distribution within human milk phases. *J Pharm Sci* 74:1071–74, 1985.

Taddio A, Klein J, Koren G. Acyclovir excretion in human breast milk. *Ann Pharmacother* 28:585–87, 1994.

Tegler L, Lindstrom B. Antithyroid drugs in milk. *Lancet* 2:591, 1980.

Tennes K et al. Marijuana: prenatal and postnatal exposure in the human. *NIDA Res Monogr* 59:48–60, 1985.

Treffers PE. Breastfeeding and contraception. *Ned Tijdschr Geneeskd* 143:1900–4, 1999.

Tunnessen WWJ, Hertz CG. Toxic effects of lithium in newborn infants: a commentary. *J Pediatr* 81:804–7, 1972.

US Nuclear Regulatory Commission. *Nuclear Regulatory Commission Guideline 8.39*. Washington, DC, April 1997.

Webster J. A comparative review of the tolerability profiles of dopamine agonists in the treatment of hyperprolactinaemia and inhibition of lactation [published erratum appears in *Drug Saf* 1996 May;14(5):342]. *Drug Saf* 14:228–38, 1996.

Webster J et al. Dose-dependent suppression of serum prolactin by cabergoline in hyperprolactinaemia: a placebo controlled, double blind, multicentre study. European Multicentre Cabergoline Dose-finding Study Group. *Clin Endocrinol (Oxf)* 37:534–41, 1992.

Weintrob N et al. Decreased growth during therapy with selective serotonin reuptake inhibitors. *Arch Pediatr Adolesc Med* 156:696–701, 2002.

Wesson DR et al. Diazepam and desmethyldiazepam in breast milk. *J Psychoactive Drugs* 17:55–56, 1985.

Whalley LJ, Blain PG, Prime JK. Haloperidol secreted in breast milk. *Br Med J (Clin Res Ed)* 282:1746–47, 1981.

White GJ, White MK. Breast feeding and drugs in human milk. *Vet Human Toxicol* 22(1):18, 1980.

White WB, Andreoli JW, Cohn RD. Alpha-methyldopa disposition in mothers with hypertension and in their breast-fed infants. *Clin Pharmacol Ther* 37:387–90, 1985.

Whitelaw AG, Cummings AJ, McFadyen IR. Effect of maternal lorazepam on the neonate. *Br Med J (Clin Res Ed)* 282:1106–08, 1981.

Wiles DH, Orr MW, Kolakowska T. Chlorpromazine levels in plasma and milk of nursing mothers [letter]. *Br J Clin Pharmacol* 5:272–73, 1978.

Wisner KL, Perel JM, Blumer J. Serum sertraline and N-desmethylsertraline levels in breastfeeding mother-infant pairs. *Am J Psychiat* 155:690–92, 1998.

Wittels B, Scott DT, Sinatra RS. Exogenous opioids in human breast milk and acute neonatal neurobehavior: a preliminary study. *Anesthesiology* 73:864–69, 1990.

Wojnar-Horton RE et al. Methadone distribution and excretion into breast milk of clients in a methadone maintenance programme. *Br J Clin Pharmacol* 44:543–47, 1997.

Work Group on Breastfeeding. Breastfeeding and the use of human milk. American Academy of Pediatrics Work Group on Breastfeeding. *Pediatrics* 100:1035–39, 1997.

Yoshioka H et al. Transfer of cefazolin into human milk. *J Pediatr* 94:151–52, 1979.

Zekoski EM, O'Hara MW, Wills KE. The effects of maternal mood on mother-infant interaction. *J Abnorm Child Psychol* 15:361–78, 1987.

VIRUSES AND BREASTFEEDING

Jan Riordan

Mother-to-child transmission (MTCT) of a viral infection is a passage of infection that can occur during pregnancy, birthing, and the postpartum period. Specific concerns about infectious diseases and possible transmission through breastfeeding include the risks from mothers who acquire an infection while breastfeeding or during or before pregnancy. Questions abound:

- Which pathogens are found in the milk of infected or seropositive women?

- What is the risk of transmission of such pathogens by breastfeeding?

- What effect does the infection have on the child?

- Do protective maternal antibodies in the milk limit transmission or reduce the severity of the viral infection in the child?

- Is there an effective treatment for the mother or the baby?

This chapter seeks to answer these questions, although we recognize that there are no simple answers to the complex puzzle of viral transmission from mother to infant.

Human milk, nature's most perfect vaccine model, plays a vital role in protecting the suckling young from viral infections. At the same time, a variety of animal and human viruses can be transmitted through mother's milk. Because breastmilk is a highly cellular fluid and viruses are intracellular (i.e., live within the cell), maternal-infant transmission by breastmilk is possible. The transmission of cytomegalovirus (CMV) through breastmilk, for example, occurs frequently and provides a natural vaccine that confers active immunity to the infant against infection. CMV primary infection during pregnancy, on the other hand, can cause serious illness in a vulnerable infant, such as a preterm baby, especially if the viral load is high (van der Strate et al., 2001).

In contrast, hepatitis B virus and rubella virus appear in human milk, but breastfeeding does not appear to be a common mode of transmission for either. The opposite is true of human immunodeficiency virus (HIV) and human T-cell lymphotropic virus type I (HTLV-1). Both are transmitted by breastmilk, with potentially adverse effects on the child.

HIV and Infant Feeding

Worldwide, approximately 800,000 children under 15 years of age are newly infected with HIV every year, most of them in sub-Saharan Africa. MTCT of

HIV accounts for approximately 90 percent of these infections. Total perinatal transmission of women who are HIV positive is about 15 to 30 percent. Intrauterine transmission accounts for about 5 to 10 percent of cases; intrapartum transmission accounts for another 10 to 20 percent. Breastfeeding increases the rate of transmission above that related to fetal and intrapartum by approximately 10 to 16 percent (De Cock et al., 2000; Dunn et al., 1992; Nduati, 2001).

At the same time, not breastfeeding in a developing country can be deadly. In a recent study (Brahmbhall & Gray, 2003) of 14 developing countries, child mortality among the offspring of women who never initiated breastfeeding was higher than among children of women who weaned (326.8 per 1000 versus 34.8 per 1000, respectively). The risk was higher both among children who were never breastfed versus children who were weaned because of preceding morbidity and among children who were never breastfed versus those who were weaned as a result of voluntary choice.

Currently, 120,000 to 160,000 US women are infected with HIV. Eighty percent of these women are of childbearing age. Routine HIV testing and counseling to all pregnant women, and AZT administration to those who are HIV positive, is now considered the standard of care in the United States. Breastfeeding by HIV-infected women in more developed countries has virtually ceased. At the same time, new antiviral drugs and the knowledge that HIV-infected women who breastfeed exclusively have a lower risk of transmitting HIV to the baby are affecting public health policy worldwide.

Antiretroviral therapy is profoundly effective in preventing perinatal transmission. Administration of short-course antiretroviral treatment to HIV-infected pregnant women and their newborns reduces the risk for perinatal transmission of HIV by approximately one half to two thirds (Connor et al., 1994; Karim et al., 2002). As a result, the overall death rate of AIDS cases in this population has decreased in recent years (Katz, 2003).

Exclusive Breastfeeding

Exclusive breastfeeding appears to also prevent HIV infection. In a seminal prospective study of 549 HIV-infected mothers in South Africa, Coutsoudis et al. (1999) examined infant feeding practices as part of a vitamin A intervention trial. After adjusting for potential confounders, they found that infants who were exclusively breastfeeding had a significantly lower risk of HIV-1 transmission. Those infants receiving supplemental formula had the same risk as infants who were not breastfeeding. The probable reasons for this all or nothing phenomenon relates to the intestinal mucosal barrier, which is maintained by reduction in dietary antigens and enteric pathogens (Smith & Kuhn, 2000). When other investigators confirm this study's findings, they will offer a major breakthrough for areas of the world where replacement feedings are not easily available (Jackson et al., 2003).

At the same time, changing existing feeding practices to exclusive breastfeeding is an enormous challenge. Worldwide, few infants are exclusively breastfed in spite of long duration of partial breastfeeding in many developing areas. In Tanzania, for example, almost half of the women in one study had introduced additional fluids to their babies after only a few days even though 85 percent started breastfeeding within the first 2 hours after birth (de Paoli et al., 2001).

What We Know

The number of AIDS cases in the developed world began to explode sometime in the late 1970s, particularly among the US male homosexual population. Formerly considered a "gay" or drug abusers' disease in the developed world, AIDS has now also emerged as a woman's disease, as evidenced by the annual increase in the number of HIV-infected women. AIDS is the most serious threat to worldwide public health since the poliomyelitis epidemics earlier in the twentieth century. Tragically, the largest impact is in the poorest countries of Africa and Asia. The United Nations estimates that about 2000 HIV-infected babies are born daily in developing countries. In parts of sub-Saharan Africa, the region hardest hit by AIDS, as many as 30 percent of pregnant women are infected. Box 6–1 presents the recommendations on infant feeding and HIV issued by the WHO Technical Consultation Task Force (World Health Organization [WHO], 2000).

BOX 6–1

WHO Recommendations for Prevention of Mother-to-Child Transmission of HIV

RECOMMENDATIONS FOR INFANT FEEDING

Risks of Breastfeeding vs. Replacement Feeding

- When replacement feeding is acceptable, feasible, affordable, sustainable and safe, avoidance of all breastfeeding by HIV-infected mothers is recommended.
- Otherwise, exclusive breastfeeding is recommended during the first months of life.
- To minimize HIV transmission risk, breastfeeding should be discontinued as soon as feasible, taking into account local circumstances, the individual woman's situation and the risks of replacement feeding (including infections other than HIV and malnutrition).
- When HIV-infected mothers choose not to breastfeed from birth or stop breastfeeding later, they should be provided with specific guidance and support for at least the first 2 years of the child's life to ensure adequate replacement feeding. Programmes should strive to improve conditions that will make replacement feeding safer for HIV-infected mothers and families.

Cessation of Breastfeeding

- HIV-infected mothers who breastfeed should be provided with specific guidance and support when they cease breastfeeding to avoid harmful nutritional and psychological consequences and to maintain breast health.

Infant Feeding Counseling

- All HIV-infected mothers should receive counseling, which includes provision of general information about the risks and benefits of various infant feeding options, and specific guidance in selecting the option most likely to be suitable for their situation. Whatever a mother decides, she should be supported in her choice.
- Assessments should be conducted locally to identify the range of feeding options that are acceptable, feasible, affordable, sustainable and safe in a particular context.
- Information and education on mother-to-child transmission of HIV should be urgently directed to the general public, affected communities, and families.
- Adequate numbers of people who can counsel HIV-infected women on infant feeding should be trained, deployed, supervised, and supported. Such support should include updated training as new information and recommendations emerge.

Breast Health

- There is some evidence that breast conditions including mastitis, breast abscess, and nipple fissure may increase the risk of HIV transmission through breastfeeding, but the extent of this association is not well quantified. HIV-infected women who breastfeed should be assisted to ensure that they use a good breastfeeding technique to prevent these conditions, which should be treated promptly if they occur.

BOX 6–1 (cont.)

Maternal Health

- HIV-infected women should have access to information, follow-up clinical care, and support, including family planning services and nutritional support. Family planning services are particularly important for HIV-infected women who are not breastfeeding.

Source: World Health Organization. *Technical Consultation on Behalf of the UNFPA/UNICEF/WHO/UNADIS Inter-Agency Task Team on Mother-to-Child Transmission of HIV.* Geneva, October 11–13, 2000: 31–36.

Treatment and Prevention

AZT and protease inhibitors block one step of the reproductive cycle of HIV and sharply reduce the risk of transmission from mother to infant. AZT given in a combined regimen to the mother during pregnancy and during labor and to the infant after birth reduces the transmission rate of HIV by two thirds; however, AZT is expensive. Nevirapine, a less expensive new AIDS drug that can be taken by breastfeeding women, is now widely used around the world. It has been estimated that widespread use of nevirapine could prevent between 300,000 and 400,000 babies a year from contracting HIV at birth. A clinical trial in Uganda showed that the rate of new infections from breastfeeding at age 6 weeks to 12 months was not increased in infants of mothers receiving nevirapine (Owor et al., 2000).

In December 2002, a new coalition was launched to promote international cooperation in expanding access to HIV treatments for all persons needing them. The International Treatment Access Coalition (ITAC) is a network of Non-Governmental Organizations (NGOs), international organizations, donors, developing countries, and research institutions. It will serve as a platform for national and international advocacy on HIV treatment access, and analyze and disseminate information and knowledge on pilot programs to guide and pool technical expertise for implementation of national programs (WHO, 2002). Risk factors that play a role in HIV transmission into human milk are listed in Box 6–2. General guidelines for avoiding perinatal transmission of HIV include the following:

- *Formula feeding if the mother is HIV-1 positive and there are safe, affordable alternatives available:* It is well established that HIV can be transmitted from mother to infant through breastfeeding. The US Department of Health and Human Services (2000) states that HIV-infected women should not breastfeed or provide their breastmilk for the nutrition of their own or other infants.

- *Exclusive breastfeeding if safe alternative supplements are not available:* If safe replacement feedings are not feasible, promotion of exclusive breastfeeding reduces risk of HIV-1 transmission to the baby. If safe replacement infant feedings are not available, the risk of HIV transmission is exchanged for the risk of diarrhea and pneumonia if fuel to boil water for replacement-feeding preparation, sterilization, nutritional additives, and equipment are not available (Savage & Lothska, 2000). Generally, the morbidity and mortality from not breastfeeding are greater than the morbidity and mortality of breastfeeding by an HIV-positive woman.

- *Deferring pregnancy:* Women who are seropositive for HIV are advised to defer pregnancy. In countries where surgical delivery is available, a cesarean section can significantly reduce mother-to-baby HIV-1 transmission. In the case of vaginal birth, premature rupture of membranes and insertion of scalp electrodes should be avoided.

- *Avoiding practices that might increase exposure to HIV:* Uninfected mothers who are breastfeeding should be especially careful to avoid high-risk practices (e.g., drug abuse or a sexual partner who is bisexual or has engaged in practices linked to HIV transmission) that might expose them to a primary HIV infection (Dunn et al., 1992; van de Perre, 1991).

- *Maintaining breast health by preventing entry of virus:* Breast conditions such mastitis, breast abscess, and nipple fissure may increase the risk of HIV transmission through breastfeeding. The extent of this association is not well documented (Smith & Kuhn, 2000).

Health-Care Practitioners

Practitioners who work with human milk or with breastfeeding women are concerned about their own protection. The Centers for Disease Control (CDC) recommends that precautions be taken when handling blood and body fluids of all patients, regardless of their infection status. These universal precautions apply to blood and other body fluids that contain visible blood (e.g., semen and vaginal secretions). Universal precautions *do not apply* to human milk unless it contains visible blood (CDC, 1988). Occupational exposure to human milk has not been implicated in the transmission of HIV. Gloves are not needed when touching the breasts (e.g., in breast assessment), and they usually are not necessary when handling breastmilk. However, if health-care workers come in frequent contact with human milk (e.g., while working in human milk banking), they may choose to wear gloves. Also, if the mother has an open wound on her breast, glove wearing is warranted for the protection of both the mother and her care provider.

Health-care workers routinely wear gloves during delivery and for newborn care. Vigorous hand washing by the care provider—both before and after any physical contact with a client or with any body fluid—is standard practice for infection control and should be performed consistently to prevent transmission of *any* infection in the mother, the child, and the health-care worker. Pasteurization of all pooled breastmilk presumably eliminates any risk of transmission of HIV, making unnecessary HIV antibody screening of donors.

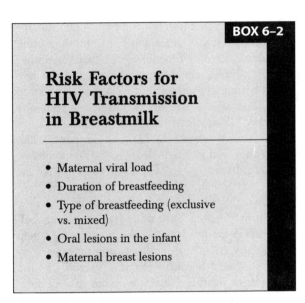

BOX 6-2

Risk Factors for HIV Transmission in Breastmilk

- Maternal viral load
- Duration of breastfeeding
- Type of breastfeeding (exclusive vs. mixed)
- Oral lesions in the infant
- Maternal breast lesions

Counseling

The WHO Technical Guidelines emphasize that all HIV-infected mothers should receive feeding counseling that includes provision of general information about the risks and benefits of various infant feeding options, and specific guidance in selecting the option most likely to be suitable for their situation (Coutsoudis, 2000). If the results of the study by Coutsoudis et al. (1999) are confirmed, a powerful new public health mandate will be to teach mothers in resource-poor settings the health benefits of practicing exclusive breastfeeding. Another mandate is working with women whose HIV status is negative or unknown and who choose not to breastfeed out of fear or misinformation—a "spillover" effect that could dissuade some women from breastfeeding (International Lactation Consultant Association, 2002).

HIV-infected women come from all walks of life; some are not drug abusers or prostitutes and are victims themselves. Whatever the direct cause of their illness, their lives are shattered by the knowledge that they are HIV positive, which may be disclosed when their babies are born or when their spouses become ill or die. Often they feel dirty, useless, unwanted, and unlovable. Few illnesses are associated with such high levels of stigma and social isolation. One woman complained that the health-care workers at the local clinic acted "like they didn't want to talk to me or touch me. It's like I have AIDS written across my forehead and they don't see anything else but that." Another noted, "I think I could be in a wreck and my arm would be hanging off and I'd be about to bleed to death, and all the doctors would see is someone with HIV" (Black & Miles, 2002).

In some areas where AIDS is rampant, white cream on a woman's face provides visible evidence that she is breastfeeding. On a visit to South Africa, I saw young women with white cream on their faces, which provided a signal to others that they were breastfeeding and thus HIV negative. Although HIV-positive women desperately need help from family, friends, and other support groups, they may be isolated because HIV is a "secret" disease. They suffer profound grief over the loss of their health, their sexuality, their chance to have more children, and their ability to breastfeed safely. Their counseling needs are necessarily complex, because these women must make difficult decisions while trying to cope with the implications of HIV for themselves and their families. When offering counseling, the care provider must recognize that children are central to many of these women's lives and they are reluctant to forgo childbearing and breastfeeding (Lindberg, 1995).

WHO has developed a 3-day HIV and infant feeding counseling course for health workers who are responsible for counseling mothers on HIV and infant feeding. The guidelines describe various feeding options for mothers who are HIV-infected, including replacement feeding, modified breastfeeding (i.e., early cessation of exclusive breastfeeding, expression and heat treatment of mother's own breastmilk), and using breastmilk from a milk bank.

Herpes Simplex Virus

The herpes simplex virus (HSV), caused by *Herpesvirus hominus*, is a common viral infection in humans. HSV Type 2 and HSV Type 1 are sexually transmitted diseases. Type 2 (HSV-2) is associated more frequently with infection of the genital area and Type 1 (HSV-1) most often occurs in the face and mouth. Herpetic lesions can erupt anywhere on the body, including the breast or the genital area, usually as a result of direct contact. The infection may be either primary or recurrent. Diagnosis is made either by culturing the lesion or by drawing serum-antibody titers.

The painful mucocutaneous blisterlike vesicles of herpes can appear within a few hours, or up to 20 days after exposure. After the lesions heal, the virus enters a dormant phase and resides in the nerve ganglia in the affected area. Usually the primary infection is the most severe. Neonatal HSV-1 infection is usually acquired when the newborn passes through an infected genital tract; congenital infection is responsible for the most serious illness in neonates. Vaginal delivery is safe in most women with a history of recurrent genital herpes unless active lesions are present at term. The American College of Obstetricians and Gynecologists (2002) officially recommends that a cesarean section be performed within six hours of rupture of membranes if active lesions are present. Cesarean delivery is not recommended when a woman with a history of recurrent infection has no obvious lesions and no symptoms of the infection.

The greatest threat of HSV-1 infection appears to be with neonates and when the mother experiences a first episode of genital herpes during pregnancy near term (Donahue, 2002). Primary infection means that the mother has insufficient antibodies that would help protect the infant from infection. Transmission rate to the newborn is 50 percent with a primary infection and only 1 to 3 percent if it is recurrent. Neonates may become seriously ill; beyond the first few weeks of the neonate's life, however, there are few adverse consequences. Despite the high prevalence of genital herpes in the general population, the incidence of neonatal herpes is low and ranges from 1 in 2000 to about 1 in 10,000 births (Brown, 1995). It is doubtful that neonatal herpes is transmitted through human milk. Transmission during breastfeeding, if it occurs, is most likely from direct contact with the herpes vesicle on the breast.

Sealander and Kerr (1989) report a case of a nursing toddler transmitting HSV to the mother through breastfeeding. In this case, the child's oral lesions (on the inner aspect of the lower lip) caused painful blisters on the mother's nipples. Culture of the child's oral lesions and the mother's nipple lesions were positive for HSV-1. After one week's cessation of breastfeeding, during which time the mother was given oral acyclovir—200 mg 5 times daily for 5 days—the mother resumed breastfeeding. The authors recommended that whenever a young child develops oral HSV lesions, the mother should be asked whether she is breastfeeding the child in order that the risk of contracting HSV from her child can be explained and appropriate intervention offered.

Sullivan-Bolyai et al. (1983) report the case of a mother with a breast lesion identified as HSV-1. Although her infant experienced an uneventful nursery course and was discharged from the hospital at 2 days of age, the mother reported developing a "skin sore" on the areola of her left breast during her postpartum stay. On the fourth day of life, the baby appeared to have pustules in the corner of his mouth and on his chin. On day 6 and 7, HSV was also isolated from the mouth of the infant; on day 7, the virus was isolated from the mother's breast lesions. The infant died at 11 days of age. This case points out the need to avoid direct infant contact with an HSV-1 lesion. Although the mother's milk may be free of the virus, the lesion itself will not be.

Although HSV-1 can occasionally be cultured from breastmilk, this appears to be rare (Oxtoby, 1988). HSV-1 has not been isolated in any of the CMV studies that used culture techniques appropriate for HSV-1 (Pass, 1986), and no role in transmitting infection in the absence of a local HSV-1 lesion has been demonstrated. Breast lesions are seldom the first clinical evidence of herpes in the family (Sullivan-Bolyai et al., 1983). The primary herpetic lesion can be manifested in other family members who then pass it on (e.g., the father through sexual contact with the mother, or a sibling who kisses a baby brother or sister). Therefore, transmission can be from mother to infant or from infant to mother; or some other family member can infect the infant, who then passes the virus on to the mother during feedings. HSV is an emotionally difficult, anxiety-producing topic. There is no way to know when a reactivation will occur. In addition, there are other issues such as disclosure of the disease to sexual partners and condom use.

Women with herpetic lesions on their breasts should refrain from breastfeeding; active lesions should be covered (AAP, 1997) to prevent contact by the suckling infant. In the absence of breast lesions, the newborn of a mother with HSV-1, if the baby is well, may breastfeed and be with the mother in her room; however, scrupulous hand washing, gowning, and covering of any lesions must be practiced to prevent possible cross-contamination. The mother does not need to wear rubber gloves while breastfeeding.

Treatment is usually directed toward symptomatic relief and prevention of a secondary infection, because there is no known cure. Acyclovir (Zovirax), valacyclovir, and famciclovir are antiviral medications used for HSV infections. Aggressive and early use of intravenous acyclovir results in apparent improvement for the mother and infant. Acyclovir can be given orally, applied topically, or given intravenously (usually when treating neonatal HSV). The routine administration of acyclovir to pregnant women with a history of recurrent infections is not recommended (Cline, Bailey-Dorton, & Cayelli, 2000). A new over-the-counter antiviral cream, docosanal (Abreva) is now available to treat cold sores/fever blisters. Cleaning affected areas with povidone-iodine (Betadine) solution is thought to help prevent a secondary infection, and applying Burrow's solution (aluminum acetate) may relieve some of the discomfort. Vitamin C or lysine and lysine supplements are frequently suggested to prevent recurrence, although their efficacy is unknown. A plan for the care of a breastfeeding mother with HSV is given in Table 6–1.

Chickenpox/Varicella

Most people have immunity to chickenpox (varicella-zoster virus); therefore the issue of whether mothers with chickenpox can breastfeed is uncommon. Those who have not had chickenpox and are not immune (5–15 percent of adults) are potentially infectious for the 10th through the 21st day after exposure. Lesions begin on the neck or trunk and spread to the face, scalp, mucous membranes, and extremities. Lesions first appear as small, flat, red blotches and progress to raised vesicles that form crusts over a period of 2 to 4 days. A vaccine (live attenuated virus) to prevent varicella was developed in 1995 and millions of doses of the vaccine have been administered since then. The CDC recommends vaccination of all susceptible health-care workers.

Table 6–1

CLINICAL CARE PLAN FOR BREASTFEEDING MOTHER WITH HERPES SIMPLEX (HSV) INFECTION

Problem	Intervention	Rationale
Seropositive for HSV	Encourage continued breastfeeding unless breast lesions are present.	Provides protective antibodies to infant
Herpes	Instruct mother to wash hands thoroughly with soap before breastfeeding.	Helps prevent spreading infection
No breast lesion	Caution mother against touching baby or breast after touching lesion from any site.	Avoid risks of shedding
	Caution mother to avoid tub bath with infant; use universal precautions (hospital staff).	Avoid risks of shedding
Breast lesion present	Discourage breastfeeding from affected breast; encourage use of breast pump to maintain comfort and milk supply; after each use, sterilize pump part that comes in contact with breast.	Prevents infant's direct contact with lesion
Pain	Administer acetaminophen.	Analgesia
	Apply Burrow's solution topically.	Soothing effect
	Employ imagery.	Distraction by focusing
Feelings of shame	Reassure mother that HSV is not uncommon.	Mothers tend to blame themselves
Secondary infection	Cleanse lesion with Betadine.	Antibacterial

Because chickenpox can occur during the reproductive years, a woman may develop this infection while she is breastfeeding. If a mother contracts chickenpox while breastfeeding, she should continue to breastfeed, because the antibodies in her milk confer immunity against chickenpox to her baby. This passive immunization may even spare the breastfed baby symptoms of chickenpox; if the disease is contracted, the course of the infant's disease is usually mild.

Congenital varicella syndrome can occur when chickenpox is contracted in the first half of pregnancy and cause serious problems for the fetus, including low birth weight and neurological problems (McCarter-Spaulding, 2001). Fortunately, this condition is very rare (1 to 6 per 100,000 births).

A mother who develops chickenpox several days before she delivers her baby or has the virus within 48 hours after birth presents a special, complex medical case that can be potentially life-threatening. Neonates of these women have a 17 to 30 percent likelihood of having a severe case of chickenpox because they do not have sufficient antibodies from their mother to lessen the severity of the infection (Cottrell & Carter, 1998). A woman with varicella who is admitted to the hospital for delivery is managed with airborne and contact infection control precautions using gowns, gloves, and masks. Following the birth, the mother and baby should be isolated from one another and from others if the neonate does not develop lesions and discharged as soon as possible; however, this decision is usually made on an individual basis (McCarter-Spaulding, 2001). The mother can maintain her breastmilk supply by pumping and discarding the milk until she is no longer infectious. The mother should express breastmilk if the baby is housed elsewhere temporarily. Antibodies appear in breastmilk within 48 hours of the onset of chickenpox manifestations. The baby should be protected from direct contact with the mother's skin lesions. If the baby has lesions, the baby can be isolated with the mother, and breastfeeding need not be interrupted. Varicella-zoster immune globulin is given as soon as possible to modify and prevent further symptoms of the disease regardless of whether the mother has already received it during pregnancy.

Frederick, White, and Braddock (1986) described two cases of varicella-zoster. In the first case, a 33-year-old mother developed classic herpetiform lesions on her left back and side. The breast was not involved. Expressed milk obtained within 24 hours of the appearance of the lesions revealed no varicella-zoster virus. Breastfeeding continued from both breasts, with slight position changes to avoid direct infant contact with the lesions. The infant remained healthy throughout the course of the mother's illness. The second case involved a mother who developed chickenpox at 40 weeks' gestation after contracting the virus from her older child. No history of chickenpox was noted, and she developed severe pulmonary problems due to varicella pneumonia. After an emergency cesarean section, this mother's healthy infant was treated prophylactically with zoster immune globulin (ZIG) and parenteral acyclovir. The mother was isolated, and her infant was not put to breast because of the mother's extensive cutaneous lesions and the danger of neonatal varicella infection from contact with the mother. During the mother's isolation, the baby remained healthy, and lactation was sustained through breast pumping. Another published case described a breastfeeding neonate who developed varicella pneumonitis when the administration of ZIG was mistakenly delayed for 60 hours (Isaacs, 2000).

Health-care workers who are not immune to varicella should not have contact with breastfeeding mothers and babies (as well as all other patients!) from day 10 to day 21 after exposure to chickenpox. If it is certain they are not pregnant, they should be vaccinated.

Cytomegalovirus

Cytomegalovirus (CMV), another herpes virus, is probably the most prevalent infection in the TORCH group, which, in addition to CMV includes toxoplasmosis, rubella, and herpes simplex virus. The CMV virus can be found in human milk and urine, and in the genital tract and pharynx, and it is transmitted by any close contact. As with other herpes viruses, it remains in host cells indefinitely. Because CMV can be transmitted through human milk, breastfeeding has proved to be an important means of conveying passive immunity to CMV, a so-called natural immunization. Although transmission though breastmilk has been documented, no serious illness or clinical symptoms in neonates secondary to breastfeeding has been reported (Bindo et al., 2001). The danger of CMV infection lies in the potential transmission to the fetus or newborn of a woman who has a primary infection during pregnancy (Damato, 2002).

Almost half of all adults have antibodies for CMV, which provide evidence of an infection at some point in their lives. The incidence of CMV antibody in young children is highest in developing countries and in countries in which communal child care and breastfeeding are common. In Japanese children whose mothers were seropositive, mother-to-child CMV transmission was 64.7 percent if the child was breastfed, as compared to 27.6 percent if bottle-fed (Minamishima et al., 1994). Breastfed children thus immunized to CMV by breastfeeding are protected later in life from symptomatic infection and from primary infection during pregnancy, which can cause intrauterine tissue damage.

Following a primary CMV infection during pregnancy, about half of the fetuses become infected (Nelson & Demmler, 1997) and about 10 percent of newborns infected with CMV will show CMV symptoms. Of these infants, a small percentage will develop some neurodevelopmental problem during early childhood (Damato, 2002). Premature infants, particularly if they are seronegative, are at risk for serious illness if they acquire CMV. Breastfed preterm infants are more likely than term infants to have a symptomatic cytomegalovirus infection (Hamprecht et al., 2001).

Pasteurization of milk appears to inactivate CMV; freezing milk at −20°C (−4°F) will decrease vital titers but does not reliably eliminate CMV; therefore, premature infants should receive only banked human milk from seronegative donors.

Rubella

Because rubella contracted during the first trimester of pregnancy causes serious birth defects, the uninformed person might be unduly concerned that rubella in human milk is likewise deleterious. Although the rubella virus can be passed through maternal milk lymphocytes to the infant, there is no evidence that the baby who acquires rubella in this manner becomes ill (Losonsky et al., 1982). As with CMV, transmission of maternal antibodies against rubella, though at lower levels, is beneficial to the infant by serving as a natural vaccine (Adu & Adeniji, 1995).

If the mother is immunized to rubella postpartum, the breastfeeding infant will develop antibodies to rubella but will not show symptoms of the disease. Buimovici-Klein et al. (1977) describe a case in which the mother developed a rash, glandular swelling, and fever 12 days after postpartum vaccination. The infant had no clear antibody response; however, 1 year later when the child was immunized, his antibody response suggested that he had sometime earlier acquired the virus. In another case (Klein, Byrne, & Cooper, 1980), a breastfeeding mother developed a rubella-like rash 8 days after a normal birth; 18 days before the onset of the rash, she was in close contact with a person who had a clinically diagnosed case of rubella. Her newborn daughter was followed for signs of rubella. The mother stopped breastfeeding for the first 2 days of her rash but resumed without incident on the third day. Her daughter remained clinically well, without sign of infection. The American Academy of Pediatrics has offered this advice: "Women with rubella, or those who have just been immunized with rubella live-attenuated virus vaccine need not refrain from breastfeeding" (1997, p. 75).

Hepatitis B

Hepatitis B virus (HBV) causes a systemic illness that involves the liver. The patient may be asymptomatic or may experience anything from mild flu-like symptoms to a fulminating illness. HBV is usually transmitted by contact with infected blood or body secretions. Contamination of the mucous membranes during birth or during sexual intercourse is another method of transmission. Approximately 5 to 15 percent of pregnant women with HBV virus will infect their babies before labor begins. The vast majority of exposure occurs during or immediately preceding labor, so that immunoprophylaxis and vaccination in the early postnatal period have an excellent chance of preventing infection. Medical and birthing centers routinely screen for HBV from umbilical-cord blood. Indicators of HBV are the presence of hepatitis B$_e$ antigen (HB$_e$Ag) in the blood, serological testing for antibody to the hepatitis B surface antigen (HB$_s$Ag), and the hepatitis B virus DNA probe (HBV DNA). Hepatitis B vaccination is recommended for all infants as part of the routine childhood immunization schedule (see Chapter 18).

Infants born to an HBV-positive mother, already exposed to maternal blood, amniotic fluid, and vaginal secretions during delivery, may breastfeed. The neonate should receive hepatitis B immunoglobulin (HBIG) within 12 hours after birth, followed by a series of three injections of HBV vaccine: during the first week of life, at 1 month, and at 6 months. All infants should undergo pediatric follow-up including repeated screening for HB$_s$Ag to rule out chronic carriers. This protocol has been successful in reducing the risk of neonatal transmission during breastfeeding. In a group of 369 infants born to women with chronic HBV, *none* of the breastfed infants and nine formula-fed infants were positive for HBV after the initial vaccination series (Hill et al., 2002).

Breastfeeding does not appear to increase the rate of infection among infants. Moreover, in areas of high prevalence of HBV and environmental exposure, lack of breastfeeding places the infant at greater risk of contracting the disease.

Hepatitis C

Hepatitis C virus (HCV), associated with later development of chronic liver disease, is today mainly acquired in childhood through vertical transmission. Perinatal transmission from mother to child is about 6 percent. Risk of transmission is related to the presence of maternal HCV at delivery and a high viral load in the mothers (Tajiri et al., 2001).

Despite the presence of the HCV RNA in some breastmilk samples, there is no evidence that breastfeeding confers risk of HCV infection (Hardikar, 2002; Tajiri et al., 2001), and no definite case of mother-to-infant transmission via breastmilk has been reported (Yeung, King, & Roberts, 2001). The overall rate of maternal-infant HCV transmission among breastfed infants is the same as that among formula-fed infants and women who are infected should be allowed to breastfeed (Fischler et al., 1996; Gibb et al., 2000; Ho-Hsiung et al., 1995). The exception is the rare case of a mother with acute HCV infection acquired after delivery, a time when no neutralizing antibodies are present (Polywka et al., 1999). It has been suggested that nipple cracks or fissures from breastfeeding may pose a risk for transmission of HCV (Buckhold, 2000; Roberts & Yeung, 2002), but this theory is hypothetical and not substantiated. The disturbing consequence of this recommendation is that it will mean *no breastfeeding* if a mother has HCV, since so many women have temporary nipple trauma postpartum.

Human Lymphotropic Virus

The human lymphotropic virus (HTLV-1), endemic in the Caribbean Islands and certain parts of Japan and Africa, is linked with adult T-cell leukemia and lymphoma. This virus is rare in the United States, but women who are seropositive are usually advised not to breastfeed (AAP, 1997). In areas of the world where many mothers are HTLV-1 positive, restrictions against these mothers breastfeeding is equivocal, and public health officials encourage an informed decision weighing risks and benefits (Hongo, 1999).

Although breastfed babies of HTVL-1-infected mothers are more likely to become infected (20–25 percent) than are artificially-fed infants (4 percent) (Kinoshita et al., 1987; Lal et al., 1993), the duration of breastfeeding appears to be critical to the child's development of the disease (Fujino & Nagata, 2000). Children who are breastfed for a long period (more than 6 or 7 months) are more likely to develop HTVL-1 infection than are those breastfed for a shorter period. Children born to seropositive carrier mothers passively acquire maternal antibodies prenatally that gradually disappear by 9 months of age. Maternal antibodies, protective in the early months after birth, are not sufficient to protect against infant infection with prolonged breastfeeding (Furnia et al., 1999; Takahashi et al., 1991).

Oddly, the seroconversion rate of infants breastfed for a short term (fewer than 7 months) is nearly equal to that of bottle-feeders: 4.4 percent (4 of 90 cases) versus 5.7 percent (9 of 158 cases) (Takahashi et al., 1991). Similarly, Oki et al. (1992) established that the seroconversion rate of short-term breastfeeders was nearly equal to that of bottle-feeders: 3.8 percent versus 5.6 percent in 885 HTLV-1-seropositive pregnant women. Hino et al. (1995) also found that antibody titers in short-term breastfeeders were about the same as those in bottle-feeders. Since 3 to 4 percent of bottle-fed babies born to HTLV-1-seropositive mothers become seropositive, there must be other HTLV-1 transmission routes from mother to child. Intrauterine transmission is one possibility (Fujino & Nagata, 2000).

West Nile Virus

In the fall of 2002, the West Nile virus was detected in breastmilk, raising the possibility that the microbe could be transmitted though breastfeeding as well as by mosquito bite and blood transfusion. The case involved a new mother who contracted West Nile virus from a blood transfusion shortly after delivery and breastfed her baby. The mother became feverish and ill after returning home. Three weeks later her baby tested positive for West Nile virus. Because of the infant's minimal outdoor exposure, the baby was most likely infected by breastmilk. Within a short period, the child was healthy and did not have symptoms of illness (CDC, 2002).

Based on this case, it appears that West Nile virus can be transmitted through breastmilk. But according to the CDC, findings from this case do not suggest a change in current breastfeeding recommendations, which include the following:

- There is no need for breastfeeding mothers to be routinely tested for West Nile virus.
- West Nile virus is not thought to be transmitted during pregnancy or birth.

- West Nile virus illnesses in young children are rare (less than 1 percent of reported cases).
- Insect repellents reduce exposure to mosquito bites.

Implications for Practice

Except for HIV and HTVL-1, viral infection in the mother rarely requires terminating breastfeeding. (See Table 6–2.) From a practical standpoint, the infant has already been exposed to the virus, usually transplacentally and during the birth process. In most cases, the only antibody protection available to the infant is from the mother's milk as a result of her infection. If the mother is well enough to care for her baby and the infant does not require special care, mother and baby should stay in the same hospital room. The concern of healthcare providers should be directed not at mothers known to have an infection but at those with an unidentified infection.

For the breastfeeding mother with a viral disease, isolation precautions should be used while she is hospitalized. If the infant's mother tests positively for HBV or other viruses, scrupulous hand washing and gowning are routinely practiced to prevent possible cross-contamination. Although antiseptic soaps for hand washing will more effectively kill organisms, no data prove that infection rates vary depending on whether plain or antiseptic soap is used. The mother does not need to wear rubber gloves while breastfeeding. The most effective ways to prevent the spread of infections among neonates, parents, and staff is for staff to maintain body-substance precautions and to teach others to do so also.

A new mother is already under stress. The news that she has a viral infection, which may or may not be considered a sexually transmitted disease, may cause her to feel pain, anger, and guilt. These feelings can be compounded by a fear that she should not breastfeed her baby. Encouraging the mother to express her fears, answering her questions, and then supporting her desires is a vital contribution that the nurse or lactation consultant can make to her care and well being.

Table 6–2

VIRUSES IN HUMAN MILK

Virus	Transmission	Recommendation
Chickenpox (varicella-zoster)	Probably not transmitted through breastmilk	Breastfeeding permitted unless mother develops chickenpox several days before delivering baby.
Cytomegalovirus	Proven	Seropositive mothers may breastfeed. Avoid breastmilk for premature infants of mothers with acute CMV infection.
Hepatitis B	Probable	Breastfeeding permitted if infant and mother have HBIG and Hb_sAg.
Hepatitis C	Proven	Breastfeeding permitted if titers not high. No reported case of MTCT through breastmilk. Individual assessment if mother has acute HVC infection.
Herpes Simplex	Probably not transmitted through breastmilk	Breastfeeding permitted if no breast lesions. Handwashing and mask if oral or genital lesion present.

Table 6–2 (cont.)		
HIV	Proven	In developed countries, breastfeeding by HIV-infected mother should be avoided.
HTLV-1	Proven	HTLV-infected mother should not breastfeed.
Rubella	Proven	Neither postpartum immunization with rubella vaccine nor rubella should prevent a mother from breastfeeding her infant.
West Nile Virus	Probable	Breastfeeding permitted.

Source: Centers for Disease Control (2002); Pass (1986); Stiehim & Keller (2001).

Summary

Toward the end of pregnancy, the fetus receives passive immunity from the mother; the baby is therefore born with the mother's immunities. Breastfed infants acquire additional antibodies to influenza, mumps, chickenpox, and other viruses, either through the mother's clinical exposure or through immunization. This passive immunity lasts from 3 to 6 months and protects the infant from childhood diseases. Concern about the risk of viral transmission through breastmilk appears to be limited to HIV and HTLV-1, and in unusual cases, for chickenpox and hepatitis. Thus, for all other viral infections, breastfeeding should continue except in the case of a mother who has a herpetic lesion on her breast.

The possibility of HIV transmission by human milk has had a negative effect on breastfeeding that is as yet unmeasured. In developing countries where replacement infant feeding is often lethal, this effect is a major concern (Coutsoudis & Rollins, 2003). Even if antiretroviral treatment is available, such medications and artificial feeding are expensive. On the basis of realistic costs, decisions must be made as to whether these high costs can be supported by individual families and national economies.

Key Concepts

- HIV-infected women should not breastfeed if safe, affordable alternatives are available. It has been well established that HIV can be transmitted from mother to infant through breastfeeding.

- If HIV-infected women have no other choice but to breastfeed, exclusive breastfeeding should be promoted and mothers should be taught about frequent emptying of the breast and breastfeeding management, including effective attachment.

- HIV-infected pregnant women should receive feeding counseling that includes general information about the risks and benefits of infant feeding options, and specific guidance in selecting the option most likely to be suitable for their situation.

- Infection control should be maintained. Gloves are usually not necessary for handling breastmilk, but if a health-care worker comes in frequent contact with human milk, she may choose to wear gloves. If the mother has an open wound on her breast, glove wearing is warranted.

- In the absence of breast lesions, the newborn of a mother with herpes simplex virus, if the baby is well, may breastfeed and be with the mother in her room; however, scrupulous hand washing, gowning, and covering of any lesions must be practiced to prevent possible cross-contamination. Women with herpetic lesions on their breasts should refrain from breastfeeding.

- If a mother develops chickenpox several days before she delivers her baby or has the virus within 48 hours after birth, she should delay breastfeeding and pump her milk. Contact infection control precautions such as using gowns, gloves, and masks are indicated. Following birth, the mother and baby should be isolated separately if the neonate does not develop lesions and discharged as soon as possible. The baby should be protected from direct contact with the mother's skin lesions. If the baby has lesions, the baby can be isolated with the mother, and breastfeeding may occur uninterruptedly. Varicella-zoster immune globulin is given as soon as possible to modify and prevent further symptoms of the disease regardless of whether the mother has already received it during pregnancy.

- Cytomegalovirus, a herpes virus found in human milk and urine, and in the genital tract and pharynx, is transmitted by any close contact. Breastfeeding is an important means of conveying passive immunity to CMV. Although transmission though breastmilk has been documented, no serious illness or clinical symptoms in neonates secondary to breastfeeding have been reported. The danger of CMV infection lies in the potential transmission to the fetus or newborn of a woman who has a primary infection during pregnancy.

- Although the rubella (measles) virus can be passed through maternal milk lymphocytes to the infant, there is no evidence that a baby who acquires rubella in this manner will become ill. Transmission of maternal antibodies against rubella, though at lower levels, is beneficial to the infant by serving as a natural vaccine. If the mother is immunized to rubella postpartum, the breastfeeding infant will develop antibodies to rubella but will not show symptoms of the disease.

- Infants who have been born to a hepatitis B-positive mother and have already been exposed to maternal blood during delivery, may breastfeed. The neonate should receive hepatitis B immunoglobulin (HBIG) within 12 hours after birth, followed by a series of injections of HBV vaccine. All infants should undergo pediatric follow-up, including screening for HB_sAg.

- There is no evidence that breastfeeding confers risk of hepatitis C (HCV) infection. The overall rate of maternal-infant HCV transmission among breastfed infants is the same as that among formula-fed infants, and women who are infected should be allowed to breastfeed. The exception is the rare case of a mother with acute HCV infection acquired after delivery, a time when no neutralizing antibodies are present.

- Women who are HTLV-1 seropositive are usually advised not to breastfeed. In areas of the world where many mothers are HTLV-1 positive, restrictions against breastfeeding are equivocal. Children who are breastfed for a long period (more than 6 or 7 months) are more likely to develop HTVL-1 infection than are those breastfed for a shorter period. Children born to seropositive carrier mothers passively acquire maternal antibodies prenatally that gradually disappear by 9 months of age.

- Mothers with West Nile virus can breastfeed.

Internet Resources

HIV/AIDS Surveillance Report: Statistics, teaching tools, PowerPoint presentations: www.cdc.gov/hiv/stats.htm

ILCA position paper on HIV and infant feeding information on West Nile virus and breastfeeding: www.ilca.org

Information from WHO on West Nile virus and breastfeeding/Counseling pregnant women and new mothers about HIV—formula-feeding counseling for children born to HIV-seropositive mothers: www.who.gov

Position papers on HIV/AIDs and breastfeeding: www.geocities.com/HotSprings/Spa/3156

References

Adu FD, Adeniji JA. Measles antibodies in the breast milk of nursing mothers. *Afr J Med Sci* 24:385–88, 1995.

American Academy of Pediatrics. *1997 Red book: report of the Committee on Infectious Diseases*, 24th ed. Elk Grove Village, IL: AAP, 1997:73–79.

American College of Obstetricians and Gynecologists. *Management of herpes in pregnancy* (ACOG Practice Bulletin, No. 8) Washington, DC: ACOG, 2002.

Bindo S et al. Transmission of cytomegalovirus. *Lancet* 357:1799, 2001.

Black BP, Miles MS. Calculating the risks and benefits of disclosure in African American women who have HIV. *JOGN Nurs* 31:688–97, 2002.

Brahmbhall H, Gray RH. Child mortality associated with reasons for non-breastfeeding and weaning: is breastfeeding best for HIV-positive mothers? *AIDS* 17:879–85, 2003.

Brown ZA. Preventing transmission of herpes simplex to newborns. *Contemp Nurse Pract* Sept–Oct:29–35, 1995.

Buckhold KM. Who's afraid of hepatitis C? *Am J Nurs* 100:26–31, 2000.

Buimovici-Klein E et al. Isolation of rubella virus in milk after postpartum immunization. *J Pediatr* 6:939–41, 1977.

Centers for Disease Control (CDC). Update: universal precautions for prevention of transmission of human immune deficiency virus, hepatitis B virus, and other bloodborne pathogens in health-care settings. *MMWR* 37:378–87, 1988.

———. West Nile virus infection and breastfeeding. Available at: http://www.cdc.gov. Accessed October 4, 2002.

Cline MK, Bailey-Dorton C, Cayelli M. Update in maternity care: maternal infections diagnosis and management. *Primary Care* 27:13–33, 2000.

Connor EM et al. Reduction of maternal-infant transmission of human immunodeficiency virus type 1 with zidovudine treatment. *N Engl J Med* 331:1173–80, 1994.

Cottrell BH, Carter C. Health care professionals: Have you had the chickenpox? *AWHONN Lifelines* 2:33–38, 1998.

Coutsoudis A. Promotion of exclusive breastfeeding in the face of the HIV pandemic [commentary]. *Lancet* 356:1620–21, 2000.

Coutsoudis A, Rollins N. Breast-feeding and HIV transmission: the jury is still out. *J Pediatr Gastroenterol* 36:434–42, 2003.

Coutsoudis A et al. Influence of infant feeding patterns on early mother-to-child transmission of HIV-1 in Durban, South Africa: a prospective cohort study *Lancet* 354:471–76, 1999.

Damato EG. Cytomegalovirus infection: perinatal complications. *JOGN Nurs* 31:86–92, 2002.

De Cock KM et al. Prevention of mother-to-child HIV transmission in resource-poor countries: translating research into policy and practice. *JAMA* 283:1175–82, 2000.

de Paoli M et al. Exclusive breastfeeding in the era of AIDS. *J Hum Lact* 17:313–20, 2001.

Donahue DB. Diagnosis and treatment of *Herpes Simplex* infection during pregnancy. *JOGN Nurs* 31:99–106, 2002.

Dunn DT et al. Risk of human immunodeficiency virus, type 1, transmission through breastfeeding. *Lancet* 340:585–88, 1992.

Fischler B et al. Vertical transmission of hepatitis C virus infection. *Scand J Infect Dis* 28:353–56, 1996.

Frederick IB, White RJ, Braddock SW. Excretion of varicella-herpes zoster virus in breast milk. *Am J Obstet Gynecol* 154:1116–17, 1986.

Fujino T, Nagata Y. HTLV-1 transmission from mother to child. *J Reproduct Immunol* 47:197–206, 2000.

Furnia A et al. Estimating the time of HTLV-1 infection following mother-to-child transmission in a breast-feeding population in Jamaica. *J Med Virol* 59:541–46, 1999.

Gibb DM et al. Mother-to-mother transmission of hepatitis C virus: evidence for preventable peripartum transmission. *Lancet* 356(9233):904–7, 2000.

Hamprecht K et al. Epidemiology of transmission of cytomegalovirus from mother to preterm infant by breastfeeding. *Lancet* 357(9255):513–18, 2001.

Hardikar W. Advances in pediatric gastroenterology and hepatology. *J Gastroenterol Hepatol* 17:476–81, 2002.

Hill JB et al. Risk of hepatitis B transmission in breast-fed infants of chronic hepatitis B carriers. *Obstet and Gynecol* 6:1049–52, 2002.

Hino S et al. Association between maternal antibodies to the external envelope glycoprotein and vertical transmission of human T-lymphotropic virus type 1. *J Clin Invest* 95:2920–25, 1995.

Ho-Hsiung L et al. Absence of infection in breast-fed infants born to hepatitis C virus-infected mothers. *J Pediatr* 126:589–91, 1995.

Hongo H. Personal communication. Tokyo, Japan, 1999.

International Lactation Consultant Association. HIV and infant feeding. Position Paper. North Carolina: Raleigh. ILCA, 2002.

Isaacs D. Neonatal chickenpox. *J Paediatr Child Health* 36:76–77, 2000.

Jackson DJ et al. HIV and infant feeding: issues in developed and developing countries. *JOGN Nurs* 32:117–27, 2003.

Karim SA et al. Vertical transmission in South Africa: translating research into policy and practice. *Lancet* 359:92, 2002.

Katz A. The evolving art of caring for pregnant women with HIV infection. *JOGN Nurs* 32:102–8, 2003.

Kinoshita K et al. Milk-borne transmission of HTLV-I from carrier mothers to their children. *Jpn J Cancer Res* 78:674–80, 1987.

Klein EB, Byrne T, Cooper LZ. Neonatal rubella in a breast-fed infant after postpartum maternal infection. *J Pediatr* 97:774–75, 1980.

Lal RB et al. Isotypic and IgG sub-class restriction of the humoral immune responses to human T-lymphotopic virus type-I. *Clin Immuo Immunopathol* 67:40–49, 1993.

Lindberg CE. Perinatal transmission of HIV: how to counsel women. *Matern Child Nurs J* 20:207–12, 1995.

Losonsky GA et al. Effect of immunization against rubella on lactation products: I. Development and characterization of specific immunologic reactivity in breast milk. *J Infect Dis* 145:661–66, 1982.

McCarter-Spaulding DE. Varicella infection in pregnancy. *JOGN Nurs* 30:667–73, 2001.

Minamishima I et al. Role of breast milk in acquisition of cytomegalovirus. *Microbio Immuol* 38:549–52, 1994.

Nduati R et al. Effect of breastfeeding on mortality among HIV-1 infected women: a randomized trial. *Lancet* 357:1651–55, 2001.

Nelson CT, Demmler GJ. Cytomegalovirus infection in the pregnant mother, fetus, and newborn infant. *Clin Perinatol* 24:151–60, 1997.

Oki T et al. A sero-epidemiological study on mother-to child transmission of HTLV-1 in Southern Kyushu, Japan. *Asia Oceania J Obstet Gynaecol* 44:371–77, 1992.

Oxtoby MJ. Human immunodeficiency virus and other viruses in human milk: placing the issues in broader perspective. *Pediatr Infect Dis* 7:825–35, 1988.

Owor M et al. The one year safety and efficacy data of the HIVNET 012 trial. Presented at: 13th International AIDS conference, Durban, South Africa, 2000.

Pass RF. Viral contamination of milk. In: Goldman AS, Atkinson SA, Hanson A, eds. *Human lactation 3: the effects of milk on recipient infant.* New York: Plenum, 1986:279–87.

Polywka S et al. Low risk of vertical transmission of hepatitis C virus by breast milk. *Clin Infect Dis* 29:1327–29, 1999.

Roberts EA, Yeung L. Maternal-infant transmission of hepatitis C virus. *Hepatology* 36:S106–13, 2002.

Savage F, Lhotska L. Recommendations on feeding infants of HIV positive mothers. *Adv Exp Med Biol* 478:225–30, 2000.

Sealander JY, Kerr CP. Herpes simplex of the nipple: infant-to-mother transmission. *Am Family Pract* 39:111–13, 1989.

Smith MM, Kuhn L. Exclusive breast-feeding: does it have the potential to reduce breast-feeding transmission of HIV-1? *Nutr Rev* 58:333–40, 2000.

Stiehm RE, Keller MA. Breast milk transmission of viral disease. *Advances Nutr Res* 10:105–22, 2001.

Sullivan-Bolyai JS et al. Disseminated neonatal herpes simplex virus type 1 from a maternal breast lesion. *Pediatrics* 71:455–57, 1983.

Tajiri H et al. Prospective study of mother-to-infant transmission of hepatitis C virus. *Pediatr Infect Dis J* 20:10–14, 2001.

Takahashi K et al. Inhibitory effect of maternal antibody on mother-to-child transmission of human T-lymphotropic virus, type 1. *Int J Cancer* 49:673–77, 1991.

US Department of Health and Human Services. *HHS blueprint for action on breastfeeding.* Washington, DC: HHS, 2000.

van de Perre P. Postnatal transmission of human immunodeficiency virus type 1 from mother to infant: a prospective cohort study in Kigali, Rwanda. *N Engl J Med* 325:593–98, 1991.

van der Strate BW et al. Viral load in breast milk correlates with transmission of human cytomegalovirus to preterm infant, but lactoferrin concentrations do not. *Clin Diag Lab Immunol* 8:818–21, 2001.

World Health Organization. New data on the prevention of mother-to-child transmission of HIV and their policy implications—conclusions and recommendations. *Technical Consultation on behalf of the UNFPA/UNICEF/WHO/UNADIS Inter-Agency Task Team on Mother-to-Child Transmission of HIV.* Geneva, October, 2000. Available at: www.who.org. Accessed March 21, 2003.

Yeung LT, King SM, Roberts EA. Mother-to-infant transmission of hepatitis C virus. *Hepatology* 34:254–29, 2001.

PRENATAL, PERINATAL, AND POSTNATAL PERIODS

A caring approach, knowledge, and clinical skills merge in the best lactation consultant services during pregnancy, the intrapartum, and the immediate postpartum.

Most breastfed infants are born at or near term and are healthy and thrive with only breastmilk. A few grow poorly when breastfed. Does this problem derive from the mother, the baby, or the hospital? How can the problem be resolved without compromising the breastfeeding relationship? Jaundice is an outcome of early extrauterine life, and how it is managed can influence the breastfeeding course. Those infants who are born early or at risk represent a small percentage of the total, yet they require extra caretaking by their mother, by the infants' caregivers, and by neonatal intensive care unit technologies.

Donor milk banks represent a means of obtaining a scarce resource, yet few of them remain in operation. The following chapters highlight the breastfeeding mother and baby's needs for donor milk and how they can be met.

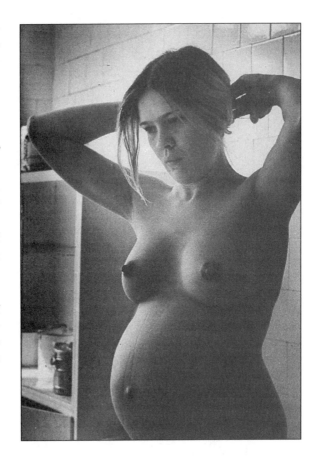

7

Perinatal and Intrapartum Care

Jan Riordan and Kay Hoover

Helping new mothers breastfeed is a rewarding experience. With a basic understanding of the anatomy and physiology of the breast and of the nutritional and immunological properties of breastmilk, the health-care worker can contribute greatly to a mother's breastfeeding experience. However, the care provider must be prepared to offer practical assistance supported by relevant research findings and to meet the urgent needs of mothers with little or no breastfeeding experience. The provider must also be able to assist new mothers who, despite previous breastfeeding experience, are still anxious. Emphasis on confident self-care is a major goal.

Breastfeeding Preparation

The best preparation for breastfeeding is for the mother to learn as much as possible before she embarks on her own lactation adventure. Learning about breastfeeding can be accomplished in any number of ways. She can attend a community-based breastfeeding support group. Groups such as La Leche League and the Australian Breastfeeding Association have regularly scheduled meetings to provide education and support for breastfeeding women. She may choose to take a prenatal breastfeeding class. Classes are offered by health-care facilities, such as hospitals or prenatal-care providers' offices and independent lactation consultants.

Some women choose to have a doula to support them throughout labor and delivery (Trainor, 2002). Doulas encourage breastfeeding and integrate breastfeeding information into their prenatal teaching. Many childbirth educators include breastfeeding in their childbirth classes. In addition to attending support group meetings or breastfeeding classes, mothers can prepare by reading books and watching videos or DVDs about breastfeeding, and talking to women who have breastfed. Discussing breastfeeding with one or more women who have had a positive experience is a good way to learn. The experienced breastfeeding mother acts as a mentor to the less knowledgeable woman. She can respond to the new mother's concerns and feelings and advise her on aspects of breastfeeding that are more difficult to address in written form or in a less personal setting.

Prenatal preparation of nipple tissue is unnecessary and is not recommended. Colostrum is produced throughout the pregnancy. In some women, colostrum spontaneously leaks during sexual intercourse and late in pregnancy. During pregnancy, the breasts begin making milk and the nipples become more elastic, which may explain why some women characterize their nipples as "flat" or "inverted" at the beginning of pregnancy, but not at the end.

How the nipple looks when the baby is not suckling bears little resemblance to its appearance in the baby's mouth, nor is it necessary for the nipple to be everted when not in the baby's mouth. Hoffmann's exercises for nipple inversion or flatness have no noticeable impact on the appearance of the nipple (Hoffmann, 1953) nor on the degree of inversion or protractility (MAIN Collaborative Group Preparing for Breast Feeding, 1994). If the nipples appear functional and are not inverted, the best preparation is to do nothing. Involving the breasts and nipples in lovemaking (except when the mother has a history of preterm labor) and washing without soap are sufficient to prepare the nipples for breastfeeding.

The most important organ for breastfeeding is the mother's brain. When it receives signals from the stimulation of the nipple and when milk is removed from the breast, the milk will be ejected and milk production will occur. Mothering is a learned role, and a mother's best "teacher" is her own baby. When reaffirmed as a person and supported in her early efforts to breastfeed, a mother will have most of what she needs to assume her new role and relish the unique joys it will provide her.

Early Feedings

Following birth, continuing assessment of the mother's physical condition and psychosocial dynamic is essential. The mother should be helped to breastfeed immediately after birth and regularly thereafter.

Several reasons support early (in the first hour after birth) and frequent breastfeeding for optimal functioning of both the infant and the mother:

- Suckling stimulates uterine contractions, aids in the expulsion of the placenta, and helps to control maternal blood loss.
- Mothers will breastfeed for a longer duration. (Lawson & Tulloch, 1995; Lothian, 1995; Wright, Rice, & Wells, 1996; Ekström, 2003).
- The infant's suckling reflex is usually intense after birth. Gratification of this reflex "im-

prints" this bio-behavior to facilitate learning to suckle (Anderson et al., 1982).
- The infant promptly receives the immunological components of the colostrum.
- The infant's digestive peristalsis is stimulated, thereby promoting elimination of the byproducts of hemoglobin breakdown. Jaundice is more likely to occur when feeding and peristalsis are delayed (see Chapter 11).
- Breast engorgement is minimized by the early and frequent removal of milk from the breast (Moon & Humenick, 1989).
- Lactation is accelerated, more milk is produced, and early and frequent intake of breastmilk lessens infant weight loss after birth (Chen et al., 1998; de Carvalho et al., 1982).
- Frequent removal of milk keeps the breast as empty as possible and stimulates the synthesis of breastmilk. The degree of emptiness of the breast is very important (Cregan & Hartmann, 1999).
- Attachment and bonding are enhanced at a time when both the mother and the infant are in a heightened state of readiness.

Some neonates will take longer to learn how to latch onto the breast and feed effectively than others because of interventions during labor and birth and the postbirth care they receive. Most women in the United States and many European countries have epidurals during labor. Such analgesia delays and diminishes neonatal suckling (Crowell, Hill, & Humenick, 1994; Riordan et al., 2000; Ransjo-Arvidson et al., 2001; Sepkoski et al., 1992; Kroeger, 2004). The baby's and the mother's body temperatures may be elevated with epidurals (Lieberman et al., 1997; Ransjo-Arvidson et al., 2001; Viscomi, 2000), resulting in separation and septic workup to determine if an infection is present. Women who have a vacuum extraction during birthing abandon breastfeeding early (Hall et al., 2002) possibly due in part to a long, drawn-out, and stressful labor and infant injury. If the birth was by cesarean, it takes longer for the mother's milk to come in. Another potential disruption is suctioning the infant's nose after birth. The suction tends to cause the infant to have nasal edema and "stuffiness." Because the baby's airway is somewhat obstructed, the baby does not feed well until the swelling subsides. Oral suctioning can lead to breastfeeding difficulties because the baby's mouth or throat may be sore (Widström et al., 1987). One pediatrician found a perforation in the soft palate due to rough suctioning with a bulb syringe (Soppas, 2003).

Newborns spend 64 percent of their time sleeping (Sadeh, Dark, & Vohr, 1996). When access to the mother is not restricted after birth, the breastfeeding neonate exhibits a sleep pattern similar to that illustrated in Table 7–1. The initial alertness for the first 2 hours after birth and eagerness of the baby to breastfeed is followed by deeper sleep and then increased wakefulness and interest in breastfeeding around 20 to 24 hours. During this period of increased wakefulness, the baby will feed frequently, alternating between relatively short periods of light sleep and quiet wakefulness (Williams & Mueller, 1989). Mothers may interpret these "cluster feedings" as indicators that the baby is not getting any milk or is getting an insufficient amount. However, they actually constitute a series of mini-feedings, snacks, or courses in a larger banquet that is part of a single breastfeeding episode. A cluster of mini-feedings by the baby is usually followed by a period of deep sleep, during which time the mother should be encouraged to sleep.

The pattern of normal infant suckling was discussed in Chapter 3. Neonates who stay with their mothers immediately after birth are more likely to learn how to suckle effectively and show increasing facility with each subsequent feeding than those who are separated. In general, full-term infants demonstrate a well-organized sequence of suckling behaviors, including bringing the hand to the mouth, rooting, and suckling within the first hours after birth (Widström et al., 1990).

The first breastfeeding should take place shortly after the infant's birth. The baby can be dried while skin-to-skin with his mother. Leaving the amniotic fluid on the baby's hands helps the baby find the breast (Varendi, Porter, & Winberg, 1996). Mother-infant body contact is as effective as supplemental heat in maintaining the healthy newborn's temperature (Johanson et al., 1992; Christensson et al., 1998). The placenta is normally expelled soon after birth, often before the infant is put to breast for the first time. If a delay occurs, breastfeeding may hasten detachment and expulsion.

With the mother on her back and slightly inclined, or propped on her side with a pillow at her back for support, the baby may breastfeed in the delivery room/birthing suite. The ambience and homey comforts of a birthing suite encourage early breastfeeding. The father can share the enjoyment of these first moments together and can help to position the mother and infant comfortably in the birthing bed.

Newborns usually lick or nuzzle the nipple at first. Given ample opportunity, the baby is able to crawl to the mother's breast, self-attach and suckle strongly within an hour (Righard & Alade, 1990; Righard, 1995). Those babies who have been affected by labor analgesia and anesthesia, and thus may suckle only minimally at this time, should still have an opportunity to lick or nuzzle the nipple. Regardless of the baby's initial suckling behavior, this interaction is advantageous, because it stimulates uterine contractions, promotes colonization of harmless bacteria on the nipple, and helps to protect the infant from pathogenic bacteria—a very pleasant method of infection control. Mothers whose infants have come in contact with their nipple/areolar complex choose to keep their babies with them for more time during the hospital stay (Widström et al., 1990). Explaining to the mother

Table 7–1

First-day Sleep Patterns of Neonates

Infant State	Time Period
Alert	Birth–2 hours
Light and deep sleep	2–20+ hours
Increasing wakefulness*	20–24 hours

*Often includes a cluster of 5 to 10 feeding episodes over 2 to 3 hours followed by deep sleep of 4 to 5 hours.

that "nuzzling" is normal behavior will help her to see this activity as a positive response rather than as disinterest in actual breastfeeding.

Sometimes the first breastfeeding takes place after the mother and her newborn are transferred from the delivery area to their room. Wherever it may be, if the mother is awake and oriented, it is best that she put her baby to breast as soon as possible because the baby is usually in an alert state for 2 hours after birth and later falls asleep (Figures 7–1 and 7–2).

A positive, satisfying birthing experience gets breastfeeding off to a good start, and parents often recall this experience in great detail many years later. The caregiver's unhurried, nurturing approach helps to establish rapport with the mother. It is important to explain to the first-time mother that breastfeeding is not as automatic for her as the suckling and rooting reflexes are for her baby. Yet the experience is new to the baby too, and the first few times at breast offer opportunities for each to learn from the other. Early breastfeeding is optimized in the following ways:

1. *Wash your hands thoroughly.* An alcohol-based hand rub may be used *in addition* to hand washing. Gloves can be worn, but universal precautions do not apply to human breastmilk so wearing gloves is a personal preference. Latex gloves should *not* be worn because of

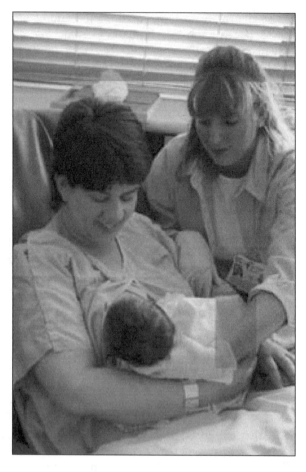

FIGURE 7–2. Baby put to breast right after delivery.

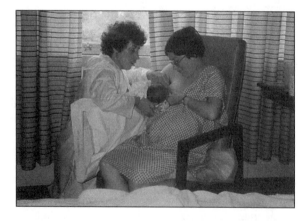

FIGURE 7–1. Lactation consultant assisting mother at eye level during first breastfeeding.

possible allergies to latex. Artificial fingernails should not be worn (Hedderwick et al., 2000; Winslow & Jacobson, 2000). Wearing these nails encourages growth of pathogens (*Candida, Staphylococcus aureus*) and their sharp edges can hurt the mother and baby.

2. *Arrange for privacy.* Concentrating on learning a new skill is easier when it is private. Ask visitors to leave as appropriate. Sometimes mothers are too polite to ask visitors to leave in order to feed the baby and it is up to the nurse or lactation consultant to make this request. Shut the door of the mother's room or pull the curtains around her bed if she wishes.

3. *Help the mother to find the most comfortable position and ensure that there are several pillows available.* Women who have had a cesarean birth often find it more comfortable to breastfeed while sitting in a comfortable chair with low arms. Almost always, the least comfortable position is leaning back in the bed, as if in a lounge chair. At the first feeding, arrange pillows on her lap, behind her back, and under her arm and shoulder on the side on which the baby is to feed. If the mother is in bed, raise the back of the bed to high Fowler's position with plenty of pillows for additional support. The mother who must remain flat may lie on her back or side with pillows at her back and between her knees. If wearing a hospital gown, open the snaps on the shoulders to pull down and expose the breast as needed.

4. *Work with the mother at her eye level.* If she is in a chair, kneel down; if she is in bed, pull up a chair; if the bed is electronically operated, raise the bed to bring her to your eye level. When an individual is engaging in a new activity, anyone standing higher than the learner provokes anxiety in the learner.

5. *Help the mother to position the baby's head.* It should be snuggled securely in the mother's arms and facing toward her. This permits the mother to easily maintain eye contact with her baby. By cradling the infant's thigh or the buttock of his lower leg with her arm, the mother can change the baby's position with ease. Be sure there is no pressure on the back of the baby's head. Other feeding positions are discussed later in this chapter.

6. *Ask the mother to support her breast with her hand.* Advise her to keep her thumb and fingers well behind the areola in a C-hold—a position in which the hand is shaped into a "C" (Figure 7–3). The mother can guide her breast to assist the baby in taking the breast into his mouth. Once latched, by lifting her breast slightly she can easily maintain the infant's airway.

7. *Help the mother to position her baby so that his nose is at the level of the mother's nipple.* Ask the mother to brush her nipple lightly against the baby's lips. When the infant opens his

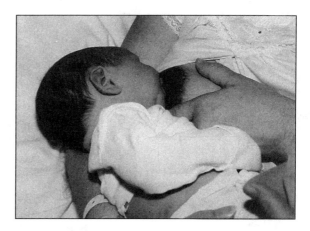

FIGURE 7–3. The C-hold.

mouth wide (rooting reflex) in response to this stimulus, help the mother bring his shoulders to her breast in one quick movement of her hand or forearm, aiming the nipple toward the soft palate. Bringing the baby to the breast at the exact moment that his mouth is at its widest gape is desirable because it maximizes the amount of breast tissue he grasps. The baby's lips should be flanged outward and his nose slightly away from the surface of the breast so that he can easily breathe (Figure 7–4). Keep in mind that at the first feeding, the baby has never breastfed before and that the suckle-swallow-breathe pattern is a relatively complex series of actions that requires learning and practice.

8. *Explain that an infant should be allowed to breastfeed as long and as often as he wants for these early feedings.* This will stimulate the need-supply response. In some cases, the neonate will take only one breast before falling asleep, but most babies will take both breasts. As long as each breast is offered frequently (at least every 2 to 3 hours), single-breast feedings of whatever duration the baby wishes are an appropriate option (Woolridge, Ingram, & Baum, 1990). "Finishing the first breast first" is an easy suggestion if the mother is concerned about when to move her baby from the first to the second breast.

9. *Teach "baby watching."* The recommendation is, "Watch the baby, not the clock." Feed the baby

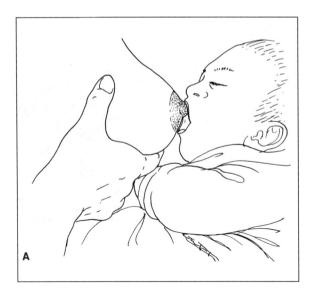

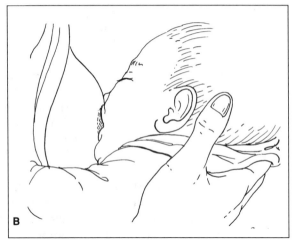

FIGURE 7–4. Latch-on. (A) Mouth gaped open. (B) Grasping breast.

at the *earliest* sign of hunger. Crying is a *late* sign of hunger. A crying baby cannot latch on; the baby needs time to be consoled and to "settle down" emotionally and physiologically before he will become interested in feeding again. With crying, both the infant's blood pressure and intracranial pressure rises causing oxygen-depleted blood to flow back into the systemic circulation rather than into the lungs (Ander-

son, 1989). Box 7–1 describes the stages of the baby readying to feed.

10. *Suggest that the mother feed until she notes cues from the infant suggesting satiety* (suckling activity ceases, baby falls asleep and lets go on his own). The length of the feedings is up to the baby. If the baby lets go of the breast within 2 to 5 minutes, suggest to the mother that she burp the baby and return the baby to the same breast. Once the baby has fallen asleep and has come off the breast on his own, she can offer the other breast when the baby gives feeding cues again. If the mother is breastfeeding for the first time and feels more comfortable with knowing an approximate length of time to feed, suggest that she feed 20 to 30 minutes on the first side until satiety and that she then offer the other side. Toward the end of the feeding, the mother will probably become relaxed to the point of sleepiness—a delightful side effect of oxytocin secretion (Mulford, 1990).

Early feedings are a critical time for learning new information, especially the first-time mother who usually asks many questions. For example, noisy breathing during feedings indicating a "stuffy" nose worries some mothers who are concerned that the baby is having trouble getting enough oxygen. If the baby is feeding well, nasal stuffiness is usually not a problem and will resolve on its own. Neonates are obligate nose breathers. In a few instances a newborn's nares are congested to the point where the baby refuses to breastfeed because he cannot breathe and feed at the same time. In this case, saline drops or a hydrocortisone solution in the nose will help alleviate the problem. Mothers also worry if the baby gets the hiccups, another normal baby behavior.

The mother should be taught how to break the infant's suction on the breast by placing her finger in the corner of his mouth between his gums so she can take him off and start over again. If the mother and baby are having problems with latching, sometimes the nurse or lactation consultant might ask permission of the mother to touch her breast and then compress her breast to assist the baby in taking more breast tissue into his mouth.

Feeding Positions

The new mother needs to know ways to position her neonate at breast. The most frequently taught techniques are the cradle (Figure 7–5), the cross-cradle (across-the-lap, Figure 7–6A), the football (or clutch, Figure 7–6B), and the side-lying position (Figure 7–7). Although there is nothing

BOX 7-1

Cues in Baby Watching

Baby Cue	Stage of Readiness to Feed
Wiggling, moving arms or legs	Early
Rooting, fingers to mouth	Early
Fussing, squeaky noises	Mid
Restless, crying intermittently	Mid
Full cry, aversive screaming pitch, color turns red	Late

Source: From Anderson (1989).

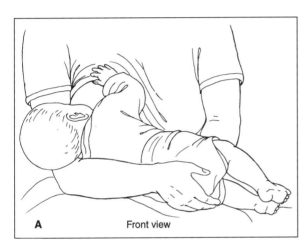

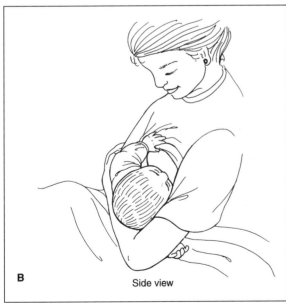

FIGURE 7–5. Madonna (cradle) position. (A) Front view. (B) Side view.

magical about a particular position, the mother may feel uncomfortable in experimenting with different positions prior to her discharge from the hospital. However, she needs to be encouraged to experiment and to use whatever position works best for her and her infant (Table 7–2). Mothers who had vaginal deliveries report less fatigue if they breastfeed in the side-lying position rather than the sitting position (Milligan, Flenniken, & Pugh, 1996).

Latch-on and Positioning Techniques

Rules for teaching new mothers the "correct" latch-on and positioning of the baby on the breast are considered fundamental in lactation clinical practice. These rules list signs of "correct nursing" and "incorrect nursing." Some even include the exact alignment that the baby's head must

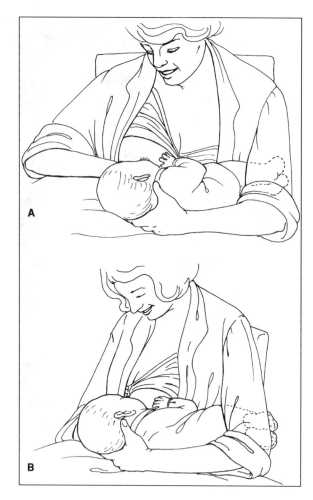

FIGURE 7–6. (A) Cross-cradle or modified clutch hold. (B) Football or clutch hold.

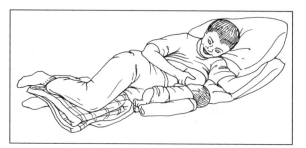

FIGURE 7–7. Side-lying position.

be with his body during a feeding. Another example of emphasis on technique is teaching the mother the mechanics of breastfeeding using the sandwich analogy:

Using the sandwich as a model, the breast must first be shaped into an oval and then it must be approached from below starting with the nose near the sandwich stuffing. The head tips back slightly and the mandible comes up and forward to fix itself well back on the sandwich. The maxilla is the last part to land on the sandwich, and it is then possible to take a large and satisfying bite (Wiessinger, 1998).

This particular teaching method and others reflects a growing interest in clinical techniques to help breastfeeding women, but for the most part, these techniques are unproven. An exception is an Australian study (Henderson, Stamp, & Pincombe, 2001) that examined teaching of correct latch-on and positioning by conducting a randomized trial on 160 first-time mothers. The mothers who received education on positioning breastfed their babies just as long as the group that did not. The mothers who had education on positioning reported less nipple pain than the control group, but the study observers who collected the data noted no observable differences in nipple trauma between the two groups suggesting a halo effect on mothers in the experimental group. Clearly, we need to be wary of assuming that "correct" latch-on is evidence-based. New evidence should change and direct our practice.

The Infant Who Has Not Latched-On

Occasionally, an otherwise healthy newborn will not latch onto his mother's breast, even after several attempts. Most nurses and lactation consultants have witnessed the frustrating situation in which a distraught mother repeatedly tries to breastfeed her neonate for the first time. Birth is a strenuous event, and it is not uncommon for a newborn baby to fall into a deep sleep.

The appropriate action in this situation is to put the baby skin-to-skin with his mother and teach her to watch for cues that the baby has cycled through the period of deep sleep and is beginning to awaken. Movement of head, arms and legs, mouthing, and

Table 7–2

POSITIVE AND NEGATIVE ELEMENTS OF INFANT FEEDING POSITIONS

Positioning	Positive Elements	Negative Elements
Cradle	"Classic" position. Most frequently pictured and most often used.	Baby's head tends to wobble around on the mother's arm. Mother has minimal control over baby's head.
Football or clutch	Provides control of baby's head. Good for low birth weight or 36–39 weekers with minimum head control. Avoids incision of Cesarean birth. Best position to be able to see the baby's mouth.	Some teaching and coaching required on how to position baby. Baby's bottom needs to be against the back of mother's chair so his head can extend back and there is room between his chin and chest.
Cross-cradle	Provides good head control. Along with football hold, allows for ease with bringing the baby to the breast.	Least familiar to caregivers. Some mothers are not comfortable holding their babies in this manner.
Side-lying	Minimizes fatigue (Milligan, Flenniken & Pugh, 1996). Enables mother to rest more completely than is possible if she is sitting up.	Not always taught in hospital. Mothers may fear smothering baby in this position. Difficult for the mother to see to assist the infant with attachment.

grimacing are all early cues that the baby is slowly awakening. This is the time to gently try to awaken him to get him to breastfeed. Teaching parents these baby cues is a valuable element in early postpartum care. Poor latch-on in this very early time is common (Dewey et al., 2003) and is not oral aversion or a breastfeeding "strike" discussed in other sections of this book. The baby's lack of interest may be due to labor-related or postbirth narcotics, or to the infant's neurological immaturity. Inappropriate timing by forcing the baby on the breast before the baby is rousable and shows active interest may result in an aversive reaction (Widström & Thingström-Paulsson, 1993).

In the unusual event of an infant who cannot attach to the breast after several attempts, a visual evaluation of the infant's mouth is appropriate. The roof of the mouth should be wide and gently domed. The tongue should be long enough to extend over the lower gum. The baby's response to a feather-light stroking of the center of the lower lip should be noted. In most cases, the alert infant will open his mouth wide and the tongue will come for-

ward in response to such stimulation, as if seeking its source. The infant's frenulum (the small tissue tag under the tongue) should be far enough away from the tip of the tongue to prevent stricture during suckling. If the frenulum appears tight, a visual examination should be performed to determine whether the frenulum prevents the tongue from elevating or extending sufficiently to produce the wavelike motion necessary for effective suckling.

Occasionally, a digital examination may be appropriate. A finger slid into the baby's mouth should identify the hard palate as being intact. The tongue should groove around the finger. When the pad of the finger lightly touches the palate, the baby usually initiates a suck response that includes massaging by the tongue on the underside of the finger from knuckle to the fingertip. In a healthy newborn, the strength of oral negative pressure is such that the examiner will feel as if the nail bed is being pulled deeper into the baby's mouth. The nature of the suckling action should be rhythmic, although some neonates quickly realize that the finger does not reward suckling and so they cease doing so after several attempts. Because the finger is not a breast, with its soft areolar and nipple tissue, suckling at the breast should be the first experience for the infant. Thereafter, a finger assessment may be attempted, although it is not necessary in most cases and should be used judiciously.

Even if the baby is found to have an anatomical variation, such variation may not interfere with effective suckling. However, infants with a cleft palate, a high palatal arch, or a short tongue may require interventions provided by a therapist knowledgeable in treating these oral problems before he can breastfeed effectively.

Most maternal and infant problems resolve with time. The full-term infant is born with additional extracellular fluid (shed in the first few days after birth) that sustains him for a short time. However, after one to two days without receiving fluid nutriment, the neonate is at risk for rapid dehydration. Most hospitals have either a written or unwritten rule that the baby must be fed if he has not latched on by 24 hours. Figure 7–8 presents a flow chart that can be used as an algorithm indicating appropriate actions for early feedings or lack of feedings. We recommend the guidelines in Box 7–2 for intervention when the infant does not latch onto the breast 12 to 24 hours after birth.

Plan for the Baby Who Has Not Latched-On Yet

The most important concern when a baby is not latching is to feed the baby. One easy technique is to teach the mother how to hand express her milk onto the spoon, and then feed her baby the drops of colostrum from the spoon. Oftentimes when staff members hear, "Feed the baby" they picture a bottle in the baby's mouth. If a baby is not latching, giving a bottle can lead to the discontinuation of breastfeeding (Howard et al., 2003). It is time for the staff to think of supplementing as using a spoon with drops of colostrum or of finger- or cup-feeding once the volume of milk has increased to 10 ml or more.

Women produce a small amount of milk during the first few days. These small amounts of colostrum give the baby an opportunity to practice suck-swallow-breathe. The baby should have lots of practice time before the milk increases in volume. After 1 week, the baby should be taking a full volume of milk. Table 7–3 lists expected breastmilk intake for the neonate's first five days after birth. The equation for milk intake based on infant weight is 2.5 times the baby's weight in pounds equals the number of ounces the baby needs in 24 hours. For example an 8-pound baby needs 20 ounces (2.5 x 8) of milk in 24 hours when he is 1 week old. This equation works for the first 10 weeks. After that, a baby eats less in proportion to his weight.

Establishing the Milk Supply

When a baby is not latching onto the breast, the mother needs to establish her milk supply. Before she leaves the hospital, a multiple-user, hospital-grade electric breast pump with a double pump kit should be made available to her. She should pump both her breasts at the same time for about 10 to 15 minutes, 8 to 10 times in 24 hours.

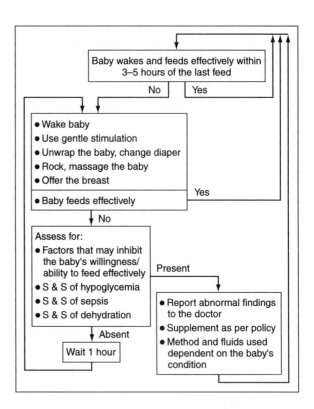

FIGURE 7–8. Breastfeeding flow chart. (From Glover J. Supplementation of breastfeeding newborns: a flowchart for decision-making. *J Hum Lact* 11:127–31, 1995. Reprinted with permission.)

BOX 7–2

Guidelines for the Infant Who Does Not Latch-On (According to Hours Postpartum)

0–24 Hours

- For full-term healthy baby, no supplement is necessary providing that the baby has periods of awake and quiet, and vital signs and blood sugar are within normal limits.
- Attempt to breastfeed during quiet, alert times or at least every 3 hr.
- Have parents hold baby skin-to-skin.
- Encourage a quiet environment.
- If not latched-on by 18–24 hr, provide electric pump and instruct in use. Pump at least 8 times in 24 hr.
- Alternative: teach mother hand expression.

24–48 Hours

- In hospital (every 3 hr) attempt to breastfeed.
- If unsuccessful after 10 minutes, feed baby with expressed breastmilk + water to equal 10–15 cc. Use formula if no breastmilk available.
- Apply nipple shield if the baby is too weak to latch or mother has flat or inverted nipple(s).
- Continue to pump.
- After discharge attempt to breastfeed every 3 hr. If unsuccessful after 10 minutes, feed baby expressed breastmilk to equal 10 to 15 cc.
- Use alternative feeding methods as appropriate: finger feed, spoon, cup, slow flow nipple.
- Continue skin-to-skin contact and quiet environment.
- Continue to pump at least 8 times/24 hr.

>48 Hours

- Attempt to breastfeed baby every 2–3 hr.
- If unsuccessful, feed baby with expressed breastmilk = 30–60 ml or expressed breastmilk + formula to equal 30–60 cc. Use formula if no breastmilk available.
- Consider nipple shield if the baby is too weak to latch or mother has flat or inverted nipple(s).
- Use alternative feeding method: cups, finger feed, slow flow nipple.
- Continue skin-to-skin contact and quiet environment.
- Continue to pump at least 8 times/24 hr.

Source: Adapted from Memorial Hospital, Breastfeeding guidelines, 2003, Colorado Springs, Colorado, with permission.

While she is pumping, she can massage her breasts. The postpartum nurses can show the mother how to hold both pump kits to her breasts with one arm, so she has a hand free to massage her breasts while pumping. The hospital should provide a form for her to keep a record of the milk expressed each time.

When a baby has not latched-on yet, it is important for them to remain skin-to-skin for as many hours a day as possible (Meyer & Anderson, 1999). Skin-to-skin contact will help the baby learn to breastfeed. Part of the discharge teaching by the postpartum nurse or lactation consultant needs to include the importance of continuing skin-to-skin

Table 7–3

NEONATAL FEEDING AMOUNTS FOR FIRST FIVE DAYS FOLLOWING BIRTH (FULL-TERM INFANTS)

Day	Per Feeding	Total in 24 Hours
1	Few drops to 5 cc (<1 tsp)	Few drops to 1 oz (2 tb)
2	5 to 15 cc (<0.5 oz or <1 tb)	1 to 4 oz (1/4 to 1/2 cup)
3	15 to 30 cc (0.5 to 1 oz or 1 to 2 tb)	4 to 8 oz (1/2 to 1 cup)
4	30 to 45 cc (1 to 1.5 oz or 2 to 3 tb)	8 to 12 oz (1.5 cup)
5	45 to 60 cc (1.5 to 2 oz or 3 to 4 tb)	12 to 18 oz (1.5 to 2 cup)

holding until the baby has learned to breastfeed well. It is important for the mother to remove as much milk as she possibly can, so once her milk supply increases in amount (usually on the third day) she needs to pump until the milk drips or spray subside, stop pumping, massage her breasts, and begin pumping again. Repeat the above two times. She should be able to complete the pumping process within 30 minutes.

Assessment of the Mother's Nipples and Breasts

When a baby is having difficulty latching, it is usually a baby problem, but the mother's nipples may be a contributing factor. On occasion the woman's nipples may be too big for the baby to accommodate all of her nipple and enough of the breast tissue to extract milk. In such a case, she will need to bring in the milk supply herself, feed her milk to her baby, and wait for the baby to grow into her nipple size.

If the mother's nipple is flat, inverted, or retracts when the baby compresses the breast with his gums, it is difficult for the baby to attach. Many babies figure out how to make their mother's breasts work for them, but other babies need some help. Teaching the mother to compress and shape her breast tissue for the baby to feel in his mouth when the nipple retracts may be just enough of a signal for the baby to continue suckling. Other techniques that have been tried, but not researched, include the following:

- Pulling back on the breast tissue so the nipples will protrude.
- Pumping the breasts just before the feed to pull out the nipples.
- Using a nipple shield (must pump or express after feed, monitor diaper output, weigh baby).
- Using a "nipple expanding" device to pull out flat or inverted nipples, such as the customized syringe (Kesaree et al., 1993) or a commercial expander (Evert-it, Niplette).
- Wearing shells between feedings to push areolar puffiness back into the breast (see section on breast edema later in this chapter) so the baby can latch.
- Expressing some milk to soften the breast for the baby if the woman is engorged.

Large-breasted women sometimes find breastfeeding challenging simply because they have difficulty dealing with their large breasts and the baby at the same time. Finding a place for the baby to be secure, so the mother can use both hands to deal with her large breast, can be the answer for these women. Care should be taken to position the baby so the weight of the breast is not resting on the baby's chest. The baby may feel his airway is being threatened with pressure on his chest. It may be just as threatening as pressure to the back of the baby's head.

Baby Problems That May Cause Difficulty with Latch-on

The baby needs an intact palate, a tongue that can cup and extend over the lower lip, lips that flange, and a mouth that does not hurt. If the baby is having any problems along these lines, he may not be able to attach well to the breast to breastfeed.

The baby needs to be able to breathe while feeding at the breast. A baby with laryngomalacia (floppy laryngeal structures pulled into the airway upon inspiration with audible stridor) or tracheomalacia (softening of the cartilaginous ring surrounding the trachea with stridor upon expiration) will need careful positioning to be able to breastfeed (McMillan et al., 1999). A prone feeding position may work well for these babies. If for any other reason (stuffy nose, swollen nares, obstructed nares, weight of the breast on his chest, etc.) the baby is having trouble breathing, he will not breastfeed.

If the baby is in pain, he may not feel like eating. Perhaps the baby could be given some pain medicine. The birth process can leave the baby with a broken clavicle, sore head, cranial sutures out of line, hematoma, forceps marks, or vacuum extraction trauma. A boy who has recently been circumcised may have shut out the world and not be interested in feeding for several hours.

Sometimes a baby will refuse one breast. This could be due to pain on one side of the body such as from a broken clavicle, an injury on one side of his head, or a painful shoulder. A few women have related stories of their children who were blind in one eye who resisted breastfeeding when the good eye was blocked.

Birth is a tiring process. Neonates may be drugged from the labor medications taken by their mothers. Some babies exhibit a hyper gag reflex. They may act as if they are backing away from the breast. Practicing sucking on a mother's clean finger may be an effective way to help these babies. If the baby has a tendency to hold his tongue in the wrong place, there are several strategies to assist the baby. If the baby is sucking the roof of his mouth, the baby may be working at stabilizing his jaw. By providing chin support, the baby may be able to lower his tongue.

If the baby holds his tongue behind the lower gum, the parents can play an imitation game with the baby and stick their tongues out at him. The baby tends to imitate the parents. Also, gently tapping a finger on the baby's lips should elicit interest on the baby's part to stick out this tongue in search of the finger.

When a baby is having difficulty latching, keep an eye, ear, and nose out for potential stimuli that could be obnoxious to the baby. The smell of perfume, soaps, body lotions, room deodorizers, etc., may disturb him. Loud noises, such as barking dogs or a mother yelling at older children, can scare the newborn. If anything is touching the baby's cheeks—such as his undershirt or a baby blanket or the mother's fingers—the baby may turn toward them and ultimately away from the breast. Removing anything that could be in the way will help the baby. The most disturbing stimulus of all is pressure on the back of the baby's head. The baby becomes very worried that his nose will become blocked. Suggest that the mother support the baby's shoulders and hold the baby's ears with her index finger and thumb. The web between these fingers make a second neck for the baby. In this way the baby knows he has control of his head and can lift his head back to free his airway if needed.

Previous negative experiences may cause aversion to the breast. If the baby's head has been pushed into the breast, the baby may start to cry when offered the breast. If the negative experience goes on, the baby shuts down when offered the breast. The parents describe the baby as falling asleep when offered the breast. When the baby has breast aversion, feeding the baby another way is important (see Chapter 10). Have the mother hold the baby skin-to-skin against her chest at nonfeeding times. Gradually move the baby, over the course of several days, to the breastfeeding position. Once the baby can be placed in the mother's arms in a breastfeeding position without the aversive behavior, the baby can be offered the breast after having been fed half of his milk for that feeding. Attempts to latch should be kept to a short time. These attempts should stop before the baby gets upset. Babies who are hypertonic or hypotonic may need the additional help of a curled/flexed position for breastfeeding.

The 34 to 38 "Weeker"

Infants born between 34 and 38 weeks gestation and treated as full-term infants pose a special situation. They fall between the cracks—i.e., they are not considered preterm infants unless they have medical problems but they often do not behave as full-term infants. In times past, these near-term babies were placed in a special nursery; now they are placed on the regular postpartum unit with their mothers. This is good for establishing breastfeeding, but as lactation consultants working in the postpartum area will testify, most 34–38-week infants require considerable time and effort before they are able to breastfeed effectively.

These babies are often neurologically disorganized and have poor state control. They can go from a highly alert state to deep sleep rapidly and the environment should be kept quiet to avoid overstimulation. Their suckle/swallow/breathe cycle may not be fully developed. Often these babies have poor muscle tone or floppiness, which requires careful positioning and extra support during feedings. The baby will need good shoulder girdle support for head control, should be placed facing the mother with the baby's arms separated and hugging the breast, and the baby's hips should be well-supported almost as high as the head (Tully, 2003). (Figure 7–9 shows a 36-week-old premature baby at breast.)

The usual pattern of these infants is to grasp the breast and suckle for a short time and then stop to rest. Once a bolus of milk is in the baby's mouth and he drops his tongue to swallow, he may not have the maturity to bring his tongue into position to initiate the next suckle. The inability of these babies to maintain sustained periods of at least 10 suck/swallows/breathe patterns limits milk transfer and puts

them at risk for high bilirubin levels, hypoglycemia, dehydration, and insufficient weight gain. Interventions for these infants must be individual; however, skin-to-skin holding, keeping them warm, allowing longer periods of rest between feedings, and limiting stimulation are all important for optimizing the baby's ability to feed well when awake.

Many of these babies feed best on approximately a 4-hour schedule until they are close to term age, at which time they go to the more usual 2- to 3-hour feeding pattern and begin to waken for feedings voluntarily. Trying to force a baby to waken before the fourth hour from the *beginning* of the last feeding may cause the baby to put a lot of energy into trying to maintain the sleep state he needs. However, at the fourth hour most of these babies will wake fairly willingly and feed vigorously taking a sufficient volume to justify 6 feedings in 24 hours. For some babies, short but frequent feedings work better.

The mother will need to pump after each breastfeeding to establish her milk production. This expressed milk can be given to the baby if the baby cannot obtain enough milk by breastfeeding. Because this small baby is learning to breastfeed, an alternative feeding method that does not provide sucking, such as cup or spoon, are options to consider. Nipple shields work well for these babies if they are having trouble maintaining latch-on and the mother has a good milk supply.

The mother/baby dyad will need extra care in such cases. Follow-up phone calls and early return for weight checks is mandatory. Mothers of 34 to 38 weekers who have breastfed a full-term baby previously need just as much help as first-time breastfeeders. They remember a vigorous baby who knows how to feed effectively. Her past experience does not prepare her for a sleepy baby who gives little feedback. Also, the mother who is engorged should be encouraged to pump or express sufficient milk to establish her milk supply.

Feeding Methods

Cup-Feeding

Babies can be fed by cup from birth and many low birth weight infants are cup-fed around the world until they are mature enough to exclusively breast-

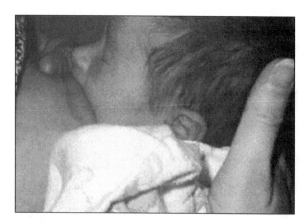

FIGURE 7–9. A 36-week-old premature baby at breast.

feed (Gupta, Khanna, & Chattree, 1999). Cup-feeding low birth weight infants was found to be at least as safe as bottle-feeding with no differences in physiological stability and the incidence of choking, spitting, apnea, and bradycardia during feeds for both feeding methods (Malhotra et al., 1999; Marinelli, Burke, & Dodd, 2001).

A study of full-term infants found cup-feeding no more stressful than bottle-feeding. However, in another study, infants took less volume and required more time to feed as they were learning to cup-feed than when learning to bottle-feed. (Dowling et al., 2002). Other drawbacks are milk spillage and that the baby is deprived of sucking. In two early cup-feeding studies (Davis et al., 1948; Freeden, 1948), full-term babies cup-fed efficiently, taking milk faster by cup than by bottle or breast. In the 1940s, newborns were in the hospital for 10 days. Given more time, they became very proficient at cup feeding.

For cup-feeding, a small cup with a rounded edge is preferred. In India, a special cuplike device called a *paladai* is used for feeding premature babies in some neonatal intensive care units. The nurses in these units prefer the *paladai* to a regular cup (Malhotra et al., 1999). Medicine cups holding small quantities are readily available in hospitals. They are thus appropriate for early feedings when volume will rarely exceed 1 to 2 oz. Commercial feeding cups are also available.

The baby should be placed in an upright, sitting position (see Figure 7–10). As the cup is brought to a position resting on his lower lip with the rim at the corners of his mouth, tipping the cup slightly to allow access to the fluid allows the baby to be fed without the risk of developing a preference for rubber nipple teats (Howard et al., 2003). As long as the caregiver does not attempt to pour too much milk into the baby's mouth, risk of aspiration is minimal and the feeding can be accomplished quickly (Lang, Lawrence, & Orme, 1994; Thorley, 1997). Babies who are poor candidates for cup-feedings are those with a poor gag reflex, neurological deficits, and respiratory problems.

Finger-Feeding

Finger-feeding with a feeding tube is an alternative feeding method for neonates (Figure 7–11). It

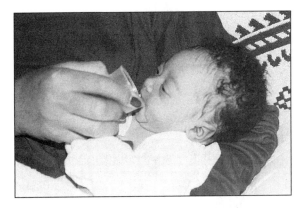

FIGURE 7–10. Baby cup-feeding. (Courtesy of Kay Hoover, MEd, IBCLC.)

is used by some lactation consultants when the baby is too sleepy to breastfeed, if the baby does not latch-on well for any reason, or if the mother and baby are separated (Newman, 2002). Proponents of finger-feeding believe that it facilitates proper use of the oral muscles, promotes optimal coordination of suck-swallow-breathe, and allows the baby to pace the feeding (Hazelbaker, 1997). Critics claim that the technique is invasive and addictive. Instructions for finger-feeding a neonate are presented in Box 7–3.

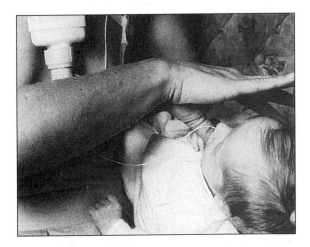

FIGURE 7–11. Finger-feeding. The technique is used to feed an infant breastmilk and avoid rubber nipple confusion when the infant is not latching onto the breast. (Courtesy of Pat Bull.)

BOX 7–3

Finger-Feeding a Neonate

- Ensure that your hands are clean and the nail on the finger or thumb you use is cut short before you begin. Wearing a latex-free glove or finger cott is preferable when the baby is finger-fed by someone other than the mother or father.
- Prop the baby, making sure his head is stable and slightly tilted back.
- If using a feeding-tube device (#5 French, 15 in. long), the tube can be held close to the end of the finger.
- Connect the feeding tube with a syringe or feeding bottle with expressed breast-milk or, if necessary, formula depending on the situation. If using a bottle, the feeding tube can be inserted through a cut made in the rubber nipple. If using a syringe, choose the size most appropriate for the circumstances (usually 10 to 30 cc).
- Select a large digit, since the breast fills the baby's mouth.
- Stroke the baby's lips gently until the baby opens his mouth. Slide your finger or allow the baby to suck the finger in

with the nail bed resting on his tongue and the pad side up. The tip of the finger needs to extend to the juncture of the hard and soft palates. The tube can be taped to the pad side of the parent's finger. In most instances, the baby will begin sucking as soon as he feels the finger pad on the hard palate.
- Push milk from the syringe into the baby's mouth ONLY if the baby is sucking.
- If the baby is sucking effectively, the person who is finger-feeding the baby will feel a pulling sensation along the nail bed with each exertion of negative pressure (suckle), as if the nail is being pulled deeper into the baby's mouth.
- Monitor color and vital signs, especially if the baby is low birth weight or has poor muscle tone or oral structural deficits.
- Record the amount of human milk (or formula) that the baby takes.
- Show the mother (and the father) how to finger-feed.

Nipple Shields

Nipple shields have a controversial history, largely due to the bad reputation of the old type of shields that were made of rubber or latex. Babies of mothers using these old type of shields were unable to ingest sufficient breastmilk often resulting in slow weight gain and failure-to-thrive. As a result, nipple shields came to be viewed as interfering with, rather than assisting, the new mother in breastfeeding. The newer ultra-thin silicone nipple shields are especially helpful for a mother with flat or inverted nipples, for preterm babies who have trouble latch-

ing and maintaining suction, or for babies who have developed a preference for a bottle nipple and thus refuse the breast.

When a woman uses a silicone nipple shield, she needs to use a multi-user electric pump (like the ones used in the hospitals) and pump her milk four to six times a day after breastfeeding to establish a milk supply. The baby needs to be weighed twice a week and diapers monitored for adequate stools and wetness. Once the baby is gaining well (about an ounce a day), the mother can stop pumping.

In many cases, the short-term use of a nipple shield will preserve the breastfeeding relationship while the baby learns to breastfeed (Meier et al., 2000; Nicholson, 1993; Wilson-Clay, 1996). A La Leche League mother movingly described how a silicone nipple shield "saved her breastfeeding relationship" with her baby (Clemmit, 2003).

Placing a feeding tube (attached to a syringe with the milk supplement) inside of the nipple shield during a feed is particularly helpful (Figure 7–12). This technique gives the baby several advantages:

- An immediate reward for latching-on and suckling
- An opportunity to stimulate the breast and remove breastmilk
- Control over the amount and flow of supplement ingested
- Nutriment (calories and fluids)

To apply a silicone nipple shield, smooth a thin layer of water inside the nipple shield brim, then flip up the brim of the shield (like that of a sombrero), center the shield directly over the nipple, and gently pat down the brim (Wilson-Clay, 2003). For additional discussion on nipple shields, see Chapter 12.

Hypoglycemia

Newborns experience a decrease in blood-glucose after birth as they adapt to the extrauterine environment and then regain blood-glucose rapidly (Eidelman, 2001). Transient asymptomatic low blood-glucose (< 30 mg/dl) in the first hours is an adaptive phenomenon as the newborn changes from the fetal state of continuous transplacental glucose feeding to that of intermittent feeding after birth. This dynamic process is self-limiting and is usually not pathologic (Haninger & Farley, 2001).

Hypoglycemia is partially a matter of definition. Whether a baby is considered to have a low blood-glucose level depends on the laboratory values used as criteria for hypoglycemia and the reliability of the methods used to measure blood glucose. Before deciding what is abnormal, one must first establish what is normal. What are normal blood sugar levels for newborns? Based on the author's experience with teaching an Internet course to graduate nurses across the United States, hypoglycemia protocols vary widely according to region, and routine glucose testing after birth is common.

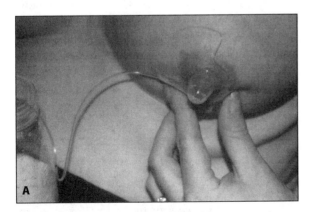 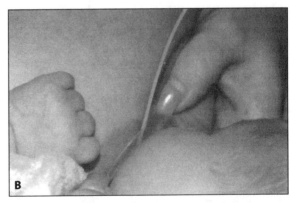

FIGURE 7–12. Feeding tube device under a silicone nipple shield. (A) Feeding tube device placed under nipple shield. Baby would need to be able to suck well in order to pull the milk out of the bottle and through the tubing. This is a good technique to keep the baby feeding at the breast until he can latch onto the breast and get out enough milk directly. It could also be used for a baby who has become accustomed to a bottle nipple. (B) Baby receives supplementation from feeding tube and breastfeeds at the same time. As soon as baby attaches, milk can be squeezed into the nipple shield to give the baby an immediate reward for any attempts made at the breast. Use with baby who has gotten used to bottle-feeding, has a weak suckle, or has had difficulty latching onto the breast. (Courtesy of Kay Hoover, MEd, IBCLC.)

On the whole, breastfed infants have lower blood sugar levels (58 mg/dL) compared with formula-fed infants (72 mg/dL), according to Hawdon, Ward-Platt, and Aynsley-Green (1992). In the same study, blood sugar levels were correlated with the intervals between the feeds—i.e, the more frequent the feeding, the higher the glucose concentration.

While there are still no universally accepted "cut-off" glucose levels for hypoglycemia, several guidelines have been recommended. On the basis of research findings from a large sample of well, full-term infants, Heck and Erenberg (1987) recommend that hypoglycemia in full-term infants be defined as serum glucose concentration of less than 30 mg/dL on the first day after birth or less than 40 mg/dL on the second day after birth. Srinivasan et al. (1986) recommended similar levels. (Table 7–4). If the higher level of 40 mg/dL were used for the first day postpartum, 20.6 percent of well, full-term infants would be considered hypoglycemic and would receive unnecessary supplements (Sexson, 1984). The Academy of Breastfeeding Medicine (2002) has published hypoglycemia guidelines on the Internet (see Box 7–4).

Table 7–4

DEFINITION OF HYPOGLYCEMIA (SERUM OR PLASMA) BY AGE

Author	Postnatal Age (hr)	Serum or Plasma Glucose mg/dL
Heck & Erenberg, 1987	0–24	<30
	24–48	<40
Srinivasan et al., 1986	0–3	<35
	3–24	<40
	>24	<45

Source: From Protocol Committee Academy of Breastfeeding Medicine, A. I. Eidelman, C. R. Howard, R. J. Schanler, and N. E. Wight. Clinical Protocol Number 1: Guidelines for Glucose Monitoring and Treatment of Hypoglycemia in Breastfed Neonates. *ABM News and Views* 5 (4): insert, 1999.

Severe neonatal hypoglycemia leads to potential brain damage and can result in serious sequelae such as seizures. Prolonged hypoglycemia can be avoided by close clinical observation of vulnerable infants while avoiding excessive invasive management (Moore & Perlman, 1999). Clinical symptoms that indicate possible hypoglycemia in neonates include the following:

- Temporary irritability
- Jitteriness
- Exaggerated reflexes
- High-pitched cry
- Seizures
- Lethargy
- Listlessness
- Rapid breathing
- Hypothermia
- Poor suck and refusal to feed

Hypoglycemia is of particular concern with certain health conditions: the infant of a mother with diabetes, a postmature neonate, or an infant who is small for gestational age. The infant of a mother with diabetes is most apt to experience hypoglycemia shortly after birth, because he continues to produce a high level of insulin, which depletes the blood glucose within hours after birth. The degree of infant hypoglycemia is usually in proportion to the success achieved in controlling the mother's blood glucose during her pregnancy. Symptomatic neonates are given 10 to 15 percent glucose intravenously immediately after birth until they stabilize.

Postmature infants also need early, frequent breastfeedings to normalize their glucose levels. Lethargy and poor feeding in these babies may contribute to hypoglycemia; thus any interest shown in feeding should be followed by immediate, unrestricted access to the breast for as often and as long as the baby wishes. Most postmature neonates, after a first breastfeeding, show increased interest in subsequent breastfeeding, thus reducing the risk of continued hypoglycemia.

The newborn who is small for his gestational age is also at risk for hypoglycemia. A prompt first breastfeeding followed by very frequent breastfeeding thereafter is usually sufficient to bring the

BOX 7–4

Recommendations on Hypoglycemia from the Academy of Breastfeeding Medicine

- Healthy term neonates do not develop symptomatic hypoglycemia as a consequence of underfeeding. Underlying illness must be excluded in such infants.
- Routine monitoring of blood glucose in asymptomatic, term neonates is unnecessary. Measure blood glucose concentration only in at-risk infants and/or those with clinical symptoms compatible with hypoglycemia. Bedside screening tests must be confirmed by true laboratory glucose measurements.
- Monitoring should begin within 30 minutes for infants of diabetic mothers and no later than 2 hours of age for infants in other risk categories. Clinical manifestations of hypoglycemia are tremors, irritability, jitteriness, exaggerated reflexes, high-pitched cry, seizure, lethargy, listlessness, rapid breathing, hypothermia, poor suck, and refusal to feed.
- Hypoglycemia can be minimized by early initiation of breastfeeding after delivery. Initiation and establishment is facilitated by skin-to-skin contact of mother and infant. Such practice will maintain normal infant body temperature and reduce energy expenditure while stimulating suckling and milk production.

Source: Adapted from Academy of Breastfeeding Medicine (2002).

baby's blood-glucose level to normal. In some cases, continued poor feeding may require a supplement. Start with the mother's own milk. If no milk can be obtained with hand expression, and there is no banked human milk, then formula may have to be used. This practice need not be repeated once the baby is breastfeeding well. The following conditions are associated with low blood sugar:

- Small for gestational age
- Postmature
- Discordant twin (smaller)
- Large for gestational age (LGA) > 90th percentile or weight
- Infants of diabetic mothers
- Low birth weight infants < 2500 gms

- Postasphyxia, cold stress, sepsis, and other stresses

Intrapartum management plays a role in the neonate's glucose level. Use of hypertonic glucose infusions during labor can lead to elevation in maternal blood glucose, which can in turn result in fetal hyperglycemia and hyperinsulinemia and eventually neonatal hypoglycemia.

Neonates' blood-glucose levels are usually measured by a heel stick to obtain blood. The blood level is then measured using Dextrostix with the glucometer or Chemstrips with an Accu-Check 11 reflectance meter. Dextrostix and Chemstrips are easily used and inexpensive; however, they are prone to many errors. A glucose electrode system is preferred because it is more accurate, especially at the "low end" of glucose values and requires no further confirmatory laboratory analysis (Haninger &

Farley, 2001). Measuring blood-glucose concentrations in asymptomatic babies in the first 2 postnatal hours is unnecessary and potentially harmful to parental well-being. It also interferes with establishing breastfeeding and can result in serious disruption of the initiation and duration of breastfeeding (Haninger & Farley, 2001).

Placing the baby skin-to-skin with his mother helps stabilize his blood sugar. Christensson et al. (1998) report average blood glucose of 57.6 mg/dl in the skin-to-skin group and 46.6 in the group cared for away from their mothers.

Cornblath et al. (2000) summarizes the problem of neonatal hypoglycemia: "At present no simple bedside measures exist that can determine these values and hence provide an absolute indication of an intervention in an individual infant. Furthermore, no data exist that define the concentration of plasma glucose or its duration that causes damage."

Problems that are most likely to be of concern in the early days of breastfeeding relate to method of birth, breast engorgement, sore nipples, and other problems that usually disappear quickly.

Cesarean Births

Over 20 percent of births in the United States are by cesarean, and the rate is rising (Lowe, 2003). Many European and South American countries have similar and even higher rates of surgical birth. The impact of cesarean birth on breastfeeding has been extensively studied. Although its effects are difficult to disentangle from other interventions, generally, breastfeeding rates and the duration of mothers who deliver by cesarean birth are about the same as those who have vaginal births (Janke, 1988; Kearney, Cronenwett, & Reinhardt, 1990; Victora et al., 1990). However, cesarean births are associated with delayed lactogenesis and, as expected, a delay in initiating breastfeeding (Chen et al., 1998; Dewey et al., 2003; Evans et al., 2003; Grajed & Perez-Escamilla, 2002; Leung, Lam, & Ho, 2002; Nissen et al., 1996; Rowe-Murray & Fisher, 2002; Wittels et al., 1997).

Cesarean births affect breastfeeding primarily by delaying the initiation and establishment of lactation but not the continuance of breastfeeding. The mother's commitment to breastfeeding plays a substantial role despite unexpected birth outcomes. A greater commitment to breastfeeding, regardless of the manner of birth, results in longer duration of breastfeeding (Janke, 1988).

Recovery from major surgery takes more time, is more painful and stressful, and represents additional risks compared to an uneventful vaginal birth, which explains why breastfeeding occurs later following cesarean birth. Women's reactions to having a cesarean birth vary. A woman may interpret an unexpected cesarean birth as a reflection on her adequacy and may be more fearful that she will fail at breastfeeding because she perceives that she failed with birthing. In balance, cesarean births are so frequent parents tend to view cesarean birth as a normal or alternative mode of delivery. Childbirth educators and others have effectively conveyed the message that cesarean birth does not have to be a threat. Parents' concerns are reduced by the knowledge that they can be awake to experience the event and that the baby's father can be present at the birth.

In working with a mother who has had a cesarean birth, the nurse or the lactation consultant needs to assess the mother's degree of physical comfort and awareness. If she is not fully conscious, she is not ready to put her baby to breast. Once the mother is alert and able to hold her baby, however, she can begin breastfeeding. The mother should be asked how she wants to hold her infant. Some mothers, particularly those still receiving intravenous pain medication or those who have had an epidural narcotic, are quite comfortable holding their babies in the cradle position using pillows for support. Others are hesitant to hold the baby at all until they have been reassured that they can do so without touching or placing any pressure near their abdominal incision. Suggest that if the mother holds her baby in a clutch position, (see again Figure 7–6B) she will avoid the sensitive incision area. As the pain of her incision decreases, the mother can be instructed and assisted in the use of positions other than the football hold, as discussed later in this chapter. By the second or third day postpartum, the side-lying position is generally comfortable, especially if the mother is adequately supported with pillows at her back and beneath her abdomen.

The baby born by cesarean may be lethargic, particularly if the birth followed a long period of exposure to analgesia or anesthesia in labor. If so, explain to the mother that a delay in feeding will not deter breastfeeding; rather, her milk supply will be established slightly later than it would be following a vaginal birth. Pumping the breasts in the immediate postpartum period neither hastens lactogenesis nor improves later milk transfer (Chapman et al., 2001).

Breast Engorgement

Breast engorgement is a major issue in the early postpartum period as the breast, under the influence of hormonal shifts, increases milk production rapidly from 36 to 96 hours postpartum. Although the gradual buildup of fluid in the breasts following parturition is a welcome sign of breastmilk, breast engorgement is a common problem in the early days after birth and a common reason for early weaning. Because women leave the hospital before their breasts become full or engorged, the situation is usually handled at home or in a postdischarge visit at a clinic or medical office.

For most women engorgement is at its height from 3 to 5 days after birth and slowly recedes but may last 2 weeks for some (Humenick, Hill, & Anderson, 1994). During normal engorgement, the mother's breast tissue usually remains compressible, thus enabling the infant to attach comfortably and efficiently, without risk of trauma to the breast or nipple tissue. Extreme breast fullness rarely lasts more than 24 hours, during which time breastfeeding can continue without discomfort. The mother with breast fullness should be encouraged to view this state as a transitory indication of milk production that will begin to regulate to meet the baby's needs as the infant breastfeeds.

Multiparous women are more likely to report more intense engorgement than primiparous women and distinct patterns of breast engorgement can be identified (Humenick, Hill, & Anderson, 1994). Severe breast engorgement, a pathologic condition, and often the consequence of mismanagement, is painful. It can be caused by any situation that allows milk stasis to occur. There are several situations that lead to uncomfortable engorgement:

- Supplements (Wright, Rice, & Wells, 1996)
- Delayed initiation of feedings at the breast
- Infrequent feedings
- Time-limited feedings
- Removing the baby from the first breast to ensure feeding from both breasts at every feeding (Lawson & Tulloch, 1995)

Breast implants can also lead to severe engorgement. Sometimes the tissue around the nipple and areola becomes so taut that the infant is unable to grasp the nipple. When the baby is unable to latch onto the breast, the mother's discomfort mounts, and her breast and nipple tissue may be so tight that even leaking cannot occur. Under such conditions, further trauma to the tissue is apt to occur when a vigorous baby attempts unsuccessfully to grasp and draw the breast into his mouth.

Various treatments for engorgement have been suggested:

- *Heat treatments*: Warm compresses, warm showers. Use warm treatments *before* breastfeeding.
- *Cold treatments*: Cold compresses, frozen vegetable bags (wrapped in a towel), cold gel packs. Use cold treatments *after* breastfeeding.
- *Cabbage compresses*: Fresh cabbages, cold or room temperature (Roberts, Reiter, & Schuster, 1995; Rosier, 1988).
- *Breast massage and milk expression*: Massaging the breast and expressing milk to relieve engorgement. This technique is commonly practiced worldwide, especially in Japan.
- *Ultrasound*: Ultrasound treatments, used for both plugged ducts and engorgement.
- *Medications*: Antiinflammatory medications.
- *Pumping*: Pumping reduces build-up of milk.

Research on engorgement is unique in that the condition slowly and inevitably resolves itself no matter what treatment is used; thus a group of mothers (preferably randomized) receiving the treatment must be compared simultaneously with a group who do not receive the treatment. Snowden, Renfrew, and Woolridge (2002) analyzed eight randomized control trials involving 424 women receiving treatments for breast engorgement in an attempt to discover which treatments were effective (see Table 7–5). They concluded that cabbage leaves, cold packs, gel packs, oxytocin, and ultrasound

Table 7–5

META-ANALYSIS OF STUDIES ON POSTPARTUM BREAST ENGORGEMENT

Treatment	Outcome
Antiinflammatory drugs	Increase total improvement rating and reduce symptoms compared with placebo. Danzen (OR 3.6, 95%, CI 1.27–10.26); Kimotab (OR 8.02, 95%, CI 2.76–23.3).
Cabbage leaves	No difference between treatment and control groups.
Cold packs	No difference between treatment and control groups.
Gel packs	No difference between treatment and control groups.
Oxytocin	No difference when compared with saline injections.
Ultrasound treatments	No benefit. Decrease in pain due to the warmth of treatment rather than ultrasound waves themselves.

Source: From Snowden, Renfrew, & Woolridge (2002).

treatments were all ineffective. Only pharmacological treatment using antiinflammatory medications (Danzen and bromelain/trypsin complex) significantly improved symptoms of engorgement.

Whatever intervention is used, the mother should be encouraged to offer the breast frequently to avoid painful engorgement. Any method that reduces the sensation of tightness in the breast tissue is likely to help the mother. If the mother is breastfeeding, how often and how long her infant is suckling should be assessed. During the first 2 weeks, the average number of minutes a baby spends breastfeeding in 24 hours is about 2.7 hours (de Carvalho, 1982). If the baby is being offered the breast fewer than eight times in 24 hours, and for less than an average of 20 minutes per feeding, it may not be enough. If the mother is unable to increase the number of feedings, she may obtain relief with the judicious use of hand expression or a fully automatic intermittent electric breast pump.

A fever of unknown origin in a mother during the first week postpartum may be another sign of breast engorgement. Occasionally, fever from engorgement can be 101 degrees F or higher. If the woman is not breastfeeding and her breasts are engorged, she can apply cold to reduce fluid filtration into the interstitium, owing to vasoconstriction. As in other areas of the body, tissue edema in the breast is reduced by cold and is increased by heat.

Breast Edema

Women who receive excessive intravenous fluids throughout labor may develop edema of their breast. This edema is different from the normal physiologic engorgement that precedes lactogenesis. The mother's breasts can be as "hard as rocks" and the nipples distended. As a result, the neonate may be unable to latch onto her breasts until the edema has subsided. Breast edema can be treated with areolar compression, a method to reduce nipple/areola edema manually by using gentle positive pressure (Miller & Riordan, 2004). The health-care provider can do the following intervention or the mother can do it herself:

- Ask mother to wash her hands thoroughly. Explain what you plan to do to the mother and ask her permission. Nails should be short and preferably unpolished. No artificial nails.

- Do a "press test" to determine areolar edema. Apply firm but gentle pressure with the index finger and thumb on either side of the areola behind the nipple. Hold it there until the edema can be felt to be giving way. Remove your fingers to see if there are finger impressions remaining in the tissue. If there are, then areolar edema is present.

- Apply pressure again slightly behind the softened spot. Hold the pressure until the area under your fingers softens. Apply, steady inward pressure toward the chest wall for 60 seconds or longer, concentrating on the areola where it joins the base of the nipple. Next, move the fingers behind the softened area to the firm tissue and apply pressure again.

- Start behind the nipple, rotate the fingers clockwise, and move back along the areola holding the pressure until the tissue is soft before moving the fingers again. If fingernails are short, press with the curved fingertips of both hands simultaneously with the nail nearly touching the sides of the nipple. The goal is to create a ring of small "dimples" or pits on the areola at the base of the nipple. (If performed by the health-care provider, the flat part of two thumbs or two fingers can also be used. This will require another 60 seconds of pressure in opposite quadrants to soften the same general area.)

- Rotate finger pressure, displacing the edema into the breast tissue until the areola is soft and the nipple is pliable.

- Plan on the procedure taking anywhere from a few minutes to 30 minutes to move the edema out enough to latch the infant onto the breast. The length of time will depend on the severity of the edema.

The effect of areolar compression, also called reverse pressure softening (Cotterman, 2004), is fourfold: (1) it moves excess interstitial fluid inward in the direction of natural lymphatic drainage; (2) it relieves overdistension of the milk ducts and reduces latch discomfort; (3) it enables the infant to draw the breast deeply into his mouth so that the stripping action of the tongue can remove the milk; (4) it stimulates the nerves supplying the nipple and areolar complex, thus triggering the milk ejection reflex (Cotterman, 2003).

Areolar compression (Color Plate 20) should be done *before* pumping the breast. Pumping the breast first before areolar compression can cause further accumulation of edema in the areola, especially when maximum settings are used. The negative pressure of a pump tends to draw excess interstitial fluid *toward* the areola and nipple instead of moving it *away* from the area, thus worsening the problem. Once edema is displaced, the nipple will stretch outward making latching easier.

Hand Expression

Although many women in the United States think first of using a breast pump to obtain milk, expressing milk by hand is a skill that has been used by many mothers for millennia. The mother's own hands represent several advantages over breast pumps:

- They cost her nothing.
- They may trigger a more effective milk ejection reflex.
- They are always available.
- They compress the breast for milk removal.

After the mother has practiced this skill, she may find she can obtain more milk more quickly than women who use an electric device for the same purpose! Techniques vary across cultures and are most effective when the breasts are compressed well behind the nipple (Figure 7–13). Every postpartum nurse and every lactation consultant should be able to instruct a mother in hand expression. Pushing back toward the chest wall with her fingers and then rolling the fingers together is recommended rather than sliding the fingers down the breast, to avoid inadvertently bruising or abrading the skin. The mother should be cautioned that she might have greater difficulty with expression if she is attempting to relieve engorgement or her breasts are very tender. She should be encouraged to be patient, to shower or use warm compresses, and to stimulate milk ejection with gentle breast massage in advance of attempting to express her milk.

If breast massage is practiced with each expression, encourage the mother to avoid creating a ritual that becomes so time consuming that it interferes with the process. This is particularly relevant if the mother is expressing her milk at work or some other site where she has only a limited time in which to accomplish it. An experienced mother who can demonstrate the tech-

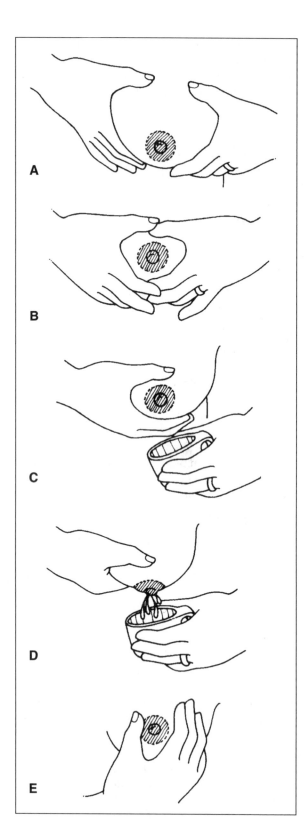

FIGURE 7–13. Hand expression.

(A) Wash hands and any collection equipment to be used. Sit comfortably, and place the collection cup under the breast. Apply warm, moist towel to enhance milk flow. Massage breasts and nipples to stimulate milk ejection reflex. Use gentle pressure using a circular motion, moving around the breast.

(B) Squeeze the breast gently, rolling the hands forward from the chest toward the nipple.

(C) Place thumb and forefingers approximately 2 to 3 cm (1 to 1 1/2 inches) behind the nipple and press into the breast.

(D) Press inward toward the chest wall squeezing gently with a slight rolling action toward the nipple. Release pressure and repeat as needed to obtain milk. If pain results, something is wrong and the mother should be observed in order to identify what may be causing the mother discomfort.

(E) Change position of the fingers around the areola to express milk from as many ducts as possible. Within 3 to 5 minutes, the milk flow may slow; this is a signal to express milk from the other breast. Both sides may be expressed as often as the mother wishes in a given session or until she tires. Particularly in the beginning, the mother should expect to spend 20 to 30 minutes expressing milk. As she becomes more adept at it, the time will decrease even as the amount of milk obtained increases.

nique to the novice can often provide the most effective teaching.

Clinical Implications

Assessment is a critical first step in working with a mother who has a newborn. For example, if the mother had maternal analgesia and her baby is sleepy and is breastfeeding infrequently, the hospital caregiver can do the following:

- Encourage and facilitate the mother to hold her baby skin-to-skin.

- Reassure the mother that the baby's sleepiness may be the result of the analgesia to which he was exposed prior to the birth.

- Encourage the mother to take every opportunity when the baby is awake to offer the breast.

- Suggest that the mother let the baby stay on the first breast until he has let go on his own before offering the second breast.

- Provide specific suggestions regarding home visitation and follow-up with a lactation consultant in private practice and a community-based breastfeeding support group. If the mother experienced difficulty in breastfeeding with an earlier baby, the caregiver may need to reassure the concerned or anxious mother that a similar condition need not recur, or if it does recur, what to do about it.

Breastfeeding Assessment

The infant's first few times breastfeeding should be assessed early in the neonatal period. Such assessment enables the health-care worker to determine how well the infant roots, latches-on, and suckles. Minor adjustments of maternal position or infant position can be made without interrupting or interfering with the mother and infant as they begin to learn how to breastfeed together.

Several assessment tools specific to feedings at the breast are available and can be found in Appendix 20-A as well as in the *Resource Guide to Breastfeeding and Human Lactation* accompanying this book.

Assessment tools are useful for evaluating infant suckling over several feedings to show mothers that their babies are learning with each feeding and are becoming more efficient at obtaining milk. They can also be used to alert the caregiver to specific "red flags." If the mother-baby dyad is not feeding effectively, they may need special attention to prevent a problem with dehydration and weight loss. Breastfeeding assessment tools also remind the mother that what her baby does is both complex and predictable and that he needs lots of opportunities to practice, just as she needs many opportunities to learn how to hold and position him for optimal breastfeeding. The ease of using these tools means that the mother can evaluate for herself what occurs at each feeding. Despite the usefulness of these tools, reliability and validity testing indicate that they need further development (Riordan & Koehn, 1997). Newer investigations are leading us closer to more valid methods of clinical prediction of breastfeeding outcomes. Of the commonly used breastfeeding indicators, audible swallowing best predicts the actual intake of breastmilk (Riordan & Gill-Hopple, 2002). We also know that certain perinatal events predict that the mother will stop breastfeeding by 7 to 10 days postpartum (Hall et al., 2002), so these mothers need extra help (see Table 7–6).

Table 7–6

MODIFIABLE PERINATAL VARIABLES PREDICTING THAT A MOTHER WILL STOP BREASTFEEDING BY 7 TO 10 DAYS POSTPARTUM

Perinatal Events	P Value	Odds Ratio
Long breastfeeding intervals	0.0001	1.1–1.3
More than 2 bottles	0.001	1.7–4.8
Vacuum vaginal delivery	0.0017	1.7–9.3
Long duration of Pitocin	0.0492	1.00–1.11

Source: Adapted from Hall et al. (2002).

Discharge Planning

Over the past 30 years the average length of a hospital stay in the United States has declined by nearly 60 percent, to 1.4 days. Mothers and infants often return home in the first 24 to 48 hours after a vaginal birth and 2 to 4 days after a cesarean birth. Early discharge from the hospital, a fact of life for most new mothers and their neonates, has had a major impact on postpartum care. It is the responsibility of the hospital caregiver to highlight critical points that the parents need to pay attention to when they are newly home with their baby. Foremost among these concerns is seeing to it that the baby feeds often and effectively. The mother needs guidelines that will help her to assess whether this is occurring and whom to contact for assistance if it does not (Hall & Carty, 1993).

Early discharge does not appear to negatively affect breastfeeding; in fact some studies indicate that mothers who leave the hospital early breastfeed longer (Edmonson, Stoddard, & Owen, 1997; Margolis & Schwartz, 2000). At the same time, early discharge may negatively influence the mother's feeling of competence in her mothering, particularly if she is unprepared or unsure of how to care for her newborn. Contact with mother-to-mother organizations can help the mother to place her experiences in the context of other women's comments about their breastfeeding course. In addition, more home health visits are being done to provide the care that used to be provided in longer-term hospitalization. Pediatricians and other physicians, cognizant of the postdischarge void in medical coverage, are routinely scheduling appointments with the family of a breastfed baby within 48 to 72 hours after discharge as recommended by the American Academy of Pediatrics.

The goal of discharge planning is twofold: to prevent common problems and to provide emotional support (Page-Goertz, 1989). With such a brief time in the hospital, the mother needs a caregiver who imparts as much basic information as possible without overwhelming her. She also needs reinforcement of her self-confidence in her role as a new mother. These two goals are mutually reinforcing and, as the caregiver instructs the mother in the prevention of problems, she is in a position to simultaneously enhance the new mother's self-esteem and self-confidence; in short, the mother is able to "take control" of her experience (Hall & Carty, 1993). The mother's perceptions of her infant not only reflect how she and the baby will interact but can also influence how long she breastfeeds.

Basic Feeding Techniques

In teaching basic feeding techniques to a new mother, priority must be given to certain guidelines:

- *Feed the baby frequently* (8 or more feedings in a 24-hour period). Using a visual aid such as the size of the baby's fist to demonstrate the size of the newborn's stomach is an excellent way to illustrate why the neonate needs frequent feedings: his stomach is simply too small to hold large quantities at a time! Additionally, the curds formed by human milk digest quickly. Artificial baby milks form large curds that take longer to digest than human milk. The formula-fed infant feeds fewer times.

- *Offer (and keep the baby on) the first breast until he has completed that side.* If he wants more, offer the second breast for as long as the baby wants. Some babies will be satiated with one breast; others prefer two, and still others may have some early marathon feedings in which they move from one to the other several times!

- *Avoid watching the clock.* The best timer of the feeding is the baby. After breastfeeding is established, the mother may identify cues that the baby is happy with one breast at each feeding or wants both breasts at each feeding.

- *Avoid the use of artificial teats, pacifiers (dummies), supplemental infant formula, water, or glucose water feeds for the first 2 to 4 weeks.* The infant may substitute nonnutritive suckling for milk intake at the breast, resulting in poor weight gain. The pacifier can also become a source of nipple confusion (Powers & Slusser, 1997) and a possible marker for other difficulties that can result in shorter breastfeeding duration. Telling the mother why these practices can interfere with early, effective breastfeeding will give her the ammunition she may need to fend off well-meaning but uninformed attempts to "assist" her with unnecessary, potentially interfering practices. The exception is preterm infants, who may benefit from nonnutritive suckling during the period that they are unable to take oral feedings (see Chapter 13).

- *Identify various ways in which the mother can recognize that her infant is getting sufficient milk.*

These include the following:

- Listening for and identifying the infant's swallows
- Baby waking on his own for at least 8 feedings in 24 hours
- Monitoring the diaper output

Signs That Intervention Is Needed

Slow infant weight gain is addressed in depth in Chapter 10. Briefly, the following signs indicate a need for health-care intervention:

- Scant, concentrated urine, brick dust urine (from urate crystals) after day 2, or no urine at all.
- Infrequent stools (fewer than four per day after day 3).
- Stools that have not turned yellow by day 4 or 5.
- Lethargy (difficult or impossible to waken for feedings).
- Extreme fretfulness (never contented after any feeding).
- No swallowing is felt or heard during feedings; when a feeding is evaluated, the clinician does not observe an "open-pause-close" pattern of suckling (Newman, 1996).
- The mother is experiencing nipple soreness that is more intense if it existed earlier, or that suddenly develops if it was previously absent.
- The mother's breasts are clinically engorged and very painful, making it difficult or impossible for the baby to breastfeed.
- A baby is not latching onto the breast.
- A baby is not waking on his own to feed at least 8 times in 24 hours.

Discharge

At discharge, the parents need clear, simply written materials that provide step-by-step information and are individualized as much as possible. Materials with drawings or photographs of positioning and other techniques are helpful. The hospital caregiver should establish a definite plan for follow-up: making a phone call to the mother at a specific time postdischarge or providing her with the phone numbers of the hospital "warm line" and of lactation consultants or La Leche League leaders in the area. If the baby has breastfeeding problems, a referral to an LC made from the mother's room prior to her discharge from the hospital is appropriate. Public health, home health, nurse case-manager, or pediatric follow-ups are other options in some communities.

Discharge packs (i.e., marketing packs) containing formula should be discouraged for the breastfeeding mother. It is logical that such a practice can undermine the mother's confidence and plant doubt about her ability to breastfeed, especially for the immigrant mother (see Chapter 24). Yet results of studies on the effects of discharge packs on breastfeeding duration are contradictory (Chezem et al., 1998; Howard & Howard, 1997; Janson & Rydberg, 1998).

To settle the question, Snowden, Renfrew, and Woolridge (2000) conducted a systematic review of nine randomized controlled trials involving 3730 North American women. The meta-analysis showed that when comparing marketing discharge packs with any of the controls (no intervention, nonmarketing pack, and combinations of these), exclusive breastfeeding was reduced at all time points in the presence of commercial hospital discharge packs but mixed feeding (nonexclusive breastfeeding) was not affected. As Howard and Howard (1997) pointed out, discharge packs may not exert as large an influence on breastfeeding duration as some other determinants, but many of the other more powerful influences such as education, race, income, martial status, or return to work are not as readily amenable to change.

The intent of health maintenance organizations (HMO) and insurers in encouraging early postpartum discharge is corporate profits since earlier discharge means greater profit. With about 4 million births annually (United States) and maternity beds averaging $1000 per day, insurers save $4 billion annually for every day they shorten the hospital stay.

Early discharge does not appear to result in earlier weaning if postpartum follow-up is integrated into care (Quinn, Koepsell, & Haller, 1997). Several studies (Lee et al., 1995; Pascale et al., 1996; Soskolne et al., 1996) link early postpartum discharge with increased hospital readmission for both jaundice and dehydration when the breastfeeding mother and baby are not followed up. Others failed to demonstrate negative effects (Edmonson, Stoddard, & Owens, 1997).

In many countries other than the United States, midwives and home health visitors routinely visit new mothers. The optimal time for a follow-up visit or call is no later than 2 to 4 days after discharge from the hospital. This is an especially crucial period because enough time has passed to make an accurate evaluation of the mother's milk supply and the infant's intake.

Summary

Consumer advocacy, the expectations of parents, childbirth and breastfeeding education, early hospital discharge, frequent cesarean births, and technologies all affect birthing and early breastfeeding. In recent years, the emphasis has changed from a management approach to support and education of childbearing families for their own self-care. No longer do we view the mother and her infant as separate entities; rather we care for them as a natural, single unit. Many hospitals now boast a family-centered birthing unit or labor-delivery room postpartum care where the mother and infant are cared for together in one room. Birthing rooms today look much like a bedroom with a comfortable reclining chair for the mother's support person; hookups for medical equipment are concealed behind wall prints and other decorations. A major benefit of this kind of mother-baby care is that families receive more comprehensive, coordinated care, which facilitates breastfeeding.

At the same time that we are seeing improvements in mother-baby care, the use of medical interventions, particularly epidural analgesia and anesthesia, has skyrocketed. Two opposing forces appear to be battling each other for control of childbirth: on one side, childbirth education, midwifery, doula services, and free-standing birthing centers; on the other, hospitals with routine epidural injections, high rates of cesarean births, and other technologies that medicalize the intrapartum experience.

Too few mothers learn enough about breastfeeding in the hospital before being asked to assume full responsibility for themselves and their babies. Only sporadically are they informed of the red flags that indicate that they should seek expert help and when to do so. Thus what should be a natural function is perceived as complicated. New mothers need reassurance that they can enjoy an uncomplicated breastfeeding experience and that common concerns can be easily managed.

As public awareness grows that breastfeeding sustains the baby's health and government and insurance companies become more aware of cost savings, breastfeeding will be promoted as the feeding of choice. Insurance companies will provide household help and visiting nurses to assess breastfeeding mothers and infants, in addition to giving substantial rebates to mothers who breastfeed. Breastfeeding will be not only socially acceptable but socially responsible.

Key Concepts

- The best preparation for breastfeeding is to learn as much as possible before the birth of the baby and find a support system.
- Nipple rolling, "toughening," and other forms of nipple preparation during pregnancy are not necessary and should be avoided.
- Neonates are initially alert for about 2 hours after birth, followed by deep sleep until 20 hours, and then increased wakefulness and interest in frequent breastfeeding.
- If there are no complications, the first breastfeeding should take place during the first hour

after the infant's birth. After the infant has been dried, the infant can be placed in the mother's arms to breastfeed skin-to-skin.

- Privacy, comfortable positioning, and optimal latch-on are all basic skills necessary to assist mothers and neonates in early breastfeeding.

- Care during labor and birth, and postbirth care, can impact on breastfeeding.

- Teaching "correct" positions for breastfeeding varies according to the practitioner. "Correct" positiong is, as yet, not evidence-based.

- When a baby is not latching onto the breast, it is important to feed the baby, establish the mother's milk supply, and find hands-on help to correct the situation and encourage skin-to-skin holding.

- If cup-feeding is done carefully, it has been found to be as safe as bottle-feeding. However, infants who are cup-fed spill more milk than infants who are bottle-fed.

- During the first 2 days infants who are breast-fed and infants who are cup-fed ingest less milk than infants who are bottle-fed

- New parents need to watch the baby, not the clock, to determine when the baby is ready to feed. Feed the baby at the *earliest* sign of hunger. Crying is a *late* sign of hunger.

- Healthy infants born between 34 and 38 weeks need special help and careful, frequent follow-up, as these babies tend to breastfeed poorly.

- Short-term use of a silicone nipple shield in certain situations (nipple inversion, low birth weight infants) can preserve the breastfeeding relationship while the baby learns to feed.

- Generally accepted guidelines for hypoglycemia in full-term infants is serum glucose concentration of less than 30 mg/dL in the first day after birth or less than 40 mg/dL after the second day. Invasive procedures for determining glucose levels can be avoided by early skin-to-skin contact between mother and baby, frequent breastfeeding, and close clinical observation.

- Generally speaking, women who deliver by cesarean birth breastfeed as frequently and for as long as those who have vaginal births. Special concerns related to breastfeeding are pain control, comfortable positioning, and early initiation of breastfeeding.

- Normal breast engorgement starts at 3 to 5 days after birth and then slowly recedes over the first 2 weeks. During normal engorgement the mother's breast tissue usually remains compressible, thus enabling the infant to suckle comfortably and efficiently. Early and frequent breastfeeding is thought to prevent severe engorgement.

- A meta-analysis of eight randomized control trials on treatments for breast engorgement concluded that only pharmacological treatment using antiinflammatory medications significantly improved symptoms of engorgement.

- Excessive intravenous fluids during labor can lead to postpartum breast edema. The technique of areolar compression can help reshape the breast/nipple area so that the neonate is able to latch onto the breast.

- Hand expression is a time-honored skill that costs nothing, is easy to learn, and is always available.

- Early discharge does not appear to affect breastfeeding if there is postpartum care and support. If follow-up care is not provided, costly readmissions to the hospital result. The goal of discharge planning is to prevent common problems and to provide emotional support. With such a brief time in the hospital, the mother needs a caregiver who imparts as much basic information as possible without overwhelming her and is able to answer her questions with researched-based information.

- Basic and priority discharge teaching includes teaching the mother her baby's feeding cues, how to latch her baby onto the breast, how to know the baby is getting enough milk, and who to call for help with breastfeeding.

- Marketing or discharge packs reduce the length of exclusive breastfeeding; however, they do not exert as large an influence on breastfeeding duration as some other determinants.

Internet Resources

Academy of Breastfeeding Medicine. Clinical protocols for hypoglycemia:
www.bfmed.org

Meta-analysis research on clinical aspects of breastfeeding:
www.breastfeedingonline.com
www.update-software.com/Cochrane/default.htm

References

Academy of Breastfeeding Medicine. Glucose monitoring and treatment of hypoglycemia in term breastfed neonates. *The Academy.* Available at: http://www.bfmed.org. Accessed October 10, 2002.

Anderson GC. Risk in mother-infant separation postbirth. *Image:J Nurs Schol* 21(4):196–199, 1989.

Anderson GC et al. Development of sucking in term infants from birth to four hours postbirth. *Res Nurs Health* 5(1):21–27, 1982.

Chapman DJ, Young S, Ferris AM, Perez-Escamilla R. Impact of breast pumping on lactogenesis stage II after Cesarean delivery: a randomized clinical trial. *Pediatrics* 107(6):E94, 2001.

Chen DC, Nommsen-Rivers L, Dewey KG, Lonnerdal B. Stress during labor and delivery and early lactation performance. *Am J Clin Nutr* 68(2):334–44, 1998.

Chezem J et al. Lactation duration: influences of human milk replacements and formula samples of women planning postpartum employment. *JOGN Nurs* 27(6):646–51, 1998.

Christensson K et al. Randomised study of skin-to-skin versus incubator care for rewarming low-risk hypothermic neonates. *Lancet* 352(9134):1115, 1998.

Clemmit S. Nipple shield perspective. *New Beginnings* 20(2):58–59, 2003.

Cornblath M et al. Controversies regarding definition of neonatal hypoglycemia: suggested operational thresholds. *Pediatrics* 105(5):1141–45, 2000.

Cotterman K. Reverse pressure softening: a simple tool for easier latching during engorgement. *J Hum Lact* 20(2): 2004.

Cotterman, KJ. Too swollen to latch on? Try reverse pressure softening first. La Leche League. *Leaven* 39(2):38–40, 2003.

Cregan M, Hartmann PE. Computerized breast measurement from conception to weaning: clinical implications. *J Hum Lact* 15(2):89–96, 1999.

Crowell MK, Hill PD, Humenick SS. Relationship between obstetric analgesia and time of effective breastfeeding. *J Nurse Midwifery* 39(3):150–56, 1994.

Davis HV, Sears RR, Miller HC, Brodbeck AJ. Effects of cup, bottle and breastfeeding on oral activities of newborn infants. *Pediatrics* 2:549–58, 1948.

de Carvalho M et al. Milk intake and frequency of feeding in breastfed infants. *Early Hum Dev* 7(2):155–63, 1982

Dewey LA et al. Risk factors for suboptimal infant breastfeeding behavior, delayed onset of lactation, and excess neonatal weight loss. *Pediatrics* 112:607–19, 2003.

Dowling DA et al. Cup-feeding for preterm infants: mechanics and safety. *J Hum Lact* 18(1):13–20, 2002.

Edmonson MB, Stoddard JJ, Owen LM. Hospital readmission with feeding-related problems after early postpartum discharge of normal newborns. *JAMA* 278(4):299–303, 1997.

Eidelman A. Hypoglycemia and the breastfed neonate. *Pediatr Clin No Amer* 48(2):377–87, 2001.

Ekström A, Widström AM, Nissen E. Duration of breastfeeding in Swedish primiparous and multiparous women. *J Hum Lact* 19(2):172–78, 2003.

Evans KC et al. Effect of caesarean section on breast milk transfer to the normal term newborn over the first week of life. *Arch Dis Child Fetal Neonatal Ed.* 88(5):F380–2, 2003.

Freeden RC. Cup feeding of newborn infants. *Pediatrics* 2:544–48, 1948.

Glover J. Supplementation of breastfeeding newborns: a flow-chart for decision-making. *J Hum Lact* 11:127–31, 1995.

Grajeda R, Perez-Escamilla R. Stress during labor and delivery is associated with delayed onset of lactation among urban Guatemalan women. *J Nutr* 132(10): 3055–60, 2002.

Gupta A, Khanna K, Chattree S. Cup feeding: an alternative to bottle feeding in a neonatal intensive unit. *J Trop Pediatrics* 45(2):108–10, 1999.

Hall RT et al. A breastfeeding assessment score to evaluate the risk for cessation of breastfeeding by 7 to 10 days of age. *J Pediatr* 141(5):659–64, 2002.

Hall WA, Carty EM. Managing the early discharge experience: taking control. *J Adv Nurs* 18(4):574–82, 1993.

Haninger NC, Farley CL. Screening for hypoglycemia in healthy term neonates: effects on breastfeeding. *J Midwifery Women's Health* 46(5):292–301, 2001.

Hawdon JM, Ward-Platt MP, Aynsley-Green A. Patterns of metabolic adaptation for preterm and term infants in the first neonatal week. *Arch Dis Child* 67(4 spec no):357–65, 1992.

Hazelbaker AK. In defense of finger-feeding. *Medela Rental Round-up* 14(2):10–11, 1997.

Heck LJ, Erenberg A. Serum glucose levels in term neonates during the first 48 hours of life. *J Pediatr* 110(1):119–22, 1987.

Hedderwick SA et al. Pathogenic organisms associated with artificial fingernails worn by healthcare workers. *Infect Control Hosp Epidemiol* 21(8):505–09, 2000.

Henderson A, Stamp G, Pincombe J. Postpartum positioning and attachment education for increasing breastfeeding: a randomized trial. *Birth* 28(4):236–42, 2001.

Hoffmann JB. A suggested treatment for inverted nipples. *Am J Obstet Gynecol* 66:346, 1953.

Howard C, Howard F. Discharge packs: how much do they matter? *Birth* 24(2):98–101, 1997.

Howard C et al. Randomized clinical trial of pacifier use and bottle-feeding or cupfeeding and their effect on breast-feeding. *Pediatrics* 111:511–18, 2003.

Humenick SS, Hill PD, Anderson MA. Breast engorgement: patterns and selected outcomes. *J Hum Lact* 10(2):87–93, 1994.

Janke JR. Breastfeeding duration following Cesarean and vaginal births. *J Nurs Midwifery* 33(4):159–64, 1988.

Janson S, Rydberg B. Early postpartum discharge and subsequent breastfeeding. *Birth* 25(4):222–25, 1998.

Johanson RB et al. Effect of post-delivery care on neonatal body temperature. *Acta Paediatr* 81(11):859–62, 1992.

Kearney MH, Cronenwett LR, Reinhardt R. Cesarean delivery and breastfeeding outcomes. *Birth* 17(2):97–103, 1990.

Kesaree N et al. Treatment of inverted nipples using a disposable syringe. *J Hum Lact* 9(1):27–29, 1993.

Kroeger M. *Impact of birthing practices on breastfeeding: protecting the mother and baby continuum.* Boston: Jones and Bartlett, 2004.

Lang S, Lawrence CJ, Orme RL. Cup feeding: an alternative method of infant feeding. *Arch Dis Child* 71(4):365–69, 1994.

Lawson T, Tulloch MI. Breastfeeding duration: prenatal intentions and postnatal practices. *J Adv Nurs* 22(5):841–49, 1995.

Lee KS et al. Association between duration of neonatal hospital stay and readmission rate. *J Pediatr* 127(5):758–66, 1995.

Leung GM, Lam TH, Ho LM. Breast-feeding and its relation to smoking and mode of delivery. *Obstet Gynecol* 99(5 pt 1):785–94, 2002.

Lieberman E et al. Epidural analgesia, intrapartum fever, and neonatal sepsis evaluation. *Pediatrics* 99(3):415–19, 1997.

Lothian JA. It takes two to breastfeed: the baby's role in successful breastfeeding. *J Nurs Midwifery* 40(4):328–34, 1995.

Lowe NK. Amazed or appalled, apathy or action? [editorial]. *JOGN Nurs* 32:281–82, 2003.

MAIN Collaborative Group Preparing for Breast Feeding. Treatment of inverted and nonprotractile nipples in pregnancy. *Midwif* 10:200–14, 1994.

Malhotra N et al. A controlled trial of alternative methods of oral feeding in neonates. *Early Hum Develop* 54(1):29–38, 1999.

Margolis L, Schwartz JB. The relationship between the timing of maternal postpartum hospital discharge and breastfeeding. *J Hum Lact* 16(2):121–28, 2000.

Marinelli K, Burke GS, Dodd VL. A comparison of the safety of cupfeedings and bottlefeedings in premature infants whose mothers intend to breastfeed. *J Perinatol* 21(6):350–55, 2001.

McMillan JA et al. *Oski's pediatrics.* Philadelphia: Lippincott Williams & Wilkins, 1999.

Meier P et al. Nipple shields for preterm infants: effect on milk transfer and duration of breastfeeding. *J Hum Lact* 16(2):106–14, 2000.

Meyer K, Anderson GC. Using Kangaroo Care in a clinical setting with fullterm infants having breastfeeding difficulties. *MCN* 24(4):190–92, 1999.

Miller V, Riordan J. Treating postpartum breast edema with areolar compression. *J Hum Lact* 20(2): 2004.

Milligan RA, Flenniken PM, Pugh LC. Positioning intervention to minimize fatigue in breastfeeding women. *Appl Nurs Res* 9(2):67–70, 1996.

Moon JL, Humenick SS. Breast engorgement: contributing variables and variables amenable to nursing intervention. *JOGN Nurs* 18(4):309–15, 1989.

Moore AM, Perlman M. Symptomatic hypoglycemia in otherwise healthy, breastfed, term newborns. *Pediatr* 103(4 Pt 1):837–39, 1999.

Mulford C. Subtle signs and symptoms of the milk ejection reflex. *J Hum Lact* 6(4):177–78, 1990.

Newman J. Decision tree and postpartum management for preventing dehydration in the "breastfed" baby. J *Hum Lact* 12(2):129–35, 1996.

———. Finger feeding. Handout #8, 2000. Available at: http//www.breastfeedingonline.com. Accessed October 2002.

Nicholson WL. The use of nipple shields by breastfeeding women. *Aust Coll Midwives J* 6(2):18–24, 1993.

Nissen E et al. Different patterns of oxytocin, prolactin but not cortisol release during breastfeeding in women delivered by Cesarean section or by the vaginal route. *Early Hum Dev* 45(1-2):103–18, 1996.

Page-Goertz S. Discharge planning for the breastfeeding dyad. *Pediatr Nurs* 15(5):543–44, 1989.

Pascale JA et al. Breastfeeding, dehydration, and shorter maternity stays. *Neonatal Network* 15(7):37–41, 1996.

Powers NG, Slusser W. Breastfeeding update 2: clinical lactation management. *Pediatrics in Review* 18(5):147–61, 1997.

Quinn A, Koepsell D, Haller S. Breastfeeding incidence after early discharge and factors influencing breastfeeding cessation. *JOGN Nurs* 26(3):289–94, 1997.

Ransjo-Arvidson AB et al. Maternal analgesia during labor disturbs newborn behavior: effects on breastfeeding, temperature and crying. *Birth* 28(1):5–11, 2001.

Righard L. How do newborns find their mother's breast? *Birth* 22(3):174–75, 1995.

Righard L, Alade MO. Effect of delivery room routines on success of first breastfeed. *Lancet* 336(8723):1105–07, 1990.

Riordan J, Gill-Hopple K. Testing relationships of breastmilk indicators with actual breastmilk intake. Presented at: National Institute of Nursing Research, State of the Science Nursing Congress; Washington, DC, September 26, 2002.

Riordan J, Koehn M. Reliability and validity testing of three breastfeeding assessment tools. *JOGN Nurs* 26(2):181–87, 1997.

Riordan J et al. The effect of labor pain relief medication on neonatal suckling and breastfeeding duration. *J Hum Lact* 16(1):7–12, 2000.

Roberts KL, Reiter M, Schuster D. A comparison of chilled and room temperature cabbage leaves in treating breast engorgement. *J Hum Lact* 11(3):191–94, 1995.

Rosier W. Cool cabbage compresses. *Breastfeed Rev* 12(1):28–31, 1988.

Rowe-Murray HJ, Fisher JR. Baby friendly hospital practices: cesarean section is a persistent barrier to early initiation of breastfeeding. *Birth* 29(2):124–31, 2002.

Sadeh A, Dark I, Vohr B. Newborns' sleep-wake patterns: the role of maternal, delivery, and infant factors. *Early Hum Develop* 44:113–26, 1996.

Sepkoski CM et al. The effects of maternal epidural anesthesia on neonatal behavior during the first month. *Dev Med Child Neurol* 34(12):1072–80, 1992.

Sexson WR. Incidence of neonatal hypoglycemia: a matter of definition. *J Pediatr* 105(1):149–50, 1984.

Snowden HM, Renfrew MJ, Woolridge MW. Commercial hospital discharge packs for breastfeeding women (Cochrane Review). In: *The Cochrane Library.* Oxford: *Update Software,* Issue 2, 2000.

———. Treatments for breast engorgement during lactation (Cochrane Review). In: The Cochrane Library. Oxford: *Update Software.* Issue 3, 2002.

Soppas P. Personal communication. June 2003.

Soskolne EI et al. The effect of early discharge and other factors on readmission rates of newborns. *Arch Pediatr Adolesc Med* 150(4):373–79, 1996.

Srinivasan G et al. Plasma glucose values in normal neonates: a new look. *J Pediatr* 109(1):114–17, 1986.

Thorley V. Cup feeding: problems caused by incorrect use. *J Hum Lact* 13(1):54–55, 1997.

Trainor C. Valuing labor support. *AWHONN Lifelines* 6:387–89, 2002.

Tully MR. Breastfeeding the 34 to 38 week infant: a challenge for the health team. International Lactation Consultant Annual Meeting. Boca Raton, Florida, July 27, 2002.

Varendi H, Porter RH, Winberg I. Attractiveness of amniotic fluid odor: evidence of prenatal olfactory learning? *Acta Pediatr* 85(10):1223–1227, 1996.

Victora CG et al. Caesarean section and duration of breast feeding among Brazilians. *Arch Dis Child* 65(6):632–34, 1990.

Viscomi CM. Maternal fever, neonatal sepsis evaluation and epidural labor analgesia. *Reg Anesth Pain Med* 25(5):549–53, 2000.

Widström AM, Thingström-Paulsson J. The position of the tongue during rooting reflexes elicited in newborn infant before the first suckle. *Acta Paediatr* 82:281–83, 1993.

Widström AM et al. Gastric suction in healthy newborn infants: effects on circulation and developing feeding behaviors. *Acta Paediatr Scand* 76(4):566–72, 1987.

Widström AM et al. Short-term effects of early suckling and touch of the nipple on maternal behavior. *Early Hum Develop* 21(3):153–63, 1990.

Wiessinger D. A breastfeeding teaching tool using a sandwich analogy for latch-on. *J Hum Lact* 14(1):51–56, 1998.

Williams J, Mueller S. A message to the nurse from the baby. *J Hum Lact* 5(1):19, 1989.

Wilson-Clay B. Clinical use of silicone nipple shields. *J Hum Lact* 12(4):279–85, 1996.

———. Nipple shields in clinical practice: a review [editorial]. *Breastfeeding Abstracts* 22(2):11–12, 2003.

Winslow EH, Jacobson AF. Can a fashion statement harm the patient? Long and artificial nails may cause nosocomial infections. *Am J Nurs* 100(9):63–65, 2000.

Wittels B et al. Postcesarean analgesia with both epidural morphine and intravenous patient-controlled analgesia: neurobehavioral outcomes among nursing neonates. *Anesth Analg* 85(3):600–06, 1997.

Woolridge MW, Ingram JC, Baum JD. Do changes in pattern of breast usage alter the baby's nutrient intake? *Lancet* 336(8712):395–97, 1990.

Wright A, Rice S, Wells S. Changing hospital practices to increase the duration of breastfeeding. *Pediatrics* 97(5):669–75, 1996.

Postpartum Care

Linda J. Smith and Jan Riordan

This chapter follows the mother-infant dyad after birth in the early postpartum period. Hospital stays following birth are short in the United States, but hospitals are required to allow mothers at least two days in the hospital after a vaginal birth and more after a cesarean birth. Early discharge offers advantages to the family. There is less time for hospital routines to interfere with early lactation and less opportunity for cross-infection. Alternatively, a disadvantage of early discharge is less time for teaching and assistance with breastfeeding. In spite of this drawback, early discharge does not seem to affect how long a mother breastfeeds (Quinn, Koepsell, & Haller, 1997).

Concerns about the baby not getting enough milk, as well as breast and nipple pain are the top reasons that mothers stop breastfeeding early (Schwartz et al., 2002). Parents are also concerned about engorgement, leaking, jaundice, and use of pacifiers during the first few weeks postpartum. This chapter addresses these topics and other common problems during the "fourth trimester" for the mother, the baby, and the family. The infant is the most vulnerable member of the dyad; therefore, assuring adequate nutrition and hydration is the most immediate goal.

Even when new mothers have adequate knowledge about breastfeeding and have social and clinical support, most still will benefit from a visit by a skillful breastfeeding advisor during the early postpartum period (Heinig & Nommsen-Rivers, 2000).

Hydration and Nutrition in the Neonate

The priority for postdischarge follow-up care of the mother-infant pair is assuring that the baby is receiving sufficient breastmilk to maintain hydration and support growth. The full-term neonate is born with additional extracellular fluid that helps maintain infant hydration in the first few days. After that time, neonates are much more likely to develop fluid and electrolyte disturbances quickly; the margin between homeostasis and overload or underload is small (Blackburn & Loper, 1992). The American Academy of Pediatrics guidelines (AAP/ACOG, 2002) for early discharge include that the baby have at least two successful feedings and be able to coordinate suckling, swallowing, and breathing while feeding.

However, in some places mothers and babies are still being discharged with a breast pump, a hope, and a prayer but without having been observed by a skilled breastfeeding helper. The AAP (1997) recommends an early postdischarge appointment with the baby's primary-care provider during the first week postpartum. Families who use health clinics should be scheduled for a postdischarge clinic visit or a home visit within 2 to 4 days after hospital release (3 to 5 days after birth). At that visit, a health professional should observe a complete feeding, weigh the baby on an electronic scale, and evaluate how mother and baby are progressing.

A healthy term infant will regain his birth weight by 14 days postpartum and, after that time, will gain at least 4 to 7 ounces (113 to 219 grams) per week or at least a pound a month. Weight loss beyond age 3 days, weight loss of more than 7 percent of birth weight, or failure to regain birth weight by age 2 weeks in the term neonate requires a careful evaluation of the feeding techniques being used and the adequacy of breastfeeding. (AAP/ACOG, 2002).

Signs of Adequate Milk Intake

The baby's nutritional needs (Table 8–1) and the mother's milk supply are rapidly changing and tightly interwoven during early infancy (see Chapter 4). When one considers that the neonate's stomach is very small, it is easy to understand why babies feed frequently.

The baby must obtain enough milk to grow and thrive. When milk transfer occurs frequently and in sufficient volumes, certain signs (Table 8–2) reassure the parents and professionals that all is proceeding normally.

Milk Supply—Too Much or Too Little

Milk supply is a major worry of many new mothers during the first few weeks postpartum. It is the almost universal reason given by mothers for early weaning and for supplementation. Mammalian survival has depended for millennia on sufficient breastmilk production to meet the needs of the young. If actual milk insufficiency occurred frequently, the species' survival would be in jeopardy.

Unrealistic expectations of infant behavior and lack of knowledge of normal breastfeeding patterns are major issues. Mothers, especially those breastfeeding for the first time, tend to believe that their infants are "nursing a lot," when they should be feeding even more frequently.

Breastfed infants typically have a sleep-wake cycle of wakefulness and frequent ("cluster") feedings in the late afternoon and early evening—an ancient pattern originating in our hunter-gatherer tribal past, according to anthropologists. This wakeful interactive period at the end of the day may be particularly trying for an inexperienced or unsure mother. She needs to be reassured that wakefulness and frequent feedings at these times are entirely normal and unrelated to mothering skills or milk supply. Milk is synthesized at a high rate at this time of day because of the baby's frequent nursing (Daly et al., 1996).

Any event, behavior, custom, or practice that keeps the baby away from the breast or causes milk to remain in the breast for long periods (> 4–6 hours) has the potential to reduce milk volume. These factors include, but are not limited to, scheduled feeds, use of bottles without corresponding expression of milk, use of pacifiers so that suckling time at the breast markedly decreases (see section on pacifiers), or maternal or infant illness.

Table 8–1

EXPECTED INFANT MILK INTAKE

Day	Milk Intake per Day (ml)	Voids and Stools (Minimum)
1	5–100 (average 30) colostrum	1 wet diaper, 1 black tarry stool
2	10–120 colostrum	2 wet
3	200	3 wet, some green stool
4	400	4 wet, 4 loose yellow stools
5	600+	6 wet, 3–4+ yellow stools
6 days to 6 months	550–950; average 750 (25 oz)	6+ wet, 3–5+ loose yellow stools

Table 8–2

Reassuring Signs of Adequate Milk Transfer

Reassuring Signs	Rationale
Baby is alert, cues for feeds, and seems satiated after feeds.	An alert baby cues the mother to indicate that he is hungry and then that he is satisfied.
Baby actively suckles a minimum of 160–180 minutes per day in the first 2 weeks.	At least that amount of time at breast is needed to obtain sufficient milk.
Audible swallowing is heard.	Swallowing reflects milk intake (Riordan & Gill-Hopple, 2002).
After feeds, mother's nipple is comfortable, wet, and intact.	Creasing, pain, and /or damage suggest poor milk transfer.
Baby and mother are satisfied with feeding.	Mother accurately reports problems with feedings (Neifert, 1998).
Baby's mucous membranes are wet and skin turgor is elastic and responsive; gently pinched skin does not remain above the normal surface (tenting).	The absence of skin tenting after pinching indicates that infant is sufficiently hydrated.
By 4 to 5 days, baby passes 3–5 or more loose, yellow stools per day.	Frequent and profuse stool output is usually the most reliable indicator of adequate nutrient intake.
By the end of the first week, baby has 6 or more soaking wet diapers per day; urine is clear (not dark or concentrated).	Voluminous urine output is an indicator of adequate hydration after the first few days.

If the baby is not removing sufficient milk, he will exhibit typical signs of hunger:

- Seems restless, fussy, irritable
- Acts "hungry all the time," especially right after a feeding
- Sucks his fists or blanket
- Moves his head rapidly from side to side at the breast
- Comes off the nipple frequently
- Cries or whimpers frequently
- Is difficult to console or is fussy right after a feeding
- Has excessively long (> 30 minutes per side) or short (< 5 minutes per side) feeds
- Eagerly takes formula or pumped milk from a bottle right after a feeding
- Falls asleep at breast but does not release the breast

Simultaneously, the mother may be uneasy because of these and other reasons:

- She does not feel the let-down (milk-ejection) reflex as strongly as she thinks she should
- She has nipples that are painful and/or damaged, especially by cracks or fissures
- Her breasts stay full and hard even after feeds OR her breasts are soft most of the time
- She is not be able to express as much milk as she thinks she should
- She thinks that frequent feeds mean "not enough milk" (and in this case she may be right)
- She has had previous breast surgery
- She thinks her breasts are too small

Most mothers have sufficient lactation capacity to synthesize at least one third more milk than their baby typically takes (Daly et al., 1996). However, if the breasts are not drained of about 75 to 85 percent of the milk most of the time by the baby's suckling or expressing, the rate of milk synthesis slows down to match the lowered demand; therefore total daily production falls. Breast storage capacity also matters. If a mother has small breasts and low milk storage capacity, her baby will need to feed more frequently to obtain all the milk he needs. Mothers with large breasts may have a large storage capacity and, as a result, may be able to provide larger feeds at longer intervals (if her baby is willing).

If a baby cannot remove sufficient milk from the breast, milk synthesis will quickly diminish unless the mother begins pumping or expressing milk. Regular milk removal will maintain the mother's milk supply while the causes of her baby's poor suck are investigated and resolved.

Temporary Low Milk Supply or Delayed Lactogenesis

The onset of lactogenesis II (the onset of copious milk secretion, or "milk coming in") occurs on days 2 to 3 after the delivery of the placenta, which causes a sharp drop in circulating progesterone. Retained placental fragments can inhibit the fall of progesterone, thereby delaying onset of lactogenesis II (Neifert, McDonough, & Neville, 1981). During lactogensis II, lactose synthesis rapidly increases, drawing water into what has been colostrum and resulting in a sweeter and less viscous fluid referred to as "transitional milk." Mothers perceive this event on average about 50 to 60 hours postbirth, after the increased rate of synthesis is underway and as their breasts fill with milk.

Delayed lactogenesis II, measured by the mother's perception, is associated with cesarean birth, and high levels of stress to the mother and fetus during birth (Chen et al., 1998; Chapman & Perez-Escamilla, 1999; Dewey, 2001). Premature delivery, insulin-dependent diabetes mellitus, obesity, cesarean birth, and endocrine disturbances can delay lactogenesis II and impede the successful establishment of lactation. Whether this delay is a maternal physiological response, or due to delayed or ineffective suckling, or a combination of factors, has

not yet been clearly established. Early, frequent, and effective breastfeeding appears to be the most important factor in establishing normal lactation. Prolactin bursts associated with the infant suckling or breast pumping support the continued growth of secretory tissue for several weeks or months after birth (Cox et al., 1999).

Very few women are unable to make sufficient milk for one baby. Neville and Morton (2001) categorize failed lactogenesis as (1) preglanduar, owing to retained placenta or lack of pituitary prolactin; (2) glandular, caused by surgical procedures or insufficient mammary tissue; or (3) postglandular, caused by ineffective or infrequent milk removal. They observe that the latter category has received insufficient attention. Studies have reported breast hypoplasia as a marker of lactation insufficiency (Huggins, Petok, & Mireles, 2000).

Effect of Pharmaceutical Agents on Milk Supply

The lactation consultant should always ask the mother if she is taking any prescription or over-the-counter drugs. Estrogen-containing contraceptives will quickly reduce milk supply. Some women will experience a reduction in supply from progestin-only preparations if they are used prior to 6 weeks postbirth (Kennedy, Short, & Tully, 1997). Smoking may reduce milk supply (Hill & Aldag, 1996), although other studies show that smoking is more apt to reduce initiation rather than duration of breastfeeding (Leung, Lam, & Ho, 2002). Anemia or hypothyroidism may cause low milk supply. In an Australian study, Aljazaf et al. (2003) found that some women's milk supply is reduced by pseudoephedrine (Sudafed). Although some claim that sage or other herbs may reduce milk supply, research has not confirmed this contention.

Dopamine antagonist drugs used for treating gastroesophageal reflux are known to raise serum prolactin levels, although circulating prolactin plays more of a permissive than regulatory role in milk synthesis. Metoclopramide (Reglan) and domperidone (Motilium) have been used to increase a mother's low milk supply, especially when she has given birth prematurely (da Silva et al., 2001). Both metoclopramide and domperidone pass into milk with no measurable effects on the infant. Unlike domperidone, metoclopramide affects the central nervous system and is associated with maternal depression in long-term (> 4 week) use. (See Chapter 5 for a detailed discussion of these drugs.)

Too Much Milk

If milk production exceeds the baby's need or ability to feed, then oversupply can be a problem. The prevalence of breastmilk oversupply seems to vary according to culture. For example, Canadian and Australian women report more oversupply problems than do women in the United States, suggesting a strong psychological or psychosocial component.

Milk supply usually adjusts itself to the baby's needs by the time the baby is about 6 weeks old, especially when mothers and babies self-regulate the pattern of feeds (Hartmann et al., 2002). During the first few weeks postbirth, an "upper limit" of potential milk synthesis is established for that particular lactation cycle (Hartmann et al., 2002; Perez-Escamilla & Chapman, 2001). Once the upper limit is set, milk volume can diminish somewhat and still be restored to the higher levels as needed.

Feeding technique may account for some cases of oversupply, such as switching the baby from the first breast before he indicates a desire for the second breast. Midwife Chloe Fisher has long advised to "finish the first side first" to avoid oversupply (Renfrew, Fisher, & Arms, 2000). A high milk supply or overfull breasts may be associated with intense sensation during the milk-ejection reflex, possibly because of overdistended tissues. There are two approaches to dealing with a baby who chokes or gags because of high breastmilk volume or rapid flow: deliberately reduce milk volume and/or investigate suck-swallow-breathe problems in the baby. Since "oversupply" can mask an infant problem, be sure to investigate the latter before addressing the former. The baby's suckling coordination almost always improves over time, and the mother's milk supply will almost always regulate itself to what the baby takes. If the baby consistently chokes when the mother's milk lets down or has difficulty handling fast-flowing milk, carefully evaluate the baby before deciding this is an oversupply issue. Choking during let-down or pulling off the breast during a feed may indicate that the baby has problems coordinating suckling, swallowing, and/or breathing. A baby with true gastroesophageal reflux may have some of the same symptoms (see Chapter 19).

If the problem truly is oversupply, the following strategies may help reduce milk supply and increase comfort for the mother and baby:

- Offer only one breast at each feeding. If the second breast becomes uncomfortably full, express enough milk to soften but not fully drain the breast. Save the milk for future use.

- Experiment with different positions for feeding. Some babies feed better vertically, with the head higher than the chest, perhaps straddling the mother's leg. Lean backward slightly so gravity helps slow the flow of milk into the infant's mouth. Side-lying may also be helpful for babies who feed better when held horizontally or supine.

- Remove the baby as the milk lets down and allow the fast-flowing milk to spray onto a towel; then put the baby back to breast.

- Use lactation-suppressing drugs only as a last resort.

These strategies should reduce total milk volume within several days. Once the milk supply has diminished and/or the suckling problem is resolved, the baby should be able to again nurse at both breasts comfortably.

Nipple Pain

During the early weeks after birth, the second most common maternal complaint is painful nipples. Nipple pain is a common, early postpartum concern and a frequent reason that mothers stop breastfeeding sooner than they intended. Most mothers have some nipple discomfort during the first 10 days postpartum that quickly resolves. The level of discomfort can range from mild tenderness to severe pain. There are two types of nipple soreness:

- *Transient soreness:* Discomfort that occurs during the first week postpartum, usually peaking between the third and sixth days and resolving after that.

- *Prolonged, abnormal pain:* Pain that persists unabated. For a few women, the term "sore nipples" does not accurately describe the reality of this sometimes agonizing condition that may be severe enough that the mother stops breastfeeding. Prolonged pain requires assessment to find out its cause and intervention to treat the problem.

Skin color, hair color, and prenatal nipple preparation are unrelated to nipple pain (Enkin et al., 2000). First-time mothers are more likely to have early nipple pain. Teaching a woman how to hold her baby for breastfeeding is a helpful preventive strategy (Heinig & Nommsen-Rivers, 2000).

Unfortunately, hospital personnel often advise mothers to limit the duration of feedings in order to prevent sore nipples. Placing a time limit on the length of each feeding has several harmful effects:

- It simply delays nipple soreness.
- Short feedings prevent the baby from receiving sufficient volumes of milk and the higher-calorie hindmilk.
- Short feedings may mean that the mother removes the baby from the breast (rather than the baby detaching himself). Repeated attempts to break the baby's suction can be painful and may damage the nipple skin.

Nipple pain that increases or remains unabated beyond the first week is abnormal. Chronic pain is a warning that something is wrong. Both mother and infant must be considered during assessment of possible causes of the pain. Nipple and breast pain—in the immediate postpartum and with older babies—can result from physical (mechanical) trauma, infection, or other conditions:

1. Mechanical pain, or physical trauma to the nipple skin or breast

   a. Poor infant positioning at breast

   b. Disorganized or dysfunctional infant suckling

   c. Friction from retracted nipples moving inside the infant's mouth

   d. Milk stasis and overfull breasts

   e. Baby's oral configuration (high palate, tongue-tie, cleft)

   f. Breaking suction improperly before repositioning baby at breast

   g. Poorly fitted device on the breast, such as breast shell or nipple shield

   h. Improper fit of a breast-pump flange or excess pump pressure

2. Pain from infections

   a. Yeast (thrush, fungus, *Candida*)

   b. Bacterial infection (usually *Staphylococcus*)

   c. Herpes simplex virus

   d. Infectious mastitis (usually *Staph* organisms)

   e. Breast abscess

3. Pain from dermatological conditions

   a. Allergy or sensitivity to topically applied preparations

   b. Eczema

   c. Psoriasis and other skin conditions

Early breast and nipple pain is nearly always "mechanical" pain, in contrast to pain caused by infection or organic conditions. Nipple pain and damage from improper placement of the nipple in the baby's mouth (Widström & Thingström-Paulsson, 1993) can occur quickly, even during the first feeding. The human nipple stretches to more than twice its resting length in the baby's mouth, and the bulbous tip rests approximately at the juncture of the hard and soft palates (Nowak, Smith, & Erenberg, 1995; Woolridge, 1986). Mothers should therefore be prepared for a stretching sensation in the nipple during feeding. When "sensation" becomes "pain" may be difficult to assess. A more objective sign of a problem is the shape of the mother's nipple postfeed. Since mechanical trauma is caused by or associated with poor latch and/or poor suck, the first remedy is correcting positioning and latch (Enkin et al., 2000; Blair, 2003). Poor latch or poor suck also compromises the infant's nutrition. Because the milk flows fastest during the downward motion of the baby's jaw (Ramsey et al., 2002), a baby who clamps her jaws tightly onto the breast may be limiting milk flow. If mechanical nipple pain or damage occurs, reassess to determine whether the infant is actually obtaining sufficient milk at the breast.

Mechanical pain is nearly always related to something the infant is doing in or with his mouth, either accidentally (as in the newborn with a tongue-tie) or deliberately (as in the older child experimenting with biting during nursing). Infant suckling patterns can be mispatterned or conditioned by a rubber teat from bottle-feeding or pacifier. Ankyloglossia (tongue-tie) is a short or tight lingual frenulum. Ballard, Auer, and Khoury (2002) diagnosed ankyloglossia in 3 percent of breastfeeding inpatients and in 13 percent of outpatients. Careful assessment of the lingual function, followed by frenuloplasty (frenotomy, or incision of the frenulum) when indicated is a successful treatment for pronounced ankyloglossia. Frenotomy is a controversial procedure; not all physicians will do it. Lactation consultants in any one area usually identify physicians or pediatric dentists who will perform this simple surgical procedure.

Other anatomic variations of the infant's oral space, of nipple size, or of nipple elasticity can cause mechanical pain and damage. Lactation consultants report nipple pain and trauma associated with a high or "bubble-shaped" palate in the infant (Snyder, 1995). Very large or fibrous nipples that are significantly bigger than the infant's oral space can cause pain or be damaged until the baby's mouth grows larger and can accommodate the mother's nipple and areola comfortably (Stark, 1993). A retracted or inverted nipple, even one that is correctly positioned in the baby's mouth, may rub on the baby's palate during feeds for a time.

When assessing a breastfeed, the LC should ask the following questions:

1. *Is the baby able to root?* Rooting indicates readiness to feed and intact nerve responses.

2. *How wide is the baby's gape?* The baby's mouth should be open to an angle at least 130—150 degrees. Pursed lips or a clenched jaw prevent deep attachment on the breast (Blair, 2001; Cadwell et al., 2001; Wilson-Clay & Hoover, 2002).

3. *What do the baby's cheeks look like?* The baby's cheeks should be full and rounded outward. Dimpling or puckering of the cheeks is related to excessive intra-oral pressure, poor latch, shallow positioning, or an unusual movement of the tongue. Verify your observations by asking the mother what she feels when dimpling of the cheeks is observed.

4. *Where is the baby's tongue?* The tongue should be barely visible over the baby's bottom lip. If the tongue is not visible, it may be curled backward or retracted, "humping" at the base.

5. *What do you hear when the baby is suckling?* A baby who is feeding effectively will make a quiet swallowing sound after every one to three sucks. Clicking or "slurping" sounds are an indication that the baby is suckling his own tongue or does not have a complete seal around the areola.

6. *How secure is the baby's seal on the breast?* The tongue should cup around the nipple, comfortably extending the nipple back into the baby's mouth (Figure 8–1). The top and bottom lip are flanged outward and rest gently on the breast—they do not create the seal (Blair, 2001). If the baby easily falls from the breast when he appears to be suckling actively, the seal is inadequate.

7. *What is the baby's suckling rhythm and rate?* Before the milk-ejection reflex, the baby has 2 to 3 rapid sucks per swallow and a slower rate toward the end of a feed (Hartmann et al., 2002). A baby who takes several sucks and then pauses for an extended period is not effectively removing milk.

8. *What does the mother feel during the feed?* She should feel her nipple elongate and a gentle massaging sensation during the feed. Although elongation may be an unusual sensation, it should not be painful.

9. *What is the appearance of the nipple and breast after the feed?* In a normal feed, the nipple should come out of the baby's mouth wet with milk,

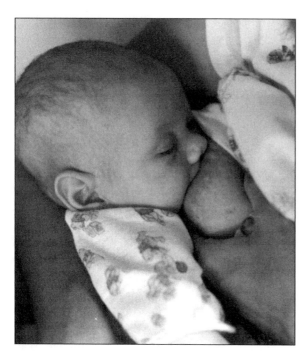

FIGURE 8–1. Breastfeeding "seal" on breast.

8–3). If there is any bruising, especially around the areola, the baby may be clenching his jaw instead of comfortably latching. The breast should be softer after a feed than before, but babies generally do not completely drain each breast at each feed (see Chapter 3).

Infant suckling patterns can contribute to nipple tenderness in the mother, particularly if the baby's first suckling has been conditioned by an artificial teat from bottle-feeding or a pacifier.

Some mothers find that their nipples become creased or misshapen during breastfeeding, yet their babies are thriving and the mothers have no discomfort. Because the goal is effective feeding and comfort for the mother and the baby, such distortions are of no concern.

More commonly, women whose nipples are distorted by breastfeeding will feel some discomfort. The distortion indicates that, *regardless of external appearance*, there is a mechanical problem that needs correction. It may require simply bringing the baby closer so that his cheek touches the breast or moving him slightly in one direction or another, it may require a frenotomy to release a short frenulum, or it may require therapy for an abnormal suckling pattern. A "normal-looking" latch that causes nipple distortion and discomfort is not a normal latch.

Nipples that remain round and undistorted during feeds despite painful breastfeeding usually indicate an infection (fungal, bacterial, viral, or—

intact, and in the same shape as before the feed began (Figure 8–2). If the nipple is flattened, creased, angled, cracked, fissured, painful, reddened, blanched or otherwise traumatized, mechanical trauma is the most likely cause (Figure

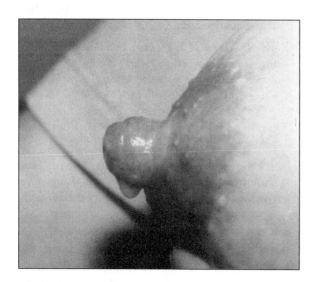

FIGURE 8–2. Normal postfeed.

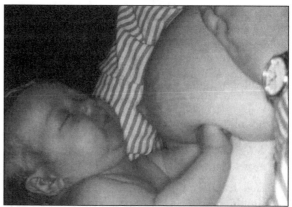

FIGURE 8–3. Creased nipple postfeed. (With permission from Linda Smith.)

very rarely—parasitic) or inflammatory process, or a skin or vascular disorder such as psoriasis, eczema, or nipple vasospasm. Mothers with moderate to severe nipple pain are more likely to have *S. aureus* on their nipples, possibly contributing to prolonged soreness (Livingstone, Willis, & Berkowitz, 1996).

The mother's breasts also need to be examined. The position of bruises on the breast may indicate the cause of the problem. For example, if too much of the top of the areola and too little of the bottom is drawn into the baby's mouth, stretching and cracking of nipple tissue on the underside of the breast is likely.

Treatments for Painful Nipples

In cases in which both a crack and a bruise are evident on the nipple and areola, rinsing the skin with clean water and bathing the crack with fresh expressed milk may aid healing and prevent bacterial infection. Usually, the crack will close and scab over before the bruise disappears. In light of a study (Livingstone, Willis, & Berkowitz, 1996) that links *S. aureus* and severe nipple soreness, topical antibiotics applied to breaks in the skin and, possibly, low-strength topical steroids for inflammation may be beneficial. Huggins and Billion (1993) report that no adverse effects were observed in any infant when thin coats of these preparations were applied to the mother's nipples.

Allowing the nipple to heal by not feeding from the breast is recommended only when the pain of suckling is intolerable or when bleeding and erosion are worsening. Rapid improvement usually follows; however, it is essential that milk continue to be removed from the breast by expressing or pumping. During this time, the infant may be fed expressed breastmilk by spoon, cup, or dropper. Placing a nipple shield (silicone) over the nipple gives the mother some relief during feedings, though there is no evidence that it hastens healing. While the nipple shield is being used, the baby should be monitored to make certain that he is receiving sufficient amounts of breastmilk for adequate growth. Some mothers have found that wearing breast shells between feedings relieves pain and promotes healing by allowing the air to circulate around the nipples.

Nipple Creams and Gels

Nipple ointments, creams, and gels are commonly used for sore nipples. There is little evidence that these products hasten nipple healing or reduce soreness, although such preparations are widely recommended and sold. Clinical research shows that an effective treatment for transient sore nipples is applying warm water (Lavergne, 1997), confirming what Niles Newton (1952) found to be true decades ago. Purified lanolin is purported to promote moist healing, which is considered to occur when a moisture barrier covers the nipple that helps prevent evaporation and drying. Hydrogels, relatively new products used to treat sore nipples, are either glycerin-based (Soothies) or water-based (Maternimates, Clear Site). Lanolin ointment and hydrogel dressings for sore nipples have been recently studied (Dodd & Chalmers, 2003). Mothers in the study were randomized to either a lanolin ointment or hydrogel dressing group. The hydrogel group had significantly greater reduction in pain score mean values by 10 days postpartum in comparison to the lanolin group. The lanolin ointment group had had eight breast infections, whereas the hydrogel dressing group had none. These results conflict with an earlier study by Brent et al. (1998) who found a high infection rate with the use of Elasto-Gel, a glycerin-based hydrogel. In the Dodd and Chalmers, a water-based hydrogel was used.

Randomized controlled trials on treatments for sore nipples are usually not done because it is difficult, if not impossible, for the mother *not* to know which treatment she is using on her nipples. Inability to "blind" the mother (and the investigator) is a consistent problem in conducting breastfeeding-related research (see Chapter 22).

The case can be made that in most cases, nipple treatments are harmless even if they have not been proved effective. They are a form of nurturing—of "mothering-the-mother." New mothers like to use creams and gels on their nipples; it makes them feel as if they are doing something to help themselves (Table 8–3).

Given the low cost of such products, it seems insensitive to discourage the use of ointment and creams for sore nipples unless some harm has resulted. A medical protocol for treating chroni-

Table 8–3

CLINICAL CARE PLAN FOR SORE NIPPLES

Assessment	Interventions	Rationale
Nipples appear slightly red and chapped; appear shiny in dark-skinned mother.	Reassure mother that discomfort is temporary and will improve.	Breast is sensitive at start of breast-feeding. Some early nipple soreness may be caused by stretching of nipple/areola.
Mother complains of soreness at latch-on or at start of pumping. Soreness subsides when milk-ejection reflex occurs.	Discontinue if soap or antiseptic is used to cleanse breasts. Apply purified lanolin or hydrogel. Use all-cotton bra.	Skin becomes dry; maintains natural skin oils and moisture.
Mother winces as infant grasps breast (or draws nipples into mouth).	Massage breast to start milk-ejection reflex and to stimulate flow. Place crushed ice in plastic bag (or a bag of frozen vegetables covered with a washcloth) to nipples.	Massage softens nipple/breast before latch-on. Cold relieves discomfort.
Nipple sticks to bra or breast pad.	Moisten bra or breast pads before removing. Wear breast shell.	Protects keratin skin layer.
Mother is using breast cream.	Discontinue using cream and note any change.	Mother may be allergic to cream.
Crescent-shaped abrasions are seen above and/or below nipple. Nipple tip is blanched after suckling. Discomfort and pain occurs throughout feeding.	Review positioning, making sure infant's mouth is open wide before latching-on and baby is held high on mother's chest with entire body facing mother. Reposition as necessary. Gently press on baby's chin to pull it downward.	Infant is gumming and pinching nipple and/or sliding up and down because of poor positioning.
Mother has sore nipples that do not heal. Baby makes clicking sound while suckling or has frequent bursts of shallow suckles. Baby's tongue feels retracted behind lower gum.	Hold infant so that breast is positioned deep in baby's mouth. Bring tongue forward. Make sure baby's lips are flanged outward.	Baby is suckling tongue and not breast. Shallow latch promotes tongue retraction. Tongue retraction prevents normal perfusion to nipple.
A bright, pinkish-red color extends beyond nipple/areola. Mother complains of pain throughout feeding.	Apply antifungal medication to nipples. Treat family for candidiasis.	Prompt treatment alleviates problem. Candidiasis spreads with warm, moist contact among family members.
Mother has persistent, painful, reddish lesions on breast that do not appear to be candidiasis.	Refer to health-care provider for possible treatment with antibiotic for bacterial infection.	Topical (or systemic in severe cases) antibiotics are effective in treating bacterial infection.

cally painful and infected nipples can be found in Chapter 9.

Table 8–4 lists some of the products used for nipple soreness. There are dozens more—for example, pawpaw cream (Australia), Bepanthen (Australia), maize oil (Kamillsoan) (Africa), Coopers

Table 8–4

Possible Risks of Nipple Creams and Gels

Product/Ingredient	Possible Risk/Drawback	Comment
Petrolatum-based products	Reduces tissue oxygenation, plugs skin pores.	No studies.
Lanolin products	May contain pesticides, wool fibers; avoid hydrous (with water) products.	Use anhydrous lanolin and highly purified products; pain less during days 6 to 10 on treated breast (Spangler & Hildebrandt, 1993).
Hydrogels (hydrocolloid dressings)	Discard if milky or cloudy; propylene glycol is a theoretical risk.	Faster wound healing (Dodd & Chalmers, 2003); use only on damaged (not intact) skin. Do not use if infection present.
Beeswax-based products	Allergies to bee pollen.	
Glycerin-based products	Should not be used for nipple wounds.	One study found mothers liked these.
Antiseptic products	May dry the skin; baby ingestion of product.	
Tea bags	Tannic acid is drying.	Conflicting studies results. Not effective in reducing pain (Buchko et al., 1994); less pain (Lavergne, 1997); messy (Riordan, 1985).
Adhesive wound dressing	May irritate or damage skin.	77% had erythemia around nipples due to dressing contact; discomfort when dressing removed (Zeimer & Pigeon, 1993).
Expressed breast milk	Causes no risks; sticky when dry.	Less nipple pain compared with air-drying or wet compresses (Akkuzu & Taskin, 2000).
Food-based oils (olive, other)	May cause possible allergy to the oil; may stain clothing.	Use sparingly; inexpensive; tasty to baby.

Source: Derived from Frantz, 1999.

Milking Salve (Africa), and Rose Calendar Cream (New Zealand). Warm water, hydrogel, and purified lanolin are the only products that have been studied and found to actually reduce soreness. Medicated creams such as neosporin, bacitracin, mupirocin clotrimazole, and hydrocortisone are used to treat infections and other nipple conditions.

In considering each item's use, keep in mind that two people are exposed to the product whenever it is used on the mother's nipples. What may be appropriate to use for the mother may expose the infant to unnecessary risk. If the product must be removed completely from the nipple to avoid infant exposure, the care provider should consider whether some other strategy might be more appropriate since removing the product may cause more damage to the nipple than any healing or pain relief from its use.

Limiting the length or frequency of feeds does not prevent nipple pain or damage, because the *quality* of the feed is more likely to cause pain and/or injury than the *quantity* of nursing sessions. Limiting time at breast reduces milk flow to the infant, resulting in underfeeding for the infant and milk retention in the breast for the mother. Use of pacifiers and feeding bottles is associated with painful nipples at hospital discharge (Centuori et al., 1999).

Engorgement + Milk Stasis = Involution

Postpartum engorgement and milk stasis are two different physiological processes. Engorgement, the marshalling of lymph and milk under hormonal influence, following birth, heralds the onset of breastmilk—a welcome sign that lactogenesis is taking place (see Chapters 3 and 7). Milk stasis or breastmilk retention, on the other hand, is an uncomfortable breast fullness that can occur at any time during lactation when the baby is not breastfeeding often enough and/or not removing milk effectively.

The best prevention for milk stasis is early, frequent, and effective breastfeeding by a well-positioned baby (Snowden, Renfrew, & Woolridge, 2003; Enkin et al., 2000). The causes of milk stasis include poor suck, scheduled feeds, milk synthesis that exceeds the baby's ability to remove available milk, and factors that keep the baby away from the breast. Regardless of the causes, the result is the same: milk is retained in the breast. Depending on the storage capacity of each individual breast, at some point the breast's capacity to store milk is exceeded, and the process of involution begins. First, components of the milk itself exert a feedback inhibition on the mammary secretory epithelial cells (lactocytes) resulting in a slower rate of milk synthesis. (Daly, Owens, & Hartmann, 1993). If milk is not removed, eventually the physical distension of the alveoli causes further disruption of milk synthesis (Cregan & Hartmann, 1999).

Removal of retained milk will reverse these processes as long as draining the breast is begun soon after stasis occurs. Unrelieved milk stasis triggers mammary involution. At some point in time involution becomes irreversible as the lactocytes, necessary for milk synthesis, are deactivated (or destroyed through apoptosis) for that particular lactation cycle (Neville & Neifert, 1983). It is unknown when the point of irreversibility is reached in women. Milk stasis can also lead to plugged ducts and inflammatory reactions in the breast, then to infectious mastitis, and then, if not corrected, to breast abscess (World Health Organization, 2000; Walker, 1999). Milk stasis is primarily a mechanical problem; therefore a mechanical solution is needed. The core strategy in addressing all forms of milk stasis is *removal of milk from the breast* by the baby, by hand expression, and/or by a pump.

Breast Massage

Massage has been used extensively and effectively during the childbearing period. It relieves the discomforts of labor and is often used for infant stimulation. Massage of the lactating breasts is common in many parts of the world and is used to stimulate milk production, to promote drainage, and relieve engorged breasts.

Breast massage is popular in Japan, where new parents and physicians are convinced that breast massage effectively increases the milk supply and relieves plugged ducts In fact, some Japanese hospitals offer mothers and fathers breast massage classes that confer certification. Figure 8–4 shows the Japanese technique for breast massage.

Massaging the mother's back to relieve discomfort from engorgement or to relax her if she has difficulty letting down her milk is an acupressure technique that La Leche leaders have recommended for years. The mother sits in a chair and someone standing behind her briskly rubs the knuckles of a fist from the base of the mother's neck to the bottom of her shoulder blades on both sides of her spine. Whether this technique has a physiological basis, or is simply comforting, has not been established.

Clothing, Leaking, Bras, and Breast Pads

Clothing worn by the breastfeeding mother should, above all else, allow her to quickly respond to her baby's cues for feeding. No special wardrobe is

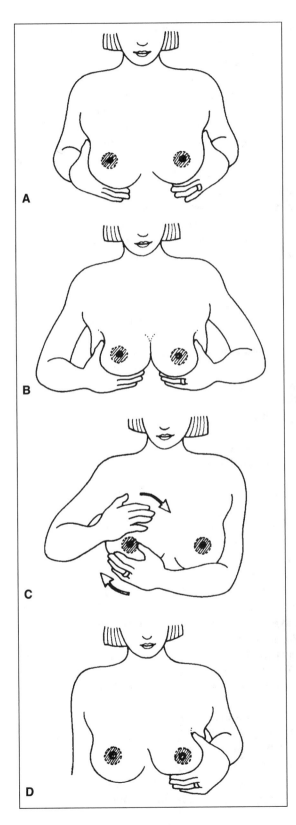

FIGURE 8–4. Japanese breast massage.

(A) Improve breastfeeding by massaging the base of the breast.

(B) Place the thumbs of both hands in armpits. The rest of the fingers support the breast from the side. Thrust the chest forward by moving the elbows back as far as possible ("chicken wing position"). Push the breasts toward the center as if trying press the nipples together. This will improve the milk flow from the base of the breast.

(C) Cup the breast with both hands and gently rotate, like making a rice ball or shaping bread dough, for 1 to 2 minutes. Repeat the first two steps two or three times.

(D) Hold one breast at a time and squeeze before putting the baby to breast.

needed. Two-piece outfits, clothing with hidden front openings, tops with loose armholes, and other fashionable designs meet this requirement and are widely available.

Bras may be worn for comfort, as long as no part of the bra is too tight or causes constriction of the milk ducts. A well-fitted nursing bra should be easily opened or removed for breastfeeding. Mothers should avoid any bras that cause discomfort, cut into the breast, press on milk ducts or glandular tissue, or are so inconvenient that the mother delays feedings because of her clothing. Mothers with large, heavy breasts especially appreciate the support of a well-fitting, comfortable bra.

Excessive leaking that requires the use of bra pads (breast pads) could be an artifact of feeds scheduled at overly long intervals. In the early weeks, most women synthesize more milk than their baby requires. By around 6 weeks, daily milk supply has adjusted itself to the baby's needs, with sufficient residual milk volume to meet short-term increased needs. The let-down reflex is triggered by infant cues and other activities associated with breastfeeding. Feeding the baby on cue and around the clock prevents most leaking, again reinforcing the importance of breastfeeding on the baby's cues.

Mothers experiencing persistent or excessive leaking may wear absorbent pads inside their bra or clothing. Whether improvised (such as a folded handkerchief) or manufactured for the purpose, pads should be comfortable, not cause irritation or inflammation of the breast, and leave no residue that could be ingested by the baby. Wet pads should be replaced with dry ones to avoid keeping the breast wet for extended periods. Direct pressure for a few seconds on a leaking breast, such as by crossed arms, is usually sufficient to temporarily inhibit leaking.

Infant Concerns

Pacifiers

"Suckling bags" and similar pacifiers have been used since the 15th century. Despite the widespread belief that pacifiers (dummies, soothers) interfere with breastfeeding and global policies that warn against routine use of these devices, pacifiers may be used by 50 to 80 percent of breastfeeding mothers (Howard et al., 1999). Their use is more common in populations of lower socioeconomic status (Mathur, Mathur, & Khanduja, 1990), in those experiencing breastfeeding problems (Righard & Alade, 1997), and if the practice is begun in the first 4 weeks (babies may refuse to accept a pacifier introduced later).

In nature, suckling is virtually always associated with food intake and a comforting touch. Even a baby who sucks his thumb in utero is getting nutrients during suckling via the umbilical cord and swallowed amniotic fluid. All suckling releases gut hormones including cholycystokinin (Uvnas-Moberg et al., 1987), insulin, gastrin, and somatostatin. Pacifiers are occasionally used therapeutically, for short periods of time, as part of an integrated therapeutic plan to establish or restore direct breastfeeding during tube-feeds by premature infants when a mother cannot be with her baby, to soothe babies after a full feed by mothers with an overabundant milk supply, and/or to repattern an infant's tongue and oral muscle contraction patterns (Barros et al., 1997). Preterm infants who practice "nonnutritive suck" on their mothers' emptied breasts or a pacifier during gavage tube-feeds gain more weight, have faster gut transit time better state organization, and can be released from the hospital earlier (Measel & Anderson, 1979). Suckling, especially skin-to-skin directly at breast, is analgesic (Gray et al., 2000, 2002) and soothes pain-elicited distress. Pain may be relieved by the act of suckling, the milk itself (Zanardo et al., 2001), or a combination of factors.

The most common use of a pacifier is to deliberately postpone or stretch out the time between breastfeeds (Barros et al., 1995). Infants who are exclusively breastfed and use a pacifier frequently have approximately one fewer breastfeeding per 24 hours ($p = <.01$) than those who did not use a pacifier (Aarts et al., 1999). Since milk supply is directly linked to frequent and effective feeds, this reduction in the infants' total time at breast is responsible for shorter and less exclusive breastfeeding among pacifier users (Aarts et al., 1999; Howard et al., 1999; Vogel, Hutchison, & Mitchell, 2001). Routine and "social" use of pacifiers has been linked to dental and orthodontic problems (Drane, 1996), accidents and injuries including fatal choking, increased oral thrush and other infections

(Mattos-Graner et al., 2001), delayed or altered speech development, behavior and brain development (Lehtonen et al., 1998; Paul, Ditrichova, & Papousek, 1996), and deficits in attachment and maturation (Barros et al., 1997; Gale & Martyn, 1996). Global policies such as Step 8 of the Baby-Friendly Hospital Initiative (see Chapter 1) and the 1997 policy statement of the American Academy of Pediatrics warn against routine (nontherapeutic) use of pacifiers.

All interventions should have a solid rationale and research basis before being suggested or recommended by lactation professionals. Given the lack of evidence of benefit and wide and diverse documented risks of pacifiers to the breastfed infant (Howard et al., 2003), parents should be cautioned to avoid pacifiers during breastfeeding except in limited therapeutic situations.

Stooling Patterns

The stools of the breastfed newborn go through several predictable, observable changes and can be used as a partial indicator of milk intake. Black, tarry stools (meconium) are passed in the first several days. With each succeeding milk feeding, the transitional stool gradually lightens in color and becomes less sticky and more liquid. The totally breastmilk stool is yellow and generally very soft or liquid (see Table 8–5). In the first weeks, the infant may pass a small, loose, sometimes explosive, unformed stool with each breastfeeding or at least 3 to 5 (average 4.2) per day by 4 to 5 days (AAP/ACOG, 2002) twice as many as those fed a cow's milk or soy preparation (Hyams et al., 1995). Stools may contain small curds, or have a mushy consistency. Color ranges from greenish-yellow to mustard-yellow; and the odor is a characteristic sweet, "yeasty," or cream cheese odor. By 2 weeks, formula-fed babies have a fecal flora very similar to that of the adult, in which coliforms and enterococci predominate, whereas the flora of the breastfed baby is dominated by lactobacilli and bifidobacteria.

In the early weeks of lactation, the whey-casein ratio of human milk is 90:10 (90 percent whey, 10 percent casein). Whey is the liquid portion of the milk, full of immune factors, and low in calcium and minerals. This early composition is perfect for the newborn's higher need for immune protection

TABLE 8–5

CHARACTERISTIC CHANGES IN BREASTMILK STOOLS WITH TIME

Time Period	Type of Stool	Number per Day	Amount
0–2 days	Meconium	1+	Scant to copious
3–4 days	Transitional	3+	
4–6 days	Milk stool	4+	
7–28 days	Milk stool	5–10+	Copious
+29 days	Milk stool	2–4+	Copious

than minerals for long bone growth. By about 6 weeks, the stools may be firmer and may be passed slightly less often, reflecting the whey-casein ratio as it has evolved to approximately 80:20. The gradual increase in casein relative to whey results in slightly thicker, more formed stools (more like toothpaste or soft peanut butter) that may be passed less often. By the middle of the infant's first year, the whey-casein ratio has evolved to 60:40 or even 50:50—exactly paralleling the infant's increasing bone and muscle development and mobility (Kunz & Lonnerdal, 1992).

Any table food or infant formula given to an infant is reflected in the infant's stools. The stool becomes darker, with larger and firmer curds, and has more odor. The formula-fed infant tends to pass larger, more copious, more odorous, but less frequent stools (Quinlan et al., 1995). As the proportion of solid foods increases, stools will likely reflect the new foods with a change in odor, color, and consistency. Sometimes portions of undigested food may be visible in the stool.

In the first 4 to 6 weeks, newborns pass stool many times a day. If more than 24 hours passes without a stool, the child should be seen by a health-care provider and adequate caloric intake assessed in other ways (Neifert, 2001). Lack of sufficient milk intake is the most common reason for lack of stooling; therefore, more attention to frequent effective breastfeeding and/or increasing milk intake should quickly increase infant output.

A healthy, thriving exclusively breastfed child over 6 weeks old may stool only a few times a week or even less. As long as the stool is soft and profuse and the infant is otherwise thriving and content, that pattern is not unusual.

If unusual stool patterns persist, the lactation consultant should collaborate with the baby's primary-care provider to investigate other diseases or conditions. Hirschsprung's disease, cystic fibrosis, cow's milk allergy (Vanderhoof et al., 2001; Daher et al., 2001), and other bowel disorders may be underlying unusual bowel patterns (see Chapter 19).

Jaundice in the Newborn

Physiological jaundice is a common clinical manifestation of all newborns. In the healthy, full-term breastfed infant, bilirubin levels rise from a level of 1.5 mg/dL (25.5 umol/L) at birth to a mean peak of approximately 5.5 mg/dL (93.5 umol/L) by the third day in white and non-Asian infants and approximately 10 mg/dL (170 umol/L) in infants of Asian origin. In the breastfed infant, this bilirubin level gradually decreases during the next 2 weeks; however, it may peak a second time around day 10 of life.

There are several points to note about physiological jaundice:

- It affects nearly all newborns.
- It manifests itself after 24 hours of age.
- It peaks on the third or fourth day of life.
- It usually declines steadily through the first month to normal levels.
- It may be more obvious in infants whose feeding is limited in frequency or duration.
- It is self-limiting in most healthy, full-term infants.
- It requires no intervention in the majority of infants.

Testing for hyperbilirubinema causes physical pain in newborns and emotional distress in parents. Nurses often order blood draws for bilirubin levels when it is not necessary. Gagnon (2001) examined 130 mother-newborn pairs and found that 91 percent of the newborns tested for bilirubin were tested unnecessarily. The nurses in this study who assessed the frequency of feedings were less likely to order bilirubin testing.

At least two thirds of all healthy, thriving breastfed infants have bilirubin levels above 5 mg/dL (85 umol/L) during the third week or even into the second month of life, a condition referred to as *breastmilk jaundice* (Gartner & Herschel, 2001). Of more concern is early exaggerated jaundice, especially in the first few days to week postpartum, which may be a warning sign that breastfeeding is not going well for the infant. Some call this "starvation jaundice" or "breast non-feeding jaundice" (see Chapter 11).

If the baby is or becomes jaundiced after hospital discharge, review the information in Chapter 11 maintaining the baby's access to the mother, ensure breastmilk transfer through proper positioning and latch, and carefully check the infant's milk intake by weighing him on an electronic scale (Meier et al., 1996). If direct breastfeeding is not providing enough milk to the baby to meet caloric needs, help the mother express or pump more milk and feed it to her baby, in addition to whatever he obtains at breast. Continue as much direct breastfeeding as possible until the baby can effectively obtain sufficient milk at breast and the jaundice has resolved.

Home phototherapy is common in the United States (Madlon-Kay, 1998). Treating the baby at home avoids the family stress and costs of hospitalizing the baby but is not without its own dollar and emotional costs. Another at-home alternative is teaching the parents to place the baby so he receives indirect sunlight, which also helps reduce bilirubin levels. Gartner reassures us that "optimal management of breastfeeding does not eliminate neonatal jaundice and elevated serum bilirubin concentrations. Rather, it leads to a pattern of hyperbilirubinemia that is normal and possibly beneficial to infants" (Gartner & Herschel, 2001).

Breast Refusal and Latching Problems

A newborn's inability to latch and suck is intensely frustrating for the mother, health professionals, and especially the baby, and it poses a uniquely difficult breastfeeding management problem. Until recently, most professionals believed that "breast refusal" was primarily due to maternal factors, including flat or inverted nipples, overfull or engorged breasts, mother not holding the baby in an effective position for latching, or "nipple confusion" resulting from the baby learning to suck on an artificial teat or pacifier. Certainly the mother's breast shape, size, and configuration play a role in the baby's ability to latch and feed comfortably. However, as knowledge and skills improve, lactation consultants have begun to look more closely at the infant's ability to latch and suck when a "breast refusal" situation occurs. Causes for early latch and suck problems include immaturity or prematurity, illness, jaundice, or facial anomalies such as tongue tie or cleft lip or palate. Other contributing factors are poorly researched, but there is growing evidence for early latch or suck problems related to epidural anesthesia/analgesia (Riordan et al., 2000; Baumgarder et al., 2003), forceps delivery, vacuum extraction, induction of labor, cesarean delivery, and/or long, difficult labor, especially with occiput posterior positioning (Kroeger & Smith, 2004).

There are several keys to preventing early breast refusal or latch problems:

1. Prenatal education, including information on nonpharmaceutical pain relief for labor and how to hold the baby comfortably for breastfeeding

2. Putting the baby to breast within the first hour after birth

3. Keeping the baby and mother together, preferably in skin-to-skin contact (Anderson, 1989; Righard & Alade, 1990), and practicing 24-hour rooming in with bedding-in under safe conditions

4. Investigating reasons for the baby's inability to latch and/or suck normally

5. Maintaining patience and gentle handling of the baby

If the baby cannot latch because of the mother's breast/nipple configuration, then gentle mechanical strategies may alter the breast/nipple shape sufficiently to allow latching and sucking. These strategies include, but are not limited to, brief use of a breast pump or "nipple expander" device to draw out the nipple, massage to soften the breast, shaping the nipple/areola complex, breast support, and short-term use of a thin silicone nipple shield. The use of such devices should be discontinued when the baby can latch and suck effectively.

If the baby cannot latch because of prematurity, illness, or facial or oral structure anomalies, collaboration with other professionals is appropriate and necessary. While diagnosis and treatment plans are pending, assist the mother to collect her milk and feed it to the baby using a device that will not exacerbate the original reason for lack of latching.

If the baby is not latching because he is sleepy or drugged from birth medications (Ranjso-Arvidson et al., 2001), patience and sufficient calories (expressed colostrum or breastmilk) will buy time until the drugs are metabolized and the baby can smoothly coordinate sucking, swallowing, and breathing. Keep the mother and baby together, skin-to-skin, as close to continuously as possible. Be patient, because the age and maturity of the baby, dosage and combination of drugs, and other birth interventions can affect the baby's ability to recover and begin to breastfeed well. Some babies need several days to several weeks to recover fully (Sepkoski et al., 1992).

If the baby can only latch in one posture or position or on one breast, then help the mother to use that posture, position, or breast at frequent intervals. Express milk from the other breast to avoid problems related to milk stasis. Again, with patience and sufficient calories, most babies will gradually improve in skill and be able to breastfeed in other postures, positions, and from both breasts within a fairly short time.

If the baby continues to be unable to latch and suck for more than a few days, the lactation consultant must collaborate with the primary-care provider and other professionals to investigate the cause and develop strategies for remediation while keeping the baby fed, assisting the mother to express and feed her milk, and providing support for the mother and family. Encourage the mother to keep the baby in nearly continuous skin-to-skin contact on her chest, continue attempts at breastfeeding, and keep the dyad together in a calm, supportive environment. The LC should carefully document these situations to assist the family and other professionals, and provide future researchers with data central to investigating the causes of and solutions to persistent breast refusal or failure to latch-on.

Later Breast Refusal

If the baby suddenly refuses one or both breasts after breastfeeding was mutually satisfying and successful, then one should consider this to be an infant-related problem, not the normal weaning process. The child could be reacting to an ear infection, injury, or pain in one arm or one side of the body, teething, sore mouth, and/or other physical or medical problem. The mother might have shouted during a nursing session, frightening the child, or rebuked (understandably) a teething child for biting her breast. The mother may have begun more frequent or longer separations from her child, or have left the child for a period of time longer than the child could comfortably tolerate. The child may be distressed with some new family situation and/or desire to exert more control over nursing sessions. The LC should evaluate the entire situation, including social factors, to determine causes and assist the mother in resuming her breastfeeding relationship with her child.

A new breast problem could also be the cause of sudden breast refusal. These problems include, but are not limited to, diminishing milk volume that changes the taste of the milk, infectious mastitis or breast abscess, a subsequent pregnancy in the mother, unpleasant taste of the milk if mother has eaten a new food or is taking a medication, or (rarely) a malignancy in the lactating breast. As with all breast problems, careful evaluation and collaboration with medical-care providers should be undertaken to identify the cause and to design a care plan that preserves breastfeeding.

The child will still need to be fed during the period of breast refusal ("nursing strike"). Overuse of bottles, teats, and pacifiers are likely to have caused or contributed to the situation. Some children will take expressed mother's milk from a cup or spoon, and other nutritious, soft family foods given by spoon and cup can provide sufficient calories and liquids during the duration of the problem. Additional attention to the child, increased skin contact,

plenty of holding, cuddling, and gentle communications are all vital to restoring the breastfeeding relationship. Some children will accept the breast at night or when dropping off to sleep, even if they refuse to breastfeed during the day. Even small amounts of human milk and short, infrequent breastfeeding sessions are beneficial, so there is no advantage in cutting off the child who breastfeeds only occasionally or for short times.

Lastly, the child may be truly ready to wean. Sudden weaning is more likely after the first year of breastfeeding. If breast refusal occurs prior to the child's first birthday, another cause is more likely. It is counterproductive and usually futile to try to coerce a child into breastfeeding who is ready to stop, because the child usually refuses to latch, bites the breast, or both. The LC may have to assist the mother in coming to terms with her growing child's reduced need to breastfeed.

Crying and Colic

An infant cries to signal a need, which may be for food, comfort, warmth, mother's presence (Christensson et al., 1995), pain, illness, or fear. When parents and caregivers promptly respond to the baby's signals, a long, secure, and trusting relationship begins to develop. The baby who is picked up and soothed quickly generally stops crying sooner (after parental response) than the infant who is allowed to cry for some time before he is picked up. Prompt response reduces the baby's stress, enhances parental enjoyment of the baby, and increases parents' confidence in their new role. With time, parents become more skilled in reading their baby's cues and cries.

Wessel's (1954) 3-3-3 definition of colic (crying more than 3 hours a day, more than 3 days a week, and lasting more than 3 weeks) helps distinguish colic from hunger or other temporary illness or conditions. Unlike other cries, colic usually is characterized by a high-pitched wail or scream, as if the baby is in severe pain (St. James-Roberts, 1999). Colic appears to be the result of sudden spasmodic abdominal cramping, with knees drawn up and sometimes a distended abdomen.

Before an assessment of colic is made, all other causes of crying should be ruled out, including hunger, illness, and injury. The baby may have an unrecognized broken arm or clavicle. Possible injury of any kind should be checked out. Crying is a *late* sign of hunger; reinforcing the mother's prompt response to her baby's feeding cues is always appropriate and may eliminate most cases of hunger-induced crying. First-time parents are more prone to have "colicky" babies. Lack of knowledge about the normal (that is, frequent and sometimes clustered) feeding patterns of the breastfed baby has led many mothers and even professionals to identify a baby's cries as colic, when in fact the child was simply hungry. Attempting to enforce a strict schedule for feeds is inappropriate (AAP, 1998) and can result in serious underfeeding, dehydration, failure to thrive (Aney, 1998), reduction in milk supply, and undermining of the mother's confidence in caring for her baby. Breastfeeding should be the first strategy to soothe infant cries, because it instantly and automatically brings the infant his mother's presence, food, comfort, warmth, natural endorphins, and immune protection (Gray et al., 2002; Carbajal et al., 2003).

Colic has been investigated extensively, yet no consensus on its causes has emerged. Possible explanations for true colic fall into two general categories: those related to gastrointestinal problems and those not related to gastrointestinal problems. Food protein hypersensitivity or allergy is the leading contender in the former group, and disturbances in parental or maternal-child interactions in the latter (Gupta, 2002). The baby's temperament may play a role. Canifet, Jackobsson, and Hagander, (2002) reported that "mothers who believe that there is a risk of spoiling an infant with too much physical contact were more likely to have infants with genuine colic and their infants were more distressed, even when given the same amount of physical contact" as other babies received. Possible causes for colic include the following:

- Allergy to cow's milk protein or cow's milk components (IgG) consumed directly, in infant formula, or passing through mother's milk

- Gastroesophageal reflux related to cow's milk protein allergy (Cavataio, Carroccio, & Iacono, 2000; Salvatore & Vandenplas, 2002)

- Allergy or sensitivity to some other food in mother's diet (Lust, Brown, & Thomas, 1996)

- Feeding problems such as overfeeding, swallowing air, or poor positioning at breast

- Smoking, including maternal smoking during pregnancy (Sondergaard et al., 2001)

Cow's milk has been shown to be the single most commonly ingested allergen in infants. Direct ingestion (from whole milk or infant formula) causes the worst symptoms; intake via mother's milk also occurs. Other less common allergens include legumes (including soy-based formula and peanuts), beef, chicken and eggs, grains such as corn and wheat, and high-acid fruits and vegetables. Babies who develop colic in response to foods in the breastfeeding mother's diet often exhibit allergic symptoms when exposed to the same foods later in life. Dietary supplements taken by the baby or mother can also cause infant distress.

After ruling out hunger and illness, the lactation consultant may help the mother identify or rule out an allergic or hypersensitive response to cow's milk. For the breastfed baby under 6 months, the following steps are helpful:

1. Purify the baby's diet. Ensure that the baby gets nothing other than mother's milk by direct breastfeeding for at least 2 to 3 weeks. Avoid all bottles (even containing mother's expressed milk), teats and pacifiers, vitamins, and supplements. If the baby has already begun to take other supplements or table foods, those items are the most likely offenders. Make sure the baby is breastfed on cue around the clock during this time.

2. At the same time, ask the mother to begin keeping a detailed written diary of her food and beverage intake, any medications or supplements taken by her or the baby, the baby's breastfeeding patterns, and the baby's behavior. Include any unusual events affecting the family. Continue keeping this diary for several weeks.

3. Examine the food and behavior diary carefully for emerging patterns, including the mother's cravings, foods avoided or disliked, large quantities or regular ingestion of common allergens (especially cow's milk or dairy products), and maternal symptoms of allergies.

4. If no discernable pattern emerges in a few weeks, consult with a professional allergist, pediatric gastroenterologist, or other specialist for further evaluation.

If the baby is truly sensitive to cow's milk protein or another component of cow's milk, it may take several days to weeks for the offending substance to be cleared from the baby's body. Estep and Kulczycki (2000) report that bovine IgG antibody levels were markedly higher in the milk of mothers of colicky babies than in the milk of mothers whose babies were not colicky. Bovine IgG has a long half-life, and its presence in high levels may require an extended period of elimination. If the mother's avoidance of cow's milk clearly relieves baby's colic symptoms, she may need to continue to avoid all dairy products while consuming nondairy sources of calcium or nondairy calcium-containing supplements (Carroccio et al., 2000; Iacono et al., 1998).

If the mother wants to reintroduce dairy products, she should start with very small amounts such as a tablespoonful of hard cheeses (cheddar, swiss) or yoghurt during the first week. If the baby shows no reactions, she can expand the trial to include small amounts of soft cheeses such as cottage cheese or gouda during the second week. If her baby is still asymptomatic, then butter, ice cream, and cooked milk can be tested, again in small quantities. The reintroduction of liquid milk should be attempted last, and in small quantities. She should continue keeping the written diary of symptoms and foods during the trial period. Some babies are so sensitive that the mother must eliminate most or all forms of dairy products for prolonged periods, even weeks or months. If the mother is also sensitive or allergic to dairy products, she may feel better as well.

Many remedies for colic (after addressing hunger and allergies, discussed above) have been suggested, including the following:

- Increased carrying on the back or chest (Barr et al., 1991)
- Carrying baby in the prone position on the parent's arm
- Swaddling
- Giving oral sucrose (Barr et al., 1999)

Mothering a baby who cries for hours a day can exhaust and undermine the confidence of any mother (Pauli-Pott, 2000). Lactation consultants should stay in close contact with mothers of colicky breastfed babies as they investigate possible causes for the baby's distress, if for no other reason than to provide the mother with emotional support during these difficult times. Reassure the mother that skin-to-skin contact, breastfeeding, and breastmilk are comforting to the baby. Even unsuccessful attempts to comfort the baby are valuable, because abandoning the baby to its pain is worse. Weaning the baby to infant formula will almost certainly make the baby's distress even worse.

Multiple Infants

An increase in the number of women delaying childbirth until after thirty and advances in techniques to treat infertility have contributed to a large increase in the number of multiple births in the last decade (Martin et al., 2002). Lactation consultants are likely to work with these families, as these women choose to breastfeed at about the same rate as women giving birth to single infants (Bowers & Gromada, 2003). LaFleur and Kiesen (1996) have even described one mother's experience of breastfeeding conjoined twins.

Many expectant parents are uncertain whether breastfeeding is possible following a multiple birth, and their decisions regarding infant feeding are often influenced by information received from health-care providers. Parents of multiples may be reassured that breastfeeding two or more infants generally is possible. Many mothers of twins, triplets, and quadruplets have breastfed for a year and longer. Research and case studies have demonstrated that most mothers of multiples are capable of producing most or all of the milk that two to four infants require (Bleyl, 2001; Auer & Gromada, 1998).

The benefits of breastfeeding are particularly advantageous for twins, triplets, and other higher-order multiples. In addition to offering optimal nutrition and immunological protection to these often preterm or otherwise compromised infants, breastfeeding helps ensure frequent mother-infant interaction with each baby. Although the frequency of feedings may be overwhelming for many new mothers, multiples' frequent feedings give a mother many daily opportunities to sit or lie down to rest while breastfeeding (Gromada, 1999) (see Figure 8–5).

Full-Term Twins or Triplets

Full-term or near-term multiple infants have the same needs as any full-term singleton; the mother's role, however, is more complex since she must meet the needs of two or more newborns. In addition, the mother of multiples is more likely to have had complications of pregnancy and childbirth, and she may require more time to recover physically.

Mothers of multiples need help and support with early feedings, as they feel overwhelmed when first trying to figure out how to manage feedings with more than one infant. Some are anxious to initiate simultaneous feedings, as they have heard it saves time. However, it is important to first assess each infant at breast separately, as it is not unusual for one or more of the babies to breastfeed poorly even when the infants are born at term or close to term.

Preterm or Ill Multiples

When multiple infants are born prematurely or have other medical complications, direct breastfeeding may be delayed for days or weeks. The LC should advise the mother to begin expressing milk for her infants within hours of giving birth (Bowers & Gromada, 2003). If a mother has had complications, she may need assistance when expressing milk (Gromada & Spangler, 1998).

Simultaneous pumping using a hospital-grade electric pump is the most effective way to obtain maximum amounts of milk and to maintain lactation (see Chapter 12). Most hospitals with neonatal intensive care units have these pumps available for mothers to use. Anticipatory guidance for any expectant mother of multiples should include helping the mother to find a breast-pump rental location in her area.

When direct breastfeeding is initiated for two or more preterm or ill newborns following days or weeks of pumping, the LC is responsible for assisting the mother in developing an individualized, evidence-based plan for transitioning each multiple to the breast (Biancuzzo, 1994). For instance, Auer and Gromada (1998) described the approach of one

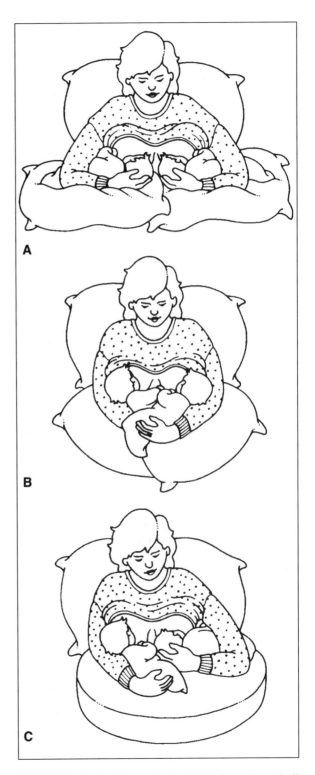

FIGURE 8–5. Feeding positions for twins. (A) Football. (B) Cross. (C) Mixed.

mother of quadruplets who used interim bottle-feedings with each baby as she gradually increased milk production. As with other aspects of breastfeeding, strategies for transitioning two or more infants to direct breastfeeding should look at each infant's signs, or cues, that the individual infant may be ready to progress. In addition, the process of transitioning multiple infants to direct breastfeeding may take time, and a mother may become discouraged. However, one study found preterm twins eventually progressed to full, direct breastfeeding at rates comparable to term infants (Liang, Gunn, & Gunn, 1995).

Putting It All Together

Caring for and breastfeeding multiple newborns require a different kind of organization by the mother than caring for a single newborn or two infants of different ages (Bowers & Gromada, 2003). The mother should be encouraged to keep simple 24-hour charts for each infant's daily activities, especially those related to feeding and intake, until weight gain for each infant is consistently normal. The charts should record the number of breastfeedings, any pumping sessions and/or alternative feedings, and the number of wet diapers and stools for each infant. Maintaining individual charts reassures the mother that all babies are receiving sufficient nutrients. Some mothers prefer to maintain daily charting after normal weight gain is established for all infants, because it allows them to observe the development of sleep-wake patterns for each.

Whether a mother or her babies are ready for simultaneous feedings in the immediate postpartum period or not, a demonstration of the various single and simultaneous feeding positions can help a mother realize that she has many choices for comfortable breastfeeding. Simultaneous feedings can save time, and many mothers feed two babies at once during the first few weeks postpartum; however, some mothers and many multiples need more time to learn to work together for simultaneous feedings (Bowers & Gromada, 2003). Also, a mother may need someone to support each infant's head during individual latch-on until she and her infants become more comfortable with simultaneous feeding. Some mothers or infants indicate a preference for individual feedings, which give a

mother the opportunity to enjoy some one-on-one time with each child. Perhaps the most common scenario is a combination of simultaneous and single feedings.

In addition to an interest in simultaneous feedings, many mothers also have questions about a feeding rotation and when to alternate breasts and babies. Almost any feeding rotation will work when all infants breastfeed on cue (Gromada, 1999). Most mothers offer one breast per feeding and then alternate breasts every feeding or every 24 hours, which often is easier to remember. Some mothers assign each baby a breast, but alternating babies and breasts appears to have more advantages unless one baby consistently cues to feed from a particular breast (Bowers & Gromada, 2003). Mothers of odd-number sets, such as triplets, may have to alternate babies and breasts more frequently than every 24 hours.

The caregiver must remain sensitive to infant differences when a mother is forming an attachment, or bond, with each infant. Because humans are designed to form an attachment with one person at a time, the attachment process is more complex. It is also more likely to be disrupted with multiples, particularly if the twin or triplet birth was not discovered until shortly before the infants' birth or if one infant is sicker than the others (Gromada, 1999). Health-care providers are in a position to help parents see and relate to each baby as an individual, rather than as part of a multiple unit. Promoting attachment behaviors, such as skin-to-skin contact, is especially important with a multiple that has been less able to interact or establish eye contact with parents because of postnatal complications or illness. The health-care provider can point out each infant's unique qualities as she helps the mother breastfeed and get to know her offspring.

Gromada (1999) contends that household help is not a luxury for mothers recuperating from a multiple pregnancy and birth who must feed and care for, and form attachments with, more than one neonate simultaneously. Another pair of hands and ongoing assistance with household chores allow a mother to spend more time and energy breastfeeding and meeting the other needs of her infants. Since taking care of babies is more fun than cleaning and cooking, the mother (and father) should make it clear that the helper is expected to assume household tasks, and that the mother feeds and takes care of the babies.

A lack of physical and emotional support, feelings of isolation, sleep deprivation, and other stressors associated with the care of multiple infants may contribute to postpartum mood or anxiety disorders (Leonard, 1998). Because of the negative effects such a problem may exert on breastfeeding and attachment, LCs and other healthcare providers should be aware of their increased likelihood and continue to assess mothers of multiples for these disorders during the entire period of lactation.

Needs, problems, and solutions vary with each multiple-birth situation. However, practical strategies to promote effective breastfeeding with multiple infants and maternal recovery may include the following ideas:

- Develop both short- and long-term breastfeeding goals with a mother to help her think of breastfeeding as a commitment and to get through the often overwhelming first few weeks or months of frequent feedings and/or pumping sessions.

- Link the mother with other women who have successfully breastfed multiples.

- Show the mother how to position and stabilize two infants for simultaneous feedings using pillows. The mother in Figure 8–5 is using a special pillow designed for feeding multiples. This pillow is longer, wider, and has a deeper "shelf" than some of the nursing pillows used for a single infant.

- Review the basics of breastfeeding, maintenance of milk production, and advantages of breastfeeding with the mother of multiples during the hectic early weeks and months of breastfeeding.

- Help the mother develop a plan to alternate infants and breasts as needed.

- Suggest that the mother create a "breastfeeding station" that she supplies with nutritious liquids and foods, breast pads, infant wipes, children's books (if she has older children), a cell or portable telephone, and a television remote.

- Emphasize the need for housekeeping help for

at least several months. Recommend she advise any helper that she expects them to be supportive of breastfeeding.

- Encourage parents to ask well-wishers who want to "do something" for the family to help by delivering a meal or sending food. The care of multiples leaves little time to prepare food, and the caloric needs of a mother breastfeeding multiple infants are greater than for a mother breastfeeding a single infant. Suggestions for nutritious "home-made fast" foods may be helpful.

Partial Breastfeeding and Human Milk Feeding

Because mothers of multiple infants are more likely to be affected by complications or other factors that may interfere with effective early breastfeeding and milk production, they are more likely to supplement or complement breastfeeding with formula. Complementing may take the form of "topping off" an occasional or daily breastfeedings, or it may involve replacing one or more breastfeedings with an alternative feeding.

With guidance from a LC who respects the overwhelming amount of infant care the mother faces daily and the lack of time to work on resolving problems, most mothers will be able to decrease the use of alternative feedings in favor of direct breastfeedings. Some mothers continue to offer an alternative feeding on a daily or weekly basis in order to have help with feedings or to sleep without interruption for a few hours. Many mothers prefer to express their own milk for such feedings. Mothers should be cautioned that milk production might decrease if the total number of breastfeedings dips below 8 to 10 in 24 hours.

Continuing to use an alternative feeding method to provide expressed human milk has been referred to as human milk feeding, and it is becoming more common with the increased availability of hospital-grade, electric breast pumps. Mothers of higher-order multiples are more likely to human milk feed, as it can be daunting to breastfeed three or more preterm infants directly (Gromada, 1999). Mothers of babies with chronic health problems that interfere with direct breastfeeding have also practiced human milk feeding. Anecdotal information indicates that many mothers have maintained lactation and human milk feeding without the use of other supplements for several months. In addition, human milk feeding leaves a door open to later direct breastfeeding. Multiples wean as individuals; they may stop breastfeeding at about the same time or one may wean before the other(s).

Breastfeeding During Pregnancy

Population studies of pregnancy occurring during full breastfeeding in the first 6 months of the baby's life reveal that this risk is extremely small (Wijden, Keijen, & Berk, 2003). The key points are "fully breastfeeding" and "in the first 6 months." Globally, over 50 percent of women will become pregnant while still breastfeeding their youngest child. When asked, many of these mothers report that the emotional needs of the child is their principal motivation to continue breastfeeding, followed by their belief in child-led weaning. The following outcomes are common when breastfeeding continues through a pregnancy:

- *Nipple tenderness and breast soreness:* Hormonal changes may cause sudden onset of nipple or breast pain that appears to be hormonal in nature. The usual remedies for breast or nipple pain are often ineffectual.

- *Maternal fatigue:* The hormones of early pregnancy often impel women to want to sleep, although this is difficult for the mother of an active toddler to do. The fatigue is related to hormonal changes of pregnancy, not to continued breastfeeding, and it will diminish as the pregnancy progresses. Pregnant women with young children, whether breastfeeding or not, should be encouraged to nap when the child naps.

- *Decline in milk supply and number of feedings:* About 70 percent of mothers report a decrease in their milk production during a subsequent pregnancy. Most nursing children breastfeed less often than they did as infants. As the pregnancy progresses, the milk volume usually declines. Sometimes the child will wean during this period. If already talking, she or he may

complain that the milk is "all gone," or that it takes "too long to get it."

- *Change in taste of milk:* As the hormones of pregnancy begin to affect the breast secretory tissue, lactose in the milk will decrease while sodium increases, changing the taste. The talking nursling may state quite clearly how the milk tastes or may simply indicate by his actions that it is not the same.

- *Uterine contractions:* Women experience uterine contractions during breastfeeding. There is no documented danger to the mother or fetus when mothers breastfeed through a healthy pregnancy, uncomplicated by risk factors for preterm labor (Moscone & Moore, 1993). Little is known about the effect of breastfeeding during pregnancy in the presence of such risk factors.

- Weaning: Many nursing children wean before their sibling is born, presumably because of the decline in milk volume, the milk's change in taste, and/or their mother's urging to wean. As the mother's body changes shape, her lap will also disappear, which may bother the nursing child. The child may wean without the mother having to do anything other than to breastfeed when asked but not to offer as she might have in the past.

A maternal history of preterm labor and birth with a previous pregnancy, repeated spontaneous abortion, "incompetent" cervix, current multiple gestation, or other risks for preterm labor and birth should be taken into consideration when contemplating continued breastfeeding through the pregnancy.

The mother who continues to breastfeed during a subsequent pregnancy will need to eat a nutritious diet; she may take supplemental vitamins as a precaution. In the study by Moscone and Moore (1993), most mothers reported continued good general health throughout their pregnancy as well as healthy outcomes in the new baby. However, the mother who breastfeeds during pregnancy faces potential criticism from her family, friends, and health-care provider. The lactation consultant may be asked for her opinion after the mother has been told by her physician that she must wean her child—even in the absence of indicators that con-

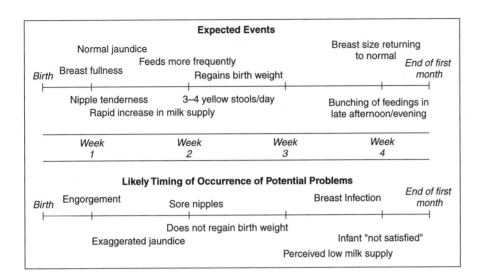

FIGURE 8–6.
Timeline of postpartum events.

tinuing to breastfeed is a risk for the mother or her developing fetus. Being told to wean by a health-care provider is especially common in developed, industrialized countries. In developing countries, traditional beliefs about weaning when the mother's pregnancy is confirmed may also reduce the frequency of breastfeeding during a subsequent pregnancy. The lactation consultant or nurse who openly accepts individual choices of breastfeeding women can be helpful in providing information and guidance that supports the mother's choice.

Clinical Implications

The first few weeks after birth are a critical time for breastfeeding. Almost all women who start off breastfeeding expect to continue for at least 6 weeks, yet approximately one fifth quit breastfeeding before their baby is 10 days old (Hall et al., 2002). Ideally, a mother starts off breastfeeding confident in her ability to meet her own and her baby's needs. Reaching this goal requires that the new mother is provided with appropriate anticipatory guidance, including what she should expect from her baby in the first few days at home, the first week, and the first month of breastfeeding. Figure 8–6 shows a timeline of events that are common in the postpartum period. This timeline can be used as a way of teaching anticipatory guidance for both mothers and health-care personnel.

Many health-care organizations pay for a postpartum office visit with the physician or for a home visit by a nurse. This health-care worker may be from the nursing staff of a hospital or birth center, from a home health agency, or a person in private practice who has been contracted to provide these services. In some cases, referrals are made directly to a private LC in the community. It is common for professionals who spot early breastfeeding difficulties at these postdischarge visits to treat the problem and then refer the mother on to a La Leche League group or similar mother-to-mother support group. Anticipatory guidance and teaching reinforces the mother's knowledge by reviewing basic breastfeeding techniques. According to adult education principles described in Chapter 23, this is the "teaching moment" in which the parents are highly receptive to information that helps them deal with practical life dilemmas.

Priority teaching for parents:

- Keep the baby close and feed on cue around the clock.

- Be sure the baby is actually getting milk. Listen for audible swallowing. Finish the first breast before offering the second so that the baby will receive the creamier milk as the feeding progresses. Watch the baby for cues that he is finished with the feed. Do not limit the frequency or duration of feeds.

- Provide a phone number to call with questions or concerns, especially if any nipple or breast pain occurs. Reinforce the mother's ability to make enough milk with comments such as

"You have lots of good milk for your baby," "Your leaking means you have lots of milk for the baby," "It looks like you could feed twins," or "What a lot of milk you have!"

Summary

The postpartum period is a time of transition from pregnancy to life with a child. Understanding normal patterns of breastfeeding helps lactation consultants identify problems and answer questions from parents and other professionals. Even when all is going well, mothers can benefit from additional support from peers, mother support groups, and lactation professionals.

Key Concepts

- Reassuring signs of adequate infant intake include 8 to 12 or more effective feeds per day, profuse daily infant stools after day 4, and comfortable maternal breasts.

- Abundant ongoing milk supply depends on frequent, thorough removal of milk from the breast by the baby or by alternative means.

- Milk supply calibrates to meet the infant's needs by about 6 weeks, and about a quarter of the milk available remains in the breasts over and above the baby's typical daily intake.

- Oversupply of milk may indicate an underlying infant suckling problem. Before reducing milk volume, rule out infant factors.

- Early-onset nipple pain is often "mechanical" pain, related to improper infant latch or suck, nipple stretching and compression, or irritation from devices.

- Sudden-onset nipple pain after comfortable breastfeeding is often a sign of infection from bacteria, yeasts, or other organisms.

- Topical preparations do not prevent nipple soreness but may offer mild relief of discomfort if no infection is present.

- Pacifiers should be avoided except in short term, therapeutic situations.

- Infant stools change from black, tarry meconium before day 3 to green transitional stools, and then to very soft, yellow stools.

- Jaundice is often a marker for poor feeding. Continued breastfeeding or feeding expressed milk is recommended for jaundiced infants.

- Crying is a late sign of distress and/or hunger.

- Sensitivity or allergy to cow's milk protein is a frequent cause of colic. Allergy to cow's milk protein or other foods calls for skilled and careful dietary management.

- Breastfeeding is particularly advantageous for twins, triplets, and other higher-order multiples. Separating "twin" issues from "breastfeeding" issues requires careful evaluation of each baby and the mother. Most mothers of multiples need practical help in caring for more than one infant.

- Breastfeeding during a subsequent pregnancy is generally not risky to the infant or the developing fetus. Mothers often experience nipple and/or breast pain, diminishing milk supply, and fatigue. Many nurslings wean themselves during a subsequent pregnancy.

Internet Resources

Academy of Breastfeeding Medicine (ABM):
www.bfmed.org

American Academy of Pediatrics (AAP):
www.aap.org

Center for Evidence-Based Medicine:
www.cebm.net

Cochrane database/reviews of research on
breastfeeding topics:
www.cochrane.org

International Lactation Consultant Association
(ILCA):
www.ilca.org

La Leche League International (LLLI):
www.lalecheleague.org

Medline/PubMed:
www.ncbi.nlm.nih.gov/entrez/query.fcgi

US Centers for Disease Control:
www.cdc.gov/breastfeeding

References

Aarts C et al. Breastfeeding patterns in relation to thumb suckling and pacifier use. *Pediatrics* 104:e50, 1999.

Akkuzu G, Taskin L. Impacts of breast-care techniques on prevention of possible postpartum nipple problems. *Prof Care Mother Child* 10(2):38–41, 2000.

Aljazaf K et al. Pseudoephedrine: effects on milk production in women and estimation of infant exposure via breast-milk. *Br J Clin Pharmacol* 56:18–24, 2003.

American Academy of Pediatrics. Work Group on Breastfeeding. Breastfeeding and the use of human milk (Policy RE9729). *Pediatrics* 100:1035–39, 1997.

———. *AAP media alert addresses scheduled feedings vs. demand feedings*. Elk Grove Village, IL: AAP, 1998.

American Academy of Pediatrics and American College of Obstetricians and Gynecologists (AAP/ACOG). *Guidelines for Perinatal Care,* 5th edition. Elk Grove Village, IL: AAP, 2002.

Anderson GC. Risk in mother-infant separation postbirth. *Image J Nurs Sch* 21:196–99, 1989.

Aney M. Babywise advice linked to dehydration, failure-to-thrive. *AAP News* 14:21, 1998.

Auer C, Gromada K. A case report of breastfeeding quadruplets: factors perceived as affecting breastfeeding. *J Hum Lact* 14:135–41, 1998.

Ballard JL, Auer CE, Khoury JC. Ankyloglossia: assessment, incidence, and effect of frenuloplasty on the breastfeeding dyad. *Pediatrics* 110:e63, 2002.

Barr RG et al. Carrying as colic "therapy": a randomized controlled trial. *Pediatrics* 87:623–30, 1991.

———. Differential calming responses to sucrose taste in crying infants with and without colic. *Pediatrics* 103:e68, 1999.

Barros FC et al. Use of pacifiers is associated with decreased breastfeeding duration. *Pediatrics* 95:497–99, 1995.

———. Breastfeeding, pacifier use and infant development at 12 months of age: a birth cohort study in Brazil. *Paediatr Perinat Epidemiol* 11:441–50, 1997.

Baumgarder DJ et al. Effect of labor epidural anesthesia on breastfeeding of healthy full-term newborns delivered vaginally. *J Am Board Fam Pract* 16:7–13, 2003.

Biancuzzo M. Breastfeeding preterm twins: A case report. *Birth* 21:96–100, 1994.

Blackburn ST, Loper DE. *Maternal, fetal and neonatology physiology*. Philadelphia: W. B. Saunders, 1992.

Blair ALC. Sore nipples and breastfeeding: assessment of the relationship between positioning and pain. Breastfeeding Review 11(2):5–10, 2003.

Bleyl JL. Breastfeeding triplets: personal reflections. In: Blickstein I, Keith LG, eds. *Iatrogenic multiple pregnancy: clinical implications*. New York: Parthenon Publishing Group, 2001.

Bowers NA, Gromada KK. *Nursing management of multiple gestation: Preconception to postpartum* [Nursing Module]. White Plains, NY: March of Dimes, 2003.

Brent N et al. Sore nipples in breastfeeding women—a clinical trial of wound dressings vs conventional care. *Arch Pediatr Adolesc Med* 152:1077–82, 1998.

Cadwell K et al. A comparison of three treatments for sore nipples in nursing mothers. Presented at: Annual Conference of the International Lactation Consultant Association; Acapulco, 2001.

Canifet C, Jackobsson I, Hagander B. Colicky infants according to maternal reports in telephone interviews and diaries: a large Scandinavian Study. *J Dev Behav Pediatr* 23:1–8, 2002.

Carbajal R et al. Analgesic effect of breastfeeding in term neonates: randomized controlled trial. *Br Med J* 326:1–5, 2003.

Carroccio A et al. Evidence of very delayed clinical reactions to cow's milk in cow's milk-intolerant patients. *Allergy* 55:574–80, 2000.

Cavataio F, Carroccio A, Iacono G. Milk-induced reflux in infants less than one year of age. *J Pediatr Gastroenterol Nutr* 30(S):36–44, 2000.

Centuori S et al. Nipple care, sore nipples, and breastfeeding: a randomized trial. *J Hum Lact* 15:125–30, 1999.

Chapman DJ, Perez-Escamilla R. Identification of risk factors for delayed onset of lactation. *J Am Diet Assoc* 99:450–54, 1999.

Chen DC et al. Stress during labor and delivery and early lactation performance. *Am J Clin Nutr* 68:335–44, 1998.

Christensson K et al. Separation distress call in the human neonate in the absence of maternal body contact. *Acta Paediatr* 84:468–73, 1995.

Cox DB et al. Breast growth and the urinary excretion of lactose during human pregnancy and early laction: endocrine relationships. *Exp Physiol* 84:421–434, 1999.

Cregan MD, Hartmann PE. Computerized breast measurement from conception to weaning: clinical implications. *J Hum Lact* 15:89–96, 1999.

da Silva OP et al. Effect of domeridone on milk production in mothers of premature infants: a randomized, double-blind, placebo controlled trial. *Can Med Assoc J* 164:17–21, 2001.

Daher S et al. Cow's milk protein intolerance and chronic constipation in children. *Pediatr Allergy Immunol* 12:339–42, 2001.

Daly SEJ, Owens RA, Hartmann PE. The short-term synthesis and infant-regulated removal of milk in lactating women. *Exp Physiol* 78:209–20, 1993.

Daly SEJ et al. The determination of short-term volume changes and the rate of synthesis of human milk using computerized breast measurement. *Exp Physiol* 77:79–87, 1996.

Dewey KG. Maternal and fetal stress are associated with impaired lactogenesis in humans. *J Nutr* 131:3012S–15S, 2001.

Dodd V, Chalmers C. Comparing the use of hydrogel dressing to lanolin ointment with lactating mothers. *JOGN Nurs* 32:486–94, 2003.

Drane D. The effect of teats and dummies on orofacial development. Presented at: National Conference of the Australian Lactation Consultant Association; Hobart, Australia, 1996.

Enkin M et al. *A guide to effective care in pregnancy and childbirth,* 3rd ed. New York: Oxford University Press, 2000.

Estep DC, Kulczycki A. Colic in breast-milk-fed infants: treatment by temporary substitution of Neocate infant formula. *Acta Paediatr* 89:795–802, 2000.

Frantz K. Breastfeeding product guide. Sunland, CA, Geddes Productions, 1999.

Gagon AJ. Indicators nurses employ in deciding to test for hyperbilirubinemia. *JOGN Nurs* 30:626–33, 2001.

Gale CR, Martyn CN. Breastfeeding, dummy use, and adult intelligence. *Lancet* 347:1072–75, 1996.

Gartner LM, Herschel M. Jaundice and breastfeeding. In: *Breastfeeding 2001, Part II: The Management of Breastfeeding,* Pediatric Clinics of North America 48(2). Philadelphia: W. B. Saunders, 2001.

Gray L et al. Skin-to-skin contact is analgesic in healthy newborns. *Pediatrics* 105:e14, 2000.

———. Breastfeeding is analgesic in healthy newborns. *Pediatrics* 109:590–93, 2002.

Gromada KK. *Mothering multiples: breastfeeding and caring for twins or more.* Schaumburg, IL: La Leche League International, 1999.

Gromada KK, Spangler AK. Breastfeeding twins and higher-order multiples. *JOGN Nurs* 27:441–49, 1998.

Gupta SK. Is colic a gastrointestinal disorder? *Curr Opin Pediatr* 14:588–92, 2002.

Hall RT et al. A breastfeeding assessment score to evaluate the risk for cessation of breastfeeding by 7 to 10 days of age. *J Pediatr* 141:659–64, 2002.

Hartmann PE et al. Innovations in breast pump research. Presented at: Annual Conference of the International Consultant Association; Boca Raton, FL, 2002.

Heinig MJ, Nommsen-Rivers L. Breastfeeding support in an ideal setting: the importance of lactation consultant services in the first month postpartum. Presented at: Annual Conference of the International Consultant Association; Washington, DC, 2000.

Hill PD, Aldag JC. Smoking and breastfeeding status. *Res Nurs Health* 19:25–32, 1996.

Howard CR et al. The effects of early pacifier use on breast-feeding duration. *Pediatrics* 103:e33, 1999.

———. Randomized clinical trial of pacifier use and bottle-feeding or cupfeeding and their effect on breastfeeding. *Pediatrics* 111:511–18, 2003.

Huggins KE, Billion SF. Twenty cases of persistent sore nipples: collaboration between lactation consultant and dermatologist. *J Human Lact* 9:155–160, 1993.

Huggins KE, Petok ES, Mireles O. Markers of lactation insufficiency: a study of 34 mothers. In: Auerbach KG, ed. *Current issues in clinical lactation 2000.* Sudbury, MA: Jones and Bartlett, 2000:25–35.

Hyams JS et al. Effect of infant formula on stool characteristics of young infants. *Pediatrics* 95:50–54, 1995.

Iacono G et al. Intolerance of cow's milk and chronic constipation in children. *N Engl J Med* 339:1100–4, 1998.

Kennedy KI, Short RV, Tully MR. Premature introduction of progestin-only contraceptive methods during lactation. *Contraception* 55:347–50, 1997.

Kroeger M, Smith LJ. *Impact of birthing practices on breastfeeding: restoring the mother-baby continuum.* Sudbury, MA: Jones and Bartlett, 2004.

Kunz C, Lonnerdal B. Re-evaluation of the whey protein/casein ratio of human milk. *Acta Paediatr* 81:107–12, 1992.

LaFleur EA, Kiesen KM. Breastfeeding cojoined twins. *JOGN Nurs* 25:241–44, 1996.

Lavergne NA. Does application of tea bags to sore nipples while breastfeeding provide effective relief? *JOGN Nurs* 26:53–58, 1997.

Lehtonen J et al. The effect of nursing on the brain activity of the newborn. *J Pediatr* 132:646–51, 1998.

Leonard LG. Depression and anxiety disorders during multiple pregnancy and parenthood. *JOGN Nurs* 27:329–37, 1998.

Leung GM, Lam TH, Ho LM. Breastfeeding and its relation to smoking and mode of delivery. *Obstet Gynecol* 99:785–94, 2002.

Liang R, Gunn AJ, Gunn TR. Can preterm twins breast feed successfully? *NZ Med Jour* 110:209-12, 1995.

Livingstone VH, Willis CE, Berkowitz J. *Staphylococcus aureus* and sore nipples. *Can Fam Physician* 42:654–59, 1996.

Lust KD, Brown JE, Thomas W. Maternal intake of cruciferous vegetables and other foods and colic symptoms in exclusively breastfed infants. *J Am Diet Assoc* 96:46–48, 1996.

Madlon-Kay D. Evaluation and management of newborn jaundice by Midwest family physicians. *J Fam Practice* 47:461–67, 1998.

Martin J et al. Births: final data for 2000. *National Vital Statistics Reports,* 50:100–102, 2002.

Mathur GP, Mathur S, Khanduja GS. Nonnutritive suckling and use of pacifiers. *Indian Pediatr* 27:1187–89, 1990.

Mattos-Graner RO et al. Relation of oral yeast infection in

Brazilian infants and use of a pacifier. *ASDC J Dent Child* 68:33–36, 10, 2001.

Measel CP, Anderson GC. Nonnutritive sucking during tube feeding: effect on clinical course in premature infants. *JOGN Nurs* 8:265–72, 1979.

Meier PP et al. Estimating milk intake of hospitalized preterm infants who breastfeed. *J Hum Lact* 12:21–26, 1996.

Moscone SR, Moore MJ. Breastfeeding during pregnancy. *J Hum Lact* 9:83–88, 1993.

Neifert MR. The optimization of breastfeeding in the perinatal period. *Clin Perinatal* 25:303–26, 1998.

———. Prevention of breastfeeding tragedies. In: Schanler RJ, ed. *Breastfeeding 2001, Part II: The management of breastfeeding.* Pediatric Clinics of North America, Vol 48:273–97 Part II, 2001.

Neifert MR, McDonough SL, Neville MC. Failure of lactogenesis associated with placental retention. *Am J Obstet Gynecol* 140:477–78, 1981.

Neville MC, Morton J. Physiology and endocrine changes underlying human lactogenesis II. *J Nutr* 131:3005S–8S, 2001.

Neville MC, Neifert MR, eds. *Lactation: physiology, nutrition and breastfeeding.* New York: Plenum Press, 1983.

Newton N. Nipple pain and nipple damage: problems in management of breastfeeding. *J Pediatr* 41:411–23, 1952.

Nowak AJ, Smith WL, Erenberg A. Imaging evaluation of breastfeeding and bottle-feeding systems. *J Pediatr* 126:S130–34, 1995.

Paul K, Ditrrichova J, Papousek H. Infant feeding behavior: development in patterns and motivation. *Dev Psychobiol* 29:563–76, 1996.

Pauli-Pott U et al. Infants with "colic"—mothers' perspectives on the crying problem. *J Psychosom Res* 48:125–32, 2000.

Perez-Escamilla R, Chapman DJ. Validity and public health implications of maternal perception of the onset of lactation: an international analytical overview. *J Nutr* 131:3021S–3024S, 2001.

Quinn AO, Koepsell D, Haller S. Breastfeeding incidence after early discharge and factors influencing breastfeeding cessation. *J Obstet Gynecol Neonatal Nurs* 26:289–94, 1997.

Quinlan PT et al. The relationship between stool hardness and stool composition in breast- and formula-fed infants. *J Pediatr Gastroenterol Nutr* 20:81–90, 1995.

Ramsey D et al. Control of breast function throughout the lactation cycle in women. Presented at: Annual Conference of the International Consultant Association; Boca Raton, FL, 2002.

Ransjo-Arvidson AB et al. Maternal analgesia during labor disturbs newborn behavior: effects on breastfeeding, temperature, and crying. *Birth* 28:5–12, 2001.

Renfrew M, Fisher C, Arms S. *Bestfeeding: getting breastfeeding right for you.* Berkeley, CA: Celestial Arts, 2000.

Righard L, Alade, MO. Effect of delivery room routines on success of first breastfeed. *Lancet* 336:1105–7, 1990.

———. Breastfeeding and the use of pacifiers. *Birth* 24:116–20, 1997.

Riordan J. The effectiveness of topical agents in reducing nipple soreness of breastfeeding mothers. *J Hum Lact* 1:36–41, 1985.

Riordan J, Gill-Hopple K. *Testing relationships of breastmilk indicators with actual breastmilk intake.* NINR State of the Science Nursing Congress. Washington, DC: Sept 26, 2002.

Riordan J et al. The effect of labor pain relief medication on neonatal suckling and breastfeeding duration. *J Hum Lact* 16:7–12, 2000.

St. James-Roberts I. What is distinct about infants' "colic" cries? *Arch Dis Child* 80:56–61, 1999.

Salvatore S, Vandenplas Y. Gastroesophageal reflux and cow milk allergy: is there a link? *Pediatrics* 110:972–84, 2002.

Schwartz K et al. Factors associated with weaning in the first 3 months postpartum. *J Fam Pract* 51:439–44, 2002.

Sepkoski CM et al. The effect of maternal epidural anesthesia on neonatal behavior during the first month. *Dev Med Child Neurol* 34:1072–80, 1992.

Snowden HM, Renfrew MJ, Woolridge MW. Treatments for breast engorgement during lactation (Cochrane Review). In: *The Cochrane Library*, Issue 1, 2003. Oxford, England: Update Software, 2003.

Snyder JB. *Variation in infant palatal structure and breastfeeding* [master's thesis]. Pasadena, CA: Pacific Oaks College, 1995.

Sondergaard C et al. Smoking during pregnancy and infantile colic. *Pediatrics* 108:342–46, 2001.

Spangler A, Hildebrandt E. The effect of modified lanolin on nipple pain/damage during the first ten days of breastfeeding. *Int J Child Educ* 8(3):15–19, 1993.

Stark Y. *Human nipples: function and anatomical variations in relationship to breastfeeding* [master's thesis]. Pasadena, CA: Pacific Oaks College, 1993.

Uvnas-Moberg K et al. Release of GI hormones in mother and infant by sensory stimulation. *Acta Pediatr Scand* 76:851–60, 1987.

Vanderhoof JA et al. Allergic constipation: association with infantile milk allergy. *Clin Pediatr* 40:399–402, 2001.

Vogel AM, Hutchison BL, Mitchell EA. The impact of pacifier use on breastfeeding: a prospective cohort study. *J Paediatr Child Health* 37:58–63, 2001.

Walker M. *Mastitis in lactating women.* Unit 2, Lactation Consultant Series 2. Schaumburg, IL: La Leche League International, 1999.

Wessel MA et al. Paroxysmal fussing in infancy, sometimes called "colic." *Pediatrics* 14:421–34, 1954.

Widström AM, Thingström-Paulsson J. The position of the tongue during rooting reflexes elicited in newborn infants before the first suckle. *Acta Paediatr Scand* 82:281–83, 1993.

Wijden C, Kleijen J, Berk T. Lactational amenorrhea for family planning. *Cochrane Database Syst Rev* (4):CD001329, 2003.

Wilson-Clay B, Hoover KL. *The Breastfeeding atlas,* 2nd ed. Austin, TX: Lactnews Press, 2002.

Woolridge MW. The "Anatomy" of infant suckling. *Midwifery* 2:164–71, 1986.

World Health Organization. *Mastitis: causes and management.* (WHO/FCH/CAH/00/13) Geneva: WHO, 2000.

Zanardo V et al. Beta endorphin concentrations in human milk. *J Pediatr Gastroenterol Nutr* 33:160–64, 2001.

Ziemer MM, Pigeon JG. Skin changes and pain in the nipple during the 1st week of lactation. *JOGN Nurs* 22:247–56, 1993.

BREAST-RELATED PROBLEMS

Jan Riordan

An ounce of prevention is worth a pound of intervention. Many difficulties women encounter while breastfeeding can be prevented by the self-care measures and breastfeeding education discussed in preceding chapters. When a woman fully understands how her body works, she is at less risk for frustration and failure when she encounters a barrier to breastfeeding. This chapter deals with specific breast problems and identifies how health professionals can help.

Clinicians who work with breastfeeding women agree that breast and nipple problems can be common barriers to breastfeeding. During prenatal visits, women should be screened for unusual-looking breasts, areolas, or nipples and lack of breast enlargement. Any of these, coupled with previous breastfeeding difficulties, are high-risk indicators for breastfeeding problems.

Before discussing the more clinical aspects of breast-related problems, including surgery, it is important to address the emotional significance of the female breasts. Breasts are part of a woman's internalized body image that she develops around adolescence and carries with her for the rest of her life. They represent a woman's deepest sense of womanhood. Any change in her breasts (e.g., breast surgery) threatens this feminine internal view of self and creates disequilibrium. When a woman's

breasts are altered by illness or infection, it can be a "double whammy": both her femininity and her ability to breastfeed can be threatened.

Nipple Variations

Inverted or Flat Nipples

There are two types of nipple inversion: (1) retractile/umbilicated where the nipple can be pulled out (everted), and (2) invaginated ("true" inversion) where the nipple cannot be everted. About 3 percent of Korean women have nipple inversion. Most of these are retractile (73–92 percent) and are bilateral (Park, Yoon, & Kim, 1999). Congenital inversion probably results from a failure of the underlying mesenchyme to proliferate and move the nipple out of its normally depressed position.

Retractile inversion sometimes resolves itself from the beginning to the end of pregnancy. In many cases, the degree of inversion is such that it does not affect the ability of the baby to grasp the areolar tissue and draw the nipple into the mouth, although this action might take longer. Lactation consultants have observed that women who have markedly inverted nipples early in their first pregnancy and who breastfeed have much less inversion with subsequent pregnancies. In some cases, these women have reported that their nipples, which initially inverted between feedings with the first baby, no longer do so with second and later infants.

The degree to which inverted nipples are an impediment to breastfeeding is partially caused by the belief that they prevent breastfeeding. How the nipple looks when it is not in the baby's mouth, however, does not always predict how well it functions. In most cases, as long as the mother positions the baby well back on the areola so that the entire nipple is placed well back in the baby's mouth, there is no reason why a mother with inverted nipples should forgo breastfeeding. During suckling, the nipple elongates to double its "resting" length (Smith, Erenberg, & Nowak, 1988). Such reactivity to infant suckling helps to explain by inference why the degree of inversion appears to lessen after weeks or months of repeated suckling by the infant.

When the clinician examines the mother's breasts and nipples in the third trimester of pregnancy, discussion about breastfeeding can continue. If the mother has flat or inverted nipples at that time, she can be taught that following birth, exercising the nipple just before latching on by a newborn appears to loosen the nipple tissue and helps to separate adhesions that cause retraction or inversion. Commercial "nipple enhancers" designed to evert flat or inverted nipples are available for purchase (Maternal Concepts, 2003). The infant also stretches the nipples during feedings.

Hoffman's exercises (exercises of the nipples during pregnancy) and breast shells, two traditional methods for treating inverted nipples, appear to be ineffective and are no longer recommended (Alexander, Grant, & Campbell, 1992).

The first intervention for treating a retractable inverted or flat nipple should be to stimulate and shape the nipple just before the feeding. For a flat nipple (not inverted), massage the nipple or apply a cold cloth to help the nipple to evert outward. For an inverted nipple, instruct the mother to shape her nipple by placing her thumb about 1 $\frac{1}{2}$ to 2 inches behind the nipple (with her fingers beneath) and pulling back into her chest. This works best in a side-lying position. Any pump can be used to help pull out the nipple immediately before the infant feeds. Placing a silicone nipple shield (described in Chapter 12) on the inverted nipple is another method of dealing with the problem of the baby not being able to latch onto the breast because of nipple inversion. The baby can usually ingest sufficient breastmilk through the thin shield, and at the same time his suckling stimulates the mother's nipples.

Absence of Nipple Pore Openings

Very rarely, duct pore openings on the mother's nipple are absent. In one case, the mother's right breast enlarged abnormally starting her third month of pregnancy. Following delivery of her baby, the breast became extremely engorged and she was unable to express any milk from that breast. An ultrasound revealed that she had no nipple pores and no ducts leading from the nipple to the larger ducts, which caused extreme enlargement of the right breast. (Her left breast was normal.) Cosmetic surgery was offered to this mother, but because she was newly emigrated from India and had no insurance, she refused the surgery (Miller, 2003).

Large or Elongated Nipples

Nipples come in assorted sizes and shapes and, like all anatomical structures, are genetically influenced. Clinicians report that Asian women are more likely to have unusually long nipples. Generally, nipples that are larger or longer than normal are less likely to cause problems in breastfeeding than are inverted or flat nipples. In fact, they are often viewed as an anatomical gift that will make breastfeeding easier. Although this is true in many cases, exceptionally long or large nipples may detract from breastfeeding, especially if the infant is small. Infants of mothers with extra-long nipples have been observed to gag after latch-on and to slide back toward the nipple tip, which in some cases causes the mother to develop sore nipples.

Plugged Ducts

No one knows the specific cause of plugged ducts, but they are usually found in mothers who have an abundant milk supply and who do not adequately drain each breast. Pathological changes within the breast that cause the plug are vaguely referred to in the literature as a stasis, clogging of milk, or local accumulations of milk or dead cells that have been shed. A plugged duct is indicated by either of these two sets of symptoms: complaints of tenderness, heat, and possible redness in one area of the breast or (if the plug is located in a duct close to the skin) a palpable lump of well-defined margins without a generalized fever. Sometimes, a tiny white milk plug can be seen at the opening of the duct on the nipple. One mother described it as "little bits of a hard white substance" that is just beneath the surface of milk duct outlets. Color Plate 11 shows a milk plug.

Clinicians are aware of a higher frequency of plugged ducts during the winter season. Although the reason for this is not clear, it may be related to the restricting effects of winter clothing or simply to the cold weather. There is also some evidence that, whereas some women are predisposed to developing plugged ducts, others never encounter it through multiple breastfeeding experiences. Plugged ducts can also lead to mastitis, especially if ignored or untreated. Box 9–1 presents self-care measures to recommend to a mother with a plugged duct.

In acute situations, briskly massaging the breast effectively dislodges the blocked milk. If a mother has chronically recurring plugged ducts, some physicians elect to open the duct with a sterile needlelike instrument. After this is done, the milk may forcibly shoot out from the duct, giving the mother relief, or strings of coalesced milk may be the "plug" that is released. It should be noted that this procedure can be followed by recurring pain in the affected area and should be done only in extreme cases.

Incomplete drainage caused by a skipped feeding or a constricting bra, poor nutrition, and stress have all been implicated in the development of plugged ducts, but a cause-and-effect relationship has never been substantiated. Assessment should include a review of these possibilities with the mother and a review of events leading up to the plugged duct, especially if the mother has a

---

BOX 9–1

Self-Care for Treating a Plugged Duct

- Continue to breastfeed often. Begin feeding on the affected breast to promote drainage.
- Depress the breast during the feed to prevent plugged ducts (Fetherston, 1998).
- Massage the affected breast before and during feeding to stimulate flow of milk. Support the breast with a cupped hand and use firm massage, starting at the periphery of the breast, using thumb to encourage flow of milk while baby suckles. (Another option is to massage the breast in a hot shower or bath.) Outside of the shower, try using an electric vibrator (on low setting).

- Soak the affected breast(s) by leaning over a basin of warm water, and gently massaging them.
- Change position of the infant during feedings to ensure drainage of all the sinuses and ductules in the breast. At least one position should result in the baby's nose being pointed toward the site of the plugged duct.
- Avoid any constricting clothing, such as an underwire bra or the straps on a baby carrier.
- Try taking lecithin, an oily substance, 1 tb/day (found in health food stores). (Lawrence & Lawrence, 1999, p. 273).

repeated problem. There is no need for an antibiotic to treat a plugged duct unless a fever and mastitis develop.

Mastitis

Lactation mastitis can develop during the early postpartum weeks after the mother leaves the hospital. Nurses and lactation consultants who practice in a clinic may be the first to speak with the mother whose symptoms suggest early indication of mastitis. The advice dispensed during this initial call can prevent the condition from advancing to an abscess, especially if the mother mistakenly thinks she should stop breastfeeding or has already done so.

Mastitis is usually a benign, self-limiting infection, with few consequences for the suckling infant. The initial symptoms of puerperal mastitis are fatigue, localized breast tenderness, headache, and flulike muscle aches (Wambach, 2003). If a breastfeeding mother complains that she has the "flu," the first consideration is to rule out infectious mastitis. Typically, fever, a rapid pulse, and the appearance of a hot, reddened, and tender area on the breast follow fatigue, headache, and muscular aching (see Color Plate 19). The infection is usually unilateral and located in one area (usually in the upper outer breast quadrant because most of the breast tissue is there), although it can occur in any area of the breast (Wambach, 2003). It can occasionally occur in both breasts simultaneously and may involve a large portion of the breast.

In worldwide studies published within the last 10 years, the incidence of lactation mastitis ranged from 4 to 27 percent depending on methods, especially subject selection, used in the study (Fetherston, 1995; Foxman et al., 2002; Vogel et al., 1999). Mastitis is most likely to occur in the first several weeks after delivery (Amir, 1999; Wambach, 2003). About one third of the cases in long-term breastfeeding mothers occur after the infant is 6 months old (Riordan & Nichols, 1990). The risk of mastitis is higher among women who have breastfed previously, especially those with a history of mastitis (Foxman et al., 2002; Wambach, 2003)—thus removing an enduring myth that mastitis results from inexperience with breastfeeding. Symptoms last approximately 2 to 5 days. Breast pain and redness peak on days 2 and 3 and return to normal by day 5. Fatigue is the slowest symptom to dissipate. A number of risk factors predispose a woman to mastitis:

- *Stress, fatigue* (Fetherston, 1998; Riordan & Nichols, 1990): Mothers who had mastitis rate stress and fatigue as major factors leading to the infection; typically they describe themselves as exhausted as a result of circumstances above and beyond the normal stresses of taking care of the infant—for example, getting ready for holiday celebrations.

- *Cracked/fissured nipples, nipple pain* (Fetherston, 1998; Foxman, Schwartz & Looman, 1994; Vogel et al., 1999): A breakdown in the epidermis provides an avenue of entry into the breast tissue, although breakdown is not a prerequisite for a breast infection. Mastitis from sore, cracked nipples usually occurs in the first few weeks postpartum.

- *Plugged/blocked ducts* (Fetherston, 1998): Some women repeatedly develop plugged ducts, some of which lead to a full-blown infection. It is not uncommon to be able to see this plug as a white "head" and to feel pressure and tenderness around the plug. Gentle massage above the area of tenderness while the baby is breastfeeding from that breast may help, particularly if the plug is newly formed.

- *Ample milk supply and/or decrease in number of feedings* (Vogel et al., 1999): Women with an abundant milk supply experience more plugged ducts (and subsequent mastitis) than those with a normal supply.

- *Engorgement and stasis:* A decrease in the frequency of feedings presents the potential for engorgement or milk stasis. Infrequent feedings and milk stasis is frequently mentioned in the literature as being associated with mastitis. But there is little evidence that this is true. In fact, at least one researcher (Foxman et al., 2002) discovered that women without a history of mastitis who fed six or fewer times a day had rate of mastitis five times lower than those who fed ten or more times a day. The daily use of a pacifier was associated with a *reduced* risk for mastitis in another study (Vogel et al., 1999)—just the opposite of conventional wisdom. Although it is logical to assume that the natural washing mechanism associated with breastmilk removal helps remove bacteria, bacteria can adhere to the epithelial cells lining the duct especially if there is trauma (Fetherston, 2001). Moreover, the presence of bacteria in milk is normal and breastmilk is not a good medium for bacterial growth.

Other conditions, such as breast trauma, constriction from tight bra or sleeping position (Fetherston, 1998), using a manual pump (Foxman et al., 2002), poor maternal nutrition, and vigorous exercise (particularly of the upper arms and chest) have been mentioned anecdotally as factors leading up to mastitis. These also should be noted in the assessment and history in the event that they predispose the mother to mastitis.

Treatment for Mastitis

The treatments for hastening recovery include continued breastfeeding, application of moist heat, increased fluids, bed rest, pain medication (acetaminophen, ibuprofen) and the judicious use of antibiotics (Table 9–1). It is well established in the medical literature that mastitis is associated with the presence of *Staphylococcus aureus*. Only rarely is a streptococcus involved; when it is, it may be present in breastmilk without causing clinical mastitis. Treatment with antibiotics can eradicate the organism from the milk (Oliver et al., 2000). Although untreated cases heal almost as quickly as treated ones, the standard antibiotic for lactation mastitis is a penicillinase-resistant penicillin or a cephalosporin that covers *S. aureus* for 6 to 10 days.

For chronic mastitis, erythromycin at low doses (regular 250–500 mg doses every 6 hours) or trimethoprim-sulfamethoxazole (Bactrim, Septra) over a longer period of time have been recommended (Cantlie, 1988). However, staphylococci rapidly develop resistance against erythromycin. Trimethoprim-sulfamethoxazole and erythromycin are also options when the mother is allergic to penicillin. In a case report, trimethoprim-sulfamethoxazole (2 tablets per day for 10 days) was effective in preventing recurrence of mastitis in a patient with multiple incidences of mastitis who was allergic to penicillin (Hoffman & Auerbach, 1986). These medications can be taken during breastfeeding without known untoward reactions in the infant.

Another less-known treatment for mastitis is a supplement of vitamin E–rich sunflower oil. Vitamin E decreases milk NaK presumably because this vitamin can decrease inflammatory cytokines and tissue damage caused by free radicals produced during inflammation (Filteau et al., 1999). In the dairy

Table 9–1

SELECTED ANTIBIOTICS FOR MASTITIS

Generic Name	Trade Name	Adult Dosage Ranges
Penicillinase-Resistant Penicillins		
Amoxicillin + clavulanate	Augmentin	875 mg 2x daily
Cloxacillin	Cloxapen, Tegopen	250–500 mg PO q6h
Dicloxacillin	Dynapen	125–250 mg PO or IM q6h
Flucloxacillin	Flucil	250–500 mg 4x daily
Oxacillin	Prostaphlin	500 mg–1 gm PO or IM q4–6h
Cephalosporins		
Cephalexin	Keflex	250–500 mg PO q6h
Cephradine	Velosef	250–500 mg PO q6h
Cefaclor	Ceclor	250–500 mg PO q8h

industry, giving antioxidants such as vitamin E to cows is commonly recognized for preventing mastitis. Echinacea, one of the most popular herbal remedies, stimulates the immune system and may help to keep the infection in check (Binns, 2000). Mothers with mastitis reported taking vitamin C supplements (Wambach, 2003) to fight infection.

Breastmilk composition changes during a breast infection. Levels of some antiinflammatory components rise to protect the baby from untoward effects from consuming mastitic milk (Buescher & Hair, 2001). Elevated levels of sodium and chloride caused by the temporary opening of the normally tight junctions between secretory cells in the paracellular pathways cause the breastmilk to taste salty. After the resolution of mastitis, the affected breast undergoes a temporary "resting" phase and usually produces less milk than it did before the infection.

A mother with mastitis feels ill and she is often discouraged. She asks, "Why does this have to happen to me?" and she may contemplate weaning. In addition, her supply of milk in the affected breast may be diminished for several weeks following the infection. She needs mothering herself, a role that the lactation consultant can assume as she reassures the mother that the infection will eventually resolve. To stop or limit breastfeeding will only increase the risk of infection or recurrence. Tender loving care goes a long way in helping her through this difficult time. She also needs specific advice and a plan for care (Table 9–2) as well as a long-term plan for self-care. A considerable number of mothers develop mastitis more than once during the course of lactation. Therefore, certain women may be prone to the condition, and prevention is important. Review with the mother all the possible factors that preceded and may have contributed to her bout(s) of mastitis. Then encourage the mother to seek medical help early if symptoms recur. Some mothers, especially if they are experienced long-term breastfeeders, do not consult their physicians, even though their mastitis warrants medical attention.

Types of Mastitis

Attempts have been made to classify types of mastitis. Generally, the distinctions are based on sever-

ity of symptoms and whether antibiotics should be started. Gibberd (1953), for instance, described two types of mastitis: cellulitis and adenitis. Cellulitis is thought to involve the interlobular connective tissue that has been infected by the introduction of bacteria through cracked nipples; it is treated with antibiotics. In adenitis, the breast ducts are presumably blocked, and the clinical symptoms are less severe. Treatment involves getting the milk flowing with heat, expression, and pumping. Antibiotics are used only if the infection is not resolving (Livingstone, 1990).

Subclinical lactation mastitis is a condition only recently described. While testing breastmilk of women in Bangladesh and Tanzania to determine vitamin A levels, Willumsen et al. (2000) found a quarter of the women tested had both a raised sodium-potassium ratio and elevated interleukin-8 (IL-8) indicating an infection without clinical symptoms. Fetherston (2001) challenged the idea of a subclinical infection by pointing out that a high sodium level in breastmilk without other symptoms is not a reliable indicator for an infection or a subclinical infection. There are known confounding factors where sodium is normally higher, such as initiation of lactation, involution, and pregnancy. Subclinical mastitis is presumably associated with an increase in the HIV load in breastmilk and could lead to higher rates of mother-to-child transmission of HIV (see Chapter 6).

Infectious versus noninfectious mastitis is another proposed classification. Noninfectious mastitis occurs when milk is not removed from the breast and milk production slows and infection results if milk stasis remains unresolved—i.e., the milk is not "washed" out of the breasts (World Health Organization, 2000). Thomsen et al. (1985) proposed three classifications of mastitis—milk stasis, noninfectious inflammation, and infectious mastitis—based on leukocyte counts in milk from the infected breast. They recommended that antibiotic treatment be used only for infectious mastitis, the most severe classification. Although this taxonomy is helpful in theory, laboratory studies on mastitic milk are seldom done in practice. By the time the mother reports the problem to a health-care provider, she usually has been ill for several hours, if not a day or two; the peak of the infectious process may have al-

Table 9–2

MASTITIS TEACHING PLAN

Content-Goal	Teaching
Prevention	
Reduction of stress and fatigue related to childbearing responsibilities	Prioritize tasks from most important to least important. Encourage other family members to assist in routine household tasks. Hire household help if possible. Delay return to job as long as possible.
	Hold one informal open house for friends and relatives to see new baby. Use voicemail to filter calls. Turn down social invitations. Ignore e-mail.
	Take day naps when infant sleeps.
Plugged ducts	Breastfeed often (at least 8 to 12 times per day). Massage any reddened area of breast, especially while breastfeeding.
Change in number of feedings	Pump or express milk if a feeding is skipped.
Engorgement-stasis	Pump or express milk if breasts become overfull or distended. Wear bras without support underwires.
Care If Mastitis Occurs	
Self-care and relief of discomfort	Recognize early signs and symptoms: redness, fatigue, fever, chills. Rest with infant and fluids at bedside. Continue frequent breast-feedings.
Medical care	Monitor oral temperature. Place moist, warm packs at place of infection and over nipple. Expect slightly reduced milk supply in affected breast postinfection. Take antibiotics if needed. (They may not be necessary if fever is already subsiding.) Take antipyretic to reduce fever.

ready passed, and she is getting well by the time she seeks medical treatment. There are other drawbacks: (1) leukocyte counts do not always correspond with bacterial counts (Fetherston, 2001), (2) the milk sample must be collected before any antibiotics are started, (3) laboratory studies take several days, and (4) the testing expense may not be covered by health insurance. Whatever the classification of mastitis, the mother suffering from symptoms clearly needs to be treated. If she has repeated mastitis, a culture of her milk and a review of risk factors are indicated.

When a lactating woman has recurrent mastitis that does not respond to antibiotic therapy, inflammatory carcinoma must be ruled out. Inflammatory breast cancer can be mistaken for mastitis because the symptoms of an inflamed, edematous breast are similar. Breast cancer is different from mastitis because inflammatory carcinoma rarely produces fever, there is no palpable mass, and the symptoms do not respond to antibiotic treatment. This woman should be referred to a surgeon experienced in this area who will perform a biopsy and other laboratory diagnostic tests to determine if inflammatory mastitis is present (Merchant, 2002). If it is, lactation is a secondary consideration, as the mother will need intensive treatments that will preclude lactation.

Breast Abscess

A small percentage of breast infections develop into an abscess. The incidence is decreasing probably because we are more educated in prevention of abscess (Vogel et al., 1999). An abscess, like a boil, is basically a collection of pus that must be drained (see Color Plates 13, 16, and 17). If the abscess is small, the pus may be aspirated with a fine needle under ultrasound guidance. According to Merchant (2002), ultrasound may be helpful but drainage is usually not performed after the ultrasound, even with symptoms of an abscess. Merchant contends that "the erythema, tenderness and induration can become worse and that breast necrosis may be considerable before adequate drainage is done." For a larger abscess, the physician makes an incision and drains the area. Love (2000) offers this advice:

Surgeons never sew up a drained abscess; that would lock bacteria into the cavity, and almost insure the infection's return. I'd tell my patients to go home and rest; then, after 24 hours, begin taking daily showers; let the water run over the breast and wash away the bacteria. Then put a dressing over it to absorb oozing fluids from the incision.

A drain is placed in the incision to promote drainage; in addition, manual expression helps to eliminate pus and milk. The incision heals from the inside out within a week or two. Treatment of abscesses varies across cultures. Efrem (1995) reported on 285 cases of breast abscess in lactating Nigerian women. Most (85 percent) grew *S. aureus*, 5 percent grew coliforms, and 10 percent grew no organism. All of the cases responded well to treatment by incision and drainage followed by packing daily with ribbon gauze soaked in magnesium sulphate solution (135 cases), Euseol (100 cases), and honey (50 cases).

Breast and Nipple Rashes, Lesions, and Eczema

Breast rashes and lesions on the nipple or areolar area are unusual and often difficult to diagnose. They are particularly distressing if they are painful. In one case (Brackett, 1988), a mother described a periodic burning sensation in the breast not related to actual breastfeeding. Most of the mother's areola was itchy, flaky, and red. The family lived without air conditioning during hot, humid weather. In addition, the mother swam in a chlorinated pool each day, often wearing her bathing suit for some time after returning home. Thrush was ruled out as a possible cause of her problem. The mother stopped swimming and her rash resolved within 2 weeks.

Eczema is a type of dermatitis with redness and crusting and oozing papules. Amir (1993) described a case in which a breastfeeding mother with celiac disease developed red, scaly, and cracked nipples. The mother appeared to have eczema, possibly infected, involving most of both breasts. A topical steroid ointment (betamethasone dipropionate 0.05% [Diprosone]) was applied four times daily and a topical antibiotic was used twice daily. Two weeks later, the eczema had resolved, and the mother was able to continue breastfeeding without pain. Box 9–2 presents interventions that will help prevent such disorders.

A more severe breast skin problem is redness and itching accompanied by tiny ulcers on the nipple and areola that resemble chickenpox. Breastfeeding is extremely painful. As the ulcers heal, they form scabs. The baby may or may not have similar perioral skin lesions. This condition requires referral to a physician, who should evaluate the mother for a possible staphylococcal or viral infection. Culture of the lesion should be taken during its early stages before the lesion begins to dry and heal over. Color Plate 8 depicts a cracked nipple with a possible bacterial infection.

Treatment will depend on laboratory results of a culture of the lesion and maternal serum antibody titers. If the lesion is herpes simplex it is advisable for the mother to wean the infant or to pump her milk until the lesions are healed. The mother will be treated with an antiviral medication.

The lactation consultant described the breast lesions from herpes (Color Plate 14) as looking like chickenpox. The healing lesions were scabbing, the active lesions were oozing ulcerations, and the new lesions were tiny, bright-red flat areas. The mother complained of extreme "razor blade–like" pain during feedings. Two physicians, who offered differing diagnoses, evaluated her. Her pediatrician suggested that it might be herpes virus, whereas her dermatologist thought the mother had a staphylococcal infection. Neither physician obtained a culture or serum antibody titers.

The woman was first treated for a staphylococcal infection, which worsened the problem, and then with an antiviral agent (Zovirax). The lesions began to resolve shortly after the mother applied Zovirax to her nipples and areola. The mother interrupted breastfeeding her 10-month-old baby for two weeks while the lesions healed. During this time, she pumped and hand-expressed her milk. She resumed full breastfeeding at the end of that time. The child had "fever blisters" every three or four months for some time after this episode, and the mother developed more breast lesions a few months after the first infection, which she again treated successfully with Zovirax. For more discussion on herpes simplex virus, see Chapter 6.

Candidiasis (Thrush)

When a mother has persistent sore nipples, candidiasis is likely. The yeast, *Candida albicans* (also called *Monilia* or thrush) is the likely cause when it occurs orally. *Candida* thrives in the warm, moist areas of the infant's mouth and on the mother's nipples. The infant's mouth can become infected during vaginal birth and can then infect the mother's breast and nipple during breastfeeding. Candidiasis should be suspected if the mother has been breastfeeding without discomfort and then rapidly develops extremely sore nipples, burning or itching, and possibly, shooting pain deep in the breast. Staphylococcal infections can be mistaken for *Candida* or the problem can be polymicrobial, i.e. both bacteria and *Candida* are involved (Smillie, 2002).

Although *Candida* is a naturally occurring yeast that lives in the mucous membranes of the gastrointestinal and genitourinary tract and on the skin, the use of antibiotics promotes overgrowth (candidiasis); consequently, infants and women who have received antibiotic therapy are more susceptible to candidiasis (Chetwynd et al., 2002). The increasing use of intrapartum antibiotic prophylaxis for group B streptococcus has contributed to rising numbers of cases of breast *Candida* overgrowth (Tanguay, McBean, & Jain, 1994).

Mothers with vaginal candidiasis and nipple trauma are also predisposed to candidiasis of the

---

BOX 9–2

Interventions for Breast and Nipple Rashes and Infections

- Discontinue irritant.
- Take frequent showers.
- Wear all-cotton bras.
- Expose breasts to sunlight (15 minutes) and to air.
- Apply a medicated cream on the affected area twice a day. (Bactroban, an antifungal, antibacterial, and hydrocortisone combination, is available over the counter). Remove cream with clean cotton swab if used on nipple-areola.
- Rinse nipple-areola area with warm water after each feeding. Pat dry, then air-dry with hair dryer on the low setting.

---

breast. In checking for candidiasis, inspect the woman's breasts for inflammation of the nipples and areola. The inflammation is usually a striking deep pink, sometimes with tiny blisters (see Color Plate 12). The mother will complain of severe tenderness and discomfort, especially during and immediately after feedings.

The baby may have a diaper rash, with raised, red, sore-looking pustules or red, scalded-looking buttocks. Also examine the child's mouth carefully for white patches surrounded by diffuse redness. The absence of symptoms in the child's mouth, however, does not rule out thrush, because the infant may be asymptomatic. On the other hand, thrush symptoms in the baby (fussiness, refusing breast) can go unnoticed or can be attributed to something else. Candidiasis is diagnosed on clinical symptoms rather than by cultures, which may take weeks to grow and are difficult to differentiate from normal skin colonization (Chetwynd et al., 2002). Whenever any woman has recurrent yeast infections, her sexual partner should be considered a potential reservoir of infection. Pacifiers and bottle nipples are another source of recurrent thrush infection; they may harbor persistent oral *Candida* colonization and should be replaced or boiled after each exposure in the infant's mouth.

Candidiasis is a "family" disease; it spreads quickly among family members, especially with intimate contact involving warm, moist areas of the body, as is the case with breastfeeding and with sexual contact. Candidiasis that develops during breastfeeding can persist and recur unless all areas of possible infection in the baby, mother, and her sex partner are treated promptly and aggressively. The infant's mouth and anal area, and the mother's breasts (nipples and areola) and vagina are prime sites for *Candida* infection; all should be treated simultaneously.

Despite the availability of antifungal medications, there are no clinical trials and very little research on their effectiveness in treating candidiasis of the lactating dyad. Treatment has been and still is more or less a "shotgun" approach of trial and error.

Treatment

Treatment of candidiasis for the infant includes placing an antifungal medication in the infant's mouth with a medicine dropper after feedings and swabbing it over the mucosa, gums, and tongue. The mother must apply an antifungal topical cream or lotion to her nipples and breast before and after each feeding and to the infant's entire diaper area if there is any redness. The mother may also have vaginal yeast infection and should simultaneously use an antifungal intravaginal preparation. Clotrimazole (Gyne-Lotrimin) is an over-the-counter drug in the United States and is available as a vaginal suppository or as a cream but is not sold as a gel. Other recommendations that can be made to the mother on a case-by-case basis include the following:

- "Air-dry" the nipples and, if possible, expose them directly to the sun for a few minutes twice a day.
- Throw away disposable breast pads as soon as they become wet.

- Dry the external genitalia with a hair dryer on a warm setting.
- Wear 100 percent cotton underpants and bras that can be washed in very hot water and/or bleach to kill spores.
- Avoid baths with other members of the family.
- Restrict alcohol, cheese, bread, wheat products, sugar, and honey.
- Take 1 tablet acidophilus daily (40 million–1 billion viable units, found at health food stores) for 2 weeks beyond the disappearance of symptoms.
- Use condoms during coitus because crossinfection with a sexual partner is possible (Wilson-Clay & Hoover, 2002).

Nystatin is the most commonly used medication for candidiasis although its effectiveness is questionable (Chetwynd et al., 2002) and can cause gastrointestinal symptoms in the baby. Its use should be limited to borderline cases of thrush. Nystatin oral suspension is painted on the baby's oral mucosa and tongue with a large cotton swab after every breastfeeding. In the case of frank thrush and persistent candidiasis, fluconazole is safe and effective. Treatment calls for oral fluconazole for both the mother and infant. The amount of fluconazole that transfers through the mother's milk is not sufficient to treat the baby. Another treatment is painting ketoconazole suspension on the breast twice a day for 5 days, followed by prolonged nystatin application. If the mother has allergies, the health-care provider must be aware that Seldane (terfenadine) should *not* be taken in conjunction with the antifungal drugs ketoconazole or itraconazole or the antibiotic erythromycin (see Chapter 5). Mixing these drugs can be life threatening.

Table 9–3 presents a listing of recommended dosages for commonly used antifungal medications. Dr. Jack Newman's All Purpose Nipple Ointment (Newman & Pitman, 2000) is a combination nipple ointment of antifungal and cortisone agents. A protocol for treating nipple infections is presented in Box 9–3.

After taking an antifungal medication, mothers need encouragement and follow-up; they may not get immediate relief from pain. In fact, after

Table 9–3

SELECTED ANTIFUNGAL PREPARATIONS

Drug Name	Preparations	Usual Dosage
Clotrimazole (Lotrimin, Mycelex)	Creams, solutions, vaginal cream, and vaginal tablets.	Skin cream: apply twice daily. Vaginal cream or tablet: 100 mg/day for 7 days or 200 mg/day for 3 days.
Gentian violet	Dilute solution 0.25% or 0.5%.	Topical: infant: 2 to 3 times over several days. Do not repeat.
Fluconazole (Diflucan)	Oral.	Adult: 400 mg loading dose, then 100 mg twice daily for at least 2 weeks until pain-free for a week. Pediatric: loading dose of 6–12 mg/kg; then 3–6 mg/kg.
Ketoconazole (Nizoral)	Oral tablets.	Adult: 200–400 mg/day, given in single dose. Pediatric: children weighing less than 20 kg, 50 mg/day; children weighing 20–40 kg, 100 mg/day.
Miconazole (Monistat)	Skin cream or lotion: creams, lotions, vaginal cream, and vaginal suppositories.	Vaginal cream or suppository: 100 mg/day for 7 days. Skin cream or lotion: apply 3 to 4 times per day.
Nystatin (Mycostatin)	Suspensions, cream, powders, ointment, and vaginal suppositories; *Candida* resistance to nystatin is growing.	Oral: for adults: 1.5–2.4 million units/day divided into 3 to 4 doses; for infants: 400,000–800,000 units/day divided into 3 to 4 doses; Topical: 1 million units applied twice a day. Duration of therapy: at least 2 days after symptoms disappear; vaginal: 1–2 million units/day.
Newman's All Purpose Nipple Ointment	Ointment mixed by a pharmacist. Clotrimazole can be left out if 10% dosage is not available. Use until pain-free.	Mupirocin 2% ointment (15 gm); Nystatin 100,000 unit/ml ointment (15 gm); Clotrimazole 10% vaginal cream (15 gm); Betamethasone 0.1% ointment (15 gm).

starting treatment the pain may become worse before it begins to fade. If nystatin does not clear the fungal infection, other antifungal medications, such as miconazole (Monistat), clotrimazole (Gyne-Lotrimin) naftifine (Naftin), or oxiconazole (Oxistat), should be tried. Johnstone and Marcinak

(1990) reported a case in which nystatin oral suspension was applied to the infant's mouth lesions with a clean cotton swab four times daily for 2 weeks, and to the mother's nipples immediately after feedings. This treatment was ineffective. The mother then applied clotrimazole gel to her nipples

BOX 9–3

Treatment for Nipple Infections (*Candida* and/or staphylococcal)

Mother:

1. Ibuprofen (Motrin, Advil, etc.) 600–800 mg, 3 to 4 times a day, around the clock; 1 prescription strength pill, or 3 or 4 "over-the-counter" 200 mg strength pills every 6 to 8 hours, around the clock, until painfree (about 2–10 days).

2. Air time! Very important

   No bra at night.
   Daytime: bra flaps open under shirt, or no bra at least some of the time.
   If you need bra for support, leave flaps open or use old bra with holes cut out for nipples.

3. After each feeding

   Rinse nipples briefly with plain water. Air-dry a few seconds, or pat dry briefly. Skin should be just moist.
   Apply a small amount of mupirocin (Bactroban) ointment to the area that the baby's mouth covers. Mupirocin is both antifungal and antibacterial.
   Rub in well until most of it disappears. It will leave a greasy film. It does not have to be scrubbed off before breastfeeding or pumping.

Baby :
(ONLY if baby has visible thrush)

1. Nystatin oral suspension: Swab tongue and inside cheeks with 1/2 cc (ml) using Q-tip or finger, 4–6 times a day, after breastfeeding/pumping.

2. If the thrush is severe or baby has already had unsuccessful nystatin treatment, use instead oral fluconazole (see below) treatment once daily.

When mother is painfree AND baby's mouth has no signs of thrush:

1. Continue using mupirocin on nipples about 3–4 times a day, for a whole pain-free week.

2. If baby has been treated, continue treating the baby's mouth with nystatin about twice a day (or fluconazole once daily) for a least 3 days after the infant's symptoms clear, and until mother has been painfree for at least 3 days.

For persistent, recurrent, severe, or complicated infections:

- If nipples are particularly red and inflamed, apply triamcinolone 0.1% ointment to inflamed area 3–4 times a day for 5–7 days. Apply the mupirocin ointment right over the triamcinolone.
- Fluconazole 400 mg orally first day, then 200 mg daily for 14 or 21 days.
- Sunshine, sunlamp, or tanning salon— 2-3 minutes max once or twice a day.
- To give rest to the healing nipples, pump and feed breastmilk via alternative method (bottle, cup, syringe) several days to a week or more.
- Gentian violet, one dot, by cotton swab, to injured/raw area only, covered by mupirocin, once a day for 3–4 days, in addition to the other regular mupirocin treatments after breastfeeding or pumping.

If mother has symptoms of staphylococcal infection (raw cracks, golden crusts):

- Dicloxacillin or cephalexin (Keflex) 500 mg orally 4 times a day, for 10 days.
- Plastic wrap over Bactroban between feedings a few hours per day. Caution: Don't use when sleeping or sleepy—remove wrap before breastfeeding!

For baby, if necessary:

- Apply nystatin or mupirocin ointment to diaper rash, 4 times a day, until clear.
- Fluconazole oral suspension: 6 mg/kg for first day; 3 mg/kg thereafter, for 5 to 10 days.

Source: Christina M. Smillie, MD, Personal communication (2002). Reprinted with permission.

and to the baby's oral lesions every 3 hours. After five applications, both mother and baby were symptom-free. In another case of persistent candidiasis and thrush, fluconazaole was the only effective treatment. For early cases, suggest that after feedings the mother try warm vinegar soaks (1 part vinegar, 4 parts water) followed by air-drying and an antifungal preparation (La Leche League International, 2000).

Gentian violet is an old-fashioned antifungal drug that is enjoying a comeback because it works well, is inexpensive, and does not require a prescription. One drawback is that gentian violet stains anything with which it comes into contact, although blotting with alcohol and then a detergent solution helps to remove the dye. In advising a mother who is using it, suggest that she keep her sense of humor and wear clothing she can throw away. She should apply the gentian violet (0.25% or 0.5% solution), using clean cotton swabs, in the baby's mouth and diaper area and on her nipples after feedings. Prolonged use of gentian violet can cause irritation and ulceration of the infant's oral mucous membrane (Utter, 1990). One to two days after the gentian violet is applied, the epidermis on both the baby's diaper area and the mother's breasts may peel and become red. A & D ointment may then be applied in the diaper area to any red areas that are not thrush-related.

A common recommendation is to wash and boil or dispose of anything that comes into contact with the baby's mouth (pacifiers, rubber nipples, teethers, or toys) or the mother's breasts (breast-pump parts, bras, breast pads) to destroy the heat-resistant spores. But considering all the work and effort involved for busy, tired mothers, it might be better to start treatment to see if the medications alone effectively treat candidiasis. Dr. Christina Smillie, a pediatrician who treats only breastfeeding patients, views *Candida* as a normal flora that is everywhere, and its treatment should be focused on regaining healthy skin so the mother can resist infection. It is not clear whether expressed milk of a mother with candidiasis should be saved and frozen for later use. Freezing deactivates yeast but does not kill it.

In one case of candidiasis infection of the breast (see Color Plate 12), the infant remained symptom-free for the entire 4-month period, whereas the mother had repeated episodes of candidiasis. Within 4 days after resolving the painful blistering and redness, she experienced a new flare-up. After four such episodes in 4 months, she obtained medication for both her infant and herself; after 5 days of treatments after *every* suckling episode, she was symptom-free and remained so (Johnstone & Marcinak, 1990).

According to conventional wisdom, when candidiasis infection is severe, it can involve the lower ducts and sinuses of the breast in addition to the outer skin of the nipples and breast. When the ducts are infected, the mother is very likely to feel a burning sensation deep in the breast, which is distinct from the burning sensation of the breast skin itself.

Often the inner burning persists several minutes after the baby has come off the breast. When the mother is treated with oral antifungal medication, the pain subsides (Chetwynd et al., 2002; Johnstone & Marcinak, 1990). It has been suggested that the more severe the candidiasis infection, the longer it takes for the treatment to work and for the pain to disappear.

Breast Pain

Breast pain that may derive from any number of sources can be both disconcerting and discouraging. Breast pain may be involved with the following conditions (Wilson-Clay & Hoover, 2002):

- Pinched nipple from poor latch-on
- Vasospasm or Raynaud's phenomenon
- Plugged duct
- Damaged nipples
- Nipple infection: bacterial, *Candida,* or both
- Engorgement
- Forceful milk ejection
- Rapid refilling of ducts
- Mastitis

In some cases, pressure on the brachial plexus can result in shooting pain in the breast. Identifying the cause of this pressure (e.g., a badly fitting bra or baby-carrier straps that are pulled too tightly across the mother's back) is a key to alleviating such pain.

Women have reported feeling shooting pain that coincided with powerful ejection of milk. Such episodes are most likely to occur in the first month of the breastfeeding course. When the milk-ejection reflex subsides, the pain often subsides as well. This temporary pain tends to occur more often in primiparous women; often the same mothers who have experienced it with a first breastfeeding baby do not experience a recurrence with later infants. This pain may reflect distention of the milk ducts, which is more obvious in the early first breastfeeding course than at later periods.

In cases in which the mother reports very intense pain coincidental with a vigorous milk-ejection response, the caregiver should encourage the mother to gently massage her breasts before putting the baby to breast to enhance the likelihood of some initial leaking of milk before the baby's active suckling stimulates milk ejection. When the milk begins to drip freely, sprays and then subsides, subsequent suckling is less likely to result in such intense discomfort. By the end of the first month, such pain is usually no longer present when the milk-ejection reflex is activated.

Plagued by recurrent plugged ducts, mastitis, and sinus infection that was treated with antibiotics, one mother eventually developed episodes of deep pain in both breasts. Although her breasts were not red or hot to the touch, and she did not have any hardness over ducts, there was a burning and shooting pain inside. Finally, a pediatric nurse practitioner suggested she take high doses of acidophilus since she thought that the problem might be ductal yeast infection. After two months of this treatment the mother had no recurrence of either breast pain or a plugged duct (Buraglio, 2003).

Women who have nipple pain are highly anxious and distressed. However, once the pain resolves, their distress also resolves (Amir et al., 1996). Heads and Higgins (1995) looked at nipple trauma in relation to nipple pain between 3 and 5 days postpartum. Visible evidence of nipple damage and nipple trauma was observed in 38 (55 percent) of the 69 women in the study. Damage occurred most commonly in the form of minor grazes (61 percent) or blisters (23 percent). Women who had a strong personal commitment to breastfeed their babies reported less nipple pain than did those who were not so strongly committed.

Treatment for breastfeeding women with unrelenting nipple/breast pain when it is not known if the problem is *Candida* or bacterial can consider using the protocol shown in Box 9-3.

Vasospasm

In breast vasospasm, the nipple appears blanched after the feeding, sometimes turning blue or red before returning to its normal color. The mother feels extreme pain during the "spasm." This cluster of symptoms is often referred to as *Raynaud's phenomenon of the nipple.* Raynaud's phenomenon (an intermittent ischemia usually affecting fingers or toes) is more prevalent in women, and there usually is a family history.

Blanching of the nipple can occur not only during feedings but also between feedings according to one report (Lawlor-Smith & Lawlor–Smith, 1997). Exposure to cold precipitates nipple blanching and pain and is relieved by warmth and covering the breast. Some mothers showed classic triphasic color change of Raynaud's phenomenon (white, blue, and red) in their nipples, or biphasic color change (white and blue).

Treatment with nifedipine (30 mg/day for 2 weeks) has been reported as effective for treating vasospasm without side effects (Garrison, 2002). Nifedipine is a calcium channel blocker used to treat hypertension; its transfer through breastmilk to the baby is not significant (Penny & Lewis, 1989). Some maternal medications, such as fluconazole and oral contraceptives, may be associated with vasospasm (Escott, 1994). Ibuprofen and warmth applied to the breasts, either by a warm shower or by covering the breasts with a heating pad, help to alleviate discomfort.

Milk Blister

Infrequently, a milk blister—a whitish, tender area—develops on the upper areola. Nipple-pore milk that has been sealed over by the epidermis and has triggered an inflammatory response probably causes a milk blister. This obstruction then prevents the duct system from draining, so milk buildup behind the occlusion causes symptoms of a blocked duct (Noble, 1991). The spot may be white or yellow, depending on how long it has been present. The skin on and around the area may be reddened (see Color Plate 11).

Persistent and very painful during feeding, a milk blister can remain for several days or weeks and then spontaneously heal by a peeling away of the epithelium over the affected area. If it does not spontaneously heal, an optional treatment is to break the epithelial tissue using a sterile needle, sometimes along with sterile tweezers and small sharp scissors to entirely remove the excess skin. Aspiration may be necessary to draw out the fluid. Compressing around the areola to express out any stringy plugs may help to prevent future blisters

from arising (Newman & Pitman, 2000). A mother who had a nipple probe for a chronically plugged duct and blister developed a lot of pain and insisted on weaning to get relief.

A less invasive treatment is rubbing the area with a damp cloth after softening the skin by immersion in warm water. With ice packs, an analgesic to relieve discomfort, and a topical antibiotic, breastfeeding can continue and healing is rapid.

In addition to the larger blister, tiny blisters that appear to have a whitish fluid, possibly milk, within may appear on nipples. These blisters are sore and painful. Vitamin E ointment (applied sparingly and wiped off before feedings) and wearing breast shells (to relieve the pressure from clothing on the nipples) relieve discomfort and possibly aid healing.

Mammoplasty

Breast augmentation and reduction are increasingly common surgical procedures. Although augmentation is performed for cosmetic effect, reduction of very large breasts is often performed to reduce discomfort from neck and back pain and the need to "feel normal" (Grassley, 2002).

Sooner or later, the clinician will see a client who has had breast augmentation or reduction and who wants to know whether she will be able to breastfeed her baby. The ability to breastfeed after these surgeries depends on the type of surgery, the specific technique used, whether neural pathways were severed, and the amount of breast tissue removed. Generally speaking, full breastfeeding is possible with augmentation surgery but usually not after reduction surgery, unless feedings are supplemented; however, exceptions occur in both instances with any breast surgery. An explanation of the differences in the operative procedures is crucial to understanding the subsequent effect on lactation.

Breast Reduction

The ability to breastfeed after breast reduction depends on whether the surgeon deliberately leaves nerve pathways and blood supply intact or the tissue is removed without regard for these structures (Soderstrom, 1993). Women with the least amount of glandular tissue removed have a greater opportunity to lactate (Marshall, Callan, & Nicholson,

1994), particularly if the fourth intercostal nerve that branches to the breast and areola is left intact (see Chapter 3).

The two techniques used for breast reduction are the *pedicle technique* and the *free-nipple technique.* The inferior pedicle technique is common for women of childbearing age. The nipple and areola remain attached to the breast gland on a pedicle, and the tissue is "reduced." A wedge is removed from the sides of the underside of the breast (Figure 9–1). Because the breast, its ducts, its blood supply, and some nerves remain intact, breastfeeding has been possible after this operation but the success of breastfeeding cannot be predicted. The free-nipple technique (autotransplantation of the nipple) involves removing the nipple-areola entirely from the breast and preserving it in saline (much like a graft) while the additional breast tissue (usually fatty tissue) is removed. Then the nipple-areola is stitched back in place. This technique is used for women with extremely large breasts and is designed to reduce risks and complications and to position the nipple approximately on the substantially resculpted breast. Breastfeeding may be possible with the pedicle technique, but it is rarely possible with the free-nipple technique, because the blood supply of the nipple-areola is completely severed and damage to the nerves occurs.

Breast reduction usually interferes with the ability to breastfeed (Grassley, 2002; Souto et al., 2003). Brzozowski et al. (2000) studied 78 women who had undergone an inferior pedicle reduction mammoplasty and subsequently had children. For the first 2 weeks postpartum, 19 percent of these women breastfed exclusively, 10 percent breastfed with formula supplementation, and 18 percent were unsuccessful in breastfeeding. Half of the sample did not even attempt breastfeeding. Others (Marshall, Callan, & Nicholson, 1994; Souto et al., 2003) found similar discouraging results. Even so, sporadic reports (Ashford, 2001) of successful breastfeeding after reduction surgery should encourage women to try breastfeeding and then supplement if it becomes necessary.

Breast scars after a reduction are illustrated in Color Plate 26. Several cases of spontaneous galactorrhea after reduction mammoplasty are reported in the literature; all of these women had not breastfed for several months before the surgery (Menendez-Graino et al., 1990; Song & Hunter, 1989).

The health professional should provide a forthright discussion about the likelihood of successful lactation and about options for supplemental feedings, especially in the later months. Plastic surgeons, though they may be sympathetic to breastfeeding, are most interested in the surgical technique and the cosmetic results; they are generally uninformed about breastfeeding. The women in one study (Souto et al., 2003) reported that almost 80 percent of their surgeons indicated that breast reduction would not affect lactation. Most of these women were young and desired to have chil-

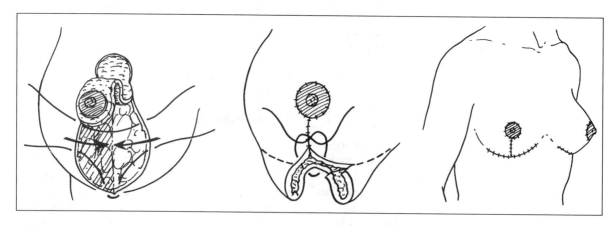

Figure 9–1. Breast reduction. (A) Wedge of breast tissue removed, areola pulled up, gap closed. (B) Excess tissue removed, skin closed with stitches. (C) Postoperative appearance.

dren in the future. Only half of them worried about not being able to breastfeed.

The breast-reduced mother's reactions to her inability to breastfeed may vary according to culture. The US mother who has had breast reduction may accept whatever extent she can breastfeed without regretting that she had the surgery. Women with heavy, pendulous breasts report back, neck, and shoulder pain. They may feel depressed and stigmatized, and experience negative comments from both men and women about their breast size, including cruel jokes during their adolescence (Grassley, 2002; Guthrie et al., 1998). Mothers who have had breast reduction surgery may feel guilty or angry about not being able to breastfeed (Engstrom, 2000).

Mastopexy

Mastopexy, like a "facelift," is a "breastlift"—cosmetic surgery where sagging breasts are uplifted and made firmer (Figure 9–2). The operation involves removing excess skin and breast tissue and elevating the nipple. It may be done either in the hospital or in the physician's office. Although there may be a slight loss of sensation in the nipple or areola, the operation "theoretically" should not affect the ability to breastfeed; however, I have worked with mothers who had this operation and thus had a

very difficult time producing sufficient milk in order to maintain adequate growth for their infants.

Breast Augmentation

Because cosmetic surgery to "augment" or enlarge the breasts is increasingly popular, lactation consultants are likely to have clients who have had this procedure (Figure 9–3). There are two types of breast implants: saline and silicone. Almost all women in the United States undergoing augmentation receive saline-filled implants. Because of public concerns about silicone leaching into the breastmilk, silicone implants can be used only for approved clinical trial research. A current consumer handbook from the Federal Drug Agency that describes problems with silicone implants is available on-line (see the list of Internet resources at the end of this chapter.).

Four techniques are used to enlarge the breasts:

- The infrasubmammary procedure calls for an incision to be made under the breast and for the implant to be placed under the breast tissue. One disadvantage is that the scar is very visible and is easily irritated by a bra.

- In the periareolar technique, an incision is made around the areola-nipple. Although the scar is less visible than in the infrasubmammary procedure, there is often a loss of sensation.

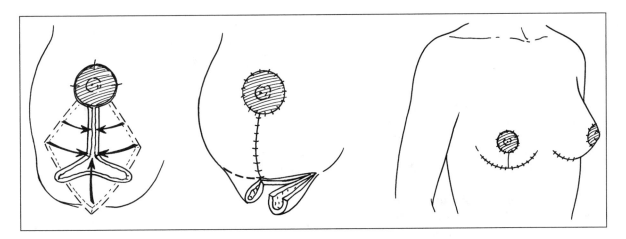

FIGURE 9–2. Breast "lift" or mastopexy. (A) Skin edges pulled together. (B) Excess tissue removed. (C) Postoperative appearance.

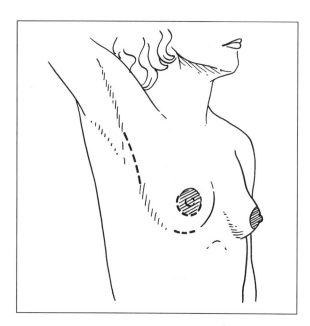

FIGURE 9–3. Breast augmentation. Incision is made through the armpit, underneath the breast, or under the areola.

- The transareolar technique involves an incision made across the areola-nipple area. This procedure is rarely done now. Full lactation is almost always impossible after this procedure, because the glandular tissue, nerve, and blood supply are extensively disrupted. This should be made clear to any woman who contemplates having this procedure.

- An axillary enlargement is done by making an incision underneath the arm and placing the implant below the gland or muscle. Although there are few scars and no interference with breast tissue and lactation, this type of implantation makes breast cancer harder to detect, and there is a possibility of contractures. It is more common for surgeons to place saline implants under the muscle where it interferes less with mammograms (Figure 9–4).

Augmentation has minimal impact on initial breastmilk production but because of the breast implants these women have greater problems with engorgement in the early days after birth. After initial engorgement, breastfeeding may go along well for days or weeks with the infant gaining weight until the rapidly growing baby's demand for milk may exceed the mother's ability to produce. The lactation consultant who works with these mothers needs to inform mothers of the possibility that supplementation may be necessary to ensure continued infant growth.

Women who had previous breast surgery have a greater than threefold risk of lactation insufficiency as compared with women who had not had surgery. Hughes and Owen (1993) interviewed 26 women with augmentation surgery and found that only one third were successful with breastfeeding. Neifert et al. (1990) and Hurst (1996) had similar findings. Women who had periareolar and transareolar incision had greater incidence of lactation insufficiency. Neifert et al. (1990) studied 319 primiparous women who were breastfeeding healthy, full-term infants. The mothers with periareolar incisions were more than four times as likely to have insufficient milk than were those with no breast surgery. Women with breast incisions in other locations had no statistically significant increase in risk compared with those who never had breast surgery. In Hurst's study of 42 women who had augmentation surgery, 64 percent had insufficient lactation. Of the women who had periareolar surgery, none lactated sufficiently, compared with 50 percent who made sufficient milk if they had submaxillary or axillary augmentation (Hurst, 1996).

Why do some women with the "right" type of incision for augmentation still have difficulty lactating? In addition to the type of incision, the pressure of the implant must also be considered. Postpartum breast engorgement can occur despite ductal damage but milk production continues only in part of the breast. Lobes that cannot empty because of severed ducts quickly undergo cellular-wall involution caused by intramammary pressure atrophy, suggesting that increased pressure, when prolonged and unrelieved, can cause an atrophy of the alveolar cellular wall and diminished milk production (Hurst, 1996; Neifert et al., 1990).

It is essential for the health-care provider to discuss the potential impact of surgery on breastmilk production. Some women who have had augmentation surgery become upset that their surgeons did not discuss with them the surgery's negative impact on breastfeeding. These women are also angry with

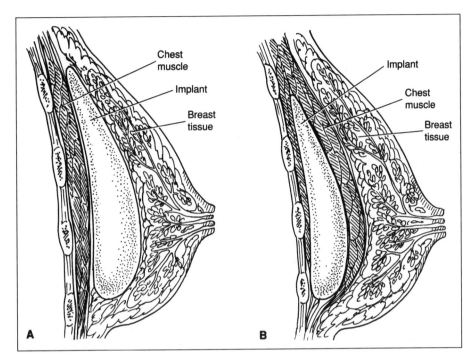

FIGURE 9–4.
Location of breast implant. (A) Implant placed between breast and muscles. (B) Implant placed under muscles.

themselves for proceeding with the surgery without having been completely informed. Because childbearing and lactation were not a priority at the time of breast surgery, many did not ask the surgeon about their future ability to breastfeed (Hughes & Owen, 1993).

Breast Lumps and Surgery

What happens if a breastfeeding mother develops a lump or nodule in her breast? Warnings by the American Cancer Society have made American women keenly aware of breast lumps, and the woman discovering one is usually anxious and perhaps frightened. However, a breast lump in a lactating woman is most often a galactocele, a milk-filled lacteal cyst caused by plugged milk in the ducts (Stevens et al., 1997). A galactocele is usually tender and will atrophy rather rapidly and disappear in a matter of days. To aspirate a cyst, the physician first cleans and anesthetizes the skin, immobilizes the mass with his or her hand and inserts a 20- to 22-gauge needle to draw out fluid. This procedure collapses the cyst and solves the problem. Cysts are almost never malignant. If the lump does

not resolve or reduce in size, the mother should be examined and biopsied. The type of biopsy will depend on the size and palpability of the lump. If a biopsy is necessary, one of the following methods are used (Love, 2000). (In the two types of nonsurgical biopsies where needles are used, a single stitch may be needed to close the incision.)

- A fine-needle biopsy draws out a few cells.
- Larger-gauged hallow needles are used to remove a small piece of the lump (called a core or "tru-cut" biopsy).
- In surgical or "open" biopsies, the surgeon takes out a large piece of the lump or removes it entirely.

Stereotactic biopsy has become standard procedure to excise microcalcifications. In this procedure, the breast is suspended through an opening on the surgical table and a mammogram is performed to locate the exact position of calcifications, which are biopsied.

Most diagnostic procedures are performed on an outpatient basis either in a freestanding ambulatory clinic or in a minor operating room. Using the lowest dosage possible of local anesthetic (usually Lidocaine) and breastfeeding just before the biopsy minimizes the amount of anesthetic the infant might ingest. When the mother resumes breastfeedings depends on her comfort level and the type of procedure used, but she certainly should be able to resume within 12 hours. Although the area will be tender, resuming feedings needs to be weighed against the discomfort of engorgement and listening to the cries of an unhappy child. If breastfeeding is not resumed within 12 hours, the mother should pump her breasts to relieve the intramammary pressure. Too much milk pressure and stasis could lead to undue stress on the surgical site and infection.

Some surgeons prefer that the mother discontinue nursing either completely before the surgery or at least stop feedings from the affected breast. Milk can leak and mix with blood, which makes a "messy" surgery. Love (2000) suggests that if the mother is thinking of weaning anyway, it is probably a good time to do so. Otherwise, the mother should look for another surgeon. One of my graduate students decided to continue breastfeeding after stereotactic biopsy but waited until the evening of the surgery. She made sure that when her daughter latched-on, she was not near the incision site. Despite some leaking of blood-tinged milk from the incision site, the incision healed cleanly and quickly (Forrester, 2001).

Day (1986) described a case in which a woman underwent biopsy of her right breast after suspicious calcifications were found by xeromammography. Biopsy was accomplished with a wedge-shaped resection at the nine o'clock position through a circumareolar skin incision with excellent cosmetic result. The pathology report indicated a benign "fibrocystic" condition. After the delivery of her next baby, the woman's breasts became engorged symmetrically. By the fourth postpartum day, she noted that her right breast remained engorged after breastfeeding, although her left breast seemed relieved of its milk supply. The client subsequently used warm packs, starting feedings on the right side only and using an electric breast pump in efforts to build up her milk supply in the treated breast. At no time was more than 2 ml of milk obtained from the right breast using the electric pump,

despite the mother's having previously breastfed her first child on both breasts.

Many mothers have shared their breastfeeding experiences after breast surgery in La Leche League's publications a rich source of clinical information. One mother (Hart, 1980) had a lump removed as an outpatient. The following day, her breast started swelling with stored milk because her baby had not nursed from that breast. After expressing by hand for 12 days, she began feeding her infant again on the affected breast. Her milk supply in the affected breast returned, though for 2 to 3 days nursing was uncomfortable.

Another woman (Paster, 1986) underwent a breast biopsy under general anesthesia for a lump that was deep within her breast. By 12 hours after the procedure, she was able to nurse on the affected side. Although painful at first, by the second or third day, breastfeeding was quite tolerable. The mother found that putting pressure (splinting) on the dressing helped to allay the feeling that the baby would pull the incision apart. At first, there was some lessening of milk production because about 25 percent of the ducts had been disturbed. Subsequently, the mother nursed another baby without noticing any difference in milk production in the affected breast.

In a third case (Resico, 1990), the nipple was cut during surgery from top to bottom and lifted to remove a golf ball-sized lump. The surgeon suggested that the mother not attempt to breastfeed when she became pregnant, because he thought he had severed milk ducts during surgery. Surprisingly, the mother was able to breastfeed from that breast. This suggests one of two possibilities: either some of the ducts were not actually severed, or it is possible for milk ducts to recanalize after having been severed.

Galactoceles

Galactoceles—milk-filled cysts in the lactating breast—are uncommon. The etiology of galactoceles is not known, but they cause multiple breastfeeding problems. Bevin and Persok (1993) described a case in which a mother had a palpable chronic galactocele behind the left areola for 10 years, during which time she breastfed several children. The left breast was the site of many plugged ducts, breast infections (some requiring antibiotics), and a breast abscess. At various stages, 10 to 20 ml of milky fluid was aspirated, but the lump refilled quickly. No single treatment was helpful. However, on one occasion, antibiotic treatment caused the galactocele to disappear temporarily. Optimal management of a galactocele has yet to be determined.

Fibrocystic Disease

Fibrocystic breast disease (benign breast disorder) is a general term that describes a number of benign breast conditions. It should not be assumed that fibrocystic disease actually refers only to a disorder in those breasts with cysts or nodules; the term is also used to include evidence of hyperplasia, metaplasia, and atypia, among other conditions (Brucker & Scharbo-DeHann, 1991). The American Cancer Society recommends that clinicians use the term fibrocystic changes; nevertheless, health-care insurers commonly use the diagnosis of fibrocystic disease because it guarantees reimbursement.

About half of all women of childbearing age will develop one of these conditions at some point. Years of menstrual cycling will eventually produce dense or fibrous breast tissue. Women usually develop cysts in their thirties. Because of its occurrence rate, the condition is sometimes referred to as a nondisease.

From 50 to 75 percent of all breast biopsies are done because of clinical diagnoses of fibrocystic disease (Norwood, 1989). About one fourth of women with fibrocystic disease develop gross evidence of a cyst or a fibroadenoma, a smooth, round lump that moves around easily when palpated. Fibroadenomas can vary from the size of a pea to the size of a lemon. A needle aspiration helps to confirm the diagnosis. If no fluid can be aspirated, a fibroadenoma is likely. Tissue is sent to the laboratory to confirm the diagnosis. Fibroadenomas are harmless in themselves and, if the woman is lactating, most surgeons choose to delay surgery at least until lactation ceases and the child is completely weaned. In middle-aged or older women, fibroadenomas are usually removed at the time they are diagnosed. A mother with persistent benign breast disease is commonly advised to reduce or eliminate caffeine (coffee, tea, cola, chocolate) and to take vitamin E supplements.

Bleeding from the Breast

Red-tinged, pink, or rusty breastmilk is relatively rare, but it does occur and causes concern because it signals the presence of blood. There are several possible antecedent factors that lead to bleeding in the milk ducts. For example, one mother with severely retracted nipples had painless bleeding from her breasts after wearing breast shells late in pregnancy. After she reduced the wearing time of the shells, the bleeding ceased.

In other cases, the etiology of the bleeding is not so clear. Chele Marmet (1990) has worked with mothers whose milk appears brown or rusty looking, like rusty water emitted from pipes that have not been used for a long while. Hence, she calls it the "rusty-pipe syndrome." This syndrome appears to occur more often in primiparous mothers during the early stages of lactogenesis and is not associated with any discomfort. O'Callaghan (1981) reported 37 cases of this syndrome in the Australian women they followed. Most of these women reported that their breast discharge was either red or brown. Its earliest appearance was during the fourth month of pregnancy and was associated with antenatal breast expression in a little over half of the mothers. Dairy farmers report similar rusty milk from cows calving for the first time and suggest that the reason is slight internal bleeding from edema during the cow's first engorgement.

Bright-red bleeding from the breast in the absence of nipple soreness or cracking indicates that the mother should be assessed for the possibility of an intraductal papilloma. This is a small, benign, wart-like growth on the lining of the duct that bleeds as it erodes. Usually no mass or tumor is palpable, and there may or may not be moderate pain and discomfort. Often the bleeding stops spontaneously without any treatment, but if bleeding continues, the woman should be medically evaluated. She can pump her breasts to maintain lactation (on low setting) until the cause of the bleeding is identified. Cytologic evaluation, mammography, and ultrasound can be useful diagnostic tools in these cases (Berens, 2001). The physician will probably remove it surgically to confirm that it is an intraductal papilloma and not something more serious such as intraductal cancer. In any case, the lactation consultant can reassure the mother that the infant is not harmed by the intake of small amounts of serosanguinous discharge. Larger amounts may lead to the infant regurgitating the blood.

Breast Cancer

Breast cancer is the most common malignancy among women. About one fourth of all women receiving diagnoses of breast cancer are premenopausal and potentially fertile. Breast cancer in lactating women is a clinical issue. New technology detects tiny precancerous calcifications that require further investigation. More women choose to breastfeed now, especially those who become pregnant later in life.

Breastfeeding is one of the few potentially modifiable factors that help to prevent breast cancer. Two recent large meta-analyses (review of many studies) on the effect of breastfeeding on the development of breast cancer concluded that breastfeeding provides a protective function against breast cancer (Bernier et al., 2000; Collaborative Group on Hormonal Factors in Breast Cancer, 2002). These studies suggest that the inverse association between breast cancer and breastfeeding exists mainly among premenopausal women (Yang et al., 1997; Katsouyanni et al., 1996; Newcomb et al., 1994) particularly among those who breastfed for a long time (Katsouyanni et al., 1996; Newcomb et al., 1994; Zheng et al., 2001; United Kingdom National Case-Control Study Group, 1993) and gave birth at an early age (Brinton et al., 1995; Yoo et al., 1992).

For a woman who is at risk for breast cancer, prolonged breastfeeding may at least delay its occurrence before menopause. On the estimates obtained from the Collaborative Group on Hormonal Factors in Breast Cancer (2002), if women in developed countries had 2.5 children on average, but breastfed each child for 6 months longer than current average, about 5 percent of breast cancers would be prevented each year, and about 11 percent of breast cancers might be prevented yearly if each child were breastfed for 12 additional months.

An older study on women in fishing villages near Hong Kong who customarily breastfeed only with the right breast is probably the most dramatic example of the protective effect of breast cancer. These women had a fourfold increased risk of cancer in the unsuckled breast (Ing, Ho, & Petrakis, 1977). Other studies suggest that breastfeeding protects not only premenopausal but also postmenopausal women against breast cancer (Romieu et al., 1996).

Breastfeeding's protective effect may be because it reduces the number of ovulations proportionally to breastfeeding duration and intensity and maintains lower estrogen levels than if the woman was menstruating. In addition, breastfeeding can reduce concentrations of endogenous and exogenous carcinogens present in the ductal and lobular epithelial cells (Helewa, Levesque & Provencher, 2002).

Although lactation has been proven to lower the risk of developing breast cancer, it *does not prevent* the rare woman from having a cancerous lump in her breast while she is breastfeeding. Unfortunately, prognosis of breast cancer found during pregnancy or lactation is less optimistic because of the delay in diagnosis and reluctance to treat patients aggressively (Hoover, 1990; Lethaby et al., 1996; Ribeiro & Palmer, 1977). The delay is due to denial, by both the physician and the mother, that it occurs in pregnant or lactating women. Breast tenderness and lobular hyperplasia hide the tumor and hinder its detection, giving it time to grow and spread. Lactating breasts are very dense (see Chapter 3), rendering mammography or sonography of little value in diagnosis.

Petok (1995) described several cases of breast carcinoma seen in her consulting practice: lobular carcinoma, ductal carcinoma, and inflammatory breast cancer. Most of these women came for treatment of what they called a plugged duct and described a large lump in the breast that had persisted for 1 to 2 weeks. The lumps were 4 to 6 cm in diameter and were irregularly shaped. One mass felt like two firm lumps clustered together. The lumps did not change after feedings or after the usual treatments for a plugged duct (hot compresses, frequent feedings, breast massage, pumping, etc.). Only one woman reported feeling pain at the site of the lump. In one woman, slight redness showed on the side of the breast opposite the lump. The redness lasted only a few days and then disappeared, although the lump did not change. This woman later developed peau d'orange (dimples on the breast similar to those on an orange peel). All of the infants were breastfeeding and gaining weight. None of the infants rejected the cancerous breast, although one did show a preference for the noncancerous breast. After diagnosis of breast cancer, two of the three women weaned their infants before beginning chemotherapy. The third woman continued to breastfeed for four months, despite the objections of her physician, before initiating chemotherapy.

Petok (1995) recommends referring the mother to a physician for evaluation for the following reasons:

- Any mass that shows no decrease in size after 72 hours of treatment

- Afebrile mastitis-like symptoms that are unresolved after a course of antibiotics

- Recurrent mastitis or plugged ducts that appear at the same location

The initial referral is usually to a primary physician, who then refers to a general surgeon. Hesitation to refer out of fear of causing unnecessary concern by mentioning referral to rule out a tumor in a breastfeeding mother is unwise.

One of the myths about breastfeeding and breast cancer is that a baby can receive cancer-causing viral particles in human milk. This is not true: there is no evidence that breastfeeding after treatment for breast cancer carries any health risk to the child (Helewa, Levesque & Provencher, 2002). There is neither an increase nor a decrease in incidence of breast cancer in breastfed daughters of women who have had breast cancer (Michels et al., 2001).

Rejection of the breast without apparent reason may be an early warning sign of breast cancer (Goldsmith, 1974; Hadary, Zidan, & Oren, 1995; Saber, 1996). Although it is true that most of the time an infant rejects the breast for another reason, close surveillance and perhaps also a search for an occult breast carcinoma in the involved breast may enable earlier diagnosis and improved prognosis.

Pregnant women diagnosed with early breast cancer are treated medically, as are nonpregnant women:

- If breast cancer is diagnosed toward the end of pregnancy, the woman will undergo diagnostic procedures, scans, and surgery.

- If the diagnosis is made during lactation, breastfeeding should be interrupted and treatment begun.

- Women receiving chemotherapy for breast cancer or for any other cancer should not breastfeed. All chemotherapeutic drugs cross into the milk. Although levels are low in milk, these compounds are potent antimetabolites, and they are potentially toxic to the infant.

Lactation Following Breast Cancer

Approximately seven percent of fertile women treated for mammary carcinoma subsequently become pregnant, usually within the first 5 years. Their survival rate is the same as for women who were never pregnant (Deemarsky & Semiglazov, 1987; Donegan & Spratt, 1988). Outcome and survival rates are similar for both pregnant and nonpregnant women who are of similar age and disease stage at time of diagnosis.

As long as the woman remains clinically free of cancer, there is no therapeutic benefit in interrupting the pregnancy. If advanced cancer is diagnosed in the first or second trimester, however, treatment often requires that the pregnancy be terminated, because chemotherapy or radiation or hormone therapy places the fetus at risk (Deemarsky & Semiglazov, 1987). Some women who have had a unilateral mastectomy breastfeed after a subsequent pregnancy. The mother should be encouraged to alter her baby's position frequently to provide optimal stimulation to all portions of the breast.

Women who have undergone treatment (surgery, radiation, chemotherapy) for breast cancer and have then become pregnant and given birth report common experiences (David, 1985; Green, 1989; Higgins & Haffty, 1994):

- There is little or no enlargement of the treated breast during pregnancy.

- The ability to lactate and breastfeed from the untreated breast is normal, but there is less likelihood of having a full milk supply from the treated breast and possible absence of lactation.

- Difficulty with latch-on sometimes occurs because the nipple on the breast may not extend as completely as might be expected.

- There is less likelihood of an absence of lactation with a circumareolar incision; lactation from the treated breast is less likely to occur in centrally located lesions (Higgins & Haffty, 1994). The interval from the time of treatment to the time of delivery does not appear to adversely affect lactation from the treated breast.

- Tamoxifen (taken to prevent breast cancer) inhibits milk production (Helewa, Levesque, & Provencher, 2002).

There are a few anecdotal case reports in the literature of women who lactated after breast-conservation surgery and postoperative radiation therapy. Green (1989) reported that a woman who received breast-radiation treatment for an infiltrating ductal carcinoma became pregnant 19 months after the irradiation treatment. After giving birth to a healthy infant, she began breastfeeding. The radiation-treated breast neither enlarged nor produced colostrum. Two days after the untreated breast began leaking milk, the treated breast also leaked milk; however, it never produced the same volume of milk as did the untreated breast, even though the baby suckled from both breasts. Approximately 4 weeks after lactation began, it ceased in the treated breast; however, lactation continued on the untreated side. Vaison and Yahalom (1991) reported a similar finding.

David (1985) also reported the lactation experience of a woman with a history of fibrocystic disease who was treated with radiation therapy for a small mass in the right breast. One year after completion of the radiation therapy, she gave birth to a healthy infant who suckled well from both breasts. The right breast enlarged during pregnancy but not as much as did the left breast. Following the baby's birth, this mother experienced near-normal lactation from the treated breast.

How does radiation therapy affect lactation? A 30-year-old woman received a dose of between 42 and 45 Gy in 20 fractions, followed by a single iridium implant of an additional 20 Gy. Three years later, the mother successfully lactated from both breasts (Rodger, Corbett, & Chetty, 1989). In a survey of radiologists who treated pregnant women with breast cancer, of 53 patients who became pregnant and delivered after radiation, 18 (34 percent) were able to lactate. Although all 18 patients were able to exhibit some level of lactation, only 13 women chose to breastfeed. Of the five who did not breastfeed, three reported insufficient milk as a reason. Of the 18, five described their treated breast as smaller (Tralins, 1995).

Clinical Implications

With abscess drainage, lump removal, or biopsy, there is usually no reason the mother should stop breastfeeding. In fact, irrigating a biopsy wound with the many antimicrobial and antiinflammatory factors in human milk may in fact facilitate healing (Forrester, 2001). Even when a breast abscess is surgically drained, the mother can breastfeed on the unaffected side and possibly on the affected side, if the incision is far enough from the nipple so that the baby's mouth does not touch it when he breastfeeds. After a biopsy, protocol at the Lactation Institute in Los Angeles calls for continued feeding on the affected breast as long as the incision and stitches are dorsal to the nipple and areola and the mother does not find this objectionable (Marmet, 1990). Sometimes, the baby feeds only from the unaffected breast while waiting for the affected breast to heal, and the mother hand-expresses or pumps milk from the affected side.

If the wound is left open to drain, breastfeeding can be "messy," because milk and other body fluids may leak from the ducts for as long as 4 weeks or more. The mother should be prepared to replace soiled dressings with clean pads. Milk leaking from the wound may slow healing. As a result, the mother is at risk for a breast infection or a milk cyst; a low-dose prophylactic antibiotic is sometimes used to avoid infection. A silicone nipple shield with the teat cut off (leaving a doughnut ring of silicone over her nipple) will hold down the bandage and keep the baby's mouth off it. Wounds closer to the nipple-areola and in the lower part of the breast usually take longer to heal. If the problems persist, gradual weaning from the affected side might be necessary while the baby feeds from the unaffected side.

Usually the mother resumes breastfeeding on the affected breast when the drain or stitches are removed and when she can tolerate it. A child's reaction to being prevented from feeding from the affected breast (sometimes his "favorite" breast) varies. Some cooperate without a fuss; others are distraught and actively fight to breastfeed there.

Any woman contemplating breast surgery needs to be fully informed about the procedure and the different techniques that are available. A chart that shows the anatomy and lactation functions of the breast is indispensable for explaining the possible effects of surgery. If the patient is highly motivated to breastfeed, it is the clinician's responsibility to counsel her and suggest techniques that are less disruptive to breastfeeding than are others. If the surgery is very likely to disrupt breastfeeding, that likelihood should be made clear to the woman before the operation. At the same time, it is almost impossible to predict whether breastfeeding will be successful. The necessity of supplements for their babies should be discussed antepartally. If supplements become necessary, a feeding tube could be used, thereby allowing the infant to suckle at the breast while receiving a supplement stimulates the milk production.

Summary

Breast-related problems constitute a substantial proportion of clinical breastfeeding counseling. The overuse of antibiotics that leads to candidiasis, the surge in the popularity of cosmetic breast surgery, and digital mammography are human-made barriers to breastfeeding unique to affluent countries.

Most of what lactation consultants do for their clients is to give of themselves—the therapeutic self. Therefore, when a mother faces surgery or other procedures on her breasts that are painful and that might also potentially alter and or scar her breasts, it is the LC's responsibility to encourage her to talk, to openly express her feelings, and to answer her questions—and perhaps anticipate her unspoken fears—as completely as possible.

Women have the right to be fully informed about any medical procedure, especially a surgical one, because the outcome is apt to be irreversible. Part of the health professional's responsibility is to act as a client advocate. The client should know all options available to her (including the right to refuse surgery) and all probable outcomes before consenting to a medical procedure.

Key Concepts

- Breastfeeding knowledge prevents problems that can be common barriers to breastfeeding.

- A woman's feminine identity is closely related to her breasts. Any changes or issues, including those due to illness, disease, or breastfeeding, hold an emotional significance to her.

- Inverted nipples need not impede breastfeeding provided a mother receives accurate information and assistance in learning effective intervention techniques. The degree of inversion typically lessens as breastfeeding continues.

- Typically, the size and length of nipples varies greatly among women and is genetically influenced. Unusually long nipples can make it difficult for a small infant to breastfeed.

- Some mothers are plagued by recurrent plugged milk ducts while other mothers never experience one. There is no conclusive evidence that shows one particular cause, but it is commonly thought that a constricting bra, poor nutrition, stress, and an inadequately drained breast are contributing factors.

- A plugged milk duct is characterized by a red, tender spot in the breast that is warm to the touch. It is a palpable lump of well-defined margins and occurs close to the surface of the skin or can be located deeper in the breast.

- A breast infection or mastitis may or may not be the result of a plugged duct. It is characterized by the symptoms of a plugged duct, but will include a flulike muscular aching and fever.

- Mastitis is usually treated with a penicillinase-resistant penicillin or a cephalosporin that covers *Staphylococcus aureus* (the bacteria usually present) for 6 to 10 days. Trimethoprim-sulfamethoxazole and erythromycin are used to treat chronic mastitis.

- Breastfeeding mothers can experience unexplained rashes, eczema, and herpes lesions on the breast that are painful and can hinder breastfeeding. Accurate diagnosis and/or use of medications help to resolve the problem.

- *Candida* is a yeast naturally found in the mucous membranes of the gastrointestinal and genitourinary tract. Use of antibiotics promotes an overgrowth that can result in symptoms that include pain in the mother's breast and vagina and symptoms in the baby's mouth and diaper area. Oral and topical antifungal medications are prescribed. Sometimes, the mother's sexual partner will require treatment too.

- A breast vasospasm causes extreme nipple pain and is often referred to as a variation of Raynaud's phenomenon, which affects fingers and toes. Exposure to the cold triggers painful nipple blanching where the nipple can experience a color change from white to blue to red. Treatment includes use of medications to reduce occurrence and topical use of heat to relieve pain.

- A milk blister can cause extreme pain when the epidermis seals over the ductal opening and prevents milk from draining. If it does not resolve naturally, it is possible to manually remove the excess skin to promote healing.

- Breast augmentation and reduction have become common in our society. Breast augmentation is less likely to impede breastfeeding than is breast reduction. Women who have had previous breast surgery have a greater than threefold risk of lactation insufficiency when compared with women who have not had surgery.

- A breast lump in a lactating woman is typically caused by a galactocele, a milk-filled lacteal cyst. Although seldom malignant, a lump that does not resolve itself should be biopsied. After the biopsy, breastfeeding can usually resume within 12 hours.

- In all women, fibrocystic disease accounts for 50 to 75 percent of all breast biopsies. About one fourth of women with fibrocystic disease develop a cyst or a fibroadenoma, a smooth, round lump that moves easily when palpated and is harmless. A needle aspiration will confirm the diagnosis.

- Slight bleeding from the breast occurs in a small percentage of women, typically with their first pregnancy or upon the birth of their baby. The breast discharge can appear pink to dark red or brown. It is painless and if it continues during lactogenesis, it is not harmful for the baby to ingest.

- Bleeding from the breast that appears bright red with no other explanation could be an indication of intraductal papilloma, a small, benign, wart-like growth on the lining of the duct. After medical evaluation, a physician may elect to surgically remove it, to confirm that it is not intraductal cancer.

- About 25 percent of all women who are diagnosed with breast cancer are in their childbearing years. Only 2 to 3 percent of breast cancer is diagnosed during pregnancy and lactation.

- Premenopausal women who breastfed have protective factors from breast cancer based on how many children they have, how long each child was nursed, and the age of the mother when she gave birth.

- Breastfeeding's protective effect may come from a reduction in the number of ovulations and lower estrogen levels. Breastfeeding also reduces the concentration of carcinogens present in the ductal and lobular epithelial cells in the breast.

- Although rare, lactating breasts can develop breast cancer. A prognosis is usually delayed due to the common myth that lactating women do not develop breast cancer. An obvious lump can be simply attributed to a plugged milk duct or a less obvious lump can be difficult to detect due to the composition of the lactating breast.

- A breastfeeding mother who has a lump that does not show change during the normal course of breastfeeding over a 72-hour period should have it evaluated.

- Breastfeeding mothers who suffer from recurring bouts of mastitis or a plugged duct that occurs in the same location should be evaluated.

- A mother diagnosed with breast cancer will not harm her baby by continuing to breastfeed. Although, when chemotherapy begins, the infant must be weaned. All chemotherapeutic drugs cross into the milk and are potentially toxic to the infant.

- Women who have been treated for breast cancer go on to have normal, uneventful pregnancies though lactation in the treated breast may be abnormal.

- After breast surgery, breastfeeding can resume as soon as the mother becomes comfortable with it. Until then, a breast pump can be used to relieve discomfort and to stimulate the milk supply.

- Breast surgery has many implications for a breastfeeding mother and baby. Health-care professionals must provide accurate and realistic information and support for the mother who must contemplate breast surgery. The lactation consultant, in particular, must act as an advocate for the breastfeeding mother and baby as the mother evaluates all possible options available to her.

Internet Resources

Breast surgery information:
www.parentsplace.com

www.breastfeed.com/resources/articles/cosmsurg.htm

www.fda.gov/fdac/departs/2001/601_upd.html

References

Alexander JM, Grant AM, Campbell MJ. Randomised controlled trial of breast shells and Hoffman's exercises for inverted and non-protractile nipples. *Br Med J* 304:1030–32, 1992.

Amir LH. Eczema of the nipple and breast: a case report. *J Hum Lact* 9:173–75, 1993.

———. An audit of mastitis in the emergency department. *J Hum Lact* 15:221–24, 1999.

Amir LH et al. Psychological aspects of nipple pain in lactating women. *J Psychosom Obstet Gynecol* 17:53–58, 1996.

Ashford T. Breastfeeding success after breast reduction. *La Leche League International: New Beginnings.* July/August, 2001:128–31.

Berens PD. *Prenatal, intrapartum, and postpartum support of the lactating mother.* In: Schanler, RJ, ed. *Breastfeeding,* Part II: the management of breastfeeding, *Pediatric Clin No Americal* 48:365–75, 2002.

Bevin TH, Persok CK. Breastfeeding difficulties and a breast abscess associated with a galactocele: a case report. *J Hum Lact* 9:177–78, 1993.

Bernier MO et al. Breastfeeding and risk of breast cancer: a meta-analysis of published studies. *Human Reproduction Update* 6:374–86, 2000.

Binns SE. Light-mediated antifungal activity of echinacea extracts. *Planta Med* 66(3):241–44, 2000.

Brackett VH. Eczema of the nipple/areola area. *J Hum Lact* 4:167–68, 1988.

Brinton LA et al. Breastfeeding and cancer risk. *Cancer Causes Control* 6:199–208, 1995.

Brucker MC, Scharbo-DeHaan M. Breast disease: the role of the nurse-midwife. *J Nurse Midwifery* 36:63–73, 1991.

Brzozowski D et al. Breast-feeding after inferior pedicle reduction mammaplasty. *Plast Reconstru Surg* 105:530–34, 2000.

Buescher ES, Hair PS. Human milk anti-inflammatory component content during acute mastitis. *Cellular Immunology* 210:87–95, 2001.

Buraglio T. Stress and deep breast pain. *New Beginnings* 20(1):9–10, 2003.

Cantlie HB. Treatment of acute puerperal mastitis and breast abscess. *Can Fam Physician* 34:2221–26, 1988.

Chetwynd EM et al. Fluconazole for postpartum Candida mastitis and infant thrush. *J Hum Lact* 18:168–71, 2002.

Collaborative Group on Hormonal Factors in Breast Cancer. Breast cancer and breastfeeding: collaborative re-analysis of individual data from 47 epidemiological studies in 30 countries, including 50,302 women with breast cancer and 96,973 women without the disease. *Lancet* 360:187–95, 2002.

David FC. Lactation following primary radiation therapy for

carcinoma of the breast [letter]. *Int J Radiat Oncol Biol Phys* 11:1425, 1985.

Day TW. Unilateral failure of lactation after breast biopsy. *J Fam Pract* 23:161–62, 1986.

Deemarsky LJ, Semiglazov VF. Cancer of the breast and pregnancy. In: Ariel IM, Cleary JB, eds. *Breast cancer: diagnosis and treatment.* New York: McGraw-Hill, 1987: 475–88.

Donegan WL, Spratt JS. *Cancer of the breast.* Philadelphia: W. B. Saunders, 1988:685–87.

Efrem SEE. Breast abscesses in Nigeria: lactational versus non-lactational. *J R Coll Surg Edinb* 40:25–27, 1995.

Engstrom BL. Women's views of counseling received in connection with breastfeeding after reduction mammaplasty. *J Adv Nursing* 32:1143–51, 2000.

Escott R. Vasospasm of the nipple: another case [letter]. *J Hum Lact* 10:6, 1994.

Fetherston C. Factors influencing the initiation and duration of breastfeeding in a private Western Australian maternity hospital. *Breastfeeding Review* 3:9–14, 1995.

———. Risk factors for lactation mastitis. *J Hum Lact* 14:101–9, 1998.

———. Mastits in lactating women: physiology or pathology? *Breastfeeding Review* 9(1):5–12, 2001.

Filteau SM et al. Milk cyotkines and subclinical breast inflammation in Tansanian women: effect of dietary red palm oil or sunflower oil supplementation. *Immunology* 97:595–600, 1999.

Forrester S. Breastfeeding after breast biopsy. Unpublished manuscript, 2001.

Foxman B, Schwartz K, Looman SJ. Breastfeeding practices and lactation mastitis. *Soc Sci Med* 38:755–61, 1994.

Foxman B et al. Lactation mastitis: occurrence and medical management among 946 breastfeeding women in the United States. *Amer J Epidemiol* 155:103–14, 2002.

Garrison CP. Nipple vasospasm, Raynaud's syndrome and nifedipine. *J Hum Lact* 18:382–85, 2002.

Gibberd GF. Sporadic and epidemic puerperal breast infections. *Am J Obstet Gynecol* 65:1038–41, 1953.

Goldsmith HS. Milk rejection sign of breast cancer. *Am J Surg* 127:280–81, 1974.

Grassley JS. Breast reduction surgery. *AWHONN Lifelines* 6:244–49, 2002.

Green JP. Post-irradiation lactation [letter]. *Int J Radiat Oncol Biol Phys* 17:244, 1989.

Guthrie E et al. Psychosocial status of women requesting breast reduction surgery as compared with a control group of large-breasted women. *J Psychosomatic Research* 45(4):331–39, 1998.

Hadary A, Zidan J, Oren M. The milk-rejection sign and earlier detection of breast cancer. *Harefuah* 128:680–81, 1995.

Hart J. Nursing after breast surgery. *La Leche League News* 22:10, 1980.

Heads J, Higgins LC. Perceptions and correlates of nipple pain. *Breastfeed Rev* 3(2):59–64, 1995.

Helewa M, Levesque P, Provencher D. Breast cancer, pregnancy, and breastfeeding. *J Obstet Gynecol Canada* 111: 164–71, 2002.

Higgins S, Haffty BG. Pregnancy and lactation after breast-conserving therapy for early stage breast cancer. *Cancer* 73:2175–80, 1994.

Hoffman KL, Auerbach KG. Long-term antibiotic prophylaxis for recurrent mastitis. *J Hum Lact* 1:72–75, 1986.

Hoover HC. Breast cancer during pregnancy and lactation. *Surg Clin North Am* 70:1151–63, 1990.

Hughes V, Owen J. Is breast-feeding possible after breast surgery? *MCN* 18:213–17, 1993.

Hurst N. Lactation after augmentation mammoplasty. *Obstet Gynecol* 87:30–34, 1996.

Ing R, Ho JHC, Petrakis NL. Unilateral breast-feeding and breast cancer. *Lancet* 2:124–27, 1977.

Johnstone HA, Marcinak JF. Candidiasis in the breastfeeding mother and infant. *JOGNN* 19:171–73, 1990.

Katsouyanni K et al. A case-control study of lactation and cancer of the breast. *Br J Cancer* 73:814–18, 1996.

La Leche League International. *Treating thrush.* Schaumburg, IL: The League, 2000.

Lawlor-Smith L, Lawlor-Smith C. Vasospasm of the nipple–a manifestation of Raynaud's phenomenon: case reports. *Br Med J* 314:644–45, 1997.

Lawrence RA, Lawrence RM. Breastfeeding: a guide for the medical profession. St. Louis: Mosby, 1999:273.

Lethaby AE et al. Overall survival from breast cancer in women pregnant or lactating at or after diagnosis. Auckland Breast Cancer Study Group. *Int J Cancer* 67:751–55, 1966.

Livingstone V. Problem-solving formula for failure to thrive in breast-fed infants. *Can Fam Phys* 36:1541–45, 1990.

Love SM. *Dr. Susan Love's breast book,* 3rd ed. Cambridge, MA: Perseus Publishing, 2000:95–100.

Marmet C. Breast assessment: a model for evaluating breast structure and function. Presented at: La Leche League International Annual Seminar for Physicians, Boston, July 11–13, 1990.

Marshall DR, Callan PP, Nicholson W. Breastfeeding after reduction mammaplasty. *Br J Plas Surg* 47:167–69, 1994.

Maternal Concepts. 130 N. Public St. Elmwood, WI 54740. Available at: www.maternalconcepts.com. Accessed November 20, 2003.

Menendez-Graino F et al. Galactorrhea after reduction mammaplasty. *Plast Reconstr Surg* 85:645–46, 1990.

Merchant, DJ. Inflammation of the breast. *Obstetrcs and Gynecol Clin No Amer* 29:89–102, 2002.

Michels K et al. Being breastfed in infancy and breast cancer incidence in adult life: results from the Two Nurses' Health Studies. *Am J Epidemiol* 153:275–83, 2001.

Miller V. Personal Communication. June 25, 2003.

Neifert M et al. The influence of breast surgery, breast appearance, and pregnancy-induced breast changes on lactation sufficiency as measured by infant weight gain. *Birth* 17:31–38, 1990.

Newcomb PA et al. Lactation and a reduced risk of premenopausal breast cancer. *N Engl J Med* 330:81–87, 1994.

Newman J, Pitman T. *The ultimate breastfeeding book of answers.* Roseville, CA: Prima Publishing, 2000.

Noble R. Milk under the skin (milk blister)—a simple problem causing other breast conditions. *Breastfeed Rev* 2:118–19, 1991.

Norwood SL. Fibrocystic breast disease. *JOGNN Nursing* 19:116–19, 1989.

O'Callaghan MA. Atypical discharge from the breast during pregnancy and/or lactation. *Aust NZ J Obstet Gynaecol* 21:214–16, 1981.

Oliver WJ et al. Neonatal group B streptococcal disease associated with infected breast milk. *Arch Dis Child Fetal Neonatal Ed* 83:48–49, 2000.

Park HS, Yoon CH, Kim HJ. The prevalence of congenital inverted nipple. *Aesthetic Plast Surg* 23:1446, 1999.

Paster BA. Surgery on the nursing breast. *New Beginnings* 2:92, 1986.

Penny WJ, Lewis MJ. Nifedipine is excreted in human milk. *Eur J Clin Pharmacol* 36:427–28, 1989.

Petok ES. Breast cancer and breastfeeding: five cases. *J Hum Lact* 11:205–9, 1995.

Resico S. Nursing after breast surgery. *New Beginnings* 6:118, 1990.

Ribeiro GG, Palmer MK. Breast carcinoma associated with pregnancy: a clinician's dilemma. *Br Med J* 2:1524–27, 1977.

Riordan J, Nichols F. A descriptive study of lactation mastitis in long-term breastfeeding women. *J Hum Lact* 6:53–58, 1990.

Rodger A, Corbett PJ, Chetty U. Lactation after breast conserving therapy, including radiation therapy, for early breast cancer. *Radiother Oncol* 15:243–44, 1989.

Romieu I et al. Breast cancer and lactation history in Mexican women. *Am J Epidemiol* 143:54–52, 1996.

Saber A. The milk rejection sign: a natural tumor marker. *Am Surg* 62:998–99, 1996.

Smillie CM. Treatment for nipple candidiasis. Personal communication. December 2002.

Smith WL, Erenberg A, Nowak A. Imaging evaluation of the human nipple during breastfeeding. *Am J Dis Child* 142:76–78, 1988.

Soderstrom B. Helping the woman who has had breast surgery: a literature review. *J Hum Lact* 9:169–71, 1993.

Song IC, Hunter JG. Galactorrhea after reduction mammaplasty. *Plast Reconstr Surg* 84:857, 1989.

Souto GC et al. The impact of breast reduction surgery on breastfeeding performance. J *Hum Lact* 19:43–49, 2003.

Stevens K et al. The ultrasound appearances of galactoceles. *Br J Radiol* 70:239–41, 1997.

Tanguay KE, McBean MR, Jain E. Nipple candidiasis among breastfeeding mothers. *Can Fam Phys* 40:1407–13, 1994.

Thomsen AD et al. Course and treatment of milk stasis, noninfectious inflammation of the breast, and infectious mastitis in nursing women. *Am J Obstet Gynecol* 149:492–95, 1985.

Tralins AH. Lactation after conservative breast surgery combined with radiation therapy. *Am J Clin Oncol* 18:40–43, 1995.

United Kingdom National Case-Control Study Group. Breast feeding and risk of breast cancer in young women. *Br Med J* 307:17–20, 1993.

Utter AR. Gentian violet treatment for thrush: can its use cause breastfeeding problems? *J Hum Lact* 6:178–80, 1990.

Vaison G, Yahalom J. Lactation following conservation surgery and radiotherapy for breast cancer. *J Surg Oncol* 46:141–44, 1991.

Vogel A et al. Mastitis in the first year postpartum. *Birth* 26:218–25, 1999.

Wambach KA. Lactation mastitis: a descriptive study. *J Hum Lact* 19:24–34, 2003.

Willumsen JF et al. Subclinical mastitis as a risk factor for mother-infant HIV transmission. *Adv Exp Med Biol* 478:211–23, 2000.

Wilson-Clay B, Hoover K. *The breastfeeding atlas.* Austin, TX: LactNews Press, 2002.

World Health Organization. *Mastitis: causes and management.* Geneva: WHO, 2000.

Yang PS et al. A case-control study of breast cancer in Taiwan—a low-incidence area. *Br J Cancer* 75:752–56, 1997.

Yoo K-Y et al. Independent protective effect of lactation against breast cancer: a case-control study in Japan. *Am J Epidemiol* 135:726–33, 1992.

Zheng T et al. Lactation and breast cancer risk: a case-control study in Connecticut. *Br J Cancer* 84:1472–76, 2001.

Low Intake in the Breastfed Infant: Maternal and Infant Considerations

Nancy G. Powers

Low intake of breastmilk relative to the infant's needs is the common denominator for a number of different clinical end points. There are numerous causes of low intake and in turn numerous outcomes. The complex interrelationship of factors is illustrated in Figures 10–1 and 10–2, which contrast the normal and abnormal situations. Table 10–1 lists various authors' methods of organizing and approaching a conceptual framework for low intake and poor growth in the breastfed infant; however, none of these frameworks are able to encompass the interactions of *all* potential factors.

Infant intake and maternal milk supply are often similar to "the chicken and the egg" problem—which comes first? "Perceived insufficient milk supply" is the erroneous belief that the mother is not producing enough milk for her infant—when in reality she is. However, delayed lactogenesis or perceived insufficient milk creates vulnerability for *actual* low milk supply if supplements are unnecessarily introduced (Chen et al., 1998). If the infant receives a low volume of intake from breastfeeding but receives supplementation, then the infant will gain weight normally, but the mother's milk supply will decline further. The mother will likely be con-

cerned about low supply, but health professionals may dismiss the concern because the infant is growing well.

If the infant does not receive supplementation, low intake will result in weight loss or abnormally slow weight gain *in addition to* low maternal milk supply. Slow weight gain in the breastfed infant is a major concern to both parents and health professionals. When the breastfed infant is not gaining normally, the infant is the "identified patient." However, in order to evaluate the situation, *both mother and infant must be assessed* for their contribution to the breastfeeding relationship. In most cases, by careful history-taking and examination, along with breastfeeding observation, the astute clinician will be able to develop a differential diagnosis for the dyad, which then allows specific management for the individual case.

Factors That Influence Maternal Milk Production

The events of lactogenesis are set in motion by the delivery of the placenta. There is wide individual variation in the rapidity of onset of copious milk

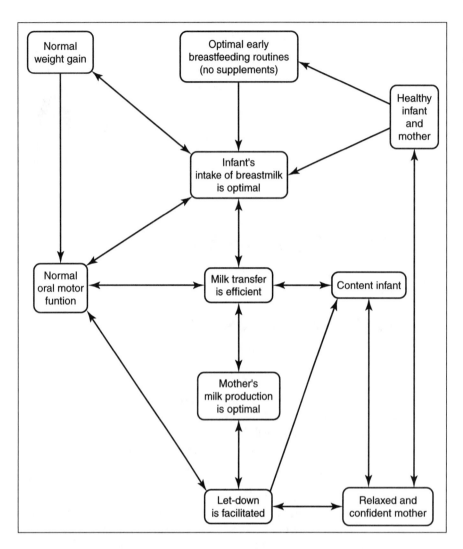

FIGURE 10–1.
Positive cycle of milk Intake and weight gain.

secretion among different women: some women take up to 2 weeks to produce the volume of milk that other women produce on the second or third day. The woman with slower onset of production will likely perceive more difficulties with supply in the early days (Chen et al., 1998), with resultant anxiety and the tendency to provide supplements, which then further limits milk supply. Risk factors for delayed lactogenesis (later than 72 hours after delivery) and supplementation are shown in Box 10–1. This vicious negative cycle becomes difficult to reverse, and continues to spiral downward. In some cases, the milk supply is so low that essentially "relactation" is required (see Chapter 16).

Ongoing milk production is stimulated by milk removal, either by the infant or by some other means of expression, such as pumping (Peaker & Wilde, 1987). In the normal situation, larger birth weight babies stimulate a larger volume of milk production than smaller babies, and the milk supply is primarily "infant driven" (Dewey & Lonnerdal, 1986; Dewey et al., 1991b). In the abnormal situation, the milk supply is not appropriately stimulated, because the infant is not feeding frequently enough, the infant is ineffective at milk removal, or (rarely) the maternal physiology is unable to respond to the stimulation of the suckling infant. The nutritional status of the mother has not been found

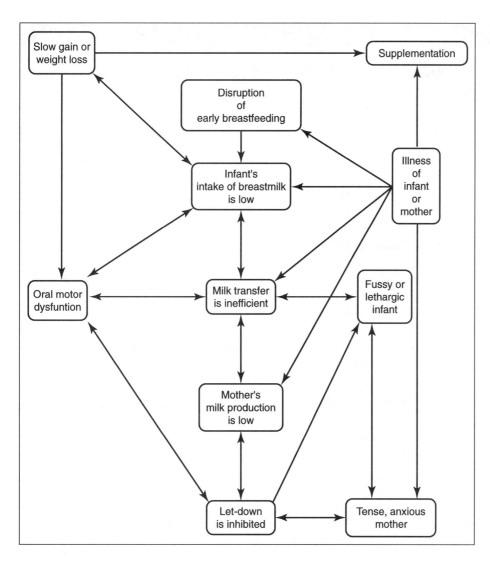

FIGURE 10–2.
Negative cycle of low intake and low milk supply.

to correlate with milk volumes in full lactation. Recently, obesity has been found to be associated with slower onset of lactogenesis (Chen et al., 1998; Chapman & Perez-Escamilla, 1999) and in a higher incidence of early cessation of breastfeeding (Hilson, Rasmussen, & Kjolhede, 1997).

Normal Milk Intake and Rate of Gain

During exclusive breastfeeding, infants around the world consume between 600–900 ml (20–30 oz) of breastmilk per day, with larger infants consuming larger amounts (see Figure 4–2 in Chapter 4). For-

mula-fed infants consume larger volumes of formula than breastfed infants consume of breastmilk, yet activity and growth are similar in the first 3 months.

Most newborns lose weight the first several days following delivery, primarily due to fluid loss as a natural consequence of declining maternal hormones. Weight loss of more than 7% from birth weight may be an indicator of breastfeeding difficulties, and requires observation and evaluation of the breastfeeding process. Weight loss of more than 10% definitely requires intervention from the physician or lactation consultant (Academy of Breastfeeding Medicine, 2001; International Lactation Consultant

Table 10–1

ASSORTED SCHEMA FOR POOR INFANT GROWTH DURING BREASTFEEDING

Scheme	Concepts	Authors
Rate of gain	Slow gain vs. impending failure-to-thrive vs. growth failure	Desmarais & Browne, 1990 Lawrence & Lawrence, 1999
Chronology	Newborn vs. infant 6 weeks to 6 months vs. infant over 6 months	Lukefahr, 1990
Energy balance	Decreased intake vs. increased losses vs. increased metabolic demands	Lawrence & Lawrence, 1999
Behavioral	Content vs. fretful	Davies & Evans, 1978 Habbick & Gerrard, 1984
Etiology	Maternal vs. infant	Lawrence & Lawrence, 1999 Neifert, 1983
Etiology	Primary vs. secondary	Desmarais & Browne, 1990
Etiology	Medical vs. psychosocial/cultural	Lawrence & Lawrence, 1999
Compartmental	Milk production (mother) vs. milk intake (infant) vs. milk transfer (both)	Lawrence & Lawrence, 1999
Occurrence	Common vs. rare	Powers, 1999
Appearance at presentation	Apparently healthy vs. known illness	Powers, 1999

Source: From Powers (1999). Reprinted with permission.

Association, 1999). Return to birth weight is expected by 14 days of age. Once gaining, the average breastfed female infant gains 34 gm/day, while the male gains an average of 40 gm/day. For both genders, the minimum expected gain is 20 gm/day (Nelson et al., 1989) (see Table 10–2).

Low volume of intake leads to low caloric intake, and subsequent compromise in weight gain. Secondarily, gains in length will be compromised, and head circumference is the last measurement to lag due to nutritional deficits. If length begins to lag prior to weight, underlying illness must be suspected and ruled out (see Box 10–2).

The American Academy of Pediatrics indicates the need for early follow-up of the breastfed infant. AAP guidelines state that an infant released from the hospital before 48 hours of age must be seen by a health professional at 3 to 5 days of age, when infant status and maternal milk production are at a critical juncture. Thereafter, the infant should be seen as necessary to reevaluate breastfeeding and monitor weight gain. Once above birth weight and gaining steadily, the baby is seen at routine health supervision intervals.

US Growth Curves

Current Growth Curves Still Underrepresent Breastfeeding

Routine measurements of weight, length (or height), and head circumference are a standard of care for infants and children. These measurements are typically plotted on a growth chart that reflects percentiles for the normal population at a given age. Growth charts that were in use in the United States between 1977 and 2000 (the 1977 National Center for Health Statistics growth charts) created confusion about the growth of many breastfed infants. The NCHS curves were derived from a pop-

BOX 10-1

Risk Factors for Delayed Lactogenesis (Later Than 72 Hours Postpartum)

Maternal Risk Factors

Primiparity (Dewey et al., 2002)

Long duration of labor (Chen et al., 1998, Dewey et al., 2003)

Prolonged duration of Stage II labor (Chapman & Perez-Escamilla, 1999, Dewey et al., 2003)

Maternal exhaustion during labor and delivery (Chen et al., 1998)

Unscheduled C-section (Chen et al., 1998, Dewey et al., 2003)

Overweight or obesity (Chapman & Perez-Escamilla, 1999, Dewey et al., 2003)

Infant Risk Factors

Infant stress (cord blood cortisol and glucose concentrations) (Chen et al., 1998)

Smaller infant size at birth (Chapman & Perez-Escamilla, 1999)

Larger infant size at birth in primiparous women (Dewey et al., 2003)

---

ulation in which the majority of subjects were *never* breastfed in the first 6 months, and few continued any breastfeeding in the second half of the first year. The growth charts, which were revised in 2000 and published by the Centers for Disease Control and Prevention, are reproduced in Figures 10–3 to 10–6 with breasfed infants' data superimposed.

The 2000 CDC growth charts addressed four major concerns with the previous charts: (1) data should be representative of the entire country; (2) data should reflect growth of the *breastfed* infant, since breastfeeding should be our reference for normal babies; (3) birth weights of the sample population should reflect a national distribution of birth weights; and (4) measurements of length must be specified as recumbent length or as standing height (stature). The new CDC growth charts include a cross section of infants and children in five nutritional surveys conducted between 1963 and 1994. Thus, the four major concerns were addressed, as shown in Box 10–3.

However, because the CDC 2000 growth charts still reflect only 50 percent of infants who were ever-breastfed (no information is provided about exclusivity), many breastfeeding authorities still judge the new charts as inadequate for an exclusively breastfed infant (Dewey, 2001) (see Figures 10–3 to 10–6). The World Health Organization (WHO) is currently coordinating a multicenter study at six sites to develop a new set of growth charts based on healthy breastfed infants. They expect the new charts to be ready for release in 2005.

In developing countries, where malnutrition, stunting, and wasting are more common than in the United States, exclusive breastfeeding for 6 months has been associated with optimal growth (World Health Organization, 2001). Faltering of weight or stature in these countries generally reflects inadequate weaning foods, prenatal maternal nutritional deficits, and genetic characteristics of the population (World Health Organization, 2000).

Table 10–2

VARIATIONS OF GROWTH IN THE NEWBORN AND YOUNG INFANT

Parameter	Normal: Follow Clinically	Of Concern: Evaluate Breastfeeding	Abnormal: Evaluate Condition and Breastfeeding
Initial weight loss (percentage below birth weight)	7% or less	Up to 10%	10% or more
Return to birth weight	By 2 weeks of age	Later than 2 weeks of age	Later than 2–3 weeks of age
Average daily weight gain (after return to birth weight)	Females 34 gm Males 40 gm	20–30 gm	Less than 20 gm
Weight loss after immediate newborn period	None		Any amount of unexplained weight loss
Growth curve—weight	Weight may cross percentiles downward *after* 3 months of age	Weight crossing percentiles downward in the first 3 months	Completely flat at any age
Growth curve—length	Length continues on a given percentile	Length crosses percentiles downward (deceleration of *rate* of growth in length)	Completely flat at any age
Growth curve—head circumference	Head size continues on a given percentile	Acceleration or deceleration of rate of growth of head	Crossing of percentiles for several consecutive measurements

Breastfed infants are leaner than formula-fed infants between 4 and 12 months of age. When growth curves do not represent the optimal situation (that is, exclusive breastfeeding for 6 months, with timely addition of complementary foods and continued breastfeeding for a year or more), then the individual plots are subject to misinterpretation. Occasionally, breastfed infants are erroneously characterized as overweight in the first 3 months if their weight exceeds the curves. More commonly, the breastfed infant is *believed* to start faltering at around 3 months of age, when, in reality, the curves are wrong for an exclusively breastfed infant (see again Figures 10–3 to 10–6). When weighing infants, it is important to remember that breastfed infants are, on average, leaner than formula-fed infants between 4 and 12 months of age. Current growth curves do not lend themselves to this interpretation.

Low Intake and Low Milk Supply: Definitions and Incidence of Occurrence

Confusing Terminology and Nonstandardized Research

Terminology surrounding abnormal growth can be confusing. Many texts have different definitions of the term "failure to thrive." Most definitions of poor growth refer to deviations on standard growth charts, which, as discussed above, are not suitable for breastfed infants. Some authors refer to "slow gain" or "growth failure." In clinical practice, the term "failure to thrive" often carries negative connotations that imply poor parenting, neglect, or abuse. For these reasons, we will refer to the guidelines that are presented in Table 10–2 and the growth plots shown in Tables 10–3 and 10–4 as opposed to any of

BOX 10–2

Infant and Maternal Conditions That May Contribute to Low Milk Supply

Infant	Maternal
Allergy	Autoimmune disease
Ankyloglossia	Breast surgery
Biliary atresia	Chronic illness of any type
Cleft lip or palate	Connective tissue disease
CNS abnormality	Eating disorder
Congenital heart disease	Hypopituitarism
Cystic fibrosis	Inverted nipples
Gastrointestinal infections	Polycystic ovary syndrome
Gastrointestinal malformations	Postpartum hemorrhage
Gastroesophageal reflux	Pregnancy
Hypocalcemia	Primary mammary glandular insufficiency
Inborn errors of metabolism	Psychiatric illness
Intestinal malabsorption syndrome	Renal failure
Oral-motor dysfunction (abnormal suck)	Retained placenta
Prematurity	Stress
Renal disease	Theca lutein cyst
Sepsis of the newborn	Thyroid disease
Thyroid disease	
Urinary tract infection	

the above jargon. If the infant falls into the category where concern is warranted, we must thoroughly evaluate the feeding process and intervene when necessary. Watchful waiting at this stage may be inappropriate, because unidentified problems often become more difficult to manage over time as the infant loses weight and the milk supply dwindles.

The Infant's Presentation

Dewey et al. (2003) prospectively studied newborn weight loss in 280 infants. Twelve percent lost 10 percent or more from birth weight. This initial excessive weight loss was correlated with delayed lactogenesis (see Box 10–1). First let us examine the problem of low intake from the perspective of the infant's presentation. Lukefahr (1990) prospectively identified 38 breastfed infants with poor growth during a 4-year period in his private practice. When the infant presented with abnormal growth at over 1 month of age, organic causes were present in 50 percent of cases. Neifert and colleagues (1990) found that 15 percent of firstborn infants gained slowly. None of the infants in their study were identified as having any underlying medical problems. It is difficult to draw conclusions because these three reports have different study designs, represent different patient selection bias, and have different definitions of "insufficient" weight gain.

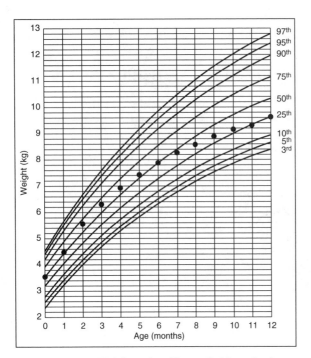

FIGURE 10–3. Weight gain of breastfed boys in the first 12 months, plotted against CDC 2000 growth charts (weight-for-age percentiles). (From Dewey, 2001. Reproduced with permission.)

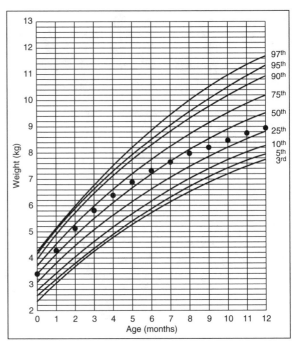

FIGURE 10–4. Weight gain of breastfed girls in the first 12 months, plotted against CDC 2000 growth charts (weight-for-age percentiles). (From Dewey, 2001. Reproduced with permission.)

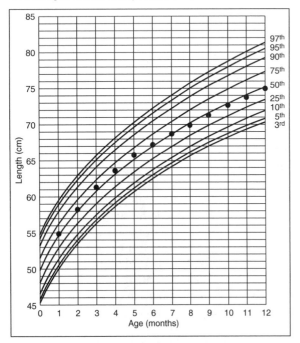

FIGURE 10–5. Growth of breastfed boys in the first 12 months, plotted against CDC 2000 growth charts (length-for-age percentiles). (From Dewey, 2001. Reproduced with permission.)

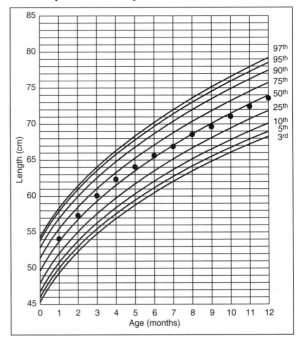

FIGURE 10–6. Growth of breastfed girls in the first 12 months, plotted against CDC 2000 growth charts (length-for-age percentiles). (From Dewey, 2001. Reproduced with permission.)

BOX 10–3

Revised Growth Charts: NCHS 1977 Versus CDC 2000. How Methodologic Concerns Were Addressed

National Center for Health Statistics 1977

Data were not representative of the entire country:
- Gathered between 1929–1975
- All infants were white and middle class
- All infants were from the state of Ohio

Majority of infants were primarily formula-fed:
- Less than 25% of infants were ever-breastfed

Birth weights were not representative of the US population

Disjunction between recumbent length and stature (standing height) for older children:
- A child did not fall in the same percentile for recumbent length as for stature

Centers for Disease Control 2000

Data are more representative of the entire country:
- Gathered between 1963–1994
- Approximately 14% were black
- Different geographic locations were represented

Reflects an average of US breastfeeding rates over the past 30 years:
- Approximately 50% of infants were ever breastfed
- Approximately 25–30% of infants were still breastfed at age 3 months

Birth weights statistically represent more closely the US population (infants with birth weights under 1500 gm are excluded; they require specialized charts)

Recumbent length was concordant with stature (standing height) for older children:
- A child falls on the same percentile if measured for recumbent length or stature

The Mother's Presentation

Approaching the issue of low intake from the maternal side is equally confusing. The definition of insufficient milk is not standardized, and there are numerous confounding variables, biological as well as cultural/psychosocial. There is also the problem of determining a meaningful control group. Selection criteria, study design, and breastfeeding definition are different for each study.

In four studies of self-selected populations of US women who decided to breastfeed exclusively for at least 3 to 4 months, only a small percentage of women were unable to produce enough milk for their infants. Parity was mixed in these studies

(Butte et al., 1984; Dewey et al., 1992; Neville et al., 1988; Stuff & Nichols, 1989). In contrast, one study of primiparous US mothers found 15 percent of women unable to produce "sufficient milk" to accomplish infant weight gain of greater than or equal to 28.5 grams per day after the fifth day of life (Neifert, Secat, DeMarzo, & Young, 1990). This cutoff point is probably too high, as the data from Nelson et al. (1989), discussed earlier, would have predicted 25 percent of normal infants gained less than 23 grams per day. Table 10–3 summarizes the results of these five studies, but caution is urged in interpreting the findings; they serve to illustrate how little data we have, and how definitions can bias study results.

Table 10–3

PERCENTAGE OF WOMEN WITH INSUFFICIENT BREASTMILK IN SELECTED REPORTS

Report	Number Insufficient of Total Number	Percentage
Dewey et al., 1992	1 of 92	1
Neifert et al., 1990	48 of 319	15
Stuff & Nichols, 1989	3 of 58	5
Neville et al., 1988	0 of 13	0
Butte et al., 1984	0 of 45	0

Source: From Powers (1999). Reprinted with permission.

The definition of insufficient milk, for the purposes of this discussion, is as follows: *insufficient breastmilk production to sustain normal infant weight gain despite appropriate feeding routines, maternal motivation to continue breastfeeding, and skilled assistance with breastfeeding problems.*

Abnormal Patterns of Growth: The Baby Who Appears Healthy

Inadequate Weight Gain in the First Month

There is limited data regarding weight loss and gain in exclusively breastfed infants during the first month of life. Dewey et al. (2003) recently published a study of infant weight loss. Twelve percent of the newborns studied lost 10 percent or more from birth weight. At this time, suggested guidelines (Academy of Breastfeeding Medicine, 2001) are as follows: the breastfed infant who loses over 10 percent from birth weight, who does not regain birth weight by 2 weeks of age, or gains less than 20 gm per day (after regaining birth weight) requires thorough medical and breastfeeding evaluation (see Table 10–2 and Tables 10–4 through 10–6). Poor feeding or poor weight gain can be signs of illness and must not be overlooked as a possible cause of

the problem (see again Box 10–2). Yet, in the first month of life, problems with the feeding process are by far a more common cause of poor weight gain than are organic illnesses (Lukefahr, 1990; Neifert, Seacat, & Jobe, 1985). When the clinician encounters a newborn with poor weight gain, detection and correction of the feeding problem should be addressed. Once feeding has improved, ongoing lack of weight gain may indicate illness. Differential diagnosis and management are discussed later in this chapter.

The Near-Term Infant

Infants delivered at 35 to 37 weeks gestation are often managed as though they are full-term infants: they usually weigh over 2500 grams, they have no medical complications, they room-in with their mothers, and they are dismissed early. However, the literature regarding early discharge of newborns points out that these infants are indeed immature. Infants between 35 to 37 weeks have five to ten times the risk for readmission due to poor feeding with resultant weight loss and/or jaundice (Edmonson, Stodddard, & Owens, 1997; Soskolne et al., 1996).

Oral-Motor Dysfunction (Ineffective Suckling)

When breastfed infants are put to breast frequently, yet fail to effectively remove milk, two problems may be responsible (separately or in combination). Either the infant is not attached properly or some form of suckling abnormality is present. The rate and pattern of suckling is flow-dependent: higher suckling rates (nonnutritive) occur with decreased flow of milk (Bowen-Jones, Thomsen, & Drewett, 1982; Glass & Wolfe, 1994). Thus ineffective suckling results in low milk supply and low flow, which further results in less efficient suckling (see again Figure 10–2).

Oral-motor dysfunction is a broad term encompassing abnormal motor tone and/or coordination of infant suck due to a variety of conditions. Oral-motor dysfunction may occur as an isolated and subtle finding in normal infants, often in conjunction with variations in motor tone and/or poor state regulation in the infant. Low-normal tone may result in weak suction and poor coordination, while

TABLE 10–4

HISTORY AND PHYSICAL FOR EVALUATION OF THE BREASTFEEDING DYAD

Infant and Maternal History	Infant Examination	Maternal Examination	Laboratory Tests
• Prenatal risk factors • Previous feeding experiences • Prenatal care • Feeding plan and education		• Prenatal breast exam	
• Perinatal history, especially labor, delivery, and first feeding			
• Medical problems • Medications • Past medical history, especially breast surgery, postpartum hemorrhage, endocrine disorders	• Weight and growth parameters • Vital signs • General physical exam • Neurological exam, especially motor tone • Oral-motor exam (detailed)	• Vital signs • General physical exam • Thyroid exam	• General laboratory tests as indicated; consider thyroid function tests and/or endocrine consultation (prolactin levels are rarely helpful)
• Postnatal feeding and elimination history	• Breastfeeding observation	• Breast and nipple examination • Breastfeeding observation	• Test-weight, if indicated
• Infant temperment and sleep patterns • Maternal sleep, fatigue, appetite	• State transition, self-calming behaviors • General appearance, alertness, attentiveness		
• Family history, especially atopy, diabetes, autoimmune diseases, cancer	• General exam	• General exam	
• Psychosocial history • Use of tobacco, alcohol, drugs	• Mother-infant interaction	• Mother-infant interaction • Signs of milk ejection reflex	• Depression screening or drug testing, if indicated

Source: From Nancy G. Powers, MD. Used with permission of the Academy of Breastfeeding Medicine, 2003.

high-normal tone results in clenching, biting, or vertical compression with the tongue. Infants with isolated oral-motor dysfunction can usually become proficient with at least one feeding method (bottle, cup, or finger-feeding). Oral-motor dysfunction will be an obvious concern when there are significant medical conditions such as neurological abnormality or cleft lip/palate. A variety of other sources (Lawrence & Lawrence, 1999; Glass & Wolfe, 1994; Drane, 1996) provide in-depth discussion of suckling disorders. Unfortunately, much of the research on this topic is based upon observations of infants

TABLE 10–5

INFANT FACTORS: PROBLEM-ORIENTED MANAGEMENT FOR LOW INTAKE/INSUFFICIENT MILK SUPPLY

Etiology	Management
Ankyloglossia (short frenulum, tongue tie)	• Arrange for careful evaluation of tongue function by lactation consultant and/or infant feeding specialist. • Consider frenotomy.
Congenital anomalies	• Express/pump milk to increase mother's production. • Facilitate maternal let-down (relaxation techniques). • Explain to mother that latch-on may be delayed due to baby's condition. • Expand definition of breastfeeding: the use of human milk by whatever feeding method is successful. • Provide consistent skilled assistance with latch-on.
Food allergy	• Follow maternal elimination diet; may take more than 1 week for results. • Arrange for maternal nutrition consultation.
Gastroesophageal reflux	• Evaluate for maternal oversupply. • Increase delivery of hindmilk (see Special Techniques for Management). • Reduce maternal supply, if applicable. • Position baby more upright during feeds. • Burp baby frequently. • Provide medical management as indicated.
Increased caloric demands	• Maximize volumes to 200 ml/kgm/day if possible. • Have the mother collect hindmilk. • Add supplemental calories/nutrients to expressed breastmilk; see "volume restriction" below.
Neurological conditions	• Express/pump milk to increase mother's production. • Use chin/jaw support. • Use supplementer tube or alternative feeding method with expressed mother's milk or formula as needed for weight gain. • Refer to lactation consultant. • Refer to infant feeding specialist.
Oral motor dysfunction	• Increas frequency of feeding. • Express/pump milk to increase mother's production. • Use supplementer tube or alternative feeding method with expressed mother's milk or formula as needed for weight gain. • Refer to lactation consultant. • Refer to infant feeding specialist.
Prematurity, stable infant	• Promote skin-to-skin contact and minimize heat loss. • Use supplementer tube or alternative feeding method with expressed mother's milk, donor milk, or formula as indicated by weight loss/gain.
Volume restriction	• Use supplemental means (commercial fortifier or carbohydrate or lipid) for additional caloric density. • Have the mother collect hindmilk or skim the fat layer from stored expressed milk. Add this fat to additional expressed milk to achieve higher caloric density per given volume (approximately 8–10 calories per ml).

Source: From Powers (1999). Adaped with permission.

Table 10–6

MATERNAL FACTORS: PROBLEM-ORIENTED MANAGEMENT FOR LOW INTAKE/INSUFFICIENT MILK SUPPLY

Etiology	Management
Acute or chronic illnes	• Provide medical management of specific entity.
Attachment difficulties; Nipple pain/trauma; inverted nipples	• Provide consistent skilled assistance with latch-on. • Express (pump) milk 8 times/24 hr.
Breast abnormalities (breast surgery, breast trauma, insufficient glandular development)	• Follow infant weight gain closely the first month. • Use supplementer tube with expressed breastmilk or formula as needed to maintain appropriate weight gain. • Maximize production by proper positioning, frequent feedings, extra pumping.
Disruption of early breastfeeding	• Increase frequency of feedings. • Nurse on both sides for sufficient lengths. • Awaken baby at night for feedings. • Arrange household help and support for mother. • Address sources of pain, anxiety, or stress.
Delayed milk ejection	• Suggest relaxation techniques. • Provide pain relief. • Arrange for household help. • Arrange for support groups or professional counseling.
Hormonal alterations (pregnancy, retained placenta, thyroid disorders, hypopituitarism)	• Continue breastfeeding; tandem nursing is an option after delivery. • Provide medical management of specific entity.
Ineffective milk removal (ineffective baby or pump)	• Review proper position, latch-on and pump function. • Use chin support, if indicated. • Improve milk expression to increase supply. • Consider evaluation by occupational, physical, or speech therapist.
Maternal medications	• Change to medications with similar therapeutic effect, but which will not affect milk supply. • Express (pump) milk 8 times/24 hr.
Nipple shields	• Express/pump milk to increase or maintain supply. • Wean from shield by removing it midfeed, or gradually cutting larger hole in tip.
Psychosocial problems	• Arrange social work involvement.
Substance use/abuse	• Determine whether continued breastfeeding is appropriate.

Source: From Powers (1999). Adapted with permission.

---

on artificial nipples, and their relevance to breastfeeding is uncertain.

Oral-motor dysfunction often presents with maternal nipple trauma and pain as well as with poor weight gain in the infant (see Figures 10–7 and 10–8). Clinically, the infants will remain calm or asleep only when at the breast. Although they appear to be asleep, when taken off the breast they cry hungrily. During active feeding, they will demonstrate a nutritive suck for only a few minutes after the initial letdown, before reverting to the nonnutritive suck. In this circumstance it is frequently difficult to deter-

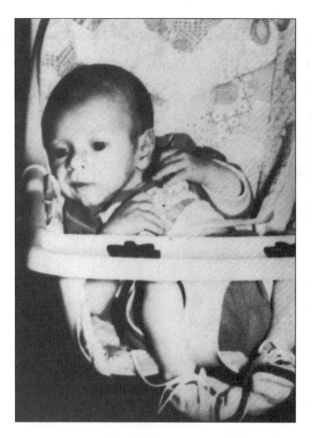

FIGURE 10–7. An infant who had low intake and slow gain at 2 months of age due to oral-motor dysfunction. (With permission of Kathleen Auerbach.)

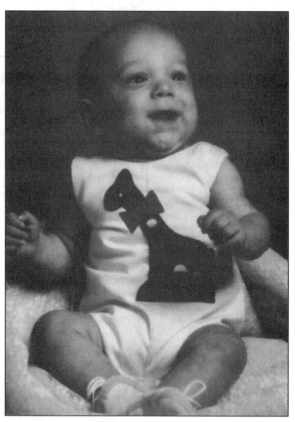

FIGURE 10–8. The same infant as in Figure 10–7 at 4 months of age, following management of low intake and low milk supply. (With permission of Kathleen Auerbach.)

mine whether the initial problem was with the infant or with the mother, but odds favor the infant. In nearly all cases, maternal milk supply is determined by the baby. An assessment of the infant's oral-motor behavior by a lactation consultant or an infant feeding specialist (e.g., an occupational, physical, or speech therapist) is required in this situation.

Gastroesophageal Reflux/Cow Milk Allergy/Oversupply

The fussy breastfed baby may have gastroesophageal reflux disease or cow's milk allergy, or symptoms may be caused by maternal oversupply. Primary care physicians encounter gastroesophageal reflux and/or milk allergy with sufficient frequency that these diagnoses are commonly made.

Sometimes gastroenterologists or allergists have entered the picture. A recent review article states that about half of infants less than 1 year of age with GER have an associated cow's milk allergy. The diagnosis of cow's-milk-induced GER is made on the basis of an elimination diet and challenge (Salvador & Vandenplas, 2002). Even though breastfed infants are less likely than formula-fed infants to have reflux and/or allergy, there are occasional severe cases in the breastfed infant. Cow's milk allergy in the breastfed infant may require a strict elimination diet by the mother, as well as nutrition consultation for both diagnosis and management of this condition. One variation of reflux in the breastfed infant is caused by oversupply of maternal milk, with delivery of high volumes of foremilk. One case report features failure to thrive

Low Intake and Low Milk Supply: A Case Study

Figure 10–7 shows a 6-week-old infant who looked and acted passive. When he went to breast, he immediately closed his eyes and appeared to be asleep; however, he could not be put down because he continually fussed and cried when not held at breast. Birth weight was 7 lb 11 oz (3.5 kg). At 2 weeks of age, the baby was 8% below birth weight, and the physician recommended formula supplementation by bottle. (Note: This is NOT the current recommendation!) The baby returned to birth weight within 1 week. The mother then made the decision to go off of supplementation, but at the 6-week visit the baby was only 6 oz (180 gm) above birth weight. The baby's physical examination did not suggest any physical problems other than weak suck. At this time, referral to a lactation consultant led to supplementation with a feeding-tube device (the amounts were calculated according to Box 10–6). The baby started at 1 oz (30 ml) in the feeding-tube device (at breast) during seven daytime feedings, and breastfed two or three times at night. The infant's appetite quickly increased to 2 oz (60 ml) per feeding (or 14 oz/320 ml per day) for approximately 2 weeks. After catch-up growth, the amount of supplement in the feeding tube gradually declined over the next 2 months. By 4 months of age, the infant was fully breastfeeding without supplementaton, as seen in Figure 10–8. This case was delayed in diagnosis and management. If proper intervention had occurred at 2 weeks, the intervention would probably have been of much shorter duration.

in such an infant who was successfully managed by measures that increased delivery of hindmilk and gradually reduced maternal milk supply (Woolridge & Fisher, 1988). Oversupply with foremilk overload rarely presents in this way with compromised weight gain. The typical scenario for oversupply is a very chubby baby who is fussy/colicky, has very frequent watery or foamy stools (lactose overload), and is fussy during feedings (see Chapter 8).

Nonspecific Neurological Problems

Infant feeding problems with resultant poor weight gain may be the earliest indicator of various neurological problems. Developmental delays and neuromuscular disorders may not become apparent for many months, but subtle abnormalities in motor tone are usually present in infancy, and may present as oral-motor dysfunction (see previous section), with resultant growth problems. In the author's experience, neurologically-based feeding problems are often characterized by disorganized feeding reflexes indicated by choking, brief apnea, or poor pacing of suck-swallow-breathe, and they occur across all feeding methods (breast, bottle, cup, finger-feeding).

Ankyloglossia (Tight Frenulum, Tongue-Tie)

A tight frenulum (Figure 10–9) may create breastfeeding problems such as low intake, low supply, or sore nipples if the frenulum prevents the tongue from coming forward past the lower gum, and prevents the upward mobility of the tip of the tongue that is necessary for peristalsis. Frequently, the infant's tongue will have a "heart shaped" indentation at the tip due to restricted movement. Given time, some of these cases will resolve with apparent stretching of the frenulum. There is limited data regarding the incidence and severity of this condition,

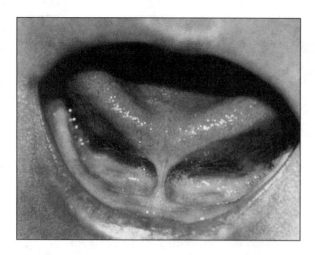

FIGURE 10–9. A tight frenulum, attached at the tip of the tongue and at the alveolar ridge, limiting full motion of the tongue for suckling. (Courtesy of Gregory E. Notestine; with permission of Kathleen Auerbach.)

and its relationship (or lack of relationship) to breastfeeding problems. It is difficult to draw conclusions about the incidence, significance, and proposed treatment of anklyoglossia because of differences in populations and study designs. Tables 10–7 and 10–8 summarize the available reports.

Abnormal Patterns of Growth: The Baby with Obvious Illness

The presence of a known medical complication, such as prematurity, infection, congenital heart disease, trisomy 21, congenital abnormalities, cystic fibrosis, and other health conditions (see again Box 10–2) put the infant at risk for poor growth. These infants often have a combination of increased metabolic demands, low endurance for feeding, and lower growth rates despite close attention to feeding routines (Combs & Marino, 1993; Jones, 1988). Despite the need for increased caloric intake, volume

Table 10–7

STUDY DESIGN, DIAGNOSTIC CRITERIA, AND INCIDENCE OF ANKYLOGLOSSIA IN SELECTED STUDIES

Study Population	Study Design	Diagnostic Criteria	Incidence	Source
2763 breastfeeding newborns in hospital	Prospective sample of all births	Hazelbaker Assessment Tool	3.2% of hospital births who are breastfeeding	Ballard & Auaer, 2002
273 outpatients with breastfeeding problems	Prospective sample of selected population; case study	Hazelbaker Assessment Tool	12.8% of outpatient breastfeeding problems	Ballard & Auaer, 2002
1041 newborns in hospital	Prospective sample of all births; control group of unaffected infants	Clinical diagnosis by study otolaryngologist (no formal criteria)	4.8% of all births	Messner, 2000
2450 newborns with breastfeeding problems identified at age 3–5 days	Prospective case study	All three: heart-shaped tongue, tongue does not cross alveolar ridge, injured nipples	0.015% of study population	Masaitis & Kaempf, 1996

Table 10–8

INTERVENTIONS AND OUTCOMES FOR INFANTS WITH BREASTFEEDING PROBLEMS AND ANKYLOGLOSSIA

Symptoms	Intervention	Outcome	Source
Poor latch or pain	Frenuloplasty performed by pediatrician at 1–12 days of age	100% improved latch and significant immediate pain reduction; no complications	Ballard & Auaer, 2002
Difficulty with breastfeeding (nipple pain lasting longer than 6 weeks or difficulty of latch-on or maintaining latch)	None	25% of affected vs. 3% of controls had breastfeeding problems	Messner, 2000
Difficulty with breastfeeding, categorized by type of abnormal frenulum	None	75% of infants with "thick frenula"; 19% of infants with "thin frenula"; 13% of infants with "notched tongue" had breastfeeding problems	Messner, 2000
Injured nipples or other breastfeeding problem	Frenotomy by otolaryngologist	100% improved range of motion of tongue; breastfeeding improved in 1 day to 3 months; no complications	Masaitis & Kaempf, 1996

restrictions may be necessary. Because such infants particularly benefit from human milk, special assistance must be provided to mothers regarding maintaining milk production while creative efforts are made to get adequate calories into the baby (see the section on special techniques for management at the end of this chapter). The goal is that with improved growth, the infant will eventually nurse completely at the breast.

Maternal Considerations: The Mother Who Appears Healthy

When there have been no previous known risk factors in the perinatal history, perhaps undiscovered risks are present, or some new disease process has arisen since delivery. What factors might be present and relatively asymptomatic except for the disruption of lactation? Box 10–2 lists maternal pathology associated with low milk production/low weight gain.

Delayed Lactogenesis

As mentioned earlier in this chapter, delayed lactogenesis may contribute to early supplementation, and subsequently, to a reduction in ultimate milk supply. (See again Box 10–1, which lists risk factors for delay of lactogenesis.)

Stress

Labor and delivery are stressful events. Chen and colleagues (1998) found that higher degrees of stress were associated with delayed onset of lactogenesis. New mothers also commonly experience a number of physical, social, and/or emotional stresses after delivery, related to the life-changing event of childbirth. These stresses are expected, and should not normally interfere with breastfeeding. Moderate to severe stress has been documented to inhibit oxytocin and subsequently interfere with milk production (see again Figure 10–2). Ruvalcaba (1987) reported some fascinating cases of sudden loss of milk and loss of milk flow in several women living in Mexico City during the 1985 earthquake. However, other mothers have been able to survive extreme circumstances while continuing to breastfeed their infants.

Inverted Nipples

Because inverted nipples can cause difficulty with proper latch-on, milk supply obviously may be adversely affected. Some experts have emphasized the importance of breast examination during the third trimester, with the intent to "treat" inverted nipples with various manual or mechanical methods. One prospective study found 6.7 percent of pregnant nulliparas ($n = 1926$) with at least one inverted or nonprotractile nipple (Alexander, Grant, & Campbell, 1992). This study is the only one performed to assess the efficacy of various treatments. There was no difference in breastfeeding outcomes between women who received treatment versus those who received none. Therefore, prenatal treatment is controversial, but knowledgeable and supportive care after delivery is essential.

Nipple Shields

Nipple shields are devices made of latex or silicon that cover the mother's nipple and areola, providing an artificial nipple for the infant while suckling at the breast. Nipple shields have been used to assist latch-on, to provide temporary relief from sore nipples, or to reduce rapid flow. Initial studies indicated that use of shields impaired milk removal and subsequent milk production. More recent case reports and editorials (Bodley & Powers, 1996; Wilson-Clay, 1996; Pessl, 1996; Sealy, 1996) indicate that knowledgeable professionals

may choose to use a silicone (not latex) shield in selected cases, after weighing the risks versus the benefits of this intervention (see Chapter 7). If a silicone nipple shield is used, the mother should pump extra milk to ensure an adequate milk supply. Eventually, the shield is removed and pumping is discontinued. Close follow-up of weight gain and milk supply are imperative until the shield has been discontinued.

Medications and Substances

In rare situations, maternal medications will impact milk supply. Although individual susceptibility varies, estrogen-containing oral contraceptives often decrease milk supply over several months. Androgen exposure will also reduce milk production. Long-acting or high doses of short-acting thiazide diuretics may suppress lactation (Hale, 2002). Bromocriptine, which reduces prolactin levels, was once used for supression of lactation but is no longer indicated for this purpose.

Several studies have demonstrated the detrimental effects of maternal smoking on milk ejection, milk volumes, infant weight gain, and total duration of breastfeeding (Hopkinson et al., 1992; Horta et al., 1997; Lawrence & Lawrence, 1999). Environmental (second-hand) smoke was shown in one study to be associated with shorter duration of breastfeeding (Horta et al., 1997).

Alcohol inhibits milk ejection in a dose-related fashion (Lawrence & Lawrence, 1999). In an experiment to analyze the effect of smell and taste upon breastmilk ingestion, Mennella (1997) found that infants ingested less breastmilk after their mothers drank an alcoholic beverage.

Hormonal Alterations

Milk production depends upon primary and supporting hormones under normal conditions. Thus, it is not surprising to find that a variety of maternal conditions characterized by hormonal alterations will affect milk supply. Pregnancy superimposed on established lactation or retained placental fragments may decrease milk supply (Lawrence & Lawrence, 1999; Neifert, McDonough, & Neville, 1981). Hormonal characteristics of polycystic ovary syndrome and theca lutein cysts are suspected of inhibiting lactation, probably due to high circulating androgen levels (Hoover, Barbalinardo, & Platia, 2002). Oral contraceptives containing estrogenic compounds will decrease milk production over several months (Hale, 2002).

Postpartum thyroiditis occurs in up to 5 percent of new mothers and may be associated with either hyper- or hypothyroidism (Wilson & Foster, 1992). Lactation experts generally agree that thyroid disorders in lactating women can affect milk supply.

Hypopituitarism (Sheehan's syndrome) following childbirth is a rare occurrence: a previous history of postpartum hemorrhage with significant hypotension causes thrombotic infarction of the anterior pituitary and loss of those hormones. Thus prolactin is not secreted, resulting in failure of lactogenesis (Lawrence & Lawrence, 1999).

Breast Surgery

If a complete medical history has been obtained, the practitioner should have learned of prior breast surgery. However, some women hide this information from their spouse or partner. Others neglect to mention biopsy when asked about any previous surgery. Cosmetic breast surgery may be difficult to detect with routine physical examination. Neifert et al. (1990) published a report that implicated breast surgery as a major risk factor for decreased milk production. Periareolar incision was associated with a fivefold increase in risk of "insufficient milk" as determined by infant weight gain. A second study confirmed these results (Hurst, 1996). Recent surgical techniques for augmentation employ an axillary incision, and placement of implants underneath the pectoral muscle, which minimizes surgical damage to mammary structures and nerves. Many women with breast implants harbor anxiety about potential problems caused by previous breast surgery (especially those with silicone implants). At this time, silicone breast implants are not considered a contraindication to breastfeeding (Hale, 2002).

Another important consideration for patients who have undergone breast augmentation is to take a careful history regarding size, shape, symmetry, and development of the breasts prior to surgery.

Unrecognized "insufficient glandular development of the breast" (see section below) may have been the reason for undergoing augmentation.

Breast reduction always involves disruption of mammary tissue, and breastfeeding outcomes are highly variable. Some reports suggest that leaving a "moderate amount" of mammary tissue attached to the pedicle of the nipple-areolar complex as it is repositioned will improve the chance of successful breastfeeding (Harris, Morris, & Freiberg, 1992; Marshall, Callan, & Nicholson, 1994; Strombeck, 1980). Close individual follow-up is required for the infants of women who have a history of breast surgery.

Insufficient Glandular Development of the Breast

In 1985, Neifert, Seacat, and Jobe reported "insufficient glandular development of the breasts" (sometimes alternatively referred to as "primary lactation failure") of three women. There were several strikingly similar features about these women. They had notable asymmetry of their breasts, and little or no breast changes during pregnancy. They were unable to nourish their infants despite maximum feeding frequency, effective milk removal, and professional breastfeeding assistance. They had normal prolactin levels. For their infants, increasing the frequency of feeding did not result in significant weight gain, and the infants required supplementation. The assumption, based on clinical findings, was that the syndrome is apparently analogous to arrested development of other organs or glands. Neifert et al. (1990) then published results of a prospective study initially designed to determine the frequency of this disorder. More than 400 women were recruited for the study, none of whom had the clinical characteristics of insufficient glandular development of the breast. The study did detect a significant number of women who had experienced breast surgery. Huggins, Petok, and Mireles (2000) published a descriptive report of 34 mothers with breast "hypoplasia." Lukefahr (2002) stated that one of the 38 mother/infant pairs in his report fit the clinical criteria for insufficient glandular development of the breast. Based upon

Neifert et al.'s (1990) study and the experience of various lactation centers, it appears that approximately 1 out of 1000 (0.01%) of lactating women may have this clinical syndrome.

Psychosocial Factors

Some women do not want to breastfeed but are being pressured to do so by a family member: breastfeeding rarely goes well under these circumstances. Classic psychosocial failure to thrive (the result of emotional/physical neglect or abuse) is rarely seen in the breastfed infant, but it does occur. Parental drug or alcohol abuse or domestic violence may be a factor in some of these cases. Moderate to severe postpartum depression may result in excessive anxiety about the baby, alienation of the mother from her infant, and occasionally in overt abuse (Wisner, Parry, & Piontek, 2002). Two cases of Munchausen syndrome by proxy have been reported in which the infant received ipecac in expressed maternal breast milk (Berkner, Kastner, & Skolnick, 1988; Sutphen & Saulsbury, 1988). Hypothyroidism must be considered in the differential diagnosis of maternal depression, and postpartum psychosis is often a manifestation of bipolar disorder (Wisner, Parry, & Piontek, 2002).

Maternal Nutrition

Several studies show no significant relationship between reduced maternal intake of calories/fluids and the volume of milk produced. Poor maternal nutrition will decrease birth weight of the infant, and smaller infants stimulate lower volumes of milk production (Institute of Medicine, 1991). The lactating woman needs to maintain good nutritional status for her own health as well as for future pregnancies. Rapid weight loss in well-nourished women requires further study to determine effects on milk volume, and much current research is focused on the effects of overweight and obesity upon lactation performance (see again Box 10–1) (Chapman & Perez-Escamilla, 1999; Hilson, Rasmussen, & Kjolhede, 1997; Dewey et al., 2003). Obviously, a woman with an eating disorder presents nutritional and psychosocial risks to the mother-infant relationship.

Maternal Considerations: Obvious Illness

Acute illnesses may temporarily decrease milk supply, but production should rebound after the initial insult, especially in full lactation. Insulin-dependent diabetes mellitus was associated with delayed lactogenesis in one small study (Neubauer et al., 1993). Occasionally, mastitis will reduce milk secretion in the affected breast for the duration of lactation. The ability of women with other chronic illnesses to breastfeed depends upon their general condition (energy level, nutritional status, motor abilities) and the medications that they are required to take. There is currently no information regarding the effect of specific illnesses upon volume of milk production. Each case must be assessed and managed individually.

History, Physical Exam, and Differential Diagnosis

History

A complete history and physical exam for both mother and infant are critical to the evaluation of low intake/insufficient milk (see again Table 10–5; see also Chapter 20). Perinatal history includes prenatal risk factors, labor and delivery, medications, interventions, and any resuscitation efforts. A complete feeding history reviews a mother's previous feeding experiences, her feeding plan for this infant, the first feeding experience after delivery, and subsequent feeding difficulties or breast problems. Maternal past medical history and review of systems must include current routine medications, history of breast surgery, postpartum hemorrhage (risk for panhypopituitarism), or endocrine disorders. Family history and psychosocial history may also provide clues to slow weight gain due to familial conditions or family stress.

Physical Examination

Physical examination for the mother is focused on areas of concern: vital signs, general skin condition, breasts, nipples, thyroid, and any other area suggested by careful history. A complete physical examination of the infant includes vital signs, weight, length, head circumference, and general examination with close attention to subtle neurological features (see Chapter 20).

A multidisciplinary approach is recommended, with input from the primary care provider (family physician, obstetrician, pediatrician, midwife) and lactation consultant. In some programs with formal feeding teams, a pediatric developmental team (developmental pediatrician, speech pathologist, occupational and physical therapists), a pediatric gastroenterologist, or a pediatric allergist may comprise part of the feeding evaluation. Selective use of laboratory tests may be helpful. Postpartum maternal thyroid disease is relatively common and may be asymptomatic aside from low milk production. However, prolactin levels do not correlate with volume of milk production and are rarely helpful.

Differential Diagnosis

After history and physical examinations have been completed, a differential diagnosis may be developed. Potential etiologies that can ultimately lead to a problem-oriented approach to management can be identified (see again Tables 10–5 and 10–6). Specific management suggestions are also included in the tables, to assist with individualizing the treatment guidelines given below.

Clinical Management

Determining the Need for Supplementation

Many cases of slow weight gain in the breastfed infant will require a decision regarding "supplementation"—a term that is frequently used but rarely defined in relationship to breastfeeding. For the purposes of this chapter, and specifically for the management guidelines below, the term will be used to indicate the practice of giving the breastfed infant additional nutriment other than what he obtains directly from the breast. Supplementation may also include additional nutrients to in-crease the caloric density of human milk feedings (e.g., human milk fortifier). There are two important facets of supplementation to keep in mind: (1) the choice of type of supplement, and (2) the choice of method for supplementation. Management guidelines in this chapter imply a hierarchy of preferences for type and method of supplementation. First choice for type of supplement is the mother's own expressed milk; pasteurized donor breastmilk (if indicated and if available) is the second choice; commercially-prepared infant formula is the third choice. First choice for method of supplementation is supplementer tube, if applicable (see Figures 10–10 and 10–11). Cup (Howard et al., 1999), syringe, spoon, and bottle-feedings provide other options, depending upon the specific circumstances of the case. Effective maternal milk expression (or pumping) is a mainstay for women who are supplementing their infants. This is best accomplished by professional electric pump or skilled hand expression (see Chapters 7 and 12 for information on breastmilk expression).

Intervention

The following management guidelines are suggested for a general approach to the slow-gaining baby. Figure 10–12 provides a flowchart of the general approach. Despite general recommendations, individualized management is required. (See again Tables 10–5 and 10–6, which give additional suggestions in this regard.)

1. Increase the frequency, duration, and effectiveness of feedings at the breast, if these factors are not optimal, and if the infant is alert and hungry. "Alternate breast massage" and "switch nursing" may be used, if the infant is suckling actively during feedings. (See the section on special techniques for management of low intake or low supply later in this chapter.)

2. Have mother express breastmilk between feedings to increase her milk supply (see Box 10–5).

3. If the infant is clinically stable and exhibiting hunger cues, suggest optional supplementation with expressed breastmilk. If immediate sup-

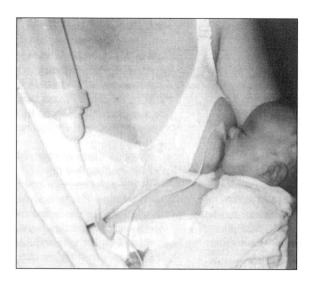

FIGURE 10–10. A mother and infant utilize a commercial feeding-tube device in order to deliver extra milk to the infant while the mother is able to feed the infant at breast and gradually increase her milk supply. (From Powers & Slusser, 1997. Reproduced with permission.)

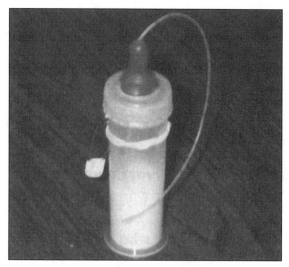

FIGURE 10–11. A homemade feeding-tube device can be made from supplies found in an office or hospital: a small bottle with slit nipple has a no. 5 French feeding tube threaded through the nipple with the hub resting in the milk; a rubber band and safety pin allow attachment of the device to the mother's clothing. (From Powers & Slusser, 1997. Reproduced with permission.)

plementation is indicated by the criteria listed in Table 10–2 or by the clinical condition of the infant, use expressed breastmilk (or another alternative) to supplement the infant during or after breastfeeding.

4. Begin with a minimum of 50 ml/kgm/24 hr, divided into 6 to 8 feedings (see Box 10–6).

5. Increase the amount of supplement as indicated by infant appetite.

6. See other specific management suggestions in Tables 10–5 and 10–6.

7. Monitor and follow-up infants under 3 months as follows:

   a. Monitor infant weight closely, every 2 to 4 days.

   b. Verify that weight stabilizes within 2 to 4 days.

   c. Verify that weight gain begins within 7 days.

   d. After 7 days, verify that the infant is gaining at least 20 gm/day.

   e. Once weight gain averages 20 gm/day or more, recheck weekly until infant establishes himself on a consistent growth curve.

8. If maternal milk supply has not increased within 1 week, do the following:

   a. Check the frequency of milk expression.

   b. Reevaluate maternal risk factors.

   c. Consider laboratory evaluation (especially maternal thyroid) as indicated.

   d. If maternal factors are involved, manage as indicated.

   e. Consider use of a galactagogue.

   f. If maternal evaluation is negative, reevaluate the infant.

9. If the infant does not gain weight as expected, consider the following:

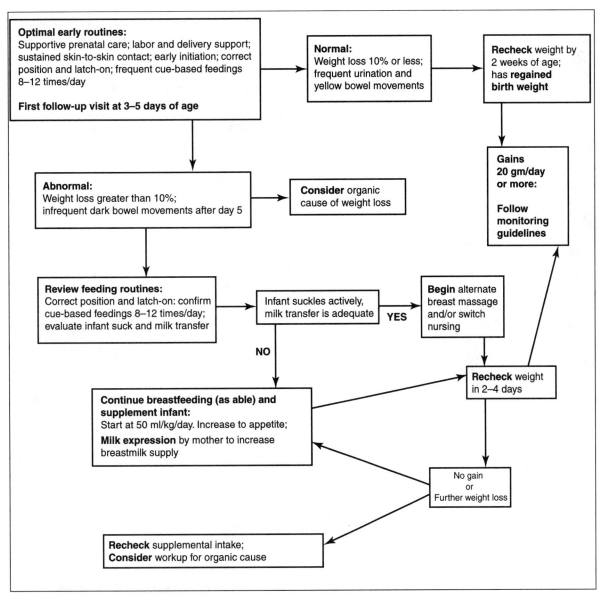

FIGURE 10–12. Flowchart for assessment and management of newborn weight loss. (Used with permission of the Academy of Breastfeeding Medicine, 2003.)

a. Verify that the infant is receiving the prescribed amount of supplemental feedings. Review specific amounts with the mother and ask her to keep written records.

b. Determine whether the infant is willing to take the minimal amount of supplementation that is recommended. If not, strongly consider an organic illness or neurological problem.

c. If the infant is actually ingesting the prescribed amount of supplement and still not gaining weight, evaluate the infant for illness or neurological problems.

d. Arrange for lab tests as indicated.

BOX 10–5

Measures That Encourage Increased Milk Production

- Apply moist heat to breasts a few minutes before feeding.
- Massage the breasts before and during feeding or pumping.
- Use relaxation techniques to reduce stress and enhance let-down.
- Feed your baby or express milk at least 8 times every 24 hours.
- Continue frequent milk removal, even if small amounts are obtained.

---

e. Treat infant illness as indicated.

f. If the recommendations above are not effective and medical work-up is underway, consider using special techniques that are discussed in the next section.

Reducing the Amount of Supplementation

As the mother's own milk production increases, the amount of other types of supplements (e.g., infant formula) will be reduced in favor of expressed breastmilk. Once maternal milk supply increases, the infant takes more milk directly from the breast and less milk by supplementary methods (infant appetite/satiety will determine this change). After the infant has attained a normal weight for age, the amount of supplementation may be reduced gradually to "stimulate" more milk production. This depends upon an increased frequency of breastfeeding

as well as the infant being effective at milk removal. Continue to monitor weight gain while supplementation is reduced or withdrawn.

Family and Peer Support

Verbal, emotional, and physical supports are very important for a mother who is stressed by a significant feeding problem. In addition to support from family members, new mothers may find peer support in the community by checking with their physician, hospital of delivery, or the Internet.

When Maternal Milk Supply Does Not Increase

Most women who seek professional help with breastfeeding are highly motivated to breastfeed their infant. Sometimes, despite appropriate intervention and conscientious attempts by the mother to follow the suggested treatment plan, her milk supply does not increase enough to fully meet the infant's needs. In some cases, her milk supply will remain at a minimal level or "dry up" completely. In these situations, the practitioner must acknowledge the emotional impact of this "failure" upon the maternal psyche: a grief reaction is common. It is often helpful for the mother to be able to talk openly with the health-care provider or a close family member regarding her loss. If possible, they should reassure her that she did everything in her power to rectify the situation. As in any other grief situation, the passage of time will allow some degree of healing.

Special Techniques for Management of Low Intake or Low Supply

Breast Massage

Breast massage during feeding, discussed in Chapter 7, is a simple method of increasing volume and fat content of the breastmilk.

Switch Nursing

In normal breastfeeding, the baby is allowed to finish one breast before the mother switches to the other side. Infant-led feeding usually results in optimal intake (Woolridge, Ingram, & Baum, 1990). For the infant who spends a large part of the feeding in a "nonnutritive" sucking pattern and is gaining weight slowly, the technique of switch nursing may be considered. This involves changing the baby frequently from breast to breast to facilitate more active swallowing and promote multiple letdowns during the feeding. The mother is taught to observe for a change from nutritive to nonnutritive suckling. At that point, she switches the infant to the other breast, and when nonnutritive sucking is again apparent, switches back. This pattern is repeated several times during a feeding. Switch nursing is not useful if the baby has low endurance (due to prematurity, illness, or weight loss) or oral-motor dysfunction with an ineffective suck.

Feeding-Tube Device

The infant can receive supplementation at the same time that he is suckling from the breast by use of a feeding-tube device which can be purchased commercially or constructed with syringes and feeding tubes (see again Figures 10–10 and 10–11). This technique provides extra volume of intake for the infant while continuing to stimulate the maternal milk supply and avoiding the potential risk of bottle preference. A feeding-tube device works well for young infants who have plenty of energy and good sucking ability but for whom the maternal milk supply has not been adequate. The mother must be carefully instructed regarding the use and cleaning of such a device (see Boxes 10–6 and 10–7).

BOX 10–6

Amount of Supplement to Use in a Feeding-Tube Device

If a feeding-tube device is used to assist the baby in gaining weight, both the caregiver and the mother need to know how much supplement to give the infant. A general rule of thumb for *normal total intake* is 150 to 200 ml/kgm/day of breastmilk or formula. Even if gaining slowly, most breastfed infants are getting *some* breastmilk from the breast, so we supplement with an amount that represents *partial* intake. Unless we use test weights, we will not know exactly how much the infant is receiving at the breast. A simple guideline is to begin with a minimum of 50 ml/kgm/day divided into 6 to 8 feedings. The table below gives some approximate guidelines per feeding. Once supplementation has started, the amounts can be increased according to infant appetite and weight gain.

Infant Weight: Kg (lb)	Total Daily Intake: 150–200 ml/kgm/day (oz per day)	Daily Supplement: 50 ml/kgm/day (oz per day)	Per Feeding Supplement 6–8 times/day: ml per feeding (oz per feeding)
2.5 kg (5 lb 8 oz)	375–500 ml (12.5–17 oz)	125 ml (4 oz)	15–20 ml (.25–.5 oz)
3.0 kg (6 lb 9 oz)	450–600 ml (15–20 oz)	150 ml (5 oz)	20–30 ml
3.5 kg (7 lb 11 oz)	525–700 ml (17.5–23 oz)	175 ml (5.5 oz)	20–30 ml (.5–1 oz)
4.0 kg (8 lb 12 oz)	600–800 ml (20–27 oz)	200 ml (7 oz)	25–35 ml (1 oz)
5.0 kg (11 lb)	750–1000 ml (25–33 oz)	250 ml (8 oz)	30–40 ml (1–1.5 oz)

BOX 10–7

Guidelines for Using a Feeding-Tube Device

1. Begin using the device when the mother and baby are most rested and when other household or family activities are unlikely to require her attention. Use will become easier with practice.

2. Refer to Box 10–6 to estimate the amount of supplement to put into the feeding-tube device. Note that most babies will take less volume per feeding in the feeding-tube device than they would from a bottle feeding.

3. Prepare the feeding and begin the feeding process before the baby becomes overly hungry or fussy. Both mother and baby should be as relaxed as possible.

4. Fill the device and position the tubing so that it extends slightly past the end of the mother's nipple. Use any kind of hypoallergenic tape to hold the tubing in place. If the baby appears to be sucking only on the end of the tubing, pull it back so that it is flush with the end of the mother's nipple.

5. Look for the appearance of air bubbles in the reservoir. This indicates that the baby is actively swallowing.

6. Be aware that most babies will take most of the fluid in the device within the first 30 minutes. Different size tubes (to increase or decrease flow) are available with some commercial devices.

7. If the baby is actively suckling but the device is flowing very slowly or not at all, look for several potential problems:

   a. The tube may be kinked so as to block the flow. Check the tubing from bottle cap to baby's mouth.

   b. The tube may be blocked inside the baby's mouth by improper placement or kinking back on itself. Re-latch the baby.

   c. The feeding-tube device may have developed a vacuum. Release the unused tube, or "prime" the device by pushing on the reservoir.

   d. The cap may be screwed on too tightly, blocking the flow. Loosen the cap and squeeze the container gently to activate the flow. If the device is working properly, there should be a steady drip from the end of the tubing.

   e. If *formula mixed from powder* is used in the device, small clumps of unmixed formula may block the tubing. Clean the tubing with hot soapy water pushed through with a syringe.

   f. The tubing was not properly cleaned and is blocked by old supplement. Try to clean the tubing again using hot soapy water pushed through with a syringe.

8. Clean the feeding-tube device soon after the feeding is finished (refer to manufacturers' instructions). The small diameter of the tubing is easily blocked.

Test Weighing

Infant test weighing has become widespread, though few practitioners understand its limitations (see Boxes 10–8 and 10–9). Test weighing involves the use of a sensitive scale (sensitivity of 2 gm or less) with digital readout and computerized integration to account for infant movement. The infant is weighed before and after feeding to determine the amount of breastmilk ingested. Weight gain in grams is approximately equal to the intake of the infant in milliliters (Woolridge et al., 1984). Test weighing on a regular office scale is not reliable and should not be done (Whitfield, Kay, & Stevens, 1981).

Test weighing should primarily be used as a research tool, because normal infants have large feed-to-feed variability. Test weighing during one feeding does not offer an adequate representation of an "average" feeding or allow calculation of overall intake (Woolridge et al., 1984). In complicated situations where infant growth is of concern, test weighing may be used at each feeding to determine the need for supplementation (Meier et al., 1990). When test weighing is used for management of individual cases, it is crucial to have an electronic scale and to use the proper protocol with each weight, and for caretakers to keep detailed records of weights and feedings. (See Box 10–9 for a sample procedure for performing infant test weights.)

Galactagogues

Galactagogues are agents that promote milk production, such as drugs, herbs, or foods. Metoclopramide (Reglan) is indicated in selected cases, when all other aspects of milk production have been maximized. The recommended dose is 10 mg three times a day for 7 to 14 days (Ehrenkranz & Ackerman, 1986; Gupta & Gupta, 1985; Kauppila et al., 1985). Prescribing metoclopramide as a galactogogue is an "off label" use of the drug. Small amounts of the drug enter into the milk but have not been associated with clinical effects in the infant (Ehrenkranz & Ackerman, 1986; Gupta & Gupta, 1985; Kauppila et al., 1985). Maternal side effects of this drug include dizziness, nausea, sweating, and agitated depression. If depression occurs, the drug must be discontinued immediately, and symptoms typically resolve within one week.

Domperidone, though not commercially available in the United States, is used as a galactagogue in other countries. The mechanism of action is similar to metoclopramide, but the advantage of domperidone is the lack of CNS side effects. Some physicians in the United States will arrange to have domperidone specially compounded for use as a galactogogue, though the cost may be prohibitive (Hale, 2002).

BOX 10–8

Principles of Test Weighing an Infant

- The scale must be accurate to 2 gm or less, with computer integration for movement and a digital read-out.
- The infant must be weighed before and after every feeding for several days to get representative values.
- Infant intake in ml is approximately equal to infant weight gain in grams.
- The typical office scale is not accurate or reliable for test weighing.
- Test weighing may be used in complicated clinical situations to monitor intake and/or adjust volume of supplementation.

Source: From Woolridge et al. (1984); Whitfield, Kay, & Stevens (1981).

BOX 10–9

Procedure for Infant Test Weighing

Definition of test weighing: Weighing a baby before and after breastfeeding to determine intake.

Equipment: Digital scale with integration function that allows for movement of the infant, accurate to 2 gm (for example, Olympic Smart Scale or Medela Baby Weigh Scale).

Procedure:

- Before breastfeeding, place baby on the scale and weigh him. This is the "before" weight. It is fine to have clothing or a blanket but the final weighing must be done with exactly the same clothing and accessories as the initial weighing.
- Mother breastfeeds the infant. Do not change diaper yet.
- Reweigh the infant, with the exact same clothes, diaper, blanket, burp cloth, etc. This is the "after" weight. (It is possible to weigh before and after each breast, if the information is useful.)
- Subtract the first (before) weight from the second (after) weight. The difference in grams is considered the "intake" in milli-

liters. (Some scales automatically store the values and compute the difference for you. Refer to manufacturers' instructions).

- If the "after" weight is smaller than the "before" weight, this means the baby has lost weight—which is possible. It also might mean that you forgot a blanket on the second weighing or that someone changed the diaper and removed weight.
- Burp cloth or clothing with any drool or emesis shall be included with the weight, to reflect original intake. (Record emesis in documentation of output.)
- If the infant receives a tube feeding at the same time as breastfeeding, subtract the amount given via tube to determine the amount of breastmilk ingested directly by breastfeeding.
- Record the intake of breastmilk and any supplement volumes.
- Parents can be taught to perform test-weights for the hospital or home setting. This allows them to start a feeding without waiting for a nurse to come and perform the test weights.

Though not strictly a galactagogue, oxytocin nasal spray (40 IU per ml) is used to stimulate milk ejection if mother's own let-down is inhibited by stress or pain. Oxytocin nasal spray is not commercially available, but like domperidone, may be specially compounded by selected pharmacies (Hale, 2002). Foods and herbs are used in many cultures to increase milk supply. Brewer's yeast and fenugreek have a long history as galactagogues, but only one abstract is available for fenugreek (Swafford & Berens, 2000) and no studies were found for brewer's yeast.

Hindmilk

Hindmilk refers to breastmilk that is obtained toward the end of the feeding episode as contrasted with the initial milk, called "foremilk." Fat content varies considerably from feed to feed, but within a given feeding, it rises steadily. There is no specific "cutoff" time for this definition, nor any specific fat percentage. The concept of foremilk and hindmilk imbalance is an artificial construct used for dyads when maternal production is significantly higher than infant intake. For example, a mother may be

BOX10–10

Patient Instructions: Hindmilk Collection

Hindmilk has been recommended for your baby in order to improve weight gain. When you start to breastfeed, there is a small amount of milk ready for your baby. Called "foremilk," this is the low-fat part of the feeding. As breastfeeding progresses, breastmilk contains more fat, and this later milk is called "hindmilk." Since hindmilk has more fat, it also has more calories than foremilk. Both foremilk and hindmilk are nutritious, so the use of hindmilk is a temporary measure. In order to obtain hindmilk, your current 24-hour milk production must be greater than the baby's 24-hour intake. To collect hindmilk for your baby, follow these guidelines:

- Review the general guidelines for breast pumping.
- Have containers ready, labeled "foremilk" and "hindmilk" (along with name and date).
- Pump for 2 to 3 minutes after the milk begins to flow.
- Stop pumping and save this milk, which should be labeled "foremilk."
- Continue pumping as usual.
- Put this milk into containers labeled "hindmilk."
- Use the containers of hindmilk for your baby until further notice.
- The foremilk may be stored in your home freezer for later use when the baby is older.

pumping 30 oz (900 ml) per day for a premature infant who is ingesting only 7 oz (210 ml) per day. If the infant is feeding at the breast, delivery of hindmilk may be increased by unlimited nursing on the first breast and/or by massage of the breast during feeding. If the mother is expressing milk for her infant, and has a generous supply (e.g., for a preterm or cardiac baby), she can fractionate her expressed milk by pumping 2 to 3 minutes after let-down (foremilk) and changing containers to finish pumping (hindmilk) and use hindmilk to feed the baby (Valentine, Hurst, & Schanler, 1994). A sample of patient instructions is presented in Box 10–10. Very low birth weight infants who receive fortified breast milk must also receive fortification in hindmilk.

Summary

Low intake of breastmilk in the breastfed infant and low maternal milk supply are significant clinical problems. Early breastfeeding follow-up by a skilled provider at 3 to 5 days after delivery would allow early detection of many correctable problems that contribute to slow gain in the first month. By the time the baby's weight gain slows, the mother's milk supply has often already declined, so that both mother and infant must be evaluated and managed with a problem-oriented approach.

Infant or maternal illness, though unusual as a cause of slow weight gain, must always be considered a possibility so as not to overlook a condition that is potentially serious and/or treatable. If infant well-being requires supplementation, it is preferable to give him expressed breastmilk at the breast with a feeding-tube device. Once the infant gains weight and the maternal milk supply improves, the amount of supplementation can gradually be decreased and the infant returned to full feedings at the breast. Rarely, maternal anatomy or physiology will preclude a full milk supply. In these cases, the mother is supported to provide as much breastmilk as possible while acknowledging the grieving process that comes with the loss of the desired breastfeeding experience.

Key Concepts

- Numerous factors, both maternal and infant, may affect infant intake and milk supply; the inter-relationships of these factors are complex.

- Removal of milk by the infant determines the amount of milk production, and maternal limitations on milk supply are rare.

- If infant intake from breastfeeding is low, then the maternal milk supply is probably also low.

- Proper positioning and latch-on are the foundation of efficient milk transfer and infant weight gain.

- During the first several weeks of breastfeeding, individual patterns of milk supply, infant intake, and growth patterns vary widely.

- Maternal nutritional status is not strongly correlated with milk production.

- Follow-up by a health professional must take place at 3 to 5 days postpartum, when breastfeeding progress is at a critical juncture: this may be an office visit or a home visit.

- Weight loss of more than 7% from birth weight warrants investigation of a potential feeding problem; weight loss of more than 10% from birth weight requires thorough assessment and intervention.

- Once gaining, the average newborn weight gain is 34 gm/day for females and 40 gm/day for males during the first 3 months.

- The *minimal* acceptable average weight gain is 20 gm/day during the first 3 months.

- If the infant is not gaining weight (not effectively removing milk), assume that the mother's milk supply has started to decline.

- In the first month of life, problems with the feeding process are more common than illness as a cause of poor weight gain.

- Illness should be suspected as a potential cause of poor feeding and poor weight gain, especially after the first month.

- Current growth charts, though updated, do not reflect the growth pattern of infants who receive exclusive breastfeeding for 6 months followed by continued breastfeeding with appropriate complementary feeding up to one year or longer.

- Using current growth charts, breastfed infants are *leaner* than formula-fed infants from 4 to 12 months of age.

- History and physical examination of both mother and infant, including breastfeeding observation, allows the clinician to develop a differential diagnosis for slow infant weight gain.

- Management of slow infant weight gain can be tailored to the suspected diagnosis.

- Two simple interventions for an actively suckling infant are breast massage during feeding and "switch nursing."

- If supplementation is indicated, start with 50 ml/kgm/day divided into 6 to 8 feedings.

- A mother's own expressed breastmilk is the preferred type of supplement.

- Supplementation can be given by feeding-tube device, cup, spoon, or bottle, depending on individual circumstances.

- As the maternal milk supply increases and the infant becomes more effective at the breast, the amount of supplementation should be decreased.

- Weighing the infant before and after feeding (test weighing) requires an electronic digital scale that is accurate to 2 gm or less.

- Test weighing is generally restricted to complicated situations where weighing is used at every feeding.

- Medications and/or herbs may be an option for increasing milk production after other measures have been tried.

- Delivery of more hindmilk to the infant is one method of increasing caloric intake.

- A few women will be unable to resolve the problem of low intake and low supply; they are likely to undergo a grieving process.

Internet Resources

Academy of Breastfeeding Medicine:
www.bfmed.org

American Academy of Pediatrics (AAP):
www.aap.org

Centers for Disease Prevention and Control (CDC):
www.cdc.gov/growthcharts

International Lactation Consultant Association:
www.ilca.org

La Leche League International:
www.lalecheleague.org

World Health Organization:
www.WHO.int

References

Academy of Breastfeeding Medicine. Clinical Protocol Number 3: Hospital guidelines for the use of complementary feedings in the healthy breastfed neonate. *ABM News and Views* [newsletter] 7(1):2, 2001.

Alexander JM, Grant AM, Campbell MJ. Randomized controlled trial of breast shells and Hoffman's exercises for inverted and non-protractile nipples. *Br Med J* 305:1030–32, 1992.

American Academy of Pediatrics. Work Group on Breastfeeding: Breastfeeding and the use of human milk. *Pediatrics* 100:1035–39, 1997.

Ballard JL, Auaer C. Ankylogossia: assessment, incidence, and effect of frenuloplasty on the breastfeeding dyad. *Pediatrics* 110(5):1001, 2002. Available at: www.pediatrics.org/cgi/content/full/110/5/e63.

Berkner P, Kastner T, Skolnick L. Chronic ipecac poisoning in infancy: a case report. *Pediatrics* 82:384–86, 1988.

Bodley V, Powers D. Long-term nipple use—a positive perspective. *J Hum Lact* 12:301–04, 1996.

Bowen-Jones A, Thomsen C, Drewett RF. Milk flow and sucking rates during breastfeeding. *Develop Med Child Neurol* 24:626-33, 1982.

Butte NF et al. Human milk intake and growth in exclusively breast-fed infants. *J Pediatr* 104(2):187–95, 1984.

Chapman DJ, Perez-Escamilla R. Identification of risk factors for delayed onset of lactation. *J Am Diet Assoc* 99:450–54, 1999.

Chen DC et al. Stress during labor and delivery and early lactation performance. *Am J Clin Nutr* 68(2):335–44, 1998.

Combs VL, Marino BL. A comparison of growth patterns in breast and bottle-fed infants with congenital heart disease. *Pediatric Nursing* 19:175–78, 1993.

Davies DP, Evans T. The starved but contented breastfed baby. *Arch Dis Child* 53:763, 1978.

Desmarais L, Browne S. Inadequate weight gain in breastfeeding infants: assessments and resolutions. In: Auerbach KG, ed. *Lactation consultant series.* Garden City Park, NY: Avery Publishing Group, 1990.

Dewey KG. Nutrition, growth and complementary feeding of the breastfed infant. *Ped Clin NA* 48:87–104, 2001.

Dewey KG, Heinig J, Nommsen LA et al. Adequacy of energy intake among breast-fed infants in the DARLING study: relationships to growth velocity, morbidity, and activity levels. *J Pediatr* 119(4):538–47, 1991a.

———. Maternal versus infant factors related to breast milk and residual milk volume: the DARLING study. *Pediatrics* 87(6):829–37, 1991b.

Dewey KG, Lonnerdal B. Infant self-regulation of breastmilk intake. *Acta Paediatr Scand* 75:893–98, 1986.

Dewey KG, Nommsen-Rivers LA, Heinig MJ, Cohen RJ. Risk factors for suboptimal infant breastfeeding behavior, Delayed onset of lactation, and excess neonatal weight loss. *Pediatrics* 112:607–19, 2003.

Dewey KG, Nommsen-Rivers LA, Heinig MJ et al. Lactogenesis and infant weight change in the first week of life. In: Davis MK et al., eds. *Integrating population outcomes, biological mechanisms, and research methods in the study of human milk and lactation.* New York: Kluwer Academic/Plenum Publishers, 2002.

Drane D. The effect of use of dummies and teats on orofacial development. *Breastfeeding Review* 4:59–64, 1996.

Edmonson MB, Stoddard JJ, Owens LM. Hospital readmission with feeding-related problems after early postpartum discharge of normal newborns. *JAMA* 278:299–303, 1997.

Ehrenkranz RA, Ackerman BA. Metoclopramide effect on faltering milk production by mothers of premature infants. *Pediatrics* 78:614–20, 1986.

Glass RP, Wolf LS. Incoordination of sucking, swallowing, and breathing as an etiology for breastfeeding difficulty. *J Hum Lact* 10(3):185–89, 1994.

Gupta AP, Gupta PK. Metoclopramide as a lactagogue. *Clin Pediatr* 24(5):269–72, 1985.

Habbick BF, Gerrard JW. Failure to thrive in the contented breastfed baby. *Can Med Assoc J* 131:765–68, 1984.

Hale T. *Medications and mothers' milk.* Amarillo, TX: Pharmasoft Publishing, 2002.

Harris L, Morris SF, Freiberg A. Is breast feeding possible after reduction mammaplasty? *Plast Reconstr Surg* 89:836–39, 1992.

Hilson JA, Rasmussen KM, Kjolhede CL. Maternal obesity and breast-feeding success in a rural population of white women. *Am J Clin Nutr* 66:1371–78, 1997.

Hoover KL, Barbalinardo LH, Platia MP. Delayed lactogenesis II secondary to gestational ovarian theca lutein cysts in two normal singleton pregnancies. *J Hum Lact* 18(3):264–68, 2002.

Hopkinson JM et al. Milk production by mothers of premature infants: influence of cigarette smoking. *Pediatrics* 90(6):934–48, 1992.

Horta BL et al. Environmental tobacco smoke and the breastfeeding duration. *Am J Epidemiol* 146:128–33, 1997.

Howard CR et al. Physiologic stability of newborns during cup- and bottle-feeding. *Pediatrics* 104:1204–07, 1999.

Huggins KE, Petok ES, Mireles O. Markers of lactation insufficiency: a study of 34 mothers. In: Auerbach KG, ed. *Current issues in clinical lactation 2000.* Boston: Jones and Bartlett, 2000.

Hurst NM. Lactation after augmentation mammaplasty. *Obstetr & Gyn* 87:30–34, 1996.

Institute of Medicine. *Nutrition during lactation.* Washington: National Academy Press, 1991.

International Lactation Consultant Association. *Evidence-based guidelines for breastfeeding management during the first fourteen days.* Raleigh, NC: ILCA Publications, 1999.

Jones WB. Weight gain and feeding in the neonate with cleft: a three-center study. *Cleft Palate J* 25:379–84, 1988.

Kauppila A et al. Metoclopramide and breast feeding: efficacy and anterior pituitary responses of the mother and the child. *Eur J Obstetr Gynecol Reprod Biol* 19:19–22, 1985.

Lawrence RA, Lawrence R. *Breastfeeding—A guide for the medical profession,* 5th ed. St. Louis: CV Mosby, 1999.

Lukefahr JL. Underlying illness associated with failure to thrive in breastfed infants. *Clin Pediatr* 29(8):468–70, 1990.

———. Frequency of insufficient glandular tissue of the breast. Personal communication. 2002.

Marshall DR, Callan PP, Nicholson W. Breastfeeding after reduction mammaplasty. *Br J Plast Surg* 47:167–69, 1994.

Masaitis NS, Kaempf JW. Developing a frenotomy policy at one medical center: a case study approach. *J Hum Lact* 12:229–32, 1996.

Meier PP et al. The accuracy of test weighing for preterm infants. *J Pediatr Gastroenterol Nutr* 10(1):62–65, 1990.

———. Nipple shields for preterm infants: effect on milk transfer and duration of breastfeeding. *J Hum Lact* 16:106–14, 2002.

Mennella JA. The human infant's suckling responses to the flavor of alcohol in mother's milk. *Alcohol Clin Exp Res* 21:581–85, 1997.

Messner AH et al. Ankyloglossia: incidence and associated feeding difficulties. *Arch Otolaryngol Head Neck Surg* 126:36–39, 2000.

Neifert MR. Failure to thrive. In: Neville MC, Neifert MR, eds. *Lactation: physiology, nutrition and breastfeeding.* New York: Plenum Press, 1983.

Neifert MR, McDonough SL, Neville MC. Failure of lactogenesis associated with placental retention. *Am J Obstet Gynecol* 140(4):477–78, 1981.

Neifert MR, Seacat JM, DeMarzo SM, Young DA. The association between infant weight gain and breast milk intake measured by office test weights [abstract]. *Am J Dis Child* 144:420–21, 1990.

Neifert MR, Seacat JM, Jobe WE. Lactation failure due to insufficient glandular development of the breast. *Pediatrics* 76(5):823–28, 1985.

Neifert M et al. The influence of breast surgery, breast appearance, and pregnancy-induced breast changes on lactation sufficiency as measured by infant weight gain. *Birth* 17(1):31–38, 1990.

Nelson SE et al. Gain in weight and length during early infancy. *Early Hum Dev* 19:223–39, 1989.

Neubauer SH et al. Delayed lactogenesis in women with insulin-dependent diabetes mellitus. *Am J Clin Nutr* 58:54–60, 1993.

Neville MC et al. Studies in human lactation: milk volumes in lactating women during the onset of lactation and full lactation. *Am J Clin Nutr* 48:1375–86, 1988.

Peaker M, Wilde CJ. Milk secretion: autocrine control. *News on Physiological Sciences* 2:124–26, 1987.

Pessl MM. Are we creating our own breastfeeding mythology? *J Hum Lact* 12:271–72, 1996.

Powers NG. Slow weight gain and low milk supply in the breastfeeding dyad. *Clinics in Perinatology* 26:399–429, 1999.

Powers N, Slusser W. Breastfeeding update 2: clinical lactation management. *Pediatrics in Review* 18(5):147–61, 1997.

Ruvalcaba RHA. Stress-induced cessation of lactation. *West J Ed* 146:228–30, 1987.

Salvador S, Vandenplas Y. Gastroesophageal reflux and cow milk allergy: is there a link? *Pediatrics* 110:972–84, 2002.

Sealy CN. Rethinking the use of nipple shields. *J Hum Lact* 12(4):299–300, 1996.

Soskolne EI et al. The effect of early discharge and other factors on the readmission rates of newborns. *Arch Pediatr Adolesc Med* 150:373–79, 1996.

Strombeck JO. Late results after reduction mammaplasty. In: Goldwyn RM, ed. *Long-term results in plastic and reconstructive surgery.* Boston: Little Brown, 1980:723.

Stuff JE, Nichols BL. Nutrient intake and growth performance of older infants fed human milk. *J Pediatr* 115:959–68, 1989.

Sutphen JL, Saulsbury FT. Intentional ipecac poisoning: Munchausen syndrome by proxy. *Pediatrics* 82:453–56, 1988.

Swafford S, Berens P. Effect of fenugreek on breast milk volume [abstract]. *ABM News and Views* 6(4):21, 2000.

Valentine CJ, Hurst NM, Schanler RJ. Hindmilk improves weight gain in low birth-weight infants fed human milk. J Ped Gastr Nutr 18:474–77, 1994.

Whitfield M, Kay R, Stevens S. Validity of routine clinical test weighing as a measure of intake of breast-fed infants. *Arch Dis Child* 56:919, 1981.

Wilson JD, Foster DW, eds. *Williams textbook of endocrinology.* Philadelphia: W. B. Saunders, 1992:441–42.

Wilson-Clay B. Clinical use of silicone nipple shields. *J Hum Lact* 12:279–85, 1996.

Wisner KL, Parry BL, Piontek CM. Postpartum depression. *N Engl J Med* 347:194–99, 2002.

Woolridge MW, Fisher C. Colic, "overfeeding" and symptoms of lactose malabsorption in the breast-fed baby: a possible artifact of feed management? *Lancet* 2(8607): 382–84, 1988.

Woolridge MW, Ingram JC, Baum JD. Do changes in pattern of breast usage alter the baby's nutrient intake? *Lancet* 336:395–97, 1990.

Woolridge MW et al. Methods for the measurement of milk volume intake of the breast-fed infant. In: Jensen RG, Neville MC, eds. *Human lactation: milk components and methodologies.* New York: Plenum Press, 1984:5–21.

World Health Organization. Working Group on the Growth Reference Protocol. Growth patterns of breastfed infants in seven countries. *Acta Paediatr* 89:215–22, 2000.

World Health Organization. Global strategy for infant and young child feeding: the optimal duration of exclusive breastfeeding. Presented at: Fifty-Fourth World Health Assembly (A54/INF.DOC./4), 2001.

11

JAUNDICE AND THE BREASTFED BABY

Marguerite Herschel and Lawrence M. Gartner

Physiologic jaundice is a common clinical condition in the majority of newborn infants that generally resolves within the first week of life in the term neonate. However, in at least one third of breastfed infants, the duration of physiologic jaundice may be prolonged for many weeks; this is normal in the healthy, thriving infant and is known as *breastmilk jaundice.* Breastmilk jaundice was recognized about 40 years ago as prolonged, exaggerated neonatal unconjugated hyperbilirubinemia that was otherwise unexplained and that often resolved within 48 hours upon discontinuation of breastfeeding. In some cases, with resumption of breastfeeding, bilirubin levels rose, but marked hyperbilirubinemia only rarely recurred. This concept appeared in the literature in collections of case reports (Newman & Gross, 1963; Stiehm & Ryan, 1965; Arias et al., 1964). With newer laboratory techniques, some cases of prolonged jaundice that might have been ascribed solely to breastmilk feeding are now recognized to have other, or associated, causes. The pathogenesis of breastmilk jaundice is currently thought to be via an as yet unidentified factor in human milk that promotes the intestinal absorption of bilirubin (Gartner, Lee, & Moscioni, 1983; Alonso et al., 1991). Because bilirubin is an antioxidant, it has been suggested that this mechanism for prolongation of physiologic jaundice may be protective for the newborn (Stocker

et al., 1987; Dore et al., 1999). To date, there is insufficient clinical evidence to support this intuitive and attractive concept, but recent animal studies strongly support the protective effect of hyperbilirubinemia in ischemic bowel injury (Hammerman et al., 2002).

Inadequate breastfeeding, particularly in the first few days of life, can as well be associated with elevated levels of bilirubin (Gartner, 2001). This manifestation is known as *breast-nonfeeding jaundice* and is the neonatal manifestation of the adult disorder, *starvation jaundice* (Whitmer & Gollan, 1983). In this condition, marked by inadequate milk and caloric intake, but not necessarily by dehydration, there may be a delay in bilirubin clearance resulting from low stool output (de Carvalho, Robertson, & Klaus, 1985) with an increase in the intestinal absorption of unconjugated bilirubin. Exaggerated jaundice due to poor breastfeeding should not be considered physiologic. It has been shown that in neonates who were adequately breastfed on demand, not according to a rigid time schedule, there was no difference in the percentage with an elevated level of bilirubin during the first days of life between those who were breastfed or those who were bottle-fed (Rubaltelli, 1993); nor was there a difference in the percentage of weight loss.

Despite the knowledge of an association between exaggerations of neonatal jaundice and breastfeeding, it would be a mistake to assume, without careful consideration, that because a neonate is breastfed and is jaundiced, breastfeeding is the sole, or main, cause of the jaundice. It would also be a mistake to believe that if the jaundice is associated with breastfeeding, it can never be harmful.

In this chapter, we will discuss neonatal jaundice, its physiologic and pathologic causes, its potential risks, and its evaluation and management.

Neonatal Jaundice

Jaundice, or icterus, is defined as a yellowish color of the sclerae and skin as a result of the deposition of bilirubin, a yellow molecule, in body tissues. Bilirubin is largely derived from red blood cell lysis and the breakdown of hemoglobin into globin and heme; subsequently, heme is degraded by the enzyme *heme oxygenase* to produce equimolar amounts of iron, biliverdin, and carbon monoxide. Biliverdin is reduced to bilirubin by biliverdin reductase (Dennery, Seidman, & Stevenson, 2001). More than half of all newborns have some degree of visible jaundice. The level of jaundice is dependent on the balance of bilirubin production and bilirubin elimination.

Serum bilirubin levels in newborns are higher than those in adults for several reasons (Gartner & Lee, 1992):

1. The fetus in utero exists in a relatively low oxygen environment and the fetal red cell mass is stimulated to be higher than in the adult in order for adequate oxygen delivery to the tissues to occur. The hematocrit of the newborn at birth will be further increased in proportion to the time between birth and clamping of the umbilical cord (Shurin, 1992). This increase in transfer of blood from the placenta to the newborn upon birth ensures an adequate volume of blood to fill the expanded vascular beds (e.g., lungs, intestine) and delivery of adequate iron for future metabolic needs. Thus the newborn has a much greater volume of red cells relative to body weight than does the adult or older child. In addition, the life span of the red cells formed in utero (about 70 to 90 days) is shorter than that of the adult (100 to 120 days). This large volume of heme combined with a shorter life span of the red cells in the circula-

tion results in synthesis of more bilirubin per unit of body weight than in the adult. In addition, the fetus produces red cells not only in the bone marrow but also in the liver and spleen. This very active erythopoiesis is driven by the hormone *erythropoietin*. Immediately after delivery of the infant into room air and the initiation of respiration, the blood oxygen level increases dramatically, resulting in complete cessation of erythropoiesis. These immature inactive red cells in the liver, spleen, and bone marrow are destroyed, producing additional bilirubin. All of the bilirubin formed in this process is insoluble in plasma, requiring that it be transported bound to serum albumin. In the fetus, the small amount of insoluble bilirubin formed was cleared from the circulation by passive diffusion across the placenta; but in the newborn, it must be eliminated by another pathway.

2. In the newborn, the insoluble bilirubin, also referred to as *unconjugated* or *indirect-reacting bilirubin*, must enter the liver cell (hepatocyte) by a process of facilitated diffusion, which in the newborn is less active than in the older child or adult, reducing the rate of clearance of bilirubin from the plasma. Once in the liver, bilirubin is conjugated with glucuronic acid via the enzyme *uridine diphosphate glucuronyl transferase* (UGT1A1) to become water soluble bilirubin glucuronide, a requirement for transfer from the liver cell into bile and movement into the small intestine and ultimately into stool. Bilirubin glucuronide is also called *conjugated* or *direct-reacting bilirubin*. Compared to adults, newborns have relative immaturity of the conjugating system as well as uptake of bilirubin. The degree of imbalance between high bilirubin synthesis and limited liver cell uptake and conjugation of bilirubin causes the varying elevation of serum bilirubin concentration in blood and body tissues and the degree of severity of jaundice.

3. In order for the conjugated bilirubin to be eliminated from the body, it must be passed in the neonatal stool. However, neonates, unlike adults, have a high level of an enzyme in the intestinal mucosa called *beta-glucuronidase*. This enzyme removes the glucuronide from the

conjugated bilirubin, making the bilirubin once again water insoluble and thus available for transport back across the intestinal lumen into the neonate's circulation. This process, called the *enterohepatic circulation of bilirubin,* contributes to neonatal jaundice. The absence of intestinal bacteria in the neonate (which in the adult convert bilirubin into other metabolites), combined with the high level of beta glucuronidase in the intestine and high concentration of unconjugated bilirubin leads to a marked increase of intestinal reabsorption of bilirubin in the neonate.

Assessment of Jaundice

Traditionally, clinicians have relied on visual inspection to determine the level of jaundice in newborns. As there is a cranio-caudal progression in

icterus of the skin with rising levels of bilirubin, the serum level of bilirubin has been inferred from the apparent level of demarcation of jaundice on the neonate's body. Newer information would suggest that the visual inspection for the estimation of bilirubin level is unreliable and inaccurate (Moyer, Ahn, & Sheed, 2000). This is particularly true in pigmented races. In this era of early hospital discharge of neonates, in which discharge commonly takes place at less than 48 hours of life, it is very hard to distinguish, simply by inspection, a pathological or concerning level of bilirubin from a normal level. For this reason, many experts now recommend that all neonates be screened by serum or transcutaneous level of bilirubin prior to hospital discharge and that this level be plotted on the nomogram of bilirubin level according to hours of age of the baby, as shown in Figure 11–1 (Bhutani, Johnson, & Sivieri, 1999). One can then readily see

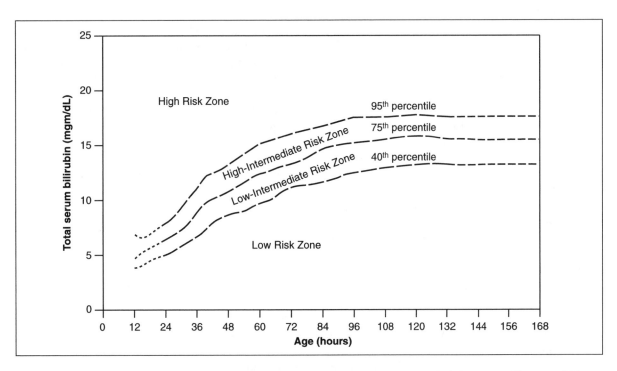

FIGURE 11–1. Risk designation of term and near-term well newborns based on their hour-specific serum bilirubin values. The high-risk zone is designated by the 95th percentile track. The intermediate-risk zone is subdivided to upper- and lower-risk zones by the 75th percentile track. The low-risk zone has been electively and statistically defined by the 40th percentile track. (Dotted extensions are based on < 300 TSB values/epoch.) (From Bhutani, Johnson, & Sivieri, 1999. Reprinted with permission.)

what risk category an infant falls in for having significant hyperbilirubinema, which is defined as bilirubin level greater than the 95th percentile at any age. This can be a guide as to what diagnostic testing may be indicated, whether or not the infant ought to be discharged to home, and when the early follow-up appointment should be scheduled.

Postnatal Pattern of Jaundice

Because of the physiological mechanisms described above, bilirubin levels rise in neonates after birth for a few days and then, typically, fall to the adult level. In the formula-fed healthy Caucasian term infant, bilirubin levels peak on day 2 to 3, which is often after hospital discharge has taken place. In preterm neonates and in infants of some racial groups—for example, in some full-term Asians—the peak may be later, day 5, and usually will be higher than in the Caucasian term newborn (Brown & Wong, 1965). Jaundice will have resolved in most infants by day 7 in the formula-fed normal term neonate, and by day 10 to 21 in the preterm neonate. The pattern of jaundice in the breastfed neonate, known as breastmilk jaundice, is more prolonged.

Breastmilk Jaundice

With its onset after the fifth day of life, in association with the appearance of transitional and mature milk, breastmilk jaundice is an extension of physiologic jaundice (Gartner & Herschel, 2001). The levels of jaundice rarely become dangerously high; if so, a careful evaluation for other causes of jaundice is essential (see below). Breastmilk jaundice is seen in healthy, thriving neonates who have good weight gain; it may persist for many weeks. However, stools will be normal yellow in color and the conjugated fraction of total bilirubin, which should be measured by 2 to 3 weeks of age in all infants who are still jaundiced, will be normal.

Breastmilk jaundice is a normal physiologic phenomenon, not a disorder (Gartner & Herschel, 2001). Two thirds of all breastfed babies have an elevation in bilirubin, and half of those have visible jaundice during the second to fourth weeks of life. As bilirubin is a potent antioxidant, modest elevations of bilirubin may possibly be beneficial, though this requires additional research.

The mechanism of breastmilk jaundice has been shown to be due to an increase in the intestinal absorption of bilirubin, not to an inhibitor of the conjugating enzyme, UGT1A1 (Alonso et al., 1991). An as yet unidentified substance in the milk of the majority of breastfeeding mothers is thought to be responsible for this increase in intestinal reabsorption of bilirubin (Gartner, 2001).

Gilbert's syndrome, a benign condition characterized by reduced activity of the bilirubin conjugating enzyme, has been associated with prolonged neonatal jaundice. Genetic studies of the promoter for the conjugating enzyme, UGT1A1, in a Scottish population (Monaghan et al., 1999) have revealed that there is a significant association between prolonged jaundice and breastfeeding in neonates who have an increase in the number of TATA box repeats. In Asians, a DNA sequence variant (Gly 71 Arg mutation) of the UGT1A1 gene has been shown to be associated with neonatal hyperbilirubinemia (Maruo et al., 1999). Fifteen of 17 Japanese infants with prolonged jaundice in association with breastfeeding had at least 1 UGT1A1 mutation (Maruo et al., 2000). Two different types of mutations of the gene for the UGT1A1 enzyme are major contributors to neonatal hyperbilirubinemia in European and Japanese populations.

Although neonatal jaundice without other signs is almost never indicative of a bacterial infection, in 7.5 percent of afebrile, asymptomatic jaundiced newborns (predominantly formula-fed) younger than 8 weeks of age (mean age of 12 days) presenting to an emergency department, a urinary tract infection was diagnosed (Garcia & Nager, 2002).

Breast-Nonfeeding Jaundice

Breastmilk jaundice will usually be identified after the neonate has been discharged home, as it generally presents as a prolongation of the earlier physiologic jaundice. On the other hand, so-called *breastfeeding jaundice*, or preferably, *breast-nonfeeding jaundice*, may be seen in the first few days after birth, but not before 24 hours (Gartner & Herschel, 2001). Again, other causes for jaundice must be considered and ruled out. Breast-nonfeeding jaundice is seen in neonates who have not established feedings because of maternal or neonatal factors or a combination of both. This is comparable to starvation jaundice, seen in adults with inadequate caloric intake, in whom bilirubin levels rise above baseline (Whitmer & Gollan, 1983); in those adults with Gilbert's syndrome, this jaundice may be particularly evident when they go without eating for more than 24 hours.

For infants who have not established effective breastfeeding, whether due to being sleepy, premature, having poor positioning and poor latch with inadequate milk transfer, or other conditions, it would be unwise to send them home until the problem is resolved (Maisels & Newman, 1998; Neifert, 1998). Breastfeeding should be formally evaluated by a trained health professional at least twice each day in the hospital with attention to position, latch, and milk transfer. Weight loss, dehydration, hypernatremia, and possibly excessive and dangerous levels of bilirubin may result, with a catastrophic outcome such as kernicterus (Johnson, Bhutani, & Brown, 2002), a permanent neurologic condition characterized by athetoid cerebral palsy and deafness. In addition to the risk of kernicterus (bilirubin encephalopathy), venous thrombosis has been reported in a few such instances (Gebara & Everett, 2001).

For neonates with jaundice and poor breastfeeding, the solution is not to stop the breastfeeding. The solution is to correct the breastfeeding problem. In some instances, expressed milk, banked human milk, or artificial milk supplementation may be required for a time. The main point is that the baby must be fed and the mother must be supported. Regardless of the etiology of the jaundice, if breastfeeding is not going well, it must be improved, not abandoned.

Infants who develop elevated bilirubin levels in the early days of life due to breast-nonfeeding jaundice are also at increased risk of developing very high bilirubin levels when they enter the stage of breastmilk jaundice. If they have developed a large bilirubin pool early, that pool will multiply with mature human milk feeding due to intestinal bilirubin absorption. Conversely, good breastfeeding practices that keep early bilirubin at lower levels will prevent later excessive levels from developing.

Hyperbilirubinemia

Levels of bilirubin that exceed the physiological parameters (7–17 mgm/dL) (Dennery, Seidman, & Stevenson, 2001) or that are at or above the 95th percentile on the nomogram of bilirubin according to hours of age of the neonate (Bhutani, Johnson, & Sivieri, 1999) represent hyperbilirubinemia. It is important that the cause of the hyperbilirubinemia be investigated, both to diagnose an underlying etiology to be able to anticipate what the clinical course may be and to assess the risk for development of bilirubin encephalopathy, also known as kernicterus, a devastating, but almost always preventable, neurological condition associated with high levels of unconjugated bilirubin.

Factors that have been associated with exaggerated hyperbilirubinemia may be categorized in the following way (Dennery, Seidman, & Stevenson, 2001), recognizing that there are often multiple reasons for hyperbilirubinemia in a given baby:

- Increased production of bilirubin (hemolysis)
    Blood group incompatibility with isoimmunization (direct antibody [Coombs'] test positive)
    Inherited red blood cell abnormalities such as enzyme deficiencies (glucose-6-phosphate dehydrogenase deficiency) and red cell membrane defects (spherocytosis, elliptocytosis)
    Birth "trauma" (ecchymoses, cephalhematoma, internal bleeding, subgaleal hemorrhage)
    Genetic factors (Greek Island extraction, Asian race)
    Induction of labor (exposure to oxytocin in hypotonic solution, prematurity)
    Polycythemia
- Decreased elimination of bilirubin
    Genetic variants/disorders of conjugation—Gilbert's syndrome, Crigler-Najjar syndromes, Asian race (Akaba et al., 1998)
    Low oral intake of feedings
    Breastmilk feedings
- Multifactorial risks
    Prematurity
    Maternal diabetes
    Urinary tract infection (Garcia & Nager, 2002)
    Hypothyroidism
    G6PD deficiency with Gilbert's syndrome (Kaplan, 2001)
    Asian race (Young et al., 2001)

Bilirubin Encephalopathy

It was believed by many that this devastating outcome of hyperbilirubinemia was no longer of concern following the introduction of preventive treatment for severe hemolytic disease of the newborn secondary to Rh incompatibility, which was a common cause of severe hyperbilirubinemia in the past. Recent reports of infants with this condition have made it evident that bilirubin encephalopathy continues to occur (Centers for Disease Control, 2001), especially in breastfed infants, in infants who may weigh as much as full-term infants but yet their gestational age is less than 38 weeks, and in those with large internal hemorrhage such as cephalhematomas.

The informal kernicterus registry at the University of Pennsylvania suggests that there is a rise in incidence of this devastating outcome (Johnson, Bhutani, & Brown, 2002). The cause of this rise is multifactorial. As a result of some articles in the pediatric literature, many pediatricians and others have adopted a more liberal and permissive approach to elevated bilirubin levels. Furthermore, it is suspected that early hospital discharge of newborns combined with an increase in the number who are breastfed, without timely follow-up within the first couple of days after discharge, is a contributing factor. Newborns are being sent home before feedings are established, without adequate assessment for the risk of significant jaundice, and without appropriate and timely follow-up (Johnson, Bhutani, & Brown, 2002).

For a given neonate, it is not known at what level of bilirubin, and for what duration of exposure to that level, kernicterus may occur. Certain factors may increase the risk, in addition to the level of serum bilirubin. The form of bilirubin that crosses into the brain is unconjugated bilirubin that is not bound to plasma proteins, so-called "free bilirubin." Thus low levels of albumin or any substance that competes with bilirubin for albumin-binding sites may increase the risk of free bilirubin being available to enter the brain. This mechanism was recognized in the 1950s (Harris, Lucey, & Maclean, 1958) when an association was found between prophylactic sulfisoxazole antibiotic usage in preterm neonates and kernicterus. Sulfisoxazole competes with unconjugated bilirubin for albumin-binding sites and can displace bilirubin, which then may enter the brain. Benzyl alcohol, which at one time was used as a preservative in parenteral medications for newborns in intensive care nurseries, may have had the same effect. The potential for displacement of bilirubin from albumin-binding sites must be considered whenever a medication is prescribed for a newborn. The commonly used antibiotic, ceftriaxone, competes for bilirubin-binding sites on albumin (Martin et al., 1993), though no cases of kernicterus are known to have been attributed to this drug.

Hemolysis also appears to increase the risk of kernicterus; the mechanism of this effect remains undefined. In addition, factors affecting the integrity of the blood-brain barrier, such as asphyxia, acidosis, sepsis, or prematurity, may increase this risk. Although one must always consider the potential effect on the jaundiced neonate of drugs in breastmilk, all drugs commonly given to mothers antepartum or postpartum are safe with regard to neonatal jaundice, with the important exception of nalidixic acid, nitrofurantoin, sulfapyridine, and sulfisoxazole in mothers of infants with G6PD deficiency, because of the risk of hemolysis in the neonate (American Academy of Pediatrics, 2001). Maternal ingestion of fava beans is also dangerous in the breastfed neonate with G6PD deficiency. Naphthalene mothballs and flakes should not be used in the home or in the clothes of any neonate because of their potential to produce hemolysis in infants with G6PD deficiency.

Evaluation of Jaundice

As noted above, it is currently recommended by experts that all neonates be screened for their level of bilirubin prior to hospital discharge (Johnson, Bhutani, & Brown, 2002). With the availability of a transcutaneous device (BiliChek, Respironics, Marietta, GA) that has been shown to be as accurate as routine laboratory methods for bilirubin screening (Rubaltelli et al., 2001), this can now be performed noninvasively and rapidly at the bedside. If the transcutaneous reading is 15 mgm/dL or higher, confirmation with a serum bilirubin level is recommended (Bhutani et al., 2000). If the bilirubin level plotted on the nomogram is at or above the 75th percentile, the neonate is at risk for significant hyperbilirubinemia and will need careful assessment; delay of hospital discharge may be appropriate.

Diagnostic Assessment

Having established that the neonate has, or is at risk for, significant hyperbilirubinemia according to the nomogram of bilirubin level for hours-of-age, consideration must be given to the cause of the jaundice. Therapy will be guided, to some extent, by the cause. Most cases of hyperbilirubinemia are due, at least in part, to increased bilirubin production (Stevenson, Dennery, & Hinz, 2001) from hemoglobin degradation (hemolysis). It is important to identify hemolysis because it may lead to very high levels of bilirubin, and/or to significant anemia. Hemolysis is also associated with an increased risk for bilirubin encephalopathy at all elevated serum bilirubin levels.

Traditional hematological tests (hematocrit, reticulocyte count, blood smear, direct antiglobulin [Coombs'] test) are generally not very helpful in making a diagnosis of hemolysis in the neonate (Newman & Easterling, 1994; Herschel et al., 2002). A clinical technique that is noninvasive and simple for estimating the rate of bilirubin production (hemolysis) is measurement of exhaled end-tidal carbon monoxide (CO), corrected for ambient CO (ETCOc) (Vreman et al., 1996).

When red blood cells break down, hemoglobin is released. The heme moiety is degraded by the enzyme, heme oxygenase, to release iron, CO, and biliverdin in equimolar amounts. Biliverdin, a water soluble compound, is reduced to unconjugated bilirubin, a fat soluble compound. CO is excreted as a component of expired breath. Since CO and bilirubin are produced in equimolar quantities, measurement of expired CO provides an indication of the rate of bilirubin production. A commercially available device (CO-Stat End-Tidal Breath Analyzer, Natus Medical, San Carlos, CA) can be used to measure ETCOc in newborns at the bedside, quickly and noninvasively. The result is immediately available on a data strip print-out and can be plotted on a nomogram of ETCOc levels for hours-of-age to identify infants with excessive hemolysis (Figure 11–2). The advantage of ETCOc over the Coombs' test is that ETCOc will identify infants with hemolysis that is not due to isoimmunization, such as G6PD enzyme deficiency or red cell membrane defects. Furthermore, a positive Coombs' test may be misleading as to the risk for hemolysis because many neonates with a positive test do not have significant hemolysis (Herschel et al., 2002). Other tests that may be diagnostic of hemolysis in adults are not usually helpful in neonates.

Since the level of bilirubin is a result of the balance between production and elimination, one must also consider deficiencies in the elimination of bilirubin in the neonate with hyperbilirubinemia. One of the more common, benign genetic causes of

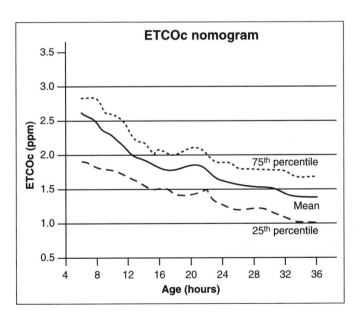

FIGURE 11–2.
End-tidal carbon monoxide level corrected for ambient air according to postnatal age in hours. (From Bhutani, Herschel, & Stevenson, 2001. Reprinted with permission.)

a delay in elimination in bilirubin, when there is a coexistent, even slight, increase in hemolysis, is Gilbert's syndrome. A common underlying cause of this syndrome is a variation in the promoter region of the gene for the conjugating enzyme, UGT1A1, resulting in decreased activity of the conjugating enzyme. By itself, people with this disorder are asymptomatic although they may have mild unconjugated hyperbilirubinemia; but in combination with some hemolysis or with starvation, bilirubin becomes significantly elevated. It has been shown that neonatal hyperbilirubinemia due to G6PD deficiency occurs in those neonates who also have Gilbert's syndrome (Kaplan, 2001).

Another reason for decreased elimination of bilirubin is an increase in the enterohepatic circulation of bilirubin (intestinal absorption), due to insufficient caloric intake (starvation jaundice) or, normally, due to breastmilk feedings.

Management of Jaundice

The management of hyperbilirubinemia will depend to some extent on the cause, but ultimately on the level of bilirubin and the condition of the neonate. If the neonate is less than 38 weeks' gestation, or has hemolysis or other medical problems, the bilirubin level for initiating phototherapy may be somewhat lower than if the neonate is full-term, healthy, and does not have any type of hemolytic disease (Table 11–1; American Academy of Pediatrics, 1994). Very high or rapidly rising bilirubin levels may need to be controlled with an exchange transfusion, in which case feedings would be temporarily interrupted for the procedure. Neonates who are treated only with phototherapy should continue to be breastfed or receive other milk feedings since good caloric intake improves the effectiveness of phototherapy.

Phototherapy of hyperbilirubinemia is based on the knowledge that light wavelength in the blue spectrum (450–500 nanometers) is absorbed by bilirubin and results in a change in the structure of the bilirubin molecule such that the fat soluble, unconjugated bilirubin becomes water soluble without having to be conjugated in the liver. This stereoisomer of bilirubin, a product of light therapy, can be excreted in the stool and urine without conjugation

Table 11–1

MANAGEMENT OF HYPERBILIRUBINEMIA IN THE HEALTHY TERM NEWBORN

Age (hours)	Total Serum Bilirubin Level, mgm/dL (μmol/L)			
	Consider Phototherapy*	Phototherapy	Exchange Transfusion If Intensive Phototherapy Fails**	Exchange Transfusion and Intensive Phototherapy
≥24†	—	—	—	—
25–48	≥12 (210)	≥15 (260)	≥20 (340)	≥25 (430)
49–72	≥15 (260)	≥18 (310)	≥25 (430)	≥30 (510)
>72	≥17 (290)	≥20 (340)	≥25 (430)	≥30 (510)

* *Phototherapy at these TSB levels is a clinical option, meaning that the intervention is available and may be used on the basis of individual clinical judgment.*

** *Intensive phototherapy should produce a decline of TSB of 1 to 2 mgm/dL within 4 to 6 hours and the TSB level should continue to fall and remain below the threshold level for exchange transfusion. If this does not occur, it is considered a failure of phototherapy.*

† *Term infants who are clinically jaundiced at ≤ 24 hours old are not considered healthy and require further evaluation.*

Source: American Academy of Pediatrics (1994).

with glucuronic acid. Phototherapy treatment of jaundice should be reserved for those infants who meet the AAP criteria for intervention (American Academy of Pediatrics, 1994; revision should be published in 2004). When phototherapy is indicated, it should be performed intensively so that it is as effective as possible (Maisels, 1996). Home phototherapy does not have a role in treating neonates with significant hyperbilirubinemia who need close and thus frequent monitoring of bilirubin levels and who would otherwise be at risk for exchange transfusion if not properly and effectively managed with light therapy. Infants under phototherapy should be fed orally and do not need intravenous fluids unless they have signs of dehydration (Boo & Lee, 2002). Breastfeeding need not be interrupted; feeding with breastmilk may still continue while a baby is in the hospital under light therapy, though the more time the infant spends under the light, the faster the bilirubin will decline. In some instances, the newborn may need to be fed while under phototherapy if the level of bilirubin is high enough that exchange transfusion might become necessary if the hyperbilirubinemia cannot be lowered. In that case, the mother could pump and feed breastmilk. For most infants under phototherapy, interruptions of light treatment for up to 30 minutes every 2 to 3 hours will not significantly reduce the effectiveness of the phototherapy.

The diagnosis, assessment, and management of neonatal jaundice should take place in the context of the breastfeeding. While it is known that there is an association between jaundice and breastfeeding, one must be very careful not to convey the wrong message to the mother and her family that breastfeeding is potentially dangerous or harmful to her baby. Mothers commonly feel guilty, believing they have caused the baby to be jaundiced (Hannon, Willis, & Scrimshaw, 2001).

As emphasized in this chapter, a careful evaluation for the etiology of the hyperbilirubinemia must be made, with jaundice associated with breastfeeding being considered as a diagnosis of exclusion. In any case, regardless of the cause, the breastfeeding must be optimized and supported. This often requires that the hospital staff be educated not to make remarks to mothers to the effect that they should supplement their babies with formula if they do not want the baby to have to remain in the hospital for treatment for jaundice. The staff on all shifts must be knowledgeable in helping babies and their mothers to have a proper latch and to feed frequently. They should also encourage mothers to speak up to get help. The staff must know the right questions to ask mothers to assess the adequacy of the breastfeeding and must be able to make useful observations of feedings, the patterns of stools, and weight loss/gain.

Neonates with jaundice who are breastfed, just as newborns with jaundice who are artificially-fed, should be approached in a global manner in the diagnostic evaluation and management of the jaundice. This will ensure the optimal outcome for the neonate and family.

Key Concepts

- Jaundice, a yellow discoloration of the sclerae and skin, is caused by the deposition of bilirubin in those tissues. Bilirubin is a product of red blood cell—specifically hemoglobin—breakdown.

- Physiologic jaundice is a common clinical condition in the majority of newborn infants that generally resolves within the first week of life in the term artificial-milk fed neonate. Approximately 60 percent of all newborns will have some jaundice in the first week of life. Nearly all will have some elevation of serum bilirubin concentration.

- Breastmilk jaundice, characterized by prolongation of physiologic jaundice, is a normal manifestation in at least one third of breastfed infants. Approximately two thirds will have an elevation of serum bilirubin concentration.

- Inadequate breastfeeding may lead to jaundice, particularly in the first few days of life but not on day 1. This is the neonatal manifestation of the adult disorder, starvation jaundice.

- Despite the known association of jaundice and breastfeeding, other causes for jaundice must be ruled out before attributing jaundice solely to breastfeeding.

- The level of bilirubin in a neonate resulting in neonatal jaundice is determined by the balance between production and elimination of bilirubin.

- Increased production of bilirubin, due to increased red cell breakdown (hemolysis), may lead to very high levels of bilirubin.

- A new bedside technique for making the often difficult diagnosis of hemolysis is measurement of exhaled breath carbon monoxide (ETCOc).

- Extreme hyperbilirubinemia may result in permanent brain damage, known as bilirubin encephalopathy (kernicterus).

- Kernicterus has become a public health problem. In order to prevent this tragic outcome, all neonates should be screened for bilirubin level prior to hospital discharge. Adequate breastfeeding must be documented prior to discharge. Follow-up with a health-care provider must take place within 3 to 5 days of age or 1 to 3 days after discharge. At that visit, jaundice and breastfeeding must be assessed.

Internet Resources

American Academy of Pediatrics Practice Guideline. Management of Hyperbilirubinemia in the Healthy Term Newborn:
http://aap.org (Keyword: jaundice)

References

Akaba K et al. Neonatal hyperbilirubinemia and mutation of the bilirubin uridine diphosphate-glucuronosyltransferase gene: a common missense mutation among Japanese, Koreans and Chinese. *Biochem Mol Biol Int* 46:21–26, 1998.

Alonso EM et al. Enterohepatic circulation of nonconjugated bilirubin in rats fed with human milk. *J Pediatr* 118:425–30, 1991.

American Academy of Pediatrics. Practice parameter. Management of hyperbilirubinemia in the healthy term newborn. *Pediatrics* 94:558–65, 1994.

American Academy of Pediatrics, Committee on Drugs. The transfer of drugs and other chemicals into human milk. *Pediatrics* 108:776–89, 2001.

Arias IM et al. Prolonged neonatal unconjugated hyperbilirubinemia associated with breast feeding and a steroid, pregnane-3(alpha), 20(beta)-diol, in maternal milk that inhibits glucuronide formation in vitro. *J Clin Invest* 43: 2037–47, 1964.

Bhutani YK, Herschel M, Stevenson DK (and the Jaundice Multinational Study Group). End-tidal carbon monoxide (ETCOc) hours-specific nomogram: for early and pre-discharge identification of babies with increased bilirubin production. *J Perinatol* 21:S01, 2001.

Bhutani VK, Johnson L, Sivieri EM. Predictive ability of a predischarge hour-specific serum bilirubin for subsequent significant hyperbilirubinemia in healthy term and near-term newborns. *Pediatrics* 103:6–14, 1999.

Bhutani VK et al. Noninvasive measurement of total serum bilirubin in a multiracial predischarge newborn population to assess the risk of severe hyperbilirubinemia. *Pediatrics* 106:e17, 2000.

Boo NY, Lee HT. Randomized controlled trial of oral versus intravenous fluid supplementation on serum bilirubin level during phototherapy of term infants with severe hyperbilirubinemia. *J Paediatr Child Health* 38:151–55, 2002.

Brown WR, Wong HB. Ethnic group differences in plasma bilirubin levels of full-term, healthy Singapore newborns. *Pediatrics* 336:745–51, 1965.

Centers for Disease Control and Prevention. Kernicterus in full-term infants, United States, 1994–1998. *MMWR* 50:491–94, 2001.

de Carvalho M, Robertson S, Klaus M. Fecal bilirubin excretion and serum bilirubin concentrations in breast-fed and bottle-fed infants. *J Pediatr* 107:786–90, 1985.

Dennery PA, Seidman DS, Stevenson DK. Neonatal hyperbilirubinemia. *N Engl J Med* 344:581–90, 2001.

Dore S et al. Bilirubin, formed by activation of heme oxygenase-2, protects neurons against oxidative stress injury. *Proc Natl Acad Sci USA* 96:2445–50, 1999.

Garcia FJ, Nager AL. Jaundice as an early diagnostic sign of urinary tract infection in infancy. *Pediatrics* 109:846–51, 2002.

Gartner LM. Breastfeeding and jaundice. *J Perinatol* 21:S25–S29, 2001.

Gartner LM, Herschel M. Jaundice and breastfeeding. *Pediatr Clin North Am* 48:389–99, 2001.

Gartner LM, Lee KS. Jaundice and liver disease. In: Fanaroff AA, Martin RJ, eds. *Neonatal-perinatal medicine: diseases of the fetus and infant.* St. Louis, MO: Mosby–Year Book, 1992: 1075–104.

Gartner LM, Lee KS, Moscioni AD. Effect of milk feeding

on intestinal bilirubin absorption in the rat. *J Pediatr* 103:464–71, 1983.

Gebara BM, Everett KO. Dural sinus thrombosis complicating hypernatremic dehydration in a breastfed neonate. *Clin Pediatr* 40:45–48, 2001.

Hammerman C et al. Protective effect of bilirubin in ischemia-reperfusion injury in the rat intestine. *J Ped Gastro Nutr* 35:344–49, 2002.

Hannon PR, Willis SK, Scrimshaw SC. Persistence of maternal concerns surrounding neonatal jaundice. *Arch Pediatr Adolesc Med* 155:1357–63, 2001.

Harris RC, Lucey JF, Maclean JR. Kernicterus in premature infants associated with low concentrations of bilirubin in the plasma. *Pediatrics* 21:875–84, 1958.

Herschel M et al. Evaluation of the direct antiglobulin (Coombs') test for identifying newborns at-risk for hemolysis as determined by end-tidal carbon monoxide concentration (ETCOc) and comparison of the Coombs' test with ETCOc for detecting significant jaundice. *J Perinatol* 22:341–47, 2002.

Johnson LH, Bhutani VK, Brown AK. System-based approached to management of neonatal jaundice and prevention of kernicterus. *J Pediatr* 140:396–403, 2002.

Kaplan M. Genetic interactions in the pathogenesis of neonatal hyperbilirubinemia: Gilbert's syndrome and Glucose-6-phosphate dehydrogenase deficiency. *J Perinatol* 21:S30–S34, 2001.

Maisels MJ. Why use homeopathic doses of phototherapy? *Pediatrics* 98:283–87, 1996.

Maisels MJ, Newman TB. Jaundice in full-term and near-term babies who leave the hospital within 36 hours. The pediatrician's nemesis. *Clin Perinatol* 25:295–302, 1998.

Martin E et al. Ceftriaxone-bilirubin-albumin interactions in the neonate: an in vivo study. *Eur J Pediatr* 152:530–34, 1993.

Maruo Y et al. Association of neonatal hyperbilirubinemia with bilirubin UDP-glucuronosyltransferase polymorphism. *Pediatrics* 103:1224–27, 1999.

Maruo Y et al. Prolonged unconjugated hyperbilirubinemia associated with breast milk and mutations of the bilirubin uridine diphosphate-glucuronosyltransferase gene. *Pediatrics* 106:e59, 2000.

Monaghan G et al. Gilbert's syndrome is a contributory factor in prolonged unconjugated hyperbilirubinemia of the newborn. *J Pediatr* 134:441–46, 1999.

Moyer VA, Ahn C, Sneed S. Accuracy of clinical judgment in neonatal jaundice. *Arch Pediatr Adolesc Med* 154:391–94, 2000.

Neifert MR. The optimization of breast-feeding in the perinatal period. *Clin Perinatol* 25:303–26, 1998.

Newman AJ, Gross S. Hyperbilirubinemia in breast-fed infants. *Pediatrics* 32:995–1001, 1963.

Newman TB, Easterling MJ. Yield of reticulocyte counts and blood smears in term neonates. *Clin Pediatr* 33:71–76, 1994.

Rubaltelli FF. Unconjugated and conjugated bilirubin pigments during perinatal development. IV. The influence of breast-feeding on neonatal hyperbilirubinemia. *Biol Neonate* 64:104–9, 1993.

Rubaltelli FF et al. Transcutaneous bilirubin measurement: a multicenter evaluation of a new device. *Pediatrics* 107:1264–71, 2001.

Shurin SB. The blood and hematopoietic system. In: Fanaroff AA, Martin RJ, eds. *Neonatal-perinatal medicine: diseases of the fetus and infant.* St. Louis, MO: Mosby–Year Book 1992:941–89.

Stevenson DK, Dennery PA, Hinz SR. Understanding newborn jaundice. *J Perinatol* 21:S21–S24, 2001.

Stiehm ER, Ryan J. Breast-milk jaundice. *Amer J Dis Child* 109:212–16, 1965.

Stocker R et al. Bilirubin is an antioxidant of possible physiological importance. *Science* 235:1043–46, 1987.

Vreman HJ et al. Evaluation of a fully automated end-tidal carbon monoxide instrument for breath analysis. *Clin Chem* 42:50–56, 1996.

Whitmer DI, Gollan JL. Mechanism and significance of fasting and dietary hyperbilirubinemia. *Semin Liver Dis* 3:42–51, 1983.

Young BWY et al. Predicting pathologic jaundice: the Chinese perspective. *J Perinatol* 21:S73–S75, 2001.

12

Breast Pumps and Other Technologies

Marsha Walker

Special devices have been used for hundreds of years to help breastfeeding mothers overcome various problems. Examples of someone, or something, other than a baby removing milk from the breasts are cited in medical literature as early as the mid-1500s (Fildes, 1986). Before breast pumps or other instruments were used to withdraw milk from the breasts, children, young puppies, or birth attendants were enlisted to do the job. By the 1500s the medical literature included discussions of "sucking glasses." These devices allowed women to remove milk themselves and were recommended for relieving engorgement or expressing milk when the nipples were damaged or when mastitis was present. Sucking glasses were also thought to help evert flat and inverted nipples. For the most part, vacuum was generated by mouth, and the devices were made of glass (Figure 12–1). Women could use a glass, glass vial, or glass bottle heated with very hot water and applied to the breast in order to draw out milk. French breast pumps in the 1700s resembled smoking pipes but were made of different materials.

As technology advanced, so did breast pump materials and design. Combinations of materials such as brass, wood, glass, and rubber were used to make pumps like the syringe pump (Figure 12–2), the long-handled lever pump (Figure 12–3) and the glass and rubber "bicycle horn" pump, all c. 1830.

The reasons why women chose to express milk also changed. Today, women pump their breasts for short periods of time to solve acute problems and for extended periods in order to provide human milk for their babies under such circumstances as employment, induced lactation, relactation, maternal or infant illness, or following a preterm birth.

Concerns of Mothers

Most mothers want a pump that works efficiently and comfortably at a reasonable cost. They want pumps that are easy to find, easy to use, and easy to clean. The amount of milk expressed and the time it takes to obtain it are the two issues most frequently mentioned by mothers when they are choosing or using a breast pump.

Satisfaction with breast pumps, however, is highly individual. In an informal survey conducted with more than 200 mothers (Walker, 1992), a pump was rated highly if it (1) worked quickly— (less than 20 minutes total), (2) obtained two or more ounces of milk from each breast, and (3) did not cause pain. The mothers in this survey suggested pumping techniques to speed the process and to increase the volume of milk per pumping session. Many mothers expressed the most milk before or after the first morning feeding when the breasts

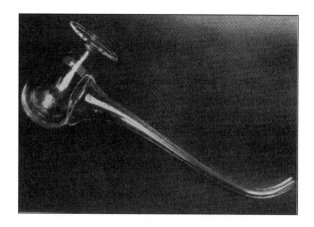

FIGURE 12–1. An American sucking glass circa 1870.

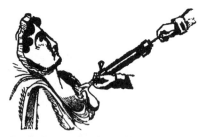

DRAWING THE BREASTS.

Where the breast is hard, swollen and painful, from inflammation, or the nipple sore from excoriation, the application of this instrument is attended with more ease to the patient than any other means, and she may without difficulty use it herself, by which she can regulate its action agreeably to her own sensations. The flat surface of the glass should be smeared with oil before it is put on, and the bulb preserved in a dependant position to receive the fluid. During the operation the small aperture in the brass socket must be closely covered with the finger, which being removed, admits air into the glass and causes it to be detached from the breast whenever it may be desired.

FIGURE 12–2. Expressing the breasts with a syringe pump, c. 1830.

were reported to be fullest (and intramammary pressure was the highest); later volumes steadily decreased throughout the day. Many mothers mentioned that if they were not relaxed, or if they were uncomfortable or felt rushed, their output dropped by one third to one half the usual amount.

The majority of mothers used one or more techniques to increase pumping efficiency. The two most frequently mentioned techniques were eliciting the milk-ejection reflex before starting to pump and massaging the breast while pumping. Both techniques increased pumping speed and milk output. Some mothers were able to double the amount pumped by using both of these techniques at each pumping session.

Stimulating the Milk-Ejection Reflex

Research conducted by the dairy industry supports the importance of eliciting the milk-ejection reflex before starting to express milk. In the dairy cow, premilking stimulation of the udder increases serum oxytocin levels (Merrill et al., 1987) and results in shorter "machine on" time and a higher average rate of milk flow (Sagi, Gorewit, & Zinn, 1980; Dodd & Griffin, 1977; Goodman & Grosvenor, 1983; Gorewit et al., 1983). In the second edition of *Dairy Science,* Petersen (1950) cited several factors that contribute to poor milking: undue excitement at milking time, improper stimulation for the let-down of milk, too long an interval between stimulation of let-down and the beginning of milking, too slow milking, and incomplete withdrawal of milk. His observations regarding proper milking techniques parallel many recommendations of professionals and the expression techniques human mothers have discovered on their own. Animal models of lactation can serve as a frame of reference from which recommendations can be drawn and applied. For example:

1. *Avoid undue excitement at milking time.* Many women use specific relaxation techniques and visual imagery before and during pumping. Feher et al. (1989) reported using a guided relaxation audiotape to increase milk output during breast pumping among mothers of preterm infants. Newton and Newton (1948) described the adverse effect of a painful or distracting stimulus during nursing on the milk-ejection reflex. Pain and psychologic stress can inhibit the milk-ejection reflex by reducing the number of oxytocin pulses during suckling episodes (Ueda et al., 1994). Opiate and B-endorphin release during stress can block stimulus-related oxytocin secretion (Lawrence & Lawrence, 1999).

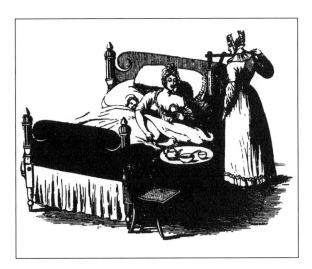

FIGURE 12–3. Expressing breastmilk with a long-handled lever pump, c. 1830.

2. *Elicit the milk-ejection reflex first, 1 to 2 minutes before pumping begins; massaging with a hot, wet cloth before milking is the most effective stimulus for let-down.* Mothers have reported using hot compresses, showers, and breast massage before expressing to obtain the best results. Some report that they are most successful if they pump one side while the baby feeds on the other breast (as with pumping in dairy cattle when all teats are milked simultaneously), if the baby elicits the milk-ejection reflex first and they then pump, or if they hand express first or massage the breast first and then pump. Upon nipple stimulation, oxytocin is released in a pulsatile nature consisting of brief 3 to 4 second bursts of oxytocin into the bloodstream every 5 to 15 minutes. This shortens and widens the lactiferous ducts, increasing the pressure inside the breast and is essential for maximum removal of milk from the breast (Neville, 2001). Correlations between oxytocin pulsatility on day two and the duration of exclusive breastfeeding suggest that the development of an early pulsatile oxytocin pattern is of importance for sustained exclusive breastfeeding (Nissen et al., 1996). Oxytocin can also be released prior to the baby being placed at breast and is not dependant solely on tactile stimula-

tion for release. It takes the baby an average of 54 seconds to elicit the milk-ejection reflex on the first side and 47 seconds on the second side. A breast pump can take up to 4 minutes to elicit the milk-ejection reflex (mean 103.2 ± 89.2 sec) (Kent et al., 2003: Mitoulas, Lai, & Gurrin, 2002a).

3. *Massage each quarter of the udder during mechanical milking.* Massaging during breast pumping can markedly increase milk yield. Breast massage may increase fat content and milk yield when a baby is at breast. Bowles, Stutte, and Hensley (1988) and Stutte, Bowles, and Morman (1988) found that infants gained greater amounts of weight and mothers experienced little nipple pain or painful engorgement when the breasts were massaged by quadrant in an alternating pattern with the baby's suckling bursts. Breast massage represents a form of positive pressure, which adds to the pressure created within the milk ducts during let-down. The diameter of the milk ducts increases by approximately 79 percent after let-down, (Hartmann, 2000) with duct diameters drifting down after a 1- to 2-minute period following let-down (Hartmann, 2002). A pump needs to remove milk quickly before the volume of milk in the ducts decreases and another let-down is necessary to reestablish the pressure gradient between breast and pump. Adding external compression probably acts as an "artificial" let-down, increasing the positive pressure within the breast and helping milk flow toward the negative pressure created in the pump. The establishment of an effective pressure gradient that can be sustained over a long enough period of time will contribute to the optimal drainage of each breast.

4. *When hand-milking, avoid point compression and digging in with the fingertips, which is likely to cause injury.* The Marmet method of hand expression (Marmet & Shell, 1980) cautioned against this technique when a mother is hand-expressing her milk.

5. *Remove the milking machine as soon as the milk stops flowing.* Stopping the pump when the milk stops flowing reduces tissue injury. Many mothers switch to the other breast when the milk flow

slows in the breast being pumped. Some mothers mention that pain is the cue for this switch, indicating a change in the pressure gradient. Auerbach (1990b) found that protracted pumping times did not significantly increase milk yield beyond a certain point. Those who pumped (sequentially or simultaneously) for longer than 16 minutes averaged total milk volumes of 55 cc or less. Mitoulas, Lai, and Gurrin (2002a) found that the rate of milk expression changed over the course of a 5-minute expression period, remaining constant the first 2.5 minutes but decreasing by 5 minutes. The variation among mothers was large, with some mothers delivering almost 2 oz in the first 30 seconds to others delivering no milk by the end of 5 minutes. If it takes a particular mother 4 minutes to elicit the milk-ejection reflex, she may need a much longer time to pump than another mother delivering 99 percent of the milk in her breasts into the pump within 5 minutes.

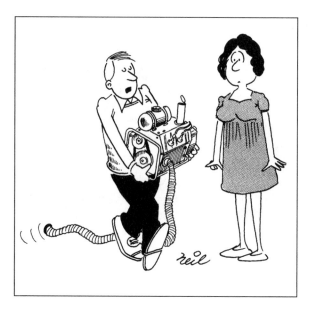

FIGURE 12–4. "They didn't actually have a breast pump. . ." (Courtesy of Neil Matteson © 1984.)

The dairy literature includes many recommendations that are applicable to human breast pumping. Even some of the modern electric breast pumps designed for mothers have similarities to the agricultural milking units. The Whittlestone pump has incorporated the design of the double-chambered teat cups. The suction and rest phases of a commercial milking unit are either 60/40 or 70/30 (percentage of suction to percentage of rest per cycle). There are usually 60 cycles generated per minute (a calf generates about 120 cycles), and negative pressure is around 375 mm Hg (similar to the higher pressures seen in many breast pumps, including hand pumps).

Breast pumps must also be easy to clean, affordable, and accessible. When recommending a pump, the caregiver should give a specific name and several places to find it to avoid acquisition of a pump that may be inappropriate or ineffective (Figure 12–4). Hospital or medical supply houses may have pumps originally designed as chest aspirators which are not as suitable for milk expression as those specifically designed for that purpose. Instructions for use may be inadequate, causing some mothers to forgo pumping and breastfeeding altogether. Many mothers have complained of the extra expense incurred if their pump broke (common with the battery pumps) and required replacement (Walker, 1992). Of 97 battery pumps used in the survey, 24 broke or stopped generating suction and had to be replaced (a 25 percent breakage rate). The life of a battery-operated pump is considered to be about 16 weeks (4 months) by some companies, a much shorter period than many employed mothers require. Batteries are a major expense for mothers who pump regularly; many purchase an A/C adapter to economize. The cost of the accessory kit and daily rental charges for an electric pump can be expensive, even with a long-term rental contract. Some insurance carriers and health maintenance organizations cover the cost of pump rentals only while a baby is hospitalized or for only a limited period of time.

Several mothers in the survey purchased a hand pump solely to cut cost. Some were dissatisfied and purchased a second, more expensive pump that worked better. Pump prices vary considerably depending upon the type of store or organization that sells them. Some breastfeeding programs provide breast pumps at cost to their clients. Many hospitals give breastfeeding mothers a high-quality hand pump upon discharge rather than formula packs. Box 12–1 summarizes recommendations for mothers using a breast pump.

BOX 12–1

Recommendations for the Nursing Mother Who Uses a Pump

General Pumping Recommendations

1. Read the instructions on the use and cleaning of a pump before expressing milk with any product.

2. Wash hands before each pumping session.

3. Frequency: For occasional pumping, pump during, after, or between feedings, whichever gives the best results. Most mothers tend to express more milk in the morning. For mothers employed outside the home, pumping should occur on a regular basis for the number of nursings that are missed. For premature or ill babies who are not at breast, the number of pumpings should total 8–10 or more each 24 hours for the 1st 14 days. Initiation of pumping should be delayed no longer than 6 hours following birth unless medically indicated. This ensures appropriate development and sensitivity of prolactin receptors. More frequent pumping will avoid the build-up of excessive backpressure of milk during engorgement.

4. Duration: With single-sided pumping, duration ranges from 10 to 15 minutes with an electric pump and 10 to 20 minutes with a manual pump. If double pumping with an electric or two battery-operated pumps, 7 to 15 minutes is optimal. Encourage mothers to tailor these times to their own situation.

5. Technique:
   - Elicit the milk-ejection reflex before using the pump.
   - Use only as much vacuum as is needed to maintain milk flow and remain comfortable.
   - Massage the breast in quadrants before and during pumping to increase intramammary pressure.
   - Allow enough time for pumping to avoid anxiety.
   - Use inserts or different sized flanges if needed to obtain the best fit between pump and breast.
   - Avoid long periods of uninterrupted vacuum.
   - Stop pumping when the milk flow is minimal or has ceased.

Recommendations for Specific Types of Pumps

1. Avoid pumps that use rubber bulbs to generate a vacuum.

2. Cylinder pumps:
   - When O rings are used, they must be in place for proper suction.
   - Gaskets must be removed after each use for cleaning to avoid harboring bacteria in the pump.
   - The gasket on the inner cylinder may be rolled back and forth to restore it to its original shape.
   - The pump stroke may need to be shortened as the outer cylinder fills with milk.
   - The mother may need to empty the outer cylinder once or twice during pumping.

BOX 12–1 (cont.)

- Hand position should be palm up with the elbow held close to the body.

3. Battery-operated pumps:

  - Use alkaline batteries, not rechargable batteries.
  - Replace batteries when cycles per minute decrease.
  - Interrupt vacuum frequently to avoid nipple pain and damage if the pump does not autocycle.
  - Use an AC adapter when possible, especially if the pump generates fewer than 6 cycles per minute.
  - Consider purchasing or renting an electric pump for pumping that will continue for longer than 1 or 2 months.
  - Use two pumps simultaneously if pumping time is limited or to increase the quantity of milk obtained.
  - Choose a pump in which the vacuum can be regulated.

  - Massage the breast by quadrants during pumping.

4. Semiautomatic pumps:

  - Vacuum may be easier to control if the mother does not lift her finger completely off the hole but rolls it back and forth rhythmically so that the vacuum is efficient but not painful.

5. Automatic electric pumps:

  - Use the lowest pressure setting that is efficient. Mothers may find that changing the vacuum and/or the cycling characteristics of the pump during each expressing session may increase milk volume.
  - Use a double setup (simultaneous pumping) when time is limited in order to increase a milk supply, as well as for prematurity, maternal or infant illness, or other special situations.

Hormonal Considerations

When milk expression using a pump is necessary, the device used must be efficient enough to activate prolactin and oxytocin release and to efficiently remove milk from the breasts.

Prolactin

A steady rise in prolactin during pregnancy prepares the breasts for lactation (Neville, 1983). Prolactin levels rise during pregnancy from about 10 ng/ml in the nonpregnant state to approximately 200 ng/ml at term. Baseline levels do not drop to normal in a lactating woman, but average about 100 ng/ml at 3 months and 50 ng/ml at 6 months. Prolactin levels can double with the stimulus of suckling. After about 6 months of breastfeeding, the prolactin rise with suckling amounts to only about

5 to 10 ng/ml. This is accounted for by the increased prolactin binding capacity or sensitivity of the mammary tissue that allows full lactation in the face of falling prolactin levels over time. The high levels of prolactin during pregnancy and early lactation may also serve to increase the number of prolactin receptors and is dependant on tactile input for stimulation and release. In spite of the importance of prolactin to lactation itself, prolactin does not directly regulate the short-term or long-term rate of milk synthesis (Cox, Owens, & Hartmann, 1996). Once lactation is well established, prolactin is still required for milk synthesis to occur but its role is permissive rather than regulatory (Cregan & Hartmann, 1999).

Prolactin concentration in the plasma is highest during sleep and lowest during the waking hours and operates as a true circadian rhythm (Stern &

Reichlin, 1990). The prolactin response is superimposed on the circadian rhythm of prolactin secretion, thus the same intensity of suckling stimulus can elevate prolactin levels more effectively at certain times of the day when the circadian input enhances the effect of the sucking stimulus (Freeman et al., 2000). Prolactin levels will only remain elevated after the first weeks postpartum if the baby is put to breast, or in the absence of breast stimulation by an infant, if a pump is used to mechanically maintain prolactin cycling. Small studies with wide variations in methodology have demonstrated the ability of various pumps to elevate prolactin levels. (Noel, Suh, & Frantz, 1974; Weichert, 1980; Howie et al., 1980; de Sanctis et al., 1981; Whitworth et al., 1984; Neifert & Seacat, 1985; Zinaman et al., 1992).

Clinical Implications

1. *The function of infant suckling (or mechanical milk removal) varies between lactogenesis II, the onset of copious milk production, and galactopoiesis (lactogenesis III), the maintenance of abundant milk production.* Lactogenesis II occurs in the absence of milk removal over the first 3 days postpartum, but milk composition and volume will not proceed along the continuum to maximum milk production and mature milk composition in the absence of frequent milk removal after that time. While suckling (or mechanical milk removal) may not be a prerequisite for lactogenesis II, it is critical for galactopoiesis. Delayed suckling by the infant, whether due to premature delivery (Cregan, DeMello, & Hartmann 2000), cesarean delivery (Sozmen, 1992), or other factors that necessitate mechanical milk removal, may affect the timing or delay the onset of lactogenesis II. Additional breast pumping after a couple of breastfeeds before the onset of lactogenesis II has not been shown to hasten the event or result in increased milk transfer to the baby at 72 hours (Chapman et al., 2001). In the absence of a baby at breast, the breasts need to be stimulated eight or more times every 24 hours. Pumping only once or twice during the day and never at night, when prolactin levels are at their peak, may contribute to delayed lactogenesis II. A faltering milk supply in the following weeks may be attributed to the lack of sufficient prolactin receptors and infrequent breast stimulation while lactation is being established.

2. *Painful overdistention of the breasts (secondary engorgement) must be prevented.* As alveolar pressure rises, lactation suppression begins. Painful engorgement lasting longer than 48 hours can potentially decrease the milk supply. Therefore, if a baby cannot keep up with a suddenly increased milk supply, the mother should express her milk. When milk production begins in the absence of a baby, pumping frequency may need to be temporarily increased to prevent involution of the alveoli caused by the back-pressure of milk and the buildup of suppressor peptides that down-regulate milk volume. Wilde, Prentice, and Peaker (1995) have identified this peptide and named it the feedback inhibitor of lactation (FIL).

3. *Early breastfeeding has a critical period during which frequent nipple stimulation and milk removal are necessary for a plentiful milk supply in later weeks.* The clinician should offer management guidelines with this in mind, especially if mother and baby are separated. Woolridge (1995) provided a practical identification of six separate stages in the lactation process:

- Priming (changes of pregnancy).
- Initiation (birth and the management of early breastfeeding).
- Calibration (the concept that milk production gets underway without the breasts actually "knowing" how much milk to make in the beginning). Over the first 3 to 5 weeks, milk output is progressively calibrated to the baby's needs, usually building up (up-regulation) but occasionally down-regulating to meet the baby's needs.
- Maintenance (the period of exclusive breastfeeding).
- Decline (the period after complementary foods or supplements are added).
- Involution (weaning).

It is the second, third, and fourth time periods that are crucial to ensuring abundant milk production. Close attention must be given to alterations that could impact the breasts' ability to calibrate their milk output to the needs of the baby.

Daly et al. (1992, 1993) have shown that the degree of breast emptying is inversely proportional to the amount of milk made to replace it; that is, the more thoroughly that a breast is drained, the more milk is made. Daly and Hartmann (1995a, 1995b) noted that breasts with smaller storage capacities may need to be expressed more frequently than breasts with larger storage capacities, even though both types of breasts are capable of synthesizing similar amounts of milk in 24 hours. Mothers with larger storage capacities are able to express a higher volume of milk with each pumping session but not necessarily more milk in a 24-hour period than mothers with smaller storage capacities. The volume of milk expressed is also related to the degree of fullness of the breast, with a fuller breast yielding more milk volume when pumped (Mitoulas, Lai, & Gurrin, 2002a). Full breasts tend to take less time to achieve the milk-ejection reflex, with a less full breast taking up to 120 seconds (Hartmann, 2002).

Oxytocin

Oxytocin is responsible for the milk-ejection reflex. By acting on the myoepithelial processes, oxytocin causes shortening of the ducts without constricting them, thus increasing the milk pressure. Cobo et al. (1967) measured milk-ejection by recording intraductal mammary pressure using a catheter placed in a mammary duct. Values were measured at 0.19 plus or minus 0.04 in/min and from 0 to 25 mm Hg on recording paper. Ductal contractions lasted about 1 minute and occurred at about 4 to 10 contractions every 10 minutes. Caldeyro-Barcia (1969) reported that intramammary pressure rose 10 mm Hg after 5 days postpartum with oxytocin release. Drewett, Bowen-Jones, and Dogterom (1982) and McNeilly et al. (1983) have shown by minute-to-minute blood sampling that oxytocin occurs in impulses at about 1-minute intervals. Thus oxytocin release is pulsatile and variable with intermittent bursts. These pressure changes cease when suckling stimulation ends. Oxytocin also responds in the same way to prenursing stimuli and mechanical nipple stimulation by a breast pump. The milk-ejection reflex, initiated by oxytocin release, serves to increase the intraductal mammary pressure and maintain it at sufficient levels to overcome the resistance of the breast to the outflow of milk. There is approximately 30 to 35 ml of milk ingested by the infant per milk-ejection (Hartmann, 2002). Milk ducts stay dilated approximately 1.5 to 3.5 minutes following let-down (Hartmann, 2002) making it beneficial to elicit multiple let-downs during the course of a pumping session.

Pumps

Mechanical Milk Removal

A pump does not pump, suck, or pull milk out of the breast. It reduces resistance to milk outflow from the alveoli, allowing the internal pressure of the breast to push out the milk. The milk-ejection reflex produces an initial rise in the intramammary pressure; because of the pulsatile nature of oxytocin release and its short half-life, periodic rises in ductal pressure maintain the pressure gradient over time.

The classic work on breast pumps conducted by Einar Egnell (1956) was based on research in dairy cattle and Egnell's own experiments with a pump that created periodic and limited phases of negative pressure. Egnell assumed that the milk-secreting alveoli of the breast and the cow udder were similar, even though the two organs are anatomically different and do not drain in the same way. He postulated that the quantity of milk secreted is regulated by the counterpressure it exerts. This counterpressure rises as milk fills the available space; secretion ceases when the pressure reaches 28 mm Hg. Egnell's pump created a maximum negative pressure of 200 mm Hg below atmospheric pressure (760 mm Hg). He based this setting on previous research done with an Abt pump (on human mothers), which produced 30 periods of negative pressure per minute and was reported to rupture the nipple skin in every third breast. Placing his settings well below this level to avoid damaging the human nipple, Egnell calculated the difference between the pressure-filled alveoli and his pump's negative pressure as $760 + 28 - 560 = 228$ mm Hg. He maintained that it was the pressure within the breast that activated milk outflow.

Egnell's original pump operated in four phases per cycle, with one cycle lasting from one initiation of suction to the next initiation of suction: (1) a period of increasing suction that is relatively short, (2) a decreasing phase of suction, (3) a resting phase, and (4) a slight amount of positive pressure when the decreased suction phase is finished. Egnell contended that mechanical pumping was safer than manual expression because he feared that the "high" positive pressure generated by "squeezing" the breast could damage the alveoli and ducts. He also speculated that manual expression would leave too much milk in the breast, a common concern in the dairy industry. However, in countries where manual expression is used to obtain mothers' milk when the baby is unavailable, increased breast damage has not been reported. Many pump manufacturers still use Egnell's pressure settings as a guide. However, various pumps are still capable of generating more suction than stated in his calculations.

The vacuum applied to the breast by an infant during suckling is not constant. The vacuum is initiated, it rises, it is released, and it is maintained with a basal resting pressure to keep the nipple in the mouth. The vacuum stretches the teat to approximately twice its resting length, with a 70 percent reduction of the teat's original diameter (Smith, Erenberg, & Nowak, 1988; Weber, Woolridge, & Baum, 1986). Speculation on the function of vacuum ranges from thoughts that (1) vacuum facilitates the refilling with milk of the ducts within the teat following each swallow, or that (2) milk is released from the teat by vacuum caused when the jaw lowers and enlarges the oral cavity (Smith, Erenberg, & Nowak, 1988). An infant feeding at breast achieves a range of 42 to 126 suck cycles per minute with a mean of 74 sucks per minute (Bowen-Jones, Thompson, & Drewett, 1982). Suction is applied over approximately half of the suck cycle (Halverson, 1944). However, vacuum or suction is not the only force that an infant employs to extract milk from the breast. A compressive force from the tongue and jaw is also applied during the suction cycle to more effectively create milk transfer from the breast to the baby.

Computer modeling that compares breastfeeding and breast pumps has shown that there is an optimal time during the suction cycle when an infant applies the compressive peristaltic force of the tongue. This results in an asymmetric compression of the teat between the tongue and hard palate.

Using a model that applied symmetric peristaltic compression of the teat during a suction cycle, Zoppou, Barry, and Mercer (1997a) found that the compressive force applied at the optimal time and speed during the suck cycle could significantly increase the mean fluid flow through the teat, while a compressive force applied at the wrong time in the pressure cycle restricted the flow of fluid. A compressive force applied by a breast pump approximately a quarter of the way through the suction cycle increased the milk volume over one suction cycle by 15 percent, while a compressive force that compressed the teat early in the suction cycle restricted milk flow into the teat, reduced milk volume (Zoppou, Barry, & Mercer, 1997b).

Compression

Whittlestone (1978) described a breast pump that not only accommodated the simultaneous pumping of both breasts but further adopted principles from the commercial dairy milking machines of providing a compressive force to the breast from a liner inside the pump flange that rhythmically contracted around the teat. He called this a physiologic breast-milker. Alekseev et al. (1998) found that adding the compressive stimulus changed the dynamics of milk expression. Using an experimental pump where the compressive stimulus could be switched on and off, it was found that in a 3- to 5-minute period of pumping, 50 percent of the milk could be removed from the breast, but when the compressive stimulus was turned off it took 1.5 to 2.0 times longer to express this volume of milk. Currently, the Whittlestone Breast Expresser (Figure 12–5) employs a compressive liner in its flanges.

The Whisper Wear breast pump (Figure 12–6) is worn under the bra and utilizes a flexible massaging cup. Some of the other pumps have a soft flange that collapses over the teat when vacuum is applied.

The Evolution of Pumps

As breastfeeding rates increased and reasons for pumping changed, mothers and professionals have demanded products that are safe, efficient, and effective in both initiating and maintaining a good milk supply. The breast pump market offers a bewildering array of devices from which to choose.

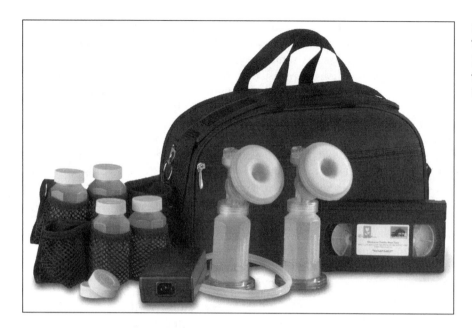

**FIGURE 12–5.
The Whittlestone
Breast Expresser. (Cour-
tesy of Whittlestone, Inc.,
Benicia, CA.)**

Three broad classifications of breast pumps will be discussed in this chapter: (1) hand pumps that generate suction manually, (2) battery-operated pumps with small motors that generate suction from power supplied by batteries, and (3) electric pumps in which suction is created by various types of electric motors. A photograph showing an example of each type of pump will be included in the chapter. There is no intent to recommend any one pump. A listing of companies that sell breast pumps can be found in Appendix 12–A. Descriptions and pictures of pumps can be found at the company Web sites.

A Comparison of Pumps

Hand pumps are popular, relatively inexpensive, and readily available. Much information on the efficiency of hand pumps is anecdotal; some pumps work quite well, whereas others suffer from poor suction, excessive suction, cylinders that pull apart during pumping, and user fatigue from the repeated motions necessary to work the pumps. A few studies have examined the efficiency of hand pumps, as well as their ability to influence prolactin levels, the volume of milk expressed, and its fat and energy content. These studies are difficult to compare because study design and methodology vary widely. The results may depend on single or random milk samples, and on measurement of milk components obtained at different postpartum times.

Zinaman et al. (1992) studied differences in the volume of milk obtained and prolactin stimulation by various types of breast pumps, as well as by the mother's baby, in 23 women who were 28 to 42 days postpartum. Their results showed that a double setup (in which both breasts are pumped simultaneously) electric pump did better in stimulating prolactin levels than did battery or manual pumps, or hand expression, when only one breast was stimulated at a time. The White River electric pump was reported to stimulate the highest prolactin levels, cycling at 40 times per minute. Milk volumes were highest with this pump. Lowest milk volume was with hand expression and the Gentle Expressions battery pump, which produced 6 to 10 cycles per minute. When mothers rated their satisfaction with the pumps, the White River electric rated as one of the more uncomfortable to use. A singular problem with this study was its comparison of double pumping to breastfeeding a single baby or sequential pumping of one breast at a time. A more reliable test of pump efficacy would be to control for breast stimulation by using mothers of twins when comparing double pumping—or using other double-pump setups or two pumps simultaneously. Neifert and Seacat (1985) has shown the greater prolactin rise when both breasts are expressed simultaneously.

Fewtrell, Lucas, and Collier (2001) compared the efficacy of the Avent Isis manual pump and

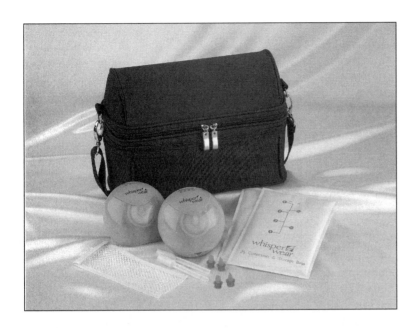

FIGURE 12–6. The Whisper Wear breast pump. (Courtesy of Whisper Wear, Marietta, GA.)

the Egnell electric pump in mothers who delivered preterm infants less than 35 weeks gestation. At 7 to 10 days, the mothers evaluated "consumer" characteristics of their assigned pump (ease of use, amount of suction, comfort, pleasant to use, and overall opinion of the pump). Mothers did not use or compare both pumps to each other. While mothers rated the Avent Isis as a more comfortable pump, mothers in both groups pumped a mean of 3 times per day with a mean volume of < 7 ounces a day (199 ml/day, range 57 to 323 ml with the Avent Isis and 218 ml/day, range 126 to 341 ml with the electric pump). It is difficult to concur with the authors' conclusions that the manual pump reflected a significant advance in pumping milk for preterm infants when milk output was so low for the amount of time spent pumping. The study did not address the ability of the pumps to initiate a milk supply or maintain milk production over a long period of time.

Fewtrell et al. (2001) compared the efficacy of the Avent Isis manual pump and the Medela Mini Electric pump in term 8-week-old babies. Each pump was tested on a single occasion with the second pump tested 2 to 3 days after the first, and the mothers rated the pumps on the same "consumer" scale as above. The rating factor for the mothers was only if the pump was pleasant to use, not the volume of milk expressed. These data also showed that irrespective of which pump was tested as the second pump, milk volumes were increased. However, when the second pump was the mini-electric, milk volume was 164 ml ±73 compared to 149 ml ±71 with the manual pump. The value of this study remains unknown, as neither of the study pumps was used over time or validated as being capable of sustaining milk production in a mother who is dependant on a pump for this purpose.

Manual Hand Pumps

The various types of hand pumps rely on differing mechanisms to generate suction.

Rubber Bulb Models. Rubber bulb pumps are seldom seen in current clinical practice. Squeezing and releasing a rubber bulb generates a vacuum in these pumps. In most "bicycle horn" pumps, the rubber bulb is attached directly to the collection container. Some manufacturers separated the bulb from the collection container by modifying the angle at which it is attached to the pump or by adding a length of tubing. These modifications were thought to reduce the high potential for bacterial contamination of the bulb caused by the easy backflow of milk. Backflow risk is reduced when the bulb is separated from the collection container. Vacuum control on these pumps is extremely difficult, thus increasing the likelihood of nipple pain and damage. Even with the use of a blood pressure-type bulb, vacuum control is left to chance.

The "bicycle horn" pumps are inexpensive, but collect only about one half ounce of milk at a time and must be emptied frequently. The other pumps collect milk in a bottle. Mothers often complain of nipple pain during pumping and low milk yields, especially if they have used these pumps for more than a few weeks. Most mothers no longer see these pumps in stores but some models may still be available and are a poor choice in any circumstance.

Squeeze-Handle Models. Squeeze-handle models (Figures 12–7 and 12–8), such as Avent Isis, Ameda One-Hand, Gerber Manual, and Evenflo ComfortEase Manual, involve squeezing and releasing a handle that creates suction in the pump. They are typically used for occasional pumping and are a type that can be used when no electricity is available. These pumps are easily cleaned but their operation may present difficulties for women with hand or arm problems, such as arthritis or carpal tunnel syndrome. The hand and wrist can tire easily with repeated use.

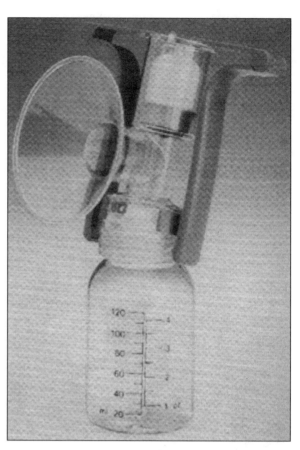

FIGURE 12–8. The Ameda One-Hand pump. (Courtesy of Hollister/Ameda-Egnell.)

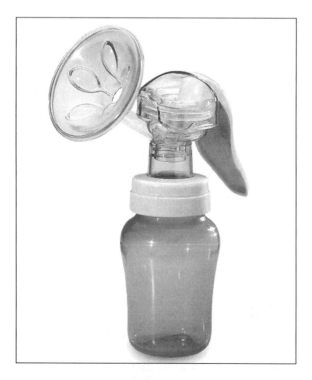

FIGURE 12–7. The Avent Isis squeeze handle manual pump. (Courtesy of Canon Babysafe Ltd., Suffolk, England.)

Cylinder Pumps. Cylinder pumps include products such as Ameda Cylinder Hand pump, Evenflo Manual, Omron Kaneson, Medela Spring Express and Manual Ease, PumpExpress, and PumpExpress Mini (CAMP Healthcare, the former White River pumps). All of these pumps, except for the Medela and Evenflo, consist of two cylinders. The outer cylinder generates vacuum as it is pulled away from the body. The inner cylinder with the flange is placed against the breast; a gasket at the other end helps form a seal with the edge of the outer cylinder. Gaskets may need to be replaced occasionally if they dry out, shrink, or lose their ability to form a seal. Gaskets can harbor bacteria and must be removed during cleaning, contrary to some user instructions. When placing the gasket back on the cylinder, roll it back and forth over the cylinder to help restore the shape. Some pumps come with extra gaskets.

Small plastic or silicone inserts can be placed in the inner opening to custom fit the pump to the breast. Silicone liners are available for some pumps; these are designed to collapse against the breast during the suction phase to provide external positive pressure. These pumps are lightweight, not too expensive, and easily cleaned.

Before recommending any of these pumps, the clinician should check if the pump automatically interrupts vacuum at a preset level, if there are adjustable vacuum settings, and if the pump has a collection bottle rather than an outer cylinder where milk accumulates during pumping. Some pumps also provide an extra cylinder for milk storage or have an angled rather than a straight flange. Some mothers report that the angled flange does not work as well as the straight pumps. As the outer cylinder fills with milk, the gasket is repeatedly dunked in the milk. Mothers who express more than 3 oz of milk at a time may have to empty these pumps more than once in a single pumping episode.

Efficiency of use varies from brand to brand. Some can also be adapted for use on the larger electric pumps. Higher vacuum is generated as the outer cylinder fills with milk. Mothers may need to shorten the outward stroke after collecting more than 1 oz.

Battery-Operated Pumps

Examples of battery-operated pumps include Evenflo Personal Comfort, Lumiscope Gentle Expressions, Omron Mag Mag, Medela Mini Electric, First Years Electric/Battery and Natural Comfort, and Gerber Battery/Electric pumps. The Whisper Wear pump is battery operated but is worn under the bra like breast shells and operates hands-free once secured in place. These pumps use a small motor with usually either size AA 1.5-volt batteries or size C batteries. Most have a vacuum adjustment mechanism. Vacuum in some pumps can take up to 30 seconds to reach maximum level and is regulated by how frequently the vacuum is interrupted.

Some of these pumps have a button to press in order to release the vacuum periodically and to simulate the rhythm of a nursing baby. All take varying periods of time for the recovery of suction following each release. This limits the number of suction/release cycles per minute to as few as 6 and may require relatively long periods of vacuum application to the nipple. To compensate for this, some mothers leave the suction on for much longer than the pump instructions recommend. Mothers in one survey mentioned 30 to 60 seconds. Four women never interrupted the suction during the entire pumping session because they could not get the milk flow restarted following vacuum interruption. Some pumps have preset automatic cycling.

Several pumps have AC adapters to decrease battery use. A major complaint about these pumps is their short battery life. This affects pumping efficiency because fewer cycles are generated as the batteries wear down. Batteries may have to be replaced as frequently as every second or third use. Rechargeable batteries are an option, but they usually require charging each night and may not produce as many cycles per minute as alkaline batteries. AC adapters usually allow the maximum number of cycles per minute that the motor can produce. Maximum suction after each vacuum release will often continue decreasing in amount throughout the pumping session. In contrast, the Medela battery pump automatically produces 32 cycles per minute with alkaline batteries, 30 cycles per minute with rechargeable batteries and 42 cycles per minute with the A/C adapter. The Evenflo pumps generate 38 cycles per minute.

Battery pumps require only one hand to operate, are lightweight, and are popular with mothers employed outside the home. Some mothers use two battery-operated pumps simultaneously to decrease pumping time when they are on a tight schedule. Mothers who plan to pump for several months while at work may consider a personal use larger pump or a long-term rental contract for an electric pump, because battery replacement can be very expensive—as can artificial formula if it must be used to substitute for breastmilk. Some of the pumps operate with a quiet hum while others are very noisy.

The Whisper Wear pump is worn under the bra and automatically cycles 30 to 70 times per minute as it has an initial rapid cycling phase as well as a flexible massaging cup that adds an element of positive pressure. The settings can be independently controlled for each breast. Battery life is up to 50 hours.

Electric Pumps

Electric breast pumps fall into one of three categories:

- Small semiautomatic pumps: Gerber, Nurture III.

- Personal use pumps: Medela Pump in Style, Ameda Purely Yours. (Figure 12–9) (lightweight portable pumps often used by employed mothers)

- Institutionally used pumps, such as those commonly rented and/or used in the hospital: Medela Lactina, Classic, and Symphony, Ameda Elite, Lact-e, and SMB, CAMP ProFlo (the former White River pump), Whittlestone Breast Expresser.

Various types of electric motors are used in this group of pumps to generate suction. Semiautomatic pumps (Figure 12–10) require the mother to cycle suction by covering and uncovering a hole in the flange base, a process that creates a pumping rhythm designed to simulate the pattern of a suckling baby. These pumps maintain a constant negative pressure. Some lack a dial or mechanism to adjust the amount

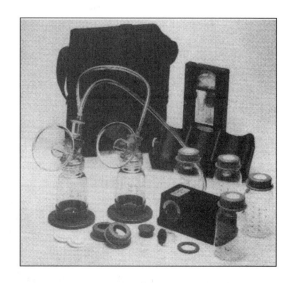

FIGURE 12–10. The Nurture III, a small semiautomatic pump. (Courtesy of Bailey Medical Engineering, Los Osos, CA.)

of suction. The actual amount of vacuum delivered to the nipple is determined by the degree of closure of the hole in the flange base. Many mothers learn to roll their finger three fourths of the way off the hole

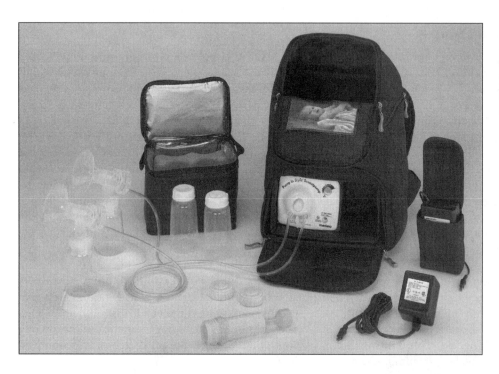

FIGURE 12–9. A personal use, pump-in-style model. (Courtesy of Medela Inc., McHenry, IL.)

rather than to lift the finger completely, to generate vacuum faster for the subsequent cycle by preventing complete interruption of vacuum. However, too much negative pressure, or negative pressure applied for too long a period, increases the risk of damage to the nipple and underlying vascular structures. The initiation of suction places the greatest pressure on the nipple; thus it is most desirable that a pump generate suction quickly.

Automatic electric pumps are designed to cycle pressure rather than to maintain it. Because Egnell (1956) observed nipple damage when cycles were 2 seconds long (30 per minute), manufacturers increased the number of cycles so that they more closely simulate that of a nursing baby. Pressure setting parameters on these large pumps also attempt to mimic that of an infant. Mean sucking pressures of most full-term infants range from -50 to -155 with a maximum of –220 mm Hg (Caldeyro-Barcia, 1969). In pumps that have a preset pulsed suction (automatic pumps), there is typically a 60/40 ratio. Negative pressure is applied for 60 percent of the cycle; 40 percent of the cycle is the resting phase. The Medela Classic/Lactina pattern has a fixed number of cycles per minute (48) with relax times becoming longer in lower vacuum ranges. The Medela Symphony (Figure 12–11) operates with a "stimulation" phase at the start of the pumping session at 120 cycles per minute with variable adjustable vacuum of 50 to 200 mm Hg. This causes a change in the "expression" phase to cycle between 54 to 78 cycles per minutes with vacuum from 50 to 250 mm Hg. The number of cycles per minute varies in this pump according to the set vacuum with higher vacuum levels resulting in lower cycles per minute. At a minimum vacuum of 50 mm Hg the Symphony applies 78 cycles per minute, and at the maximum vacuum of 250 mm Hg, 54 cycles per minute are applied. The maximum pressure that these pumps will generate at their normal (high) setting is approximately 220 to 250 mm Hg. By comparison, the Nurture III semiautomatic pump produces 220 mm Hg after about 2.5 seconds using a single collecting kit (approximately 24 cycles per minute). With the double collecting kit, this same pump takes about 3.25 seconds to achieve this level, generating about 18 cycles per minute.

Negative pressure—a function of the volume of air in the accessory kit—increases as the bottle fills with milk. The pressure generated varies with different sized bottles (collecting containers) and from one manufacturer to another. When double-pump setups are used (with two collecting containers being filled simultaneously), the potential for very

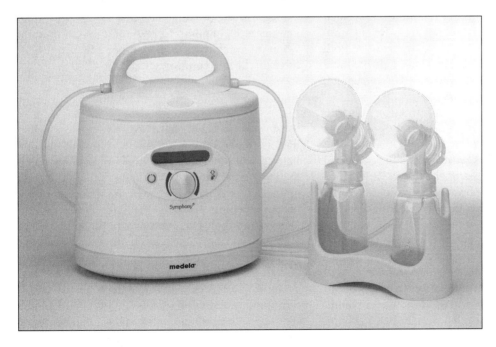

FIGURE 12–11. The Medela Symphony Pump. (Courtesy of Medela Inc., McHenry, IL.).

low negative pressure exists when the containers are empty; negative pressure increases as the bottles fill. Most accessory kits attempt to compensate for this by separating the collection containers from the power source so that the amount of air in the system remains constant regardless of the amount of fluid in the collection container. If a mother is using an accessory kit or pump without a similar feature, she can compensate by using a smaller collection bottle (Vol-u-feeders fit on some pumps), turning down the vacuum as the bottle fills, emptying the bottle more frequently, or cycling the suction more frequently on the hand, battery-operated, or semiautomatic pumps.

The Whittlestone Breast Expresser does not use alternating vacuum pulses but generates about 147 mm Hg on a constant basis with the inner flange liners rhythmically compressing the breast 45 times per minute.

Simultaneous and/or Sequential Pumping

All of the automatic electric pumps and a few of the battery-operated pumps have collection kits that allow pumping both breasts at the same time. Neifert and Seacat (1985) reported the experiences of 10 mothers who were 2 to 7 months postpartum. The women alternated between sequentially pumping each breast for 20 minutes and then pumping both breasts simultaneously for 10 minutes. Milk yield was about the same with both techniques but was obtained in one half the time with lower pump suction (320 mm Hg versus 260 mm Hg) when pumping was simultaneous. They also found a significantly higher prolactin rise with double pumping. This is similar to Tyson's report (1977) of a doubling in prolactin rise when two infants were put to breast simultaneously and echoes the findings of Saint, Maggiore, and Hartmann, (1986), who reported larger milk volumes in mothers of twins (up to double that of singleton mothers).

Auerbach (1990b) studied 25 mothers with babies between 5 and 35 weeks of age. She investigated the amount of milk obtained with single and double pumping, whether it takes longer to pump with a single setup compared to a double setup, and whether the milk fat varies between the two methods of pumping. Results showed that highest milk yields with single pumping occurred over 10 to 15 minutes. With double pumping, maximum milk volumes were seen in 7 to 12 minutes. The maximum yield overall occurred with double pumping. Milk fat concentrations were only slightly higher for double pumping sessions with no time limits. However, the mothers preferred double pumping three to one. Mothers' preferences regarding pumping regimens usually predicted how they obtained the highest yields. Groh-Wargo et al. (1995) studied 32 preterm mothers, half of whom pumped each breast in sequence; the other half pumped both breasts simultaneously. Daily frequency of pumping in both groups ranged from three to nearly five times. The single pumping group averaged 24 minutes for each pumping session; the bilateral pumping group expressed milk for an average of 16 minutes per session. Other aspects of simultaneous (SIM) versus sequential (SEQ) pumping have been studied, helping the clinician to construct pumping guidelines tailored to maximizing milk output for mothers encountering a variety of problems or situations (Table 12–1).

A number of factors combine to result in optimum milk expression: vacuum generated by the pump, cycling patterns of the vacuum, compressive forces from the pump flange, compressive forces external to the pump, oxytocin pulses, sequential or simultaneous pumping, number of times per day and per week of pumping sessions, time postpartum when pumping was initiated, type of flange, proper fit of the flange, comfort, etc. (Table 12–2).

Flanges

Most pumps have hard plastic shields called flanges. Some may have softer plastic or silicone flanges, soft inner liners, soft inserts, projections on the flange that compress the breast when vacuum is applied, or inserts that change the diameter of the nipple opening. The CAMP Healthcare ProFlo electric and their two manual pumps (formerly the White River pumps) use a silicone flange available in one size that varies in thickness over the flange and down into the shank. The thinner areas and projections collapse more deeply over the breast during the vacuum phase.

The Whittlestone Breastmilker Pump, developed in New Zealand, is a double-pumping flange

Table 12–1

METHODS OF MILK EXPRESSION: SELECTED STUDIES

Study	Findings
Neifert & Seacat, 1985 n=10 term infants	Milk yield similar, volume obtained in half the time with SIM with lower vacuum levels; increased prolactin rise with SIM.
Auerbach, 1990b n=25 5–35 weeks postpartum term infants	SIM = highest milk yields in 7–12 minutes; higher milk volume SEQ = 10–15 minutes to reach maximum milk yield
Groh-Wargo et al., 1995 n=32 Preterm infants Pumped 3–5 times/day	SIM = 16 minutes/session; 7.6 ± 3 hours/week SEQ = 24 minutes/session; 11.1 ± 3.1 hours/week Average 28 pumping sessions/week = 400 ml/day of milk did not see increased prolactin.
Hill, Aldag, & Chatterton, 1996 n=9 Preterm infants Pumped 5 times/day during hospital stay Pumped 8 times/day at home through day 42	SEQ 5x5x5x5 20 minutes total; milk volumes decreased after 25 days; proportion of prolactin at day 42 was 52% of level at day 21. Milk yield ranges 158.4 g day 3–505.8 g day 20; SIM milk volumes continued to rise over entire study time; prolactin at day 42 was 85% of level at day 21. Milk volume ranges 41.4 g day 3 to 741 g on day 41.
Hill, Aldag, & Chatterton, 1999 n=39 Preterm infants Pumped 8 times/day	SIM 10 minutes; milk weights higher each week of the study in SIM; pumping frequency=31 + 11.93 times/to 45 + 10.88 times. SEQ 5x5x5x5 for 20 minutes; pumping frequency=28 ± 8.9 times/week to 41 ± 9.05 times/week. Hours from birth to initiation of pumping: 　SEQ-9.7 hours to 101 hours (4.2 days) 　SIM-28.28 hours to 84.3 hours (3.5 days) Milk weights inversely correlated to number of hours from birth to initiation of pumping. Milk weights positively correlated with weekly frequency of pumping and Kangaroo Care.
Hill, Aldag, & Chatterton, 2001 n=39 Preterm infants 2–5 weeks postpartum	Studied median number of hours from birth to initiation of pumping and median frequency of pumping over weeks 2–5 to categorize subjects into high and low pumping frequency and early and late pumping initiation. Early initiation = 30.9 ± 11.4 hours post delivery. Late initiation = 82.0 ± 37.9 hours post delivery. Low pumping frequency group = 4.9 times/day; range = 2.6–6.14 times/day. High pumping frequency = 7.0; range 6.25–8.10 times/day. Mothers with both late initiation and low frequency had lowest milk weights. Frequency of pumping was primary influence on milk weights.
Jones, Dimmock, & Spencer, 2001 n=36 Preterm infants 4 days total study time	Compared simultaneous and sequential pumping on milk volume and energy yield. Secondary aim: measure the effect of breast massage on milk volume and fat content. Milk yield per expression: 　SEQ with no massage = 51.32 ml 　SEQ with massage = 78.71 ml 　SIM with no massage = 87.69 ml 　SIM with massage = 125.08 ml Fat concentrations were not affected.

SIM Simultaneous (double) pumping
SEQ Sequential pumping

Table 12–2

COMPARISON OF PRESSURE, HORMONAL RESPONSES, AND MECHANICS AMONG VARIOUS METHODS OF BREASTMILK REMOVAL

Negative Pressure Ranges

Baby	Hand Expression	Hand Pump	Battery Pump	Electric Pump
50–241 mm Hg 50–155 mm Hg average Basal resting pressure to keep nipple in mouth 70–200 mm Hg	None	0–400 mm Hg	50–305 mm Hg	10–500 mm Hg

Positive Pressure Ranges

Baby	Breast and Milk-Ejection Reflex	Hand Expression	Hand Pump	Battery Pump	Electric Pump
Tongue .73–3.6 mm Hg	28 mm Hg when breast is full	Theoretically could exert >760 mm Hg, which is atmospheric pressure	None to minimal	None to minimal	Without compression stimulus, none to minimal
Jaw 200–300 mm Hg	10–20 mm Hg with milk-ejection reflex				With compression stimulus

Hormonal Response Ranges

	Baby	Hand Expression	Hand Pump	Battery Pump	Electric Pump
Prolactin Basal levels up to 200 ng/ml first 10 days	55–550 ng/ml	67 ng/ml 28–42 days postpartum	67 ng/ml 28–42 days postpartum	59.7 ng/ml 28–42 days postpartum	46–405 ng/ml Single pumping 92.1 ± 29.2 ng/ml
10–90 days 60–110 ng/ml					Double pumping 136 ± 31.6 ng/ml
90–180 days 50 ng/ml					
180 days to 1 year 30–40 ng/ml					
Oxytocin	5–15 units/ml 100 mU released during 10 minutes				

Mechanics

	Baby	Hand Expression	Hand Pump	Battery Pump	Electric Pump
Cycles per minute	36–126 cycles	Variable	Variable	5–60 cycles	2–84 cycles
Duration of vacuum	.7 seconds	None	Variable	1–50 seconds	1–3 seconds
Duration of rest	.7 seconds	Variable	Variable		
Volume of milk per suck	.14 ml/suckle at the beginning of a feeding				
	.01 ml/suckle at end of feeding				

design based on milking techniques used by the dairy industry. The Whittlestone design was an answer to early mechanical milking devices used on domestic animals, which consisted of a single-chambered teat cup attached to a vacuum source that withdrew milk by simple suction (Woolford & Phillips, 1978). This design was inefficient, and the cows objected to the discomfort. The teat cup that is now used consists of a metal case lined with soft rubber. The milking apparatus produces a regular collapsing of the rubber liner against the teat to cause stimulation. The Whittlestone breast cups consist of a solid casing attached to a pulsating vacuum source. A foam pad in the cup case is held in place by a liner. When negative pressure occurs in the cup case, the liner moves against the pad, and the nipple and areola are drawn down into the conical portion of the liner (Whittlestone, 1978). Mothers reported that this pump is comfortable and efficient with a full milk supply. The current Whittlestone Breast Expresser uses a silicone liner and a lower vacuum level. The Whisper Wear pump utilizes a flexible massaging cup.

Johnson (1983) measured several aspects of flanges, including the diameters of the outer opening (flare), the inner opening, the depth of flare, and the length of the shank. She measured negative pressure at the inner opening of the flange and reported that the smaller the nipple cup the greater the pressure exerted on the tip of the nipple. The larger and deeper flanges may provide greater stimulation of the areolar region of the breast. Zinaman (1988) repeated the same measurements on 11 manual pumps, 4 battery pumps, and 7 electric pumps. Comparing these measurements among pumps highly rated in the other studies showed that the diameter of the flange ranged from 60 to 69 mm, depth ranged from 25 to 30 mm, and the inner opening was between 21 and 26 mm for the manual pumps. A woman with a large or wide nipple may have difficulty with a flange that has a small opening or a narrow slope.

Because one size of flange does not fit all breasts, some manufacturers provide a choice of different sized flanges (Table 12–3), silicone flange liners, or small plastic inserts that are placed at the level of the inner opening to change the diameter of the shank and inner opening. Silicone or soft plastic flange liners are supposed to cushion the pumping forces and are purported to "massage" the

Table 12–3

FLANGE SIZES

Company	Flange Options	Nipple Tunnel Diameter
Avent	One standard flange with projections	22.2 mm
Whisper Wear	One size	22.0 mm
Ameda	Custom flange	30.5 mm
	Custom flange with insert	28.5 mm
	Standard flange	25.0 mm
	Standard flange with reducing insert	23.0 mm
	Standard flange with Flexishield	21.0 mm
Medela	Personal Fit small	21.0 mm
	Personal Fit standard	24.0 mm
	Personal Fit large	27.0 mm
	Personal Fit extra large	30.0 mm
	Blown glass flange	40.0 mm

breast or mimic external compressive forces. Inserts placed in the flanges are designed to provide a better fit between pump and breast.

When vacuum is applied, the nipple and part of the areola elongate and are drawn past the inner opening and down into the shank or nipple tunnel (Biancuzzo, 1999). In general, the pump is more likely to be effective when the flange accommodates the anatomic configuration of the particular breast. However, mothers have various sized nipples. Zeimer and Pidgeon (1993), Stark (1994), and Wilson-Clay and Hoover (2002) measured nipple diameters that ranged from <12 mm at base to >23 mm at base. Wilson-Clay and Hoover (2002) also observed that nipples swell during pumping. Thus a mother with large nipples may find that a standard size flange is too small to accommodate both the large nipple and subsequent swelling. Clinicians have observed damage on the areola presenting as suction rings or cracks at the junction of the nipple and areola from flanges that are too small. Such a misfit between flange and breast could endanger milk production if the teat were strangulated to the point where little to no milk could be expressed. Wilson-Clay and Hoover (2002) speculate that if a mother has a nipple size of approximately 20.5 mm (or the size of a US nickel) or larger she may benefit from using a larger than standard size pump flange. Lacking a clinical algorithm for nipple size and flange selection that would provide a path for decision making, some health professionals who have access to autoclaving or similar sterilizing facilities offer mothers the opportunity to try several different brands of breast pumps and flange sizes in order to ascertain optimal fit before they purchase or rent a pump.

Miscellaneous Pumps

Pedal Pumps

Medela, Inc., and BreastPump.Com, Inc., manufacture breast pump pedals that generate vacuum by pressing a foot down on a pedal. The leg muscles tend to be stronger than are hand and arm muscles; thus this type of a pump may be useful for women with a compromised upper body, arms, or hands. The pumps run without electricity and may accommodate a number of different flange and tubing sets. Their effectiveness in comparison to other pumps on the market is not known.

Clinical Implications Regarding Breast Pumps

The concerns of health professionals may vary considerably from those of mothers and typically center around safe collection techniques and the maintenance of low bacteria counts in the expressed milk. Of equal importance are choosing the right pump for each individual situation, providing appropriate pumping instructions, and tempering all this with a consideration of the emotional toll that pumping can sometimes exact.

The professional literature includes reports of bacterial contamination of breastmilk and breast pumps. Factors related to nipple cleansing, hand washing, collection technique, type of pump, feeding method of preterm infants, pump-cleaning routines, and gestational age of the baby have all been identified as contributing to concern over high bacteria counts in expressed milk. Expressed breast milk is not sterile (el-Mohandes et al., 1993b). There is considerable disagreement over what constitutes an acceptable bacteria count, especially if the recipient of the milk is a preterm infant (el-Mohandes et al., 1993a). Caution must be exercised in reviewing the literature because certain institutional practices may actually increase the likelihood of contamination problems with expressed milk.

With the increased use of both hand and electric pumps in the 1970s, many reports described contaminated milk as one source of bacteremia, but the reports lacked conclusive epidemiology. Hand expression of breastmilk showed lower bacteria counts than breastmilk obtained by manual or electric pumps when pumps first began to be commonly used. Donowitz et al. (1981) reported an outbreak of *Klebsiella*-caused bacteremia in a neonatal intensive care unit (NICU). The electric breast pump was grossly contaminated and lacked proper bacterial surveillance. Once gas sterilization of pump parts was required between each mother's use of the equipment, the problem disappeared. However, all five affected babies in the report were fed milk by the nasoduodenal route, which delivers the milk directly to the small bowel, thus bypassing the protective action of gastric acid in the stomach. Four of the five infants had received broad-spectrum antibiotic therapy prior to the contaminated feedings, and therefore received contaminated milk in a bowel with altered protective gastrointestinal flora. Such a practice predisposes an infant to infection given even small challenges of bacteria.

Gransden et al. (1986) reported an outbreak of *Serratia marcescens* in a NICU via inadequately disinfected breast pumps (Kaneson manual and Egnell electric models). Kaneson pump parts (after being washed) were soaked in a solution of hypochlorite. Egnell pump parts were washed with the metal parts soaked in a solution of 0.5 percent chlorhexidine in 70 percent ethyl alcohol. The pumps were soaked for 1.5 hours in a 1 percent hypochlorite solution, and the solution was changed every 24 hours. Bacteria were isolated from the soaked pump parts as well as from the hypochlorite solution itself. When the Egnell pump parts were autoclaved and the Kaneson pumps were washed at 80° C, the problem was resolved. Often, the available chlorine in these chemical solutions is readily inactivated by small amounts of organic matter. The original disinfection technique in this study had several faults, including failure to completely dismantle the hand pump completely, failure to remove the rubber gasket, and failure to totally immerse the pump components.

Moloney et al. (1987) reported isolation of *Serratia marcescens, Staphylococcus aureus,* and *Streptococcus faecalis* from hand-operated and electric breast pumps. The pumps were disinfected in a hypochlorite solution as in the previous study. It is well known that there are infection risks from electrically-operated breast pumps. With proper surveillance and sterilizing by autoclaving, gas (ethyline oxide), or high temperature washing—rather than chemical sterilization—the risk of overgrowth and transmission of pathogenic bacteria can be substantially reduced. If pumps or pump parts are heat sensitive, consideration should be given to using pumps that do not depend on chemical sterilization.

Asquith, Sharp, and Stevenson (1985) compared Medela hand and electric pumps to manual expression in order to measure the amount of bacterial contamination. Boiling the personal use kits for 10 minutes worked well. The disposable kits were washed in hot soapy water and used for only 1 day. In some hospitals a fresh sterile kit is used for each pumping session but this has not been shown to be a requirement for bacteriologically safe breastmilk.

Other approaches to reducing the bacterial count in expressed breastmilk have included expressing techniques and various breast-nipple cleansing routines. Asquith et al. (1984) noted that the bacterial content of milk is high when expression is first begun, regardless of collection technique. Asquith and Harod's earlier work (1979) recommended that stripping and discarding the first 10 ml of expressed milk would decrease total bacteria counts. They observed that bacterial contamination was high within the first 24 hours after birth or after initiation of pumping, whether or not the first 10 ml were discarded. Asquith and colleagues (1984) suggest that delayed expression of breastmilk is associated with high bacterial counts of nonnursing mothers of NICU infants: "Milk stasis and breast engorgement may provide an opportunity for bacteria, including 'normal flora' or pathogenic species, to incubate in the breast." Their recommendations for mothers of hospitalized newborns include initiation of expression as soon as possible on a frequent and regular basis, thereby avoiding excessive engorgement, and the discarding of the first 10 ml of milk with each pumping. Some mothers may get only 10 ml of colostrum or milk at first, so care should be taken to determine the necessity of discarding this early milk. Most NICU milk expression instructions no longer carry this recommendation.

Pittard et al. (1991) found no difference in the number of heavily contaminated (>10,000 colony-forming units/ml [cfu/ml]) milk cultures when a clean versus a sterile collection container was used, or when manual versus mechanical collection techniques were employed. They did not observe increased levels of bacteria in the initial milk removed from the breast.

According to Meier and Wilks (1987), acceptable bacteria levels in expressed breastmilk are difficult to define and vary between healthy full-term infants and preterm, high-risk babies. Healthy term infants can tolerate some pathogens and relatively high levels of nonpathogenic bacteria (>104 cfu/ml of milk). Preterm or high-risk infants with immature immune systems who are not nursing directly from the breast may be at greater risk from the same level of bacterial growth. The investigators' criteria for acceptable bacteria levels for preterm infants are the absence of any pathogens and a maximum concentration of 104 cfu/ml. Mothers in their study were instructed in hand washing, especially under and around the fingernails. The nipples and areolae were cleaned with pHisoDerm soap before each pumping session. Increased nipple soreness was not noticed in this study but the number of weeks of pumping was not specified. Using these guidelines, 74 out of 84 expressed milk specimens had concentrations of <104 cfu/ml. It is not known whether this type of cleansing increases the risk for problems other than topical soreness, such as dry areolar skin that is susceptible to breakdown and infection, or a change in the pH of the skin, which affects the secretions of the glands of Montgomery.

Costa (1989) showed significantly lower bacterial counts when preterm mothers washed their nipples and areolae with pHisoDerm soap prior to each pumping session. Although Costa noticed no skin breakdown with this routine, it is unknown what adverse affects would be encountered from using this soap six to eight times a day over an extended period of time.

Thompson et al. (1997) demonstrated that pre-expression breast cleaning with pHisoDerm and tap water were no more effective than plain tap water in producing expressed milk that was free from bacterial contamination. No control group that refrained from breast cleaning preparations provided a basis for comparison. Because breastmilk is not sterile, some bacteria will always be present, even if it is nonpathologic. In a larger study by Law et al. (1989), no cases of infant sepsis could be linked to the particular bacteria present in expressed breastmilk feedings received by an infant who was either colonized or septic.

Wilks and Meier (1988) describe guidelines for care of hospital breast pump equipment that include scrubbing collection kits and tubing with instrument cleaning solution after each use and autoclaving each item. The exterior of the pump should be cleaned with antiseptic solution each day and the pump cultured monthly. They also described other factors that may influence the amount of nonpathogens that a preterm baby can tolerate. These include the baby's clinical condition; the use of bolus feedings every 2 hours rather than continuous feedings; the use of refrigerated rather than frozen milk to retain active antiinfective properties; and feeding the baby directly from the breast as much as possible to receive unaltered antiinfective properties, thereby further decreasing the risk of infection.

Nwankwo et al. (1988) showed that colostrum inhibited bacterial growth more than did mature milk-full-term colostrum even more so than preterm colostrum. At room temperature (27–32° C/ 74–96° F), mature milk from full-term mothers could be stored without significant increase in bacterial counts for 6 hours. Preterm milk could be stored for 4 hours at room temperature before bacterial counts exceeded 104 cfu/ml, or became significantly higher than initial counts at the time of ex-

pression. Colostrum was obtained within 6 days of delivery and mature milk at 6 weeks or more postpartum. The authors suggest caution in the storage of preterm milk. This should also be kept in mind for situations of continuous versus bolus tube feedings. Milk storage guidelines for term infants (Tully, 2000), particularly for employed mothers are a little more lenient (Table 12–4).

Arnold (1999) has summarized recommendations for collecting, storing, bacteriological screening, transporting, warming, and feeding expressed breastmilk for preterm or ill infants (see Chapter 14). Staff caring for such vulnerable infants must exercise care and caution in the proper handling of this milk.

Each year many pumps change or add features that reduce the chance of milk backflow and contamination. Some models now have in-line air

---

Table 12–4

BREASTMILK STORAGE GUIDELINES FOR HEALTHY INFANTS

- 38° C (100° F) ambient temperature—safe storage for less than 4 hours.
- 29° C (84.2° F) ambient temperature—safe storage for at least 3 hours.
- 25° C (77° F) ambient temperature—safe storage for up to 4 hours.
- 15° C (59° F)—safe storage for 24 hours (equivalent to a styrofoam box with blue ice).
- 4° C (39° F)—safe storage in a refrigerator 72 hours and probably longer.
- Previously thawed milk in a refrigerator—24 hours.
- Freezer inside refrigerator compartment—2 weeks.
- –20° C (–4° F) freezer separate from refrigerator—3-6 months, up to 12 months (milk should be stored in the back of the freezer, not in shelves on the door. Storage containers should be placed on a rack above the floor of the freezer to avoid warming during the automatic defrost cycle in freezers above the refrigerator compartment).
- –70° C deep freezer (–94° F)— > 12 months.

Source: Derived from Hamosh et al. (1996); Williams-Arnold (2000); Eteng et al. (2001).

filters in the pump; some use overflow bottles, and others have filters and/or protection against overflow in the accessory kit. Some have a completely closed collection system, deemed the optimal manner in which to prevent contamination (Slusser & Frantz, 2001). When choosing a pump for milk collection for term or preterm babies, the professional should know whether and how the pump or accessory kit guards against contamination. This is especially important if the pump is operated by more than one user.

Morse and Bottorff (1988) observed 61 nursing mothers and their emotional experiences related to expressing milk. Many were surprised that the ability to express their milk was not automatic. They often found that verbal and written instructions were unclear and confusing; many learned by trial and error. Mothers in this study stressed that "instructions for one mother did not necessarily work for all." Some were embarrassed and others were frustrated when they obtained only small amounts of milk. Although success with expression increased a mother's self-confidence, women who perceived expression to be an important aspect of breastfeeding, but who were unable to express milk, displayed heightened feelings of inadequacy. The authors suggest modifying how expression is taught to include not only explicit how-to's but the encouragement of private exploratory practice and the use of humor by the instructor (when appropriate) to reduce embarrassment.

Many mothers receive only the instructions that come with the pump to use as a guide in learning milk expression and handling. These instructions vary widely in their recommendations on pumping techniques and even on the cleaning of the pump. Further confusion is possible if a mother uses more than one type of pump, especially if she fails to read all of the instructions carefully or if the instructions from one manufacturer conflict with those from another.

The concerns of mothers are rarely addressed in the professional literature on breast pumps and milk expression. Clinicians must remember that the best pump will do little for a mother whose emotional needs are not met and who lacks the guidelines necessary to use the equipment properly for optimal results.

When Pumps Cause Problems

Breast pumps are considered to be a medical device by the US Food and Drug Administration (FDA) and as such are regulated within the FDA's Center for Devices and Radiological Health. The FDA maintains a medical product reporting program, called MedWatch, that enables consumers and health-care providers to report problems with these devices. Problems with breast pumps could include defective parts, poor labeling, a malfunction of the pump, nipple damage or pain, or being ineffective at removing milk, and should always be reported to the manufacturer. In addition, problems can be reported to the FDA online at the FDA's Web site, www.fda.gov. Clinicians can also access reports of problem devices through two databases:

1. Manufacturer and User Facility Device Experience (MAUDE) (www.accessdata.fda.gov/scripts/cdrh/cfdocs/cfMAUDE/Search.cfm) which represents reports of adverse events involving medical devices. The data consist of all voluntary reports since June 1993, user facility reports since 1991, distributor reports since 1993, and manufacturer reports since August 1996.
2. The Medical Device Reporting database (www.accessdata.fda.gov/scripts/cdrh/cfdocs/cfmdr/search.CFM) allows you to search the Center for Devices and Radiological Health's database information on medical devices that may have malfunctioned or caused a death or serious injury during the years 1992 through 1996. It is no longer being updated.

Some mothers give their used pumps to other mothers, borrow used pumps, or purchase previously used breast pumps to save money. This practice has the potential for improper functioning and cross-contamination (Box 12–2). Multiple use of single-user devices also typically invalidates the manufacturer's warranty (Box 12–3).

Sample Guidelines for Pumping

The health-care professional needs to base pumping recommendations on many factors and to take

BOX 12–2

Policy on Used Breast Pumps

The concern of buying a used pump is something many breastfeeding moms encounter. Although a used pump may be more affordable than a new one, there are real health implications involved. The FDA's position on the matter of reuse of breast pumps labeled for a single user is as follows:

> The FDA does not regulate the sale of individual breast pumps by individuals to other individuals. Rather, we regulate these medical devices when they are in interstate commerce. We have not said that this practice is legal or illegal. Instead, we have the following position, which recommends that if the pump cannot be adequately disinfected between uses by different mothers, that the pump not be used by different mothers (FDA, 2001).

The FDA advises that there are certain risks presented by breast pumps that are reused by different mothers if they are not properly cleaned and sterilized. These risks include the transmission of infectious diseases or the risk of improper function. The FDA believes that the proper cleaning and sterilization of breast pumps requires the removal of any fluid that has entered the pumping mechanism itself. If proper sterilization of the breast pump cannot be achieved, the FDA recommends that it not be reused by different mothers.

If you are considering buying a used breast pump, determine whether or not the pump is a "single user" pump before purchasing it.

into account each mother's situation. For example, a mother whose premature infant is younger than 30 weeks of gestation and is not taking oral feedings needs instructions very different from those of a mother who is pumping during her hours of employment, or one who is only occasionally expressing milk. The mother of the premature infant needs a pump that has the following characteristics:

- Removes milk quickly
- Pumps both breasts simultaneously
- Promotes physiologic prolactin cycling
- Obtains milk with a high energy content
- Has an easily controlled vacuum
- Permits the vacuum to be applied for short periods of time to avoid tissue damage
- Produces high milk yield
- Is easy to use

- Is heat resistant for sterilization
- Has a collection kit that is easily assembled and cleaned
- Is durable (will not stop working or break easily)
- Is economical
- Is accessible

A reasonable option for long-term pumping is an electric pump with a double collecting kit that is leased on a long-term basis. The mother should begin pumping as soon after the birth as possible and do so at least eight times each 24 hours (Hill, Aldag, & Chatterton 1996).

The mother who has a healthy 2- to-3-month-old infant and is returning to full-time employment outside the home may have different needs. Although battery pumps are popular, using an AC adapter will help increase efficiency and decrease the cost of replacement batteries. This mother might

BOX 12–3

Pumps Labeled for Single Use

The following pumps are labeled as "single user" devices:

Avent Isis

Nurture III

Double Up

Evenflo Press and Pump

Evenflo Manual Breast Pump

Gentle Expressions Mini Electric

Gerber Precious Care

Hollister/Ameda Purely Yours

MagMag Mini Electric

Medela Pump In Style Breastpump

Medela Pump In Style Traveler

Medela Pump In Style Companion

Simplicity

The following pumps are designed and FDA approved to be used by multiple users:

Hollister Elite

Hollister Lact-e

Hollister SMB Breastpump

Medela Classic Breastpump

Medela Lactina Breastpump

Source: Cindy Curtis, RN, IBCLC. Frequently asked questions about used breastpumps. Available at: http://www.breastfeedingonline.com/

also consider a long-term lease on an electric pump or the purchase of a personal-use pump. If this mother chooses to use a manually-operated cylinder pump, instructions should include proper hand positioning in order to avoid developing lateral epicondylitis, (i.e., tennis elbow; Williams, Auerbach, & Jacobi, 1989). These instructions emphasize shoulder adduction, with the elbow lying against the body, the forearm in supination (turned up), and the wrist slightly flexed. A mother with carpal tunnel syndrome, arthritis, or other hand, wrist, arm, or shoulder problems may need to use an electric pump rather than a manual or battery-operated pump to avoid exacerbation of her symptoms.

A mother who expresses only small amounts of milk or who has a low milk supply should be advised to elicit the milk-ejection reflex by baby suckling, looking at a picture of her baby, listening to guided relaxation tapes, or practicing slow chest breathing before applying the pump, and to massage the breast by quadrants throughout the pumping session. She may need to sit in a quiet area that permits relaxation with a minimum of interruptions. Pumping early in the morning or on the opposite breast while the baby is nursing may also prove helpful. In the absence of an abundant milk supply and reliable milk-ejection reflex, the use of a battery-operated pump may not prove to be the best choice. She could also be advised to pump after each breastfeeding to drain the breasts as much as possible. Some mothers find the use of synthetic oxytocin nasal spray helpful in eliciting the milk-ejection reflex. This preparation can be obtained by prescription from a compounding pharmacy.

Common Pumping Problems

The most common pumping problems seen by clinicians are sore nipples, obtaining only small amounts of milk per pumping session, erratic or delayed milk-ejection reflex, and dwindling milk supply over a long-term course of pumping. (Walker, 1987). Sore nipples caused by breast pumps can be minimized by using the lowest amount of vacuum that works to obtain milk; applying vacuum only after the breast has begun to release its milk; interrupting the vacuum frequently to avoid or decrease pain while still maintaining milk flow; switching from side to side frequently as the milk flow slows (when using single-sided pumping); ensuring proper flange fit with an inner opening that is not too small for the nipple entering it or too large to be effective; and pumping for shorter periods of time.

Obtaining only small amounts of milk per pumping session occurs most often when the milk-ejection reflex has not been elicited. Mothers complain that the milk drips but does not spray out and that it takes more than 45 minutes to accumulate $1/2$ to 1 oz. As a result of this frustration, pump vacuum levels are often increased or left on for long, uninterrupted periods of time. This contributes more to sore nipples than to increased milk yields. To elicit the milk-ejection reflex, some mothers have reported using a hot shower or hot compresses, using breast massage or hand expression, or establishing a pumping routine (activities performed prior to each pumping session that elicit milk flow).

Increasing fluid intake does not usually increase milk yield. Some mothers pump whenever they experience a spontaneous milk-ejection. Timing pumping sessions may also help, particularly if some women find it difficult to obtain much milk immediately after the baby has fed. Pumping midway between feedings may help this situation. Morning pumping sessions also tend to yield more milk. Mothers who are employed full-time report that pumping sessions early in the week also tend to yield more milk than pumping sessions later in the week (Auerbach & Guss, 1984).

Oxytocin (Syntocinon) has been used prior to each pumping session as a temporary boost to milk-ejection. While it is no longer available as a nasal spray, compounding pharmacies can purchase oxytocin and mix it into the nasal spray form (Gross, 1995). Oxytocin has been used by mothers during the first week of pumping following a preterm birth with significant results. In one study, milk production increased by a factor of 3.5 for primiparous mothers and 2.5 for multiparous mothers compared to mothers not using oxytocin nasal spray prior to each pumping session (Ruis et al., 1981).

Medicine and technology are saving infants as young as 23 weeks gestational age. Mothers wishing to breastfeed extremely preterm infants will be pumping milk for many months. They can encounter difficulties maintaining an optimal milk supply through artificial means. A flexible pumping plan should be developed for optimal milk production (Auerbach & Walker, 1994; Hill, Aldag, & Chatterton, 1999). Faltering milk production is not unusual with extended pumping. In addition to the guidelines in this chapter, additional interventions (Gabay, 2002) include the use of metaclopromide (Ehrenkranz & Ackerman, 1986; Toppare et al., 1994), acupuncture (Clavey, 1996), domperidone (da Silva et al., 2001), and human growth hormone (Gunn et al., 1996).

Factors other than the type of equipment used also affect milk flow. Morse and Bottorff (1988) have stated that "understanding the complex feelings towards expressing and the experimental nature of learning to express has important implications for the way that expression is taught." An erratic or delayed milk-ejection reflex is common when a mother must respond to a mechanical device rather than her baby, particularly when she is first learning to use a pump. If the milk-ejection reflex is not triggered quickly, the nipples and breast tissue are exposed to high levels of vacuum over an inefficient pressure gradient. This can result in low milk yields, sore nipples, and frustration with the pumping process.

Although pumps are capable of eliciting milk-ejection and their instructions often advise applying the pump for this purpose, some women will have difficulty releasing their milk. This may be caused by inhibitory messages received by the hypothalamus. Embarrassment, tension, fear of failure, pain, fatigue, and anxiety may block the neurochemical pathways required for milk-ejection. If these factors appear to interfere with milk-ejection, ask the mother how she feels about pumping. A negative attitude does little to contribute to milk flow. One mother, when offered the option of double pumping, said it made her feel like a cow. Single-sided pumping was more appealing to her. When the clinician knows the mother's feelings and attitudes about pumping, guidelines can be individually created for each situation.

It is not unusual for the milk-ejection reflex to take longer to trigger as the lactation course increases. This is common both with a baby at breast and with long-term pumping. What works early in lactation may change over time. Some mothers report improved results later in lactation, after they change to a different pump or use a different flange that fits the breast better.

Expressing milk has different meanings for each mother. Some see it as a way to continue providing breastmilk in their absence, especially in families with a history of allergies. Some mothers prefer to express milk by hand because they obtain as much milk in as quick a time as they do when using a pump. Other mothers view pumping as part of a grieflike reaction that is reinforced every 2 to 3 hours when they must use a pump in the absence of a baby at breast. Sound pump recommendations, pumping instructions based on a clear understanding of the anatomy and physiology of the breast, and knowledge of the lactation process will enable many women to give their infant the best possible nutritional and emotional start.

Nipple Shields

Nipple shields appeared in the medical literature as early as the mid-1600s. Scultetus, an early physician, described shields made of silver and used so that "nurses may suckle the infants without trouble which, when children were breast-fed until long after their front teeth were cut, must have been very necessary" (Bennion, 1979). Shields were first used to evert flat nipples and protect nipples from the cold and rubbing against clothing between feedings. Between the 16th and 19th centuries, a variety of other functions for shields were also described:

- To cover flat nipples
- To prevent sore or ulcerated nipples
- To treat cracked, sore, or infected nipples
- To protect clothing from milk leakage
- To be used as a base for attaching an artificial nipple or cow's teat

Shields were made of lead (which caused brain damage in babies), wax, wood, gum elastic, pewter, tin, horn, bone, ivory, silver, and glass. The gum elastic shield in Figure 12–12 was used for babies to nurse on. Maygrier (1833) stated that, "This mode is difficult and generally the child is unwilling."

The design of nipple shields has changed little since the 1500s. By the 1800s rubber shields began appearing. The Maw's shield (Figure 12–13) was constructed with a rubber lining, a glass shank, and a rubber teat. In the 1980s this design was still used with a glass or plastic shank and a rubber teat (Davol). Rubber versions of the silver and wood shields also began appearing. The early shields were composed of thick rubber with a firm nipple cone (The Mexican Hat, Macarthy's Surgical, Ltd.). One US version, the Breast-Eze, was a modified

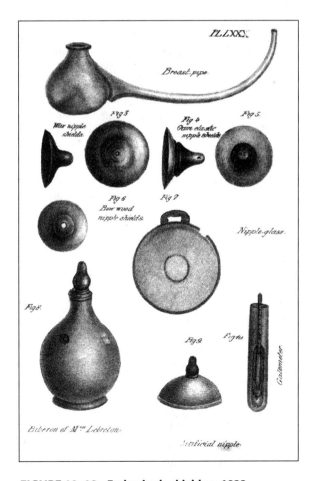

FIGURE 12–12. Early nipple shields, c. 1833.

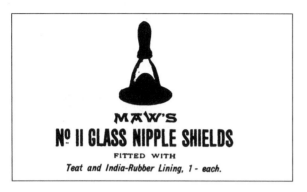

FIGURE 12–13. Nipple shield and breast glass, c. 1864.

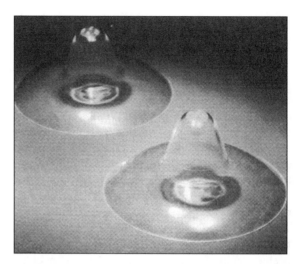

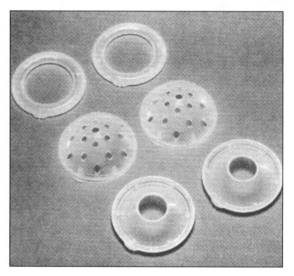

FIGURE 12–14. Modern silicone nipple shields (above) and breast shells (below).

rubber nipple on a rubber base with thick rubber ribs lining the inside to help "stimulate" the breast. This design was reported to be very painful to use. The rubber shields gradually became thinner (Evenflo) and were replaced with thin latex (Lewin Woolf, Griptight, Ltd.) and ultra-thin silicone (Cannon Babysafe, Medela, Ameda, Avent) seen today (Figure 12–14).

Early nipple shield use generated poor outcomes in many babies due to misuse, misunderstanding, the very thick nature of the device that prevented mothers from feeling the baby at breast (which probably reduced prolactin levels), and overall poor milk transfer. The barrier that the thick shield created between the baby's mouth and teat exceeded the limits of the mechanical requirements for milk removal. They became destructive to the course of lactation and risky to the health of the baby (Desmarais & Browne, 1990).

Review of Literature

Woolridge, Baum, and Drewett (1980) studied the effect of the all rubber shield (Macarthy-Mexican Hat) and a thin latex shield on the suckling patterns and milk intake of five-to-eight-day-old babies of mothers with problem-free lactation experiences. The Macarthy-Mexican Hat reduced milk transfer by 58 percent and changed infant suckling patterns by increasing the suckling rate and the time spent pausing. This is a pattern typically seen when milk flow decreases. The thin latex shield reduced milk intake by 22 percent and had no significant effect

on suckling patterns. This thin shield was being tested as part of an apparatus in a new system for measuring milk flow and composition during breastfeeding. The babies observed in this study had no difficulty latching onto mothers' nipples, and no nipple soreness was reported by the mothers in the study. Theoretically, if these problems existed, milk transfer and suckling patterns could be further compromised with the continued use of a thick shield. Using the same thin latex shield, Jackson et al. (1987) showed a 29 percent decrease in milk transfer during their study of nutrient intake in healthy, full-term newborns.

Amatayakul et al. (1987) measured plasma prolactin and cortisol levels in mothers, with and without a thin latex nipple shield in place. They found that prolactin and cortisol levels were unaffected by the shield but that milk transfer was decreased by 42 percent when the shield was in place during feedings. They postulate that this effect on milk volume is attributable to an interference with oxytocin release.

Auerbach (1990a) studied changes in pumped milk volume with and without the use of a thin silicone shield (Cannon Babysafe). Twenty-five mothers used a breast pump (Medela electric model) to provide milk samples, which prevented any change in infant suckling patterns from affecting milk volume amounts. Milk volume was significantly reduced when a shield was in place. Seventy-one percent of the total milk obtained was recorded when no shield was used. Pumping without a shield resulted in mean volumes five to seven times greater than when a shield was in place.

Nipple shield use has yielded more beneficial outcomes. Key to such outcomes is the use of ultra-thin silicone shields, critical assessment by a skilled lactation consultant, and continuous follow-up. Babies who otherwise may have been unable to breastfeed have benefited from the judicious use of this device. However, there still remain drawbacks to much of the published research as it lacks prospective, randomized controlled trials of shield use; it refers to old studies conducted with thick rubber shields; it contains samples of babies with no feeding problems; it uses small sample sizes; and it often measures only a single feeding (Table 12–5).

Types of Shields

Rubber Shields. Rubber shields are seldom seen today and should not be used.

Standard Bottle Nipples or Bottle Nipples Attached to a Glass or Plastic Base. These types of shields place the baby and his mouth one to two inches away from the mother's nipple, significantly altering positioning at breast. This does not permit compression of the milk sinuses or skin-to-skin stimulation of the nipple/areolar complex and may alter prolactin cycling. Milk may pool in the base, which

Table 12–5

NIPPLE SHIELD RESEARCH

Study	Description
Brigham, 1996	Reviewed 51 mothers, with 81% reporting positive outcomes in resolving breastfeeding problems.
Bodley & Powers, 1996	In 10 cases weight gain was appropriate during and following the period of nipple shield use.
Woodworth & Frank, 1996	Shield used for breast refusal.
Wilson-Clay, 1996	Experiences of 32 mothers using shields to resolve breastfeeding problems.
Clum & Primomo, 1996	9 of 15 preterm infants consumed 50% more milk at breast with an ultra-thin shield than without a shield.
Meier, Brown, & Hurst, 2000	34 preterm infants showed increased milk transfer with a shield; 3.9 ml without the shield and 18.4 ml with the shield.

holds the artificial nipple, and never reach the baby, or simply leak out the sides. These too are seldom seen and should not be used, nor should an artificial nipple itself be placed over a mother's nipple.

Latex and Silicone Shields. These are extremely thin, flexible shields with the nipple portion being firmer. Because the silicone is so thin, more stimulation reaches the areola, and milk volume is not as seriously depleted as with the other designs (Auerbach, 1990a). Because of the increasing reports of latex allergy in the general population, latex-containing shields should be avoided. Silicone shields are available in a number of sizes (Table 12–6).

Shield Selection and Instructions

There is little in the literature regarding shield selection and instructions for use. Wilson-Clay and

Table 12–6

Silicone Shields

Product	Diameter (in.)	Height of Nipple (in.)	Width of Nipple (in.)	Number of Holes
Avent	2 6/8	7/8	5/8 at tip, 1 at base	3
Medela				
Standard	2 6/8	7/8	5/8 at tip, 1 at base	4
Extra Small	2 6/8	6/8	3/8 at tip, 5/8 at base	3
Ameda	2 5/8	7/8	4/8 at tip, 7/8 at base	5

Hoover (2002) state that "the teat height must not exceed the length of the infant's mouth from the juncture of the hard and soft palates to lip closure. If the height of the teat of a shield is greater than this length, the infant's jaw closure and tongue compression will fall on the shaft of the teat, and not over the breast." Wilson-Clay and Hoover also recommend that the base diameter should fit the mother's nipple and that better results occur with the shortest teat height and smallest base diameter. A summary of instructions includes the following:

- Apply the shield by turning it almost inside out.
- Moisten the edges to help it adhere better.
- Drip expressed milk onto the outside of the teat to encourage the baby.
- Hand express a little milk into the teat if necessary.
- Use alternate massage to help drain breast.
- Run tubing inside or outside of shield for supplementation.
- The baby's mouth must not close on the shaft of the teat.
- The latch should be checked to see that the baby is not just suckling on the tip of the teat.
- The shield should be washed in hot soapy water after each use and rinsed well.
- If yeast is present on the areola, the shield should be boiled.
- Some mothers may need more than one shield.

- Weight check about every 3 days until milk supply is stable and baby is gaining well.
- Check breasts for plugged ducts and areas that are not draining well.

Weaning from the Shield

- No set time; extended use of the ultra-thin silicone shield has not been shown to be detrimental.
- Mothers start by just skin-to-skin next to nipple, starting the feed with the shield and removing it, and gradually trying feeds without the shield.
- The shield should not be cut.

Responsibilities

The health-care professional has the following responsibilities regarding breastfeeding women and nipple shields:

- Document all of your encounters and instructions and communicate these to the primary healthcare provider.
- Understand the risks and advantages (Box 12–4) of using such a device.
- Assess the situation before recommending a shield (Auerbach, 1989). Shields used as a quick fix to ensure infant feedings before early discharge act as "band-aid therapy." They cover up the problem without addressing the cause. Identify and take steps to correct the problem rather than issuing a shield as the initial therapy.

BOX 12–4

Quick Guide to Nipple Shield Use

What Shields Do

- Therapeutically supply oral stimulation not provided by mother's nipples
- Create a nipple shape in infant's mouth
- Allow extraction of milk by expression with minimal suction and negative pressure
- Help compensate for weak infant suction
- Present a stable nipple shape that remains during pauses in suckling bursts
- Maintain the nipple in a protruded position
- Raise the rate of milk flow

What Shields Will Not Do

- Correct milk transfer problems or weight gain if the mother has inadequate milk volume
- Fix damaged nipples if the cause is not discovered and remedied
- Replace skilled intervention and close follow-up

Advantages of Nipple Shields

- Permit learning to feed at breast
- Allow supplementation at breast (i.e., thread tubing under or alongside of the shield)
- Encourage nipple protractility
- Will not overwhelm mother with gadgets
- Prevent baby fighting the breast

Disadvantages of Nipple Shields

- Used as a substitute for skilled care
- Used as a quick fix
- May exacerbate original problem
- May lead to insufficient milk volume, inadequate weight gain, weaning
- Prevent proper extension of the nipple back into the baby's mouth (Minchin, 1985)
- May pinch the nipple and areola, causing abrasion, pain, skin breakdown, and internal trauma to the breast if not applied properly
- Create nipple shield addiction (DeNicola, 1986), after which the baby will not feed at breast without the shield in place
- Predispose the nipple to damage when the baby is put to breast without the shield, as he may chew rather than suckle
- Discarded as a useful intervention in selected situations

Possible Indications for Nipple Shield Use

Latch Difficulty

- Nipple anomalies (flat, retracted, fibrous, inelastic)
- Mismatch between small baby mouth and large nipple
- Baby from heavily medicated mother
- Birth trauma (vacuum extraction, forceps)
- Oral aversion (vigorous suctioning)
- Artificial nipple preference (pacifiers, bottles)
- Baby with weak or disorganized suckle (slips off nipple, preterm, neurological problems)
- Baby with high or low tone
- Delay in putting baby to breast

BOX 12–4 (cont.)

Oral Cavity Problems

- Cleft palate
- Channel palate (Turner's syndrome, formerly intubated)
- Bubble palate
- Lack of fat pads (preterm, SGA)
- Low threshold mouth
- Poor central grooving of the tongue
- Micrognathia (recessed jaw)

Upper Airway Problems

- Tracheomalacia
- Laryngomalacia

Damaged Nipples

- When all else fails and mother states she is going to quit breastfeeding

---

- Consider written informed consent. The mother and the provider who is recommending the shield sign the consent form. This ensures that everyone knows the risks of using a shield, as well as how to use it so that its dangers are minimized. It also serves as a teaching aid to professionals who are unaware of potential long-range problems. A copy should be given to the mother, another copy is retained in the medical record, and a third copy is sent to the pediatrician (Kutner, 1986).

- Ensure that the mother will receive close follow-up during the time the shield is in use.

- Realize that the risks of nipple shield use have legal implications for the hospital and/or professional who recommend them (Bornmann, 1986).

- Provide proper instructions and referrals if a shield is used as an interim recommendation to assist with breastfeeding. If a mother is discharged from the hospital using a shield, a community referral must be made to a lactation consultant or the nurse practitioner at the pediatrician's office for daily follow-up. Weight checks may need to be obtained twice a week. The pediatrician should be alerted to the problem that required use of the shield in the first place and should be aware of suggestions for discontinuing its use.

Breast Shells

Breast shells are two-piece plastic devices worn over the nipple and areola to evert flat or retracted nipples. Historically, these shells were called nipple glasses (center device in Figure 12–12) and were used to protect the mother's clothing from leaking milk, or applied if the mother had "too much" milk. Some brands are still marketed as a device for catching leaked milk between feedings. Currently, shells are not recommended for this use, although many mothers find them helpful for collecting drip milk from one breast while nursing or pumping on the opposite side. Some clinicians also recommend their use for engorgement, as their gentle pressure encourages milk to leak. The milk collected between feedings must be discarded because of potential high bacteria counts. If drip milk is collected during a feeding or pumping session, it can be stored as usual.

Inverted nipples are identified when the areola is compressed behind the base of the nipple and the nipple retreats into the surrounding skin. This is caused by the presence of the original invagination of the mammary dimple. Prenatally, breast shells were worn for increasingly longer periods throughout the day and removed at night. The constant gentle pressure around the base of the nipple was thought to release the adhesions anchoring the nipple, thus allowing it to protrude when the baby latches onto the breast. Shells can be worn between feedings, after the baby is born, if nipple flattening or retraction is identified postpartum or if the nipples still need correction. Concern about this practice arises if the areola is edematous. Current information shows that little correction of the nipple actually takes place prenatally and that some women do not like using these devices (Alexander et al., 1992).

Several brands of shells are available, all of which have a dome that is placed over a base through which the nipple protrudes when worn under a bra. Depending on the brand, the dome may have one or many ventilation holes. The domes with only one or two holes may not provide adequate air circulation to the nipple and areola. The retained moisture and heat (especially in hot weather) can create a miniature greenhouse effect that promotes soreness and skin breakdown. Extra holes can be drilled in the top of the dome. Some brands have many holes in the dome to help with this problem. Another form of breast shell with a wider base has been used for sore nipples to keep air circulating around them and to prevent them from adhering to a bra. Currently, most clinicians seldom recommend these devices.

Feeding-Tube Devices

Judicious use of feeding-tube devices enables many mothers and babies to breastfeed who otherwise would have lost this unique opportunity. Such devices consist of a container to hold breastmilk or formula and a length of thin tubing that runs from the container to the mother's nipple. The tube is secured in place by nonallergenic tape or run under the nursing bra and as the baby suckles at breast, supplement is simultaneously delivered. Providing milk in this manner may be a novel idea to the mother. Careful explanations should include how the feeding-tube device is used and the expected outcomes. Some mothers are put off by the thought of feeding their babies in what they consider a "nonnatural" way that at first appears complicated. Explaining that the device is a temporary aid in establishing the baby at breast while ensuring adequate nutrition helps the mother to accept tube feeding. Several commercial devices are on the market; in addition, noncommercial devices can be constructed from bottles or syringes and tubing (see Chapter 10.)

Lact-Aid (USA). Developed in 1971 for nursing the adopted baby, the Lact-Aid device created a breastfeeding experience for those mothers and babies who previously had no choice in terms of feeding methods. It is a closed system consisting of a presterilized, disposable four-ounce bag to hold milk—with a cap through which a length of fine tubing extends to the nipple. The bag hangs around the mother's neck on a cord. Air is squeezed out of the bag to facilitate milk flow. Powdered formulas will not flow readily through the device.

Supplemental Nutrition System (USA) Medela, Inc. The SNS device consists of a 5-oz plastic bottle with a cap through which a length of tubing is secured to each breast. This two-tube unit allows the tubing to be set up on both breasts at the same time and comes with three different sizes of tubing. It is a vented system with a cap that has notches for pinching off both tubes while setting up the unit and securing one tube while the baby is feeding from the other side. Flow rates are influenced by the size of the tubing used (small, medium, large), the height of the bottle, and whether or not the opposite tube is pinched off during the feeding. A smaller version is also available with only one tube.

Situations for Use

Feeding-tube devices can be recommended and used in many situations where other measures have failed or in order to prevent further complications.

Infant Suckling Problems. Babies with weak, disorganized, or dysfunctional suckling are candidates for feeding-tube devices. Health problems where feeding-tube devices are helpful are discussed in detail in Chapter 19.

Maternal Situations. Mothers can benefit from the use of feeding-tube devices in the following situations:

- Adoptive nursing (induced lactation) mothers (Auerbach & Avery, 1981; Sutherland & Auerbach, 1985)

- Relactation—i.e., inducing a milk supply after a separation or interruption of breastfeeding (Bose et al., 1981; Auerbach & Avery, 1980)

- Breast surgery, especially breast reduction mammaplasty that involved moving the nipple

- Primary lactation insufficiency—i.e., not enough functional breast tissue to support a full milk supply (Neifert & Seacat, 1985)

- Severe nipple trauma

- Illness, surgery, or hospitalization

Generally, a feeding-tube device is used to maintain a mother's milk supply, to deliver sufficient or extra nutrients to the baby, and to create a behavior-modification situation that shapes the baby's suckling pattern to one suitable for obtaining milk from the breast (or prevents the suckling pattern from changing). These devices allow feedings to be done at breast when formerly, in certain situations, bottles with artificial nipples were used. Because these devices are used only in special situations, it is imperative that the professional who recommends their use follow-up closely (daily if necessary) to ensure adequate milk intake by the baby, to validate correct use by the mother, and to wean from the device when it is appropriate to do so.

A baby using a feeding tube at breast must be able to latch-on and execute some form of suckling. For babies who are unable at first to do this because of complete nipple confusion, strong extensor positioning, hypotonia, or lethargy, finger-feeding with the device can be used as an interim measure (Bull & Barger, 1987), followed by attempts to feed at breast. The mother can place a tube on the pad of her index finger or whichever finger is closest in size to her nipple. She allows the baby to draw the finger into his mouth. Correct suckling will cause the milk to flow and will reward the desired behavior; no milk is removed if the baby bites the finger like an artificial nipple. While this also allows the father or other caregiver to feed the baby, some babies become unable to feed at breast because of the strong stimulus that the firm finger provides. Finger-feeding in this manner may prevent improper suckling patterns from being reinforced and move the baby to breast faster than if artificial nipples are used to feed the baby, but care must be taken that babies do not become so accustomed to this form of feeding that they are unwilling to suckle at breast.

When considering feeding-tube devices, the clinician should note the following guidelines:

- They can be used to temporarily assist the baby at breast but are generally not necessary if the baby is gaining weight adequately.

- In situations of adoptive nursing, breast reduction surgery, primary lactation insufficiency, and certain genetic, anatomic, or neurologic problems in an infant, these feeding devices may require long-term use with or without breast pumping.

- Close follow-up is mandatory with short- or long-term use.

- Because the baby controls the flow, he will not aspirate or be overwhelmed by the fluid he receives. When he swallows or releases the vacuum, the milk flows backward and the baby must initiate another suckle to start the flow. If he cannot initially do this, the bottle or bag of supplement can be squeezed or the plunger of the syringe can be pushed slightly. The milk will not continuously drip or flow as with a bottle and artificial nipple.

- Risks of use include "addiction" to the device by the clinician, mother, and/or baby. The mother and baby should be weaned from the device as quickly as is appropriate. Some mothers may have difficulty believing that they can support a milk supply without the device and not trust themselves to provide for the baby. The clinician should avoid routine use of tube-feeding devices except where necessary. Some clever babies learn to suckle only on the tube, in which case it should be placed so it does not extend beyond the end of the mother's nipple. If the baby has become accustomed to the feel of the tubing, it can be moved to the corner of his mouth and gradually removed. One mother finally taped a one inch length of the tube to her areola and withdrew it after her baby latched-on.

- One or both tubes can be secured on either side of the areola or the top or bottom, whichever gives the best results.

- The "football-hold" or clutch position may be easier to use at first because the mother has greater control of the infant's head.

- A gavage setup with a No. 5 feeding-tube can also be used as a feeding device.

- Tubing from a butterfly needle can also be used as it is smaller and softer than gavage tubing (Edgehouse & Radzyminski, 1990).

- A baby can also be fed by dropper, spoon, cup, or bowl if tubing is not available.

- Powdered formulas and special formulas may clog the smaller tubes if the formula is not mixed well. Larger sizes of tubing may be necessary to prevent clogging.

- The device should be rinsed in cold water after each use and then filled with warm soapy water which is squeezed through the tubing and rinsed well. Sterilization can be done once a day, usually by placing it in boiling water for 20 minutes. In the hospital some of the devices can be steamed or autoclaved (Rental Roundup, 1986).

- Feeding in public may be more difficult or obvious. The mother may prefer to use alternatives to tube feeding when she is away from home.

Summary

Just as the health-care professional must base recommendations for use of breast pumps on various factors, the same holds true for the temporary use of other breastfeeding technologies. Too often a breastfeeding mother may see a device advertised as an aid to breastfeeding and assume that she needs to use it. If she then attempts to do so without thoroughly understanding its risks and benefits, actual and presumed, she could unwittingly interfere with the lactation course and/or the baby's ability to breastfeed. This is particularly true if she obtains the device from a person or institution that lacks a specialist in lactation management.

Nipple shields are most apt to be used when they are not necessary—in part because of their wide availability and in part because of their attractiveness in busy hospitals or practices, where health-care workers offer the devices because they appear to "make the baby nurse." Thus, when a health-care provider considers offering the device to a mother, careful instructions and emphasis on the temporary nature of the use of the device must be offered.

Feeding-tube devices are more complex and therefore potentially more off-putting than either breast shells or nipple shields. Mothers who insist upon using the device because they are convinced that their own milk supplies are inadequate to support appropriate infant growth need careful follow-up. Too often, the mother misinterprets the instructions or reads only enough to know how to put the device together and to clean it. The manner in which the device should be used is rarely completely understood from a single reading of the instructions that accompany the device. Health-care providers or counselors who recommend the inappropriate use of feeding-tube devices can potentially interrupt the breastfeeding relationship or cause further problems. In addition, observation and assessment of the mother and infant as they breastfeed both with and without the device is a necessity if the health-care provider is to make appropriate recommendations for an optimal outcome. In most cases, the nature of the problem that requires assistance of a feeding-tube device is such that the mother's anxiety level is high and the need to provide additional nutrition for the baby is critical. The lactation consultant, nurse, or other health-care worker can expect that working with such a mother and baby will be time-consuming and will require many more hours of follow-up time than is the case for other situations.

In all cases where any breastfeeding device or pump is used, the benefits of such technology must be weighed against the risks of interfering in the breastfeeding relationship. Anticipating the emotional response of mothers to devices and discussing them in a straightforward manner will assist the health-care provider in determining whether and when to suggest a particular technology, as well as how to help the mother stop using it when it is no longer necessary. As with all other care, the use of a breastfeeding device of any kind must first be found to "do no harm."

Key Concepts

- Examples of mothers using a device to remove milk from the breasts are cited in medical literature as early as the mid-1500s. The various devices were typically used to relieve engorgement or to express milk because of damaged nipples or mastitis.

- Today women express breastmilk on a short-term basis to solve acute problems, but they also pump on a long-term basis to provide human milk for their babies following a preterm birth or during periods of employment, illness, induced lactation, or relactation.

- Mothers list the following criteria as important when choosing a breast pump: (1) quick and effective in removing milk, (2) comfortable to use, (3) reasonably priced, and (4) easy to find, use, and clean.

- To increase pumping efficiency, mothers use two techniques: (1) elicit milk-ejection reflex before pumping, and (2) massage the breasts while pumping. Research and literature from the dairy industry support both techniques.

- Other factors that contribute to pumping efficiency include using relaxation techniques and visual imagery, and applying warm, moist heat to the breasts before and during pumping. To avoid breast or nipple injury, it is recommended that the pump be removed as soon as the milk stops flowing. When hand expressing, fingertip compressions deep in the breast tissue should be avoided.

- Considering the bewildering array of breast pumps in the marketplace today, a caregiver recommending one should give a specific name and several places to find it. Prices vary considerably depending upon where it is purchased.

- When expressing milk, the device used must be efficient enough to activate prolactin and oxytocin release. The volume of milk expressed is also related to the degree of fullness of the breast, with a fuller breast yielding more milk volume when pumped. Full breasts tend to take less time to achieve the milk-ejection reflex, with a less full breast taking up to 120 seconds.

- Stage III of lactogenesis is dependent upon early and regular stimulation of the nipple and regular removal of milk from the breasts. Lactogenesis II occurs in the absence of milk removal, but lactogenesis III can be inhibited without regular milk removal. The amount of milk produced is dependent upon the rate the breast is emptied.

- A breast pump does not pump, suck, or pull milk out of the breast. It reduces resistance to milk outflow from the alveoli, allowing the internal pressure of the breast to push out the milk.

- Einar Egnell was the pioneer in breast pump design and based his design on research from the dairy industry. He designed a pump that created periodic and limited phases of negative pressure. It operated in four phases per cycle. Many pump manufacturers still use Egnell's pressure settings as a guide in current breast pump design.

- W. G. Whittlestone found that by providing a compressive force to the breast from a liner inside the pump flange, it enhanced the dynamics of milk expression. The compression is analogous to a baby's tongue and jaw compress the teat between the tongue and hard palate during the suction cycle. Some pumps currently offer a soft flange that collapses over the teat when suction is applied while others with a hard plastic flange offer an insert or liner that is intended to serve the same purpose.

- Breast pumps are divided into three broad classifications: (1) manual hand pumps, (2) battery-operated pumps, and (3) electric pumps.

- Manual hand pumps are easy to find, easy to use, and inexpensive. Some are more effective than others in expressing milk. These pumps are typically used in the short-term or occasionally. The hand and wrist can tire easily with repeated use. Because of nipple pain and low milk yields, the old-fashioned "bicycle horn" pump is not recommended.

- Battery-operated pumps use a small motor to create a vacuum that is usually adjustable. Most have a button the mother presses to release the vacuum in a rhythmic pattern to simulate the rhythm of a nursing baby. They are lightweight, easy to find and use, and are relatively inexpensive. One disadvantage of these pumps is the short battery life. Some have AC adapters. The time each pump takes to achieve optimal suction varies, and those that require up to 30 seconds can cause nipple pain.

- Electric pumps include some that are small and semiautomatic and use a small motor to create a vacuum that is adjustable. Most have an open hole in the flange that the mother covers and uncovers with her fingertip to create a rhythmic pattern to simulate the rhythm of a nursing baby. These pumps are moderately priced and most can do double pumping.

- Automatic electric pumps are designed to cycle pressure rather than maintain it. Pressure setting parameters are set to mimic a nursing infant. Pumps are now designed with adjustable cycling rates up to 120 cycles per minute. Vacuum pressure adjusts up to 250 mm Hg. These pumps are considered the most effective of all pumps and use the double collection kits. They cost more and are heavier than their handheld counterparts.

- All automatic electric pumps and some of the smaller semiautomatic pumps offer double collection kits that allow both breasts to be pumped simultaneously. When researched, prolactin levels were significantly higher and maximum milk yield occurred with double pumping.

- Product manufacturers offer flanges in different sizes to accommodate the anatomic configuration of a particular breast. If a nipple swells during pumping, the mother with a larger nipple may find that a standard size flange is too small to accommodate both the large nipple and subsequent swelling. Those mothers whose nipples are larger than 20.5 mm (the size of a US nickel) may benefit from a larger sized flange.

- Expressed breastmilk is not sterile and there is considerable disagreement over what constitutes acceptable bacteria count, especially when pumping for a preterm infant. Many factors play a part in the bacteria level, including nipple cleaning, hand washing, collection techniques, type of pump, feeding method of preterm infant, pump-cleaning routines, and gestational age of infant. Some bacteria will always be present and are nonpathogenic. Healthy term infants can tolerate some pathogens and relatively high levels of nonpathogenic bacteria. Yet, preterm or high-risk infants may be at greater risk from the same levels of bacterial presence.

- There are infection risks from electric breast pumps with multiple users and health-care facilities must take the necessary precautions to prevent contamination.

- Colostrum and breastmilk inhibits bacterial growth at different rates in both full-term and preterm milk. Milk storage guidelines and practices differ depending on the health of the infant.

- Mothers who chose to discontinue pumping for their hospitalized infants cited insufficient milk collection as the first reason and complained that pumping was too time-consuming.

- Mothers pumping for a hospitalized infant need much clinical encouragement and emotional support to ease embarrassment and frustration and gain understanding of the significance of collecting breastmilk for their hospitalized infant.

- Breast pumps are considered to be medical devices by the US Food and Drug Administration and as such are regulated within the FDA's Center for Devices and Radiological Health. They maintain a medical product reporting program to record problems with breast pumps as encountered by consumers and clinicians.

- The issue of mothers selling and buying used breast pumps remains pertinent. The FDA advises that there are certain risks presented by breast pumps that are reused by different mothers if they are not properly cleaned and sterilized. It is not recommended that a pump that is labeled as a "single user" pump be reused or resold.

- Common pumping problems include sore nipples, low milk yield, erratic or delayed milk-ejection reflex, and dwindling milk supply over a long-term course of pumping.

- An erratic or delayed milk-ejection reflex can have an overwhelming impact on effective milk expression. A mother's feeling about pumping such as embarrassment, tension, fear of failure, pain, fatigue, and anxiety can inhibit the neurochemical pathways required for milk-ejection. When a clinician knows a mother's feelings and attitudes about pumping, guidelines can be individually created for her specific situation.

- Early use of nipple shields generated poor outcomes. The thickness of material created a barrier that prevented a mother from feeling her baby at the breast and inhibited milk transfer.

- Nipple shields fell into disfavor when the ramifications of use became destructive to the course of lactation and risky to the health of the baby.

- Recent research and discussions of nipple shields have yielded more beneficial outcomes with the use of the ultra-thin silicone shields. Use of all other shields, including latex, is not recommended. Critical assessment and continuous follow-up by a skilled lactation consultant is essential. Babies who otherwise may have been unable to breastfeed have benefited from the judicious use of this tool.

- Nipple shields can therapeutically supply oral stimulation not provided by mother's nipples, create a nipple shape in an infant's mouth, and allow extraction of milk by expression with minimal suction. With negative pressure inside the shield tip keeping milk available, the shield may compensate for weak infant suck, present a stable nipple shape that remains during pauses in sucking bursts, maintain the nipple in protruded position, and impact the rate of milk transfer.

- The disadvantages of nipple shields include use as a substitute for skilled care or a quick fix. Their use may lead to insufficient milk volume, inadequate weight gain or weaning, and a nipple shield addiction after which the baby will not feed without the shield in place. They may also predispose the nipple to damage when the baby is put to breast without the shield, as he may chew rather than suckle.

- The proper size of nipple shield must be used. The teat height should not exceed the length of the infant's mouth from the juncture of the hard and soft palates to lip closure. The base diameter should fit the mother's nipple and better results occur with the shortest teat height and smallest base diameter.

- Breast shells are two-piece plastic devices worn over the nipple and areola to evert flat or inverted nipples. Historically, these shells were called nipple glasses and were used to protect the mother's clothes from leaking milk, or used if the mother had "too much milk." Milk collected in the shells must be discarded due to potential bacterial growth.

- When worn prenatally, breast shells were designed to create a constant gentle pressure around the base of the inverted nipple and were thought to release the adhesions anchoring the nipple. Current information shows little correction of the nipple actually happens prenatally.

- Although breast shells have been used to provide air circulation around sore nipples and to keep a bra from adhering to the nipple, most clinicians today seldom recommend these devices.

- Designed to supplement feedings at the breast, feeding-tube devices can enable many mothers and babies to breastfeed when they would otherwise have to use an alternate feeding method without the baby at the breast.

- Feeding-tube devices consist of a container to hold breastmilk or formula and a length of thin tubing that runs from the container to the mother's nipple. The tube is secured in place with nonallergenic tape.

- The use of a feeding-tube device is indicated for babies with weak, disorganized, or dysfunctional sucking. A partial list includes those babies who are preterm, hypertonic, hypotonic; babies who have Down syndrome, cardiac problems, nipple-preference, neurologically impairment, or cleft lip or palate; infants who have experienced perinatal asphyxia, low, slow, or no weight gain, or weight loss due to ineffective suckling.

- The feeding-tube device is useful in maternal situations such as adoptive nursing and for mothers who are relactating, have had breast surgery, suffer from primary lactation insufficiency, have severe nipple trauma, are suffering from an illness, or are undergoing surgery or hospitalization.

- With finger-feeding, a mother places the tube on the pad of her index finger or whichever finger is closest in size to her nipple. The baby draws the finger into his mouth and with cor-

rect suckling, causes the milk to flow. This method also allows the father or other caregiver to feed the baby.

- Finger-feeding can also be used to take the edge off the baby's hunger before putting him to the breast and to help transition a baby to nursing at the breast.

- With the use of a feeding-tube device, the clinician must closely follow the progress in short- or long-term use. Risks of use include "addiction" to the device by the clinician, mother, and/or baby. The mother and baby should be weaned from the device as quickly as is appropriate.

- Health-care professionals must employ judicious use of devices and other technology that are designed to aid in breastfeeding. As with all care, the use of a breastfeeding device of any kind must be found to "do no harm;" thereafter its benefits must outweigh the risks it represents in order for the breastfeeding relationship to be truly supported.

Internet Resource

Breast pumps and supplies:
www.medela.com
www.hollister.com
www.breastpumps-etc.com
www.lalecheleague.org/catalog/pump96.html

For reporting problems with breast pumps and other technologies go to the FDA's web site:
www.fda.gov

For detailed information on breast pumps:
www.geddesproduction.com

References

Alekseev NP et al. Compression stimuli increase the efficacy of breast pump function. *Eur J Obstet Gynecol Reproduct Biol* 77:131–39, 1998.

Alexander JM et al. Randomized controlled trial of breast shells and Hoffman's exercises for inverted and nonprotractile nipples. *Br Med J* 304(6833):1030–32, 1992.

Amatayakul K et al. Serum prolactin and cortisol levels after suckling for varying periods of time and the effect of a nipple shield. *Acta Obstet Gynecol Scand* 66:47–51, 1987.

Arnold LDW. *Recommendations for collection, storage and handling of a mother's milk for her own infant in the hospital setting.* Denver, CO: Human Milk Banking Association of North America, 1999.

Asquith M, Harod J. Reduction of bacterial contamination in banked human milk. *J Pediatr* 95:993–94, 1979.

Asquith M, Sharp R, Stevenson D. Decreased bacterial contamination of human milk expressed with an electric breast pump. *J Calif Perin Assoc* 4:45–47, 1985.

Asquith M et al. The bacterial content of breast milk after early initiation of expression using a standard technique. *J Pediatr Gastroenterol Nutr* 3:104–7, 1984.

Auerbach KG. Using nipple shields appropriately. *Rental Roundup* 6:4–5, 1989.

———. The effect of nipple shields on maternal milk volume. *JOGNN* 19:419–27, 1990a.

———. Sequential and simultaneous breast pumping: a comparison. *Int J Nurs Stud* 27:257–65, 1990b.

Auerbach KG, Avery JL. Relactation: a study of 366 cases. *Pediatrics* 65:236–42, 1980.

———. Induced lactation: a study of adoptive nursing by 240 women. *Am J Dis Child* 135:340–43, 1981.

Auerbach KG, Guss E. Maternal employment and breast-feeding: a study of 567 women's experiences. *Am J Dis Child* 138:958–60, 1984.

Auerbach KG, Walker M. When the mother of a premature infant uses a breast pump: what every NICU nurse needs to know. *Neonatal Network* 13:23–29, 1994.

Bennion E. *Antique medical instruments.* Berkeley, CA: University of California, 1979:271.

Biancuzzo M. Selecting pumps for breastfeeding mothers. *JOGNN* 28:417–26, 1999.

Bodley V, Powers D. Long-term nipple shield use—a positive perspective. *J Hum Lact* 12:301–4, 1996.

Bornmann P. *Legal considerations and the lactation consultant—USA,* Unit 3 (Lactation Consultant Series). Garden City Park, NY: Avery Publishing Group, 1986.

Bose C et al. Relactation by mothers of sick and premature infants. *Pediatrics* 67:565–68, 1981.

Bowen-Jones A, Thompson C, Drewett RF. Milk flow and sucking rates during breast-feeding. *Dev Med Child Neurol* 24:626–33, 1982.

Bowles B, Stutte P, Hensley J. Alternate massage in breast-feeding. *Genesis* 9:5–9, 1988.

Brigham M. Mothers' reports of the outcome of nipple shield use. *J Hum Lact* 12:291–97, 1996.

Bull P, Barger J. Fingerfeeding with the SNS. *Rental Roundup* 4:2–3, 1987.

Caldeyro-Barcia R. Milk-ejection in women. In: Reynolds M, Folley S, eds. *Lactogenesis, the initiation of milk secretion at parturition.* Philadelphia: University of Pennsylvania Press, 1969.

Chapman et al. Impact of breast pumping on lactogenesis stage II after cesarean delivery: a randomized clinical trial. *Pediatrics* 107(6), e94 2001. Available at: http://www.pediatrics.org/cgi/content/full/107/6/e94.

Clavey S. The use of acupuncture for the treatment of insufficient lactation (Que Ru). *Am J Acupuncture* 24:35–46, 1996.

Clum D, Primomo J. Use of a silicone nipple shield with premature infants. *J Hum Lact* 12:287–90, 1996.

Cobo E et al. Neurohypophyseal hormone release in the human: II. Experimental study during lactation. *Am J Obstet Gynecol* 97:519–29, 1967.

Costa K. A comparison of colony counts of breast milk using two methods of breast cleansing. *JOGNN* 18:231–36, 1989.

Cox DB, Owens RA, Hartmann PE. Blood and milk prolactin and the rate of milk synthesis in women. *Exp Physiol* 81:1007–20, 1996.

Cregan MD, De Mello TR, Hartmann PE. Preterm delivery and breast expression: consequences for initiating lactation. *Adv Exp Med Biol* 478:427–28, 2000.

Cregan MD, Hartmann PE. Computerized breast measurement from conception to weaning: clinical implications. *J Hum Lact* 15:89–96, 1999.

da Silva OP et al. Effect of domperidone on milk production in mothers of premature newborns: a randomized double-blind, placebo-controlled trial. *Can Med Assoc J* 164:17–21, 2001.

Daly SEJ, Hartmann PE. Infant demand and milk supply. Part 1: Infant demand and milk production in lactating women. *J Hum Lact* 11:21–26, 1995a.

———. Infant demand and milk supply. Part 2: The short-term control of milk synthesis in lactating women. *J Hum Lact* 11:27–37, 1995b.

Daly SEJ et al. The determination of short-term breast volume changes and the rate of synthesis of human milk using computerized breast measurement. *Exp Phys* 77:79–87, 1992.

———. The short-term synthesis and infant regulated removal of milk in lactating women. *Exp Phys* 78:209–20, 1993.

de Sanctis V et al. Comparison of prolactin response to suckling and breast pump aspiration in lactating mothers. *La Ric Clin Lab* 11:81–85, 1981.

DeNicola M. One case of nipple shield addiction. *J Hum Lact* 2:28–29, 1986.

Desmarais L, Browne S. *Inadequate weight gain in breastfeeding infants: assessments and resolutions,* Unit 8 (Lactation Consultant Series). Garden City Park, NY: Avery Publishing Group, 1990.

Dodd F, Griffin T. *Milking routines, machine milking.* Reading, England: National Institute of Research on Dairying, Shinfield, 1977:179–200.

Donowitz L et al. Contaminated breast milk: a source of *Klebsiella* bacteremia in a newborn intensive care unit. *Rev Infec Dis* 3:716–20, 1981.

Drewett R, Bowen-Jones A, Dogterom J. Oxytocin levels during breastfeeding in established lactation. *Horm Behav* 16:245–48, 1982.

Edgehouse L, Radzyminski S. A device for supplementing breast-feeding. *MCN* 15:34–35, 1990.

Egnell E. The mechanics of different methods of emptying the female breast. *J Swe Med Assoc* 40:1–8, 1956.

Ehrenkranz RA, Ackerman BA. Metoclopramide effect on faltering milk production by mothers of premature infants. *Pediatrics* 78:614–20, 1986.

el-Mohandes AE et al. Aerobes isolated in fecal microflora of infants in the intensive care nursery: relationship to human milk use and systemic sepsis. *Am J Infect Control* 21:231–34, 1993a.

———. Bacterial contaminants of collected and frozen human milk used in an intensive care nursery. *Am J Infect Control* 21:226–30, 1993b.

Eteng MU et al. Storage beyond three hours at ambient temperature alters the biochemical and nutritional qualities of breast milk. *Afr J Reprod Health* 5:130–34, 2001.

Feher S et al. Increased breastmilk production for premature infants with a relaxation/imagery audiotape. *Pediatrics* 83:57–60, 1989.

Fewtrell MS, Lucas P, Collier S. Randomized trial comparing the efficacy of a novel manual breast pump with a standard electric breast pump in mothers who delivered preterm infants. *Pediatrics* 107:1291–97, 2001.

Fewtrell M et al. Randomized study comparing the efficacy of a novel manual breast pump with a mini-electric breast pump in mothers of term infants. *J Hum Lact* 17:126–31, 2001.

Fildes V. *Breasts, bottles, and babies.* Edinburgh: Edinburgh University, 1986:141–43.

Freeman ME et al. Prolactin structure, function, and regulation of secretion. *Physiological Rev* 80:1523–631, 2000.

Food and Drug Administration (FDA). Personal Communication. June 1, 2001.

Gabay MP. Galactogogues: medications that induce lactation. *J Hum Lact* 18:274–79, 2002.

Goodman G, Grosvenor C. Neuroendocrine control of the milk-ejection reflex. *J Dairy Sci* 66:2226–35, 1983.

Gorewit R et al. Current concepts on the role of oxytocin in milk-ejection. *J Dairy Sci* 66:2236–50, 1983.

Gransden W et al. An outbreak of *Serratia marcescens* transmitted by contaminated breast pumps in a special care baby unit. *J Hosp Infec* 7:149–54, 1986.

Groh-Wargo S et al. The utility of a bilateral breast pumping system for mothers of premature infants. *Neonat Network* 14:31–36, 1995.

Gross MS. Letter. *ILCA Globe* 3:5, 1995.

Gunn AJ et al. Growth hormone increases breast milk volumes in mothers of preterm infants. *Pediatrics* 98:279–82, 1996.

Halverson HM. Mechanisms of early infant feeding. *J Gen Psych* 64:185–223, 1944.

Hamosh M et al. Breastfeeding and the working mother: effect of time and temperature of short-term storage on proteolysis, lipolysis, and bacterial growth in milk. *Pediatrics* 97:492–98, 1996.

Hartmann P. *Human lactation: current research and clinical implications.* Presented at: Australian Lactation Consultants' Association Conference, Melbourne, Australia, October 12–15, 2000.

———. New insights into breast physiology and breast expression and development of the Symphony breastpump. In: *Human lactation-the science of the art series*, CD, Baar, Switzerland: Medela AG, Medical Technology, 2002.

Hill PD, Aldag JC, Chatterton RT. The effect of sequential and simultaneous breast pumping on milk volume and prolactin levels: a pilot study. *J Hum Lact* 12:193–39, 1996.

———. Effects of pumping style on milk production in mothers of non-nursing preterm infants. *J Hum Lact* 15:209–16, 1999.

———. Initiation and frequency of pumping and milk production in mothers of non-nursing preterm infants. *J Hum Lact* 17:9–13, 2001.

Howie P et al. The relationship between suckling-induced prolactin response and lactogenesis. *J Clin Endocrinol Metab* 50:670–73, 1980.

Jackson D et al. The automatic sampling shield: a device for sampling suckled breast milk. *Early Hum Dev* 15:295–306, 1987.

Johnson CA. An evaluation of breast pumps currently available on the American market. *Clin Pediatr* 22:40–45, 1983.

Jones E, Dimmock PW, Spencer SA. A randomized controlled trial to compare methods of milk expression after preterm delivery. *Arch Dis Child Fetal Neonatal Ed* 85:F91–5, 2001.

Kent JC et al. Response of breasts to different stimulation patterns of an electric pump. *J Hum Lact* 19:179–86, 2003.

Kutner L. Nipple shield consent form: a teaching aid. *J Hum Lact* 2:25–27, 1986.

Law BJ et al. Is ingestion of milk-associated bacteria by premature infants fed raw human milk controlled by routine bacteriologic screening? *J Clin Microbiol* 27:1560–66, 1989.

Lawrence RA, Lawrence RM. *Breastfeeding: a guide for the medical profession.* St. Louis: Mosby, 1999.

Marmet C, Shell E. *Marmet technique of manual expression of breastmilk.* Encino, CA: The Lactation Institute, 1980.

Maygrier J. *Midwifery illustrated.* Philadelphia: Carey & Hart, 1833:173.

McNeilly AS et al. Release of oxytocin and prolactin response to suckling. *Br Med J* 286:646–47, 1983.

Meier PP, Brown LP, Hurst NM. Nipple shields for preterm infants: effect on milk transfer and duration of breastfeeding. *J Hum Lact* 16:106–14, 2000.

Meier P, Wilks S. The bacteria in expressed mothers' milk. *MCN* 12:420–23, 1987.

Merrill W et al. Effects of premilking stimulation on complete lactation, milk yield and milking performance. *J Dairy Sci* 70:1676–84, 1987.

Minchin M. *Breastfeeding matters.* Victoria, Australia: Alma Publications, 1985:142–45.

Mitoulas LR, Lai CT, Gurrin LC. Efficacy of breast milk expression using an electric breast pump. *J Hum Lact* 18:344–52, 2002a.

Moloney A et al. A bacteriological examination of breast pumps. *J Hosp Infec* 9:169–74, 1987.

Morse J, Bottorff J. The emotional experience of breast expression. *J Nurse Midwifery* 33:165–70, 1988.

Neifert M, Seacat J. *Milk yield and prolactin rise with simultaneous breast pumping.* Presented at: Ambulatory Pediatric Association Meeting, Washington, DC, May 7–10, 1985.

Neville M. Regulation of mammary development and lactation. In: Neville M, Neifert M, eds. *Lactation: physiology, nutrition and breast-feeding.* New York: Plenum, 1983:118.

Neville MC. Anatomy and physiology of lactation. *Pediatr Clin North Am* 48(1):13–34, 2001.

Newton M, Newton N. The let-down reflex in human lactation. *J Pediatr* 33:698–704, 1948.

Nissen E et al. Different patterns of oxytocin, prolactin, but not cortisol release during breastfeeding in women delivered by cesarean section or by the vaginal route. *Early Hum Dev* 45:103–18, 1996.

Noel G, Suh H, Frantz A. Prolactin release during nursing and breast stimulation in postpartum and nonpostpartum subjects. *J Clin Endocrinol Metab* 38:413–23, 1974.

Nwankwo M et al. Bacterial growth in expressed breast-milk. *Ann Trop Paediatr* 8:92–95, 1988.

Petersen W. *Dairy science: principles and practice.* Philadelphia: Lippincott, 1950:373–87.

Pittard W et al. Bacterial contamination of human milk: container type and method of expression. *Am J Perinatol* 8:25–27, 1991.

Rental Roundup. New product, SNS. 3:1–3, 1986.

Ruis H et al. Oxytocin enhances onset of lactation among

mothers delivering prematurely. *Br Med J* 283:340–42, 1981.

Sagi R, Gorewit R, Zinn S. Milk-ejection in cows mechanically stimulated during late lactation. *J Dairy Sci* 63:1957–60, 1980.

Saint L, Maggiore P, Hartmann P. Yield and nutrient content of milk in eight women breast-feeding twins and one woman breast-feeding triplets. *Br J Nutr* 56:49–58, 1986.

Slusser W, Frantz K. High-technology breastfeeding. Part II: the management of breastfeeding. *Ped Clin North Am* 48:505–16, 2001.

Smith W, Erenberg A, Nowak A. Imaging evaluation of the human nipple during breastfeeding. *Am J Dis Child* 142:76–78, 1988.

Sozmen M. Effects of early suckling of cesarean-born babies on lactation. *Biol Neonate* 62:67–68, 1992.

Stark Y. Human nipples: function and anatomical variations in relationship to breastfeeding [master's thesis]. Pasadena, CA: Pacific Oaks College, 1994.

Stern JM, Reichlin S. Prolactin circadian rhythm persists throughout lactation in women. *Neuroendocrinology* 51:31–37, 1990.

Stutte P, Bowles B, Morman G: The effects of breast massage on volume and fat content of human milk. *Genesis* 10:22–25, 1988.

Sutherland A, Auerbach KG. *Relactation and induced lactation,* Unit 1 (Lactation Consultant Series). Garden City Park, NY: Avery Publishing Group, 1985.

Thompson N et al. Contamination in expressed breast milk following breast cleansing. *J Hum Lact* 13:127–30, 1997.

Toppare MF et al. Metoclopramide for breast milk production. *Nutr Res* 14:1019–29, 1994.

Tully MR. Recommendations for handling of mother's own milk. *J Hum Lact* 16:149–51, 2000.

Tyson J. Nursing and prolactin secretion: principle determinants in the mediation of puerperal infertility. In: Crosignani P, Robyn C, eds. *Prolactin and human reproduction.* New York: Academic, 1977:97–108.

Ueda T et al. Influence of psychological stress on suckling-induced pulsatile oxytocin release. *Obstet Gynecol* 84:259–62, 1994.

Walker M. How to evaluate breast pumps. *MCN* 12:270–76, 1987.

———. Breast pump survey. Unpublished manuscript, 1992.

Weber F, Woolridge MW, Baum JD. An ultrasonographic study of the organization of sucking and swallowing by newborn infants. *Dev Med Child Neurol* 28:19–24, 1986.

Weichert C. Prolactin cycling and the management of breastfeeding failure. *Adv Pediatr* 27:391–407, 1980.

Whittlestone W. The physiologic breastmilker. *NZ Fam Phy* 5:1–3, 1978.

Whitworth N et al. The effect of fetal genotype on the human maternal PRL response to labor, delivery and breast stimulation. *Abst Proc Int Cong Prolactin* 4:60, 1984.

Wilde CJ, Prentice A, Peaker M. Breast-feeding: matching supply with demand in human lactation. *Proc Nutr Soc* 54:401–6, 1995.

Wilks S, Meier P. Helping mothers express milk suitable for preterm and high-risk infant feeding. *MCN* 13:121–23, 1988.

Williams J, Auerbach K, Jacobi A. Lateral epicondylitis (tennis elbow) in breastfeeding mothers. *Clin Pediatr* 28:42–43, 1989.

Williams-Arnold LD. *Human milk storage for healthy infants and children.* Sandwich, MA: Health Education Associates, 2000.

Wilson-Clay B. Clinical use of silicone nipple shields. *J Hum Lact* 12:279–85, 1996.

Wilson-Clay B, Hoover K. *The breastfeeding atlas.* Austin, TX: LactNews Press, 2002.

Woodworth M, Frank E. Transitioning to the breast at six weeks: use of a nipple shield. *J Hum Lact* 12:305–7, 1996.

Woolford M, Phillips D. Evaluation studies of a milking system using an alternating vacuum level in a single chambered teatcup. *Proceedings of the international symposium on Machine Milking.* National Mastitis Council, 1978:125–49.

Woolridge MW. Breastfeeding: physiology into practice. In: Davies DP, ed. *Nutrition in child health. Proceedings of conference jointly organized by the Royal College of Physicians of London and the British Paediatric Association.* RCPL Press, 1995:13–31.

Woolridge M, Baum J, Drewett R. Effect of a traditional and of a new nipple shield on sucking patterns and milk flow. *Early Hum Dev* 4:357–64, 1980.

Ziemer M, Pidgeon J. Skin changes and pain in the nipple during the first week of lactation. *JOGNN* 22:247–56, 1993.

Zinaman M. Breast pumps: ensuring mothers' success. *Contemp Obstet Gynecol* 32:55–62, 1988.

Zinaman M et al. Acute prolactin, oxytocin response and milk yield to infant suckling and artificial methods of expression in lactating women. *Pediatrics* 89:437–40, 1992.

Zoppou C, Barry SI, Mercer GN. Dynamics of human milk extraction: a comparative study of breast feeding and breast pumping. *Bull Math Biol* 59:953–73, 1997a.

———. Comparing breastfeeding and breast pumps using a computer model. *J Hum Lact* 13:195–202, 1997b.

Appendix 12–A

MANUFACTURERS/DISTRIBUTORS OF BREAST PUMPS

Avent America, Inc., 475 Supreme Drive, Bensenville, IL 60106 (www.aventamerican.com)

Bailey Medical Engineering, 2020 11th Street, Los Osos, CA 93402 (Nurture III small semiautomatic breast pump) (www.baileymed.com)

BreastPump.com, Inc., P.O. Box 18475, Tucson, AZ 85731 (VersaPed pedal pump)

Camp Healthcare, 2010 East High Street, Jackson, MI 49203 (former White River breast pumps)

Evenflo Products Co., P.O. Box 1206, 771 North Freedom Street, Ravenna, OH 44266

The First Years, One Kiddie Drive, Avon, MA 02322

Gerber Products Co., 445 State Street, Fremont, MI 49412

Hollister Inc., 2000 Hollister Drive, Libertyille, IL 60048-3781 (www.hollister.com)

Lact-Aid, P.O. Box 1066, Athens, TN 37303 (feeding-tube device)

Lumiscope Company, Inc., 400 Raritan Center Parkway, Edison, NJ 08837 (Gentle Expressions battery pump)

Medela, Inc., P.O. Box 660, McHenry, IL 60051 (www.medela.com)

Omron Marshall Products, Inc., 300 Lakeview Parkway, Vernon Hills, IL 60061 (Kaneson cylinder and Mag Mag battery pumps)

Whisper Wear, 2221 Newmarket Parkway, Suite 136, Marietta, GA 30067 (www.whisperwear.com)

Whittlestone, P.O. Box 2237, Antioch, CA 94531 (www.whittlestone.com)

Breastfeeding the Preterm Infant

Nancy M. Hurst and Paula P. Meier

The importance of human milk in the management of preterm infants is well recognized (American Academy of Pediatrics [AAP], 1997) and has been reported to improve host defenses, digestion and absorption of nutrients, gastrointestinal function, neurodevelopmental outcomes, and enhanced maternal psychological well-being (Schanler, 2001). Yet mothers of preterm infants encounter numerous, well-documented barriers to breastfeeding that are not experienced by mothers of healthy term infants. Recent studies suggest that these barriers exist in both developed and developing countries, as reflected in lower worldwide rates of breastfeeding initiation and duration for preterm and/or low birth weight infants than for healthy term babies (Meier, 2001). Lower breastfeeding rates for this vulnerable population are of particular concern because preterm infants and their mothers receive unique benefits from breastfeeding that cannot be duplicated in the feeding of commercial infant formulas.

In order to improve these breastfeeding outcomes, clinicians must use research-based strategies that target specific barriers to breastfeeding initiation and duration for mothers and their preterm infants. In the past decade, numerous scientific reports have focused on delineating and studying these barriers (Baker & Rasmussen, 1997; Blaymore-Bier, 1997; Cregan et al., 2002; Hedberg

Nyqvist & Ewald, 1999; Hurst, Myatt, & Schanler, 1998; Jaeger, Lawson, & Filteau, 1997; Killersreiter et al., 2001; Nyqvist, Sjoden, & Ewald, 1999; Ortenstrand et al., 2001; Pietschnig et al., 2000; Pinelli, Atkinson, & Saigal, 2001; Wheeler et al., 1999). Cumulatively, these studies indicate that preterm infants are not just "small term infants" with respect to breastfeeding management. Instead, they have maturity-dependent physiologic and metabolic differences that require integration. Similarly, mothers of preterm infants experience unique physiologic and emotional challenges, such as maintaining lactation for several weeks, and coping with extreme vulnerability about infant intake during breastfeeding. These barriers adversely affect breastfeeding initiation and duration rates for this population.

Suitability of Human Milk for Preterm Infants

Evidence for the benefits of human milk feeding for preterm infants continues to accumulate (Table 13–1). Specific bioactive factors, such as, secretory IgA, lactoferrin, lysozyme, oligosaccharides, nucleotides, cytokines, growth factors, enzymes, antioxidants, and cellular components present in human milk have been implicated in reports of decreased rates of infections in premature infants fed human milk compared with those fed commercial formula (Hamosh, 2001). Gastrointestinal effects of feeding human milk include enhanced intestinal lactase activity (Shulman et al., 1998b), more rapid gastric emptying (Ewer et al., 1994), and a decrease in intestinal permeability early in life (Shulman et al., 1998a), compared with preterm formula. The feeding of human milk has been associated with improved cognitive and motor development at 3, 7, and 12 months (Bier et al., 2002), greater intellectual performance scores at 7.5 to 8.0 years of age (Lucas, Morley, & Cole, 1998), and faster brainstem maturation (Amin et al., 2000) compared with formula-feeding in former premature infants. Human milk-fed infants have been found to have enhanced visual acuity (Birch et al., 1992) and less incidence and severity of retinopathy of prematurity (Hylander et al., 2001) compared to preterm formula-fed infants—possibly due to the presence of very long-chain polyunsaturated fatty acids and antioxidant activity in human milk (Koletzko et al., 2001). Finally, the provision of mother's own milk to her infant allows the mother a distinct role in the care of her infant, at a time when many of the infant's needs are met by the nursing and medical NICU staff.

Studies comparing human milk composition of mothers delivering prematurely compared to those delivering at term have shown specific differences, at least during the first few weeks following delivery (Gross et al., 1980). There were higher concentrations of several components in preterm compared to term milk, including the following: sIgA and other anti-infective properties (Britton, 1986), oligosaccharides (Miller et al., 1994) protein (Butte et al., 1984), fat (Luukkainen, Salo, & Nikkari, 1994), sodium, chloride, and iron (Lemons et al., 1982; Trugo et al., 1988) has led some to speculate that the mother adapts to the higher needs of her preterm infant. Yet more recent studies examining the influence of gestational age at delivery and duration of lactation on the changing macronutrient composition of preterm milk theorize that these compositional differences are a result of the interruption of the gestational developmental processes

occurring in the mammary gland (Maas et al., 1998). Whatever the etiology of these compositional differences, the clinical significance of these gestationally dependent differences in milk composition is apparent when short- and long-term health outcomes are compared for preterm infants receiving either human milk or formula-feedings. These outcomes, summarized in Table 13–1, suggest that human milk may provide optimal "nutritional programming" for preterm infants, and may be protective against several prematurity-related health conditions (Dvorak et al., 2003; Furman et al., 2003; Schanler & Atkinson, 1999).

Yet despite these profound benefits, studies have shown the rate of linear growth and bone mineralization is negatively effected in preterm infants fed unfortified human milk (Nicholl & Gamsu, 1999; Schanler, Shulman, & Lau, 1999). Commercial fortifiers providing mineral supplementation of a mother's own milk have shown a normalization of these indices (Kuschel & Harding, 2000; Schanler, 1998). Given these recent findings, current recommendations include the provision of fortified mothers' own milk as the preferred feeding for preterm infants (Canadian Pediatric Society [CPS], 1995; Schanler, 2001).

Mothers of Preterm Infants

Breastfeeding has been described as a contribution to infant care that only the mother can make and as one aspect of "natural" caregiving that is not forfeited because of preterm birth. These clinical impressions were confirmed and extended in a qualitative study of 20 mothers of preterm infants who were interviewed in the home 1 month after infant discharge from the NICU (Kavanaugh et al., 1997). These women, who received research-based in-hospital breastfeeding services (Meier et al., 1993), reported that "the rewards outweigh the efforts" in describing their breastfeeding experiences during the first month that their infants were home.

The mothers from Kavanaugh's study (1997) delineated and exemplified five rewards of breastfeeding their preterm infants. Most frequently reported was "knowing that they had given their infants a good start in life," with references to the

Table 13–1

BENEFITS OF HUMAN MILK FOR PRETERM INFANTS

Host Defense

- Cellular functions (Garofalo & Goldman, 1998; Hanson, 1999)
- Bioactive factors (Akisu et al., 1998)

    Secretory IgA (Eibl et al., 1988)

    Cytokines (Fituch et al., 2001; Srivastava et al., 1996)

    Lactoferrin (Goldblum et al., 1989; Goldman et al., 1990; Hutchens et al., 1991)

- Enzymes (Henderson et al., 2001)
- Reduced risk and severity of infections (Contreras-Lemus, 1992; Furman et al., 2003; Hylander, Strobino, & Dhanireddy, 1998; Kosloske, 2001; Lucas & Cole, 1990; Schanler, Shulman, & Lau, 1999)

Gastrointestinal

- Hormones (Armand et al., 1996)
- Lactase activity (Rudloff et al., 1996; Shulman et al., 1998b)
- Growth factors (Burrin & Stoll, 2002; Diaz-Gomez, Domenech, & Barroso, 1997)

    Epidermal growth factor (Xiao et al., 2002)

- Improved feeding tolerance (Moody et al., 2000; Schanler, Hurst, & Lau, 1999; Shulman et al., 1998b; Weaver & Lucas, 1993)

Nutrition

- Amino acids (Moro et al., 1989)
- Lipid profile (Genzel-Boroviczeny, Wahle, & Koletzko, 1997; Heird, 2001; Peterson et al., 1998)
- Antioxidants (Ostrea et al., 1986; Zheng et al., 1993)
- Glutamine, Taurine (Bernt & Walker, 1999; Rassin et al., 1983)

Neurodevelopment

- Omega 3 fatty acids (Farquharson et al., 1995; Luukkainen et al., 1995)
- Cholesterol (Boehm et al., 1995; Woltil et al., 1995)
- Improved visual acuity (Birch et al., 1992; Uauy et al., 1992)
- Enhanced neurocognitive outcomes (Bier et al., 2002; Lucas et al., 1994; Lucas, Morley, & Cole, 1998)
- Maternal/infant bonding (Aguayo, 2001; Brandt, Andrews, & Kvale, 1998; Wheeler et al., 1999)

---

health benefits of breastfeeding for premature babies, followed by the mothers enjoyment of the physical closeness and intimacy of breastfeeding, and their perception that their infants "preferred" the breast to bottle-feedings of expressed milk. A fourth reward was "making a unique contribution to infant care," but mothers circumscribed this reward to the NICU stay, when other caretaking opportunities were limited. Finally, the mothers felt that, even with the extra effort of feeding and continued milk expression in the home, breastfeeding was "convenient" for them.

Thus the literature suggests that breastfeeding affords unique advantages for this vulnerable population that are in addition to the health benefits of breastfeeding for mothers of healthy term infants. These important findings provide scientific justification for the allocation of resources to improve breastfeeding outcomes for this vulnerable population.

Rates of Breastfeeding Initiation and Duration

Although breastfeeding statistics vary for individual countries, worldwide data suggest that mothers of preterm infants initiate and sustain breastfeeding at rates lower than the general population (Furman, Minich, & Hack, 1998; Jaeger, Lawson, & Filteau, 1997). Several conclusions and practice priorities can be drawn from this body of worldwide studies.

First, breastfeeding initiation rates appear to be increasing for this population (Adams et al., 2001; Wagner et al., 2002), presumably because promotion efforts have made mothers aware of the health benefits of human milk. Second, the duration of breastfeeding for mothers and preterm infants is typically shorter than the mothers' initial goals. Third, rates for breastfeeding initiation and duration can be improved if mothers are provided with research-based, comprehensive breastfeeding services. Thus a prerequisite for research and practice is to address the documented barriers to breastfeeding for mothers and preterm infants through the use of evidence-based strategies.

Research-Based Lactation Support Services

In recent years several publications have provided models for provision of breastfeeding services in the NICU (Hurst, Myatt, & Schanler, 1998; Jones, 1995; Meier et al., 1993), which included specific interventions within a four-phase temporal model: expression and collection of mothers' milk; gavage feeding of mothers' milk; in-hospital breastfeeding; and postdischarge breastfeeding management. A central feature of this model is that breastfeeding services are directed and/or coordinated by a nurse and/or physician with expertise in both lactation and intensive preterm infant care.

The Decision to Breastfeed

Until recently, health-care providers took the position that preterm infant feeding was a matter of parental "choice." Professional responsibility was limited to implementing a parent's decision. However, this perspective has been challenged by emphasizing the importance of sharing research-based health benefits of breastfeeding with parents, so that they can make informed decisions about feeding method (Meier, 2001; Meier & Brown, 1997). Specifically, this information should include factual verbal and written materials and alternatives to exclusive, long-term breastfeeding for women who do not want to make these commitments.

Facilitating an Informed Decision

All mothers who are hospitalized for preterm labor should be approached by a health professional to provide this specific information. If the mother has already given birth, breastfeeding should be discussed as soon after delivery as the mother is able to converse. The clinician should use specific information about the baby—such as maturity or health condition—and share with the mother breastfeeding research that is relevant to her baby's situation.

One barrier to providing mothers with this information is concern among some health-care providers that mothers will be made to feel guilty if they elect not to breastfeed. However, in other areas of NICU care, professionals do not withhold factual information that may influence a parent's decisions about infant management plans. Withholding such information would be considered unethical if it involved respiratory care or a surgical procedure. Providing parents with research-based options for infant feeding should be handled in a manner consistent with NICU policies for other decisions about infant management.

Alternatives to Exclusive, Long-Term Breastfeeding

Many mothers, especially those who had not intended to breastfeed, remain indecisive and/or reluctant to begin milk expression if they feel they must make a commitment to exclusive breastfeeding for several months. Additionally, healthcare providers or family members may have advised them that breastfeeding is "too much" for them at a time when they are consumed with discomfort, anxiety, stress, and fatigue. These women should be encouraged to begin milk expression immediately after birth when the hormonal milieu is optimal, so their infants can receive colostrum. Mothers should be told that they could cease milk expression at any time if they desire, and that professional help is available to help them discontinue pumping.

When women are indecisive and their initial plans include a day-by-day commitment to breastfeeding, several issues can help women make these important choices. For example, mothers who are unenthusiastic about pumping often ask how long they must provide milk for their infants. The practitioner can use infant milestones to make the recommendations more "real" for mothers. For example, a mother can be told that the most important time for the preterm infant is the introduction and advancement of early feedings, and that her colostrum is ideal for this purpose. This translates into milk expression for approximately 1 week. The clinician can further explain that providing milk until term, corrected age for the infant is especially beneficial because of the unique nature of the lipids in preterm milk. Most mothers are willing to consider short-term "contracts" of this nature when they understand the day-by-day importance of their milk for their infant.

Some mothers will express milk with a breast pump, but do not want to feed their infants at the breast. The practitioner can introduce this option by stating: "Some women decide that they will use a breast pump to express milk and then feed it to their babies by bottle. Is this something that you would consider?" This approach informs mothers and reassures them that other women have chosen this option.

When the mother of a preterm infant selects an alternative to exclusive, long-term breastfeeding, the breastfeeding specialist and NICU staff must not imply that her choice is "second best." Instead, the previously indecisive mother should be praised for her commitment and respected for her choice. The mother should be made aware of resources to help her if she changes her breastfeeding goals in the future.

Models for Hospital-Based Lactation Support Services

A variety of hospital-based breastfeeding support services have been developed in recent years and serve as models for clinical areas choosing to improve their services. The Lactation Support Program and Mothers' Own Milk Bank at Texas Children's Hospital in Houston was established in 1984 to provide support to mothers of hospitalized infants and improved quality control in the handling of expressed breastmilk (Hurst, Myatt, & Schanler, 1998). Registered nurses with additional certification in lactation management provide mothers and their infants with instruction and support in milk volume maintenance and breastfeeding. The Mothers' Milk Club at Rush-Presbyterian Hospital in Chicago utilizes a peer-support group model in providing breastfeeding support to mothers of hospitalized, preterm infants (Meier, 2001). Mothers meet once a week to discuss issues related to breast pumping, expressed breastmilk feeding and initiation, and progression of breastfeeding in the hospital and postdischarge. This support extends into the neonatal unit where mothers assist each other in their breastfeeding efforts.

Regardless of the model or combination of approaches used in a specific clinical environment, strong support from the neonatal physician and nursing staff will facilitate the progress of the program. Without the provision of evidence-based rationale for specific lactation management and breastfeeding policies and procedures to all staff involved, compliance will be less than optimal. Establishing early in the neonatal period the mother's feeding plans and goals will allow for individualized strategies to ensure that these goals are realized and to allow for timely modifications when warranted.

Finally, a primary source of support for breastfeeding comes from other family members. A recent qualitative study examined the management styles observed in breastfeeding families of preterm infants (Krouse, 2002). Families were described as facilitating (positive and proactive), maintaining (passive and adaptive), or obstructing (negative and feeling out of control) in their management styles related to breastfeeding. Although this small sample of families received intensive breastfeeding support services, the diversity in management styles observed highlights the complexity in providing effective interventions to assist mothers in obtaining their breastfeeding goals.

Initiation of Mechanical Milk Expression

Mothers of preterm infants must initiate and maintain lactation with a breast pump until their infants are able to regulate intake from the breast. This universally frustrating experience may last from several days to a few months, and mothers need research-based advice and support to persevere with their breastfeeding goals during this time.

Principles of Milk Expression

Few studies have focused on a mother's physiologic response to exclusive, long-term breast pump use (Chatterton et al., 2000; Cregan et al., 2002; Hartmann & Cregan, 2001). Thus the principles of lactation that have been studied for the healthy population are commonly applied to the mother who initiates and maintains lactation with a breast pump. Although giving birth prematurely does not appear to limit milk production, several factors surrounding the birth experience—prolonged bedrest, maternal complications, fatigue, stress, and irregular breast emptying—are documented prolactin-inhibitors and can adversely affect milk volume. Additionally, the close infant contact most frequently experienced by mothers following term delivery is limited after preterm birth. This maternal-infant proximity has been implicated in the enhancement of the neurohormonal stimulus of the lactogenic hormones, specifically, oxytocin and prolactin (Carter & Altemus, 1997; Uvnas-Moberg, 1998).

The available research supports the practice of beginning milk expression with a hospital-grade electric breast pump as early as possible after delivery (Hill, Aldag, & Chatterton, 1999). Factors shown to optimize milk yield include frequent milk expression of adequate duration to promote complete breast emptying (Hill, Aldag, & Chatterton, 2001). Some studies (Groh-Wargo et al., 1995) but not all (Fewtrell et al., 2001; Hill, Aldag, & Chatterton, 1999) have shown an advantage to simultaneous compared to sequential breast pumping. Clinically, advising mothers to express milk more frequently—e.g., 8 to 10 times daily during the first week to 10 days postbirth—may result in a milk volume approximating 750 to 1000 ml per day. Theoretically this practice may stimulate mammary alveolar growth during a time when circulating lactogenic hormones are elevated (Cox et al., 1999). Informing mothers of this rationale for frequent milk expression during this optimal time may provide abundant milk yield acting as a "reserve" against diminishing milk volume later in lactation. Achievement of a daily milk volume between 800 and 1000 ml at the end of the second week following delivery ensures that even if the mother's milk volume decreases by 50 percent during the infant's hospitalization, she will still have enough milk to feed her preterm infant at discharge.

Selecting a Breast Pump

Until recently evaluation of the efficacy of breast-milk expression using an electric breast pump had been limited to anecdotal reports (Auerbach & Walker, 1994; Biancuzzo, 1999). Recent studies have provided objective determination of major parameters of breast pump efficacy—namely, time to milk-ejection, amount of milk removed, and rate of milk removal (Daly et al., 1993; Daly et al., 1996; Mitoulas et al., 2002b). Mothers who initiate long-term milk expression need a hospital grade electric breast pump and as some studies have demonstrated (Hill, Aldag, & Chatterton, 1999) may benefit from a double collection kit.

The clinical challenge is ensuring that these breast pumps are available to mothers who need them. These pumps may be rented through pharmacies, lactation consultants, and home health agencies, but low-income mothers may be unable to incur the rental expense. A letter, such as the one shown in Figure 13–1, should be prepared on hospital letterhead, signed by a neonatologist and/or the NICU lactation specialist, and given to mothers for reimbursement purposes. Even with such a letter, the rental expense may be rejected by third-party payers, with an explanation that the mother

RUSH-PRESBYTERIAN-ST. LUKE'S MEDICAL CENTER 1653 WEST CONGRESS PARKWAY, CHICAGO, ILLINOIS 60612-3833 · 312.942.6640
RUSH UNIVERSITY RUSH MEDICAL COLLEGE

RUSH
SECTION OF NEONATOLOGY
DEPARTMENT OF PEDIATRICS

Date

Insured:

Policy Number:

Re: Electric Breast Pump Rental

To Whom It May Concern:

Dr. _____, a neonatologist in the Special Care Nursery at Rush-Presbyterian-St. Luke's Medical Center has prescribed human milk feedings for _____, who was born on _____, and whose parents are _____. Because this infant is too small and/or ill to feed at the breast, the mother must remove her milk with an electric breast pump, store it, and transport it to the Special Care Nursery so that it can be fed to her infant using a gavage tube.

A hospital grade electric breast pump with a double collection kit is necessary for extracting milk under these circumstances. Randomized controlled trials have shown that manual and/or battery-operated pumps, intended for occasional use by mothers of healthy infants, are inadequate for mothers who must initiate and maintain lactation in the absence of a nursing infant. Although hospital grade electric pumps can be purchased (approximately $900), they are more economical to rent on a short-term basis. We estimate that this mother will require use of the pump for approximately _____.

I trust that this information will expedite insurance coverage of the electric pump rental for this mother and infant. Should there be additional questions, please contact me at the above address/telephone.

Sincerely,

Paula P. Meier, RN, DNSc, FAAN
NICU Lactation Program Director

FIGURE 13–1.
Sample letter to request third-party payment for breast pump.

can use a less expensive battery-operated model or that breastfeeding is "elective," and formula-feeding is cheaper.

It is helpful to have a packet of research-based materials, such as the following documents, that parents can use to challenge these decisions: (1) an official letter on institutional letterhead that is specific to the infant's condition and the mother's breastfeeding needs; (2) research reports that demonstrate the superiority of electric breast pumps (Mitoulas et al., 2002a); and (3) official statements and/or data that endorse the importance/health outcomes of human milk feeding for preterm infants.

Milk-Expression Technique

The mother's milk-expression technique can influence the composition and the bacterial count of the milk to be fed to her infant. For this reason, mothers need detailed verbal and written information about the specific components of the procedure and the underlying rationale.

Mothers should be informed of how their expression technique can influence the amount of lipid and calories in their milk. Because lipids provide at least 50 percent of the calories in human milk, and lipid concentration increases over a single milk expression (Daly et al., 1993; Woodward, Rees, & Boon, 1989), it is essential that mothers be instructed to pump until all milk droplets cease flowing. The last few drops of milk are very high in lipid, and can contribute a substantial proportion of the calories in the entire milk sample. The duration of time to achieve breast emptying usually takes approximately 10 to 15 minutes, but this time may vary from woman to woman, and once lactation is established, some mothers may find that less time is required to achieve breast emptying.

Similarly, mothers should understand that all milk from a single milk expression should be thoroughly mixed before it is placed into sterile containers for storage. Mothers who produce large volumes of milk may have to empty the collection containers during milk expression to avoid overflow of the bottles. Typically, the first part of the expression will have lower fat and calories than will the latter. If the specimens are not mixed, the infant can receive feedings with markedly different fat and caloric values, affecting metabolic processes and overall weight gain (Valentine, Hurst, & Schanler, 1994). An exception to this principle is the intentional feeding of hindmilk-only, which is discussed later in this chapter.

Milk Expression Schedule

Mothers must be informed of the importance of frequent milk expression during the early days and weeks postbirth when the lactation hormones support optimal milk production. The actual number of daily milk expressions will depend upon each mother's breastfeeding goals. Mothers who need to produce maximal volumes of milk to achieve their goals should plan to express milk 8 to 10 times daily. Included in this group are women who want to breastfeed exclusively at the time of infant discharge, provide hindmilk for infant feedings, and/or have given birth to multiples. Mothers who plan to provide milk for a limited time—for example, until an infant's expected birth date—or those who plan to combine formula and breastfeeding, can pump less frequently. Instructing "short-term" breastfeeding mothers to express milk more than

five or six times daily is unnecessary and may discourage them from pumping at all.

The NICU staff can make it possible for mothers to accomplish frequent milk expression by modifying the nursery environment to meet mothers' needs. Mothers who must spend time traveling to and from the NICU often prefer to be with their infants rather than in a separate room where they can express milk. As a result, these mothers may pump only before leaving home and after returning home, and several hours elapse when their breasts are not stimulated. Enabling mothers to remain at their infants' bedside while expressing milk with the electric breast pump (Meier, 2001) promotes frequent stimulation and sends a strong message to the mother regarding the importance placed (by the staff) on providing her milk to her infant. Allowing mothers to pump at the infant's bedside provides an opportunity for the mother to see, touch, or hold her infant while expressing milk. Mothers use the pump upon arrival in the NICU, every two hours thereafter, and immediately before departure. Bedside pumping incorporates the scientific literature on the use of relaxation and imagery in enhancing milk volume (Feher et al., 1989), and is convenient for the mother and staff. Additionally, the expectation that mothers will provide milk while in the NICU highlights their indispensable role in infant care. Anecdotally, mothers have reported that they express more milk at their babies' bedsides, and combined with skin-to-skin care and nonnutritive sucking at the breast, that bedside pumping gives them a purpose for frequent and lengthy NICU visits.

Written Pumping Records

Keeping a written log of pumping frequency and milk volumes expressed is useful for the mother to monitor her lactation progress. Pumping records that document the time, duration, and amount of milk expressed provide useful information to the mother that can be shared with the NICU staff for assessment of milk volume maintenance (Figure 13–2). Evaluation of pumping frequency and milk volumes obtained allows the NICU staff to assist the mother in modifying her pumping schedule (to

PUMPING RECORDS

Your name:_____Your infant's medical record #_____

Use the table below to keep track of the date, time, and volume of milk expressed from each breast for every pumping session.

TIPS FOR INCREASING YOUR MILK SUPPLY	
• Pump frequently—at least 6 to 8 times a day • Rest and sleep whenever you can • Hold your baby skin-to-skin whenever possible	• Completely empty both breasts • Use relaxation techniques while pumping • Breathe deeply while pumping

If you have any questions, please contact one of the lactation consultants.

Today's date:_____

Time of day	Volume from left breast	Volume from right breast	Circle where you pumped
1.			Hospital / Home / Work / Other
2.			Hospital / Home / Work / Other
3.			Hospital / Home / Work / Other
4.			Hospital / Home / Work / Other
5.			Hospital / Home / Work / Other
6.			Hospital / Home / Work / Other
7.			Hospital / Home / Work / Other
8.			Hospital / Home / Work / Other
9.			Hospital / Home / Work / Other

♥ **Only you can provide the wonderful gift of breastmilk for your baby** ♥

Texas Children's Hospital
Lactation Support Program, 2003
www.texaschildrenshospital.org

FIGURE 13–2. Sample of pumping records. *Source:* Texas Children's Hospital, Lactation Support Program, 2003. www.texaschildrenshospital.org.

be explained later) based on her individual milk synthesis rate.

Maintaining Maternal Milk Volume

Expressed Milk Volume Guidelines

An arbitrary guideline categorizing levels of 24-hour milk volume is useful in order to determine the need for appropriate intervention (see Box 13–1). The volume of 500 ml/24 hrs was set as a cutoff point since most preterm infants will require at least this amount upon discharge from the hospital. "How much milk should I be expressing?" is a question frequently asked by mothers of hospitalized infants. Providing specific guidelines will help each mother assess her individual breast-feeding goals and the need for more (or less) frequent pumping. As previously mentioned, encouraging mothers to maintain a written pumping record will allow an accurate accounting of each mother's individual milk expression pattern and the need for appropriate interventions. In the event that a mother does not achieve a minimum milk volume of 350 ml/24 hrs by 10 to 14 days following delivery, strategies to stimulate milk syn-

thesis should be initiated in order to take advantage of the optimal hormonal milieu present during the early postpartum period.

Based on research demonstrating the variability from mother to mother regarding the rate of milk synthesis (Daly & Hartmann, 1995b), mothers can be advised whether extending the nonpumping interval at night is appropriate or not. Calculating the volume attained at a pumping and dividing that volume by the interval (in hours) between milk expressions provides an estimate of the rate of milk synthesis. Calculating milk synthesis rates over a 24-hour period provides a picture of the mother's overall milk synthesis rate. Milk synthesis rates are calculated by taking the volume obtained divided by the number of hours since the last milk expression (i.e., 90 cc divided by 3 hours = 30 cc/hr). Mothers with large milk storage capacities are able to maintain fairly consistent milk synthesis rates despite longer intervals between breast emptying (Kent et al., 1999). This is an invaluable strategy for mothers who must maintain their milk volumes over a long period of time.

Preventing Low Milk Volume

Milk expression guidelines as previously described are based on observational studies demonstrating that mothers who pump early and often following delivery experience higher milk yields (Hill, Aldag, & Chatterton, 1999). Yet despite the best efforts of some mothers, persistent low milk volumes occur—or milk production decreases over the many weeks following preterm delivery. Due to the lack of research, little is known about the physiology of long-term milk expression for mothers who are separated from their infants for extended periods following delivery. Therefore, strategies to manage low milk volume for mothers of preterm infants have focused on pharmacologic and non-pharmacologic enhancement of prolactin secretion (Budd et al., 1993; da Silva et al., 2001; Emery, 1996; Milsom et al., 1998). Obtaining a thorough history from the mother is vital in order to provide appropriate interventions to manage low milk volume. Information regarding maternal medication use, history of breast surgery, infertility, thyroid conditions, polycystic ovarian syndrome, extended

BOX 13–1

Guideline for Expressed Milk Volumes for Mothers of Hospitalized Infants

Milk volume by day 10 to 14 following delivery

Ideal	> 750ml/24 hr
Borderline	350–500 ml/24 hr
Low	> 350 ml/24 hr

bedrest prior to delivery, and previous breastfeeding experience, will provide a clearer picture of potential risk factors and possible effective interventions. Table 13–2 summarizes various strategies to increase maternal milk volume.

The use of certain maternal medications, including oral contraceptives, may diminish milk volume in mothers of preterm infants who are expressing milk with a breast pump. Although obstetricians usually advise women that progestin-only contraceptives will not interfere with lactation, reports indicate that this may not be true for a less-established "vulnerable" milk supply. Anecdotally, mothers report that milk volume diminishes markedly within days of starting oral contraceptives and returns to baseline shortly after they are discontinued. This phenomenon needs to be explored in controlled studies. But in the interim, clinicians should ask about oral contraceptive use if mothers report a rapid decline in a previously adequate volume. Some nonprescription medications such as pseudoephedrine have been associated with a 30 percent decrease in maternal milk volume. Since some mothers do not consider oral contraceptives and over-the-counter medications of concern when breastfeeding, it is best to ask about these groups of medications specifically.

Table 13-2

STRATEGIES TO INCREASE LOW MILK VOLUME

- Frequent milk expression (> 6 times/day)
- Periodic breast massage prior to and during pumping
- Pumping at the infant's bedside
- Holding the infant skin-to-skin
- Getting uninterrupted sleep of 5 to 6 hours
- Ensuring proper fit of pump flange/efficiency of pump
- Taking some medications (i.e., metoclopramide, domperidone)
- Taking some galactogogues (i.e., Fenugreek)

Most mothers of preterm infants experience a decrease in milk volume during the second month of milk expression (Hill, Brown, & Harker, 1995; Hurst, Myatt, & Schanler, 1998). Although no published studies have examined the physiology of this phenomenon, data from studies of term infants may offer some insight. Studies (Daly & Hartmann, 1995a, 1995b) have documented that maternal milk volume is limited primarily by infant demand rather than by a finite capacity of the mother to produce milk. These findings suggest that, over days or weeks, the milk expression procedure may be ineffective in stimulating an optimal milk supply for mothers of preterm infants. In particular, a breast pump does not mimic the infant's physical closeness and responsiveness that may be essential for optimal hormonal regulation of milk volume. Thus, encouraging infant contact during and after milk expression in the NICU may represent a promising intervention in preventing and improving low milk volume.

Skin-to-Skin (Kangaroo) Care

A series of worldwide studies have documented the safety of skin-to-skin (STS; Kangaroo) care and its effectiveness in promoting physiologic stability in preterm and high-risk infants (Bauer et al., 1997; Bier et al., 1996; Bohnhorst et al., 2001; Cattaneo et al., 1998; Gazzolo, Masetti, & Meli, 2000; Tornhage et al., 1998; Whitelaw & Liestol, 1994). Although the relationship between STS care and lactation has been studied less systematically, the duration of breastfeeding appears to be higher for STS infants than for incubator controls (Charpak et al., 2001; Ludington-Hoe et al., 1994).

Furthermore, it has been speculated that STS holding may trigger the production of maternal milk antibodies to specific pathogens in the infant's environment through mechanisms in the entero-mammary pathway (Hurst et al., 1997). In this study, mothers' milk volume at 1, 2, 3, and 4 weeks after delivery was compared for two groups of women: 8 mothers who participated in STS holding; and 15 mothers who did not. Even with just 30 minutes daily of STS holding, mothers in the STS group had a significantly greater increase in milk volume between 2 and 4 weeks than did mothers in the control group. At 4 weeks after delivery, when data collection ended, mothers in the STS group produced significantly more milk each day than did control mothers (647 ml vs. 530 ml, respectively).

Mothers whose infants are in STS care have reported observing their infants' rooting and mouthing movements, and moving toward the nipple during STS sessions (Hurst et al., 1997). Mothers frequently note feelings of milk-ejection and leaking, and many report that they express the largest milk volumes immediately following STS care. Yet milk-ejection is but one of the effects of oxytocin that occurs during the developing maternal-infant relationship. Emerging evidence reveals that oxytocin coordinates both the causes and effects of positive social interactions (Uvnas-Moberg, 1997). During social interactions, oxytocin can be released by sensory stimuli perceived as positive, including touch, warmth, and odors (Uvnas-Moberg, 1998). Oxytocin also may mediate the consequences of positive social interactions, such as reduced sympathoadrenal activity and enhanced parasympathetic-vagal activity (Nelson & Panksepp, 1998; Nissen et al., 1998). Because the release of oxytocin can become conditioned to emotional states and mental images, the actions of this peptide may provide an additional explanation for the long-term benefits of positive experiences. However, the conditioning of this response for the mother of a preterm infant, at least initially, is related to experiences far removed from her infant, such as entering the neonatal intensive care unit (NICU), turning on an electric breast pump, or walking into the entry of the hospital. How best to "normalize" this conditioning to its proper maternal-infant orientation is one of the challenges clinicians are faced with when working with this vulnerable population—and STS holding may provide an early antidote (Feldman et al., 2002).

Although a complete review of procedures for STS holding is beyond the scope of this chapter, several principles can be summarized. First, infants can be safely placed in STS care while very small and mechanically ventilated (Gale, Franck, & Lund, 1993; Legault & Goulet, 1995; Tornhage et al., 1999). Second, there is no scientific reason to restrict the duration of STS care, unless an infant becomes physiologically unstable while on the mother's chest. Typically, a STS care session is

ended based upon the mother's availability rather than infant criteria. Third, the position of the infant in STS care is important in maintaining physiologic stability, and recliners are ideal in achieving this position. The infant should be placed upright between the mother's breasts, with the side of the face against the internal surface of one breast (Figure 13–3). The recliner is angled back to allow the infant's body to remain at a 45 to 60° angle from the floor. A mirror positioned to allow the mother to observe her infant's face is helpful during these sessions. STS sessions of two or more hours are ideal, and it is not uncommon for infants to display behaviors that suggest autonomic instability when returned to the incubator following STS care (Kirsten, Bergman, & Hann, 2001).

Evidence-Based Guidelines for Milk Collection, Storage, and Feeding

Guidelines for Collection and Storage of Expressed Mothers' Milk (EMM)

The collection and storage of EMM for later use by the mother's own infant has an impact on milk composition and various constituents. Several factors should be considered, including the type of collection container and storage conditions. Even with meticulous technique, no mother's milk is sterile (el-Mohandes et al., 1993; Thompson et al., 1997). A mother's attention to hand washing and cleaning of milk expression equipment is extremely important in reducing colonization by pathogens other than normal skin flora (Tully, 2000). Milk collection and storage guidelines are summarized in Table 13–3 and place special emphasis on ensuring that anything coming in contact with the milk or the breast be thoroughly cleaned prior to each pumping session. Special attention should be placed on disassembling all pump parts following each collection for washing to avoid harboring of bacterial growth. Glass (Pyrex) and hard plastic (polypropylene) containers are recommended for storage of human milk—as both provide stability of water-soluble constituents and immunoglobulin A and are easy to handle (Goldblum et al., 1981; Williamson & Murti, 1996). Flexible, polyethylene bags are not recommended for milk collection and storage due to significantly greater loss of cells (Goldblum et al.,

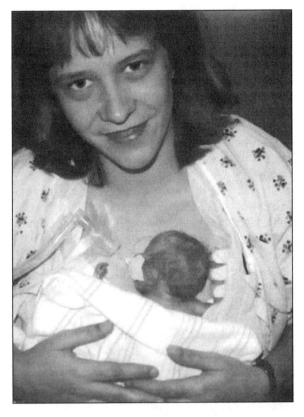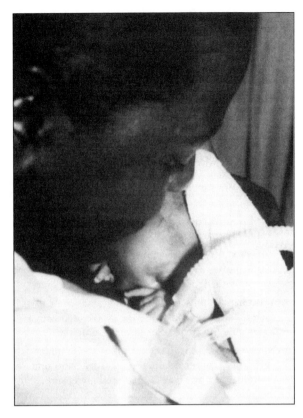

FIGURE 13–3. Mothers and their preterm infants during skin-to-skin holding. (With permission, The Lactation Support Program and Mothers' Own Milk Bank, Texas Children's Hospital, Houston.)

1981) and chance of leakage during storage and handling. The temperature at which milk is stored is based on the duration of time until the infant receives the milk for feeding. Table 13–4 summarizes the criteria to determine storage temperature to be used for human milk.

Preparing Expressed Mother's Milk for Infant Feeding

In most countries, preterm infants receive their mothers' milk by gavage until they are able to consume feedings directly from the breast. At this time, infants are small and vulnerable to problems that can occur when EMM is handled unnecessarily. Proper procedures should be developed and adhered to in order to minimize bacterial growth and possible changes in milk constituents during storage and feeding. Table 13–4 describes the situational and environmental opportunities for bacterial cont-

amination and guidelines for minimizing/preventing bacterial growth.

NICU Area Used for Milk Preparation. Attention to the environment designated in the NICU for milk storage/preparation is important in ensuring optimal quality control in the provision of EMM for infant feeding. Utilization of similar procedures used for storage of perishable food items should be adhered to, such as monitoring of refrigerator/freezer temperatures and routine cleaning and maintenance of storage units and milk preparation spaces. Input from the hospital infection control department can be useful in developing appropriate guidelines for establishing an optimal environment for the storage and preparation of EMM.

Quality Control. Mothers of hospitalized infants play a vital role in this process by ensuring correct labeling of each milk container with the infant's

Guidelines for Collection and Storage of Mother's Own Milk for Preterm Infant Feeding

1. All milk-collection equipment coming in contact with the breast and breastmilk should be thoroughly cleaned prior to and following use. Disassemble all parts prior to cleaning.

2. Sterilize milk collection equipment once a day by boiling the parts in water for 15 to 20 minutes.

3. Collect/store expressed milk in glass (Pyrex) or hard plastic (polypropylene) containers. Plastic bags are not recommended for milk storage for preterm infants.

4. Wash hands and scrub under fingernails prior to each milk expression. Wipe the nipple area with water only (no soap) prior to each pumping.

5. Following pumping, label each bottle with infant's name, medical record number, and date and time of pumping. List any current maternal medications on the label.

---

name, medical record number, date and time of collection, and use of any maternal medications. If the milk is to be transferred to another container by the nurse or other designated NICU staff prior to feeding, each individual syringe/bottle should be labeled appropriately. Human milk is a living fluid, not unlike blood, and should be handled as such. Proper hand washing and/or wearing gloves during handling should be practiced to avoid potential bacterial contamination of the EMM. Countertops/surfaces used for milk preparation should be wiped down with an appropriate antibacterial cleaner prior to preparation activities.

All milk that is to be used for infant feeding should be stored in the hospital under controlled conditions. All too often, mothers are told to store their expressed milk at home because of insufficient storage space in the NICU freezer. However, this approach would not be recommended for medications or blood; expressed milk should be no exception. When milk is out of sight of the NICU staff, there is no assurance that it has remained com-

pletely frozen and/or unopened before it is subsequently fed to small preterm infants. A final consideration is ensuring that EMM in the NICU is not subject to tampering. There are no clear guidelines as to whether refrigerators and freezers should be locked and/or have restricted access, but this is a very important issue. Anecdotally, NICU staff and parents have expressed concern that suggests that EMM should be kept in an environment that eliminates the potential for tampering.

Every effort should be made to provide stringent quality control standards to minimize potential errors in which infants receive another mother's milk. Considering the host-defense nature of human milk and the extent to which viruses can be transferred via milk, administering the wrong milk to an infant is a serious error. Proper labeling of milk collection/preparation containers with infant's name and medical record number and verification of this information (checked with another nurse) against infant's name band before feeding is an effective procedure to avoid potential errors. The NICU staff should never administer a container of unlabeled milk to an infant under any circumstances.

Warming EMM for Feeding.   Rapid heating, especially microwaving, has been demonstrated to adversely affect both the immunologic and nutritional properties of EMM (Hamosh, 1996; Quan et al., 1992). Refrigerated EMM should be gradually warmed (over 30 minutes) to approximately body temperature before being fed to small preterm infants (Gonzales et al., 1995). For the smallest infants, the feeding volume can be withdrawn into a syringe that is placed in the infant's incubator for gradual warming.

Special Issues Regarding the Feeding of EMM

The scientific literature supports feeding of fresh (unfrozen) milk when possible, because the anti-infective properties are maximally preserved (Hamosh, 1996, 2001). Ideally, preterm infants should receive at least one daily feeding of milk that has been pumped at the bedside and fed without refrigeration. This milk retains all of the anti-infective properties, and has been subjected to minimal handling and temperature changes. Many mothers will ensure that their infants have fresh milk available

Table 13–4

GUIDELINES TO MINIMIZE/PREVENT BACTERIAL GROWTH IN MOTHER'S OWN MILK FOR INFANT FEEDING

Milk Collection

- Instruct mother on proper collection technique including hand washing and maintenance of pumping equipment (see Table 13–3).

Milk Storage

- Use fresh, unrefrigerated milk within 1 hour of milk expression.
- Refrigerate milk immediately following expression when the infant will be fed within 24 to 48 hours.
- Freeze milk when infant is not being fed or the mother is unable to deliver the milk to the hospital within 24 hours of expression.
- Store each collection in a separate bottle. When pumping both breasts at the same time, two bottles can be combined into one.
- Ensure fresh/frozen milk is transported to the hospital on ice, in an insulated cooler to avoid thawing/warming.
- Do not refreeze any milk that has thawed.

Thawing

- Thaw milk gradually in a warm water bath, for no longer than 20 minutes.
- Ensure milk collection bottle caps are tightly secured to prevent contamination during water-bath process.
- Do not leave milk unattended under a running faucet.

Milk Preparation

- Designate optimal physical space in the NICU for milk preparation.
- Gloves should be worn by staff when preparing/handling milk.
- When preparing feedings for more than one infant at a time, wash hands/change gloves, and wipe down counter between preparations.

Fortification

- Add fortification per physician's order, ensuring complete mixing.
- Avoid vigorous shaking of milk to prevent disruption of milk fat membrane integrity (can result in adherence of milk fat to feeding tubes, bottles, etc.).
- Feed milk within 24 hours of addition of fortifier to EMM.

Warming

- Warm EMM to room temperature (27° C) prior to feeding.
- Milk containers can be placed in the infant's incubator 30 minutes prior to feeding to warm.
- Use of unattended warm water baths for warming purposes should be discouraged as milk could be warmed to high temperatures resulting in changes in milk constituents.

Feeding

- For continuous milk infusions, limit infusion time to 4 hours.
- Avoid use of additional extension tubing for gavage feeding of EMM.

for feedings if they understand the rationale behind this practice. The staff can support this plan by developing a sequence of feeding the milk so it can be used within 48 hours of expression, and/or alternated with frozen milk when necessary. In addition, it is important to emphasize to the mother that frozen milk still retains most of the anti-infective properties and is nutritionally superior to formula.

Volume Restriction Status

Special considerations regarding the feeding of EMM to preterm infants are based on the infant's fluid restrictive status at a time of greatest nutritional need. Although full feeding volume status for preterm infants is routinely considered to be a daily volume of 150cc/kgm/d, human milk-fed infants usually tolerate volumes much higher—up to 200 cc/kgm/d (Schanler, 2001). The ability to handle a greater volume has been attributed to the faster gastric emptying rates observed with human milk (Moody et al., 2000). However, in order to achieve optimal bone mineralization at a vulnerable time in the preterm infant's development, human milk fortifiers are routinely mixed with the milk to provide greater intake of specific minerals, such as calcium and phosphorous (Sankaran, et al., 1996; Wauben et al., 1998).

Commercial Nutritional Additives

Unfortified EMM is deficient in protein and selected minerals to support optimal growth and bone mineralization for small preterm infants (Schanler, 1998; Schanler, Hurst, & Lau, 1999; Schanler, Shulman, & Lau, 1999; Simmer, Metcalf, & Daniels, 1997). Thus, for most preterm infants, these additional nutrients are provided in the form of commercial milk fortifiers. However, recent studies have raised concern that these commercial liquids and powders may affect the bioavailability and function of human milk components (Ewer & Yu, 1996; Jocson, Mason, & Schanler, 1997; Lucas et al., 1996; Quan et al., 1994; Schanler, 1998). Studies evaluating the effects of nutrient fortification on some of the general host defense properties of human milk have shown no affect on the concentrations of IgA (Jocson, Mason, & Schanler, 1997; Quan et al., 1994), however, bacterial colony counts increased over time during storage of fortified human milk. The overall increase in bacterial counts under simulated nursery conditions was not significantly different after 24 hours' storage in the refrigerator, suggesting that current practice should include limiting storage to 24 hours once fortification is added to the milk.

Hindmilk Feeding

The feeding of the hindmilk-only fraction of EMM has received considerable interest among clinicians (Griffin et al., 2000; Valentine, Hurst, & Schanler, 1994). The lipid and caloric content of hindmilk is greater than that of foremilk or composite milk (e.g., a full pumping that includes fore- and hindmilk). By fractionating the hindmilk portion of a milk expression, mothers can provide high-lipid, high-calorie milk that promotes accelerated infant growth (Valentine, Hurst, & Schanler, 1994). Although hindmilk feeding holds remarkable potential for preterm infant nutrition, the technique has not yet been subjected to randomized controlled trials.

There is tremendous within and between mother variations in lipid content. Thus a standard procedure for collection of hindmilk does not ensure a standard outcome. Clinically, the lipid and caloric content of milk can be estimated with the creamatocrit, a technique that involves centrifuging a milk specimen that has been drawn into a capillary tube (Lucas et al., 1978; Polberger & Lonnerdal, 1993). The creamatocrit, or the percentage of total volume in the capillary tube that is equivalent to lipid, can be converted to an estimate of lipid and caloric content using one of the published regression graphs (Table 13–5). However, creamatocrits performed in this manner represent only a relative estimate of lipid and calories. A more accurate quantification of lipid and caloric content requires that the creamatocrit be standardized with one of the direct measures of total milk lipid, such as the Folch technique (Jensen, 1989).

Hindmilk and commercial fortifiers/additives are not interchangable, a point that is often misunderstood. Although commercial fortifiers provide small amounts of calories in the form of carbohydrates, their primary purpose is to supplement essential minerals, such as calcium and phosphorus, which are needed in higher concentrations than are present in human milk. In contrast, hindmilk does not "concentrate" these nutrients (Valentine, Hurst, & Schanler, 1994), but does provide an extremely efficient energy source by concentrating the endogenous milk lipids. Thus the use of hindmilk does not replace the need for mineral supplementation, and commercial fortifiers are a relatively inefficient means of supplying extra calories.

Finally, the needs of the mother must be considered whenever her composite milk is not used exclusively. It is easy for mothers to infer that their

Table 13–5

CREAMATOCRIT READINGS AND ASSOCIATED LIPID/CALORIC CONTENT OF HUMAN MILK

Creamatocrit	3	4	5	6	7	8	9	10	11
Cal/oz	15.7	17.8	20	22.1	24.3	26.4	28.5	30.7	32.8
% of calories—fat	22	37	44	48.2	52.1	56	58.2	60.4	62.6

Source: From Lucas et al. (1978).

milk is not "adequate" for their infants when it must be fortified or fractionated for hindmilk feedings. Mothers should be informed that their milk is ideal with respect to immunologic and nutritional properties—but the rapid growth of their very small infants requires temporary supplementation with commercial fortifiers and/or hindmilk.

Lactoengineering of own mother's milk (OMM) through a combination of hindmilk and creamatocrit measures can be empowering for mothers of preterm infants (Griffin et al., 2000; Jennings, Meier, & Meier, 1997). Specifically, mothers are assisted in expressing milk with a creamatocrit value that meets their individual infant's growth needs. When their infants demonstrate the desired weight gain pattern, mothers recognize that their milk modifications supported the desired growth.

Methods of Milk Delivery

A series of studies provides strong scientific support for the administration of EMM by intermittent rather than slow-infusion continuous gavage (Brennan-Behm et al., 1994; Schanler, Shulman, & Lau, 1999). In particular, milk lipids that comprise 50 to 60 percent of the calories in EMM adhere to the lumen of infusion tubings, and their loss results in a relatively dilute, low-calorie feeding (Brennan-Behm et al., 1994). The greatest lipid loss occurs during the slowest infusion rates (Greer, McCormick, & Loker, 1984; Stocks et al., 1985). Clinically, this means that the smallest babies, for whom caloric requirements are the highest, will receive EMM by the slowest infusion rates, resulting in a low-calorie milk. For this reason, EMM should be administered by slow intermittent bolus, rather than by continuous gavage infusion.

Maternal Medication Use

When small preterm infants receive their OMM by gavage, extra care must be taken to ascertain that maternal medications in the milk can be tolerated safely. Preterm infants, especially those who are extremely low birth weight, have immature metabolic and excretory pathways. As a result, drugs that may be safely given to mothers of term healthy infants may have adverse consequences for more vulnerable infants. Although a detailed description of these issues is beyond the scope of this chapter, several principles should be considered when a mother of a preterm infant must take medications:

- The medication should be considered "safe" for healthy term infants (AAP, 2001); if this is not the case, the medication should not be considered safe for the small preterm infant.

- If the medication or its metabolites has been shown to accumulate in newborn body tissues, its accumulation may be even more exaggerated for the preterm infant.

- Many mothers of preterm infants will have had complicated births and/or health conditions that necessitate a combination of medications.

- The infant may be receiving medications and/or other therapies that could interact with the maternal medications. The safety of these combinations—rather than the individual medications—must be considered.

- Extra caution is needed when lipid-rich hind-milk is being fed: medications that are lipophilic may cross readily into the milk.

Only health-care professionals who have expertise in lactation, pharmacology, and neonatal care should provide advice concerning the safety of medications for small preterm infants. When in doubt about a specific medication, or a combination of medications, a national expert should be consulted. In all instances any information about maternal medications should be reviewed with the neonatologist who is responsible for the infant's care, and mothers should record any medications consumed on the individual milk container.

Feeding at Breast in the NICU

Early oral experiences may influence later oral feeding development. Many clinicians specializing in feeding disorders report a high percentage of their patients as former preterm infants. This is not surprising given the amount of oral insults experienced by these infants, such as intubation, suctioning, and insertion of feeding tubes. Thus the provision of positive oral experiences early in their development may counteract some of the effects of these negative but necessary procedures. Nonnutritive suckling and suckling at the emptied maternal breast provides a positive experience for preterm infants.

Suckling at the Emptied Breast

There are no universally established criteria for the initiation of breastfeeding (or bottle-feeding for that matter) for preterm infants. Although a minimum body weight or gestational age (commonly 34 weeks) has been used, more recent practice has been to consider each infant's individual abilities when determining the initiation of oral feeding, be that breast or bottle (Lau & Hurst, 1999; Medoff-Cooper, 2000). Whereas judging the ability to breastfeed on the infant's achievement of consuming a prescribed milk volume by bottle, evidence-based research as previously described prove this practice inappropriate. In neonatal units whereby

infants are allowed nonnutritive suckling at the emptied breast (Meier, 2001; Narayanan et al., 1991), the idea of "when to initiate" breastfeeding has been reconceptualized.

Controlled clinical trials have demonstrated many benefits of nonnutritive suckling (NNS) with a pacifier for preterm infants (Pinelli & Symington, 2000). Theoretically, these same benefits should extend to the preterm infant's suckling at the mother's recently pumped breast, an experience that may also maximize the mother's milk production. Initiating NNS at the emptied breast provides a maternal stimulus that is different from routine breast pump use, and as such, may increase milk yield. Additionally, mothers receive instant reinforcement from infants' behaviors that reflect enjoyment and physiologic stability while at the breast. For the infant, the ability to "taste" the milk allows for optimal oral stimulation during a time whereby the oral cavity is bypassed via oral-gastric tube feedings.

For small (<1000 gm) infants, the mother completely expresses milk from the breast just prior to the infant being placed in STS care at the breast. The infant should be supported in the football hold or across the chest, so that the infant's entire ventral surface is in direct contact with the lateral aspect of the mother's breast. The infant's temperature can be monitored noninvasively if this is a concern—however the same criteria and outcomes utilized for STS holding should apply during suckling at the emptied breast (Bell & McGrath, 1996). Although the infant should be held in proximity with the breast, no attempt should be made to "position" the infant's mouth and gums over the nipple and areola. Instead, licking and suckling on the nipple tip is all that is expected of very small preterm infants. In one NICU, NNS is begun as soon as small infants are extubated (Meier, 2001). Infants on Neonatal Continuous Positive Airway Pressure (NCPAP) can participate in NNS; positioning across the lap with NCPAP tubings directed upward and over the breast is most effective (Figure 13–4). For larger infants, the mother can combine NNS at the emptied breast with administering her freshly expressed milk by gavage (Figure 13–5).

These early opportunities for the infant to suckle at the emptied breast allows the mother to

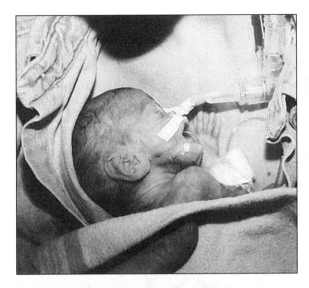

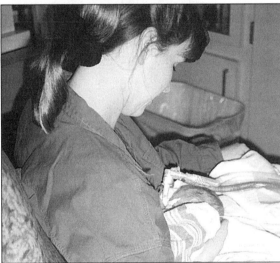

FIGURE 13–4. Infants with NCPAP tubes positioned across mother's lap.

observe the infant's behavior and developing signs for readiness to oral feeding. In this way the mother can provide invaluable input into the plan of care as it relates to advancement of oral feeding. For this reason, a specific postnatal/gestational age or body weight is not used as the criteria for advancing oral feedings (Sidell & Froman, 1994). Observations made by the mother and nursing staff during early STS holding and suckling sessions allows for the

development of an individualized plan of care regarding initiation and progression of oral feeding. As feeding at breast advances in the NICU, two principal topics should be discussed: the science and practice of initiating and advancing direct breastfeedings; and the measurement and facilitation of milk transfer.

The Science of Early Breastfeeding

Studies have demonstrated that preterm infants serving as their own controls had more stable measures of transcutaneous oxygen pressure and body temperature during breastfeeding compared to bottle feeding (Blaymore-Bier, 1997; Meier, 1988; Meier & Anderson, 1987) but less milk was transferred during breastfeeding than measured during bottle feeding (Blaymore-Bier, 1997; Martell et al., 1993; Meier & Brown, 1996). Table 13–6 represents the body of work present in the literature to date regarding breastfeeding behavior in preterm infants. These data suggest that the more stable patterns of oxygenation for breastfeeding than for bottle-feeding are a result of less interruption of breathing during breastfeeding—possibly as a result of a slower rate of milk flow during breastfeeding. To safely project a bolus of milk through the pharynx, an infant must coordinate sucking, swallowing, and breathing. Infant oral-motor skills must not only be adequate for sucking, but sucking must be intricately coordinated with both swallowing and breathing (Gewolb, 2001). Considering the preterm infant's novice skills, the restricted milk flow experienced during breastfeeding may be a more optimal environment for development of oral-motor skills.

To test this theory, Meier and Brown (1996) studied a cohort of clinically stable preterm infants who served as their own controls for serial breastfeeding and bottle-feedings from the time of oral feeding initiation until NICU discharge. The following variables were monitored and recorded continuously on an 8-channel polygraph: sucking event; respiratory event; body temperature; and oxygen saturation during each feeding session. Volume of milk intake was measured by test weighing. Previous research in Meier's lab had validated the instruments that were used for the measure-

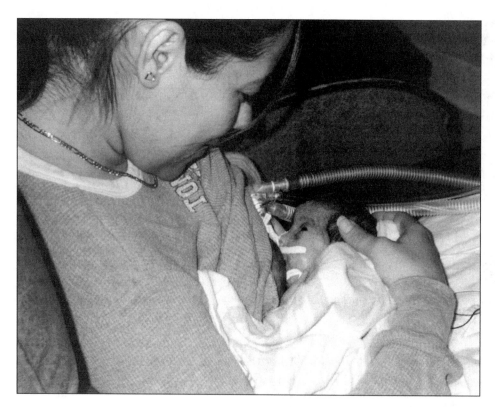

FIGURE 13–5. Suckling at the emptied breast. (With permission, Rush Mother's Milk Club, Rush-Presbyterian St. Luke's Medical Center, Chicago.)

ment of sucking (deMonterice et al., 1992) and milk intake (Kavanaugh, Meier, & Engstrom, 1989; Meier et al., 1990) in this research. Results revealed that during bottle-feedings preterm infants frequently did not breathe during sucking bursts; instead they alternated short bursts of sucking with pauses during which they breathed rapidly. Oxygen saturation measures in response to this suck-breathe patterning varied. For most, but not all, infants who maintained short sucking bursts (e.g., minimal durations of not breathing), oxygen saturation remained relatively stable. For infants who attempted longer sucking bursts, or for those who demonstrated long durations of suspended breathing followed by short sucking bursts, oxygen saturation declined significantly. Examples of these patterns of suck-breathe coordination are depicted in Figure 13–6. During breastfeeding episodes, these same infants integrated breathing within sucking bursts (Figure 13–7). A maturational trend was seen in which less mature infants demonstrated brief episodes of suspended breathing within long

sucking bursts. As the infants approached 34 to 35 weeks of gestation, the suck-breathe patterning approximated a ratio of 1:1.

These findings are consistent with those of previous researchers who described more stable patterns of oxygenation during breastfeedings than during bottle-feedings for preterm infants. However, these findings explain the mechanism for this stability: less interruption in breathing during breastfeeding. Meier concluded that differences in suck-breathe patterning for bottle- and breastfeeding may be due to the infant's ability to control the flow of milk during breastfeeding by subtle alterations in the suck mechanism. These alterations, consisting of the infant's manipulation of intra- and intersuck intervals to accommodate breathing, may not be clinically apparent but were detected during this research. Infants did not demonstrate similar suck-breathe patterning during bottle-feedings until they were several weeks older.

More recently, a large cohort ($n = 71$) of preterm infants was studied prospectively from the

Table 13–6

Studies Related to Physiologic Effects of Breastfeeding in Preterm Infants

Reference	Design/ Sample (*n*)	Measures	Findings	Limitations
Meier, 1988	Crossover; healthy preterm infants (5)	Respiratory rate PaO_2 Heart rate Temperature	Oxygenation patterns were more stable and body temperature increased during breastfeeding compared to bottle-feeding.	Small sample size; milk intake was not measured.
Martell et al., 1993	Crossover; preterm infants Breastfed (16) Bottle-fed (46)	Test weighing at 3-minute intervals for breastfeeding; for bottle-feeding an observer counted number of SU and ingested volume during each suction period	Shorter feeding duration w/ bottle compared to breastfeeding.	Of the 16-mother/infant breastfeeding dyads studied, only 6 were studied at all the time periods—no reason is given for this; one possibility is that the other 10 infants were unable to sustain an adequate attachment to the breast for the initial attempts.
Bier, 1993	Crossover; preterm (20); 9 infants w/ one or more morbidities associated w/prematurity	Respiratory rate PaO_2 Heart rate Temperature Test weights NOMAS scores	No difference in PaO_2 during breastfeeding; lower incidence of O_2 desat (<90%) (21% and 38% in breastfeeding vs. bottle); milk intake during breastfeeding was less than during bottle-feeds; no differences in temp, duration of feeds, and NOMAS scores between bottle and breastfeeding groups.	
Nyqvist, Sjoden, & Ewald, 1999	Observational; healthy preterm infants (71)	Describe the development of feeding behavior; time to full oral feeds	First experience breastfeeding at a median PMA of 33.7 wks; 51% of infants were observed on the 1st day of breastfeeding intro (all but 2 of these infants showed rooting behavior).	Total duration of latching-on and sucking during each session and vigor of sucking behavior were not assessed; focus of study was infant behavior, not milk intake.
Dowling, 1999	Crossover; healthy preterm infants (8)	Sucking parameters Respiratory rate PaO_2 Heart rate Test weight	Sucking bursts longer for bottle than breastfeeding; decreased late in feed when compared with early	Only one type of bottle nipple was tested; did not examine the effect of the use of the orthodontic nipple on

Table 13–6	*(cont.)*			
Reference	**Design/ Sample (n)**	**Measures**	**Findings**	**Limitations**
			in feed for both bottle- and breastfeeding; no difference in sucking rate between bottle- and breastfeeding; 10 breastfeeding and 1 bottle-feeding were not included due to no milk intake.	the time to full breastfeeding or the duration of breastfeeding; small sample size.
Meier, 2000	Crossover, healthy preterm infants (34)	Milk transfer as measured by test weights w/ and w/o nipple shield (NS); duration of NS use; duration of breastfeeding	Mean milk transfer was significantly greater for feedings w/ NS (18.4 vs. 3.9 ml), with all infants consuming more milk w/NS in place; mean duration of NS use 32.5 days; mean duration of breastfeeding 169.4 days; no significant association between the percentage of time the NS was used and total breastfeeding duration.	Maternal nipple characteristics were not reported.
Chen et al., 2000	Crossover, healthy preterm infants (25)	PaO_2 Heart rate Respiratory rate Body temperature	PaO_2 and body temperature were significantly higher during breastfeeding; 2 episodes of apnea and 20 episodes of PaO_2; < 90% during bottle and none during breastfeeding.	Milk intake was not measured.
Nyqvist et al., 2001	Observational; preterm infants (26)	Sucking (SU) and swallowing (SW) behavior as measured by electromyography (EMG)	Agreement between direct observations of SU and EMG data were high; there was considerable variation between infants in the extent of mouthing; no association with maturational level appeared for any of the components in oral behavior.	Milk intake was not measured.

initiation of breastfeeding in the hospital until discharge (Hedberg Nyqvist & Ewald, 1999). In this Swedish hospital setting where early maternal contact was encouraged, infants demonstrated rooting, areolar grasp, and latching-on as early as 28 weeks, nutritive sucking (as defined by ≥ 5 ml intake) from 30.6 weeks, and repeated swallowing at 31 weeks. In a smaller cohort ($n = 26$) Nyqvist et al. (2001) used surface electrodes to record the oral behavior during breastfeeding of preterm infants

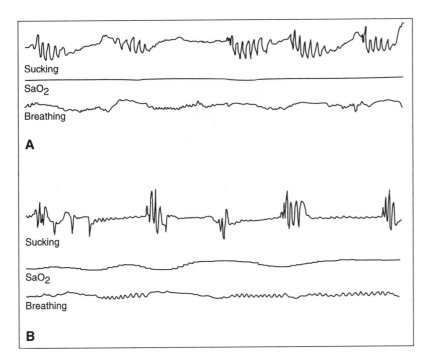

FIGURE 13–6.
(A) Polygraphic recording demonstrating suck/breathe patterning and oxygenation during bottle-feeding for a preterm infant. In this recording, the infant alternates short sucking bursts with breathing but does not breathe within sucking burst. Oxygen saturation remains stable. (B) Polygraphic recording demonstrating suck/breathe patterning and oxygenation during bottle-feeding for a preterm infant. Oxygen saturation fluctuates, with values as low as 78 percent during short sucking bursts.

(mean gestational age 32.5 ± 2.1, range 26.7 to 36). These infants showed a wide variation in sucking behavior, both in duration and intensity. Analyses of possible factors influencing the infants' oral feeding behavior revealed only one significant association—that is, infants with a higher postnatal age had a higher mean duration of sucks ($r = 0.39$, $p < 0.05$).

The results of these studies demonstrate the infant's sucking ability at the breast and physiologic stability during breastfeeding. Thus, waiting to initiate breastfeeding until the infant demonstrates the ability to consume entire bottle-feedings is not a research-based criterion of readiness to breastfeed. For clinical purposes, all infants should be

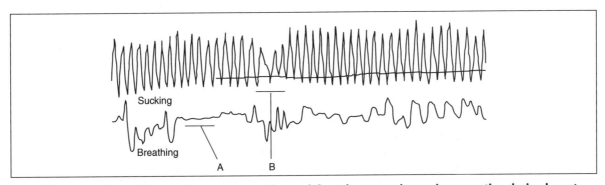

FIGURE 13–7. Polygraphic recording demonstrating suck/breathe patterning and oxygenation during breastfeeding for an infant of 33 weeks' gestational age. The infant breathes within this long (104 sucks) suckling burst until phase A, when breathing is interrupted for several sucks. In phase B, the infant alters the duration and amplitude of individual sucks, apparently to reinstitute a more regular breathing pattern, which continues through the remainder of the burst.

monitored for physiologic stability during early oral feedings regardless of method.

Progression of In-Hospital Breastfeeding

When infants are placed at the breast for daily non-nutritive sucking opportunities, the transition to "nutritive feedings" can be a natural progression appropriate to the infant's individual abilities. When it is determined that the infant should consume some "low-flow" milk, the mother can express some, but not all, of the milk from the breast. In this way, the preterm infant is introduced to small droplets of milk that do not necessitate prolonged closure of the airway for swallowing. As the infant matures, the mother can regulate the milk flow by pumping the amount of milk necessary to reduce the post–milk-ejection flow. When the infant demonstrates the ability to coordinate sucking and breathing, the mother no longer needs to express milk prior to the feeding. This progressive increase in the rate of flow during breastfeeding is consistent with observations from a study in which suction and expression pressures were measured during low-flow bottle-feedings for low birth weight infants (Lau et al., 1997). Data from this study suggested that less mature preterm infants could initiate feedings safely provided that milk flow was restricted.

The preterm infant should be breastfed in a position that affords support to the head and neck, such as the football or the across-the-lap hold. The head of the preterm infant is heavy in relation to the weak musculature of the neck, and undirected head movements can easily collapse the airway, with resultant apnea and bradycardia. Use of these positions will also compensate for the preterm infant's disadvantage in extracting milk from the breast. Specifically, the data from nonnutritive sucking and bottle-feeding studies reveal that suction pressures are maturationally dependent (Hafstrom & Kjellmer, 2000; Lau et al., 2000). With this limitation, the small preterm infant needs to be "placed" and "kept" on the nipple, because the limited suction pressures do not permit the infant to draw the nipple into the intraoral cavity to achieve milk extraction (Figure 13–8).

Mothers of preterm twins use additional strategies for successfully initiating breastfeeding, includ-

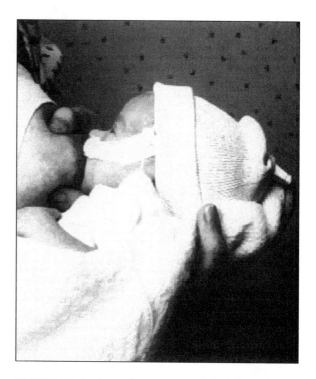

FIGURE 13–8. Providing support of the infant's head and support of the breast during breastfeeding. (With permission, The Lactation Support Program and Mothers' Own Milk Bank, Texas Children's Hospital, Houston.)

ing the following: synchronizing feeding with the twins' behavioral states; twin co-bedding; obtaining adequate information about lactation physiology and milk expression; early introduction of simultaneous breastfeeding; use of appropriate armchairs and breastfeeding pillows; experimenting with breastfeeding positions (particularly the football hold); the spontaneous assistance of nurses; and the father's presence in the NICU (Nyqvist, 2002).

Milk Transfer During Breastfeeding

Factors Influencing Milk Transfer During Breastfeeding. Milk transfer during breastfeeding is dependent upon sufficient maternal milk secretion and ejection concurrent with proficient infant oral-motor skills. Table 13–7 provides an algorithm of the various components essential to achieve milk transfer during breastfeeding and the

Table 13–7

ALGORITHM OF ESSENTIAL COMPONENTS OF MILK TRANSFER DURING BREASTFEEDING

	Essential Components							Outcome
	Maternal Components				Infant Components			
MS*	+	ME	+	MA →	SU	+	SW	=	MT

Clinical States

	MS*	ME	MA	SU	SW		Outcome
1.	+	+	+	+	+	=	Adequate
2.	–	+	+	+	+	=	Insufficient*
3.	+	–	+	+	+	=	Insufficient
4.	+	+	–	+	+	=	Insufficient**
5.	+	+	+	–	+	=	Insufficient†
6.	+	+	+	+	–	=	Insufficient†

Clinical interventions

No intervention required (1)

Interventions to increase MS required (2)

Strategies to elicit ME are required to facilitate milk flow (3)

Interventions to facilitate attachment to the maternal nipple (i.e., nipple shield) (4)

Strategies to improve infant SU response (5)

Strategies to improve infant SW ability (6)

MS: milk synthesis
ME: milk ejection
MA: maternal nipple/areolar attributes
SU: infant expression or suction or combination of both
SW: infant swallow
MT: milk transfer
* May be sufficient for the preterm infant considering lower milk volume needs.
** May be sufficient if infant can achieve sustained attachment despite MA.
†May be sufficient if attachment to breast and MS + ME are adequate.

possible outcomes in the absence of each of these components. In examining this diagram it is apparent that the mother contributes important elements (milk synthesis/ejection and maternal nipple/areolar attributes) and the infant equally vital components (effective suck/swallow). Mothers and their preterm infants may experience problems with any or all of these components. Conversely, because these components are interactive, a problem with one, such as ineffective suckling, can be compensated for by adequacy in the other components. Application of this framework to intake-related questions and problems is essential in determining the appropriate clinical intervention.

For example, most but not all preterm infants have ineffective and/or marginally effective suckling during early breastfeeding experiences. Typically, these infants suckle in short bursts and fall asleep quickly at the breast (Kavanaugh et al., 1995; Nyqvist, Sjoden, & Ewald, 1999; Nyqvist, Ewald, & Sjoden, 1996). However, some infants can still consume an adequate quantity of milk during breastfeeding because the mothers have a copious milk volume that flows readily. Thus milk volume and ejection can compensate for marginally effective suckling. Anecdotally, it is not uncommon for some mothers, whose milk-ejection response has become conditioned to the higher suction pressures experienced with the mechanical breast pump, to have difficulty eliciting milk-ejection during early breastfeeding attempts.

To document the progression of breastfeeding behavior observed for each individual mother/infant dyad, several tools have been used, varying from simple approximation based on the observer's assessment to detailed observations using checklists or coding forms. The Preterm Infant Breastfeeding Behavior Scale (PIBBS) is a tool developed specifically for mothers of preterm infants (Nyqvist, Ewald, & Sjoden, 1996). The PIBBS was developed from observations of preterm behavior in collaboration between observers and mothers. By observing her infant in a more systematic way using the PIBBS, the mother develops greater sensitivity to her infant's behavioral pattern at the breast and is able to develop his capacity for nutritive suckling without restrictions of breastfeeding frequency or duration of breastfeeding sessions, irrespective of maturational level or age (see Appendix 13-A).

The PIBBS measures rooting, areloar grasp, duration of latching on sucking, longest sucking burst, and swallowing. Scores range from 1 to 20. Hedberg Nyqvist and Ewald (1999) tested reliability of the PIBBS by comparing scores among the preterm infants' mothers and the nurses. The study found acceptable levels of agreement between the two nurses (.64–1.00), both in percentage of observed agreement and kappa values (.30–1.00), but agreement between the nurses and the mothers was not as satisfactory. Apparently this method works. The maturational level at the time when infants reach exclusive breastfeeding in this Swedish neonatal unit is today still decreasing, and the number of infants who are discharged exclusively breastfeeding at 33, 32, and even 31 weeks is increasing (Nyqvist, 2003).

A checklist such as the one shown in Figure 13–9 can be used to document specific behaviors and observations made by the nurse/lactation consultant during a breastfeeding session in the NICU. This form summarizes the key components necessary to effectively evaluate the infant and maternal contributions to the dyad in the preterm population. Inclusion of this documentation in the infant's medical record provides pertinent information regarding the preterm infant's progress with breastfeeding that is then conveyed to the entire health-care team. This checklist of key components provides an evaluation of the infant's sucking behavior and activity as well as the mother's milk-ejection response and average pumped milk volume. However, this tool should not be used to place a "score" on the feeding session; it should merely provide information as to relevant aspects of the contributions made by each member of the breastfeeding dyad, allowing for appropriate interventions to be utilized.

Methods to Estimate Milk Transfer. Along with these key components observed during the feeding, it is important to evaluate milk transfer once the preterm infant has been introduced to unrestricted milk flow during breastfeeding. Mothers and health-care professionals are unable to use clinical indices to accurately estimate milk intake for preterm infants (Kavanaugh et al., 1995; Meier et al., 1996). However, clinicians are concerned that more accurate measures of milk intake are either too stressful for mothers or unnecessary for preterm infants (Meier, 1995; Walker, 1995). Similarly, many health-care providers are unaware that accurate measurement of milk intake for preterm infants is possible.

Test weighing procedures, whereby the clothed infant is weighed pre- and postfeed (the difference in weight equals the volume consumed) provides an accurate measure of milk intake for clinical and research settings (Meier et al., 1994, 1996; Scanlon et al., 2002) Using test weights, 1 gm of weight gain approximates 1 ml of milk intake. When performed correctly, test weighing is accepted as the technique of choice in clinical situations whereby milk intake needs to be measured accurately (Scanlon, 2002).

Test weighing should be introduced in the NICU when it appears that milk transfer has occurred and/or discharge is imminent. For smaller preterm infants, the test weight estimate permits individualized complementation of breastfeedings, so that 24-hour fluid and caloric requirements can be

PREMIE Breastfeeding Assessment

Recent Oral Feeding

Number of PO feeding attempts/d during previous 24 hours (circle one): None 1 3–5 8

Type of PO feeding attempt: Breast (#)_____ Bottle (#)_____

If bottle-fed, % of prescribed volume taken_____

If breastfed, was additional milk given via bottle or gavage pc: Yes___ No___

Maternal Nipple Attributes (Prior to Feeding)

(Check appropriate items.)

☐ Prominent

☐ Flat

☐ Inverted

☐ Other, describe:_____

Assessment of Breastfeeding Session:

(Check appropriate items.)

Predominant infant behavior	☐ Quiet/active alert
	☐ Drowsy
	☐ Deep sleep/crying
Rooting	☐ Obvious rooting w/ minimal stimulation
	☐ Some rooting w/ stimulation
	☐ No rooting
Effective latch-on	☐ Maintains effective latch
	☐ Attempts latch, slips off or holds nipple in mouth
	☐ No latch achieved
Milk ejection	☐ Obvious objective or subjective signs
	☐ Possible signs, uncertain or not noticed
	☐ No objective or subjective signs
Infant suck	☐ Rhythmic sucking
	☐ Arrhythmic sucking
	☐ No sucking
Evident swallowing	☐ Smooth swallowing
	☐ Strained swallowing
	☐ No swallowing

Nipple shield used? If so, which size: ☐ Small ☐ Newborn

Maternal Milk Volume

Average pumped volume nearest to the time of the current feeding session_____(ml)

Milk Transfer

Infant weight prior to feeding_____(gm) Following feeding_____(gm)

Total milk transfer during feeding (postfeed weight – prefeed weight)_____(gm)

FIGURE 13–9. An assessment document for preterm infants. (With permission, The Lactation Support Program, Texas Children's Hospital.)

met. For larger infants awaiting NICU discharge, test weights can be used to diagnose milk-transfer problems. For example, the infant may suckle marginally, but the mother's milk volume is adequate. It is impossible to know whether the mother's milk flow can compensate for the infant's suck unless volume of intake is measured.

Strategies to Facilitate Milk Transfer. Seldom does significant milk transfer occur during the first few breastfeeding sessions for preterm infants. However, as NICU discharge approaches, consistently small volumes of intake become a concern that must be evaluated. Selected problems of milk transfer are particularly common among preterm infants.

The single most important factor for mothers who will be breastfeeding a preterm infant at home is maintaining a milk supply that exceeds the baby's requirements at hospital discharge (Hill, Ledbetter, & Kavanaugh, 1997; Lawrence, 2001; Meier, 2001). With an adequate milk supply, the infant's immature suckling may be less problematic. Mothers can plan for this by expressing their milk an extra time or two in the week before their baby's discharge. For mothers who have a borderline milk supply as NICU discharge approaches, the clinician should consider a regimen of metoclopramide (Emery, 1996) or domperidone (da Silva et al., 2001) to augment the milk yield. Theoretically, the prolactin stimulus from the medication will be maintained by the infant's direct breastfeeding in the home.

Mothers should be reminded to express milk with the electric breast pump after each breastfeeding in the hospital. NICU staff and mothers seldom appreciate that a preterm infant cannot substitute for the breast stimulation provided by the electric breast pump, especially if the infant consumes only small milk volumes. Mothers frequently question how to coordinate milk expression with demand feedings because they are concerned their breasts will be empty when their infants awake to feed. An appropriate strategy in this situation is to emphasize the priority of maintaining the milk yield. Unlike a term infant, the preterm infant's suck is unlikely to extract milk that remains after breast pump usage.

Many mothers of preterm infants deny feeling the sensations of milk-ejection both when using the electric pump and when feeding their infants at breast. Thus it is often difficult to evaluate the synchronization of milk-ejection and infant suckling. One strategy that may be useful in evaluating the milk-ejection response is to instruct the mother to uncover the opposite breast during a breastfeeding session in order to observe the spontaneous dripping of milk during milk-ejection. Typically, mothers experience a delay in milk-ejection when infants are placed at the breast because the women are conditioned to the sensations of the breast pump. It is not uncommon for milk flow to begin just as the preterm infant falls asleep at the breast. If this situation persists for more than a few feedings, the mother can use the electric breast pump to initiate the milk flow. This can be done by placing the infant at one breast and the pump at the other, or by first initiating the milk flow with the breast pump and then placing the infant at breast.

Sustaining Attachment to the Maternal Breast. The sucking pattern of the healthy term infant is characterized by the rhythmic alternation of two types of pressure, negative (suction) and positive (compression) pressure (Dubignon & Campbell, 1969; Sameroff, 1968). Suction defines the negative intraoral pressure generated as the infant draws milk into the mouth whereas compression denotes the positive pressure resulting from the compression and/or stripping of the nipple between the tongue and the hard palate as milk is ejected into the mouth (Ardran, Kemp, & Lind, 1958; Nowak, Smith, & Erenberg, 1994, 1995; Waterland et al., 1998). The majority of milk transfer problems for preterm infants can be related to immaturity and inconsistency in suckling (Kavanaugh et al., 1995; Meier & Brown, 1996). The relatively low suction pressures and the infants' inconsistent, irregular sucking bursts do not sustain the milk flow needed for effective milk transfer or in many cases allow for sustained attachment to the maternal breast. These phenomena appear to be maturationally dependent. Until the infant achieves term, corrected age, strategies to increase the effectiveness of sucking to achieve sustained attachment to the breast are often necessary.

Weak sucking pressures (- 2.5 to - 15 mm Hg) measured in preterm infants may result in difficulties maintaining attachment to the maternal breast (Lau et al., 1997). Bottle-feeding studies (Lau et al.,

2000; Lau et al., 1997) have concluded that sucking ability does not need to be at a mature level before preterm infants are introduced to oral feeding. These preterm infants were able to transfer milk during bottle-feeding via compression only—using little or no suction pressure. Therefore the provision of a rigid nipple may allow the infant the ability to transfer milk without the need to generate suction pressure, utilizing instead the compression component of infant feeding.

It is this theoretical basis that may explain reports of improved milk transfer during breastfeeding in preterm infants using a thin, silicone nipple shield placed over the mother's nipple to facilitate sustained attachment (Clum & Primomo, 1996; Meier et al., 2000). A study of 34 preterm infants (Meier et al., 2000) revealed a significantly greater increase in milk transfer with the shield than for the previous breastfeeding without the shield (18.4 ml vs. 3.9 ml, $p = 0.0001$). In a retrospective study of 15 preterm infants, the nipple shield was introduced following at least five failed attempts to achieve breast attachment or milk transfer without the nipple shield (Clum & Primomo, 1996). Nine of the 15 infants consumed at least half or greater of the prescribed feeding amount with the nipple shield. Clinical indications for nipple shield use among this group included the inability of the infant to sustain attachment to the breast, holding the nipple in the mouth while falling asleep, and maternal nipple characteristics.

The results of these studies (Clum & Primomo, 1996; Meier et al., 2000) raise further questions as to the underlying etiology of the nipple shield's effect on infant and maternal breastfeeding responses. One possible explanation could be the nipple shield provides a uniform rigid structure that extends deeper into the infant's oral cavity, thus allowing greater tactile stimulation (Figure 13–10). As a result of this stimulation the infant responds by compression and or compression/suction and sustained breast attachment. Consequently, sustained attachment and compression of the shield results in stimulation of the underlying nipple/areolar tissue providing a stimulus for activation of the maternal milk-ejection reflex and improved milk flow and transfer. However these responses are only speculative since maternal nipple/areolar attributes and/or infant suction pressures were not measured in these

studies. Although an ideal nipple shield for preterm infants has yet to be designed, the smallest, thinnest shield available is indicated for these babies.

The nipple shield is extremely well-accepted by mothers because it often represents the first breastfeeding experience in which the infant remains awake, sucks eagerly, and consumes measurable volumes of milk. However, mothers are concerned about providing the gentle pressure necessary to keep the infants correctly positioned over the areola, because of the plastic nature of shield. Thus mothers need to be shown how to support the breast with the shield in place so that the infant can achieve an effective sucking position while keeping the shield away from the nares.

Clinicians often assume that preterm infants do not take as much milk with the shield in place as they would without its use. This concern seems to be based on the data collected by Auerbach (1990), which demonstrated reduced milk transfer when mothers of term infants expressed milk with a breast pump with a nipple shield in place. Although this study addressed an important concept, the findings cannot be applied indiscriminately to infants since milk transfer was measured for milk expression—not infant feeding. Preterm infants who are unable to transfer milk during breastfeeding prior to nipple shield use actually increase milk intake

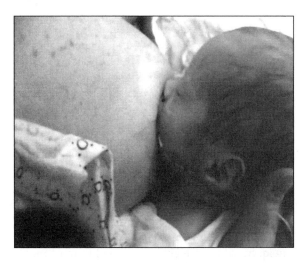

FIGURE 13–10. Preterm infant at breast with nipple shield in place. (With permission, The Lactation Support Program, Texas Children's Hospital.)

when the shield is in place. Similarly, concern that use of the shield will reduce the milk yield over time is not applicable in this situation. Preterm infants who feed longer and more eagerly with the shield in place provide considerably more breast stimulation than breastfeeding without the shield.

In addition, clinicians suggest that other feeding techniques, such as cup- or finger-feedings be used as an alternative to the nipple shield. This approach appears to reflect an unscientific bias against the nipple shield and is especially problematic because use of the shield means that the infant can feed at the breast. Mothers of preterm infants who have spent weeks or months expressing milk prefer to feed their babies at the breast, even if it entails temporary nipple shield use. The use of a shield also saves time for mothers, because they do not need to offer a complement after breastfeeding, as is the case with a cup- or finger-feeding.

Finally, the duration of nipple shield use is a common concern, in that clinicians frequently ask how to "wean" babies from the shield. Recent data indicate that for a sample of preterm, low birthweight infants who received the same research-based breastfeeding services, duration of breastfeeding was twice as long for the group of infants who were breastfed with the shield (Meier et al., 2000). Thus common concerns that use of the nipple shield decreases the milk supply and shortens the duration of breastfeeding are not supported by the available research for preterm infants.

If the nipple shield is effective in correcting milk transfer problems in the hospital, its use should be continued after NICU discharge. Additionally, there is no scientific reason for recommending that infants be "weaned" from the shield as soon as possible. Typically, the infant will require the shield for adequate milk transfer until approximately term, corrected age. For most mothers, this coincides with 2 to 3 weeks of nipple shield use, over which time the infant's intake and weight gain can be monitored regularly. Mothers have described their individual approaches to discontinuing the shield, but in no case should they be advised to "cut back" or tamper with the integrity of the shield. Serial test weights are helpful to most mothers as they transfer from the shield to feeding at the breast without the shield.

In addition to the nipple shield, other breastfeeding devices are frequently recommended to measure and facilitate milk transfer. A supplemental nurser can be helpful for the mother who has a limited milk supply and the infant is able to achieve sustained attachment and sucking mechanism at the breast. This device is especially helpful for borderline preterm infants (i.e., > 34 weeks gestation) who are still premature with respect to the ability to extract adequate volumes of milk. Providing they are able to sustain attachment, these infants can receive the extra milk they need with a supplemental nurser while feeding at the breast.

Discharge Planning for Postdischarge Breastfeeding

Unlike healthy term infants, preterm infants do not demonstrate predictable demand-feeding behaviors until close to term, corrected age (Kavanaugh et al., 1995; Nyqvist, Sjoden, & Ewald, 1999). Thus infants may consume minimal volumes at a breastfeeding and still sleep for several hours, if undisturbed. The use of test weights permits the emergence of demand-feeding behaviors, while retaining a safeguard against slow weight gain and/or dehydration in the days before NICU discharge.

When the infant has demonstrated the ability to consume all feedings orally, the neonatologist or neonatal nurse practitioner can prescribe a 24-hour minimal milk intake for the infant. The 24-hour volume can then be subdivided into 6- or 8-hour volumes to permit a modified demand-feeding schedule. For example, if an infant weighing 1700 gm needs a minimum of 300 ml per day, the mother and nurse can plan to feed 100 ml every 8 hours. The infant is then allowed to "demand," but must receive the prescribed 100 ml volume within an 8-hour period. Test weights are measured with each breastfeeding and the volume of complements and/or supplements is recorded. Thus, if the infant consumes 15 ml, 12 ml, and 18 ml within a period of 2 hours, the infant has been given the opportunity to self-regulate sleep and feeding. However, the infant still must consume the remaining 55 ml over the next 6 hours. NICU nurses can help mothers implement this plan in the days before infant discharge, so that mothers develop an understanding of how the infant coordinates sleep and feeding.

Many mothers of preterm infants, both borderline babies and those who are smaller, find it reassuring to measure milk intake and/or serial weight gain in the first days after infant discharge. A portable, battery-operated scale that mothers can rent and perform test weights and/or daily weights in the home is ideal for this purpose. The scale, which weighs to the nearest 2 gm and automatically calculates milk intake from the prefeed and postfeed weights, has been demonstrated to measure milk intake accurately for term and preterm infants (Meier et al., 1994). This scale can be a useful adjunct to breastfeeding management for mothers and preterm infants during the first week or two after discharge. However, mothers should be introduced to the proper use of the scale during the days prior to NICU discharge.

In the United States, preterm infants are typically discharged from the NICU before their expected birth dates, whether or not breastfeeding has been well-established. In contrast, preterm infants in most European countries are discharged only when weight gain on exclusive breastfeeding has been documented, which may be several weeks later than discharge dates in the United States (Nyqvist, Sjoden, & Ewald, 1999). In developing countries, preterm infants are frequently discharged at lower weights, but many of these infants are small-for-gestational age, (Ramasethu, Jeyaseelan, & Kirubakaran, 1993), and/or maintained in skin-to-skin care in the home (Bergman & Jurisoo, 1994; Cattaneo et al., 1998; Charpak, Ruiz-Pelaez, & Charpak, 1994; Whitelaw & Liestol, 1994).

When these data are considered in combination, it appears that preterm infants remain at risk for underconsumption of milk by exclusive at-breast feeding until approximately term corrected age (Meier & Brown, 1996). This is suggested by the low incidence of exclusive at-breast feeding in the early weeks after NICU discharge in the United States (Furman et al., 1998; Hill, Ledbetter, & Kavanaugh, 1997); the longer hospitalization in European countries so that exclusive at-breast feeding is established (Nyqvist, Sjoden, & Ewald, 1999); and the slow weight gain on exclusive breastfeedings in the first 2 to 4 weeks after hospital discharge in developing

countries. This commonality probably reflects a problem with the maturationally-dependent "infant suckling" component of milk transfer, often expressed by mothers as "getting enough."

Getting Enough: Determining Need for Extra Milk Feedings

Studies from the United States have examined the phenomenon of "getting enough" for mothers and preterm infants (Hill, Ledbetter, & Kavanaugh, 1997; Kavanaugh et al., 1995). However, clinicians who work primarily with healthy term infants do not always comprehend the difference between "getting enough" and "insufficient milk supply." As a result, mothers of preterm infants are frequently told to breastfeed their babies and/or pump more frequently, interventions that are focused upon the milk volume component of milk transfer. These recommendations are inappropriate for most mothers of preterm infants who describe problems with "getting enough." These women report that they can express adequate volumes of milk with the breast pump, but perceive that their infants do not take all of the milk available to them. Thus, effective interventions must focus on the infant suckling component of milk transfer. This distinction has important research and practice implications.

The most fundamental research issue is that accepted nomenclature for describing and classifying amount of breastfeeding does not fit the breastfeeding patterns for this population (Meier & Brown, 1997). For example, most mothers of preterm infants complement at-breast feedings with their own expressed milk during the early weeks at home, but the Labbok and Krasovec (1990) schema does not accurately capture this pattern. If this pattern is categorized as "exclusive breastfeeding," it overestimates mothers' successes and misrepresents data on duration of breastfeeding. Thus research-based criteria to categorize the amount of breastfeeding for these mothers must be developed and standardized.

Research addressing the early postdischarge period must also include methods that accurately and reliably distinguish between insufficient maternal milk supply and the infant's ability to consume adequate milk volumes (Hill, Ledbetter, & Kavanaugh, 1997; Meier & Brown, 1997). These studies must incorporate available technology to measure milk volume and infant intake during breastfeeding, rather than relying on checklists or clinical indices that have been demonstrated to be inaccurate and/or unreliable. Similarly, other studies in which milk intake during breastfeeding was not measured have related slow weight gain and/or the need for continued milk fortification postdischarge to deficiencies in the mothers' milk (Chan, Borschel, & Jacobs, 1994; Hall, Wheeler, & Rippetoe, 1993; Wauben et al., 1998). Thus, future postdischarge studies for preterm infants must include accurate instrumentation to differentiate among milk supply, milk "quality," and infant intake.

Methods to Deliver Extra Milk Feedings Away from the Breast

Alternative feeding devices are frequently recommended by clinicians to avoid "nipple confusion" (Lang, Lawrence, & Orme, 1994; Newman, 1990; Stine, 1990). Although the phenomenon of "nipple confusion" has received little systematic study, it is likely that selected risk factors make it difficult for some infants to alternate breast- and bottle-feedings (Cronenwett et al., 1992; Neifert, Lawrence, & Seacat, 1995). Reports from clinicians suggest that these alternative feeding methods are safe when performed by experts (Lang, Lawrence, & Orme, 1994), but few controlled clinical trials have established either safety or effect on breastfeeding outcome for these devices (Dowling et al., 2002; Rocha, Martinez, & Jorge, 2002). An interesting finding revealed in a recent study showed the oral mechanisms used by preterm infants during cup-feeding as "sipping" rather than "lapping" in the majority of the 15 cup-feeding sessions for 8 preterm (mean gestational age at birth 30.6 wks) infants (Dowling et al., 2002). Additionally, a significant amount (38.5 percent) of milk taken from the cup was drooled by the infants onto the feeding bib, suggesting that a significant volume of milk is spilled during cup-feedings.

Postdischarge Breastfeeding Management

Preterm infants are vulnerable to underconsumption of milk during the first weeks after discharge. Clinicians who are accustomed to helping mothers of healthy term infants must acknowledge this phenomenon. Several key principles must be understood and incorporated into postdischarge breastfeeding plans for preterm infants:

- The practitioner must recognize that the clinical indices of intake used for healthy term infants—for example, breastfeeding behaviors, wet diapers, frequency of stools, and sleep patterns—are not accurate or reliable for preterm infants. For example, a preterm infant may remain "hydrated," but still not consume enough milk to grow.

- Preterm infants may not consistently "demand," so mothers should not be given instructions such as "You'll know when your baby is hungry."

- Preterm infants should not be awakened more frequently than every 3 hours to breastfeed because sleep interruption interferes with growth hormone release, retarding weight gain.

- Mothers of preterm infants are not reassured with nonspecific comments such as "Trust your body." It is important to accept that mothers' concerns about intake are real, not just a reflection of their NICU experience.

In summary, mothers of preterm infants need a "safety net" during the first weeks at home, until their infants have demonstrated the ability to gain weight on exclusive breastfeedings. Milk transfer must be monitored regularly—every 48 to 72 hours—and accurately at this time, either through frequent visits to the primary care provider for serial growth measures or by in-home test weighing.

Care must be taken to listen to these women and their feelings of vulnerability with respect to infant intake. They must not be hurried through these processes or told that they are not breastfeeding "correctly." For example, if a mother feels that she needs to give bottle supplements of her expressed milk in the first few days, she should not be warned about "nipple confusion," or told that alternative feedings should be used. Instead, her ability to determine and advocate what she feels is best for her infant must be interpreted as a sign of strength. It is important to remember that breastfeeding is only one activity that these women must deal with; their babies are vulnerable to many conditions, and mothers need time to sort out care priorities.

Similarly, mothers should be encouraged to continue the breastfeeding strategies that worked in the hospital until their infants have demonstrated an acceptable pattern of growth for at least a week or two. For many women, these devices will include a nipple shield and/or in-home weighing, and there are no data to support withdrawing these aids before the mother is ready. Finally, the mother needs access to both consumer support groups and a professional who is experienced with breastfeeding for preterm infants when discharge approaches.

Summary

Breastfeeding for preterm infants and mothers is different from breastfeeding for healthy populations in many important ways. The vast body of research in this area suggests that these differences are physiologic, biologic, metabolic, and emotional, and that they are common across a variety of national boundaries and cultures. The challenge to researchers and clinicians who work with mothers and preterm infants is to continue to generate new studies and practices that incorporate findings from these scientific publications. Only research-based practices can address the many barriers to breastfeeding initiation and duration for this at-risk population.

Key Concepts

- Studies indicate that preterm infants are not just "small term infants" with respect to breastfeeding management, which means that research-based strategies that target specific barriers for this vulnerable population should be used.

- Human milk may provide optimal "nutritional programming" for preterm infants and may be protective against several prematurity-related conditions.

- Based on current research related to the superiority of human milk for preterm infants, parents should be provided accurate information in order to make an informed choice in providing a mother's own milk for a preterm infant.

- Mothers providing breastmilk for their preterm infants should be praised for their efforts regardless of the length of time of their commitment.

- Although giving birth prematurely does not appear to limit milk production, several factors surrounding the birth experience are documented prolactin-inhibitors and can adversely affect milk volume.

- The mother's milk expression technique can influence the composition and the bacterial count of the milk to be fed to her infant.

- Documenting the time, duration, and amount of milk expressed provides useful information to the mother that can be shared with the NICU staff for assessment of milk volume maintenance.

- It has been speculated that skin-to-skin holding may trigger the production of maternal milk antibodies to specific pathogens in the preterm infants' environment through mechanisms in the enteromammary pathway.

- Proper NICU procedures should be developed and adhered to in order to minimize bacterial growth and possible changes in milk constituents during storage and feeding.

- Special consideration regarding the feeding of expressed mothers' milk to preterm infants is based on the infant's fluid restrictive status at a time of greatest nutritional need.

- Unfortified expressed mothers' milk is deficient in protein and selected minerals to support optimal growth and bone mineralization for small preterm infants.

- Lactoengineering of expressed mother's milk through a combination of hindmilk and creamatocrit measures can impact the caloric density of the milk provided to preterm infants, as well as empowering their mothers.

- Early oral feeding experiences may influence later oral feeding development in preterm infants.

- There are no universally established criteria for the initiation of breastfeeding (or bottle-feeding for that matter) for preterm infants.

- NICUs in which infants are allowed nonnutritive suckling at the emptied breast provide mothers with valuable observation of their infants' behavior and developing signs for readiness to oral feeding.

- Delaying to initiate breastfeeding until the infant demonstrates the ability to consume entire bottle-feedings is not a research-based criterion of readiness to breastfeed.

- Milk transfer during breastfeeding is dependent upon sufficient maternal milk secretion and ejection concurrent with proficient infant oral-motor skills.

- Test weighing procedures provide the most accurate measure of milk intake for clinical and research settings.

- The single most important factor for mothers who will be breastfeeding a preterm infant at home is maintaining a milk supply that exceeds the infant's requirements at hospital discharge.

- The majority of milk transfer problems for preterm infants can be related to immaturity and inconsistency in suckling.

- For preterm infants who are unable to sustain attachment to the maternal breast and/or transfer milk, the nipple shield has proven an effective strategy as a milk transfer device.

- It appears that preterm infants remain at risk for underconsumption of milk by exclusive at-breast feeding until term corrected age.

- Mothers' concerns regarding their preterm infants ability to "get enough" milk during breastfeeding are real and should not be dismissed.

Internet Resources

American Association for Premature Infants (AAPI), founded in 1992, an organization dedicated to improving the quality of health, developmental and educational services for premature infants, children, and their families:
www.aapi-online.org

Congenital Heart Information Network (CHIN), an international organization that provides reliable information, support services, and resources to families of children with congenital heart defects and acquired heart disease:
www.tchin.org

iVillage Web site, a unique discussion board designated for mothers who are exclusively pumping their breastmilk for their infants:
http://boards2.parentsplace.com/messages/get/pp exclusivelypumping88.html
or go to the main website and put in the search term, "exclusively pumping":
www.ivillage.com

La Leche League International, parent and professional materials on breastfeeding a preterm infant:
www.lalecheleague.org

National Organization of Mothers of Twins Clubs, Inc. (NOMOTC), founded in 1960, a group providing support, education, and information for mothers of twins:
www.nomotc.org

Parents of Premature Babies, Inc. (Preemie-L), a Web site offering support to families of premature infants while the babies are hospitalized and following discharge:
www.preemie-l.org

Preemie Place, an online resource providing answers to questions, or information for a specific topic regarding prematurity:
www.thepreemieplace.org

Premature Baby Premature Child, a volunteer Web site providing parents with information to care for premature infants:
www.prematurity.org

Texas Children's Hospital newsletter for parents of preterms and professionals:
www.texaschildrenshospital.org/lactationstation

References

Adams C et al. Breastfeeding trends at a community breastfeeding center: an evaluative survey. *J Obstet Gynecol Neonatal Nurs* 30:392–400, 2001.

Aguayo J. Maternal lactation for preterm newborn infants. *Early Hum Dev,Suppl* 65:19–29, 2001.

Akisu M et al. Platelet-activating factor levels in term and preterm human milk. *Biol Neonate* 74:289–93, 1998.

American Academy of Pediatrics (AAP). Breastfeeding and the use of human milk. Work Group on Breastfeeding. *Pediatrics* 100:1035–39, 1997.

———. Transfer of drugs and other chemicals into human milk. *Pediatrics* 108:776–78, 2001.

Amin SB et al. Brainstem maturation in premature infants as a function of enteral feeding type. *Pediatrics* 106:318–22, 2000.

Ardran GM, Kemp F, Lind J. A cineradiographic study of breastfeeding. *Br J Radiol* 31:156–62, 1958.

Armand M et al. Effect of human milk or formula on gastric function and fat digestion in the premature infant. *Pediatr Res* 40:429–37, 1996.

Auerbach KG. The effect of nipple shields on maternal milk volume. *J Obstet Gynecol Neonatal Nurs* 19:419–27, 1990.

Auerbach KG, Walker M. When the mother of a premature infant uses a breast pump: what every NICU nurse needs to know. *Neonatal Netw* 13:23–29, 1994.

Baker BJ, Rasmussen TW. Organizing and documenting lactation support of NICU families. *J Obstet Gynecol Neonatal Nurs* 26:515–21, 1997.

Bauer K et al. Body temperatures and oxygen consumption during skin-to-skin (kangaroo) care in stable preterm infants weighing less than 1500 grams. *J Pediatr* 130:240–44, 1997.

Bell RP, McGrath JM. Implementing a research-based kangaroo care program in the NICU. *Nurs Clin North Am* 31:387–403, 1996.

Bergman NJ, Jurisoo LA. The 'kangaroo-method' for treating low birth weight babies in a developing country. *Trop Doc* 24:57–60, 1994.

Bernt KM, Walker WA. Human milk as a carrier of biochemical messages. *Acta Paediatr Suppl* 88:27–41, 1999.

Biancuzzo M. Selecting pumps for breastfeeding mothers. *J Obstet Gynecol Neonatal Nurs* 28:417–26, 1999.

Bier JA et al. Comparison of skin-to-skin contact with standard contact in low-birth-weight infants who are breastfed. *Arch Pediatr Adolesc Med* 150:1265–69, 1996.

———. Human milk improves cognitive and motor development of premature infants during infancy. *J Hum Lact* 18:361–67, 2002.

Bier JB. Breast-feeding of very low birth weight infants. *J Pediatr* 123:773–78, 1993.

Birch EE et al. Dietary essential fatty acid supply and visual acuity development. *Invest Ophthalmol Vis Sci* 33:3242–53, 1992.

Blaymore-Bier JA. Breastfeeding infants who were extremely low birth weight. *Pediatrics* 100:E3, 1997.

Boehm G et al. Fecal cholesterol excretion in preterm infants fed breastmilk or formula with different cholesterol contents. *Acta Paediatr* 84:240–44, 1995.

Bohnhorst B et al. Skin-to-skin (kangaroo) care, respiratory control, and thermoregulation. *J Pediatr* 138:193–97, 2001.

Brandt KA, Andrews CM, Kvale J. Mother-infant interaction and breastfeeding outcome 6 weeks after birth. *J Obstet Gynecol Neonatal Nurs* 27:169–74, 1998.

Brennan-Behm M et al. Caloric loss from expressed mother's milk during continuous gavage infusion. *Neonatal Netw* 13:27–32, 1994.

Britton JR. Milk protein quality in mothers delivering prematurely: implications for infants in the intensive care unit nursery setting. *J Pediatr Gastroenterol Nutr* 5:116–21, 1986.

Budd SC et al. Improved lactation with metoclopramide: a case report. *Clin Pediatr (Phila)* 32:53–57, 1993.

Burrin DG, Stoll B. Key nutrients and growth factors for the neonatal gastrointestinal tract. *Clin Perinatol* 29:65–96, 2002.

Butte NF et al. Longitudinal changes in milk composition of mothers delivering preterm and term infants. *Early Hum Dev* 9:153–62, 1984.

Canadian Paediatric Society (CPS). Nutrient needs and feeding of premature infants. Nutrition Committee, Canadian Paediatric Society. *Cmaj* 152:1765–85, 1995.

Carter CS, Altemus M. Integrative functions of lactational hormones in social behavior and stress management. *Ann N Y Acad Sci* 807:164–74, 1997.

Cattaneo A et al. Kangaroo mother care for low birthweight infants: a randomized controlled trial in different settings. *Acta Paediatr* 87:976–85, 1998.

Chan GM, Borschel MW, Jacobs JR. Effects of human milk or formula feeding on the growth, behavior, and protein status of preterm infants discharged from the newborn intensive care unit. *Am J Clin Nutr* 60:710–16, 1994.

Charpak N et al. Kangaroo Mother Program: an alternative way of caring for low birth weight infants? One year mortality in a two cohort study. *Pediatrics* 94:804–10, 1994.

———. A randomized, controlled trial of kangaroo mother care: results of follow-up at 1 year of corrected age. *Pediatrics* 108:1072–79, 2001.

Chatterton RT et al. Relation of plasma oxytocin and prolactin concentrations to milk production in mothers of preterm infants: influence of stress. *J Clin Endocrinol Metab* 85:3661–68, 2000.

Chen CH et al. The effect of breast- and bottle-feeding on oxygen saturation and body temperature in preterm infants. *J Hum Lact* 16:21–27, 2000.

Clum D, Primomo J. Use of a silicone nipple shield with premature infants. *J Hum Lact* 12:287–90, 1996.

Contreras-Lemus J. Morbidity reduction in preterm newborns fed with milk of their own mothers. *Bol Med Hosp Infant Mex* 49:671–77, 1992.

Cox DB et al. Breast growth and the urinary excretion of lactose during human pregnancy and early lactation: endocrine relationships. *Exp Physiol* 84:421–34, 1999.

Cregan MD et al. Initiation of lactation in women after preterm delivery. *Acta Obstet Gynecol Scand* 81:870–77, 2002.

Cronenwett L et al. Single daily bottle use in the early weeks postpartum and breastfeeding outcomes. *Pediatrics* 90: 760–66, 1992.

Daly SE, Hartmann PE. Infant demand and milk supply: Part 1. Infant demand and milk production in lactating women. *J Hum Lact* 11:21–26, 1995a.

———. Infant demand and milk supply: Part 2. The short-term control of milk synthesis in lactating women. *J Hum Lact* 11:27–37, 1995b.

Daly SE et al. Degree of breast emptying explains changes in the fat content, but not fatty acid composition, of human milk. *Exp Physiol* 78:741–55, 1993.

———. Frequency and degree of milk removal and the short-term control of human milk synthesis. *Exp Physiol* 81:861–75, 1996.

da Silva OP et al. Effect of domperidone on milk production in mothers of premature newborns: a randomized, double-blind, placebo-controlled trial. *Cmaj* 164:17–21, 2001.

deMonterice D et al. Concurrent validity of a new instrument for measuring nutritive sucking in preterm infants. *Nurs Res* 41:342–46, 1992.

Diaz-Gomez NM, Domenech E, Barroso F. Breast-feeding and growth factors in preterm newborn infants. *J Pediatr Gastroenterol Nutr* 24:322–27, 1997.

Dowling DA. Physiological responses of preterm infants to breast-feeding and bottle-feeding with the orthodontic nipple. *Nurs Res* 48:78–85, 1999.

Dowling DA et al. Cup-feeding for preterm infants: mechanics and safety. *J Hum Lact* 18:13–20, 2002.

Dubignon J, Campbell D. Sucking in the newborn during a feed. *J Exp Child Psychol* 7:282–98, 1969.

Dvorak B et al. Maternal milk reduces severity of necrotizing enterocolitis and increases intestinal il-10 in a neonatal rat model. *Pediatr Res* 53:426–33, 2003.

Eibl MM et al. Prevention of necrotizing enterocolitis in low-birth-weight infants by IgA-IgG feeding. *N Engl J Med* 319:1–7, 1988.

el-Mohandes AE et al. Bacterial contaminants of collected and frozen human milk used in an intensive care nursery. *Am J Infect Control* 21:226–30, 1993.

Emery MM. Galactogogues: drugs to induce lactation. *J Hum Lact* 12:55–57, 1996.

Ewer AK, Yu VY. Gastric emptying in pre-term infants: the effect of breastmilk fortifier. *Acta Paediatr* 85:1112–15, 1996.

Ewer AK et al. Gastric emptying in preterm infants. *Arch Dis Child Fetal Neonatal Ed* 71:F24–27, 1994.

Farquharson J. Effect of diet on the fatty acid composition of the major phospholipids of infant cerebral cortex. *Arch Dis Child* 72:198–203, 1995.

Feher SD et al. Increasing breastmilk production for premature infants with a relaxation/imagery audiotape. *Pediatrics* 83:57–60, 1989.

Feldman R et al. Comparison of skin-to-skin (kangaroo) and traditional care: parenting outcomes and preterm infant development. *Pediatrics* 110:16–26, 2002.

Fewtrell M et al. Randomized study comparing the efficacy of a novel manual breast pump with a mini-electric breast pump in mothers of term infants. *J Hum Lact* 17:126–31, 2001.

Fituch CC et al. Interleukin-10 concentration in milk of mothers delivering extremely low birth weight infants. *Pediatr Res* 49:398A, 2001.

Furman L, Minich NM, Hack M. Breastfeeding of very low birth weight infants. *J Hum Lact* 14:29–34, 1998.

Furman L et al. The effect of maternal milk on neonatal morbidity of very low-birth-weight infants. *Arch Pediatr Adolesc Med* 157:66–71, 2003.

Gale G, Franck L, Lund C. Skin-to-skin (kangaroo) holding of the intubated premature infant. *Neonatal Netw* 12: 49–57, 1993.

Garofalo RP, Goldman AS. Cytokines, chemokines, and colony-stimulating factors in human milk: the 1997 update. *Biol Neonate* 74:134–42, 1998.

Gazzolo D, Masetti P, Meli M. Kangaroo care improves post-extubation cardiorespiratory parameters in infants after open heart surgery. *Acta Paediatr* 89:728–29, 2000.

Genzel-Boroviczeny O, Wahle J, Koletzko B. Fatty acid composition of human milk during the 1st month after term and preterm delivery. *Eur J Pediatr* 156:142–47, 1997.

Gewolb IH. Developmental patterns of rhythmic suck and swallow in preterm infants. *Dev Med Child Neurol* 43:22–27, 2001.

Goldblum RM et al. Human milk banking I: Effects of container upon immunologic factors in mature milk. *Nutrition Research* 1:449–59, 1981.

———. Human milk feeding enhances the urinary excretion of immunologic factors in low birth weight infants. *Pediatr Res* 25:184–88, 1989.

Goldman AS et al. Molecular forms of lactoferrin in stool and urine from infants fed human milk. *Pediatr Res* 27:252–55, 1990.

Gonzales I et al. Effect of enteral feeding temperature on feeding tolerance in preterm infants. *Neonatal Netw* 14:39–43, 1995.

Greer FR, McCormick A, Loker J. Changes in fat concentration of human milk during delivery by intermittent bolus and continuous mechanical pump infusion. *J Pediatr* 105:745–49, 1984.

Griffin TL et al. Mothers' performing creamatocrit measures in the NICU: accuracy, reactions, and cost. *J Obstet Gynecol Neonatal Nurs* 29:249–57, 2000.

Groh-Wargo S et al. The utility of a bilateral breast pumping system for mothers of premature infants. *Neonatal Netw* 14:31–36, 1995.

Gross SK et al. Nutritional composition of milk produced by mothers delivering preterm. *J Pediatr* 96:641–44, 1980.

Hafstrom M, Kjellmer I. Non-nutritive sucking in the healthy pre-term infant. *Early Hum Dev* 60:13–24, 2000.

Hall RT, Wheeler RE, Rippetoe LE. Calcium and phosphorus supplementation after initial hospital discharge in breast-fed infants of less than 1800 grams birth weight. *J Perinatol* 13:272–78, 1993.

Hamosh M. Bioactive factors in human milk. *Pediatr Clin North Am* 48:69-86, 2001.

———. Breastfeeding and the working mother: effect of time and temperature of short-term storage on proteolysis, lipolysis, and bacterial growth in milk. *Pediatrics* 97: 492–98, 1996.

Hanson LA. Human milk and host defence: immediate and long-term effects. *Acta Paediatr Suppl* 88:42–46, 1999.

Hartmann P, Cregan M. Lactogenesis and the effects of insulin-dependent diabetes mellitus and prematurity. *J Nutr* 131:3016S–20S, 2001.

Hedberg Nyqvist K, Ewald U. Infant and maternal factors in the development of breastfeeding behaviour and breastfeeding outcome in preterm infants. *Acta Paediatr* 88: 1194–203, 1999.

Heird WC. The role of polyunsaturated fatty acids in term and preterm infants and breastfeeding mothers. *Pediatr Clin North Am* 48:173–88, 2001.

Henderson TR et al. Gastric proteolysis in preterm infants fed mother's milk or formula. *Adv Exp Med Biol* 501: 403–38, 2001.

Hill PD, Aldag JC, Chatterton RT. Effects of pumping style on milk production in mothers of non-nursing preterm infants. *J Hum Lact* 15:209–16, 1999.

———. Initiation and frequency of pumping and milk production in mothers of non-nursing preterm infants. *J Hum Lact* 17:9–13, 2001.

Hill PD, Brown LP, Harker TL. Initiation and frequency of breast expression in breastfeeding mothers of LBW and VLBW infants. *Nurs Res* 44:352–55, 1995.

Hill PD, Ledbetter RJ, Kavanaugh KL. Breastfeeding patterns of low-birth-weight infants after hospital discharge. *J Obstet Gynecol Neonatal Nurs* 26:189–97, 1997.

Hurst NM, Myatt A, Schanler RJ. Growth and development of a hospital-based lactation program and mother's own milk bank. *J Obstet Gynecol Neonatal Nurs* 27:503–10, 1998.

Hurst NM et al. Skin-to-skin holding in the neonatal intensive care unit influences maternal milk volume. *J Perinatol* 17:213–17, 1997.

Hutchens TW et al. Origin of intact lactoferrin and its DNA-binding fragments found in the urine of human milk-fed preterm infants. Evaluation by stable isotopic enrichment. *Pediatr Res* 29:243–50, 1991.

Hylander MA, Strobino DM, Dhanireddy R. Human milk feedings and infection among very low birth weight infants. *Pediatrics* 102:E38, 1998.

Hylander MA et al. Association of human milk feedings with a reduction in retinopathy of prematurity among very low birthweight infants. *J Perinatol* 21:356–62, 2001.

Jaeger MC, Lawson M, Filteau S. The impact of prematurity and neonatal illness on the decision to breast-feed. *J Adv Nurs* 25:729–37, 1997.

Jennings T, Meier W, Meier P. High lipid and caloric content in milk from mothers of preterm infants. *Pediatr Res* 41:233A, 1997.

Jensen RG. *The lipids of human milk.* Boca Raton, FL: CRC Press, 1989.

Jocson MA, Mason EO, Schanler RJ. The effects of nutrient fortification and varying storage conditions on host defense properties of human milk. *Pediatrics* 100:240–43, 1997.

Jones E. Strategies to promote preterm breastfeeding. *Mod Midwife* 5:8–11, 1995.

Kavanaugh K, Meier PP, Engstrom JL. Reliability of weighing procedures for preterm infants. *Nurs Res* 38:178–79, 1989.

Kavanaugh K et al. Getting enough: mothers' concerns about breastfeeding a preterm infant after discharge. *J Obstet Gynecol Neonatal Nurs* 24:23–32, 1995.

———. The rewards outweigh the efforts: breastfeeding outcomes for mothers of preterm infants. *J Hum Lact* 13:15–21, 1997.

Kent JC et al. Breast volume and milk production during extended lactation in women. *Exp Physiol* 84:435–47, 1999.

Killersreiter B et al. Early cessation of breastmilk feeding in very low birthweight infants. *Early Hum Dev* 60:193–205, 2001.

Kirsten GF, Bergman NJ, Hann FM. Kangaroo mother care in the nursery. *Pediatr Clin North Am* 48:443–52, 2001.

Koletzko B et al. Long chain polyunsaturated fatty acids (LC-PUFA) and perinatal development. *Acta Paediatr* 90: 460–64, 2001.

Kosloske AM. Breastmilk decreases the risk of neonatal necrotizing enterocolitis. *Adv Nutr Res* 10:123–37, 2001.

Krouse AM. The family management of breastfeeding low birth weight infants. *J Hum Lact* 18:155–65, 2002.

Kuschel C, Harding J. Multicomponent fortification of human milk for premature infants. *Cochrane Database Syst Review* (2) CD000343, 2000.

Labbock M, Krasovec K. Toward consistency in breastfeeding definitions. *Studies in Family Planning* 21:226–30, 1990.

Lang S, Lawrence CJ, Orme RL. Cup feeding: an alternative method of infant feeding. *Arch Dis Child* 71:365–69, 1994.

Lau C, Hurst N. Oral feeding in infants. *Curr Probl Pediatr* 29:105–24, 1999.

Lau C et al. Oral feeding in low birth weight infants. *J Pediatr* 130:561–69, 1997.

Lau C et al. Characterization of the developmental stages of sucking in preterm infants during bottle feeding. *Acta Paediatr* 89:846–52, 2000.

Lawrence RA. Breastfeeding support benefits very low-birth-weight infants. *Arch Pediatr Adolesc Med* 155:543–44, 2001.

Legault M, Goulet C. Comparison of kangaroo and traditional methods of removing preterm infants from incubators. *J Obstet Gynecol Neonatal Nurs* 24:501–6 1995.

Lemons JA et al. Differences in the composition of preterm and term human milk during early lactation. *Pediatr Res* 16:113–17, 1982.

Lucas A, Cole TJ. Breastmilk and neonatal necrotising enterocolitis. *Lancet* 336:1519–23, 1990.

Lucas A, Morley R, Cole TJ. Randomised trial of early diet in preterm babies and later intelligence quotient. *Br Med J* 317:1481–87, 1998.

Lucas A et al. Creamatocrit: simple clinical technique for estimating fat concentration and energy value of human milk. *Br Med J* 1:1018–20, 1978.

———. A randomised multicentre study of human milk versus formula and later development in preterm infants. *Arch Dis Child* 70:F140–46, 1994.

———. Randomized outcome trial of human milk fortification and developmental outcome in preterm infants. *Am J Clin Nutr* 64:142–51, 1996.

Ludington-Hoe SM et al. Kangaroo care: research results, and practice implications and guidelines. *Neonatal Netw* 13:19–27, 1994.

Luukkainen P, Salo MK, Nikkari T. Changes in the fatty acid composition of preterm and term human milk from 1 week to 6 months of lactation. *J Pediatr Gastroenterol Nutr* 18:355–60, 1994.

Luukkainen P et al. Fatty acid composition of plasma and red blood cell phospholipids in preterm infants from 2 weeks to 6 months postpartum. *J Pediatr Gastroenterol Nutr* 20:310–15, 1995.

Maas YG et al. Development of macronutrient composition of very preterm human milk. *Br J Nutr* 80:35–40, 1998.

Martell M et al. Suction patterns in preterm infants. *J Perinat Med* 21:363–69, 1993.

Medoff-Cooper B. Multi-system approach to the assessment of successful feeding. *Acta Paediatr* 89:393–94, 2000.

Meier PP. Bottle- and breast-feeding: effects on transcutaneous oxygen pressure and temperature in preterm infants. *Nurs Res* 37:36–41, 1988.

———. Caution needed in extrapolating from term to preterm infants: author's reply. *J Hum Lact* 11:91, 1995.

———. Nipple shields for preterm infants: effect on milk transfer and duration of breastfeeding. *J Hum Lact* 16:106–14, 2000.

———. Breastfeeding in the special care nursery. Prematures and infants with medical problems. *Pediatr Clin North Am* 48:425–42, 2001.

Meier PP, Anderson GC. Responses of small preterm infants to bottle- and breast-feeding. *MCN Am J Matern Child Nurs* 12:97–105, 1987.

Meier PP, Brown LP. State of the science. Breastfeeding for mothers and low birth weight infants. *Nurs Clin North Am* 31:351–65, 1996.

———. Defining terminology for improved breastfeeding research. *J Nurse Midwifery* 42:65–66, 1997.

Meier PP et al. The accuracy of test weighing for preterm infants. *J Pediatr Gastroenterol Nutr* 10:62–65, 1990.

———. Breastfeeding support services in the neonatal intensive-care unit. *J Obstet Gynecol Neonatal Nurs* 22:338–47, 1993.

———. A new scale for in-home test weighing for mothers of preterm and high risk infants. *J Hum Lact* 10:163–68, 1994.

———. Estimating milk intake of hospitalized preterm infants who breastfeed. *J Hum Lact* 12:21–26, 1996.

Miller JB et al. The oligosaccharide composition of human milk: temporal and individual variations in monosaccharide components. *J Pediatr Gastroenterol Nutr* 19:371–76, 1994.

Milsom SR et al. Potential role for growth hormone in human lactation insufficiency. *Horm Res* 50:147–50, 1998.

Mitoulas LR et al. Effect of vacuum profile on breastmilk expression using an electric breast pump. *J Hum Lact* 18:353–60, 2002a.

———. Efficacy of breastmilk expression using an electric breast pump. *J Hum Lact* 18:344–52, 2002b.

Moody GJ et al. Feeding tolerance in premature infants fed fortified human milk. *J Pediatr Gastroenterol Nutr* 30:408–12, 2000.

Moro G et al. Growth and plasma amino acid concentrations in very low birthweight infants fed either human milk protein fortified human milk or a whey-predominant formula. *Acta Paediatr Scand* 78:18–22, 1989.

Narayanan I et al. Sucking on the "emptied" breast: non-nutritive sucking with a difference. *Arch Dis Child* 66:241–44, 1991.

Neifert M, Lawrence R, Seacat J. Nipple confusion: toward a formal definition. *J Pediatr* 126:S125–29, 1995.

Nelson EE, Panksepp J. Brain substrates of infant-mother attachment: contributions of opioids, oxytocin, and norepinephrine. *Neurosci Biobehav Rev* 22:437–52, 1998.

Newman J. Breastfeeding problems associated with the early introduction of bottles and pacifiers. *J Hum Lact* 6:59–63, 1990.

Nicholl RM, Gamsu HR. Changes in growth and metabolism in very low birthweight infants fed with fortified breast milk. *Acta Paediatr* 88:1056–61, 1999.

Nissen E et al. Oxytocin, prolactin, milk production and their relationship with personality traits in women after vaginal delivery or Cesarean section. *J Psychosom Obstet Gynaecol* 19:49–58, 1998.

Nowak AJ, Smith WL, Erenberg A. Imaging evaluation of artificial nipples during bottle feeding. *Arch Pediatr Adolesc Med* 148:40–42, 1994.

———. Imaging evaluation of breast-feeding and bottle-feeding systems. *J Pediatr* 126:S130–34, 1995.

Nyqvist KH. Breast-feeding preterm twins: development of feeding behavior and milk intake during hospital stay and related caregiving practice. *J Pediatr Nurs* 17:246–56, 2002.

———. Personal communication. June 2003.

Nyqvist KH, Ewald U, Sjoden PO. Supporting a preterm infant's behaviour during breastfeeding: a case report. *J Hum Lact* 12:221–28, 1996.

Nyqvist KH, Sjoden PO, Ewald U. The development of preterm infants' breastfeeding behavior. *Early Hum Dev* 55:247–64, 1999.

Nyqvist KH et al. Development of the preterm infant breastfeeding behavior scale (PIBBS): a study of nurse-mother agreement. *J Hum Lact* 12:207–19, 1996.

Nyqvist KH et al. Early oral behaviour in preterm infants during breastfeeding: an electromyographic study. *Acta Paediatr* 90:658–63, 2001.

Ortenstrand A et al. Early discharge of preterm infants followed by domiciliary nursing care: parents' anxiety, assessment of infant health and breastfeeding. *Acta Paediatr* 90:1190–95, 2001.

Ostrea EM et al. Influence of breast-feeding on the restoration of the low serum concentration of vitamin E and beta-carotene in the newborn infant. *Am J Obstet Gynecol* 154:1014–17, 1986.

Peterson JA et al. Milk fat globule glycoproteins in human milk and in gastric aspirates of mother's milk-fed preterm infants. *Pediatr Res* 44:499–506, 1998.

Pietschnig B et al. Breastfeeding rates of VLBW infants—influence of professional breastfeeding support. *Adv Exp Med Biol* 478:429–30, 2000.

Pinelli J, Atkinson SA, Saigal S. Randomized trial of breast-feeding support in very low-birth-weight infants. *Arch Pediatr Adolesc Med* 155:548–53. 2001.

Pinelli J, Symington A. Non-nutritive sucking for promoting physiologic stability and nutrition in preterm infants. *Cochrane Database Syst Rev* (2) CD001071, 2000.

Polberger S, Lonnerdal B. Simple and rapid macronutrient analysis of human milk for individualized fortification: basis for improved nutritional management of very-low-birth-weight infants? *J Pediatr Gastroenterol Nutr* 17:283–90, 1993.

Quan R et al. Effects of microwave radiation on anti-infective factors in human milk. *Pediatrics* 89:667–69, 1992.

———. The effect of nutritional additives on anti-infective factors in human milk. *Clin Pediatr* 33:325–28, 1994.

Ramasethu J, Jeyaseelan L, Kirubakaran CP. Weight gain in exclusively breastfed preterm infants. *J Trop Pediatr* 39:152–59, 1993.

Rassin DK et al. Feeding the low-birth-weight infant: II. Effects of taurine and cholesterol supplementation on amino acids and cholesterol. *Pediatrics* 71:179–86, 1983.

Rocha NM, Martinez FE, Jorge SM. Cup or bottle for preterm infants: effects on oxygen saturation, weight gain, and breastfeeding. *J Hum Lact* 18:132–38, 2002.

Rudloff S et al. Urinary excretion of lactose and oligosaccharides in preterm infants fed human milk or infant formula. *Acta Paediatr* 85:598–603, 1998.

Sameroff AJ. The components of sucking in the human newborn. *J Exp Child Psychol,* 6:607–23, 1968.

Sankaran K et al. A randomized, controlled evaluation of two commercially available human breastmilk fortifiers in healthy preterm neonates. *J Am Diet Assoc* 96:1145–49, 1996.

Scanlon KS et al. Assessment of infant feeding: the validity of measuring milk intake. *Nutr Rev* 60:235–51, 2002.

Schanler RJ. The role of human milk fortification for premature infants. *Clin Perinatol* 25:645–57, 1998.

———. The use of human milk for premature infants. *Pediatr Clin North Am* 48:207–19, 2001.

Schanler RJ, Atkinson SA. Effects of nutrients in human milk on the recipient premature infant. *J Mammary Gland Biol Neoplasia* 4:297–307, 1999.

Schanler RJ, Hurst NM, Lau C. The use of human milk and breastfeeding in premature infants. *Clin Perinatol* 26:379–98, 1999.

Schanler RJ, Shulman RJ, Lau C. Feeding strategies for premature infants: beneficial outcomes of feeding fortified human milk versus preterm formula. *Pediatrics* 103:1150–17, 1999.

Schanler RJ et al. Feeding strategies for premature infants: randomized trial of gastrointestinal priming and tube-feeding method. *Pediatrics* 103:434–39, 1999.

Shulman RJ et al. Early feeding, antenatal glucocorticoids, and human milk decrease intestinal permeability in preterm infants. *Pediatr Res* 44:519–23, 1998a.

———. Early feeding, feeding tolerance, and lactase activity in preterm infants. *J Pediatr* 133:645–49, 1998b.

Sidell EP, Froman RD. A national survey of neonatal intensive-care units: criteria used to determine readiness for oral feedings. *J Obstet Gynecol Neonatal Nurs* 23:783–89, 1994.

Simmer K, Metcalf R, Daniels L. The use of breastmilk in a neonatal unit and its relationship to protein and energy intake and growth. *J Paediatr Child Health* 33:55–60, 1997.

Srivastava MD et al. Cytokines in human milk. *Res Commun Mol Pathol Pharmacol* 93:263–87, 1996.

Stine MJ. Breastfeeding the premature newborn: a protocol without bottles. *J Hum Lact* 6:167–70, 1990.

Stocks RJ et al. Loss of breastmilk nutrients during tube feeding. *Arch Dis Child* 60:164–66, 1985.

Thompson N et al. Contamination in expressed breast-milk following breast cleansing. *J Hum Lact* 13:127–30, 1997.

Tornhage CJ et al. Plasma somatostatin and cholecystokinin levels in preterm infants during kangaroo care with and without nasogastric tube-feeding. *J Pediatr Endocrinol Metab* 11:645–51, 1998.

———. First week kangaroo care in sick very preterm infants. *Acta Paediatr* 88:1402–4, 1999.

Trugo NM et al. Concentration and distribution pattern of selected micronutrients in preterm and term milk from urban Brazilian mothers during early lactation. *Eur J Clin Nutr* 42:497–507, 1988.

Tully MR. Recommendations for handling of mother's own milk. *J Hum Lact* 16:149–51, 2000.

Uauy R et al. Visual and brain function measurements in studies of n-3 fatty acid requirements of infants. *J Pediatr* 120:S168–80, 1992.

Uvnas-Moberg K. Physiological and endocrine effects of social contact. *Ann N Y Acad Sci* 807:146–63, 1997.

———. Oxytocin may mediate the benefits of positive social interaction and emotions. *Psychoneuroendocrinology* 23:819–35, 1998.

Valentine CJ, Hurst NM, Schanler RJ. Hindmilk improves weight gain in low-birth-weight infants fed human milk. *J Pediatr Gastroenterol Nutr* 18:474–77, 1994.

Wagner CL et al. Breastfeeding rates at an urban medical university after initiation of an educational program. *South Med J* 95:909–13, 2002.

Walker M. Test weighing and other estimates of breastmilk intake. *J Hum Lact* 11:91–92, 1995.

Waterland RA et al. Calibrated-orifice nipples for measurement of infant nutritive sucking. *J Pediatr* 132:523–26, 1998.

Wauben IP. Moderate nutrient supplementation of mother's milk for preterm infants supports adequate bone mass and short-term growth: a randomized, controlled trial. *Am J Clin Nutr* 67:465–72, 1998.

Wauben IP et al. Growth and body composition of preterm infants: influence of nutrient fortification of mother's milk in hospital and breastfeeding post-hospital discharge. *Acta Paediatr* 87:780–85, 1998.

Weaver LT, Lucas A. Development of bowel habit in preterm infants. *Arch Dis Child,* 68:317–20, 1993.

Wheeler JL et al. Promoting breastfeeding in the neonatal intensive care unit. *Breastfeed Rev* 7:15–18, 1999.

Whitelaw A, Liestol K. Mortality and growth of low birth weight infants on the Kangaroo Mother Program in Bogota, Colombia. *Pediatrics* 94:931–32, 1994.

Williamson MT, Murti PK. Effects of storage, time, temperature, and composition of containers on biologic components of human milk. *J Hum Lact* 12:31–35, 1996.

Woltil HA et al. Erythrocyte and plasma cholesterol ester long-chain polyunsaturated fatty acids of low-birth-weight babies fed preterm formula with and without ribonucleotides: comparison with human milk. *Am J Clin Nutr* 62:943–49, 1995.

Woodward DR, Rees B, Boon JA. Human milk fat content: within-feed variation. *Early Hum Dev* 19:39–46, 1989.

Xiao X et al. Epidermal growth factor concentrations in human milk, cow's milk and cow's milk-based infant formulas. *Chin Med J (Engl)* 115:451–54, 2002.

Zheng MC et al. Alpha-tocopherol concentrations in human milk from mothers of preterm and full-term infants in China. *Biomed Environ Sci* 6:259–64, 1993.

APPENDIX 13-A

THE PRETERM INFANT BREASTFEEDING BEHAVIOR SCALE (PIBBS)

The PIBBS is used to describe the infant's behavior, as defined by the scale. It does not assess the infant's breastfeeding behavior capacity in a way that can be quantified by a total score.

Scale Items	Maturational Steps	Score
Rooting	Did not root	0
	Showed some rooting behavior	1
	Showed obvious rooting behavior	2
Areolar grasp	None, the mouth only touched the nipple	0
(How much of the	Part of the nipple	1
breast was inside	The whole nipple, not the areola	2
the baby's mouth?)	The nipple and some of the areola	3
Latched-on and	Did not latch on at all so the mother felt it	0
fixed to the breast	Latched on for 5 minutes or less	1
(scored on a	Latched on for 6–10 minutes	2
continuous scale)	Latched on for 11–15 minutes or more	3
Sucking	No sucking or licking	0
	Licking and tasting, but no sucking	1
	Single sucks, occasional short sucking bursts (2–9 sucks)	2
	Repeated short sucking bursts, occasional long bursts (≥ 10 sucks)	3
	Repeated (2 or more) long sucking bursts	4
Longest sucking burst	1–5	1
(in consecutive sucks,	6–10	2
scored on a continuous scale)	11–15	3
	16–20	4
	21–25	5
	26–30 or more	6
Swallowing	Swallowing was not noticed	0
	Occasional swallowing was noticed	1
	Repeated swallowing was noticed	2

Definition of Terms

1. Rooting: some rooting (mouth opening, tongue extension, hand-to-mouth movements) and obvious rooting (simultaneous mouth opening and head turning). Examples of suggestions to mothers for stimulation of rooting are touching the infant's lips with the nipple and expressing some milk on the lips.

2. Areolar grasp: part of the nipple, whole nipple, or nipple and part of the areola. The mother can facilitate this by encouraging the infant to continue rooting until he shows a wide open mouth, by shaping her breast into a form that fits the infant's mouth, and then letting the infant latch-on and pulling him close to her body; in order for successful latching-on to take place the mother should sit in an upright position, with proper support for her back, arms, and feet, and with a pillow under the infant that supports a comfortable position in front of the breast.

3. Duration of latching-on: momentarily, less than a minute, or several minutes. The infant is assisted in staying fixed at the breast by adjustment of the mother's and infant's position and of the areolar grasp.

APPENDIX 13–A (cont.)

4. Sucking: occasional sucks, short or long (10 consecutive sucks or more) sucking bursts, occasional or repeated bursts. The mother can encourage sucking by talking to the infant and by gently depressing the breast tissue in front of the infant's mouth, which makes the nipple touch the hard palate.

5. The longest sucking burst: maximum number of consecutive sucks, a measure of sucking maturity.

6. Swallowing: occasional or repeated. When swallowing is noticed, the mother can be asked to commence test weighing (if this is included in the unit policy) and the milk given by alternative methods can be reduced.

Source: From Nyqvist (1996). Reprinted with permission.

Donor Human Milk Banking

Lois D. W. Arnold

In the absence of breastmilk from an infant's own mother (the preferred feeding choice, with very few exceptions), banked donor milk can be lifesaving and enhancing. Health professionals caring for mothers and children need to understand donor human milk banking—from its safety and standardization as a product to its clinical uses and accessibility. With more complete knowledge and understanding of donor human milk, more individuals in need will be able to access this valuable public health resource.

This chapter discusses donor human milk banking and the issues surrounding its clinical use, including the state of the art milk banks in North America, as represented by the Human Milk Banking Association of North America member milk banks. Comparisons with countries around the world, the need for further research, and how donor milk banking should be positioned in public health policy are also discussed in this chapter.

Defining Donor Milk Banking

Donor human milk banking is the collection, processing, storage, and dispensing *on prescription* of human milk that is donated by healthy nursing mothers who have an overabundance of milk for their own infants. All donors are thoroughly screened, all milk is pasteurized, and donor milk banks operate within standardized guidelines to ensure a safe product.

A Brief History of Human Milk Banking

Foundations of Donor Human Milk Banking: Pre-1975

In eighteenth-century Europe, foundling hospitals with an infant feeding practice of routine dry-nursing (i.e. hand- or artificial-feeding) had much higher rates of mortality than did those hospitals that either provided wet nurses in house or sent their infants out to supervise wet nurses (Fildes, 1988). Even though wet nurses gained reputations for transmitting diseases such as syphilis and tuberculosis to the infants in their care, studies showed that, during the late nineteenth and early twentieth centuries in Europe and the United States, infants breastfed by their own mothers or wet nurses had mortality rates lower than those of artificially-fed infants. The benefits of breastfeeding for infant health and the difficulties of formulating artificial infant milk spurred the development of donor human milk banks.

In the early twentieth century, a study conducted in Boston showed that babies who were not

409

breastfed were six times more likely to die of diarrhea and enteritis in the first year of life than were breastfed babies (Davis, 1913). Wet nurses also became exceedingly difficult to find during this period. Two Boston physicians, Fritz Talbot and Francis Parkman Denny, developed the idea of stockpiling human milk, separating the "product" from the "producer." Both were medical directors of the Massachusetts Infant Asylum, which employed wet nurses to feed sick foundlings, and both were concerned about the quality of the stored product (Golden, 1988). Donors were screened for tuberculosis, syphilis, and other contagious diseases and the milk was pasteurized (Talbot, 1911). This processed milk was fed to hospitalized infants. Hospitals in other cities quickly followed suit and developed their own milk banks.

At the turn of the twentieth century, many poor women in urban areas returned to work to supplement family incomes. One result was a greatly shortened duration of breastfeeding in urban areas. Physicians tried to alter cow's milk to make this substitute as good for babies as human milk, but there were few regulations and standards for this milk and its handling. The urban supply was stored in large open vats, was shipped in unrefrigerated railroad cars, and was delivered to the city "dirty, spoiled, easily adulterated, and loaded with pathogens." (Wolf, 2001, p. 42). More often than not, the milk also came from sick animals. Many cities mounted campaigns to teach mothers how to store the milk and care for it properly, and legislative agendas attempted to regulate milk collection, storage, and handling, with much resistance from the dairy industry. Cities began to establish human milk "stations" to provide nutrition for sick infants recovering from disease caused by spoiled cow's milk. By 1929, at least 20 of these human milk stations existed around the country. In some cities, such as Chicago, mothers were carefully screened and were paid for their milk, milk collection was supervised in hospital, and the collected milk was bottled, pasteurized, and dispensed. The Chicago Board of Health required that the Breast Milk Station furnish milk to a hospital "immediately upon request" with no charge for the milk supplied (Wolf, 2001, p. 153). Some of these milk stations existed through World War II, but as ac-

ceptance and use of formula increased, milk banks fell out of favor. The first official recognition of donor milk banking from the American Academy of Pediatrics (AAP) occurred in 1943 with its recommendations for operating donor human milk banks (AAP, 1943).

Donor Human Milk Banking in the United States: Post-1975

In the 1970s, rapid advances in neonatal intensive care included recognition that human milk's special properties improved survival and decreased complications in preterm infants. Milk banking gained in popularity once again and many hospitals established milk banks. However, screening procedures for donors were not uniform and most milk was dispensed raw. In the mid- to late 1980s, milk banking declined in North America with the development of special formulas for preterm infants and increased concern about viral transmission, particularly the human immunodeficiency viruses (HIV). Many milk banks closed when HIV was first reported in human milk because of fear of transmission and because of the additional cost of having to serum-screen all donors. In 1985 the Human Milk Banking Association of North America (HMBANA) was formed to respond to these concerns. One organizational goal of HMBANA was to formulate standards for donor milk banking operations.

The first edition of HMBANA's *Guidelines for the Establishment and Operation of a Donor Human Milk Bank* was published in 1990. Guidelines were developed in consultation with the Centers for Disease Control and Prevention (CDC), the Food and Drug Administration (FDA), and other medical experts, and they are reviewed and revised annually (HMBANA, 2003). These guidelines require thorough donor screening, pasteurization of all milk, and bacteriological quality control of all dispensed milk. Adherence to the guidelines was voluntary until 2000, when HMBANA decided to make adherence to the guidelines mandatory for member milk banks. However, as of this writing, there is no regulation or monitoring of milk banks by the FDA and no method for enforcing compliance with the guidelines by HMBANA. Only New York and California have state regulations for donor human milk banks. Milk cannot be legally shipped into these states unless it comes from a milk bank licensed in that state, nor can milk from women in New York State be shipped out of state unless it goes to a milk bank licensed in New York.*

Through the 1990s distributing milk banks continued to decline in number in the United States. However, the few that remain have dispensed an increasing number of ounces since 1992 (see Table 14–1). Since 1997 two older milk banks have closed, and two new ones have opened, leaving the United States with five milk banks as of this writing. Current status of North American milk banks and their contact information may be found at the HMBANA Web site.

Additionally in the United States, the National Commission on Donor Milk Banking was formed specifically to address research and policy issues regarding donor human milk banking.

Potential Hazards of Informal Sharing of Human Milk

Donor milk banks conduct thorough screening of all donors for disease and for other health behaviors such as smoking, alcohol consumption, and medication usage (HMBANA, 2003). Donor milk banks provide additional safeguards through bacteriological screening and pasteurization. When access to banked donor milk is difficult or availability of the service is not known, mothers may resort to obtaining milk from a friend or relative. Some women have resorted to purchasing milk over the Internet or through an advertisement in a local newspaper. In an era of incurable viral diseases, these practices should be discouraged. There is no way of guaranteeing that a potential donor is disease-free. The donor may be unaware of her partner's behavior that might place her at risk. Even if parents are knowledgeable about issues related to

---

[In New York see Subpart 52–9, Part 52 (Tissue Banks and Nontransplant Anatomic Banks), Title 10 (Health) of the Official Compilation of Codes, Rules and Regulations of the State of New York, effective December 31, 2000. In California see California Health and Safety Code, Section 1635–1644.5. Chapter 4.1 Tissue Banks; Chapter 4.2 Donations of Organs, Tissues, or Body Fluids.]

Table 14–1

ANNUAL STATISTICS: MILK DISPENSED BY HMBANA MILK BANKS*

Year	Number of Ounces	Liters	Number of Milk Banks
1986	266,000	7,988	14
1989	177,000	5,315	8
1991–1992	133,700	4,015	9
1992–1993	144,200	4,330	8
1993–1994	163,000	4,895	8
1994–1995	182,400	5,477	8
1995–1996**	203,500	6,111	8
1996–1997**	180,100	5,408	8
1997–1998	280,000	8,408	7
1999	322,700	9,691	7
2000	410,100	12,315	6
2001	511,700	15,366	5
2002†	501,100	15,186	6

Source: Human Milk Banking Association of North America, Inc., 2003.
Rounded to the nearest 100 oz or nearest whole liter.
**Figures incomplete or missing for one milk bank.*
†Iowa milk bank opened as of August 2002, but did not dispense milk.

sharing of body fluids, they may receive incomplete information. While a single bottle pasteurizer (maximum volume = 200 cc [6.7 oz]) is on the market and is currently being used in Africa and Eastern Europe, primarily by mothers who are HIV-positive, the availability of this product elsewhere is unknown. There are no published tested protocols for home pasteurization of larger batches of milk, and the potential for doing unnecessary damage to the milk through excessive heating and imprecise methodology may outweigh any benefits of the milk.

Although the World Health Organization (WHO) still recommends use of a "healthy wet nurse" in developing countries where milk banking services are not available (WHO, 2002), in developed countries with sound infrastructures, donated human milk should come from a milk bank that practices according to established guidelines. Lactation consultants should consider their liability and the ethics of assisting women with informal milk sharing or purchasing arrangements without the safeguards of a donor human milk bank. Legal issues also exist in many states and consent is required from the biological mother before an adoptive mother can breastfeed or use donor milk (Tagge, 2001).

Donor Milk Banking Beyond North America

Donor milk banking thrives in many countries outside North America. However, there is no parent organization to which all milk banks belong, nor is there a central repository for data about existing milk banks internationally. Many milk banks exist solely as a result of the commitment of a particular individual or group of individuals.

Donor milk banking is a common practice in much of Europe. The first human milk bank in Germany was founded in 1919. In 1952, the former East German government decreed that every city with a population over 55,000 was required to have its own milk bank. Both East and West Germany had a great interest in donor milk banking until the early 1970s when aggressive marketing of specialty milks in West Germany prompted closure of all West German milk banks. In East Germany, the economy dictated that these specialty milks could not be used and donor milk banks flourished. The number of milk banks rose and the volume dispensed increased. By 1989, 60 milk banks were operating in East Germany. With German reunification in 1990, many of these milk banks closed. In 1998, the remaining 15 milk banks (9 of them regional) supplied 8000 L (266,400 oz) of donor milk. (Springer, 1997; Springer, 2000; see also Arnold, 2001). In Leipzig, community acceptance of donor milk banking has resulted in some families having a third generation of women providing donated milk (Springer, 1997).

European countries have developed standards for milk banking practices. In France, standards for operation are incorporated into public health law. These laws and regulations dictate donor-screening procedures, pasteurization methods, and bacteriological standards (Arnold, 1994; Arnold & Courdent, 1994). The United Kingdom Association of Milk Banks (UKAMB) also has developed standards for establishing and operating a donor milk bank. While not part of public health law, these guidelines are supported by the Royal College of Paediatrics and Child Health (formerly the British Paediatric Association), which publishes them (Balmer, 1995; Balmer & Wharton, 1992; UKAMB, 2003). Donor milk banks have existed for many years in Scandinavian countries (Siimes & Hallman, 1979; Arnold, 1999a). Poland also has a large milk bank in Lodz, the main purpose of which is to increase the number of premature infants receiving human milk as first feedings (Penc, 1996). The Human Milk Bank in Sofia, Bulgaria, was founded in 1989 as an "independent socially oriented health institution" funded and staffed by the Municipality of Sofia (Sotirova, 2002).

Countries in Central America and the Caribbean have developed donor milk banks as part of their national campaigns to promote breastfeeding and the benefits of human milk feedings. Support for equipment as well as training has come from UNICEF in many cases. Almeida (2001) describes a "new paradigm" for milk banking in Brazil where the milk banking association has taken the lead in protecting, promoting, and supporting breastfeeding. Milk banking has influenced legislation and has become an integral part of the training of health-care providers on the importance of breastfeeding. Milk banking experts and administrators are responsible for implementing the Baby-Friendly Hospital Initiative in Brazil as well.

As late as 1996, donor milk banking was being practiced in China in some maternity hospitals as an extension of Step 6 of the Baby-Friendly Hospital Initiative (i.e., to "give newborn infants no food or drink other than breastmilk, unless medically indicated"). Donor milk was collected from postpartum mothers while they were in the hospital (average stay, 7 days). The milk was processed and dispensed to healthy newborns whose mothers were too ill to nurse immediately or who had insufficient milk to meet the infant's needs in the first 5 to 7 days of life (Arnold, 1996). By 2001 there was an increased demand for information about donor milk banking, its clinical uses, and how to dispense it. The Ministry of Health also incorporated guidelines for establishment and operation of donor milk banks into its policies based on a copy of the HMBANA guidelines given to a representative of the Ministry of Health (Hong, 2001).

The Impact of Culture on Donor Milk Banking

Cultural issues impact the way donor milk banking is practiced. Even when health-care providers accept the use of donor milk, opposition may exist from both donors and parents of recipients. Among Africans, it is widely believed that diseases and genetic and personality traits can be transferred through human milk. The author encountered similar beliefs in a nursing school in Moscow in 1997. In a survey conducted in Nigeria, 70 percent of mothers were unwilling to accept donated human milk for their infants because of these fears and because of sociocultural and religious beliefs (Ighogboja et al., 1995). The other 30 percent of mothers surveyed would accept donor milk only if it came from a close relative. Similar reasons would prevent 40 percent of women from donating milk.

Narayanan et al. (1980) noted that some Muslim women objected to their babies receiving milk from Hindu women, although the converse was not true. The Koran treats human milk as altered blood; children suckled by the same woman become blood relations or "milk siblings" and they are forbidden to marry each other to avoid the possibility of incest from a consanguineous marriage (Ighogboja et al., 1995). There are ways of dealing with this issue, and AL-Naqeeb et al. (2000) describe a donor milk bank in Kuwait. Wet-nursing full-term babies is an acceptable practice in Kuwait. The solution to establishing a milk bank in a Kuwait NICU was to introduce the mother of the recipient to the donor mother so that their offspring could avoid the potential of a consanguineous mar-

riage. In most other countries milk bank donors remain anonymous and donor information is confidential.

The Benefits of Banked Donor Human Milk

The benefits of donor milk are similar to those for breastfeeding/human milk in general:

- Species specificity
- Ease of digestion
- Promotion of growth, maturation, and development of organ systems
- Immunological benefits

All are related to the unique composition of human milk and the dual and synergistic functions of many milk components.

Species Specificity

Occasional references appear in the literature regarding the theoretical potential for a graft-versus-host reaction to donor milk by the recipient when fresh milk is used (AAP, 1980; Xanthou, 1987). Young animals fed fresh milk containing live white blood cells from a *different species* exhibit this type of reaction. However, this has not been shown to occur in humans when human milk is given to members of the same species (Xanthou, 1987). The success of wet-nursing and cross-nursing throughout human history also negate the graft-versus-host theory. Current milk banking practice includes pasteurization of all milk prior to dispensing. Thus there are no live cells in the final product and therefore no potential for a graft-versus-host reaction.

Ease of Digestion

Donor milk is advantageous to premature infants and infants and children with certain digestive and metabolic conditions because it is easy to digest and creates minimal metabolic stress to organs and tissues. There is very little gastric residual left when infants are fed banked human milk, making it the ideal postsurgical feeding after gastrointestinal surgery for gastroschisis repair, necrotizing enterocolitis, or Hirschsprung's disease (Rangecroft, de San Lazaro, & Scott, 1978; Riddell, 1989; Springer, 1997). Every effort is made to match the lactational stage of the donor with the age of the infant to further improve digestibility with an appropriate whey-casein ratio. Efforts are also made to provide premature infants with milk donated by mothers of other premature infants to better meet the premature infant's protein requirements.

Promotion of Growth, Maturation, and Development of Organ Systems

Many components of human milk are heat stable at the temperatures used during pasteurization (Fidler et al., 2001; McPherson & Wagner, 2001; Goes et al., 2002). The nutrient composition is rarely affected. Other components include growth factors and essential fatty acids that enhance neurological development in the infant. For premature infants who have been deprived of the full complement of developmental factors *in utero*, the presence of these factors in donor milk is highly advantageous. These components do not occur in formulas. When infants and children have suffered tissue damage (e.g., damage to the mucosal epithelial lining of the digestive tract as a result of allergies to formulas), donor milk allows healing and maturation of the tissues and enzyme systems so that other foods can be tolerated as the child matures.

The unique nutrients and growth factors in human milk are implicated in the improved developmental outcome of infants who are fed human milk (Lucas et al., 1992). These advantages are particularly strong in premature infants, as shown in a meta-analysis of published studies (Anderson, Johnstone, & Remley, 1999). The essential fatty acids found naturally in human milk, arachidonic acid and docosahexanoic acid, are not affected by pasteurization (Luukkainen, Salo, & Nikkari, 1995) and may promote better visual acuity by promoting better development of neurological synapses and impulse conduction. One cannot achieve the same results by taking reagents off the shelf and adding them to a foreign environment (formula). Finnish neonatologists have concluded that the use of

banked donor milk is preferable to formula because it is a good source of these long-chain polyunsaturated fatty acids (Luukkainen, Salo, & Nikkari, 1995).

Immunological Benefits

Immune factors such as IgA, lactoferrin, and lysozyme are important to infants and children whose immune systems are either too immature to function or have been compromised in some way by disease or genetics. Equally important are the anti-infective nutrients in human milk. For example, human milk is the optimal source of IgA for patients with IgA-deficiency. A reduction in the incidence of necrotizing enterocolitis in premature infants fed donor milk has been documented by Lucas and Cole (1990). Other anti-infective factors include the mucin complexes, lipids with antiviral properties (Isaacs & Thormar, 1990), carbohydrates that prevent bacterial, and parasitic adhesion. Donor milk is an ideal way to acquire many of these factors that are not present in formulas or other animal milks.

Clinical Uses

Distribution of Banked Donor Milk: Setting Priorities

In the World Health Organization's hierarchy of feeding choices, a mother's own milk is always the first choice for feeding infants. Donor milk is the second choice when a mother's own milk is unavailable and is usually preferred to formula use (Savage, 1998). Donor milk may be used to supplement a mother's supply, primarily in cases when an infant is ill or has some medical condition where the use of banked donor milk is beneficial. Donor milk may be provided for certain maternal conditions in which breastfeeding by the biological mother would be contraindicated. In the United States, examples of such conditions include HIV-positive status of the mother or a mother undergoing chemotherapy treatments. Donor milk may also be used when the mother is healthy and the baby is adopted, or in cases where the mother dies and the baby is healthy. Other uses are being considered more frequently in the United States. Donor milk can be used to "buy time" until a diagnosis is made.

Donor milk will "first do no harm" and is frequently part or all of a solution to a problem. The use of banked donor human milk is meant to be temporary, although the definition of temporary may vary according to the needs of the individual recipient.

In order to meet the increasing demands for donor milk from a disparate population of individuals, the milk banks in the United States and Canada have developed a list prioritizing uses. In a case of short supply, milk banks first collaborate to see if a shortage in one geographic area can be covered by another milk bank. If a short supply continues, individuals with the lowest priority are denied access to donor milk so that those with the highest priority will continue to receive it. A prioritization list can be found in Table 14–2 (HMBANA, 2003; Tully, 2002).

In 1986, approximately 72 percent of donor milk dispensed in the United States went to infants in neonatal intensive care units (NICUs), 23 percent to infants in the home, and 2 percent to patients in pediatric units of hospitals (Arnold, 1988). In 1994, a survey of 7 HMBANA milk banks was conducted. Findings of this survey indicated that the distribution pattern had shifted, with only 40 percent going to premature or ill infants in the NICU and the balance going to older infants (Arnold, 1997b). A list of diagnoses for which donor milk was dispensed between January 2001and December 2002 can be found in Table 14–3.

Milk banks in Europe and Scandinavia reserve their donor milk primarily for use by premature infants. Banked donor milk is routinely used as first feedings in many NICUs when a mother's own milk is unavailable (Arnold, 1991, 1999a). At the Triangle Lactation Center and Mother's Milk Bank in Raleigh, North Carolina, where 70 to 80 percent of mothers of preterm infants express their milk, the donor milk bank is a psychologically reassuring entity. Mothers relax and are thought to be more successful in producing milk when they know that the option of donor milk is available should their milk supplies falter (Tully, 1996).

Classifying Clinical Uses: Is Donor Milk Food or Medicine?

The clinical uses of banked donor human milk may be arbitrarily divided into nutritional, medicinal or

Table 14-2

RECIPIENT PRIORITIZATION IN ALLOCATION OF BANKED DONOR MILK

1. Premature infants who are ill
2. Healthy premature infants
3. Infants less than 1 year of age with medical conditions that will respond to use of donor milk
4. Individuals over 1 year of age with medical conditions that will respond to use of donor milk
5. Milk designated for well-designed clinical research studies
6. Persons over 1 year of age with chronic medical conditions, "high normal functioning," and low dosage needs
7. Persons over 1 year of age with chronic medical conditions, "high normal functioning," and high dosage needs
8. Persons over 1 year of age with chronic medical conditions, "low level function," and low dosage needs
9. Persons over 1 year of age with chronic medical conditions, "low level function," and high dosage needs
10. Infants with no specific medical condition for short-term use (can be a maternal problem such as illness, death, low milk supply)
11. Laboratory research (uses milk that cannot be used for clinical consumption due to incomplete donor screening, medications consumed by donor, or age of milk)

Source: Adapted from HMBANA (2003) and Tully (2002).

therapeutic, and preventive uses. However, in practice donor milk may serve several purposes for the same recipient. For example, a preterm infant receives *nourishment* when fed donor human milk. The infant also receives *therapy* in the form of immune substances and growth factors, and disease is *prevented*—e.g., necrotizing enterocolitis (NEC). The younger the recipient the larger the role of nutrition: in an adult recipient, the role of donor milk may be almost exclusively therapeutic or medicinal.

Table 14–3

DIAGNOSES FOR WHICH DONOR MILK WAS DISPENSED IN 2001 AND 2002

ABO incompatibility/formula intolerance

Adopted: cystic fibrosis; drug exposure; failure to thrive (FTT); formula intolerance; history of allergies

Adopted/surrogate: healthy; illness

Adult: cancer (included brain, breast, lung, prostate, rectal, skin); dialysis; FTT/eating disorder; IgA deficiency; irritable bowel syndrome; other immune deficiency; immune deficiency/pneumonia; ulcerative colitis

Alcohol exposure

Allergies (including family history)

Bone marrow transplant

Cardiac defect

Cat's eye syndrome

Cerebral palsy/formula intolerance

Chronic diarrhea

Congenital anomalies

Congestive heart failure/reflux

Developmental delays

Down syndrome/formula intolerance

Epidermylosis bullosa

Failure to thrive

FTT/fetal alcohol syndrome

Formula intolerance

Foster care

GI problems

High LFTs/possible hepatitis B exposure

Hirschsprung's disease/formula intolerance

HIV-positive mother

Hospital NICU—general use

Hypoglycemia

Hypoplastic left heart

Immune deficiency—infant

Infection/formula intolerance

Insufficient milk supply

Jaundice/dehydration

Liver damage/formula intolerance

Low white blood cells/brain bleed

Low/slow weight gain

Maternal Rx/illness (includes mastectomies, chemotherapy)

Metabolic condition

Multiple births (term/near term twins, triplets)

Necrotizing enterocolitis (NEC)

Older child—feeding problems

Oomphalitis

Pearson syndrome

Pediatric inpatient service

Pierre Robin syndrome

Pneumonia

Postoperative: cardiac; cleft lip/palate; GI; nutrition

Preterm: adopted; adopted/FTT; cardiac anomalies/seizures; FTT; formula intolerance; foster care; gastroschisis; lung disease; GI; maternal Rx/illness; multiple births (twins, triplets); NEC

Renal failure

Respiratory distress syndrome

Respiratory syncytial virus

Ruben Taybi syndrome

Seizures

Short gut syndrome

Swallowing impairment

Trisomy 13/defect chromosome 13 and formula intolerance/allergies

VATER syndrome

Source: Human Milk Banking Association of North America, Inc. (2002, 2003, unpublished data).

Clinical Use in Preterm Infants. The most widely accepted use of donor milk is for feeding the preterm infant, despite the fact that preterm infants do not grow as rapidly when they are fed human milk, either maternal or donor, compared with infants fed formula substitutes. However, this result may derive from an inadequate quantity of human milk given to these infants. Term infants allowed to feed at the breast on demand will feed every 2 hours or less because human milk is so digestible and gastric emptying times are short. Yet preterm infants are rarely fed on demand and volumes are frequently restricted. Hamosh recommends avoiding use of restricted volumes when feeding preterm infants (Hamosh, 1994; see also Arnold, 2002b). Sharpe (2002) believes that many preterm infants could be fed more frequently and larger volumes per kilogram per day. Thureen and Hay (2001) propose that earlier and larger quantities be fed to preterm infants. Ziegler, Thureen, and Carlson (2002) also note that preterm infants frequently grow at a slower rate than they did *in utero* because their nutrient intakes are deficient when compared to nutrient uptakes of the fetus. Ziegler et al. advocate "aggressive practice" or practice that exceeds standard practice. For the premature infant, early enteral nutrition (trophic feedings) with human milk should be started on the day of birth to stimulate gut maturation. A mother's own colostrum is preferred, but if her milk supply does not increase rapidly, then "greater use should be made of donated breast milk, which is available from milk banks. Gastric residuals should not be allowed to interfere with feeding. Infants with cardiovascular instability should be fed" (Ziegler, Thureen, & Carlson, 2002, p. 240). Sharpe points out that the mucins inherent in human milk generate a mucus-like substance in the gut that is slow to break down. This substance is often mistaken for feeding residual when it is actually a protective coating. Frequent checking for residuals can injure the mucosa of the gut and interrupt a baby's progress (Sharpe, 2002).

In their large prospective multicenter study of the effect of early diet on the development of premature infants, Lucas and Cole (1990) found that NEC was six to ten times more likely to develop in exclusively formula-fed infants than in those infants fed only human milk. NEC was three times more common when the exclusively formula-fed infants were compared to those receiving both human milk and formula. Furthermore, pasteurized donor milk was as protective as was unheated maternal milk. Schanler, Shulman, and Lau (1999) found that preterm infants fed fortified human milk had a lower incidence of infection and NEC compared to formula-fed infants and infants who received alternate feedings of fortified human milk and preterm formula.

Potential methodological problems may exist when studying human milk-fed infants when there is no clear separation of feeding groups. Maternal and donor milk may be fortified with cow's milk products or formula in one study while none were fortified in another. Narayanan et al. (1984) found that supplementary formula feedings (used as fortifiers) inhibited the protective effect of pasteurized donor milk. The fortification of all human milk in some studies (Schanler et al., 2002) and the lack of definition of study groups may also obscure differences.

Eibl et al. (1988) found that giving oral immunoglobulins to formula-fed infants was prophylactic against NEC. Lucas and Cole (1990) believe that human milk protects against NEC by providing IgA to the lumen of the gut. Most IgA remains intact in donor milk during the pasteurization process, and banked milk continues to be effective prophylaxis. With a decrease in the use of human milk—both maternal and donor—in British neonatal units in the 1980s, Lucas and Cole (1990) estimated that exclusive formula feeding could account for approximately 500 cases of NEC each year and 100 additional infant deaths per year in the United Kingdom.

Lucas and Cole also found that delay in starting feedings was associated with a significant reduction in the incidence of NEC among formula-fed infants. This was not the case with infants fed human milk. These infants could start enteral feedings much earlier without serious consequences. Neonatologists at the University of Leipzig attributed their low rate of NEC (0.2 percent) to early enteral feedings of fresh human milk, both maternal and/or donor milk, at 1, 2, or 3 days postpartum (Springer, 1997). Similar low rates of NEC were reported by the NICU at Ostra Sjukhuset in Göteborg, Sweden. Infants are fed either maternal or banked milk for the first time within the first 6 to 12 hours of life. They are fed 2 to 3 ml every 3 hours, increasing the amount slowly until the infant is on full enteral feedings, usually at 5 to 6 days of age. This NICU averages 800 to 900 admissions each year. However, its population of premature infants is somewhat different from that found in a US NICU. In Göteborg, all surgical cases, sick term newborns, and cardiac-care patients go to other hospitals. Nevertheless, the Göteborg NICU sees only one or two cases of NEC a year, also a rate of 0.2 percent (Arnold, 1999a), compared to an average United States NEC rate of about 10 percent. While some may view a 10 percent NEC rate as negligible and too small for concern, any rate of NEC over what would naturally occur in an exclusively human milk-fed population is unacceptable. Physicians constantly work toward reducing rates of NEC in their NICUs because of its added costs and its short- and long-term impact on growth and development in the infant.

Donor Milk Fortification. Low birth weight (LBW) and very low birth weight (VLBW) infants have nutritional requirements different from those of full-term infants because of nutrient malabsorption secondary to immaturity of their digestive systems. The composition of milk from preterm mothers differs from that of term mothers for about the first 2 to 4 weeks postpartum (Atkinson, Anderson, & Bryan, 1980; see also Chapter 3). HMBANA guidelines define preterm milk as the "milk pumped within the first month postpartum by a mother who delivered at or before 36 weeks gestation" (HMBANA, 2003; Luukkainen, Salo, & Nikkari, 1994). There has been a long-standing debate on whether LBW and VLBW infants can achieve proper growth on banked donor human milk obtained from mothers of term infants be-

cause of these compositional differences (AAP, 1985).

There are several mechanisms by which donor milk can better meet the nutritional needs of the preterm infant:

- *Efforts are made by donor milk banks to match gestationally appropriate milk to the recipient.* When preterm milk is donated, most milk banks separate it from the milk of mothers of term infants, so that it is available for younger preterm infants. Several milk banks can also supply colostrum separately.

- *Nutritional content or availability of nutrients in donor milk can be manipulated.* Milk banks in Scandinavia routinely use infrared analysis of each batch of donor milk (as well as maternal milk) to determine the protein, fat, and carbohydrate content of donor milk (see Figure 14–1) (Michaelsen et al., 1990; Arnold, 1999a). Individual milk donations can then be analyzed and pooled to produce milk with the desired levels of protein, fats, and carbohydrates to

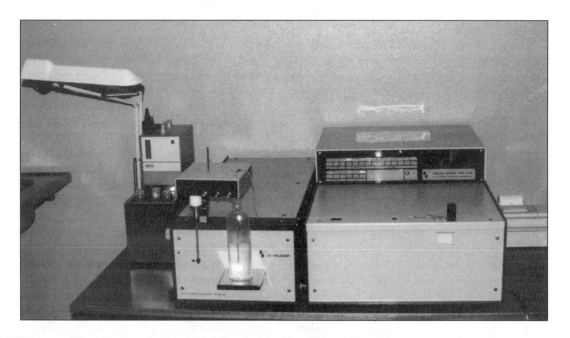

FIGURE 14–1. The MilcoScan infrared analyzer used in the milk bank in Hvidovre, Denmark. Small samples are warmed to maintain the flow of fat through the analyzer. As the milk passes through the analyzer from left to right, the scanner generates a printout of the carbohydrate, protein, and fat content of each batch of pasteurized milk. (From Arnold, 1999a. Reprinted with permission of Sage Publications.)

meet the requirements of preterm infants. Two milk banks in the United States also have the capacity to scan donor milk and can label batches nutritionally so that fortification can be individualized.

Martinez et al. (1987) used ultrasonic homogenization of expressed milk to prevent fat from adhering to feeding tubes. Premature Brazilian infants with an average birth weight of 1400 gm were fed pasteurized ultrasonically homogenized banked donor milk; they gained an average of 5 gm/day more than their counterparts receiving milk that had not been homogenized (Martinez, 1989). The group receiving the homogenized donor milk also had significantly greater gains in length, tricipital skinfold, and subscapular skinfold (Rayol et al., 1993; Martinez & Desai, 1995). Furthermore, they achieved intrauterine growth rates and hospital stays were shortened (Martinez, 1989). Martinez and Desai (1995) also report the use of a human milk "formula," a modification of banked donor milk from term mothers in which excess lactose is precipitated out, while leaving other nutrients in concentrated form. These are then diluted, homogenized, and pasteurized for later use.

- *More aggressive nutrition practices can be instituted as described above* (Ziegler, Thureen, & Carlson, 2002). Infants can be fed larger volumes of milk on demand. (See earlier discussion under Clinical Uses.)

- *Fortifiers can be added to or used separately from donor milk.* Human milk fortifiers are made from cow's milk and are not made out of human milk components as the name might imply. These fortifiers are in a powdered or liquid form, depending on the manufacturer. The "ready to feed" variety replaces the volume of human milk fed; therefore, infants fed this product receive smaller doses of human milk and its beneficial properties. Other types of fortification can be found in vegetable oils (sources of essential fatty acids), Polycose (carbohydrates in liquid form), and simple minerals such as calcium and phosphorus, which are added to improve bone mineralization. However, addition of some types of fortifiers to

human milk may increase its osmolality after storage and warming to levels that exceed current recommended limits of osmolality for premature infants (Fenton & Belik, 2002).

In addition to the risk of enterobacterial infection, the use of commercial bovine preparations to fortify human milk can impair the anti-infective properties of the milk. Quan, Mason, and Schanler, (1997) found significant decreases in lysozyme content and IgA specific for *E. coli* when fortifiers were added to fresh frozen milk. Jocson, Mason, and Schanler (1997) also noted an increase in bacterial growth during 24 hours of refrigeration when commercial fortifier was added to human milk, although this increase was not large. Differences were statistically significant, however, when fortified milk was refrigerated for 72 hours.

Many European milk banks have the ability to fractionate and lyophilize (i.e., freeze dry) human milk. Recent work has focused on using these fractionated and lyophilized components to fortify either maternal or donor milk on an individualized basis. (Hylmo et al., 1984; Polberger et al., 1999). Polberger et al. (1999) analyzed maternal and donor milk feedings daily for protein content, then either a bovine whey protein fortifier or a human milk protein fraction was added to bring the total protein content for each infant to 3.5 g/kg. Both groups demonstrated similar biochemical and growth results.

In Athens, Greece, mothers of healthy term newborns express their milk while they are in the hospital (average hospital stay, 4 to 5 days). This milk is pooled, pasteurized, and fed to premature infants. Mothers of preterm infants also express their milk. The milk fed to preterm infants thus consists primarily of unfortified colostrum and transitional milk from term mothers and milk from mothers of premature infants. In a study of 44 infants born weighing less than 1500 grams, infants fed the pooled pasteurized donor milk, their mother's own milk, or preterm formula were compared. All groups gained more than the intrauterine daily growth rate. The investigator concluded that the quality of banked milk determines appropriate growth (Zachou, 1996; see also Arnold, 2002c, p. 170).

Other Neonatal and Pediatric Uses. Other pediatric uses of banked donor human milk include cases of malabsorption and feeding intolerances (Asquith et al., 1987). Malabsorption is a well-recognized complication of neonatal surgical short gut. Banked milk is beneficial following surgery to repair damage from NEC and following surgery to repair congenital anomalies of the gastrointestinal tract, such as gastroschisis, tracheoesophageal fistulas, intestinal atresia, intestinal obstruction, anorectal abnormalities, and diaphragmatic hernias (Brink, 1977; Rangecroft, de San Lazaro, & Scott, 1978; Riddell, 1989). Historically, donor milk has also been used to control an outbreak of diarrhea in a NICU when antibiotics failed to stem the infection (Svirsky-Gross, 1958).

Infants who fail to thrive benefit from the use of donor milk, which helps them heal, gain weight, and gradually wean to foods they can tolerate without adverse effects (Arnold, 1995a). Subtle and sometimes unrecognized feeding intolerances may lead to failure to thrive or slow weight gain. Other feeding intolerances and allergies are more obvious, with gastrointestinal bleeding, projectile vomiting, wheezing, and skin rashes. Donor milk has been used in a number of cases where gastrointestinal bleeding was severe. Within 24 hours of starting exclusive donor milk feedings, bleeding ceased and the infant began to show improvement (Tully, 1996).

Donor milk has also been used in infants with the following conditions: cardiac problems (Radcliffe, 1995); chronic renal failure (Anderson & Arnold, 1993) and bronchopulmonary dysplasia (BPD) (Buchter & Wright, 1996); a glycolytic pathway defect (Arnold, 1995b); intractable diarrhea (Asquith et al., 1987); gastroenteritis and ulcerative colitis (Asquith et al., 1987); infantile botulism (Asquith et al., 1987); allergies to bovine proteins (Asquith et al., 1987); and IgA deficient patients (Asquith et al., 1987; Tully, 1990).

Donor milk is a metabolically ideal feeding medium for severely burned infants and children. Complications from stress ulcers are fewer when elemental formulas (e.g., formulas that have fats, proteins, and carbohydrates broken down into their simplest elements) are added to the diet of burn victims (Young, Motil, & Burke, 1981). However, elemental formulas are hyperosmolar, formulated for adults, and not meant for long-term pediatric use (Brady et al., 1986). Burn victims have an increased metabolism and therefore greater energy requirements, but they do not utilize glucose efficiently. They also have a higher rate of sepsis and would benefit from more immune factors (Young, Motil, & Burke, 1981). Human milk provides lactose as a more easily metabolized source of energy, immunoglobulins and other bacteriostatic protection, and growth factors for wound healing.

Other Uses. Merhav et al. (1995) use donor milk to supply IgA to adult liver transplant patients who are IgA-deficient. Donor milk has also been used in patients with immuno-depressed states related to bone marrow transplants or leukemia therapy (Asquith et al., 1987). Wiggins and Arnold (1998) describe the use of donor milk in the case of a young adult male with episodes of severe gastroesophageal reflux. Banked donor milk is also being used in some prostate cancer patients. More research needs to be done to determine the effectiveness of banked donor milk on tumors of various types. Banked donor milk has been used as hospice care in infants, children, and adults who are dying to provide them with amelioration of symptoms and a better quality of life remaining.

Current Practice

The HMBANA, in consultation with the FDA and the CDC, has developed guidelines to standardize donor milk banking operations. These guidelines follow the US Public Health Service recommendations for tissue and organ transplant banks (Centers for Disease Control, 1994) and are reviewed and revised annually. How milk banks in North America operate has been reviewed elsewhere (Arnold, 1997a, 1997b). Individuals interested in starting a milk bank may find the article by Tully (2000) helpful.

Donor Selection and Screening

Current guidelines do not allow payment of donors in the United States, although some European countries do allow paid donors (Arnold, 1999a). Williams et al. (1985) offer two reasons why mothers should not be paid: (1) to avoid the need for surveillance of milk for water dilution or addition of cow's milk to increase volume and therefore payment; and (2) to ensure that the mother's own infant is receiving adequate nutrition and is not being deprived of milk so that the mother can earn more money. When Brazil had a system of financial rewards to encourage donation of milk, a population of poor women often jeopardized their own infants' health to earn more income (Almeida, 2001). This type of collection system did not promote and protect breastfeeding. When the shift was made to an unpaid donation, the volume of milk collected increased, as did the number of donors.

Donors must be healthy, lactating women, usually of healthy full-term infants (Arnold & Borman, 1996). Mothers of preterm infants often donate their excess pumped milk, although some milk banks do not use this milk until the infant has either been discharged or is nursing well, to ensure sufficient maternal milk for this infant. Occasionally, a mother whose baby has died will donate milk that she has pumped. She may elect to continue pumping and donating after the infant's death as part of the grieving process. The process of donating this milk may help women to "feel like a mother" and give meaning to the infant's short life (Tully, 1999). The author has also worked with donors who have suffered fetal demises at 19 or 20 weeks gestation. With the drop in progesterone from delivery of the placenta these mothers produce milk. Unless they can turn the milk supply into something positive through donation, they go through the physical pain of engorgement as well as the emotional pain of having a constant reminder of their loss and how things might have been if the baby had survived. One young woman gave her term baby up for adoption, and expressed milk for 6 weeks until she returned to work. She commented to the author that the donation process made her "feel like a mother" and was very helpful in combating her depression over relinquishing her baby. Lactation supporters should be aware of this opportunity to donate.

Donor screening begins with a preliminary phone conversation and a few basic questions. Each donor is asked to complete a detailed health history that follows the American Association of Blood Banks guidelines for blood donor screening as well as some issues unique to breastfeeding. A current list of reasons why donors may be excluded from donating is found in Table 14–4.

Banked donor human milk is the only human donor tissue with three layers of protection for the recipient. Thorough donor screening is the

---

Table 14–4

REASONS FOR EXCLUDING POTENTIAL MILK DONORS

Women wishing to donate milk will be excluded from doing so for the following reasons:

- Receipt of a blood transfusion or blood products (with the exception of RhoGam) within the year prior to donating
- Receipt of an organ or tissue transplant within the last year
- Application of permanent make-up or tattooing applied with a needle, piercing of any body part, or accidental stick with a contaminated needle within the last year
- Regular use of more than 2 oz of hard liquor or its equivalent on a daily basis
- Regular use of over-the-counter medications or other systemic preparations
- Regular use of herbal products used as medication (including vitamin-herb combinations, and mega-doses of vitamins)
- Vegan diet, if not supplemented with vitamins
- Use of illegal drugs
- Use of tobacco products (cigarettes, cigars, snuff, chewing tobacco, etc.)
- History of chronic infection (e.g., HIV, HTLV, active TB, malaria), history of hepatitis, or history of cancer (except nonmelanoma skin cancer or cervical cancer *in situ*)
- History of a sexual partner during the last year who is at risk for HIV, HTLV, or hepatitis (including hemophiliacs or anyone who has used a needle for injection of illegal or nonprescription drugs)
- History of a sexual partner in the last year who has had tattoos, body piercings, application of permanent make-up using needles, or accidental stick with a contaminated needle
- History of receiving human pituitary derived growth hormone, or dura mater (brain covering) graft, or having a family history of Creutzfeldt-Jakob disease
- Residence outside North America since 1980, according to the American Association of Blood Banks guidelines

---

Source: Adapted from HMBANA (2003).

first layer. After answering the health question-naire, donors are also serum-screened for a panel of viruses. The current screening includes HIV-1 and HIV-2 antibody and antigen; human T-cell Leukemia Virus (HTLV-1) antibody; hepatitis B surface antigen; hepatitis C antibody; and syphilis. As new viruses and problems emerge, new serum tests will be added as deemed necessary by the US Public Health Service, the FDA, and/or the CDC.

Collection

Milk banks may supply donors with sterile collection containers for milk collection if they are continuous donors. In recent years, many donors in the United States have been women who make a one-time-only donation: They have a stockpile of hundreds or thousands of frozen ounces that their baby is never going to use and donate this stockpile in a single transaction. While milk banks welcome this sort of milk because of the need for volume, some quality control is lost because the donor has not been instructed in careful collection techniques nor been given sterile containers. The type of container the donor has chosen may also affect the quality of the milk, and the duration of storage in the home setting may also lead to greater compromise of milk composition (Goldblum et al., 1981). (See also Appendix 14-A for an outline of storage and handling recommendations for both home and hospital.)

Differences in collection methods can affect nutrient content, especially the amount of fat in the milk. Milk that is passively collected from one breast while the infant feeds at the other (drip milk) may be low in fat. Pumped milk contains a higher fat content than drip milk because of the negative pressure exerted by the pump (Arnold, 1997c). Drip milk also tends to be more contaminated (Gibbs et al., 1977). Milk banks rarely use drip milk now, but older studies in which donor milk was used may have used drip milk. This is the case for Lucas's prospective longitudinal study of diet in preterm infants (Lucas et al., 1984). Lack of fat as well as restricted feeding volumes may explain some of the less than favorable growth outcomes in studies using drip milk. Despite this loss of fat, the donor milk proved to be beneficial for the infants that received it (Lucas & Cole, 1990).

Pasteurization

The second level of protection is pasteurization of banked donor milk. Fresh-frozen milk may be provided in those rare circumstances where an individual recipient does not tolerate pasteurized milk, and then only with informed consent.

Milk from several different donors is thawed and pooled to make a batch. Pooling mixes milks of various fat concentrations to ensure a more even distribution of fat from one batch to another (AAP, 1980). Once a batch is thoroughly mixed and poured into small bottles (Figure 14–2) the containers are tightly capped and submerged in a constant

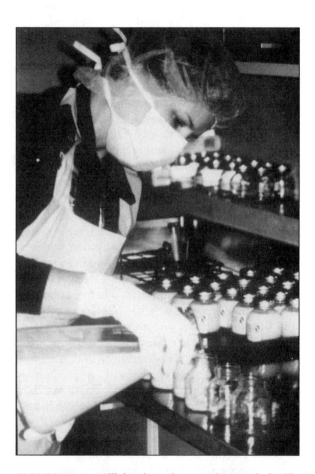

FIGURE 14–2. Milk bank worker pouring pooled milk into bottles for pasteurizing. (With permission from the Mothers' Milk Bank, Denver, Colorado, USA.)

temperature water bath (Figure 14–3). Some milk banks use human milk pasteurizers designed specifically for this purpose. A control bottle is also placed in the water bath so that the temperature of the milk can be monitored. When the control bottle reaches 62.5°C, the batch is held at that temperature for 30 minutes. This is called Holder pasteurization. Because cytomegalovirus is reliably destroyed at this temperature, North American milk banks have opted to use 62.5°C as the only acceptable temperature for pasteurization (Dworsky et al., 1982; Friis & Andersen, 1982). When the pasteurization process is complete, the bottles are removed from the water bath and chilled rapidly. Once the bottles are thoroughly chilled and a culture sample taken, they are frozen pending the results of bacterial culture (Figure 14–4) and dispensed *only on prescription* (Arnold, 1998).

The third layer of safety guarantees quality assurance of the final product. One bottle from each batch is chosen at random and a small sample is drawn for bacteriological culture. No milk is dispensed unless the bacteria counts after pasteurization are at 0 CFU (colony-forming units) per milliliter. Better quality assurance could be achieved if milk banks tested the pool of milk from each donor prior to pasteurization so that collection techniques among ongoing donors could be improved through education. Another method of quality control is to conduct bacterial assays of the pool of milk prior to pasteurization. There is a risk of release of toxins by certain bacteria as they undergo pasteurization, so the potential to know what the milk contains prior to pasteurization might be valuable. However, the level of toxin release in relation to bacterial counts is not known, nor is it known what level of toxin is a potential threat to an infant. Milk banks in the United Kingdom are required by their guidelines to have prepasteurization and postpasteurization cultures. If prepasteurization

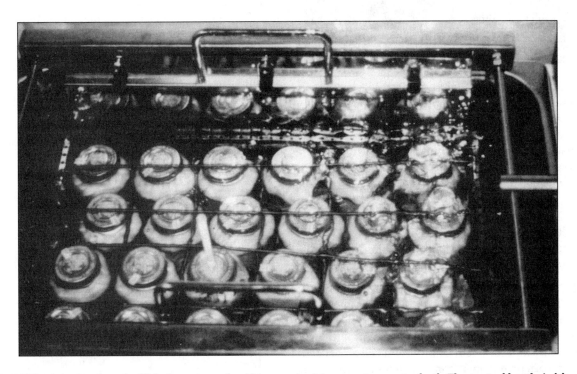

FIGURE 14–3. Bottles of milk being pasteurized in a constant temperature water bath. The control bottle (with the thermometer) indicates when the temperature of the milk reaches 62.5°F, and pasteurization time of 30 minutes is counted from that point. (With permission from the Mothers' Milk Bank, Denver, Colorado, USA.)

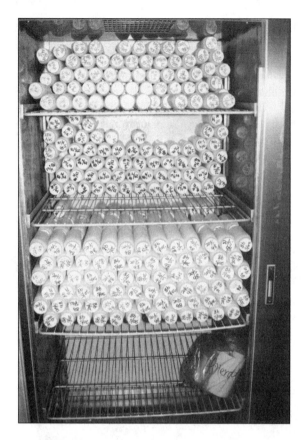

FIGURE 14–4. Bottles of pasteurized milk in the freezer waiting to be dispensed by the Hvidovre milk bank. This milk bank has had special bottles designed with a triangular cross section which allows a more stable stacking method to optimize utilization of freezer space. (From Arnold, 1999a. Reprinted with permission of Sage Publications.)

cultures show evidence of pathogens or colony counts exceed 10^5 CFU/ml, then the milk is discarded (Balmer, 1995; UKAMB, 2003).

Effects of Pasteurization. In 1989, using donor milk banking procedures, the FDA and the CDC conducted experiments to see whether pasteurization at 62.5°C destroyed HIV. Donor milk was spiked with HIV (both cell-free and cell-associated) and pasteurized in a constant temperature water bath. Destruction of the virus was rapid, and no virus could be recovered through culturing after processing at 62.5°C (Orloff, Wallingford, & McDougal, 1993). These results confirmed those of Eglin and Wilkinson (1987). As new viruses are identified, it will be important to assess each virus using this standard laboratory technique.

Heat treatment affects various milk components. The general rule of thumb is that the higher the temperature the greater the loss. As part of the FDA/CDC study above, Eitenmiller (1990) looked at various components of human milk and analyzed what was left after employing milk banking processing protocols. His results are listed in Table 14–5. Other studies as cited in Tully, Jones, and Tully (2001) have found smaller losses, citing 70 percent retention of IgA and 40 percent retention of lactoferrin. Growth factors are heat stable (Wallingford, 1987), as are fatty acids, including the long-chain polyunsaturated fatty acids so important to neurological development (Tully, Jones, & Tully, 2001; see also Lawrence, 2002). However, despite these losses banked donor human milk retains its antibacterial and antiviral activity. Formula has no IgA; retention of 70 percent of human milk IgA during pasteurization gives the edge to donor milk.

The effects of freezing, heating, and handling of human milk are cumulative. Garza, Hopkinson, & Schanler (1986) reported that freezing affects lipids in human milk by breaking down fat-globule membranes, thereby decreasing the size of the fat globules and increasing the surface available for lipase

Table 14–5

EFFECTS OF HOLDER PASTEURIZATION ON HUMAN MILK COMPONENTS*

Bacterial Markers	
Staphylococcus aureus	100% killed
Escherichia coli	100% killed
Components	
Lactoferrin	22%
IgA	51%
Folic acid	57%
Lysozyme	100%
Phosphatase	1.4%

Source: From Eitenmiller (1990).
Expressed as percentage retained after 30 minutes at 62.5°C

activity. This may lessen the digestibility and availability of fat to the patient. The counterargument might be that as the fat-globule membrane breaks down, more of the fat globule core contents of triglycerides may be released. This might be an advantage to the infant with immature enzyme systems, especially since the lipases in human milk (lipoprotein lipase and bile salt activated lipase) are very sensitive to heat and do not survive pasteurization (Hamosh, 1997; Tully, Jones, & Tully, 2001).

To avoid some of these losses, lyophilization and irradiation to reduce bacterial and viral content have been explored. However, early reports indicated that both these methods also lowered the concentration of immune substances (Liebhaber et al., 1977; Raptopoulou-Gigi, Marwick, & McClelland, 1977). Oxtoby (1988) also reports that they may not be effective in destroying HIV.

Packaging and Transport

Milk can be shipped over great distances by bus or airline. For long-distance shipping of frozen milk dry ice should be used. Containers may be styrofoam boxes, picnic coolers, insulated boxes used to ship blood or frozen chemicals, etc. Overnight shipping companies can successfully move milk from one location to another without having it thaw.

Costs of Banked Donor Milk

Banked donated human milk is not sold in the United States, but all US milk banks charge a processing fee to help cover some of the costs of production. As of this writing, the average cost per ounce is $3.50 plus shipping of the milk. While this may appear expensive at first glance, there are accrued cost benefits when banked donor human milk is used. Wight (2001) estimates that for every $1 spent in the NICU on donor milk there are savings of between $11 and $37 in NICU costs. Using several models, Arnold (2002a) calculated the approximate cost of using banked donor human milk for a hypothetical preterm infant. The cost of donor milk plus fortifier was estimated to be about $1350. When one considers that the cost of a nonsurgical case of NEC adds approximately $73,700 to the cost of caring for a preterm infant, $1350 is a very small price to pay for prevention of NEC (Bisquera, Cooper, & Berseth, 2002).

Policy Statements Supporting the Use of Banked Donor Human Milk

The World Health Organization has a remarkably consistent policy with regard to human milk banking. In 1979, WHO and UNICEF issued a joint resolution on infant and young child feeding that was fully endorsed by the World Health Assembly in 1980. The "first alternative" when a mother is unable to breastfeed should be human breastmilk, using banked donor milk where appropriate and available (WHO/UNICEF, 1980). In 1992 banked donor milk was included as an acceptable feeding alternative when the biological mother tests positive for HIV (WHO/UNICEF, 1992). In 1998 banked donor milk was presented as an option in a publication on HIV and infant feeding (WHO, 1998). In 2002 the World Health Assembly unanimously endorsed the Global Strategy for Infant and Young Child Feeding, which recommends banked donor milk as an option when an infant cannot breastfeed and/or the mother's own expressed milk is unavailable. Savage (1998) has shared a WHO Feeding Hierarchy for Low Birth Weight Infants, which includes donated human milk as part of the hierarchy (Arnold, 2002b).

WHO has also affirmed the importance of donor milk banking in the awarding of the prestigious Sasakawa Prize for 2001 to Dr. Joao Aprigio Guerra de Almeida of Brazil for his work in organizing the largest and most important donor milk banking system in the world. At last count, more than 180 milk banks distribute banked donor human milk in Brazil. For the year 1999–2000, the milk banks of Brazil collected and processed more than 218,000 liters of donated milk and distributed it to over 300,000 premature and low birth weight infants, saving the country's Ministry of Health more than $540 million per year (INFACT Canada, 2001; IBFAN, 2001). The entire community is involved in this project and firemen pick up the donated milk from the mothers in their communities. The use of donor milk in Brazil is part of a comprehensive public health policy aimed at reducing infant mortality.

UNICEF supports a role for banked donor human milk. Banked donor milk usage is implied in the GOBI Initiative (the acronym stands for Growth, Oral rehydration, Breastfeeding, and Immunization). Breastfeeding (human milk) is an integral part of oral rehydration, growth, and immunization (Arnold, 2002b). The Baby-Friendly Hospital Initiative (BFHI) through the Ten Steps to Successful Breastfeeding has a place for donated human milk. If the mother's own milk is unavailable, donor milk is the next choice.

Professional associations also issue policy statements concerning donor human milk banks. A recent example is that of the Royal Australasian College of Physicians (2003). The German Pediatric Society also has a statement in support of donor milk banking (as cited in Springer, 1997). In the United States the last statement specifically addressing donor milk banking from the American Academy of Pediatrics was published in 1980 (AAP, 1980). However, subsequent publications such as the *Pediatric Nutrition Handbook* (1998), the AAP *Red Book* (2003), and the *Guidelines for Perinatal Care* (2002) are considered statements of policy and standards of practice. In a departure from previous editions and other policy statements issued by the American Academy of Pediatrics, the 2002 edition of the *Guidelines for Perinatal Care* states, "The use of pooled human milk is the least satisfactory regimen for feeding newborns and should be discouraged" (p. 230). However, not a single supporting reference is offered to back this opinion. It is discouraging to see such an austere group basing policy statements on opinions rather than scientific evidence. The 2003 edition of the *Red Book* contradicts the 2002 edition of the *Guidelines for Perinatal Care*. In 1997, the AAP issued this statement in "Breastfeeding and the Use of Human Milk" (AAP, 1997): "Human milk is the preferred feeding for all infants, including premature and sick infants, with rare exceptions" (p. 1036). While not mentioned specifically, donor milk banking has its place in this statement. The Academy of Breastfeeding Medi-

cine published clinical protocols that specifically recommend the use of banked donor milk for supplementing healthy term infants in the hospital. "If the volume of mother's own colostrum does not meet her infant's feeding requirements, pasteurized donor human milk is preferable to other supplements" (Academy of Breastfeeding Medicine, 2002).

Some countries have established regulations and policies concerning banked donor human milk. France and Germany have operating procedures that are governed by public health law. Beyond that, however, the process depends on how banked donor milk is treated within the medical system and whether it is an item that is covered by the healthcare system. In Canada and in Scandinavia and other European countries, parents do not have to pay out of pocket for donor milk; it is covered as a benefit by national health plans. In the United States, because of the lack of a single-payer healthcare system, the processing fee charged to recipients or their families is not always covered by health insurance. (This processing fee is not a charge for the milk itself but a fee to defray the expense of screening donors and the labor involved in pasteurizing the milk.) Private insurers do not always cover the cost of banked donor milk. Some of the large insurers have policies concerning coverage for donor milk that differ from one state to another.

In some states, Medicaid covers qualifying infants and children. The CDC considers donor milk a tissue transplant and has provided valuable advice on developing guidelines that acknowledge this (CDC, 1994). In general, the expansion of milk banking services in the United States is hampered by a lack of governmental policy and a contradiction in how different governmental agencies perceive donor milk.

Summary

The availability of banked donor human milk is essential to a small but needy population. Without it, some patients would not survive. For others, donor human milk may help to prevent long-term medical problems. Although some experts agree on the effi-

cacy of donor human milk as therapy, much of the data are in anecdotal form.

The challenge in North America is to educate the health-care provider who will be writing the prescription so that any patient who needs banked donor human milk will be able to receive it rapidly. In the absence of the biological mother's own milk, banked donor human milk should be considered by physicians in the treatment plan for certain infants, children, and adults.

Key Concepts

- Donor human milk banking is a highly controlled method of supplying human milk to recipients that differs substantially from wet nursing.
- Cultural beliefs may affect the availability of donors as well as clinical uses of banked donor human milk.
- Protective policies at the governmental level are essential to the survival and growth of donor milk banking.
- Little "residual" is found in donor milk-fed infants owing to the digestibility of banked donor milk.
- Banked human milk promotes growth, maturation, and healing of tissues and organ systems.
- Use of banked donor human milk provides immunological protection to ill recipients who have weakened immune systems.
- Where supplies of donor human milk are low, prioritization of clinical uses favor the ill infant for whom there is no feeding alternative.

- Banked donor human milk is more than just a food: it is a therapeutic agent and preventive medicine.
- Internationally, the use of banked human milk for feeding premature infants in the absence of maternal milk is the primary clinical use.
- There are a wide variety of clinical uses of banked donor milk.
- Banked donor human milk is dispensed only by prescription.
- All donors to a milk bank are screened verbally and serologically.
- All banked human milk is pasteurized and bacteriologically tested prior to distribution, unless there is a medical reason why the recipient cannot tolerate pasteurized milk.
- Pasteurization does not destroy all beneficial components in human milk.
- Considerable cost savings can be realized from the reduction in mortality and morbidity in recipients of banked human milk.

Internet Resources

Ace-Intermed (a source for single-bottle human milk pasteurizer):
www.ace-intermed.com/products.htm

The Human Milk Banking Association of North America (HMBANA):
www.hmbana.com

United Kingdom Association of Milk Banks (UKAMB):
www.ukamb.org

References

Academy of Breastfeeding Medicine. ABM Clinical Protocol Number 3: hospital guidelines for the use of supplementary feedings in the healthy term breastfed neonate. *ABM News & Views* 8(2):10–11, 2002.

Almeida JAG. *Breastfeeding: a nature-culture hybrid.* Rio de Janeiro, Brazil: Editora FIOCRUZ, 2001.

AL-Naqeeb NA et al. The introduction of breast milk donation in a Muslim country. *J Hum Lact* 16:346–50, 2000.

American Academy of Pediatrics (AAP), Committee on Fetus and Newborn, and American College of Obstetricians and Gynecologists, Committee on Obstetric Practice. *Guidelines for perinatal care.* 5th ed. Elk Grove Village, IL: American Academy of Pediatrics, 2002.

American Academy of Pediatrics (AAP), Committee on Infectious Diseases. *2003 red book.* 26th Edition. Elk Grove Village, IL: American Academy of Pediatrics, 2003.

American Academy of Pediatrics (AAP), Committee on Mother's Milk. Recommended standards for the operation of mothers' milk bureaus. *J Pediatr* 23:112–28, 1943.

American Academy of Pediatrics (AAP), Committee on Nutrition. Human milk banking. *Pediatrics* 65:854–57, 1980.

———. Nutritional needs of low-birth-weight infants. *Pediatrics* 75:976–86, 1985.

———. *Pediatric nutrition handbook.* 4th ed. Elk Grove Village, IL: American Academy of Pediatrics, 1998.

American Academy of Pediatrics (AAP), Work Group on Breastfeeding. Breastfeeding and the use of human milk. *Pediatrics* 100:1035–39, 1997.

Anderson A, Arnold LDW. Use of donor breastmilk in the nutrition management of chronic renal failure: three case histories. *J Hum Lact* 9:263–64, 1993.

Anderson JW, Johnstone BM, Remley DT. Breast-feeding and cognitive development: a meta-analysis. *Amer J Clin Nutr* 70:525–35, 1999.

Arnold LDW. Milk bank survey—Preliminary report of findings and discussion. *HMBANA Newsl* 3:7–9, 1988.

———. The statistical state of human milk banking and what's in the future. *J Hum Lact* 7:25–27, 1991.

———. The lactariums of France: Part 1. The Lactarium Docteur Raymond Fourcade in Marmande. *J Hum Lact* 10:125–26, 1994.

———. Use of donor human milk in the management of failure to thrive: case histories. *J Hum Lact* 11:137–40, 1995a.

———. Use of donor milk in the treatment of metabolic disorders: glycolytic pathway defects. *J Hum Lact* 11:51–53, 1995b.

———. Donor milk banking in China: the ultimate step in becoming Baby Friendly. *J Hum Lact* 12:297–99, 1996.

———. How North American donor milk banks operate: results of a survey, Part 1. *J Hum Lact* 13:159–62, 1997a.

———. How North American donor milk banks operate: results of a survey, Part 2. *J Hum Lact* 13:243–46, 1997b.

———. A brief look at drip milk and its relation to donor human milk banking. *J Hum Lact* 13:323–24, 1997c.

———. How to order banked donor milk in the United States: what the health care provider needs to know. *J Hum Lact* 14:65–67, 1998.

———. Donor milk banking in Scandinavia. *J Hum Lact* 15:55–59, 1999a.

———. *Recommendations for collection, storage and handling of a mother's milk for her owni infant in the hospital setting.* 3rd ed. Raleigh, NC: Human Milk Banking Association of North America, 1999b.

———. Trends in donor milk banking in the United States. In: Newburg D, ed. *Bioactive components of human milk.* New York: Kluwer Academic/Plenum Publishers, 2001:509–17.

———. The cost-effectiveness of using banked donor milk in the neonatal intensive care unit: prevention of necrotizing enterocolitis. *J Hum Lact* 18:172–77, 2002a.

———. Human milk for fragile infants. In: Cadwell K, ed. *Reclaiming breastfeeding for the United States: protection, promotion and support.* Boston: Jones and Bartlett, 2002b: 137–59.

———. Using banked donor milk in clinical settings. In: Cadwell K, ed. *Reclaiming breastfeeding for the United States: protection, promotion and support.* Boston: Jones and Bartlett, 2002c:161–78.

Arnold LDW, Borman LL. What are the characteristics of the ideal human milk donor? *J Hum Lact* 12:143–45, 1996.

Arnold LDW, Courdent M. The lactariums of France: Part 2. How association milk banks operate. *J Hum Lact* 10:195–96, 1994.

Asquith MT et al. Clinical uses, collection, and banking of human milk. *Clin Perinatol* 14:173–85, 1987.

Atkinson SA, Anderson GH, Bryan MH. Human milk: comparison of the nitrogen composition in milk from mothers of premature and full-term infants. *Am J Clin Nutr* 33:811–15, 1980.

Balmer SE. Donor milk banking and guidelines in Britain. *J Hum Lact* 11:221–23, 1995.

Balmer SE, Wharton BA. Human milk banking at Sorrento Maternity Hospital, Birmingham. *Arch Dis Child* 67:556–59, 1992.

Bisquera JA, Cooper TR, Berseth CL. Impact of necrotizing enterocolitis on length of stay and hospital charges in very low birth weight infants. *Pediatrics* 109:423–28, 2002.

Brady MS et al. Specialized formulas and feedings for infants with malabsorption or formula intolerance. *J Am Diet Assoc* 86:191–200, 1986.

Brink S. The successful use of human breast milk in a premature infant with the surgical short gut syndrome. *Am J Dis Child* 131:471, 1977.

Buchter S, Wright L. Use of donor milk for the treatment of severe formula intolerance in a preterm infant with chronic lung disease and failure to thrive: a case presentation. Presented at: Annual meeting of the Human Milk Banking Association of North America, Raleigh, NC, March 1, 1996.

Centers for Disease Control. Guidelines for preventing transmission of human immunodeficiency virus through transplantation of human tissue and organs. *MMWR* 43(RR-8): 1–17, 1994.

Davis WH. Statistical comparison of the mortality of breast-fed and bottle-fed infants. *Am J Dis Child* 5:234–47, 1913.

Dworsky M et al. Persistence of cytomegalovirus in human milk after storage. *J Pediatr* 101:440–43, 1982.

Eglin RP, Wilkinson AR. HIV infection and pasteurisation of breast milk. *Lancet* 1:1093, 1987.

Eibl MM et al. Prevention of necrotizing enterocolitis in low-birth-weight infants by IgA-IgG feeding. *NEJM* 319:1–7, 1988.

Eitenmiller R. An overview of human milk pasteurization. Presented at: Annual meeting of the Human Milk Banking Association of North America, Lexington, KY, October 15, 1990.

Fenton TR, Belik J. Routine handling of milk fed to preterm infants can significantly increase osmolality. *J Pediatr Gastroenterol Nutr* 35:298–302, 2002.

Fidler N et al. Fat content and fatty acid composition of fresh, pasteurized, or sterilized human milk. In: Newberg D, ed. *Bioactive components in human milk.* New York: Kluwer Academic/Plenum Press, 2001:485–495.

Fildes V. *Wet nursing: a history from antiquity to the present.* Oxford: Basil Blackwell, 1988.

Friis H, Andersen HK. Rate of inactivation of cytomegalovirus in raw banked milk during storage at –20°C and pasteurization. *Brit Med J* 285:1604–5, 1982.

Garza C, Hopkinson J, Schanler RJ. Human milk banking. In: Howell RR, Morriss RH, Pickering LK, eds. *Human milk in infant nutrition and health.* Springfield, IL: Charles C. Thomas, 1986: 225–55.

Gibbs JH et al. Drip breast milk: its composition, collection and pasteurization. *Early Hum Devel* 1:227–45, 1977.

Goes HCA et al. Nutrient composition of banked human milk in Brazil and influence of processing on zinc distribution in milk fractions. *Nutrition* 18:590–94, 2002.

Goldblum RM et al. Human milk banking I: effects of container upon immunologic factors in mature milk. *Nutr Res* 1:449–59, 1981.

Golden J. From wet nurse directory to milk bank: the delivery of human milk in Boston, 1909–1927. *Bull Hist Med* 62:589–605, 1988.

Hamosh M. Digestion in the premature infant: the effects of human milk. *Sem Perinatol* 18:485–94, 1994.

———. Digestive enzymes in human milk: stability at suboptimal storage temperatures. *J Pediatr Gastroenterol Nutr* 24:38–43, 1997.

Hong Y. Personal commmunication. 2001.

Human Milk Banking Association of North America: (HMBANA). *Guidelines for the establishment and operation of a donor human milk bank.* Tully M, ed. Raleigh, NC: HMBANA, 2003.

Hylmo P et al. Preparation of fat and protein from banked human milk: its use in feeding very-low-birth-weight infants. In: Williams AF, Baum JD, eds. *Human milk banking.* Nestle Nutrition Workshop Series Vol. 5. New York: Vevey/Raven Press, 1984:55–61.

Ighogboja IS et al. Mothers' attitudes towards donated breastmilk in Jos, Nigeria. *J Hum Lact* 11:93–96, 1995.

IBFAN. Brazil leads world in human milk banks. *IBFAN INFO* 3(4):5, November, 2001.

INFACT Canada: Brazil wins prestigious WHO Sasakawa prize. *INFACT* 2001:10.

Isaacs CE, Thormar H. Human milk lipids inactivate enveloped viruses. In: Atkinson SA, Hanson LA, Chandra RK, eds. *Human Lactation 4: breastfeeding, nutrition, infection and infant growth in developed and emerging countries.* St. John's, Newfoundland: ARTS Biomedical Publisher, 1990:161–74.

Jocson MAL, Mason EO, Schanler RJ. The effects of nutrient fortification and varying storage conditions on host

defense properties of human milk. *Pediatrics* 100:240–43, 1997.

Lawrence RA. Milk banking: the influence of storage procedures and subsequent processing on immunologic components of human milk. In: Woodward B, Draper HH, eds. *Immunological properties of milk*, vol. 10, *Advances in Nutritional Research.* New York: Kluwer Academic/Plenum Publishers, 2002:389–404.

Liebhaber M et al. Alterations of lymphocytes and of antibody content of human milk after processing. *J Pediatr* 91:897–900, 1977.

Lucas A, Cole TJ. Breast milk and neonatal necrotising enterocolitis. *Lancet* 336:1519–23, 1990.

Lucas A et al. Multicentre trial on feeding low birthweight infants: effects of diet on early growth. *Arch Dis Child* 59:722–30, 1984.

———. Breast milk and subsequent intelligence quotient in children born preterm. *Lancet* 339:261–264, 1992.

Luukkainen P, Salo MK, Nikkari T. Changes in the fatty acid composition of preterm and term human milk from 1 week to 6 months of lactation. *J Pediatr Gastroenterol Nutr* 18:355–60, 1994.

———. The fatty acid composition of banked human milk and infant formulas: the choices of milk for feeding preterm infants. *Eur J Pediatr* 154:316–19, 1995.

Martinez FE. Growth of premature neonates fed banked pasteurized human milk homogenized by ultrasonication. Presented at: Annual meeting of the Human Milk Banking Association of North America, Vancouver, British Columbia, October 15, 1989.

Martinez FE, Desai ID. Human milk and premature infants. In: Simopoulos AP, Dutra de Oliveira JE, Desai ID, eds. *Behavioral and metabolic aspects of breastfeeding*, vol. 78, World Rev Nutr Diet. Basel: Karger, 1995:55–73.

Martinez FE et al. Ultrasonic homogenization of expressed human milk to prevent fat loss during tube feeding. *J Pediatr Gastroenterol Nutr* 6:593–97, 1987.

McPherson RJ, Wagner CL. The effect of pasteurization on transforming growth factor alpha and transforming growth factor beta 2 concentrations in human milk. In: Newberg D, ed. *Bioactive components in human milk.* New York: Kluwer Academic/Plenum, 2001:559–66.

Merhav HJ et al. Treatment of IgA deficiency in liver transplant recipients with human breast milk. *Transplant Int* 8:327–29, 1995.

Michaelsen KM et al. Variation in macronutrients in human bank milk: influencing factors and implications for human milk banking. *J Pediatr Gastroenterol Nutr* 11:229–39, 1990.

Narayanan I et al. Partial supplementation with expressed breast-milk for prevention of infection in low-birth-weight infants. *Lancet* (September 13):561–63, 1980.

———. Randomised controlled trial of effect of raw and holder pasteurised human milk and of formula supplements on incidence of neonatal infection. *Lancet* (November 17):1111–13, 1984.

Orloff SL, Wallingford JC, McDougal JS. Inactivation of human immunodeficiency virus type I in human milk:

effects of intrinsic factors in human milk and of pasteurization. *J Hum Lact* 9:13–17, 1993.

Oxtoby MJ. Human immunodeficiency virus and other viruses in human milk: placing the issues in broader perspective. *Pediatr Infect Dis J* 7:825–35, 1988.

Penc B. Organization and activity of a human milk bank in Poland. *J Hum Lact* 12:226–29, 1996.

Polberger S et al. Individualized protein fortification of human milk for preterm infants: comparison of ultrafiltrated human milk protein and a bovine whey fortifier. *J Pediatr Gastroenterol Nutr* 29:332–38, 1999.

Quan R et al. The effect of nutritional additives on anti-infective factors in human milk. *Clin Pediatr* 33:325–328, 1994.

Radcliffe A. Personal communication. 1995.

Rangecroft L, de San Lazaro C, Scott JES. A comparison of the feeding of the postoperative newborn with banked breast-milk or cow's-milk feeds. *J Pediatr Surg* 13:11–12, 1978.

Raptopoulou-Gigi M, Marwick K, McClelland DBL. Antimicrobial proteins in sterilized human milk. *Br Med J* 1:12–14, 1977.

Rayol MRS et al. Feeding premature infants banked human milk homogenized by ultrasonic treatment. *J Pediatr* 123:985–88, 1993.

Riddell DG. Use of banked human milk for feeding infants with abdominal wall defects. Presented at: Annual meeting of the Human Milk Banking Association of North America, Vancouver, British Columbia, October 15, 1989.

Royal Australasian College of Physicians. Paediatric policy: human milk banking. Available at: http://www.racp.edu.au/hpu/paed/milkbank/index.htm. Accessed January 15, 2003.

Savage F. Personal communication. 1998.

Schanler RJ, Shulman RJ, Lau C. Feeding strategies for premature infants: beneficial outcomes of feeding fortified human milk versus preterm formula. *Pediatrics* 103:1150–57, 1999.

Schanler RJ et al. Pasteurized donor human milk vs. preterm formula if mother's own milk is unavailable for the extremely premature infant: a randomized trial. [Abstract #PL2] *ABM News & Views* 8:18, 2002

Sharpe G. Donor milk in the NICU. Presented at: 20th Annual Breastfeeding Conference, "Breastfeeding Premature Infants: A Blueprint for Success," Brigham and Women's Hospital, Natick, MA, May 31, 2002.

Siimes MA, Hallman N. A perspective on human milk banking, 1978. *J Pediatr* 94:173–74, 1979.

Sotirova V. Personal communication. 2002.

Springer S. Human milk banking in Germany. *J Hum Lact* 13:65–68, 1997.

———. News about human milk banking in Germany. In: Koletzko B et al., eds. *Short and long term effects of breast feeding on child health.* New York: Kluwer Academic/Plenum, 2000:441–442.

Svirsky-Gross S. Pathogenic strains of coli (0,111) among prematures and the use of human milk in controlling the outbreak of diarrhea. *Ann Paediatr* 190:109–115, 1958.

Tagge ME. Wet nursing 2001: old practice, new dilemmas? *J Hum Lact* 17:140–41, 2001.

Talbot FB. A directory for wet-nurses: its experiences for twelve months. *JAMA* 56:1715–17, 1911.

Thureen PJ, Hay WW. Early aggressive nutrition in preterm infants. *Sem Neonatol* 6:403–15, 2001.

Tully DB, Jones F, Tully MR. Donor milk: what's in it and what's not. *J Hum Lact* 17:152–55, 2001.

Tully MR. Banked human milk in the treatment of IgA deficiency and allergy symptoms. *J Hum Lact* 6:75, 1990.

———. Personal communication. 1996.

———. Donating human milk as part of the grieving process. *J Hum Lact* 15:149–151, 1999.

———. Cost of establishing and operating a donor human milk bank. *J Hum Lact* 16:57–59, 2000.

———. Recipient prioritization and use of human milk in the hospital setting. *J Hum Lact* 18:393–96, 2002.

United Kingdom Association for Milk Banking (UKAMB). *Guidelines for the establishment and operation of human milk banks in the UK.* 3rd ed. London: Royal College of Paediatrics and Child Health, 2003.

Wallingford J. Nutritional and anti-infective consequences of pasteurization of breast milk. Presented at: Annual meeting of the Human Milk Banking Association of North America, Raleigh, NC, October 15, 1987.

Wiggins PK, Arnold LDW. Clinical case history: donor milk use for severe gastroesophageal reflux in an adult. *J Hum Lact* 14:157–58, 1998.

Wight NE. Donor human milk for preterm infants. *J Perinatol* 21:249–54, 2001.

Williams AF et al. Human milk banking. *J Trop Pediatr* 31:185–90, 1985.

Williams-Arnold LD. *Human milk storage for healthy infants and children.* Sandwich, MA: Health Education Associates, 2000.

Wolf JH. *Don't kill your baby: public health and the decline of breastfeeding in the 19th and 20th centuries.* Columbus, OH: Ohio State University Press, 2001.

World Health Organization (WHO). *HIV and infant feeding. A guide for health care managers and supervisors.* Geneva: WHO. WHO/FRH/NUT/CHD/98.2. 1998. Available at: http://www.who.int/nut/publications.htm#inf. Accessed February 5, 2003.

———. Infant and young child nutrition: global strategy on infant and young child feeding. 55th World Health Assembly, A55/15, 16 April, 2002. Available at: http://www.who.int/gb/EB_WHA/PDF/WHA55/ea5515.pdf. Accessed February 5, 2003.

World Health Organization/United Nations Children's Fund (WHO/UNICEF). Meeting on infant and young child feeding. *J Nurs-Midwif* 25:31–38, 1980.

———. *Concensus statement from the WHO/UNICEF consultation on HIV transmission and breast-feeding.* Geneva, 2 pp., April 30, May 1, 1992.

Xanthou M. Immunology of breast milk. In: Stern L, ed. *Feeding the sick infant.* New York: Raven Press, 1987: 101–17.

Young VR, Motil KJ, Burke JF. Energy and protein metabolism in relation to requirements of the burned pediatric patient. In: Suskind RM, ed. *Textbook of pediatric nutrition.* New York: Raven Press, 1981:309–40.

Zachou T. Growth in preterm infants fed different types of feedings. Presented at: Annual meeting of the Human Milk Banking Association of North America, Raleigh, NC, March 1, 1996

Ziegler EE, Thureen PJ, Carlson SJ. Aggressive nutrition of the very low birthweight infant. *Clin Perinatol* 29:225–44, 2002.

Appendix 14-A

STORAGE AND HANDLING OF EXPRESSED HUMAN MILK

This appendix is based on the following two publications: (1) *Recommendations for Collection, Storage and Handling of a Mother's Milk for Her Own Infant in the Hospital Setting* (Arnold, 1999b) and (2) *Human Milk Storage for Healthy Infants and Children* (Williams-Arnold, 2000). The latter publication also provides recommendations for storage of human milk in the workplace and in child-care settings.

Depending on the health and age of the infant, expressed human milk should be handled with different degrees of safety precautions. Banked donor milk requires the highest level of safety precautions because it is used to feed and treat infants and children who are biologically unrelated to the donor and who are already ill. An intermediate level of safety should be observed in handling a mother's milk for her hospitalized or sick infant. For milk that is expressed for a healthy full-term infant or older baby in child care, less stringent precautions are necessary. The goal in all cases is to supply a human milk feeding that will (1) not make the infant sick and (2) provide milk that is as close in quality as possible to that nursed directly from the breast. This goal is accomplished by minimizing the losses involved in storing and handling expressed milk and minimizing the potential for contamination of the expressed milk.

The general recommendations listed here are conservative. When making a public health recommendation, it is important to be conservative so that the safety net is as broad as possible. The following recommendations can be accessed in their entirety in a more thorough fashion by referring to the above referenced publications.

General Principles of Milk Expression

- *Human milk should be treated with respect.* Mother's milk is extremely valuable to her infant's well-being and development. For this reason, expressed milk should be treated with respect and provided with proper storage facilities. Health-care providers working with mothers should be aware of the sometimes subtle and potentially discouraging messages that they give, such as placing "Biohazard" stickers on refrigerators used for human milk. Expressed human milk has economic, nutritional, and medical/health value. It is wasteful to throw away expressed human milk because of improper collection, storage, and handling.

- *The more expressed milk is "handled," the greater the loss of components and the higher the risk of contamination from outside sources.* When milk is poured from container to container, exposed to light or air, chilled, frozen, thawed, left to sit on counters, warmed or heated, the composition of the milk is changed and beneficial components may be lost or destroyed. The goal is to minimize these losses. The more frequently milk is handled, the greater the opportunity for introduction of contamination from outside sources and for bacterial growth.

- *Human milk is an extremely robust fluid.* Despite losses during storage and handling, human milk can withstand a great deal of mishandling and still protect the infant from infection and provide superior nutrition.

- *Human milk is not a sterile fluid.* The assumption that unpasteurized human milk should contain no bacteria, even when fed to sick infants, is unreasonable. However, mothers should be carefully instructed in methods of expressing to minimize bacterial contamination. Too many colony-forming units of bacteria in milk may begin to deplete the nutrient content of the milk as the bacteria grow. It is also inappropriate to view expressed human milk as a source of disease transmission and a danger to the person feeding the milk. Only when human milk is being used as a donated banked tissue should precautions be taken to protect the handler.

- *Keep it simple.* Instructions for mothers need to be kept as simple as possible to ensure compliance with a procedure. Too many detailed protocols may discourage mothers from expressing milk at all or force them to take shortcuts that may not be safe for their infants.

Recommendations

For the Hospitalized Infant

A. Collection: Getting Started
1. Wash hands thoroughly.
2. Wash pumps/kits thoroughly before each use. Sterilization is not necessary.

B. Choosing a Pump
1. Each mother should have her own personal kit for use with hospital grade pumps.

C. Storage Containers
1. Storage containers should be aseptic, hard-sided containers with lids that will provide an airtight seal.
2. Do not use polyethylene bags for storage of expressed milk in the hospital setting.

D. Storage Times and Temperatures
1. Fresh milk
   a Room temperature: Refrigerate within 1 hr of expression (exception: refrigerate within 4 hr when milk is fed continuously rather than by bolus).
   b. Refrigeration: Refrigerate at 4°C (39°F) for 48 hr
2. Milk frozen at −20°C (−4°F)
   a. 3 months (use of older milk preferred to not using human milk at all).
   b. Hospital settings should have dedicated freezers for human milk that are large enough to hold milk from a number of mothers in separate bins.
3. Thawed milk
   a. Use within 24 hr

E. Thawing and Warming Milk
1. Never thaw milk in a microwave oven.
2. Thaw milk by placing the bottle in lukewarm water, being careful not to allow the water to touch the edge of the container.
3. Thaw the milk for one infant separately from the milk for another infant to avoid mix-ups.
4. Warm human milk only to approximately body temperature (37°C/98.6°F). Avoid overwarming.

For the Healthy Infant/Child

A. Collection: Getting Started
1. Wash hands thoroughly.
2. Wash pumps/kits thoroughly before each use.

B. Choosing a Pump
1. There is no one pump that is ideal for every mother in every situation.
2. Hand expression is frequently faster and cleaner than a pump.

C. Storage Containers
1. Storage containers should be clean and airtight. Hard-sided containers are preferred for long-term storage and freezing.

D. Storage Times and Temperatures
1. Fresh milk
   a. Room temperature: ≤25°C (77°F)–4 hr
   b. In a cooler: 15°C (59°F)–up to 24 hr
   c. Refrigeration: 4°C (39°F)–72 hr
2. Milk frozen at −20°C (−4°F)
   a. 2 weeks if freezer is inside refrigerator compartment.
   b. 3–6 months in a frost-free refrigerator/freezer with separate outside door for freezer compartment.
   c. 6–12 months in a separate manual defrost deep freeze.
3. Thawed milk
   a. Use within 24 hr

E. Thawing and Warming Milk
1. Never thaw milk in a microwave oven.
2. Thaw milk in the refrigerator overnight or by placing the bottle in a pan of lukewarm water.
3. Do not subject milk to excessive heat; warm milk only to body temperature (37°C/98.6°F).
4. Warm only the volume that will be fed to the infant.

5. Discard any milk that has been warmed for a feeding and not used.

6. Pasteurizing a mother's own milk is not recommended except in rare medical situations.

F. Miscellaneous

1. *Portion sizes:* Milk should be stored in feeding-sized portions where possible.

2. *Layering:* If a single expression is not enough for a complete feeding, especially colostrum and transitional milk, amounts may be combined. Newly expressed milk should be chilled prior to adding to already expressed and stored milk. As expression amounts become greater, it is advisable to use a new clean container for each expression and to combine amounts immediately before feeding.

3. *Labeling expressed milk:* Labels should be waterproof and written in indelible ink. They should contain the date of expression, the baby's name, and the mother's name if last names differ.

4. *Routine bacteriological screening:* This is an unnecessary procedure for maternal milk and wastes health-care funds.

5. *Caring for shared pumps:* Pumps should be cleaned and checked on a regular basis by hospital staff. Pumps that are contaminated internally should be removed from use and serviced completely according to protocols for hospital equipment.

6. *Feeding errors:* Policies and procedures should be in place to prevent and deal with feeding errors. If the wrong milk is fed to an infant, both the inadvertent donor and the recipient should be serologically tested.

F. Miscellaneous

1. *Portion sizes:* Milk should be stored in feeding-sized portions.

2. *Layering:* Milk may be added to that of another expression to reach the desired amount for a single feeding. Milk should be chilled at least 1 hr in the refrigerator prior to adding to another bottle. Only expressions from a single day should be combined.

3. *Labeling expressed milk:* Labels should be waterproof and written in indelible ink. They should contain the date of expression, the baby's name, and the mother's name if last names differ.

4. *Refeeding milk:* Milk left over from a feeding should be discarded. It should not be fed at a later point.

5. *Emergency portions:* Smaller portions of only 1 to 2 oz may be just enough to pacify a frantic baby in child care when the mother is expected imminently.

6. *Prioritizing use:* Oldest milk by dates should be used first.

7. *Wearing/not wearing gloves:* It is not necessary for child-care providers or others who feed infants to wear plastic gloves when feeding expressed human milk.

BEYOND
POSTPARTUM

Most women are healthy during their childbearing years, and it is rare that a mother's nutritional status is detrimental to her health and ability to lactate. With adequate social support and health care, pregnancy, birth, and breastfeeding usually go well. Nonetheless, some mothers encounter difficulties, many of which are preventable and nearly all of which can be resolved in a manner that preserves breastfeeding. Major concerns for the breastfeeding woman include her child's health, her employment outside the home, and concerns relating to her fertility and resumption of sexual activity after the birth of her infant. Infant assessment provides the baseline for assisting both the healthy and the ill breastfeeding child.

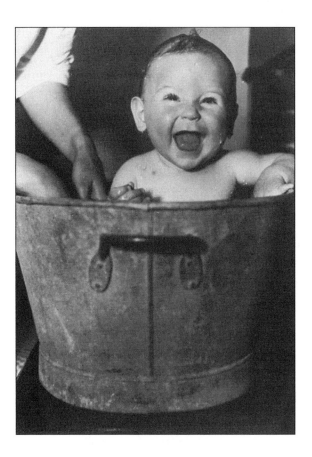

Maternal Nutrition During Lactation

Yvonne L. Bronner and Kathleen G. Auerbach

As the rates of breastfeeding continue to increase, this method of infant feeding is becoming the norm in the United States. The American Dietetic Association, the American Academy of Pediatrics, the American College of Obstetricians and Gynecologists, the American Academy of Family Physicians, the Women, Infants, and Children (WIC) supplemental food program, and other public and private organizations strongly encourage breastfeeding. In an effort to clarify nutritional issues related to breastfeeding, this chapter discusses common concerns that lactating women bring to dietitians such as weight change, exercise, and vegetarian diets. In addition, we examine the effect of supplements (used to maintain or add to nutrient intake in the childbearing woman), caffeine, and food flavorings on both mother and breastfeeding baby, and explore the development of allergic reactions during lactation. We offer counseling suggestions related to the questions most frequently asked by mothers who are planning to breastfeed or who already are breastfeeding their babies. Finally, we warn against being rigid about the lactating mother's diet and instead incorporate cultural food habits into healthy eating patterns that she enjoys.

Women are beginning to relate nutritional intake to the entire continuum of childbearing—from the preconceptional phase through lactation. Pregnant women have traditionally been more motivated to eat a more healthful and more varied diet than they ate before they were pregnant. Based on recommendations in the Institute of Medicine (IOM) report on *Nutrition During Pregnancy and Lactation: An Implementation Guide*, more women and health-care practitioners recognize the benefits of improving nutritional intake during the preconception period and maintaining these improved habits throughout the cycle (Institute of Medicine, 1992). Thinking about optimal nutrition during pregnancy and lactation is similar to the transition seen in the use of the word "diet" to "weight management," a change that is targeted to improved health status throughout life. Pregnancy is a "teachable moment" in the continuum for encouraging good nutrition for a lifetime.

Although the emphasis on achieving and maintaining a "good" diet is important, this message must be tempered by an understanding that the breastfeeding woman can still breastfeed even if her diet is not optimal. Why? Because the body efficiently uses nutrients that are available in the mother even if the mother's diet is limited. Under conditions of chronic malnutrition, nutrients to synthesize breastmilk can be mobilized from maternal stores at the mother's expense (Dewey, 1997; Alam et al., 2003).

Worldwide studies support the finding that maternal nutrition has only a modest effect on milk production and milk composition. For example, during the "hunger winter" in Holland between 1944 and 1945, women were severely undernourished as a result of wartime conditions. Dutch infants born during this period were found not to be affected by their mothers' inadequate nutritional intake. Slightly less maternal milk was produced than in previous years when the food supply was more ample, but neither duration of breastfeeding nor infant growth patterns were affected (Smith, 1947). Malnourished Brazilian women produce milk with a slightly higher fat content than do more well-nourished women (Spring et al., 1985). Nepalese women with protein-calorie malnutrition breastfed babies who were in the low-normal range of weight and length for age yet who appeared healthy. And Bangladeshi women who are considered "marginally nourished" maintain an average daily milk production of 750 gm (Brown et al., 1986).

Maternal Caloric Needs

The amount of energy intake needed by lactating mothers continues to be debated. The lactating mother need not maintain a markedly higher caloric intake than that maintained prior to pregnancy: in most cases, 400 to 500 calories in excess of that which is needed to maintain the mother's body weight is sufficient. Even though Recommended Dietary Allowance (RDA) levels are thought by many to exceed the levels that women actually need, the RDA is based on the average energy expenditure of moderately active women with an additional 500 calories allowed for lactation. For several reasons, a woman might ingest fewer calories during lactation than are stipulated in the RDA for lactating women:

- She is attempting to return to her prepregnancy weight while breastfeeding her infant.

- She does not have access to sufficient food in a given day.

- She does not wish to gain weight.

- She did not eat this amount of calories before she became pregnant.

- She is less active than the level used to estimate daily caloric intake.

Basal metabolic rates are higher during lactation but are lower than those during the latter months of pregnancy (Piers et al., 1995). Metabolic efficiency increases during pregnancy, enabling women to use fewer calories more efficiently. This energy efficiency has not been demonstrated as well for lactation although women with a wide variety of energy intakes adequately breastfeed their infants. Two studies make the case for recommending fewer calories as a base against which to evaluate maternal energy intake during the childbearing years (Murphy & Abrams, 1993; Todd & Parnell, 1994). Other studies using new techniques for measuring energy expenditure are now being conducted on lactating women; thus more, and perhaps better, data will be used for future energy intake recommendations.

In their prospective study of 458 pregnant women followed for one year, Murphy and Abrams (1993) found that women with lower incomes and African-American women—as compared to women with higher incomes and whites—take in fewer calories, whether they are preconception, pregnant, or lactating. Only if they were not breastfeeding did poorer or African-American mothers have higher energy intake than the other women with whom they were compared. For lactating women in this study, the mean energy intake was considerably lower than recommended levels. Among white and higher-income mothers lactating beyond 3 months postpartum, energy levels were lower than in the earlier postpartum period. This pattern was reversed among African-American and lower-income women, who increased their energy intake as the infant aged.

Most striking in this study is the substantial difference between RDAs and reported energy intake, averaging 700 to 900 kcal lower than levels routinely recommended. Murphy and Abrams (1993) offer the following explanation for this disparity: pregnant and postpartum women (whether lactating or not) have lower energy requirements than were previously computed as a result of their lower average energy expenditures. Additional studies are needed to track the energy intake of pregnant and lactating women, and to note the health outcomes of their infants over time. Only with such studies can we be assured that women are able to adequately sustain lactation with lower energy levels at no risk to themselves or the babies for whom they are producing milk.

Todd and Parnell (1994) followed 73 women who provided nutrient intake information with 24-hour recalls for 3 months. Most of the women in this study reported dietary intakes approximately two thirds the level of the Australian Recommended Nutrient Intake (RNI) for zinc, calcium, folate, and vitamin A. The authors concluded that lactation can be maintained on lower levels of energy intake than currently are recommended, and they suggest reassessment of RNI levels. It should be noted that recommendations are usually set higher than average need and therefore it is not surprising that reported intakes are less than those recommended.

The efficiency of conversion of food energy into breastmilk appears to be higher than the 80 percent assumed by the FAO/WHO/UNU joint expert consultation (1985), according to Piers et al. (1995). Frigerio et al. (1991) propose that the figure of 95 percent is more appropriate to calculate the energy cost of lactation. However, the consensus of opinion still suggests that 80 percent is the efficiency value of conversion.

Maternal Fluid Needs

Increased fluids also aid the lactating mother's milk production but should not be overemphasized, because excess fluid intake also may result in reduced milk production (Dusdieker et al., 1994). What the mother drinks will not markedly affect the fluid content of breastmilk. If the mother drinks to meet her own thirst needs, she will drink enough to sustain lactation. One easy way to ensure adequate fluid intake is to suggest that the mother have something to drink each time she sits down to breastfeed the baby. If a busy mother forgets to drink enough fluids as she rushes through her day, she may experience more constipation, one of the first signs of dehydration. Additionally, she can check the color of her urine as she voids throughout the day. With the exception of the first-morning urination, if the mother is drinking enough liquid, her urine will be clear to light yellow.

A woman should be encouraged to follow a diet appropriate to her culture, eating foods of different colors, flavors, and textures, and in as natural a state as possible. It should be noted that water intake includes the water present in food.

Stumbo et al. (1985) found that on average, about 22 percent of the usual water intake came from the foods that lactating women ate. She should avoid processed foods as much as possible, particularly those containing refined sugars. If the mother does not overeat and maintains a low intake of animal fat, she is unlikely to gain weight while she is breastfeeding, particularly in the early weeks when she is using more energy to make milk for her infant who is breastfeeding exclusively and nursing frequently.

Weight Loss

Teleologically speaking, fat storage during pregnancy is a normal physiologic adaptation in order to give new mothers a nutrient reserve during times of food deprivation. A portion of the energy stored during pregnancy will be mobilized to accommodate milk production. For example, if a woman gains 24 to 26 lb (11 to 12 kg) during pregnancy, she can expect that a reserve of about 4 to 7 lb (2 to 3 kg) is used at the rate of 100 to 150 kcal/day to support lactation (Institute of Medicine, 1989). If all goes well, this mobilized fat will be associated with a gradual but steady weight loss until the client reaches her prepregnant weight or "healthy weight" (the weight achieved when the client is eating wholesome foods and engaging in at least 30 minutes of physical activity on most days of the week (Meisler & St. Jeor, 1996).

Because being thin is often equated with feminine attractiveness, new mothers are concerned about their weight. They also may want information about dietary regimens that are compatible with breastfeeding, advice about when they can begin an exercise program, and how strenuously they can exercise.

The true effect of lactation on maternal weight after delivery is still unclear despite dozens of international studies on the topic. However, we can make the following evidence-based conclusions about postpartum weight loss and breastfeeding:

- Breastfeeding women appear to lose slightly more weight postpartum than do their non-breastfeeding counterparts (Bradshaw & Pfeiffer, 1988; Dugdale & Eaton-Evans, 1989; Kramer et al., 1993) although the evidence is conflicting—i.e., some studies show no correlation of lactation with weight loss after delivery (Thorsdottir & Birgisdottir, 1998; Walker & Freeland-Greaves, 1998) possibly because of inconsistencies in the definition of breastfeeding and also due to confounding factors that were not taken into consideration (Fraser & Grimes, 2003).

- Maternal weight loss is greater in the first 12 months postpartum if mothers breastfed; the weight-loss pattern is most marked in the second 6 months postpartum and is related to both breastfeeding frequency and duration (Dewey et al., 1993). The longer the mother breastfeeds, the more weight she is likely to lose (up to a point) (Dugdale & Eaton-Evans, 1989).

- During the recuperative postpartum period, mothers tend to eat less and to be less active than they were prior to delivery. This pattern of lessened activity is more pronounced among breastfeeding than among bottle-feeding mothers. In spite of these differences, breastfeeding women lose more weight than bottle-feeding women throughout the first 6 months postpartum (Dugdale & Eaton-Evans, 1989).

- Even moderate dieting during breastfeeding can achieve a 4 to 5 lb weight loss per month (Dewey & McCrory, 1994).

- Breastfeeding women begin losing body fat from the 15th day postpartum (Fornes & Dorea, 1995).

Gradual weight reduction has no deleterious effect on lactation and is attainable with lower energy intakes than usually are recommended (Butte et al., 1984; van Raaij et al., 1991). Women with a caloric intake of 2600 kcal/day had no weight loss, whereas those taking in fewer than 2200 kcal/day gradually lose weight. Mothers with less than 20 percent body fat do not produce less milk than do heavier mothers; however, they do consume more energy. In addition to weight loss from stored energy reserves, weight loss during lactation is best achieved by lowering the fat content of the diet and exercising (Dewey, 1998; McCrory et al., 1999). Weight loss is more likely to occur when the fat content represents no more than 20 to 25 percent of

total calories. Modest weight loss (approximately 1 lb/week) appears to have no adverse effect on the quantity or quality of the breastmilk (Dusdieker et al., 1994). Strode et al. (1986) reported that a modest intake of 1500 kcal/day in the first 6 months postpartum did not adversely affect milk production. With this nutritional intake, prolactin levels remained unaffected, and the nursing mothers lost approximately 1 lb/week.

The mother who chooses to diet while lactating should be encouraged to avoid crash or fad diets that promise marked, rapid weight loss. Fat-soluble environmental contaminants and toxins stored in body fat are released into the milk when caloric intake is severely restricted. Additionally, a marked reduction of caloric intake can result in fussiness in some babies. Modest food intake (1500 kcal/day) does not adversely affect milk production; however, a rapid, severe weight loss will negatively affect infant weight gain.

Motil et al. (1994) reported a case in which a breastfed infant failed to thrive as a result of the mother's seriously fat-restricted dietary regimen. The volume of milk declined markedly, although milk composition was unaffected. A safe maternal weight-loss regimen includes careful analysis of the mother's prepregnancy caloric needs accompanied by a plan that enables her to maintain her own nutritional needs while total calories are gradually reduced. In most cases, a weight loss of no more than 1 to 1.5 lb/week can be sustained during lactation without compromising the baby's total milk supply or cream content.

Exercise

Regular exercise is healthy at any time during life, including during lactation. Exercise does not interfere with the mother's milk supply (Lovelady et al., 2001; Larson-Meyer, 2002; Rooney & Schauberger, 2002) or with the baby's feeding pattern (Dewey et al., 1994; Dewey, 1998). Lovelady et al. (2000) followed 40 overweight breastfeeding women beginning 4 weeks after they gave birth. About half were assigned to a diet-and-exercise group and half to a control group. Women in the diet-and-exercise group lost an average of 10 pounds by the end of 10 weeks. They reported that they seemed to be producing enough milk and that the exercise sessions gave them more energy. Women in the control group, on the other hand, lost an average of only 2 pounds.

In an earlier study, Lovelady et al. (1990) followed eight exercising and eight sedentary women who were exclusively breastfeeding their 9- to 24-week-old infants. No differences in plasma hormones or milk energy, lipid, protein, or lactose content of the milk was noted between the groups. However, the subjects who were exercising gained less weight during their pregnancy, made more milk, expended more energy, and ate more than the nonexercising women. In no way was lactation adversely affected by these women's moderate exercise regimen.

Alternatively, exercising to exhaustion may increase lactic acid levels to the point at which the baby refuses to breastfeed (Wallace et al., 1992). Removing milk from the breasts prior to exercise and giving this milk to the baby might be one way to reduce the likelihood of infant refusal or even difficulty accepting milk with elevated lactic acid. The authors speculated that, when the breasts are not emptied in advance of vigorous exercise, lactic acid increases rapidly and then decreases steadily throughout the postexercise recovery period. Dewey and Lovelady (1993) noted that such elevated lactic acid levels are not seen when moderate exercise is practiced.

Calcium Needs and Bone Loss

Some women fear that breastfeeding will cause sufficient bone loss and place them at risk for developing osteoporosis later in life. These concerns are unfounded. In fact, the opposite is true: bone density is restored after weaning, although the mother suffers slight bone loss while she is lactating (King, 2001; Carranza-Lira & Mera, 2002; Ensom et al., 2002).

Prentice (1994) reviewed the RDAs for calcium in different countries and found that they vary widely. Similarly, calcium intake varies widely with women in Finland having the highest levels, whereas black women in South Africa have the lowest calcium intakes. Clearly, these findings reflect dietary differences in these countries. Prentice points out that for postmenopausal osteoporosis to occur, the woman must not have achieved maximum bone mass during her young adult life. Fur-

thermore, calcium intake by the mother is not closely related to her breastmilk calcium secretion. In fact, no relationship has been found between breastmilk calcium concentrations and maternal calcium intake through food or calcium supplements (Kirksey et al., 1979; Vaughan, Weber, & Kemberling, 1979). Increasing calcium intake may result in increased risk of kidney stones and urinary tract infections and may result in reduced absorption of other minerals, including iron, zinc, and magnesium (Prentice, Goldberg, & Prentice, 1994). In fact additional calcium intake from diet or supplements does not prevent bone loss during lactation nor does it influence the recovery of calcium status after weaning (Kalkwarf, & Specker, 2002).

Outcomes of bone loss studies during lactation are relatively consistent and favor breastfeeding. There is little evidence to justify therapeutic intervention. Specker, Tsang, and Ho (1991) compared 26 lactating women with 32 nonlactating postpartum controls over the first year postpartum. Lactating women were more likely to mobilize bone during lactation and to recover bone mass during and after weaning, whether that occurred before or after 6 months postpartum. Cumming and Klineberg (1993) asked whether there was a relationship between parity, breastfeeding, age at menarche and menopause, and the risk of hip fracture among Australian women aged 65 years and older. As duration of breastfeeding increased, the risk of hip fracture decreased in a dose-response relationship ($p = < .01$). Additionally, parous women who breastfed all their children were at lower risk for hip fracture than were parous women who had never breastfed their children.

In another study (Sowers et al., 1993) women who breastfed longer than 6 months had mean bone mineral density (BMD) losses of 5.1 percent of the lumbar spine and 4.8 percent of the femoral neck. Women who breastfed 1 month or less lost no BMD at either site. Among the women who breastfed 6 months or longer, there was a return to baseline BMD levels at 12 months postpartum. The authors stated that transient bone loss occurs with several months of lactation but this bone loss is recovered following lactation.

Sowers et al. (1995) reported 5 percent short-term bone loss among breastfeeding women, followed by recovery of lost bone within the first 18 months after parturition. Predictive factors were lactation status and the number of months to resumption of menses. These authors concluded that menstrual activity, rather than diet, dietary calcium intake, or physical activity, is the primary factor in bone mass recovery after initial bone loss during lactation.

Kalkwarf and Specker (1995) followed 65 lactating women and 48 nonlactating women for 5 to 6 months postpartum. The breastfeeding women lost significantly more bone in the total body (2.8 percent versus 1.7 percent) and lumbar spine (3.9 percent versus 1.5 percent) than did the nonbreastfeeding women. However, after weaning, the breastfeeding women gained significantly more bone in the lumbar spine (5.5 percent versus 1.8 percent) than the nonbreastfeeding women. These investigators also found that earlier resumption of menses was associated with small amounts of bone loss during lactation and with greater increase of bone after weaning. They concluded that lactation may result in a transient loss of bone and that compensation may exceed the level of loss.

Although dietary calcium intake does not explain calcium recovery after lactation, Kalkwarf et al. (1996) suggest that calcium and phosphorus levels are higher in breastfeeding women and that this becomes apparent after weaning and resumption of menses. These researchers suggest that serum calcium concentrations are maintained or elevated by calcium that is metabolized from bone owing to low blood estrogen concentrations. King (2001) contends that calcium needs for milk production are met by decreased urinary excretion of calcium and increased bone resorption.

Vegetarian Diets

Vegetarianism as a nutritional practice continues to be popular in the United States. People choose vegetarianism for religious, economic, cultural, and ecologic reasons. Lacto-ovo vegetarians eat milk, eggs, and plant food. Lacto-vegetarians eat milk and plant food. Usual vegetarian diets supply a balance of nutrients but may be low in energy owing to their low fat and high fiber content. The vegan

diet generates the greatest concern because it is very restricted (Sanders, 1999; Ciani et al., 2000; Shaikh et al., 2003). Some practitioners of this diet are called fruitarians; they eat only fruits, nuts, and honey. Women practicing this diet should be encouraged to take in adequate calories and complementary protein combinations and to consume foods rich in iron, calcium, and vitamins D, B_{12}, and riboflavin to ensure adequate intake. Special attention should be given to vitamin B_{12} intake because it is available only from animal sources, fortified soy, and meat analogues, or B_{12} supplements (Institute of Medicine, 1989). The milk of breastfeeding vegetarians is generally nutritionally adequate. However, women on a macrobiotic diet who avoid meat, poultry, dairy products, and sometimes fish may produce milk with decreased levels of calcium, magnesium, and vitamin B_{12}.

Dietary Supplements

Nutrient needs during lactation vary by the volume of breastmilk produced and the mother's postpartum nutritional status. Generally, if the mother is consuming the recommended calories from a variety of foods, her nutrient needs will be met from food alone. If insufficient resources to purchase food of adequate quantity or quality is a problem, WIC and similar programs should be recommended and referrals made. For women whose income level qualifies them, WIC provides food supplements for lactating mothers. This program supports breastfeeding by providing additional food to the breastfeeding mother through the first year of the baby's life, should the mother breastfeed that long. In addition to food, nutrition education and suggestions about how to select and prepare foods for optimal food value are offered. If the mother is restricting her caloric intake to fewer than 1800 kcal/day in order to lose weight while nursing, she should be encouraged to eat nutrient-dense foods—that is, foods that supply a large proportion of nutrients relative to their calorie content. Vegetables and legumes are good examples of nutrient-dense foods.

If a nutrient deficiency is identified, a balanced multivitamin supplement that supplies iron to 100 percent of RDAs may be recommended on an individual basis. Women who avoid dairy products and other calcium-rich food sources may need a calcium supplement of 600 mg/day of elemental calcium taken with meals. Likewise, the mother's avoidance of vitamin D-enriched foods and the baby's limited exposure to sunlight may lead to inadequate levels of vitamin D in the baby (Specker, et al., 1985, 1987a). In this case vitamin D supplement for the infant is indicated (5 to 7.5 mcg/day) (Dawodu et al., 2003).

Foods That Pass Into Milk

Caffeine

Caffeine-containing foods or fluids have been questioned as an appropriate item for breastfeeding mothers. Some mothers report that their very young babies seem to react when caffeinated beverages or foods are part of the maternal diet. Measurable amounts of caffeine pass into breastmilk. However, the amount of caffeine available to the infant is minimal, only 0.06 to 1.5 percent of the maternal dose and no caffeine is detected in the infants' urine (Berlin et al., 1984). Breastfeeding women who ingest caffeine in moderate amounts present no significant dose to the normal full-term infant.

Ryu's findings (1985a, 1985b) are also reassuring for parents who regularly consume caffeinated beverages. For young neonates, even 5 cups of coffee ingested daily by the mother over a 5-day period altered neither infant heart rate nor sleep time. Concentrations of caffeine in the term infants' serum were slightly elevated but, by day 9, caffeine levels in the mothers' milk and their babies' serum were below the limits of detectability. LeGuennec and Billon (1987), however, caution that babies born prematurely exhibit a delay in eliminating caffeine. Maternal intake of caffeine may have variable effects on preterm or sick infants.

Food Flavorings

Food flavorings are often the first and most lasting cultural cues that infants receive, potentially expanding the sensory experience of feeding. Mennella and Beauchamp (1991) examined the effects of maternally ingested garlic and reported that breastfeeding babies suckled longer and obtained more milk when it was garlic-flavored. They speculated that formula feeding might represent a deficient sensory experience in that the milk always tastes the same. Sullivan and Birch (1994) (see also Mennella & Beauchamp, 1997) reported that breastfed babies were more accepting of solids at their introduction than were formula-fed infants. These investigators suggested that the varied flavor cues to which breastfeeding babies are exposed might facilitate acceptance of new foods. Furthermore, "learning" the taste of foods acceptable to the mother may also facilitate later independent appropriate food selection by the young child (Mennella, 1995).

Vanilla, a potent food flavoring, also alters infant feeding behavior (Mennella & Beauchamp, 1996). Breastfeeding babies suckled longer when first exposed to vanilla-flavored milk. Bottle-feeding babies similarly exposed fed longer when the milk was flavored but did not continue to do so over time, suggesting that the change in flavor, but not the flavor itself when repeated, may trigger altered feeding behavior. For the breastfeeding baby, continued flavor changes enable the child to become familiar with the flavors represented in his family's foodways.

Allergens in Breastmilk

Now and then, infants who are exclusively breastfed and are receiving no solids develop allergic symptoms that appear to be from something they have ingested. In this case, the baby is probably reacting to foods or substances taken by the mother that are being passed through the breastmilk. The most common allergic-producing offenders are cow's milk and milk products. Other foods that tend to produce allergic responses in Western cultures are chocolate, cola, corn, citrus fruits, wheat, and peanuts. Peanut allergy can result in severe, even life-threatening reactions in susceptible babies (Vadas et al., 2001).

Health professionals are beginning to realize that some breastfeeding infants have a sensitivity to certain foods transmitted into breastmilk. When exclusively breastfeeding mothers in a study were asked what foods they ate that they believed caused fussy behavior in their infants, they identified broccoli, cabbage, cauliflower, chocolate, cow's milk, and onion (Lust, Brown, & Thomas, 1996). Allergies and breastfeeding are discussed in greater detail in Chapter 4.

The Goal of the Maternal Diet During Lactation

The goal of the maternal diet during lactation is optimal nutritional intake. Certain demographic, lifestyle, and environmental factors may place a client at increased nutritional risk during lactation. The most important of these factors are listed in Box 15–1.

BOX 15–1

Nutritional Risk Factors During Lactation

1. *Maternal age younger than 17 years:* Teens may often have less-than-adequate dietary habits. Therefore, a careful assessment of their food intake is important. Often such assessment will reveal low intake of calcium-rich food as well as fruits and vegetables rich in vitamins and fiber.

2. *Economic deprivation:* The WIC program, the Commodity Supplemental Food Program, food stamps, and the Expanded Food and Nutrition Education Program (EFNEP) are examples of federally funded food and nutrition programs that may meet the needs of economically deprived mothers.

3. *Past restrictive dietary practices or unsound current dietary practices:* Some women severely restrict caloric intake in order to lose weight shortly after pregnancy, even while they are breastfeeding. Screen for less-than-adequate food intake, especially the omission of an entire group of foods (grains, fruits, vegetables, protein rich foods, and dairy products).

4. *Multiple babies:* The mother of multiples should be encouraged to eat to appetite and drink to thirst while getting as much rest as possible.

5. *Maternal weight less than 85 percent of suggested height and weight:* Data are provided by the Institute of Medicine (1989).

6. *Suboptimal weight gain during pregnancy:* This will result in a low postpartum body mass index ($<$ 19.8).

7. *Rapid weight loss while breastfeeding:* May indicate inadequate caloric intake.

8. *Pregnant while breastfeeding:* Breastfeeding one infant while pregnant with another necessitates that the mother eat to appetite and drink to thirst while getting as much rest as possible.

Note: Items 5 through 7 in this list relating to weight should receive careful assessment by the health-care team. The screening questions in Box 15–2 might be useful.
Source: Adapted from the American Dietetic Association (1996).

In 1992, the Institute of Medicine published *Nutrition During Pregnancy and Lactation: An Implementation Guide*, a key document that was developed to help deliver high-quality nutritional care during lactation (Institute of Medicine, 1992).* This guide contains a variety of information:

- A sample nutrition questionnaire to help identify women at nutritional risk (see Box 15–2)

- Answers to questions in the nutrition questionnaire

- General strategies for providing effective nutritional care

- Dietary assessment and nutritional guidance

Single copies of this guide are available from the National Maternal and Child Health Clearinghouse, 8201 Greensboro Drive, Suite 600, McLean, VA 22102; 703-821-8955.

- Guidance for assessing weight change using the body mass index chart (which helps in evaluating whether the lactating woman is underweight, overweight, or in the average weight range)

- A chart of indications for vitamin and mineral supplementation

- Supplementary information for nutrition referrals and resources to help the clinician meet the comprehensive nutritional needs of clients

The nutrition questionnaire will help to evaluate the client's (1) eating behavior (meal patterns, food intake patterns); (2) food security (the ability to get enough food); (3) actual food intake; and (4) lifestyle issues related to nutritional status (smoking, alcohol, and other drug use). Answers provided on the questionnaire will help to focus nutrition coun-

---

BOX 15–2

Screening Questions Assessing Maternal Nutritional Risk

1. Do you have trouble getting adequate food on a regular or periodic basis? For example, do you run out of food before the end of the month? Do you have problems getting to the store to purchase food? Do you use money allocated for food for other purposes?

2. Does your diet contain calcium-rich foods such as dairy products, fish with edible bones, greens (collards, turnip, etc.), tofu, and broccoli?

3. Are you restricting your food intake in order to lose weight?

4. If you practice vegetarianism, indicate which of the following foods you exclude from the diet: meat, fish, poultry, eggs, and dairy products.

5. Are you on some type of special diet that causes you to limit your food intake?

6. Within a week, do you regularly eat 5 fruits and vegetables?

7. Are you exposed to sunlight on a regular basis? If not, do you regularly consume vitamin D-fortified milk or cereal products?

8. How would you describe your weight status—underweight, overweight, average weight?

Source: Adapted from the Institute of Medicine (1992).

seling. After reviewing the steps to successful dietary counseling in Box 15–3, the lactation consultant can begin the counseling session. She should bear in mind that certain factors place mothers and babies at nutritional risk during lactation.

Nutrition Basics

The term *nutrition* has multiple meanings but consists of several different elements, including energy; macronutrients, such as carbohydrates, protein, and fat; and micronutrients such as vitamins and minerals.

BOX 15–3

Steps to Successful Dietary Counseling

1. Acknowledge that the client is doing something right.

2. Help the client identify areas of the diet that need to be improved.

3. Let the client help develop a plan to improve her food intake.

4. Work with the client to determine exactly how the plan will be implemented.

5. Identify facilitators to more appropriate food intake and barriers to same.

6. Determine a time for follow-up so that progress toward meeting the dietary goals can be evaluated.

Energy

Energy is the capacity to do work. The sun provides the source of energy through plant photosynthesis. Humans gain energy by eating plants or animals that have eaten plants. Several factors influence the total daily amount of energy needed by the body: (1) the basal metabolic rate (BMR), which represents the amount of energy needed for mechanical activities of the body, such as breathing, heart muscle activity, and maintaining body temperature; (2) physical activity; and (3) the thermal effects of food, such as digestion and metabolism. Energy needs are individualized, and studies suggest that there may be some adaptive conservation adjustments in energy expenditure during lactation (Illingsworth et al., 1986; Paul, Muller, & Whitehead, 1979; Schutz, Lechtig, & Bradfield, 1980). The RDA for energy during lactation is specified by age and represents the average energy expended for light to moderate activity (Institute of Medicine, 1989). The following quick method may be used to calculate energy need:

1. Convert "desirable" body weight in pounds to kilograms (kg) by dividing weight in pounds by 2.2.

   Example: Desired body weight = 130 pounds/2.2 = 59 kg

2. Use Table 15–1 to select the factor that represents the client's activity level or energy expenditure factor. For this example, let us assume a moderate activity level: moderate energy expenditure factor (MEEF) = 37. Add 500 kcal/day during lactation. Using this figure and the client's "desirable" body weight in kilograms, calculate the caloric estimate for the day.

   Example: 59 kg x 37(MEEF) = 2183 kcal/day + 500 kcal (lactation) = 2683 kcal/day

The 500 additional calories recommended during lactation can be obtained in the form of a sandwich (~300 to 350 kcal), fruit (60 to 80 kcal), and a glass of skim milk (90 kcal). This calculation assumes 10 hours of rest and 14 hours of moderate activity.

Table 15–1

TOTAL ENERGY NEEDS OF WOMEN (AGED 19–50 YEARS) AT VARIOUS LEVELS OF PHYSICAL ACTIVITY

Level of General Activity	Energy Expenditure (kcal/kg, body wt/day)
Very light	30
Light	35
Moderate	37
Heavy	44
Exceptional	51

Source: Adapted from the Institute of Medicine (1989).

The preceding commonly used calculation may require more calories than most women need while avoiding weight gain. This formula may assume an activity level higher than is applicable to most women in the early postpartum weeks. The health-care worker must keep this variability in mind when recommending caloric intake. In addition, the recommendation of an additional 500 kcal during lactation, to account for energy needs in making milk, is now considered the *upper* level of a range of additional calories.

Macronutrients

Carbohydrates

Food intake during lactation is designed to provide for the nutritional needs of the mother while enabling her to produce adequate milk for the baby. Therefore, most nutritional needs increase during lactation. Carbohydrates are the main energy source for all body functions and are classified as monosaccharides (glucose, fructose, galactose), disaccharides (sucrose, lactose, maltose), and polysaccharides (starch, glycogen, dietary fiber, dextrin). Low carbohydrate intake is associated with fatigue, dehydration, and energy loss. Carbohydrates provide 4 kcal/gm. When carbohydrate is in short supply, protein is broken down to take its place as a source of energy (Mahan & Escott-Stump, 1996).

Carbohydrates should make up 55 percent of total calories, with a minimum intake of 100 gm/day for lactating women. Lactating women should obtain their carbohydrates from foods such as whole-grain breads and cereals, fresh fruits, and vegetables and avoid simple sugars found in soft drinks and juice products labeled as "drinks."

The diet should also contain 25 gm/day of dietary fiber. The carbohydrates just recommended, in the form of soluble or insoluble fiber, will help lactating women reach this goal. Soluble fiber such as pectins and gums (found in fruits—apples, citrus fruits, strawberries, etc.) helps to reduce serum cholesterol levels and cardiovascular disease. Insoluble fiber, such as cellulose and hemicellulose (found in fruit and vegetable pulp and skins) helps to prevent constipation and to reduce the incidence of colon cancer.

Protein

Proteins are the highly complex substances in the body that build muscle tissue, enzymes, hormones, and antibodies. They are made up of 22 amino acids, eight of which are essential for adults. The body cannot produce adequate quantities to meet physiological needs; therefore, they must be supplied from the diet. Food proteins are considered complete and of high quality when they contain all eight of the essential amino acids. Protein from animal sources contains all of the essential amino acids; protein from vegetable sources may be low in one or more of the essential amino acids. Eating at one meal combinations of cereals and legumes—which are low in lysine and methionine, respectively—results in a mixture of amino acids that are adequate for protein synthesis. When caloric intake is adequate, vegetarian diets containing a variety of nutrient-dense foods provide sufficient essential amino acids for protein metabolism.

Rice contains all of the essential amino acids although in less-than-optimal quantities. When rice is mixed with small quantities of meat or fish, amino acids become adequate for protein synthesis. Complete proteins can be mixed with incomplete proteins or with each other to provide adequate amounts of the essential amino acids. Adding milk to cereal is an example (Mahan & Escott-Stump, 1996).

The average daily dietary protein requirement is influenced by many factors such as age, digestibility, rate of protein synthesis, and carbohydrate and fat levels (DeSantiago et al., 1995). The current recommendation is 65 gm/day of protein intake for the mother during lactation during the first 6 months and 62 gm/day during the second 6 months (Institute of Medicine, 1984). Protein, like carbohydrates, provides 4 kcal/gm.

Fat

Of all the nutrients in human milk, lipids are most affected by the mother's food intake (Butte et al., 1984; Nommsen et al., 1991). Fats carry the fat-soluble vitamins A, D, E, and K, as well as the essential fatty acid linoleic and the long-chain omega-3 polyunsaturated fatty acid—docosohexaeonoic acid (DHA). DHA is important to brain development in infants and has been noted to be low in American women (Al et al., 1995, 1997; Francois et al., 1998; Horwood & Fergusson, 1998; Benisek et al., 2000). During a recent National Institute of Health workshop, a group of experts recommended an intake of 300 mg/day of DHA as adequate intake for lactating women. This intake is related to adequate DHA levels in breastmilk (Specker et al., 1987b; Simopoulos et al., 1999). DHA supplements are associated with higher breastmilk levels (Jensen et al., 2000). These supplements are being marketed to US women. Fats provide elements for tissue structure, cell metabolism, and nerve impulse transmission. They are a concentrated source of energy—9 kcal/gm, as compared to 4 kcal/gm from carbohydrates and protein. Fat should comprise no more than 30 percent of the total calories consumed daily. No more than 7 to 10 percent of calories should be from saturated fat (available primarily from animal sources such as milk and meat, as well as coconut and palm oils), more than 10 percent should be monounsaturated, and 10 percent should be polyunsaturated fat (from vegetable sources, nuts, and seeds) (Mahan & Escott-Stump, 1996). The overall recommended distribution of

calories from the macronutrients for lactating women is as follows:

Carbohydrates: 50 to 55% of calories
Protein: 12 to 15% of calories
Fat: < 30% of calories

Macronutrients are required in large amounts, and they compose most of the body's weight, whereas micronutrients are required in smaller quantities and make up a small percentage of body weight.

Micronutrients

Vitamins

Traditionally, vitamins have been best known by diseases deriving from their deficiencies (e.g., vitamin A deficiency causes blindness; vitamin C deficiency causes scurvy) More recent recommendations for vitamin intake are based on principles of health promotion and disease prevention. An example is increasing folate during the periconceptional period to protect against neural tube defect.

Vitamins are organic, noncalorigenic food substances that are required by the body in small quantities and contribute to the regulation of metabolic processes. Fat-soluble vitamins (A, D, E, and K) are stored by the body in fatty tissue, whereas water-soluble vitamins (B complex and C) are not stored for long periods and need to be supplied in the diet more frequently. As a mother's intake of water-soluble vitamins increases, the vitamin level in her milk will also increase, but it will reach a plateau that is not raised by giving additional vitamin supplements. Water-soluble vitamin levels in human milk are more likely to be associated with maternal diet or supplement intake than are fat-soluble vitamins or minerals. For example, vitamin B_6 is essential to normal neurological development. Concentrations in breastmilk vary with the vitamin B_6 nutritional status of the mother. Therefore, mothers whose dietary intake of vitamin B_6 is low may be at risk of secreting milk with less-than-adequate quantities (Borschel, Kirksey, & Hannemann, 1986; West & Kirksey, 1976).

Even though vitamin K is fat-soluble and passes more slowly into human milk, oral supplements of vitamin K in exclusively breastfed infants elevate plasma levels and may be an alternative method of supplementation in situations in which parents refuse intramuscular newborn vitamin K prophylaxis shortly after birth. In addition, maternal oral supplements postpartum should be considered, given the decreased intake of breastmilk during the first few days of life and the risk of hemorrhagic disease of the newborn (Greer et al., 1997).

Minerals

Minerals are inorganic substances that build body tissues and that activate, regulate, and control metabolic processes. They also transmit neurological messages. There is no consensus regarding the exact amount of calcium required during lactation (Prentice et al., 1995). The recommendation for calcium is 1200 mg/day, an amount that can generally be achieved with generous quantities of dairy products and green, leafy vegetables. Since calcium need is linked to level of protein consumption, low levels of calcium intake may be adequate in cultures and circumstances where protein intake is low. Even in countries in which calcium intake is chronically low, Fairweather-Tait et al. (1995) report no effect on the efficiency of calcium absorption by type or amount of calcium supplementation or stage of lactation. This finding suggests that body calcium may be mobilized to meet additional needs during lactation if necessary.

Clinical Implications

Optimal food patterns to maintain health emphasize intake of grains, fruits, vegetables, and small amounts of low-fat meat and legumes and low-fat dairy products. When making recommendations related to eating, the lactation consultant must consider such factors as the client's or family's culture, environment, socioeconomic status, and energy and nutrient needs. Food labels help mothers to apply the principles from the US Dietary Guidelines for Americans when purchasing food and planning meals. These guidelines emphasize seven general recommendations, each of which applies to all members of the family:

1. *Eat a variety of foods.* Different foods are rich in varying nutrients. Therefore, it is important to eat foods from each of the five food groups (grains, fruits, vegetables, protein-rich foods, and dairy products) and to explore new foods to increase their variety. Vegetarians can obtain adequate nutrients if they eat a variety of foods and take in adequate calories. Vegans, who eat only foods from plant origin, need to ensure that they take a vitamin B_{12} supplement or eat foods fortified with the vitamin.

2. *Balance the food eaten with physical activity.* Physical activity will help to maintain appropriate weight. Although it is important to select foods wisely, it is also necessary to watch portion sizes. For example, a hamburger roll is 2 servings of bread; 1 cup of raw or cooked vegetable equals 1 serving; 3 oz of meat (about the size of the palm of the adult hand) equals 1 serving. People who restrict their total calorie intake need to eat nutrient-dense foods (high portion of nutrients per calories). Lactating women need to eat a diet rich in calcium (low-fat dairy products, dark-green, leafy vegetables, tofu, canned fish with soft bones) and iron (low-fat meat, fish, and poultry, leafy greens, legumes, and iron-enriched grain products). To maintain a healthy weight, food intake should be balanced with exercise.

3. *Choose a diet with plenty of grain products, vegetables, and fruits.* Most calories should come from grain products, fruits, and vegetables. These foods are high in nutrients and fiber and low in fat.

4. *Choose a diet low in fat, saturated fat, and cholesterol.* Total and saturated fat is highly correlated with serum cholesterol. Therefore, eating low-fat dairy products and meat and increasing the number of meatless meals by using legumes as the main dish are recommended. Monounsaturated and polyunsaturated fats found in olive and canola oils are recommended over butter and fats that are hard at room temperature (such as lard). Limit the number of meals containing egg yolks, organ meats, and other meats to decrease cholesterol intake. Total cholesterol intake should be kept below 300 mg/day.

5. *Choose a diet moderate in sugar.* Sugars alone are not associated with diabetes or becoming overweight, but people who eat large quantities of sweets (foods that are often also high in fat) will

consume too many calories, which can lead to obesity.

6. *Choose a diet moderate in salt and sodium.* Processed and prepared foods often contain high amounts of salt and sodium. In addition, some people add salt at the table and during food preparation. Encourage women to enjoy the natural taste of food by eating fresh fruits and vegetables rather than versions that have added salt or sugar. If a client is salt-sensitive, ask her to limit her intake. The daily value for sodium is 2400 mg/day. Reading food labels can help you to determine when a food is high in sodium.

7. *If you choose to consume alcoholic beverages, do so in moderation.* Any alcohol taken during lactation can cross into the milk; the effect on the infant is dose-related. Alcohol is not recommended during lactation but, if it is taken, it should be ingested in small amounts, with meals, and at a time when breastfeeding is less likely to be compromised.

Dietitians have extensive education in infant and maternal nutrition and so are well-equipped to educate lactating women; yet they remain a rarely tapped resource in breastfeeding management (Helm, Windham, & Wyse, 1997). The dietitian or clinician who is assisting the breastfeeding family to eat in an optimal fashion may wish to refer to one or more of many nutrition information resources. In the United States, these resources include the following:

- Institute of Medicine: *Nutrition During Lactation: Report and Summary.* Washington, DC: National Academy Press, 1991
- Institute of Medicine: *Nutrition During Pregnancy and Lactation: An Implementation Guide.* Washington, DC: National Academy Press, 1992
- USDA/DHHS: *US Dietary Guidelines for Americans, 1995*

Questions that mothers commonly ask about nutrition and lactation are reviewed in Box 15–4.

BOX 15–4

Questions Mothers Often Ask About Nutrition and Lactation

1. *Am I at risk for osteoporosis from calcium loss when I breastfeed my baby?* No. Breastfeeding for 6 months or longer is the best protection against bone loss. Although calcium is mobilized during breastfeeding, hormones increase calcium absorption and limit the amount of calcium that is excreted. A diet that includes low-fat dairy products and green, leafy vegetables will provide adequate calcium; taking in plenty of sunshine will ensure an adequate supply of vitamin D, which also is important in bone health.

2. *Can I provide sufficient vitamin D to protect my breastfeeding baby against rickets?* Human milk contains small amounts of vitamin D, and some sunshine exposure is usually sufficient to maintain appropriate levels of vitamin D in the breastfeeding baby However if you live in an area where sunlight may be severely limited for several months of the year or if your baby's clothing restricts the amount of sunlight he receives, your health care provider will probably recommend a vitamin D supplement for your baby.

3. *I am a teen mother. Can I make enough milk for my baby?* Yes. Only minimal differences exist between milk samples from teenage mothers and older mothers (Lipsman, Dewey, & Lönnerdal, 1985). If you are capable of sustaining a pregnancy, you can also make sufficient milk to nourish your baby.

4. *What about folic acid? I have been told this is important for the growing infant.* Folate deficiency and subsequent anemia is highly unlikely in the breastfeeding baby. Breastfeeding babies nearly always have higher folate levels than their formula-feeding age-mates (Salmenpera, Perheentupa, & Siimes, 1986).

5. *If I eat high-fat foods, will I also produce high-fat milk?* To some degree. The specific dietary fatty acids that you consume will be reflected in the milk your baby receives. However, foods low in fat will not prevent you from making milk with sufficient creamy portions.

6. *If I have low levels of vitamin B_6, will this affect my milk supply?* Vitamin B_6 deficiency in a mother may contribute to lethargy in her infant. In one study, a baby with this deficiency also was difficult to console when distressed (McCullough et al., 1990).

7. *What if I am anemic? Will this mean that my baby will have low iron levels too?* Breastfed babies use the iron in their mother's milk more efficiently than do babies who are fed iron-fortified commercial formulas; thus your baby is at lower risk for anemia when breastfed (Duncan et al., 1985).

8. *Is it true that caffeine makes breastfed babies jittery?* Most studies do not support this expectation. The amounts of caffeine found in infants are usually very small; in other cases, they are undetectable (Berlin et al., 1984).

9. *Will I make enough milk if I don't eat "right"?* Your diet does not have to be perfect in order for you to breastfeed. Caloric intake is what enables a mother to make milk. Even if you eat foods high in sugar or fats, you will still make milk that can nourish your baby. Nonetheless, it is to your advantage to select foods wisely not only because you are breastfeeding, but because you are feeding yourself, your body, and your future, and because you are responsible for modeling healthful eating for your baby.

10. *How will I know my milk is "rich" enough or "not too rich" for my baby?* Nature has made the nutritional composition of your breastmilk just right for your baby. In particular, your milk has an abundant supply of the fatty acids that will lead to optimal nerve and brain development in your child. The milk you make will vary slightly from one feeding to the next, throughout the day, and throughout the baby's entire breastfeeding period. Some feedings will be richer than others, but all will meet the baby's needs.

11. *I am a vegetarian. Can I still breastfeed?* People who practice vegetarianism eat a variety of foods, and most of them are healthful. Nutritionists and other health professionals recommend five or more fruit and vegetable servings per day for everyone. As long as you consume enough calories to maintain an appropriate weight and you use a variety of foods, including legumes and other forms of protein, you will do well. If you are a vegan—consum-

BOX 15–4 (cont.)

ing only plant foods—you may need to take a vitamin B_{12} supplement. If you express milk after eating a large amount of dark green vegetables, your milk may have a slight green tinge, but the baby will not care!

12. *I hate to drink milk. Does this mean I cannot breastfeed?* Drinking milk and making breastmilk are not related. Think about the nutrients available from milk and get them from other foods. You can get calcium, for example, from other low-fat dairy products, green, leafy vegetables, and canned fish with soft bones.

13. *What do you mean by "drink to thirst?" How much should I drink?* This depends in part on where you live. A hot, dry climate may cause you to drink more than another climate. Your body needs water to make optimal use of the foods you eat. If you drink sufficiently, your urine will be pale in color. If you are thirsty, drink water; it is a thirst-quencher. Sugar-added fluids tend to make you feel more, not less, thirsty.

14. *How soon can I resume my previous exercise plan now that I am breastfeeding? Is it true that exercise will make my milk sour?* You can begin a previous exercise plan as soon as you feel ready to do so. However, it is wise to breastfeed shortly before doing any exercise that causes the breasts to bounce. Wear a support bra. Your milk will not be affected by exercise unless you are exercising to exhaustion; most women report no effects whatsoever (Dewey & McCrory, 1994).

15. *I was told I could not begin a weight-reduction program while breastfeeding, but*

I need to lose weight—and more than a few pounds too! Some of the weight you gained during pregnancy is designed to be used during lactation. Most of the reputable weight-reduction programs have a plan geared to pregnant and breastfeeding women. They are safe. Increasing fiber and the number of fruit and vegetable servings, using low-fat cooking methods, and decreasing the number of meals that are high in fat, sodium, and calories but low in fiber will also help you lose weight. In addition, daily exercise helps with weight reduction. Frequent breastfeeding has been shown to help women lose weight, particularly in the early weeks and months when the baby is most likely to be fully breastfeeding (Dewey et al., 1993).

16. *I have never been one to take pills, even vitamins. How important are extra vitamins if I breastfeed?* If you eat a healthful diet and you and your baby get plenty of sunshine (30 minutes per week), there should be no need to take extra vitamins.

17. *What special foods should I eat in order to breastfeed?* You do not need to eat any special foods in order to breastfeed. Eating a variety of nutrient-dense foods should be your goal—before, during, and after you are pregnant or lactating.

18. *What foods should I avoid in order to breastfeed?* Most babies and mothers do well with most foods. Sometimes babies will react to certain foods in the mother's diet. Experiment if this happens to you: eliminate the suspected food to determine whether the difficulty goes away. If so, eliminate this

food for a while. In most cases, a baby who seems to react to a food when he is very young may not have a problem with that same food when he is older, even if still breastfeeding. Remember too that babies have been found to like highly flavored milk, such as occurs when the mother uses garlic (Mennella & Beauchamp, 1991). Do not be afraid to enjoy highly flavored foods when you eat. Variety seems to be the spice of life for breastfed babies too!

Summary

Nutrition during the pregnancy continuum has been highlighted as an opportunity to keep in place or begin healthy food intake habits that will lead to optimal health for a lifetime. During pregnancy, what a woman eats will influence her physical well-being and that of her growing fetus. During lactation, how well she eats has less effect on her ability to make milk than on her well-being. Nevertheless, it is appropriate for clinicians who are offering suggestions pertaining to food intake to encourage the breastfeeding mother to eat in a manner that will support her optimal health.

At the same time it is not necessary to emphasize that the lactating mother must stick to a rigid diet of the "right foods" in order to breastfeed. Overemphasis on diet adds to the mother's stress level, and places an unnecessary burden on her; it will likely result in reluctance by some to breastfeed their babies out of fear that their own eating habits are not adequate. Food choices that the client is already making that support and sustain adequate energy intake and optimal health deserve praise; suggestions for change need to be offered within the context of established food patterns.

Food intake—including food selection, meal planning and preparation, and serving size—reflects a social behavior that has significance far beyond its nutritional and life-sustaining roles, Remaining sensitive to this understanding will enable the clinician to make suggestions more likely to be accepted and acted on by the client. Enabling a new mother to breastfeed by encouraging her to view her milk as the optimal food for her growing baby and child may help her to make changes in her own dietary choices that will sustain her health as well as that of her children.

Key Concepts

- Optimal nutrition during pregnancy and lactation encourages good nutrition for a lifetime.

- Although the emphasis on achieving and maintaining a "good" diet is important, the breastfeeding woman can still breastfeed even if her diet is not optimal.

- The lactating woman needs only an extra 400 to 500 calories per day.

- If the mother drinks enough fluids to meet her own thirst needs, she will drink enough to sustain lactation.

- A portion of the energy stored during pregnancy will be mobilized to accommodate milk production. This mobilized fat will be associated with a gradual but steady weight loss. Breastfeeding women lose slightly more weight postpartum although the evidence is conflicting.

- Gradual weight reduction has no deleterious effect on lactation and is attainable with lower energy intakes (fewer than 2200 kcal/day) to gradually lose weight. Modest weight loss (approximately 1 lb/week) appears to have no adverse effect on the quantity or quality of the breastmilk.

- Exercise does not interfere with the mother's milk supply or with the baby's feeding pattern; however, exercising to exhaustion may increase lactic acid levels to the point at which the baby refuses to breastfeed.

- Women have slight bone loss during lactation; this bone density is restored after weaning.

- Breastfeeding women who are vegetarians should consume foods rich in iron, calcium, and vitamins D, B_{12}, and riboflavin to ensure adequate intake. Special attention should be given to vitamin B_{12} intake.

- A balanced multivitamin supplement may be recommended on an individual basis. Women who avoid dairy products and other calcium-rich food sources may need a calcium supplement of 600 mg/day.

- Breastfeeding babies suckle longer and obtain more milk when breastmilk retains the flavor of vanilla or garlic that the mother has eaten. The varied flavors of breastmilk to which babies are exposed contrasts with a deficient sensory experience of babies who are fed formula that always tastes the same.

- Cow's milk and milk products are the most common allergens in breastmilk. Others are chocolate, cola, corn, citrus fruits, wheat, and peanuts. Peanut allergy can result in severe, even life-threatening reactions.

- Alcohol consumed during lactation crosses into the milk; the effect on the infant is dose-related. If taken, alcohol should be ingested in small amounts.

- The lactating mother need not stick to a rigid diet of the "right foods" in order to breastfeed. Overemphasis on diet can cause some mothers to be reluctant to breastfeed out of fear that their eating habits are inadequate.

Internet Resources

American Dietetic Association, Breastfeeding promotion:
www.eatright.org/adap0697.html

The decade's progress in 44 developing countries, 1989–1999:
www.childinfo.org/eddb/brfeed/probl3/htm

References

Al MDM et al. Maternal essential fatty acid patterns during normal pregnancy and their relationship to the neonatal essential fatty acid status. *British J Nutr.* 74:55–68, 1995.

———.Relation between birth order and the maternal and neonatal docosahexaenoic acid status. *Eur J Clin Nutr* 51:548–53, 1997.

Alam DS et al. Energy stress during pregnancy and lactation: consequences for maternal nutrition in rural Bangladesh. *Eur J Clin Nutr* 57:151–56, 2003.

American Dietetic Association. *Manual of clinical dietetics.* Chicago: Chicago Dietetic Association and the South Suburban Dietetic Association, 1996.

Benisek D et al. Dietary intake of polyunsaturated fatty acids by pregnant or lactating women in the United States. *Obstet Gynecol* 95 (4 Suppl 1):S77–S78, 2000.

Berlin CM et al. Disposition of dietary caffeine in milk, saliva, and plasma of lactating women. *Pediatrics* 73:59–63, 1984.

Borschel MW, Kirksey A, Hannemann RE. Effects of vita-

min B_6 intake on nutrition and growth of young infants. *Am J Clin Nutr* 43:7–15, 1986.

Bradshaw MK, Pfeiffer S. Feeding mode and anthropometric changes in primiparas. *Hum Biol* 60:251–61, 1988.

Brown KH et al. Lactation capacity of marginally nourished mothers: infants' milk nutrient consumption and patterns of growth. *Pediatrics* 78:920–27, 1986.

Butte NF et al. Effect of maternal diet and body composition on lactational performance. *Am J Clin Nutr* 39:296–306, 1984.

Carranza-Lira S, Mera JP. Influence of number of pregnancies and total breast-feeding time on bone mineral density. *Int J Fertil Womens Med* 47:169–71, 2002.

Ciani F et al. Prolonged exclusive breast-feeding from vegan mother causing an acute onset of isolated methylmalonic aciduria due to a mild mutase deficiency. *Clin Nutr* 19:137–39, 2000.

Cumming RG, Klineberg RJ. Breastfeeding and other reproductive factors and the risk of hip fractures in elderly women. *Int J Epidemiol* 22:684–91, 1993.

Dawodu A et al. Hypovitaminosis D and vitamin D deficiency in exclusively breastfeeding infants and their mothers in summer: a justification for vitamin D supplementation of breastfeeding infants. *J Pediatr* 142:169–73, 2003.

DeSantiago S et al. Protein requirements of marginally nourished lactating women. Unidad de Investigacion en Nutricion, Hospital de Pediatria, Centro Medico Nacional. *Am J Clin Nutr* 62:364–70, 1995.

Dewey KG. Energy and protein requirements during lactation. *Annu Rev Nutr* 17:19–36, 1997.

————. Effects of maternal caloric restriction and exercise during lactation. *J Nutr* 128:386S–89S, 1998.

Dewey KG, Lovelady C. Exercise and breast-feeding: a different experience [letter]. *Pediatrics* 91:514–15, 1993.

Dewey KG, McCrory MA. Effects of dieting and physical activity on pregnancy and lactation. *Am J Clin Nutr* 49(suppl):446s–48s, 1994.

Dewey KG et al. Maternal weight-loss patterns during prolonged lactation. *Am J Clin Nutr* 58:162–66, 1993.

————. A randomized study of the effects of aerobic exercise by lactating women on breast-milk volume and composition. *N Engl J Med* 330:449–53, 1994.

Dugdale AE, Eaton-Evans J. The effect of lactation and other factors on post-partum changes in body-weight and triceps skinfold thickness. *Br J Nutr* 61:149–53, 1989.

Duncan B et al. Iron and the exclusively breast-fed infant from birth to six months. *J Pediatr Gastroenterol Nutr* 4:421–25, 1985.

Dusdieker LB et al. Is milk production impaired by dieting during lactation? *Am J Clin Nutr* 59:833–40, 1994.

Ensom MH et al. Effect of pregnancy on bone mineral density in healthy women. *Obstet Gynecol Survey* 57:99–111, 2002.

Fairweather-Tait S et al. Effect of calcium supplements and stage of lactation on the calcium absorption efficiency of lactating women accustomed to low calcium intakes. *Am J Clin Nutr* 62:1188–92, 1995.

FAO/WHO/UNU. *Report of a joint expert consultation: energy and protein requirements* (Tech. Rep. series 724). Geneva: WHO, 1985.

Fornes NS, Dorea JG. Subcutaneous fat changes in low-income lactating mothers and growth of breast-fed infants. *J Am Coll Nutr* 14:61–65, 1995.

Francois CA et al. Acute effects of dietary fatty acids on the fatty acids of human milk. *Am J Clin Nutr* 67:301–8, 1998.

Fraser A, Grimes DA. Effect of lactation on maternal body weight; a systematic review. *Obstet Gynecol Surv* 58:265–69, 2003.

Frigerio C et al. Is human lactation a particularly efficient process? *Eur J Clin Nutr* 45:459–62, 1991.

Greer F et al. Improving the vitamin K status of breastfeeding infants with maternal vitamin K supplements. *Pediatrics* 99:88–92, 1997.

Helm A, Windham CT, Wyse B. Dietitians in breastfeeding management: an untapped resource in the hospital. *J Hum Lact* 13:221–25, 1997.

Horwood LJ, Fergusson DM. Breastfeeding and later cognitive and academic outcomes. *Pediatrics* 101:E9, 1998.

Illingsworth PJ et al. Diminution in energy expenditure during lactation. *Br Med J* 292:437–41, 1986.

Institute of Medicine (IOM), Committee on Nutritional Status During Pregnancy and Lactation, Food and Nutrition Board. *Nutrition during pregnancy and lactation: an implementation guide.* Washington, DC: National Academy Press, 1992.

Institute of Medicine (IOM), Food and Nutrition Board, National Research Council. *Recommended dietary allowances.* 9th ed. Washington, DC: National Academy of Sciences, 1984.

Institute of Medicine (IOM), Food and Nutrition Board, National Research Council, National Academy of Sciences. *Recommended dietary allowances.* 10th ed. Washington, DC: National Academy Press, 1989.

Jensen CL et al. Effect of docosahexaenoic acid supplementation on lactating women on the fatty acid composition of breast milk lipids and maternal and infant plasma phospholipids. *Am J Clin Nutr* 71:292s–99s, 2000.

Kalkwarf HJ, Specker BL. Bone mineral loss during lactation and recovery after weaning. *Obstet Gynecol* 86:26–32, 1995.

————. Bone mineral changes during pregnancy and lactation. *Endocrine* 17:49–53, 2002.

Kalkwarf HJ et al. Intestinal calcium absorption of women during lactation and after weaning. *Am J Clin Nutr* 63:526–31, 1996.

King JC. Effect of reproduction on the bioavailability of calcium, zinc and selenium. *J Nutr* 131:1355S–58S, 2001.

Kirksey A et al. Influence of mineral intake and use of oral contraceptives before pregnancy on the mineral content of human colostrum and of more mature milk. *Am J Clin Nutr* 32:30–39, 1979.

Kramer FM et al. Breast-feeding reduces maternal lower-body fat. *J Am Diet Assoc* 93:429–33, 1993.

Larson-Meyer DE. Effect of postpartum exercise on mothers and their offspring: a review of the literature. *Obstet Res* 10:841–53, 2002.

LeGuennec J-C, Billon B. Delay in caffeine elimination in breast-fed infants. *Pediatrics* 79:264–68, 1987.

Lipsman S, Dewey KG, Lönnerdal B. Breast-feeding among teenage mothers: milk composition, infant growth, and maternal dietary intakes. *J Pediatr Gastroenterol Nutr* 4:426–34, 1985.

Lovelady CA et al. Lactation performance of exercising women. *Am J Clin Nutr* 52:103–9, 1990.

————. The effect of weight loss in overweight lactating women on the growth of their infants. *N Engl J Med* 342:449–53, 2000.

————. Effect of energy restriction and exercise on vitamin B_6 status of women during lactation. *Med Sci Sports Exerc* 33:512–18, 2001.

Lust KD, Brown JE, Thomas W. Maternal intake of cruciferous vegetables and other foods and colic symptoms in exclusively breast–fed infants. *J Am Diet Assoc* 96:46–48, 1996.

Mahan LK, Escott-Stump S. *Krause's food, nutrition, and diet therapy.* 9th ed. Philadelphia: Saunders, 1996.

McCrory MA et al. Randomized trial of the short-term effects of dieting compared with dieting plus aerobic exercise on lactation performance. *Am J Clin Nutr* 69:959–67, 1999.

McCullough AL et al. Vitamin B_6 status of Egyptian mothers: relation to infant behavior and maternal-infant interaction. *Am J Clin Nutr* 51:1067–74, 1990.

Meisler JG, St. Jeor S. Summary and recommendations from the American Health Foundation's Expert Panel on Healthy Weight. *Am J Clin Nutr* 63(suppl):474s–77s, 1996.

Mennella JA. Mother's milk: a medium for early flavor experiences. *J Hum Lact* 11:39–45, 1995.

Mennella JA, Beauchamp GK. Maternal diet alters the sensory qualities of human milk and the nursling's behavior. *Pediatrics* 88:737–44, 1991.

———. The human infants' response to vanilla flavors in mother's milk and formula. *Infant Behav Dev* 19:13–19, 1996.

———. Mothers' milk enhances the acceptance of cereal during weaning. *Pediatr Res* 41:188–92, 1997.

Motil KJ et al. Case report: failure to thrive in a breast-fed infant is associated with maternal dietary protein and energy restriction. *J Am Coll Nutr* 13:203–8, 1994.

Murphy SP, Abrams BF. Changes in energy intakes during pregnancy and lactation in a national sample of US women. *Am J Public Health* 83:1161–63, 1993.

Nommsen LA et al. Determinants of energy, protein, lipid, and lactose concentrations in human milk during the first 12 months. *Am J Clin Nutr* 53:457–65, 1991.

Paul AA, Muller EM, Whitehead RG. The quantitative effects of maternal dietary energy intake on pregnancy and lactation in rural Gambian women. *Trans R Soc Trop Med Hyg* 73:686–92, 1979.

Piers LS et al. Changes in energy expenditure, anthropometry, and energy intake during the course of pregnancy and lactation in well-nourished Indian women. *Am J Clin Nutr* 61:501–13, 1995.

Prentice A. Maternal calcium requirements during pregnancy and lactation. *Am J Clin Nutr* 59(suppl):477s–83s, 1994.

Prentice A et al. Calcium requirements of lactating Gambian mothers: effects of a calcium supplement on breast-milk calcium concentration, maternal bone mineral content, and urinary calcium excretion. *Am J Clin Nutr* 62:58–67, 1995.

Prentice AM, Goldberg GR, Prentice A. Body mass index and lactational performance. *Eur J Clin Nutr* 48(suppl 13):S78–S89, 1994.

Rooney BL, Schauberger CW. Excess pregnancy weight gain and long-term obesity: one decade later. *Obstet Gynecol* 100:245–52, 2002.

Ryu JE. Caffeine in human milk and in serum of breast-fed infants. *Dev Pharmacol Ther* 8:329–37, 1985a.

———. Effect of maternal caffeine consumption on heart rate and sleep time of breast-fed infants. *Dev Pharmacol Ther* 8:355–63, 1985b.

Sanders TAB. Essential fatty acid requirements of vegetarians in pregnancy, lactation and infancy. *Am J Clin Nutr* 70:555S–59S, 1999.

Salmepera L, Perkeentupa J, Siimes MA. Folate nutrition is optimal in exclusively breast-fed infants but inadequate in some of their mothers and in formula-fed infants. *J Pediatr Gastroenterol Nutr* 5:283–89, 1986.

Schutz Y, Lechtig A, Bradfield RB. Energy expenditures and food intakes of lactating women in Guatemala. *Am J Clin Nutr* 33:892–902, 1980.

Shaikh MG et al. Transient neonatal hypothyroidism due to a maternal vegan diet. *J Pediatr Endocrinol Metab* 16:111–13, 2003.

Simopoulos AP et al. Workshop on the essentiality of and recommended dietary intakes for omega-6 and omega-3 fatty acids. *J Am Coll Nutr* 18:487–89, 1999.

Smith CA. Effects of maternal undernutrition upon the newborn infant in Holland (1944–45). *J Pediatr* 30:229–43, 1947.

Sowers MF et al. Changes in bone density with lactation. *JAMA* 269:3130–35, 1993.

———. Biochemical markers of bone turnover in lactating and nonlactating postpartum women. *J Clin Endocrinol Metab* 80:2210–16, 1995.

Specker BL, Tsang RC, Ho ML. Changes in calcium homeostasis over the first year postpartum: effect of lactation and weaning. *Obstet Gynecol* 78:56–62, 1991.

Specker BL et al. Effect of race and diet on human-milk vitamin D and 25-hydroxyvitamin D. *Am J Dis Child* 139:1134–37, 1985.

———. Effect of vegetarian diet on serum 1,25-dihydroxyvitamin D concentrations during lactation. *Obstet Gynecol* 70:870–74, 1987a.

———. Differences in fatty acid composition of human milk in vegetarian and non-vegetarian women: long-term effect of diet. *J Ped Gastroent Nutr* 6:764–68, 1987b.

Spring PCM et al. Fat and energy content of breast milk of malnourished and well nourished women, Brazil 1982. *Ann Trop Paediatr* 5:83–87, 1985.

Strode MA et al. Effects of short-term caloric restriction on lactational performance of well-nourished women. *Acta Paediatr Scand* 75:222–29, 1986.

Stumbo PJ et al. Water intakes of lactating women. *Am J Clin Nutr* 42:870–76, 1985.

Sullivan SA, Birch LL. Infant dietary experience and acceptance of solid foods. *Pediatrics* 93:271–77, 1994.

Thorsdottir I, Birgisdottir BE. Different weight gain in women of normal weight before pregnancy: postpartum weight and birth weight. *Obstet Gynecol* 92:377–83, 1998.

Todd JM, Parnell WR. Nutrient intakes of women who are breastfeeding. *Eur J Clin Nutr* 48:567–74, 1994.

US Department of Agriculture Department of Health and Human Services. *US dietary guidelines for Americans.* Washington, DC: USDA, 1995.

Vadas P et al. Detection of peanut allergens in breast milk of lactating women. *JAMA* 285:1746–48, 2001.

van Raaij JM et al. Energy cost of lactation, and energy balances of well-nourished Dutch lactating women: reappraisal of the extra energy requirements of lactation. *Am J Clin Nutr* 53:612–19, 1991.

Vaughn LA, Weber CW, Kemberling SR. Longitudinal changes in the mineral content of human milk. *Am J Clin Nutr* 32:2301–6, 1979.

Walker LO, Freeland-Greaves J. Lifestyle factors related to postpartum weight gain and body image in bottle- and breastfeeding women. *JOGN Nurs* 27:151–60, 1998.

Wallace JP et al. Infant acceptance of postexercise breast milk. *Pediatrics* 89:1245–47, 1992.

West KD, Kirksey A. Influence of vitamin B_6 intake on the content of the vitamin in human milk. *Am J Clin Nutr* 29:961–69, 1976.

CHAPTER 16

WOMEN'S HEALTH AND BREASTFEEDING

Jan Riordan

This chapter discusses acute and chronic maternal health problems that have an effect on lactation. The health of a mother has a direct impact on her ability (both emotional and physical) to care for her infant. For example, mothers of preterm infants are particularly vulnerable to decreases in their immune function postpartum and have greater anxiety and depression compared to mothers of term infants. The normal immunosuppression of pregnancy recovers slowly over the months postpartum, exacerbating immune-mediated diseases such a rheumatoid arthritis and lupus (Gennaro et al., 1997).

   Most lactating women are healthy and fit. Illness is usually episodic: a head cold or a case of influenza. Breastfeeding empowers women to stay healthy by providing a variety of such health benefits as a reduction in the likelihood of carcinoma-in-situ of the uterine cervix (Brock et al.,1989), ovarian cancer (Rosenblatt & Thomas, 1993; Siskind et al., 1997), endometrial cancer (Rosenblatt & Thomas, 1995), breast cancer (Newcomb et al., 1999), rheumatoid arthritis (Brun et al., 1995), osteoporosis (Paton et al., 2003), and obesity (Hammer et al., 1996). Even plasma concentrations of both cholesterol and triglycerides remain significantly lower in breastfeeding mothers than in bottle-feeding mothers during postpartum (Qureshi et al., 1999).

The health-care provider usually does not see the more serious health conditions described in this chapter. When she does, she needs a working knowledge of these conditions and the ability to develop a plan of care based on the wishes and needs of the breastfeeding mother who has a health problem.

Alterations in Endocrine and Metabolic Functioning

Anything that affects control of the endocrine system can also affect the production of breastmilk. The following discussion of diabetes mellitus, thyroid problems, and pituitary dysfunction explains uncommon conditions that may affect the breastfeeding mother's milk supply. Any woman with symptoms that suggest she might have an altered metabolic functioning should be referred to a physician for further evaluation and treatment.

Diabetes

Diabetes is a chronic disease of impaired carbohydrate metabolism caused by insufficient insulin or the inefficient use of insulin. Pregnant women with diabetes mellitus can be classified into two main categories: women who have (1) prepregnancy diabetes (type I or II), or (2) gestational diabetes. Type

I diabetes is a serious disease where insulin is not being produced as a result of autoimmunity directed at the ß cells of the pancreas. Type II diabetes used to be seen infrequently in pregnancy because the age of diagnosis was usually made after the reproductive years. It is much more common in pregnant women today and is part of a metabolic syndrome commonly seen with hypertension, obesity, and dyslipidema.

Gestational Diabetes. Gestational diabetes, a glucose intolerance that occurs in 4 percent of all pregnancies, manifests itself only during pregnancy (American Diabetes Association, 2000). Gestational diabetes is far more common than a decade ago because more women (as well as the rest of the population) are obese today. Gestational diabetes is detected in the same ways as other forms of diabetes. Most women with gestational diabetes will revert to normal status. Breastfeeding should be encouraged and proceed normally in these women. In fact, women with gestational diabetes are twice as likely to develop type II diabetes later on if they do not lactate following the birth of the baby whose pregnancy provoked gestational diabetes (Kjos et al., 1993). Lactation—even for a short duration—improves glucose metabolism and is a low-cost intervention that may reduce or delay diabetes in these women.

Type I Diabetes. With improvement in the monitoring and control of maternal blood sugar, women with type I diabetes who have well-controlled glucose levels can usually look forward to a safe and relatively healthy pregnancy and birth. It is commonplace today for a woman with diabetes to experience a normal delivery and for the infant to be with the mother from birth and to breastfeed without the need for special care. The current use of subcutaneous insulin infusion pumps and multiple daily insulin doses has decreased the erratic glucose levels once seen, resulting in fewer perinatal complications. During pregnancy, her blood glucose levels should be maintained below 130 mg/dl as much as possible. During labor, delivery, and for some time after delivery, blood glucose levels are closely monitored.

The woman with type I diabetes not only can, but should, be encouraged to breastfeed her infant. Colostrum helps to stabilize the infant's blood sugar and, although breastfeeding should begin as soon after birth as possible, this is usually not the case. Infants of mothers with diabetes are occasionally placed in the special care unit after delivery. If breastfeeding is delayed, the mother should be encouraged to begin expressing or pumping her milk as soon as she feels able.

Lactating women with type I diabetes have lower milk prolactin concentrations than do women without diabetes (Ostrom & Ferris, 1993); causing a delay of about one day in lactogenesis II, or "coming in," of the milk for mothers (Arthur, Kent, & Hartman, 1994; Bitman et al., 1989; Miyake et al., 1989; Murtaugh et al., 1998). These mothers and their neonates need additional attention and care to establish lactation. In addition to early, frequent feedings, pumping to stimulate the milk supply is advised as well. It may be necessary to supplement the neonate during the first 2 to 3 days. Formula is often given in the interim until the mother's milk comes in, which brings up the issue of a potentially destructive autoimmune response in an infant. Rather than give artificial milk supplements, one pregnant mother with type I diabetes stored donor breastmilk that she later used to supplement her baby during the first few days postpartum.

During the immediate postnatal period, sudden but normal hormonal changes cause marked fluctuation in maternal blood glucose levels. Maternal hypoglycemia can be expected to occur immediately postbirth, lasting 5 to 7 hours after delivery. In addition, lactose excretion in the urine drops to a low level 2 to 5 days after birth and then rises rapidly. These sudden metabolic shifts of erratic blood glucose levels and an increase in insulin reaction require close monitoring. Juggling the feeding schedule of the infant and the amount of milk taken at each feeding are factors to be considered in maintaining good diabetic balance. Nighttime feedings present special challenges to the breastfeeding mother with diabetes. The mother should be encouraged to test her glucose levels during the night. She may need an additional snack at night.

Lactose is reabsorbed from the breast and is normally excreted in the urine; therefore nurses and mothers should be aware that in testing the urine after delivery, the presence of lactose may result in a false-positive test if copper-reducing urine testing (Clinitest) is used. For this reason, testing with Testape or Diastix, which measure only glucose, are the preferred methods. Once she is physiologically stable, the patient can return to subcutaneous injection insulin or to injection via a portable infusion pump.

Blood glucose meters are reliable for testing blood glucose by the mother at home. By keeping a daily record of blood glucose levels, the mother can self-monitor day-to-day changes. Once the blood glucose level stabilizes, it is generally lower during lactation. Ferris et al. (1988, 1993) compared 30 mothers with type I diabetes with 30 controls and found that fasting plasma glucose levels during the exclusive breastfeeding period were significantly lower than were the glucose levels of the women with type I diabetes who had stopped breastfeeding or who had never breastfed, even in the face of markedly higher caloric intake by the breastfeeding mothers. Women with type I diabetes usually take insulin by injection. Insulin, a large peptide that does not pass into breastmilk, is not a problem medication with breastfeeding.

Given the continuous conversion of glucose to galactose and lactose during milk synthesis, less insulin is required when the mother breastfeeds. Davies et al. (1989) showed that women with diabetes may need to reduce their prepregnancy insulin dose by about 27 percent to avoid hypoglycemic reactions. Breastmilk nutrients, especially lactose, vary slightly during the first several days postpartum (Lammi-Keefe et al., 1995) but these changes do not affect the mother's ability to produce breastmilk.

In addition to providing the known physiological advantages of breastfeeding for the infant, breastfeeding helps to fulfill the mother's need to feel normal in spite of her diabetic condition. An advantage of working with these women is their keen awareness of their body functions and the importance of diet. They are more knowledgeable than the average woman about physiology and are quick to notice changes that may forewarn of problems.

Mothers with diabetes may be more susceptible to mastitis, especially if they are not well controlled (Ferris et al., 1988; Gagne, Leff, & Jefferis, 1992). Any infection will quickly raise the level of blood glucose. Self-care teaching should emphasize recognizing early symptoms of mastitis and seeking prompt treatment while continuing to breastfeed.

Mothers with diabetes are also at risk for candidiasis if blood glucose levels are elevated. Preventing this problem involves careful control of blood glucose, drying the nipple after breastfeeding, and being aware of the early symptoms (see Chapter 15).

Once lactation is established, most women who have diabetes report that their breastfeeding experiences are no different from those of mothers without diabetes. The mother with diabetes needs additional calories while breastfeeding. As her child begins to wean, the mother will again need to make alterations in her diet and insulin intake to compensate for a decrease in milk production. If weaning is gradual, fewer problems and adjustments arise.

Thyroid Disease

The thyroid gland controls the body's metabolism and promotes normal growth of central nervous system development. It produces three hormones: thyrosine (T_4), triiodothyronine (T_3), and calcitonin. T_3 and T_4 are chemically similar and are known as thyroid hormones. Postpartum thyroid dysfunction is a common event, occurring in some 17 percent of women. Thyroid disease is considered an immune-mediated dysfunction. Its connection to the postpartum changes of the immune system is not yet clear (Gennaro et al., 1997). Breastfeeding women who develop disorders of the thyroid gland can be treated and continue to breastfeed.

Hypothyroidism. Maintaining full-term pregnancy is rare in untreated women who suffer from hypothyroidism; therefore, most breastfeeding women with a history of hypothyroidism are on replacement therapy. For the untreated breastfeeding woman, hypothyroidism can result in a reduced milk supply. Other symptoms in the mother are thyroid swelling or nodules (goiter), cold intolerance, dry skin, thinning hair, poor appetite, extreme fatigue, and depression. When the thyroid deficiency is not known, these problems are often attributed to postpartum hormonal changes and changes in lifestyle (notably, constant care of the baby) and remain undiagnosed—at least for a time. When the infant of one mother suddenly and completely weaned, the mother, subsequently receiving a diagnosis of hypothyroidism, reported that she "never experienced any fullness in the breast—it was as though I'd dried up overnight."

These complaints, sometimes coupled with the infant's failure to gain weight satisfactorily on breastmilk alone, should alert the nurse or lactation consultant to the possibility of thyroid deficiency and to the reality that the mother needs further medical diagnostic evaluation. If replacement therapy of thyroid extract with synthetic T_4 (thyroxine, sodium levothyroxine, or Synthroid) or other thyroid preparation is adequate, the relief of the symptoms and an increase in the milk supply can be quite dramatic. The daily replacement dose of thyroid is 0.25 to 1.12 mg of sodium levothyroxine or equivalent doses of other thyroid preparation. Women whose replacement therapy was determined before pregnancy should be reevaluated after the baby's birth to determine whether adjustment is necessary.

Postpartum Thyroiditis. Postpartum thyroiditis is an autoimmune disorder that affects women worldwide. Its symptoms—fatigue, depression, and anxiety—may go unrecognized in the postpartum period.

Hyperthyroidism. An excess of thyroid hormone is characterized by loss of weight (despite an increased appetite), nervousness, heart palpitations, and a rapid pulse at rest. A well-developed case of hyperthyroidism with exophthalmos (bulging eyes) is called Graves' disease. Hyperthyroidism, a common disorder thought to affect 2 percent of women typically in their mid-twenties or thirties, can develop for the first time postpartum. The ability to lactate does not appear to be affected, although the mother's nervousness may complicate her ability to cope with the daily caregiving of her infant.

Generally, laboratory diagnosis of hyperthyroidism can be established by values from just two laboratory tests: serum TSH and serum free T_4 index. When evaluation of the thyroid using a radioactive substance is deemed essential, technetium-99m pertechnetate is the preferred agent. A listing on the safety of use of isotopes in breastfeeding women from the Nuclear Regulatory Commission can be found at http://neonatal.ttuhsc.edu/lact/html/radio.html.

Pituitary Dysfunction

Severe postpartum hemorrhage and hypotension may result in the pituitary gland's failure to produce gonadotropins, which leads to a condition known as *panhypopituitarism* or *Sheehan's syndrome.* Along with lactation failure, the woman has loss of pubic and axillary hair, intolerance to cold, breast tissue atrophy, low blood pressure, and vaginal tissue atrophy. Milder cases of pituitary disruption may occur, with less severe symptoms and delay in milk synthesis. DeCoopman's report (1993) that lactation continued following pituitary resection suggests that the role of the pituitary gland may be temporary in the early establishment of lactation rather than an essential requirement throughout its course. Prolactinomas (prolactin-secreting adenomas) are pituitary tumors that stimulate the secretion of prolactin and produce secondary amenorrhea and galactorrhea. Women with prolactinomas may breastfeed without restriction.

Polycystic Ovarian Syndrome

Polycystic ovarian syndrome (PCOS) is a common endocrine-metabolic disorder in women in which the presence of multiple cysts interferes with ovarian function. The prevalence of PCOS is anywhere from 3 to 20 percent. Originally called Stein-Leventhal syndrome, women with polycystic ovarian syndrome are also likely to have amenorrhea and hirsutism (unusual hair growth), and to be obese. Maracso, Marmet, and Shell (2000) describe three cases of breastfeeding women with PCOS who had insufficient milk supply.

There is a strong possibility that the high level of testosterone associated with PCOS interferes with the hormones necessary for full lactation; however, results of a study of one such hormone, insulin, showed no differences between breastfeeding women with and without PCOS (Maliqueo et al., 2001). The LC working with a mother who is experiencing a delay with her milk coming is wise to ask questions about menstrual problems, infertility, miscarriages, and ovarian cysts.

Theca Lutein Cysts

Theca lutein cysts are an unusual condition in which, during pregnancy, both ovaries are enlarged by multiple cysts that produce a high level of testosterone. Several weeks postpartum, the cysts resolve and the testosterone level returns to normal. Women with this condition usually have delayed lactogenesis II. After testosterone drops (~300 ng/dl), milk production begins and the mother is able to breastfeed (Hoover, Barbalinardo, & Pia Platia, 2002).

Cystic Fibrosis

Cystic fibrosis (CF) is a generalized hereditary disorder of infants, children, and young adults. It is associated with the widespread dysfunction of the exocrine glands and is marked by signs of chronic pulmonary disease, obstruction of the pancreatic ducts, and pancreatic enzyme deficiency. In the past, children with the disease rarely lived to adulthood. Early treatment has enabled young women with CF to grow up, marry, give birth, and breastfeed.

Generally, mothers with CF should be encouraged to breastfeed as much as any other mother. Concern about breastfeeding involves the possible risk to the mother's own health status while breastfeeding and caring for a young infant, rather than the quality of the breastmilk. Although there are some differences in lipid composition, the breastmilk of mothers with CF contains nutrients sufficient to supply the energy needs of the nursing infant.

Although these women may breastfeed, they need close nutritional monitoring. Because the nutritional status of the person with CF is already compromised, the extra calories needed for breastmilk production may cause excessive weight loss. Breastfeeding is an acceptable option for women with the disease as long as the maternal diet is closely monitored and vitamin and caloric supplementation is offered when necessary.

Shiffman et al. (1989) reported two cases in which the mothers breastfed for 1 month and 2 months respectively, during which time the babies grew at appropriate rates. In both cases, the concentrations of milk sugar, electrolytes, sodium, potassium, and chloride were within normal limits. At the same time, concentrations of milk proteins, fat, and IgA appeared to decrease during periods of pulmonary exacerbations. In another study (Michel & Mueller, 1994) on five women with cystic fibrosis who breastfed, four of their five infants maintained adequate growth. The mother of the fifth infant who exclusively breastfed him for 6 months added supplemental foods when it became apparent that his growth slowed.

Although these women may breastfeed, they need close nutritional monitoring. Because the nutritional status of the person with CF is already compromised, the extra calories needed for breastmilk production may cause excessive weight loss. One early case presentation (Welch, Phelps, & Osher, 1981) discussed the breastfeeding course of a 20-year-old woman with CF. Her early breastfeeding course was normal, and the baby grew appropriately through the first 10 weeks postpartum. Thereafter, the mother continued to lose weight and her respiratory status began to worsen. She began antibiotic therapy and stopped breastfeeding. Another case report documented the normal growth of an infant through 6 weeks of exclusive breastfeeding by a 24-year-old mother with CF. These authors concluded that breastfeeding was an "acceptable option" for women with the disease, as long as the maternal diet was closely monitored and vitamin and caloric supplementation was offered when necessary (Golembeski & Emergy, 1989).

Breastfeeding has another advantage for the mother with CF. Because individuals with CF are chronic carriers of bacterial pathogens (such as *Staphylococcus aureus* and *Pseudomonas*), breastmilk lymphocytes, sensitized to the bacterial pathogens carried by the mother protect the infant against these infections.

Acute Illness and Infections

Common illnesses, such as colds and upper-respiratory tract infections or gastroenteritis, are not contraindications for breastfeeding. For most infections, the key word is self-limiting. Usually, such infections are not life-threatening; furthermore, the infected mother provides antibody protection to her infant through continued breastfeeding, thereby decreasing her baby's exposure or modifying the illness. Interruption of breastfeeding renders the infant more susceptible to the maternal illness, exposes him unnecessarily to the hazards of artificial baby milks, and removes an important source of comfort for him (Coates & Riordan, 1992).

Postpartum infections expose the breastfeeding dyad to potential delayed breastfeeding, prolonged hospital stay, and possible separation. Urinary tract infection (UTI) is the most common problem in women seen by primary care providers. Many women, especially if they are sexually active, suffer from multiple recurrence of UTIs. *Escherichia coli* is the most common pathogen associated with UTIs. Breastfeeding women with a UTI are treated with antibiotics; thus concern relates to the safety of taking a medication while they are breastfeeding.

Timethroprim (100 mg every 12 hours for 3 days) is an effective and commonly prescribed treatment for UTIs. Quinolones (norfloxacin, ciprofloxacin), used to treat a broad spectrum of gram-positive and gram-negative infections, are also used to treat UTIs. Both drugs are considered safe during breastfeeding (Hale, 2002). Women should ask their physician for a "standing" prescription at home that will allow them to begin medication as soon as they experience symptoms. Uro-sticks, which detect white cells in the urine, can be purchased for women to use in self-diagnosis. Self-treatment also includes drinking at least 6 to 8 glasses of water a day, drinking cranberry juice, avoiding caffeine, and urinating immediately after having sex.

Antibiotics are commonly used to treat postpartum infections. When given to the mother, they usually pose no danger to the infant and thus should not be used to justify an unnecessary interruption or cessation of breastfeeding (Chapter 5). In addition to UTIs, other postpartum infections that are treated with antibiotics are mastitis (see Chapter 9 for a detailed discussion), puerperal infections (puerperal fever, mastitis), wound infections from cesarean incisions, and episiotomies.

Tuberculosis

Approximately one third of tuberculosis (TB) cases in the United States occur in people younger than 35 years of age (Centers for Disease Control, 2000). Tuberculosis in women in their childbearing years reflects other coexisting influences, such as drug abuse associated with conditions of urban poverty and the influx of immigrants from areas of the world where there is a high prevalence of tuberculosis (Simpkins, Hench, & Bhatia, 1996). Women with tuberculosis who have been treated appropriately for 2 or more weeks (and who are otherwise considered to be noncontagious) may and should breastfeed (American Academy of Pediatrics,

1997a; World Health Organization, 1998). Separation of the mother from her infant is rarely justified.

A latent TB infection during pregnancy is usually treated with a 9-month course of isoniazid. Active TB is treated with isoniazid, rifampin, and ethambutol for 9 months (Lake, 2001). Drug therapy for women with active cases may be initiated in the second trimester of pregnancy. The risk of drug toxicity to an infant breastfed by a mother taking antituberculosis medication is minimal. A breastfeeding newborn might receive 6 to 20 percent of the therapeutic dose of isoniazid and 1 to 11 percent of other drugs, such as rifampin, ethambutol, and streptomycin (Snider & Powell, 1984). Moreover, infants exposed to tuberculosis are themselves treated with a therapeutic dose of isoniazid.

The 1998 policy of the Global Program for Vaccines and Immunization states that "infants in situations where they are at-risk of TB infection should be immunized with BCG (Bacillus Calmette-Guérin) as soon after birth as possible" (WHO, 1998). Thus, women who have moved to the United States from countries where TB is endemic and have been vaccinated with BCG will probably have a positive purified protein derivative (PPD) test. PPD, an intradermal injection on the forearm, is a screening test for TB. If it is positive, it will appear as a reddened induration. There is no reliable way to tell if a positive PPD is from BCG vaccination or infection (Lake, 2001) and this mother will need to be followed-up with more testing.

If a breastfeeding mother becomes acutely ill with TB, breastfeeding may have to be interrupted. The mother's breasts should not be allowed to become engorged; a staff member should arrange for the mother to express her milk so that the woman's breasts remain comfortable.

Group B Streptococcus

Group B streptococcus (GBS) is the leading cause of neonatal sepsis. From 15 to 30 percent of women are carriers of the GBS (American Academy of Pediatrics, 1997b). US women are routinely screened for GBS during pregnancy. Women at-risk for GBS infection are given antibiotics intravenously during labor. There is a possibility that GBS can be passed to the infant through breastmilk (Dinger et al., 2002).

Questions may arise about the transfer of the antibiotic into mothers' milk and the effect on the baby. None of the antibiotics commonly used (penicillin, ampicillin, or if penicillin-allergic, clindamycin or erythromycin) are contraindicated in pregnant or nursing mothers. In fact, antibiotics to prevent GBS are directly given to infants. At the time of this writing, it is not known if the frequent antibiotics administration for GBS leads to greater exposure to candidiasis in breastfeeding mothers.

Dysfunctional Uterine Bleeding

Normal uterine bleeding (lochia) following birth ceases in about 3 to 5 weeks. The median duration of lochial flow for breastfeeding women is 27 days (Visness, Kennedy, & Ramos, 1997). Nearly half of women who fully breastfeed experience some vaginal bleeding or spotting between 6 and 8 weeks postpartum (Visness, Kennedy, & Ramos, 1997). Abnormal bleeding can inhibit breastmilk synthesis. Willis and Livingstone (1995) described ten cases of insufficient milk following severe postpartum hemorrhage. In the early weeks, excessive bleeding may be due to placental fragments retained in the uterus (Neifert, McDonough, & Neville, 1981).

Bleeding caused by a relaxed uterus occurs less often in the breastfeeding woman, because the oxytocin released by the suckling infant causes the uterus to contract during each suckling episode. Later bleeding may result from miscarriage or the irregular onset of hormonal function. Treatment includes hormonal therapy or nonsteroidal anti-inflammatory drugs (NSAIDs). If bleeding is excessive, prolonged, or unexplained, curettage of the uterine lining may be necessary.

For excessive postpartum bleeding, the physician usually orders intravenous oxytocin and then methylergonovine maleate (Methergine), a derivative of an ergot alkaloid, if the uterus fails to respond. Unlike crude ergot preparations, no adverse effects have been reported following the use of methylergonovine by nursing mothers. Prostaglandin may also be given. None of these medications suppress lactation.

Anxiety always accompanies excessive bleeding. Intervention should focus on relieving the mother's anxiety and assisting in determining the cause of the bleeding while maintaining breastfeeding. The mother should be referred to a physician for an immediate appointment or, if the bleeding is especially severe and a physician is not available, she should be taken to the hospital emergency room. Because leaving her alone only increases her fear, someone should stay with her until she can be medically evaluated. A dilation and curettage (D&C) if required, can usually be performed in an outpatient setting, which reduces the likelihood and duration of mother-infant separation.

Maternal Immunizations

Health care workers tend to be reluctant to immunize breastfeeding women. Standard immunizations with killed or attenuated vaccine can usually be given to breastfeeding women without any problem. Immunization with a live vaccine is an exception to this rule. For example, nasal influenza vaccine or smallpox vaccine should not be given to breastfeeding women. If a breastfeeding woman lives with a person recently vaccinated with a live vaccine, she should take precautions. Guidelines for breastfeeding and emerging infections are changing rapidly and the health care provider should go to the Internet (www.cdc.gov) to retrieve the most recent guidelines from medical experts.

Surgery

Surgery of any kind is a stressful experience. Surgery that is scheduled when the mother is breastfeeding and caring for a small child or infant raises the possibility of separation from the baby and the inability to care for him. The mother who enters the hospital in advance of a surgical procedure may have sufficient time to make plans. If she knows on which floor she will be housed, she can learn the visitation policy for that floor in that hospital (whether her baby and other minor children will be allowed to visit her), how long she will be in the hospital, the availability of a fully automatic breast pump, and the staff's knowledge and experience with breastfeeding mothers.

Getting in touch with a lactation consultant in the hospital ensures that someone knowledgeable is aware of her concerns about preserving lactation and the breastfeeding relationship. This person may be able to arrange for a breast pump to use in advance of the surgery (and immediately thereafter if needed). Guidelines for helping the breastfeeding mother who undergoes surgery are summarized in Box 16–1.

Generally, surgery is likely to result in a temporary reduction in a woman's milk supply as measured by expressing. However, once the mother is fully awake, she may feel uncomfortably full. If the surgery involved the breast, pumping should begin as soon as possible to avoid putting further pressure on the operative site from engorgement and to relieve the mother's discomfort. A mother who donated her kidney to her sister continued to breastfeed and pump while in the hospital. If the staff has limited experience in assisting breastfeeding women, a referral should be made to the in-hospital lactation consultant so that she can provide care for the mother. Most hospitals allow a breastfeeding infant to stay with the mother after the surgery if another adult is present to take care of the infant. If this is not possible, the baby can be brought to the hospital to be breastfed.

During her hospitalization, the mother may be receiving one or more medications. If she must be separated from her baby, she needs to determine whether she will express and discard her milk or send it home with a family member to be given to the baby. Once the mother is at home, how her baby will react to her depends on several factors, including the length of time the mother was absent, how the baby was fed in her absence, and the baby's age at the time of the separation.

Donating Blood

Is it a good idea for a breastfeeding woman to donate blood? It depends upon the circumstances. For example, it would not be a good idea for a mother to give blood soon after childbirth. The American Red Cross says that lactating women may donate blood if they wish to do so but they suggest waiting at least 6 weeks after an uncomplicated term delivery or cesarean birth. If a blood transfusion was

---

BOX 16–1

Surgery and the Breastfeeding Mother: Guidelines for Care

- Encourage the mother to plan for help at home after surgery to allow time to recuperate.
- Use an outpatient surgical facility rather than an inpatient facility.
- Arrange for breastfeeding of the baby immediately before the surgery.
- Assist the mother in breastfeeding as soon as she awakes from anesthesia.
- Make rooming-in arrangements for the breastfeeding child if an inpatient facility is required. (Most hospitals require that another adult be present to care for the baby.)

- Express and freeze a supply of breastmilk before the surgery (if needed).
- Aid the mother in conditioning the baby to cup-feedings before surgery if it is determined that temporary supplementary feedings will be necessary.
- Encourage the mother to take postoperative analgesia to alleviate pain. (The infant will receive only a small dose through breastmilk.)
- Show the mother how to "splint" the surgical area with pillows if abdominal surgery is performed. Cover the incision area with dressings.

necessary during delivery, the mother should wait for 12 months. If a breastfeeding mother does give blood, she should eat especially well, stay hydrated, and avoid lifting her baby or heavy items with the arm used to donate the blood (La Leche League International, 2001b).

Relactation

Relactation is the process of restimulating lactation. It can occur days, weeks, or months after lactation has ended. In developing countries, relactation is routinely initiated as part of the rehydration therapy that is offered to ill and seriously malnourished infants and young children whose nutritional difficulties start after weaning from the breast, when the baby develops diarrhea after bottle-feedings are introduced. In these centers, the mothers receive additional foods, the babies are put to breast frequently and for long periods, and they are fed other foods only after suckling. The mothers live at the center with other mothers receiving the same assistance, and they become a mutual support system along with the staff, who strongly support the importance of reestablishing breastfeeding. In nearly all cases, the mothers relactate fully, and the babies' health status is improved.

In the developed world, the purpose of relactation and induced lactation is to enable breastfeeding after an untimely weaning or to initiate breastfeeding that has been delayed by neonatal or maternal illness or prematurity (Seema & Satyanarayanan, 1997; Thompson, 1996). Relactation is also an option for a mother who bottle-feeds at first but has a change of mind or discovers that her infant cannot tolerate infant formula.

Generally, relactation is easier for the mother to accomplish if the interval between the end of the pregnancy or the last day of previous breastfeeding (or pumping) is short. A milk supply can be reestablished with sufficient, regular stimulation. Although metoclopramide, domperidine, and hormones have been used to assist mothers, hormonal preparations are not necessary in all cases. Furthermore, an important but often neglected consideration is the baby's willingness to accept the breast. In situations in which the baby has never been put to breast, the age of the infant at the time this is attempted makes

a difference. The younger the baby, the greater the likelihood that he will be willing to suckle, particularly within the first 3 months of life. If the baby has previously breastfed, the chances are greater.

The reason for relactation is important. If the baby is intolerant of all or most of the available human milk substitutes, the mother may be more committed to resuming breastfeeding or to increasing her milk supply. However, placing emphasis only on her milk as evidence of success can result in increasing her anxiety and thereby inhibiting her milk production and ejection reflex. Thus the clinician needs to weigh carefully—with plenty of discussion with the mother—both the benefits and the more problematic elements of relactation.

Generally, a baby younger than 3 months old can usually be coaxed back to the breast. Between 3 and 6 months of age, individual infants may be more or less willing to do so; after 6 months, most babies cannot be convinced that the breast will provide either nutrition or nurturing. This fact points out poignantly that breastfeeding is a two-person activity; failure to keep this point continuously in mind in assisting the mother to relactate is likely to result in disappointment and a sense of failure that is avoidable. Realistic expectations are especially important with relactation, because many unknowns characterize the situation.

Induced Lactation

Induced/adoptive lactation is becoming more common and accepted as a cultural practice. Adopting couples, including lesbian couples, aware of the benefits of breastfeeding, seek assistance in breastfeeding their adopted baby. Health-care workers in hospitals where these babies are born are expected to be knowledgeable about inducing lactation and be able to refer the mother to a LC in the community who is an expert in this area.

Induced lactation is the process of stimulating lactation when a woman has not had the benefit of the hormones of pregnancy and has not lactated in the recent past. After the milk supply is established, ongoing production or "galactopoiesis" depends upon supply and demand (autocrine system) through the emptying of the breasts by breastfeeding or pumping (see Chapter 3 for a review of hormonal mechanisms). Examples of induced lactation include the following: breastfeeding an orphan for survival purposes (Abejide et al., 1997); a nulliparous woman who wants to breastfeed an adopted infant for nurturing and bonding in addition to providing some breastmilk; or a woman with biological children who has previously lactated and now wants to breastfeed an adopted child. Induced lactation attempts to increase proliferation of ducts and growth of the mammary via artificial means. Stimulation of the endogenous hormones prolactin and oxytocin can be accomplished by suckling an infant, by hand expression and nipple stimulation, or by pumping. Administration of exogenous hormones such as estrogen and progesterone, along with galactagogues has been the subject of anecdotal reports. The uterus and ovaries are not necessary for induction of lactation.

As an example, an adoptive mother (Cheales-Siebenaler, 1999) with a history of bilateral oophorectomy due to benign ovarian tumors initiated induced lactation with hormone replacement therapy. She discontinued the hormones when she began pumping to stimulate the milk production. After receiving notice that her baby was ready for placement, she began pumping her breasts every 3 to 4 hours and took metoclopramide to raise her prolactin levels. Syntocinon nasal spray was used before pumping. After a few weeks, she was able to discontinue the supplement and breastfeed on her own, the infant gaining weight normally.

The use of *exogenous* hormones and galactagogues as preparation for induced lactation has not been subjected to any scientific study. A detailed protocol for inducing lactation is provided in Box 16–2.

Inducing lactation is not a new phenenomen. For example, preliterate peoples have long known that it is possible to induce lactation. Most clinical studies on this topic are descriptive and were done over 20 years ago by Auerbach and Avery (1980, 1981) who surveyed adoptive mothers. More recent publications on this topic are case studies. As a result, some information presented in this chapter is anecdotal and is not evidence-based. For example, the treatment protocols for inducing lactation have not been tested in clinical trials. Searching the Internet reveals numerous Web sites on induced lac-

tation by women who have relactated or induced lactation and want to share their stories.

Adoptive mothers do not have the benefit of the hormones of pregnancy; therefore, induced lactation involves taking hormones to mimic pregnancy and stimulate their breasts through proliferation of ducts and growth of the mammary epithelium. The uterus and ovaries are necessary for pregnancy but this is not the case for induced lactation. Once the mother delivers, her progesterone and estrogen levels drop and prolactin "takes over" resulting in lactation. After the milk supply is established, it works on supply and demand (autocrine system) through the emptying of the breasts by breastfeeding or pumping. This process is described in detail in Chapter 3.

Domperidone, Metoclopramide, and Sulpride

Domperidone, metoclopramide, and sulpride are galactagogues that are used to help stimulate milk production. All three medications significantly raise prolactin levels by suppressing dopamine, and they subsequently increase breastmilk volume (Hale, 1999). Domperidone (Motilium) is a popular galactagogue in Canada. Unlike metoclopramide, it has minimal transfer across the blood-brain barrier and is not known to cause depression. Domperidone is not available in the United States but it is legal for a US physician to prescribe it. A Canadian pharmacy can ship domperidone with a prescription from a US physician or other practitioner with prescriptive authority.

Metoclopramide is commonly used in the United States to treat nausea and gastroesophageal reflux. The average interval between the first dose of metoclopramide and improvement in lactation is about 3 days. It increases breastmilk volume by inducing prolactin release and blocking dopamine but, unfortunately, it has a side effect of depression and should not be used over a long period.

Sulpride is an antidepressant and antipsychotic. Its use results in only moderate increases in breastmilk and is used less often for increasing breastmilk supply than the other two drugs.

Domperidone is the best choice as a galactogogue. Most adopting mothers will need to re-

BOX 16–2

Induced Lactation Protocol

Regular Protocol: Approximately 6 Months to Prepare Before Baby Arrives

- *6 months before baby is expected:* Start combination progesterone/estrogen birth control pills equivalent to Ortho 1/35 (1 mg norethindrone + 0.035 mg ethinyl estradiol) to stimulate breast development (must contain at least 1 mg of progesterone (2 to 3 mg is better) and no more than 0.035 mg of estrogen). Take continuously (without stopping for 1 week a month).

- *5 months before baby is expected:* Start taking domperidone, 10 mg 4 times daily increasing to 20 mg 4 times daily after 1 week. (See details on domperidone below.)

- *2 months before baby is expected:* Stop the combination progesterone/estrogen pill. There will be vaginal bleeding. Continue the domperidone at maximum dosage of 20 mg 4 times daily.

- Begin expressing milk preferably using an electric pump with a double setup for pumping both breasts. Pump every 3 hours and once during the night. Encourage the mother if at first very little (or no) milk is expressed. Freeze any pumped milk. Once pumping has started, the mother can take herbs considered to be galactagogues.

- Put the baby to breast immediately after arrival. Use a supplementer with formula or breastmilk to ensure that the baby receives sufficient nutriment for hydration and growth. Types of supplementers (commercial and "homemade") are described in Chapters 10 and 12.

- The amount of daily infant milk intake varies according to the weight and age of the baby. A baby who is over 7 pounds (3.7 kg) and over 1 week old should be receiving at least 600 ml/day (see Chapter 10).

- Continue taking the domperidone 20 mg 4 times daily until satisfactory milk supply is achieved. The dosage can be slowly dropped to see if the milk volume can be maintained with a lower dose

Accelerated Protocol: When There Is Little Time to Prepare

- Start combination oral progesterone/estrogen birth control pills to stimulate breast development. Take continuously (without stopping for 1 week a month).

- Start taking domperidone 20 mg 4 times daily the same time as the combination oral contraceptive pills.

- If significant breast changes occur within 30 days, stop taking the birth control pill while continuing to take domperidone.

- Begin pumping breasts and continue domperidone (see Regular Protocol above).

Source: Adapted from Goldfarb & Newman (2002); Newman & Pittman (2000).

main on the galactagogues for the entire time the baby is breastfeeding to maintain a milk supply. Domperidone and metoclopramide are approved by the American Academy of Pediatrics for use with breastfeeding women. Sulpride is under review.

Taking herbs in an attempt to increase breast-milk volume is a time-honored practice. Despite the popularity of blessed thistle herb and fenugreek seed to increase breastmilk supply, almost no scientific evidence thus far supports their effectiveness. The placebo effect, however, is very strong. If lactating women take herbs thinking that it will increase the volume of their breastmilk, and if there is no harm from taking them, then it is positive activity that enhances the lactation experience.

In some cases, the adopted baby will switch from bottle to breast fairly easily. In others, however, adopted babies will not go to breast. One mother who obtained a baby from an overseas agency was told that her new daughter had been suckled by her birth mother. Although the baby was then housed for 5 months in an orphanage and bottle-fed before being placed with her adoptive family, her new mother offered the breast. She reported that her baby reacted "in horror, as if she remembered having been nursed, but not by me!" It became clear that breastfeeding would not work. This mother continued to offer as much body contact and touching during bottle-feedings as possible.

With a newborn or a baby younger than 1 month, the usual experience is that the baby will, with little encouragement, root at and accept the breast using a feeding-tube device that enables the mother to feed the baby at (if not from) the breast. Many such mothers often report mild to moderate changes in menstrual cycling, some breast changes (including a feeling of fullness, a change in breast shape, and occasional leaking of milk), and other indicators of increasing milk production in the early adoptive nursing period when breastfeeding occurs very frequently.

Another obvious indication of an increasing supply of breastmilk is the change in infant stooling: less stool odor, a softening of the stool so that it more closely resembles the nearly liquid breastmilk stool, and a resultant lightening of the color from dark brown to mustard yellow. Because these stool changes usually occur gradually, the health-care worker assisting the adoptive mother needs to remind her that they are an indication of an increase in the proportion of human milk versus artificial formula that the baby is receiving.

In a few instances, mothers have reported a cessation of menstrual bleeding, although such a response is rare; it probably reflects a highly responsive mother and a baby whose suckling pattern is both vigorous and frequent. One mother laughingly reported, "If *your* baby sucked like a vacuum cleaner, you'd get milk in a week, too!" Often the adoptive mother will find that as solid feedings increase in frequency and volume, the amount of necessary supplemental fluid declines.

Even the highly motivated adoptive mother cannot be assured that she will produce milk. To do so without the benefit of a pregnancy that prepares her breasts for milk production, she more obviously depends on the suckling style of her baby: the frequency with which he is put to breast, the strength of his suckling, and the duration of each suckling episode.

Keeping one's priorities clear from the outset can provide the mother and baby with a unique relationship built on the special closeness that characterizes the breastfeeding experience. The clinician who assists a family with relactation or induced lactation is in a position to observe how mother and baby must truly work together to enjoy that which cannot be duplicated with any other method of feeding. Even if the mother never produces a single drop of milk, the closeness and intimacy that mother and baby derive from this special relationship cannot be underestimated (Davis, 2001).

Autoimmune Diseases

Systemic Lupus Erythematosus

Systemic lupus erythematosus (SLE), an autoimmune disease of the connective tissues, primarily affects women of childbearing age; therefore, lactation consultants not infrequently are called upon to care for women with this problem. The clinical presentations of lupus are remarkably diverse and include headaches, arthritic symptoms of joint, redness and swelling, and a butterfly rash on the cheeks and nose. Women with lupus have higher rates of miscarriage and infant prematurity. Raynaud's phenomenon is present in about 30 percent of cases. Fatigue is a major symptom, and the diagnosis of chronic fatigue syndrome and fibromyalgia may also be made concomitantly.

Lupus may be exaggerated after delivery, so close observation for lupus flares is needed. Some of these women report having an insufficient milk supply. One mother who has lupus stated that she "had never had enough milk" with all of her four children and always found it necessary to supplement feedings. Moreover, well-intentioned advice that she would have enough breastmilk if only she would breastfeed more often was frustrating to her because she was already breastfeeding frequently. Another mother who had plenty of breastmilk for her first two children was diagnosed with lupus after the birth of her third child. This infant, unlike her other children, failed to gain adequate weight despite the fact that he was able to suckle effectively at the breast. With supplementation using a feeding-tube device, the infant started gaining weight. The mother continued supplementing her baby's breastfeedings until he was about 5 months old, when he began taking solid foods.

There is no single medication appropriate for lupus patients; their health problems are managed in a problem-oriented fashion. NSAIDs and corticosteroids are a widely prescribed mainstay of therapy.

Multiple Sclerosis

Multiple sclerosis (MS) is a progressive degenerative neurological disorder that includes such symptoms as weakness, fatigue, incoordination, paralysis, and speech and visual disturbances. It affects twice as many women as men, and the diagnosis usually is made during the reproductive years (ages 20 to 40). The condition is known for its unpredictability and the variability of its prognosis and symptoms; the cause is unknown. Breastfeeding for these mothers is especially important, because some element of breastmilk, perhaps the essential fatty acids, appears to protect their children from subsequently developing multiple sclerosis (Pisacane et al., 1994).

Pregnancy and the number of births a woman has experienced have no effect on long-term disability from MS. Studies consistently report remission of symptoms during pregnancy followed by substantially increased exacerbation (deterioration) in the postpartum period, especially in the first 3 months (Worthington et al., 1994). The presence of an immunosuppressive factor in the maternal serum during the pregnancy may be protective; the subsequent drop in serum hormonal levels after birth may provoke exacerbations.

Women with MS who breastfeed are no more likely than women who do not breastfeed to alter the risk or timing of the exacerbation in the postpartum period. Fatigue and exhaustion from care of the infant is a particular problem in all cases, regardless of feeding method. One mother includes this report from Kirshbaum (1990):

I was nursing every two-and-one-half hours around the clock; I was totally exhausted. Also I had insomnia and sometimes couldn't get back to sleep after nursing . . . I had a bad exacerbation and my doctor prescribed a nurse who took care of both of us for two months. After that I used a babysitter, and now day care. I've recovered but I'm still more fatigued than before my pregnancy (p. 864).

Disrupted sleep, compromised nutrition, excess weight, and lack of supportive household help—all risks during the postpartum period—are more likely to result in a worsening of the disease, regardless of how the mother is feeding her baby. These mothers, especially, need support of all kinds including help with household work and child care. The concern the disabled woman has for her children and the consequences of living with a disability in a socially isolating and stigmatizing environment may lead to depression (Harrison & Stuifbergen, 2002). Interferon Beta-1B (Betaseron) is the current drug given to women with MS. Because of the large molecular weight, transfer of this drug into breastmilk is limited. Its lactation risk category is moderately safe (Hale, 2002). Acute exacerbations are treated with adrenocorticotropic hormone and methylprednisolone. Both drugs appear in breastmilk in low concentrations.

Rheumatoid Arthritis

Rheumatoid arthritis (RA) is a chronic inflammatory disease thought to be caused by a genetically influenced autoimmune response. Symptoms include pain and swelling of the joints, pain on movement, and fatigue. RA symptoms usually go into remission during pregnancy and then relapse postpartum. The problem is greater for breastfeeding women, probably owing to their hyperprolactinemic state; prolactin has been shown to act as an immunostimulator (Brennan & Silman, 1994). The most severe symptoms occur after a first pregnancy; symptoms are less severe following subsequent pregnancies (Barrett et al., 2000).

NSAIDs are used as first-line therapy to decrease pain and inflammation. Due to their erosive effect on the gastrointestinal tract, the mother may also be anemic from blood loss. Methotrexate therapy, used for severe cases, is contraindicated with breastfeeding, according to the American Academy of Pediatrics (see Chapter 5). However, only very small amounts of this drug are secreted into breastmilk (Hale, 2002). Women with RA often feel overwhelmed with fatigue both during pregnancy and postpartum (Carty, Conine, & Wood-Johnson, 1986). If the mother's hands and fingers are stiff, breastfeeding is simpler than is artificial feeding, which requires more complex movements. Although this mother needs additional rest, she still needs to continue range-of-motion exercises. Periodic rest periods and the wearing of removable braces or splints to support joints will help to reduce fatigue (Carty, Conine, & Hall, 1990).

Physically Challenged Mothers

Increasing numbers of women who are physically impaired are choosing to become pregnant and to breastfeed. For physically impaired women, breastfeeding is more than the giving of good nutrition; it helps to normalize this aspect of their life experience. Breastfeeding builds the mother's confidence and self-esteem by proving that her body is capable of nourishing her baby even though she may be able to do little else quite as easily. Using the mother's knowledge of her health problem and the breastfeeding specialist's expertise in breastfeeding can lead to some ingenious solutions. (Minami, 2000).

In a study of women who had spinal cord injury, 67 percent reported having sexual intercourse after injury (Jackson & Wadley, 1999). As a rule, the lower the injury the less loss of function (Cesario, 2002). A woman with a spinal cord injury should be able to breastfeed her baby if her injury is below the sixth cervical lumbar vertebrae (C6) (Craig, 1990; Halbert, 1998). The point of origin for the nerves

that innervate the breast and nipples (see Chapter 3) is the fourth to sixth thoracic vertebrae (T4–T6), well above C6. If she can breastfeed, chances are that the mother has function of her upper extremities and can position the baby for breastfeeding and perform other baby care activities, but she may need help.

In some disorders involving impaired mobility, especially those that are immunologically mediated (e.g., RA, MS, and myasthenia gravis), pregnancy may bring a period of remission followed by postpartum relapse. Often, women suffering from such a disease feel so good during their pregnancy that they take it for granted that their condition has improved. When the condition worsens after birth, it is doubly difficult because additional energy is now required to care for a new baby.

Physcially challenged parents are adaptive and even ingenious in devising ways to carry out basic baby care activities. A case study (Thomson, 1995) of a mother with a congenital below-elbow limb absence describes how the mother positioned her baby at the breast. "Using her right hand, she held her breast between her thumb and fingers in the same plane as the baby's mouth, when closed. She then placed her breast in the baby's mouth by leaning forward. This mother had her older daughter help her to attach for about 4 months. After this, the baby was able to 'hop on' by herself."

The lesson for the nurse and lactation consultant assisting mothers with disabilities is simple: creativity counts. Often the mother with a disability knows better than anyone else how important flexible thinking is in solving a problem or overcoming a problem that may seem to be insoluble. Ask for the mother's help in thinking through the situation. Together, a solution may be found. For example, 3 years before her baby's birth, one mother suffered a debilitating stroke, one outcome of which was substantial loss of arm and hand control and strength. She and her lactation consultant experimented with a variety of slings that the mother could put on with one hand and wear to keep her baby close to her. This was especially important when the mother had to move the baby from one room to another or out of the house, for she was fearful when she could not hang onto a handrail when going down stairs, for example. After practicing with several different positions, the mother identified alternate ways to present the breast to the baby that enabled both to be comfortable and required a minimum of movement by the mother. By the time the baby was 3 months old, he had learned to help his mother by scooting up to the breast himself when placed on the bed next to her.

Good parenting occurs even when a mother is severely disabled. Generally, these mothers find that breastfeeding is more convenient than is bottlefeeding. Breastfeeding also renders caring for the infant simpler, because there is nothing to measure, prepare, pour, or sterilize. Yet friends and relatives may react negatively, concerned that the mother should not breastfeed due to her limited energy or abilities. These mothers need compassionate support and guidance more than those with normal mobility. Suggestions for the physically disabled mother and her family on breastfeeding and baby care are listed in Box 16–3.

Because the physically challenged mother is usually under continuing medical care and has so many needs, the health professional working with the disabled breastfeeding mother may find her role expanding to that of a case manager; she coordinates medical, family, and community support and services. If the mother has someone to help her with the physical tasks, diplomatically arrange for that person to take over the household jobs and care of older children and let the mother take care of her baby. Many of these mothers are already on medications and their physicians should be consulted about the safety of taking specific medications while breastfeeding. Most medications are compatible with breastfeeding (see Chapter 5), especially with short-term use. If the physician recommends weaning, the health-care provider should research the drug using up-to-date references and, if necessary, act as an advocate for the mother in her desire to continue to breastfeed.

For peer support, set up group sessions that include any woman who has a disability and has given birth in the last 5 years. The purpose of these sessions is to provide information about coping with the demands placed on them by pregnancy, birthing, and early infant care, and about allowing the more experienced women to serve as mother-to-mother role models for those women having a first child.

Nurses and health professionals can learn a great deal from the mother who has developed extraordinary survival skills to work around inconveniences. For example, one mother has no left hand and lower arm, yet she tends to breastfeed her baby on her left side, propping her baby against her upper-left arm so that her right hand is free. This mother also needs a battery or electric pump, not a hand-operated device, to express her milk.

For mothers who are blind and cannot rely on visual cues, breastfeeding is a way to communicate with their infant nonvisually through touch, smell, sound, and even intuitive sensitivity (Martin, 1992).

Until recently, limited information was available regarding breastfeeding (and all other aspects of childbearing) among women with disabilities. Unfortunately, society's general view remains that women with a physical disability are not capable of having or caring for a child. Even now, only a few resources for these families exist. Two such resources are La Leche League International and the Australian Breastfeeding Association. Both organizations have educational materials, including audiocassette tapes and Braille material, for the physically disabled mother who is breastfeeding. These organizations will also refer the mother to another woman who has had a similar experience.

Seizure Disorders

Seizure disorders are classified into two major groups: partial and generalized. Partial or focal seizures begin in a specific area of the brain and produce symptoms ranging from simple repetitive movements to more complex abnormal movements and bizarre behavior. Generalized seizures have no specific point of origin in the brain. The most common type is a major motor seizure, formerly called grand mal epilepsy.

Seizure disorders can be so well controlled by medications that seizures are rarely a problem for the lactating mother. However, nurses need to know about the effect of the medication on the breastfed infant. The physician will prescribe antiseizure medications on the basis of diagnosis of the seizure and its pattern of occurrence, and on the tolerance and response of the mother to the prescribed drug.

BOX 16–3

Baby Care Guidelines for Physically Disabled Breastfeeding Mothers

- Mothers with some upper-body strength who are confined to a wheelchair can use a harness or a wide belt with a long strip of Velcro to lift and retrieve a crawling baby from the floor.
- One or two special "feeding nests" for breastfeeding that are easily accessible and comfortable for the mother can be set up. Group together a crib or other sleeping place for the infant, diaper-changing supplies, and a comfortable place to breastfeed.
- If the baby is small, he can be laid diagonally across the mother's knees on a pillow to breastfeed. Put other pillows under the mother's arms for support. Elevate the mother's feet on a footrest to keep the infant secure during the feeding.
- A mother who cannot elevate her feet can rest her forearm holding the infant on a pillow placed across her knees. This arrangement ensures that if the infant rolls, he will roll toward the mother.
- Changing tables and cribs can be adapted so that they are accessible to a wheelchair, and the room can be arranged so that moving about is minimized. A low-sided pram or baby stroller makes it easier to slide the baby out onto the mother's lap without requiring much lifting.
- A baby sling allows the mother's arms to be free while ensuring that the baby is safe and supported during breastfeeding. This is also helpful when the mother has unilateral weakness or paralysis (e.g., as from a stroke).
- A bell tied to the baby's shoes keeps track of where the mobile child is.
- A toddler will quickly learn to climb on his mother's knee for a ride and to sit still while the chair is moving.
- The baby can be given extra cuddling, such as touching at night in bed, if there are barriers to physical contact during the day.
- A baby clothed in overalls with crossed straps can be picked up fairly easily.
- The mother's use of a nursing bra that opens in the front instead of the back, one with an easy-to-fasten clip or Velcro that can be handled with one hand, will facilitate breastfeeding. The usual clip for opening and closing the bra flap can be replaced with Velcro. Some all-elastic bras are easily pulled down to allow the baby to breastfeed.
- Maternity clothes can be altered to incorporate Velcro openings or large ring zippers. Antique buttonhooks are helpful to manipulate the small buttons found on many garments.
- The mother should plan rest periods during the day and should sit to work whenever possible.
- The mother can sleep with the infant or have the father or someone else bring the baby to her to nurse during the night.
- Use of an intercom system that picks up the sound of the baby crying is helpful. If the mother is deaf, the sound can be transformed into flashing light signals.
- If the mother cannot lift both the baby and herself, she might care for her baby on the floor (preferably carpeted), feeding, changing, and playing with him. This enables her to roll the baby to her, instead of lifting him, when he needs attention. A beanbag will provide support for breastfeeding.

Common medications for seizure disorders are phenytoin (Dilantin), carbamazepine (Tegretol), primidone (Mysoline), and phenobarbital. Phenobarbital taken in higher-than-average amounts (50 to 100 mg two or three times daily), however, may cause drowsiness in infants or mothers; primidone may also cause sedation in the infant. For example, an estimated maximal dose of carbamazepine that the breastfed baby would consume in breastmilk is 3 to 5 percent of the weight-adjusted maternal dose, an amount similar to other drugs, such as phenytoin and valproic acid. Consensus guidelines among neurologists state that taking antiepileptic drugs (except for such sedatives as phenobarbital, primidone, or benzodiazepine) does not constitute a contraindication for breastfeeding (Delgado-Escueta & Janz, 1992). Although monitoring the infant is important for detecting idiosyncratic reactions, the risk of these reactions appears to be outweighed by the benefits of breastfeeding (Ito et al., 1995).

In the unusual case in which the mother has seizures, breastfeeding is in no way contraindicated. Dropping or harming the infant during a seizure is no more probable during breastfeeding than it is during bottle-feeding. Usually, a prodromal warning (aura) alerts the mother of an impending seizure, and she is able to take safety precautions to protect her infant (Box 16–4).

Headaches

Migraine headaches, hormonally sensitive headaches of an episodic nature, tend to lessen through the course of pregnancy and menopause (Sances et al., 2003; Silberstein, 1993). Postpartum headaches can be caused by oral contraceptives or by having epidural or spinal anesthesia during childbirth, or they can occur for no apparent reason. Breastfeeding delays the postpartum recurrence of migraine headaches.

Some women have a brief but intense headache when they have an orgasm. It is thought that rise in blood pressure and heart rate during sexual activity are similar to the physiological process that produces migraine. Thorley (2000) identified two types of lactational headaches:

- Type 1 occurs on the first let-down during a feed and is linked to the surge of oxytocin from the let-down.

BOX 16–4

Guidelines for a Breastfeeding Mother with a Seizure Disorder

1. On each level of the house, make sure there is a playpen in which to quickly place the baby when a seizure seems imminent.

2. Pad the arms of the rocker or chair where the mother usually breastfeeds with extra pillows and cushions.

3. Place guardrails padded with pillows around the mother's bed if she customarily takes her infant to bed to breastfeed.

4. Attach to the baby and to the stroller or baby carrier tags stating that the mother has a seizure disorder, along with other pertinent information, whenever she is away from home.

- Type 2 is triggered by overfullness of the breast and is relieved by breastfeeding and/or pumping.

In addition to oxytocin surge at let-down and breast overfullness, trigger factors for headaches in lactating women include the baby sleeping through the night (Thorley, 1997) and breastfeeding twins (Wall, 1992). A family history of lactational headaches that disappear with weaning can also be a factor (Walker, 1999). Rest and ice packs should be tried before resorting to medications. Propranolol (Inderal), sumatriptan succinate (Imitrex), and NSAIDs—the standard drugs used for migraine headaches—are listed as being compatible with breastfeeding. Ergotamine alkaloids (Cafergot, DHE-45) are contraindicated in breastfeeding mothers due to their suppression of prolactin (Hale, 1999).

Postpartum Depression

Postpartum depression is a generic term that describes three types of disorders (the word depression is probably a misnomer, because anxiety and agitation are just as common with postpartum mood disorder as are typical signs of depression, such as withdrawal and lethargy):

- *Postpartum "blues":* About 70 to 80 percent of women experience a transient depression following birth, usually starting on the third postpartum day and lasting for a few days. The "blues" is temporary, accompanied by lability of mood, tearfulness, and negative feelings and is more common in women having their first child.

- *Postpartum depression:* As many as 20 percent of postpartum women have mild to moderate depression. Symptoms are tearfulness, despondency, feelings of inadequacy, suicidal ideation, sadness, reduced appetite, insomnia, feelings of helplessness and hopelessness, anxiety, and despair. Because every new mother experiences at least some of these symptoms that may be wrongly interpreted as clinical depression, this percentage may be inflated. This type of depression lasts at least 2 weeks but is usually longer.

- *Postpartum psychosis:* The most severe of the postpartum disorders, psychosis, typically begins within 2 to 4 weeks postpartum. The mother with postpartum psychotic depression may have insomnia, irrational ideas, feelings of failure, self-accusatory thoughts, depression, fatigue, and hallucinations; sometimes, she may threaten to commit suicide.

New mothers with high levels of life stress and few supportive relationships (especially with husband or partner) suffer more from postpartum depression. There is no consistent evidence that the mother's age, the number of children she has, or complications during the pregnancy and delivery are associated with the appearance of depression. Depressed new mothers have a 1.25 times greater risk of stopping breastfeeding than new mothers who have not developed depression (Henderson, 2003).

Postpartum hormonal shifts, although dramatic, appear to play no clear role in postpartum depression. Maternal hormonal levels during lactation represent the *normal postpartum state;* thus breastfeeding women should be at no greater risk for postpartum depression because their hormone levels are different from those in nonlactating women, particularly if this pattern of mothering is supported. Kangaroo Care, where the infant is placed skin-to-skin with his mother (Anderson et al., 2003), has been reported to lessen post-partum "blues" by hastening the return of the hypothalamic-pituitary-adrenal axis to its prepregnant state (Dombrowski et al., 2001). Prolonged maternal depression has an adverse effect on children's general behavior and developmental functioning.

Beck (1992) conducted a phenomenological study of the lived experience of women with postpartum depression. Eleven themes emerged from interviews with mothers:

- Loneliness
- Obsessive thinking
- Insecurities
- Anxiety attacks
- Loss of control
- Guilt
- Diminished concentration
- Fear that life would never be normal again
- Loss of interest in hobbies or goals
- Lack of all positive emotion
- Contemplation of death

Through further study, Beck (1993) found that loss of control was the basic social psychological problem in postpartum depression. One mother said, "I had absolutely no control and that was the scariest thing because I always had control." Another woman said of her feelings, "I just couldn't get out of the pain. It's like you hurt so bad and you don't want to be that way and yet you lost all control of everything."

Women who experienced postpartum depression attempted to cope with the problem of loss of control through a four-stage process: (1) encountering terror, (2) dying of self, (3) struggling to survive, and (4) regaining control. When depression started, these mothers felt trapped with no foreseeable escape. "One night I had my first severe panic attack, I felt like everything was closing in on me. Something just snapped in me and there was no going back." Mothers described this period as "going to the gates of hell and back," and "your worst possible nightmare." As the mothers regained control, gradually the number of good days experienced increased; yet they mourned the lost time they would not be able to recapture with their infants. When the mothers recovered, they talked about how their symptoms just eventually faded away. "When I was sick, I didn't want my baby. I didn't love my husband. I didn't want to work. I hated everything. When I got better, it all melted away" (Beck, 1993).

Ugarriza (2002) reported similar findings from studying 30 women with postpartum depression. These mothers had sleep deprivation, and they were confused, overwhelmed, and guilty about thoughts of hurting their babies. They described the illness as severe, long lasting, and causing marital discord.

Postpartum psychosis is rare, occurring in about one or two of every 1000 women who have a child. The onset of the psychosis occurs within a few days to 2 weeks after delivery, and symptoms peak at about 6 weeks postpartum. Hardly any problem is more distressing to all concerned than a mother suffering from postpartum psychosis. The family is in a state of severe crisis and disequilibrium and suffers from lack of sleep. If the mother is breastfeeding, the consulting therapist often insists that she wean her baby because of undue concern about a prescribed medication passing through the breastmilk. If the mother needs constant observa-

tion, there is the threat of hospitalization and separation. The decision about whether to hospitalize a psychotic mother and to separate her from her baby is agonizing. Care of the infant and possibly other children is an immediate concern.

Clinical Implications

Postpartum depression tends to occur when the maternal-infant bond is being formed. Every effort should be made to foster this crucial bond and breastfeeding as well. The mother with depression suffers a loss of maternal identity and self-esteem. Mothers at risk for postpartum depression usually display emotional problems very soon after the birthing experience. In fact, experienced maternity nurses can usually identify the mothers who are likely to become depressed. Typically, this mother has difficulty bonding with her baby and will make self-accusatory remarks, such as, "I am a terrible person" or "I have a lovely baby, a lovely house and a lovely husband, and I know I should be happy, yet I feel awful." Kitzinger (1989) offers this reminder:

Few women are prepared for the resentment, the sense of inadequacy, the guilt, anger and murderous feelings we have as mothers. There is delight, discovery and joy, and sometimes sheer ecstasy, too, and that makes it all worthwhile. But the trouble is that the image of motherhood is romanticized.

Health professionals vary in their knowledge about postpartum depression. Nurses tend to be more aware of postpartum depression than are physicians in that they better understand the disorder's impact on the mother and her family. Table 16–1 presents a clinical care plan for postpartum depression. If the mother has severe symptoms, she should be referred to a psychiatrist, psychologist, or advanced practice nurse who will probably initiate drug therapy. Most of these medications do not pass into the breastmilk in quantities sufficient to harm the infant. Weight gain of infants of breastfeeding women taking antidepressant medications is normal unless the mother has relatively long-lasting episodes of major depression (Hendrick et al., 2003).

Table 16-1

CLINICAL CARE PLAN FOR POSTPARTUM DEPRESSION*

Assessment	Intervention	Rationale
Previous history of postpartum depression	Listen to mother describe her feelings	Postpartum depression is likely to recur with subsequent births
Beyond first week postpartum: Tearfulness	Maintain a supportive and nonjudgmental attitude	Clinical depression occurs in about 20% of mothers
Mood swings Feelings of failure	Maintain mother's privacy and let her cry	Role changes and increased responsibilities cause stress
Insomnia and fatigue Anxiety and suicidal thoughts	Assist in providing social support and physical help for mother and infant	
Possible disinterest in baby	Monitor baby's weight gain and general well-being	Infant may not be receiving adequate nurturing and care due to mother's depression
Depression worsens	Refer to therapist for counseling and evaluation for medication therapy	Antidepressant and/or antianxiety drugs are effective in treating depression.
Mother taking medication for depression and wishes to continue breastfeeding	Research the effect of the medications upon the breastfeeding infant. Recommend optional medications	Most medications are safe to take while breastfeeding

Nursing diagnosis: Coping, ineffective individual, related to stress or potential complications of perinatal period and to life changes

Medications and Herbal Therapy for Depression

Women who suffer from severe postpartum depression should be medicated. The first-choice medications commonly used to control symptoms of postpartum depression in breastfeeding mothers are sertraline (Zoloft) and paroxetine (Paxil). These drugs are selective serotonin reuptake inhibitors (SSRIs) that control neuronal reuptake of serotonin. Their advantages include wide therapeutic range, a greater margin of safety, and fewer side effects than other drugs used to treat depression. Unlike tricyclics, which have an ascending dose curve, the SSRIs have a flat dose curve; thus the starting dose is often the same as the therapeutic dose. Sertraline (Zoloft) has the least drug-interaction potential among the SSRIs. Venlafaxine (Effexor), another drug often used in postpartum depression,

combines the SSRI action with that of norepinephrine reuptake inhibitors, such as desipramine. A list of medications used in postpartum depression is found in Table 16-2.

Such phenothiazines as perphenazine (Trilafon), such antianxiety drugs as alprazolam (Xanax), and such tricyclic antidepressants as imipramine (Trofanil) or nortriptyline (Pamelor) are also used for postpartum depression. With the exception of monoamine oxidase (MAO) inhibitors, these medications appear to be relatively safe for short-term therapy. The dosage of tricyclics is slowly increased over several days to minimize side effects. Sedation and other side effects may begin at once, but the antidepressant response occurs only after 10 to 21 days at full therapeutic dosage. MAO inhibitors may produce a mild stimulation effect almost at once, but again, full therapeutic benefit may take 2 to 6 weeks. Antidepressants need not be continued

Table 16–2

DRUGS USED FOR POSTPARTUM DEPRESSION

Drug Name	Usual Daily Oral Dosage (mg)	Use in Breastfeeding Mother and Safety Level
Selective Serotonin Reuptake Inhibitors (SSRI)		
fluoxetine (Prozac)	10–40	Dose transferred to breastmilk is high—from 1/5 to 1/4 of maternal dose. Problems reported; use alternate SSRI while breastfeeding
paroxetine (Paxil)	20	Infant receives about 1% of maternal dose; considered safe for breastfeeding
sertraline (Zoloft)	50–200	No apparent adverse effects reported; considered safe for breastfeeding
Serotonin-Norepinephrine Reuptake Inhibitors (SSNI)		
venlafaxine (Effexor)	75–200	Dose transferred to breastmilk is high—about 4% of maternal dose; use with caution
Tricyclics		
amitriptyline (Elavil)	50–300	Safe; no effects on infants reported; no apparent accumulation in nursing infant
desipramine (Norpramin)	50–300	Relatively safe
imipramine (Tofranil)	50–300	Relatively safe; infant would receive approximately .04 mg/kg/day; recommended therapeutic dosage for children is 1 mg/kg/day
nortriptyline (Pamelor)	25–100	Safe; not detected in serum of infant
MAO Inhibitors		
phenelzine (Nardil)	15–90	Contraindicated; inhibits lactation
tranylcypromine (Parnate)	10–30	Should not use
Phenothiazines		
chlorpromazine (Thorazine)	30–1000	Relatively safe if average dosage; one report of infant drowsiness with high dosage; may increase mother's milk supply
mesoridazine (Serentil)	100–400	Relatively safe
perphenazine (Trilafon)	4–6	Safe; dose passed to child through milk is only 0.1% that given the mother
thioridazine (Mellaril)	150–800	Relatively safe

Source: Adapted from Hale (2002).

indefinitely, and the drug will be discontinued after the mother has been asymptomatic for several weeks. Both tricyclics and MAO inhibitors are highly toxic in overdose. As a general rule, the health-care provider will limit the prescription to a 7- to 10-day supply.

Saint-John's-wort is a popular but controversial herb used for postpartum depression. Does it help alleviate depression? It may with mild depression but not when the depression is severe. The first large-scale multicenter randomized, placebo-controlled trial of Saint-John's-wort in patients with *major* depression revealed that the herb is no more effective than a placebo in treating the disorder (Shelton et al., 2001). To rely on herbal therapy when the breastfeeding mother is severely depressed is dangerous.

Support for the Mother with Postpartum Depression

Support of the breastfeeding woman with postpartum depression is critical. A support group of women with postpartum depression introduces the mother to women who have recovered from postpartum depression and helps to counter the isolation and loneliness these mothers feel (Maley, 2002). This support is especially crucial for mothers who are relatively housebound and likely to be drained by the demands of child care. Reducing the social isolation of the depressed mother reinforces her identity and ability to cope. A friend of the mother, a neighbor, a La Leche League chapter, or a church group are all possible supports. The quality of the marital relationship is of primary importance in the mother's postpartum adaptation, especially for first-time mothers. Because the father plays a key role, he should also be counseled and supported. If the mother and/or father are sleep deprived, every effort should be made to devise a plan by which they may sleep for at least 6 hours and thus benefit from the restoration of sleep.

Asthma

Between 1 and 7 percent of pregnant women have active asthma that may improve, worsen, or remain unchanged during pregnancy (Simpson & Creehan, 2002). Women with family history of asthma should be encouraged to breastfeed exclusively, because of the long-term protective effect of breastfeeding on asthma (see Chapters 4 and 18).

The main concern is the effect of medications taken by the mother to control her asthma. Asthma therapy should be continued during lactation and generally does not have to be altered. The two central classes of antiasthmatic medications are corticosteroids and bronchodilators, including beta-agonists (albuterol, terbutaline, metaproterenol). Beta-agonists are used to treat acute exacerbations and to prevent exercise-induced asthma. Most anti-asthma medications are administered by metered-dose inhalers that avoid systemic side effects by delivering the drug directly to the lungs. Metered aerosol inhalers deliver a given amount of a drug, and the likelihood of overdose is small. Halogenated corticosteroids given by inhalation provide selective topical effects that lessen the amount of corticosteroids transferred into breastmilk (see Chapter 5 for more information). Theophylline (Theo-Dur, Slo-BID, Slo-phyllin) is used less frequently now. The infant receives only a small percentage (< 10 percent) of the maternal dose (Ellsworth, 1994) but the drug may occasionally cause infant irritability and insomnia.

Smoking

Women who smoke are less likely to intend to breastfeed, less likely to initiate breastfeeding, and likely to breastfeed for a shorter period of time than nonsmokers (Amir & Donath, 2002). The fat content of breastmilk of smoking mothers is lower than nonsmokers and contains nicotine. The mother who smokes also exposes her infant to second-hand smoke that raises inhaled carbon monoxide to unsafe levels, aggravates allergies, and increases his risk of respiratory illnesses (Horta et al., 1997). Maternal cigarette smoking is associated with a 20 to 35 percent increase in respiratory illnesses. The breastfeeding smoker is also at greater risk for breast abscess (Bundred et al., 1992) and breast periductal inflammation (Furlong et al., 1994).

Despite the damning evidence about the detrimental effects of smoking, Amir and Donath (2002) maintain that the reasons smokers breastfeed less often and for a shorter period are psychological, not physiological. Their study shows that some women who smoke can and do breastfeed for a long duration of time, debunking a consistent negative physiological effect on lactation. Our concern about smoking and breastfeeding begs the question: When we insist that women do not smoke and breastfeed, do we invite the possibility that some mothers will give up breastfeeding rather than stop smoking?

Poison Ivy Dermatitis

Breastfeeding mothers, like everyone else, can develop a painful dermatitis from poison ivy, especially during summer months. Poison ivy is caused by contact with an oil in the sap of plants called urusion. A contact dermatitis, poison ivy can be spread by contact. Nursing mothers who contact poison ivy can continue to breastfeed but they should avoid contact between the area of the dermatitis and the baby, especially around his mouth (La Leche League International, 2001a). Poison ivy is usually treated with 1 percent hydrocortisone ointment applied to the affected area or by oral prednisone.

Diagnostic Studies Using Radioisotopes

The degree of interference with lactation from radioactive drugs depends in part on the proposed dose and on the radioactive element to be used. Such elements as iodide are selectively concentrated in human milk; thus their use may interrupt breastfeeding for a longer period (Romney, Nickoloff, & Esser, 1989). Studies using radioactive isotopes usually require that breastfeeding be interrupted until nearly all radioactivity is excreted in order to avoid its passage to the infant. Most studies use an isotope such as technetium 99, which has a short half-life (4 hours) (Evans et al., 1993). Iodine isotopes (123I and 131I) have much longer half-lives, and breastfeeding has to be interrupted for a longer period (Robinson et al., 1994).

Gallium 67 requires 2 weeks before nursing is safe to resume. In one study, pumping the breasts did not appreciably reduce the radioactivity of the milk during the period when the mother had to interrupt breastfeeding for her baby's protection against the radioisotopes to which the mother was exposed (Weiner & Spencer, 1994). In some cases, transmission can occur directly from the mother even when she cuddles the baby (Coakley & Mountford, 1985). Ways to reduce the effects of radiation therapy are presented in Box 16–5. More information can be obtained from the Nuclear Regulatory Commission at http://neonatal.ttuhsc.edu/lact/html/radio.html.

BOX 16–5

Reducing an Infant's Radiation Exposure from the Breastfeeding Mother

1. Ensure that the investigation is essential; avoid unnecessary tests.
2. Request that the physician reduce the dose to the minimum required to obtain a diagnostic result.
3. Change the radiopharmaceutical to one with less concentration in the milk or other more favorable dosimetric properties, including a shorter half-life.
4. Balance the inconvenience and disadvantage of interrupting breastfeeding against the potential risk of exposure to the infant.
5. Consider interruption of breastfeeding rather than weaning baby from the breast.

Source: Adapted from Coakley & Mountford (1985).

The Impact of Maternal Illness and Hospitalization

Hospitalization of a mother is a traumatic experience for all members of the family. A mother faced with separation from her infant, whether brief or prolonged, is a mother in crisis. For the breastfeeding woman and her infant, it is essential that ongoing, intimate, and regular contact be maintained. A mother with an acute illness is now more likely to be treated as an outpatient rather than to be hospitalized. As a result, separation because of hospitalization is not as frequent a barrier to breastfeeding as it was a few years ago.

If hospitalized, the baby should be allowed to room-in with the mother or at least be brought to her for breastfeeding at frequent intervals. Nurses and lactation consultants can be advocates for changing polices and for relaxing hospital restrictions that place an unnecessary additional hardship on families.

A mother who is chronically or acutely ill may find that the decisions about her health care and advice regarding breastfeeding are divided among her obstetrician, the baby's pediatrician, and the medical specialist. Additional health-care professionals such as a dietitian, nurse practitioner, or physician's assistant may be involved. Even when all agree that breastfeeding is desirable, childbirth may be riskier for the mother and infant, and they are more likely to be separated postpartum. Although it is possible to establish breastfeeding after an initial separation, it can be more difficult, especially if the separation lasts more than a few days (Coates & Riordan, 1992). Moreover, when an illness is associated with a reduced milk supply, the mother is further traumatized when she is lectured about breastfeeding more often and about "supply and demand" when the care provider does not first assess the total picture and the possibility that she is already breastfeeding frequently.

Chronic illnesses present a somewhat different potential dilemma for the breastfeeding mother and the clinician assisting her. Not surprisingly, women with disabilities are likely to be depressed. They also worry about their children more than other mothers (Harrison & Stuifbergen, 2001). In some cases, the nature of the chronic illness and its effect on the mother's functioning may interfere to a greater or lesser extent with her ability to breastfeed. In other cases, creative alternatives to "usual" solutions are all that is needed to give the mother the opportunity to experience the same infant feeding as do those mothers who do not have a chronic illness. Additionally, drug therapy, particularly because it is likely to be long-term, may pose risks to the breastfeeding infant that are not an issue if the mother has an acute, self-limiting illness. Thus the clinician needs to look beyond the illness itself and examine how the condition is being managed and what the mother wants to do, given complete information relating to the risks and benefits of breastfeeding to herself and her baby in light of her chronic illness. In many cases, the therapy of choice need not be changed because it poses no dangers for the suckling infant.

Care must be taken to accurately interpret the mother's desire to begin or to continue breastfeeding when faced with uncommon difficulties or situations. Occasionally, when an illness or a breastfeeding problem occurs, health professionals may be asked to give permission to wean to a woman who no longer wants to continue breastfeeding. Even if there is no reason to wean, a relatively minor difficulty can occasionally present a mother with a socially acceptable "out" from a situation that she finds emotionally uncomfortable or finds inconvenient for her lifestyle. The comment—that the physician, lactation consultant, or nurse "told me to wean" because of a problem—may partially reflect the mother's own desires. Avoiding judgmental responses and encouraging her to air conflicting feelings may enable the mother to place her breastfeeding experience in context, so that she can focus on the positive aspects of her experience rather than on its more problematic elements.

Summary

This chapter reviewed health conditions that relate to the lactating mother and suggested interventions that facilitate the lactation process. Admittedly, this discussion does not include the full range of acute or chronic disease that the health professional will find in practice. To find information on other health problems that the mother may develop while she is lactating, we recommend gynecological and medical-surgical texts for physicians and nurses that more thoroughly discuss the conditions described here and others not addressed.

Key Concepts

- Women with type I diabetes should be encouraged to breastfeed their infants. If breastfeeding is delayed, the mother should be encouraged to begin expressing or pumping her milk as soon as she feels able.

- Lactating women with type I diabetes have lower milk prolactin concentrations than do women without diabetes, causing a delay of about one day in lactogenesis II.

- For the untreated breastfeeding woman, hypothyroidism can result in a reduced milk supply. If replacement therapy (0.25 to 1.12 mg of sodium levothyroxine or equivalent doses of other thyroid preparation) is adequate, the relief of the symptoms and an increase in the milk supply can be dramatic.

- Polycystic ovarian syndrome can interfere with the production of hormones necessary for full lactation and lead to high levels of testosterone.

- Theca lutein cysts, an unusual condition where ovaries are enlarged by multiple cysts that produce a high level of testosterone, usually delays lactogenesis. Several weeks postpartum, the cysts resolve and the testosterone level returns to normal.

- Mothers with cystic fibrosis can breastfeed. The breastmilk of these mothers contains nutrients sufficient to supply the energy needs of the nursing infant despie some differences in lipid composition. The mother's diet should be closely monitored to avoid excessive weight loss.

- Women with tuberculosis who have been treated appropriately for 2 or more weeks (and who are otherwise considered to be noncontagious) may and should breastfeed (American Academy of Pediatrics, 1997a; World Health Organization, 1998). If the mother is acutely ill with TB, breastfeeding may have to be interrupted.

- US women are routinely screened for group B streptococcus (GBS), a leading cause of neonatal sepsis. Those at-risk for GBS infection are given antibiotics intravenously during labor and can breastfeed.

- Excessive postpartum bleeding can inhibit lactogenesis. Breastfeeding is encouraged, especially because suckling causes the uterus to contract. In addition to packed red blood cell transfusion, the mother usually receives intravenous oxytocin and then Methergine.

- Relactation is restimulating lactation days, weeks, or months after lactation has ended. In developing countries, relactation is done to enable breastfeeding after an untimely weaning as part of rehydration therapy for seriously malnourished infants. Relactation is easier if the interval between the end of the pregnancy and relactation is short. A milk supply can be reestablished with sufficient, regular stimulation. Hormonal preparations are not necessary in all cases.

- Induced lactation involves taking hormones to mimic pregnancy and stimulate production of breastmilk. Protocol for induction typically begins with an oral combination hormones (progesterone/estrogen), followed by Domperidone or Reglan, regular pumping of the breasts, and finally suckling by the infant.

- Blessed thistle and fenugreek seed are popular herbs taken to increase breastmilk supply, although almost no scientific evidence supports their effectiveness.

- Women with autoimmune conditions should be encouraged to breastfeed. Rheumatoid arthritis and lupus symptoms usually go into remission during pregnancy and then relapse postpartum. Women with lupus sometimes have a reduced milk supply.

- In the case in which a mother has seizures, breastfeeding is in no way contraindicated. Dropping or harming the infant during a seizure is no more probable during breastfeeding than during bottle-feeding. With a few exceptions, antiepileptic drugs do not constitute a contraindication for breastfeeding although the infant is monitored for idiosyncratic reactions.

- Women who suffer from severe postpartum depression should be supported, closely monitored, and medicated. First-choice medications

for breastfeeding women with severe depression are sertraline (Zoloft) and paroxetine (Paxil). Sertraline has the least drug-interaction potential. Saint-John's-wort is no more effective than a placebo in treating major depression (Shelton et al, 2001).

Internet Resources

Information on domperidone:
www.bflrc.com/newman/breastfeeding/
domperid.htm

Information on radiotherapeutics and breastfeeding from the Nuclear Regulatory Commission:
http://neonatal.ttuhsc.edu/lact/html/radio.html.

National Women's Health Information Center:
www.4women.gov

References

Abejide OR et al. Non-puerperal induced lactation in a Nigerian community: case reports. *Ann Trop Paed* 17:109–14, 1997.

American Academy of Pediatrics, Committee on Infectious Diseases. *1997 red book, report of the Committee on Infectious Diseases.* 24th ed. Elk Grove Village, IL: AAP, 1997a:73–79.

———. Revised guidelines for prevention of early-onset group B streptococcal (GBS) infection. *Pediatrics* 99:489–96, 1997b.

American Diabetes Association. Clinical practice recommendations. Gestational diabetes mellitus; definition, detection, and diagnosis. *Diabetes Care* 23:77–82, 2000.

Amir LH, Donath SM. Does maternal smoking have a negative physiological effect on breastfeeding? The epidemiological evidence. *Birth* 29:112–23, 2002.

Anderson GC et al. Mother-newborn contact in a randomized trial of Kangaroo (skin-to-skin) care. *JOGN Nurs* 32:604–11, 2003.

Arthur PG, Kent JC, Hartman PE. Metabolites of lactose synthesis in milk from diabetic and nondiabetic women during lactogenesis II. *J Pediatr Gastroenterol Nutr* 19:100–8, 1994.

Auerbach KG, Avery JL. Relactation: a study of 366 cases. *Pediatrics* 65: 236–42, 1980.

———. Induced lactation: a study of adoptive nursing by 24 women. *Am J Dis Child* 135:340–43, 1981.

Barrett JH et al. Breast-feeding and postpartum relapse in women with rheumatoid and inflammatory arthritis. *Arthritis* 43:1010–15, 2000.

Beck CT. The lived experience of postpartum depression: a phenomenological study. *Nurs Res* 41:166–70, 1992.

———. Teetering on the edge: a substantive theory of postpartum depression. *Nurs Res* 42:42–48, 1993.

Bitman J et al. Milk composition and volume during the onset of lactation in a diabetic mother. *Am J Clin Nutr*

50:1364–69, 1989.

Brennan P, Silman A. Breast-feeding and the onset of rheumatoid arthritis. *Arthritis Rheum* 37:808–13, 1994.

Brock KE et al. Sexual, reproductive and contraceptive risk factors for carcinoma-in-situ of the uterine cervix in Sydney. *Med J Aust* 150:125–30, 1989.

Brun JF et al. Breast feeding, other reproductive factors and rheumatoid arthritis: a prospective study. *Br J Rheumatol* 34:542–46, 1995.

Bundred NJ et al. Breast abscesses and cigarette smoking. *Br J Surg* 79:548–59, 1992.

Carty E, Conine TA, Hall L. Comprehensive health promotion for the pregnant woman who is disabled. *J Nurse Midwifery* 35:133–42, 1990.

Carty E, Conine TA, Wood-Johnson F. Rheumatoid arthritis and pregancy: helping women to meet their needs. *Midwives Chron* 99:254–57, 1986.

Centers for Disease Control and Prevention (CDC). Prevention and control of influenza: recommendations of the advisory committee on immunization practices. *MMWR* 52(RR-8), 2003.

Cesario SK. Spinal cord injuries: nurses can help affected women and their families achieve pregnancy and birth. *AWHONN Lifelines* 6:225–32, 2002.

Cheales-Siebenaler NJ. Induced lactation in an adoptive mother. *J Hum Lact* 15:421–23, 1999.

Coakley AJ, Mountford PJ. Nuclear medicine and the nursing mother. *Br Med J* 291(6489):160, 1985.

Coates MM, Riordan J. Breastfeeding during maternal or infant illness. *Clin Iss Perin and Wom Health Nurs* 3(4):683–94, 1992.

Craig D. The adaptation to pregnancy of spinal cord injured women. *Rehab Nurs* 15:6–9, 1990.

Davies HA et al. Insulin requirements of diabetic women who breastfeed. *Br Med J* 298:1357–58, 1989.

Davis M. Breastfeeding my adopted baby. *New Beginnings*

La Leche League International, May-June 2001:88.

DeCoopman J. Breastfeeding after pituitary resection: support for a theory of autocrine control of milk supply? *J Hum Lact* 9:35–40, 1993.

Delgado-Escueta AV, Janz D. Consensus guidelines: preconception counseling, management, and care of the pregnant woman with epilepsy. *Neurology* 42(suppl 5):149–60, 1992.

Dinger J et al. Breast milk transmission of group B streptococcal infection. *Pediatr Infect Dis J* 21:567–68, 2002.

Dombrowski MA et al. Kangaroo (skin-to-skin) care with a postpartum woman who felt depressed. *Am J Matern Child Nurs* 26:214–46, 2001.

Ellsworth A. Pharmacotherapy of asthma while breastfeeding. *J Hum Lact* 10:39–41, 1994.

Evans JL et al. Secretion of radioactivity in breast milk following administration of 99Tc^m -MAG3. *Nucl Med Commun* 14:108–11, 1993.

Ferris AM et al. Lactation outcome in insulin-dependent diabetic women. *J Am Diet Assoc* 88:317–22, 1988.

———. Perinatal lactation protocol and outcome in mothers with and without insulin-dependent diabetes mellitus. *Am J Clin Nutr* 58:43–8, 1993.

Furlong AJ et al. Periductal inflammation and cigarette smoke. *J Am Coll Surg* 179:417–20, 1994.

Gagne MG, Leff EW, Jefferis, SC. The breast-feeding experience of women with type I diabetes. *Health Care Wom Int* 13:249–60, 1992.

Gennaro S et al. Lymphocyte, monocyte, and natural killer cell reference ranges in postpartal women. *Clin Diagnostic Lab Immunol* 4:195–201, 1997.

Goldfarb L, Newman J. Protocol for induced lactation. Unpublished manuscript. 2002.

Golembeski DJ, Emergy MG. Lipid composition of milk from mothers with cystic fibrosis (letter). *Pediatrics* 31(suppl):631–32, 1989.

Halbert L. Breastfeeding in women with a compromised nervous system. *J Hum Lact* 14:327–31, 1998.

Hale T. *Clinical therapy in breastfeeding patients*. Amarillo, TX: Pharmasoft Medical Publishing, 1999.

———. *Medications and mothers' milk*. 10th ed. Amarillo, TX: Pharmasoft Medical Publishing, 2002.

Hammer R et al. Low-fat diet and exercise in obese lactating women. *Breastfeed Rev* 4:29–34, 1996.

Harrison T, Stuifbergen A. Disability, social support, and concern for children: depression in mothers with multiple sclerosis. *JOGN Nurs* 31:444–53, 2002.

Henderson J. Impact of postnatal depression on breastfeeding duration. *Birth* 30:175–80, 2003.

Hendrick V et al. Weight gain in breastfed infants of mothers taking antidepressant medications. *J Clin Psychiatry* 64:401–12, 2003.

Hoover K, Barbalinardo L, Pia Platia M. Delayed lactogenesis II secondary to gestation ovarian theca lutein cysts in two normal singleton pregnancies. *J Hum Lact* 18:264–68, 2002.

Horta BL et al. Environmental tobacco smoke and breastfeeding duration. *Am J Epidemiol* 146:128–33, 1997.

Ito S et al. Initiation and duration of breast-feeding in women receiving antiepileptics. *Am J Obstet Gynecol* 173:881–86, 1995.

Jackson AB, Wadley V. A multicenter study of women's self-reported reproductive health after spinal cord injury. *Arch Phys Med Rehabil* 80:1420–28, 1999.

Kirshbaum M. The parent with a physical disability. In: Auvenshine JM, Enriques MG, eds. *Comprehensive maternity nursing: perinatal and women's health*. Boston: Jones and Bartlett, 1990.

Kitzinger S. *The crying baby*. New York: Penguin Books, 1989.

Kjos SL et al. The effect of lactation on glucose and lipid metabolism in women with recent gestational diabetes. *Obstet Gynecol* 82:451–55, 1993.

La Leche League International. Helping a breastfeeding mother with poison ivy dermatitis. *Leaven* 37:29–31, 2001a.

———. Question from breastfeeding mothers: should lactating women donate blood? *New Beginnings* 18(4):227, November/December, 2001b.

Lake MF. Tuberculosis in pregnancy. *AWHONN Lifelines* 5:35–41, 2001.

Lammi-Keefe CJ et al. Vitamin E in plasma and milk of lactating women with insulin-dependent diabetes mellitus. *J Pediatr Gastroenterol Nutr* 20:305–9, 1995.

Maley B. Creating a postpartum depression support group. Out of the blue. *AWHONN Lifelines* 6:6205, 2002.

Maliqueo M et al. Resumption of ovarian function during lactational amenorrheoea in breastfeeding women with polycystic ovarian syndrome: metabolic aspects. *Hum Reprod* 16:1598–602, 2001.

Marasco L, Marmet C, Shell M. Polycystic ovary syndrome: a connection to insufficient milk supply? *J Hum Lact* 16:143–48, 2000.

Martin DC. LLL and the mother who is blind. *Leaven*, Sept–Oct 1992:67–68.

Michel SH, Mueller DH. Impact of lactation on women with cystic fibrosis and their infants: a review of five cases. *J Am Diet Assoc* 94:159–65, 1994.

Minami J. Helping mothers with chronic illness. *Leaven* 36:5–6, 2000.

Miyake A et al. Decease in neonatal suckled milk volume in diabetic women. *Eur J Obstet Gynecol Reprod Biol* 33:49–53, 1989.

Murtaugh MA et al. Energy intake and glycemia in lactating women with type 1 diabetes. *J Amer Dietetic Assoc* 98: 642–52, 1998.

Neifert M, McDonough S, Neville M. Failure of lactogenesis associated with placental retention. *Am J Obstet Gynecol* 140:477–78, 1981.

Newcomb PA et al. Lactation in relation to postpmenopausal breast cancer. *Am J Epidermiol* 150:174–82, 1999.

Newman J, Pittman T. *The ultimate breastfeeding book of answers*. Roseville, CA: Prima Publishing, 2000.

Ostrom KM, Ferris AM. Prolactin concentrations in serum and milk of mothers with and without insulin-dependent diabetes mellitus. *Am J Clin Nutr* 58:49–53, 1993.

Paton LM et al. Pregnancy and lactation have no long-term deleterious effect on measures of bone mineral in healthy women: a twin study. *Am J Clin Nutr* 77:707–714, 2003.

Pisacane A et al. Breast feeding and multiple sclerosis. *Br Med J* 308:1411–12, 1994.

Qureshi IA et al. Hyperlipidaemia during normal pregnancy, partuition and lactation. *Ann Acad Med Singapore* 28:217–21, 1999.

Robinson PS et al. Iodine-131 in breast milk following therapy for thyroid carcinoma. *J Nucl Med* 35:1797–801, 1994.

Romney BM, Nickoloff EL, Esser PD. Excretion of radioiodine in breast milk. *J Nucl Med* 30:124–26, 1989.

Rosenblatt KA, Thomas DB. Lactation and the risk of epithelial ovarian cancer. WHO Collaborative Study of Neoplasia and Steroid Contraceptives. *Intl J Epidemiol* 22:192–97, 1993.

———. Prolonged lactation and endometrial cancer. *Int J Epidemiol* 24:499–503, 1995.

Sances G et al. Course of migraine during pregnancy and postpartum: a prospective study. *Cephalalgia* 23:197–205, 2003.

Seema PAK, Satyanarayanan L. Relactation: an effective intervention to promote exclusive breastfeeding. *J Trop Pediatr* 43:213–16, 1997.

Shelton RC et al. Effectiveness of St. John's Wort in major depression: a randomized controlled trial. *JAMA* 285:1978–86, 2001.

Shiffman ML et al. Breast-milk composition in women with cystic fibrosis: report of two cases and a review of the literature *Am J Clin Nutr* 49:612–17, 1989.

Silberstein SD. Headaches and women: treatment of the pregnant and lactating migraneur. *Headache* 33:533–40, 1993.

Simpkins S, Hench CP, Bhatia G. Management of the obstetric patient with tuberculosis. *JOGN Nurs* 25:305–12, 1996.

Simpson KR, Creehan P. *Perinatal nursing.* New York: Lippincot, 2002.

Siskind V et al. Breastfeeding, menopause, and epithelial ovarian cancer. *Epidemiology* 8:188–91, 1997.

Snider DF, Powell KE. Should women taking antituberculosis drugs breastfeed? *Arch Intern Med* 144:589–90, 1984.

Thompson NM. Relactation in a newborn intensive care setting. *J Hum Lact* 12:233–35, 1996.

Thomson VM. Breastfeeding and mothering one-handed. *J Hum Lact* 11:211–15, 1995.

Thorley V. Lactation and headaches. Presented at: Breastfeeding—The Natural Advantage Conference. Sydney, Australia, October 1997.

———. Headaches in breastfeeding women. *Birth Issues* 9(3):85–88, 2000.

Ugarriza DN. Postpartum depressed women's explanation of depression. *J Nurs Schol* 34:226–33, 2002.

Visness CM, Kennedy KI, Ramos R. The duration and character of postpartum bleeding among breast-feeding women. *Obstet Gynecol* 89:159–63, 1997.

Walker J. Lactational headaches. *Nurs Mothers Assoc Australia Talkabout* 39(1):12–13, 1999.

Wall VR. Breastfeeding and migraine headaches. *J Hum Lact* 8:209–12, 1992.

Weiner RE, Spencer RP. Quantification of gallium-67 citrate in breast milk. *Clin Nucl Med* 19:7653–65, 1994.

Welch MJ, Phelps DL, Osher AB. Breast-feeding by a mother with cystic fibrosis. *Pediatrics* 67:664–66, 1981.

Willis CE, Livingstone V. Infant insufficient milk syndrome associated with maternal postpartum hemorrhage. *J Hum Lact* 11:123–26, 1995.

World Health Organization (WHO). Breastfeeding and maternal tuberculosis. *WHO Division of Child Health and Development* 23:1–3, February 1998.

Worthington J et al. Pregnancy and multiple sclerosis—a 3-year prospective study. *J Neurol* 241:228–33, 1994.

MATERNAL EMPLOYMENT AND BREASTFEEDING

*Karen A. Wambach and Wilaiporn Rojjanasrirat**

The decision to return to work soon after childbirth and to continue breastfeeding presents a unique challenge for women, and it is becoming an increasingly common choice in the United States and other industrialized countries. Women who desire to continue to breastfeed when they return to work may face difficulties, especially if their worksite lacks a supportive environment and their work duties and schedule lack flexibility. This chapter focuses on breastfeeding and working women, and the influence of maternal employment on breastfeeding practice and duration. Strategies for continued breastfeeding and employment for the individual will be described, as well as workplace and community strategies.

Why Women Work

Women have always worked, either paid or unpaid. The focus of this chapter is on paid work outside

the home in combination with breastfeeding. The majority of women work in order to earn the money needed to support their families (US Department of Labor, 1996). However, many more women today than in previous years are the sole supporter of their families; some are married to men who are underemployed, and others are putting their partners through school. Many women also work because they gain self-esteem by being valued for their marketable skills. In addition, the social rewards of the time spent with other adults on the job help women to feel good about themselves—to feel as if they are improving the skills for which they have been educated (at whatever level) and that they (and their skills) are not going to stagnate or become outdated from lack of use. The most common reasons that women give for returning to employment during the first few months postpartum are financial constraints, self-fulfillment, workplace policy, work-motivation, and family/baby-motivation (Killien, 1993). In a qualitative study of factors influencing single mothers' employment status, women expressed a sense of obligation to their children and responsibility for providing a nice home, food, and clothing (Youngblut et al., 2000).

* The authors acknowledge Kathleen Auerbach, the chapter's original author, and thank Amal Omer-Salim for her contribution on the International Labour Organization.

Historical Perspective

Work has played a prominent role in women's lives for centuries. Prior to the Industrial Revolution, women played two active roles: raising a family and working predominantly in the home. In 1800, only 5 percent of white women worked outside the home (Begun, Blair, & Quiram, 1998). Factors influencing married women to seek employment during the early industrial period were due to wartime demand for labor, mandatory schooling for young children, a decline in fertility rates, and inadequate earnings by men. The proportion of women in the labor force went from 9.7 percent in 1870 to 20 percent in 1940. The proportion of *married women* in the labor force increased from 5.6 percent in 1900 to 15.2 percent in 1940 (Marshall & Paulin, 1987). By 1951, women comprised one third of the working population (Myrdal & Klein, 1956).

In 1978, working wives contributed only 26 percent to family income. Employment rates for women have increased considerably since 1960 for both single and married women.

The reported numbers of working women varies with age of the youngest child, marital status, and race. Rates of employment were highest among married women with young children. In 2001, 51 percent of married women returned to the labor force while their children were under the age of one, with 67 percent of those women working full-time (US Bureau of Labor Statistics, 2001). Working wives and mothers are the rule rather than the exception, and many of these women will return to work during the period when they are most likely to be breastfeeding. In spite of this reality, women continue to complain that the workplace culture neither supports nor respects families. Many women report that neither their employers nor public policy adequately recognizes or supports women's family responsibilities (Killien et al., 2001).

The patterns of women's employment have changed in the last four decades, as shown in Table 17–1. In the 1960s and 1970s, the employment of married women tended to be intermittent, with women more often working until they began bearing children. Women would then return to work after their children reached school-age.

Table 17–1

LABOR FORCE PARTICIPATION RATE OF MARRIED WOMEN WITH CHILDREN UNDER 6 YEARS OF AGE

Year	Participation Rate (%)
1960	18.6
1970	30.3
1980	45.1
1990	57.4
2000	65.3

Source: US Census Bureau (1998, 2000).

The Effect of Work on Breastfeeding

The findings of the most recent Ross Laboratories Mothers Survey (RLMS) indicate that the prevalence of breastfeeding initiation and breastfeeding to 6 months of age in the United States has reached its highest recorded levels, 69.5 percent and 32.5 percent, respectively (Ryan, Wenjun, & Acosta, 2002). The high employment rates among women with infants under 1 year of age indicate that many mothers will attempt to combine breastfeeding and employment.

For many women in the United States, the workplace seems to be incompatible with breastfeeding for a longer period. The RLMS reported that women started off breastfeeding at about the same rate whether or not they were employed (66 percent versus 69 percent), but by 6 months postpartum continued breastfeeding differed substantially between these groups. Only 25 percent of full-time employed women versus 36 percent of unemployed women continued to breastfeed at 6 months. Other studies confirm the RLMS findings (Chezem, Montgomery, & Fortman, 1997; Dodgson & Duckett, 1997; Fein & Roe, 1998; Visness & Kennedy, 1997). Among mothers who return to work while continuing to breastfeed, those who exclusively breastfeed (no formula supplementation) are more likely to continue any amount of breast-feeding longer (Hills-Bonczyk, 1994; Piper & Parks, 1996). In addition, when a mother viewed breast-feeding as a special time with the baby that she did not want to give up, she was more likely to breast-feed longer. Research also indicates that working full-time or more than 20 hours per week compared to part-time, has a significant negative influence on breastfeeding duration (Hills-Bonczyk, 1993; Lind-berg, 1996; Ryan, Wenjun, & Acosta, 2002). Most international studies, particularly those conducted in developing countries, report that working nega-tively affects breastfeeding (Rea et al., 1999; Yimyam, 1998; Yimyam & Morrow, 1999).

Lindberg (1996) used a role-incompatibility model to explain why some employed women breastfeed and others do not. She noted that women working part-time were more likely than full-time workers to breastfeed, and that more women quit breastfeeding in the same month that they returned to work, supporting her contention that these two behaviors—breastfeeding and work-ing—are viewed by many as being incompatible. The longer women delayed their return to work, the lower the negative effect of employment on their breastfeeding experience.

Types of occupations were also associated with duration of breastfeeding. Women who were classi-fied as professional, administrative, or managerial had a longer duration of breastfeeding than did women in the lower-skill occupations such as cleri-cal and service jobs (Hills-Bonczyk, 1993; Piper & Parks, 1996). In general, there is a need for more re-search into the experiences of clerical, industrial, and service workers with combining breastfeeding and employment.

Strategies to Manage Breastfeeding and Work

Prenatal Planning and Preparation

Just as pregnancy is a time of planning that focuses on caring for and feeding a baby, pregnancy is the best time to plan for one's return to the employ-ment scene. Some women have already thought about a plan, often before they become pregnant. They must sort out the many myths that exist about

breastfeeding, especially those saying that combin-ing breastfeeding and employment is difficult and not worth the effort. Thus the health-care worker who has contact with the employed pregnant woman does her a great service simply by asking how she plans to combine breastfeeding and return to work. In some cases, the mother's reply to such a question will identify fallacies that need to be de-bunked and areas of information that need to be shared. For mothers who are ambivalent or unde-cided about continued breastfeeding after returning to work, health-care workers can share what Neifert (1998) and Bocar (1997) suggest as benefits: (1) op-timal infant health, growth, and development; (2) fewer work absences due to infant illness; (3) lower expenses for infant health care; (4) improved per-sonal health and well-being; (5) lower expenses for infant nutrition; (6) less energy and time spent for purchasing, storing, and preparing formula; (7) feel-ing more connected to the baby during the work-day when pumping; (8) periodic lactation breaks that restore mother's perspective; and (9) the op-portunity to restore feelings of closeness while nurs-ing the baby when back together.

The health-care worker should begin by en-couraging the pregnant woman, especially the first-time mother or breastfeeder, to learn as much as she can about breastfeeding and how to get off to a smooth start when breastfeeding after returning to work. This includes learning about infant feeding patterns, breast pump alternatives, milk expression and storage, and maintaining the optimal milk sup-ply (Meek, 2001). Various books, pamphlets, and Web sites may also provide the woman with helpful information (see the Internet Resources and other sources of information listed at end of this chapter).

The woman should also talk with women who have combined breastfeeding and employment to learn practical tips. Breastfeeding classes, especially those with an emphasis on planning for return to work while breastfeeding, can be very helpful and can boost a mother's knowledge and confidence about breastfeeding. Rojjanasrirat (2000) tested a prenatal educational intervention to prepare pri-miparae to combine breastfeeding and employ-ment. The education focused on an individual plan for combining breastfeeding and employment along with involvement of the partner/significant other, and role modeling by employed, breastfeeding women. The researcher found a favorable trend among the experimental group, indicating they breastfed for longer durations than those in the control group.

The health-care provider can next help the mother to begin planning for breastfeeding when she returns to work. The timing of the return to work should be decided before the baby arrives and in most cases is planned with her family and her employer. The constraints of official maternity leave and family financial needs often determine the timing. However, the longer that a mother can stay at home after birth the better, as demonstrated by research showing a detrimental effect of shorter maternity leave on breastfeeding duration (Duckett, 1992; Lindberg, 1996; Piper & Parks, 1996).

The employed pregnant woman will want to determine whether her workplace is supportive of breastfeeding so that she can use her work breaks to nurse her baby or to express milk. She must also determine if there is a private and clean space to express her milk and facilities to store it (see Figure 17–1). An open discussion with the employer about the benefits of continued breastfeeding after return to work—for example, reduced absenteeism (Cohen, Mrtek, & Mrtek, 1995)—may be useful in gaining employer support. There is further discussion about worksite considerations later in this chapter.

Another area that the health-care provider should inquire about is child-care decisions. Has a child-care provider been chosen or is there on-site day care in the workplace? Is the child-care provider supportive of continued breastfeeding after return to work? Is the child-care provider knowledgeable about breastfeeding and human milk qualities (e.g., rapid digestibility)? Is the child-care provider familiar with how to store and warm human milk? In addition, the mother needs to ask how babies are fed at the day-care center—specifically, are they given a bottle to hold while lying alone in a crib or on a pad on the floor, or are they held? Information sources such as La Leche League International's pamphlet, *The Balancing Act*, addresses issues that many employed mothers face while breastfeeding and includes tips on how to prepare the child-care provider for the breastfeeding infant. Further discussion on child-care issues is found later in this chapter.

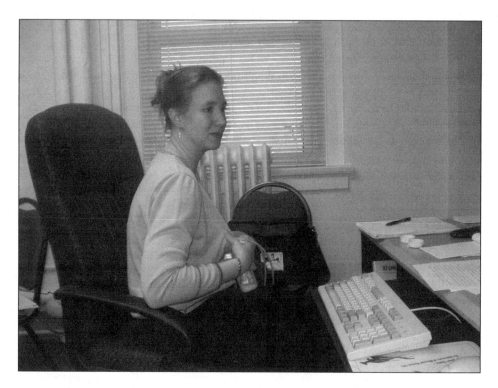

FIGURE 17–1. Expressing breast-milk in the workplace.

Finally, the health-care provider should discuss different work options and the woman's specific plans or goals for breastfeeding while employed. Will she work full-time or part-time? Women who work part-time breastfeed longer (Hills-Bonczyk, 1993; Lindberg, 1996; Ryan, Wenjun, & Acosta, 2002). Working at home is an option for some mothers, particularly where electronic linking to the job via computer modems and fax machines is possible. Telecommuting offers an opportunity for parents who previously worked elsewhere to continue employment while remaining at home with an infant or young child. It also enables the new mother to resume an organized way of life while she learns that a freer form to the day that recognizes when a baby's needs come into play has its own rewards. However, even these workers go into the workplace at least part of the week to attend meetings and to share their work with others in face-to-face encounters. When preparing to engage in telecommuting, mothers are often asked to retain established child-care arrangements in order to maintain some degree of separation between home and work activities, even if the site is the same.

Yet another employment option is job-sharing. Advantages to the employer may include greater productivity, greater worker satisfaction, and lower turnover. One study of two community-based private practice physician groups with 13 years of job-sharing (Vanek & Vanek, 2001) found that job-sharers perceived their situation as successful and most wanted to continue. They had significantly higher job satisfaction than their counterparts who did not job-share. The flexibility of job-sharing may be appropriate for an employee who wishes to maintain work skills while avoiding stress and burnout, which may occur with having young children.

Return to Work

The day on which a mother returns to work, even when she has prepared for it throughout her time at home after the baby's birth, is often characterized by the emotional and physical tugs she feels, the tears that slide unbidden down her cheeks, and the many times she pulls out pictures of the baby to share with her coworkers. Rarely is this day one in which she is as productive as she was prior to the baby's birth.

Informing the mother that her first day back is one for showing off the baby photos and straightening her desk so that her infant's picture is prominently displayed is one way to let her know that things will not be the same and that however prepared she thinks she is, it may be one of the most difficult days she will experience. The depth of her attachment to the baby means that regardless of the baby's age, this day simply will be one to "get through."

The timing of return to work—particularly if it is full-time employment—will influence the specific problems that the breastfeeding mother encounters and the length of time that she may have to deal with them. Breastfeeding problems typical of the early postpartum include the following:

- Concern about an inadequate or fluctuating milk supply
- Engorgement
- Leaking
- Baby's need for frequent feedings
- Baby's frequently changing feeding patterns, including appetite spurts and nighttime nursing

Added to these difficulties is the mother's low reserve of energy and fatigue (Wambach, 1998). The helping professional should inform the mother that each of these difficulties will resolve over time and that the longer she is home with the baby, the less likely is it that any of these issues will prove insurmountable. None of these issues are major obstacles after the baby is older than 4 months; pointing this out may encourage her to see that these difficulties need not reduce breastfeeding duration when the mother returns to work very soon after her baby's birth. This information may also assist her in making decisions about the length of her leave from work, if she has an opportunity to extend it beyond the usual 4 to 6 weeks.

Helping the mother to maintain realistic expectations about her first days on the job will enable her to see that most of the problems that she encounters will not be specific to breastfeeding (Thompson & Bell, 1997) but rather will be specific to the overworked woman with a family. However, how she plans to breastfeed can make a difference. For example, women who practiced exclusive breastfeeding in the first postpartum month and whose postpartum behaviors were consistent with their prenatal intention to fully or partially breast-feed were more likely to breastfeed longer than 6 months after returning to work (Piper & Parks, 1996). Hills-Bonczyk (1993) reported that women who returned to work and provided only breast-milk to their infants made their return earlier, and worked fewer hours, than those women who breast-fed and used supplemental formula.

There are many ways in which breastfeeding can be continued after the mother returns to work: hand expressing breastmilk, breast pumping, having the baby brought to the mother during meal breaks, or substituting formula for those feedings that occur during the mother's workday. Each of these alternatives represents an option that deserves discussion. In cases in which a family history of allergies has been identified, formula use should be avoided for as long as possible.

Hand Expression and Pumping

Prior to the mother's return to work, the lactation consultant or other health-care worker who is counseling the mother will want to discuss the need to express milk when she is away from her baby. Decisions must be made regarding how much breastmilk the mother desires for her baby's diet: all breastmilk or a combination of breastmilk and commercial formula. This decision and the baby's age upon return to work will determine the need and frequency for milk expression, either by hand or pump.

Based on their now classic research, Auerbach and Guss (1984) suggested that 7 to 10 days before the mother returns to work is a good time for her to begin practicing expression and pumping and to begin stockpiling milk. Other authors suggest that 2 weeks is needed to become proficient at pumping and to start building a supply of milk (Bocar, 1997; Wyatt, 2002).

As a general rule, the earlier in the postpartum period the mother returns to full-time work, the more frequently she will need to express or pump her breasts. Expressing milk at work to give the baby human milk feedings in the mother's absence is only one reason for doing so. The mother is also protecting her baby from infections and allergies. In addition, the mother who is comfortable is a more efficient worker. Painful engorgement contributes to embarrassing leaking, an increased risk of mastitis from milk stasis (Hager & Barton, 1996; Fetherston, 1998; Thompson, Espersen, & Maigaard, 1984), and reduction of the milk supply from overfull breasts.

For a baby who is younger than 2 months old, 1 to 2 oz for each feeding will usually be sufficient. When the mother begins expressing milk, she may be dismayed that she obtains so little (sometimes barely enough to cover the bottom of a small 4-oz bottle). However, each time she expresses, she will probably obtain more milk. Just as she had to learn to breastfeed, her body needs to learn to respond to the stimulation of hand expression or breast pumping in order to trigger milk ejection. Mothers should expect no more than half an ounce with the first several pumping or expression sessions.

During practice sessions, the mother should express or pump in the morning, when she is more likely to feel rested and when she may have more residual milk volume, rather than later in the afternoon or evening. Usually two practice sessions, timed about 1 hour after two consecutive morning feedings, are sufficient to develop her milk-expression skills. Mothers who feel particularly full late in the evening have also found that expressing at this time helps to build up a sizable stockpile of milk. Remind the mother that the milk she obtains in this way is "excess," not an indication of the amount of milk the baby obtains. Furthermore, milk is still present in the breasts after all breastfeedings, regardless of the rate at which the baby is growing (Daly & Hartmann, 1995).

When planning pumping sessions at work, the employed mother may choose to practice the 5–15–5 rule. The fives refer to two very short, pump-for-comfort sessions in the midmorning and midafternoon. Rarely do such periods last longer than 5 minutes. Some mothers will choose simply to express briefly until the breast fullness that they are feeling has subsided and discard the milk. Other women will save this milk and combine it with milk from a later, longer pumping session. At a meal break, the mother then expresses or pumps her breasts for 10 to 20 minutes and saves this milk for later use. As the mother becomes adept at expressing or pumping and as her baby gets older, she may find that she can reduce the duration of each expression period or the number of pumping sessions to two and then to one per day. Some women have combined the midmorning and midafternoon coffee breaks into a single longer period that is more conducive to breast expression.

When babies are cared for near the workplace, mothers may use this time, as well as lunchtime, to go to the baby for a relaxed midday nursing or sometimes they have the baby brought to them. In either case, breastfeeding stimulates the breasts more effectively than do the best electric pumps or the accomplished mother who hand expresses her milk. Furthermore, both parties enjoy their time together; the baby is nourished and nurtured at the breast, and the mother may also grab a quick sandwich at the babysitter's house or child-care center.

Although hand expression is an option, most mothers in our technology-focused culture choose to use a mechanical pump of some kind (automated or nonautomated). She will need to rent or purchase this equipment. Many mothers actually purchase a pump prior to giving birth—a good way to avoid making decisions about the best pump for them during the very busy time following birth and leading up to returning to work. The questions in Box 17–1 are a useful guide for the mother who is planning to pump her breasts.

There is a pump that is best suited for each mother's needs, including how negative pressure is exerted, maintained, and released; how easily the pump can be cleaned; and its comfort, cost, and convenience (Biancuzzo, 1999, p. 420). An important consideration in selecting a breast pump is that it must be easy to clean. If the user cannot be assured that cleaning is possible at home or work, with or without a dishwasher, the pump should not be purchased.

The pump should be easy and comfortable to use. Comfort depends upon closeness of fit of the pump flange on the mother's breast, to the angle of "pull" of cylinder-style pumps, and other factors as yet undetermined. The angle of the flange varies from one pump to another, as do the shape, size, and degree of fullness of each mother's breasts. Optimally, the mother should experiment with several pumps before purchasing one. The next best alternative is for her to talk with other mothers who are successfully pumping and compare the efficiency and reported comfort of different pumps, keeping

in mind that what works for one person may not work for another. The health-care worker who assists the mother should be familiar with the many types of pumps available and criteria for choosing the pump that best fits the mother's needs. Additionally, pump instructions should be reviewed to determine whether the pictures demonstrating use of the equipment are accurate.

If the mother cannot obtain replacement parts or extra pieces without purchasing an entirely new kit, the cost of using the pump may become prohibitive. The same is true if she plans to use a battery-operated pump with cost-effective batteries or a rechargeable battery pack. The least expensive breast pumps tend not to have replacement parts. Because double pumping is more effective in obtaining milk quickly than is pumping each breast separately (see Figure 17–2), electric pumps that do not offer this option should be carefully considered (Auerbach, 1990b).

Efficiency of the pump is a factor of importance. Efficiency needs to be gauged by whether the mother is comfortable with the pump during its use, whether her breasts feel softer after using the pump, and whether, over time, the amount of milk she obtains tends to increase. When she begins offering solid foods, breastfeedings become less frequent or shorter. At that time, the amount obtained by pumping usually declines. If the foregoing efficiency criteria are met, the pump can be considered efficient. See Chapter 12 for an in-depth discussion of breastpumps.

Human Milk Storage

Human milk is a dynamic substance that kills bacteria. This ability is highest in the first several hours after expression, even when it is not refrigerated (Ogundele, 2000), and some investigators have reported that colony counts remain low in such milk for at least 48 hours (Hamosh et al., 1996). For this reason, when women use careful hand washing and clean containers in which their own fresh milk is stored for less than 6 to 8 hours prior to refrigeration, they are not endangering their healthy babies (see Box 17–2). Other mothers who prefer to refrigerate their milk should do so in a clean, capped, glass or plastic container and use the milk within 8 days after it has been refrigerated (Pardou et al.,

BOX 17–1

Questions to Ask a Mother Who Is Planning to Use a Breast Pump

1. Is there a pump available for expressing her milk in the workplace?

2. What is the experience of other women who have used the breast pump in the workplace?

3. Is an automated or nonautomated pump needed based on frequency of use?

   - *For occasional use (once a week)*—hand expression or nonautomated pump (suck/release totally regulated by mother)

     - Cylinder pumps

     - Trigger or handle pumps

   - *For part-time (once a day) or dependent (frequent pumping)*—automated pump

     - 20 cycles per minute

       Partially or fully automated

       Battery-operated or battery-electric

     - 21–40 cycles per minute

       Partially or fully automated

       Compression component with some

       Electric

     - More than 40 cycles per minute

       Fully automated

       Bilateral pumping possible

       Most effective in mimicking infant sucking

4. Is the pump easy to clean? Are washable parts dishwasher safe?

5. Is the pump easy to assemble, disassemble, and use?

6. Is the pump physically comfortable to use?

7. Is the pump effective in obtaining milk quickly? Can the suck/release mechanism be adjusted easily? Is the pump self-cycling? Is the suction adequate?

8. Are the instructions accompanying the pump understandable, accurate, and easy to follow?

9. What is the cost (initial investment and daily, weekly, or monthly rental fee) of using the pump?

10. Are extra or replacement parts available without having to purchase a new kit?

11. Are both single and double pumping options available if desired?

12. What have other mothers reported about using specific equipment?

13. What size and weight is the pump?

14. How much noise does it make?

15. Can standard bottles be used to collect the milk?

16. Does the mother feel emotionally and psychologically comfortable pumping her milk? If she does not, has she considered expressing her milk by hand or breastfeeding without expressing her milk for the periods when she is separated from her baby?

Source: Adapted from Auerbach (1990a); Biancuzzo (1999); Bocar (1997).

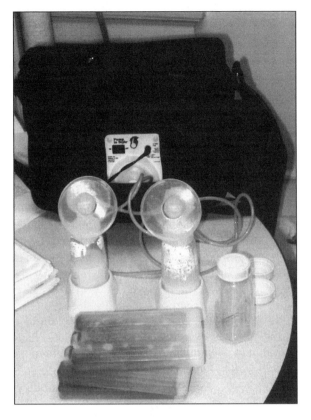

FIGURE 17–2. Double pump set-up with blue ice for chilling expressed milk in the workplace.

1994). Polyethylene bags designed for milk collection and storage are also appropriate; however there can be fat loss in these bags (Tully, 2000).

If a mother plans to use the milk before 8 days, it should be refrigerated rather than frozen, as suggested by Pardou et al. (1994) who found that antimicrobial properties were better preserved with refrigeration rather than freezing. With regard to vitamin C content in milk, longer storage equates to greater loss, as found by Buss et al. (2001) who recommended using milk in the refrigerator within 24 hours or under 1 month in a freezer. Milk stored in the freezer compartment of a refrigerator (top, bottom, or side models) should be placed as far away from the door as possible; most mothers use frozen milk within 1 month of the date when it was expressed. If a deep-freezer is used to store the milk, it can be used up to 6 months after the date of expression. The mother should be reminded that human milk is a substance that is matched to the baby's age: milk obtained when the baby was 3 months old will not as completely meet that same baby's needs when he is 6 months old. Therefore she should label the milk with the date expressed and use the milk that was expressed first.

If the mother finds that her milk changes in odor or consistency after storage, or if the baby

---

BOX 17–2

General Guidelines for Storing Human Milk

- Always use a clean container.
- Label each container with date and time of the earliest contribution to the container, particularly if "layering" different expressions into the same container.
- Store milk in the approximate quantities that the baby is likely to need for one feeding.
- If refrigerated within 6 to 8 hours, store in a clean, tightly capped container for the unrefrigerated interim period.
- If refrigerated, use within 8 days.*
- If frozen in a refrigerator freezer section, use within 1 month.*

- If frozen in a deep-freezer, use within 6 months.*
- Discard any remaining milk that was not used at the feeding for which it was thawed and warmed.
- Match the "age" of the milk as closely as possible to the baby's age in order to optimize the degree of fit between the baby's needs and the properties of the milk.

Shake while thawing to remix the creamy portion that separates during storage.

begins to refuse it, the mother may need to reduce the storage time and freeze rather than refrigerate in order to avoid possible adverse reactions. Once the milk has been refrigerated or frozen, it should be thawed and warmed to body temperature by placing it under the faucet in a sink and running gradually warmer water over the container. It is inappropriate to thaw milk at room temperature; this practice enables bacteria to multiply in the milk. Neither should it be heated very quickly on a stove or in a microwave oven. Although some research (Carbonare et al., 1996; Ovesen et al., 1996) suggests that microwave heating does not negatively impact immunoglobulins (IgA) and nutrients (vitamins B_1 and E, linoleic and linolenic acids), microwave heating nearly always results in uneven distribution of the heat. This can go unnoticed because the container rarely feels as warm as the center portion of the fluid; thus the milk can be too hot in some spots and substantially cooler in others. Even water-warmed milk should be mixed well and tested on the inside of the caregiver's wrist before offering it to the baby. Mixing should be done not only for heat distribution but also to ensure that the creamy portion of the milk is redistributed.

The fat content of milk is altered with refrigeration as well as when the milk is frozen and then thawed for reuse (Pardou et al., 1994; Hamosh et al., 1996). Loss can be minimized when the container is shaken gently before offering its contents to the baby, and single-serving amounts should be stored to prevent wastage. When giving thawed milk, the unused portion should be discarded to prevent bacterial colonization. Mothers should be told not to refreeze thawed milk. However, small amounts of fresh milk can be added to frozen milk.

Fatigue and Loss of Sleep

Fatigue is an issue for all parents. In comparison to women who bottle-feed their infants, fatigue among breastfeeding women in the first 3 months postpartum is more pronounced (Pugh & Milligan, 1993). Using Pugh and Milligan's childbearing fatigue framework in a small pilot study ($N = 41$), Wambach (1998) examined fatigue levels among breastfeeding primiparae over the first 9 weeks postpartum. Fatigue levels were found to be moderate during the first 3 weeks postpartum and decreased to mild levels at 6 and 9 weeks. When the mothers returned to work, it was found that the more difficulty women experienced with combining working and breastfeeding, the greater their fatigue.

Sleep deprivation is a fact of life for nearly all parents of very young infants. Many employed breastfeeding mothers who work during the day find that their babys' sleep patterns change after their return to work. Instead of taking short naps during the day and sleeping longer at night, the baby begins to sleep for very long periods during the day and remains awake later into the evening. Called "reverse-cycle breastfeeding," this is a coping behavior that enables the baby to tolerate many hours away from his mother. Often, the baby's waking time with his mother may alternate between short breastfeeding episodes and simply nestling in her arms. Such behavior need not mean that the mother loses still more sleep. In fact, what better built-in "excuse" than breastfeeding does a mother have for lying down on the couch when she gets home? Sleep-saving techniques that families have found work well include any one of a variety of co-sleeping arrangements:

- Keeping the baby's cradle or crib in the parents' room
- Creating an extension on the parents' bed
- Graduating from a double to a queen- or even king-size mattress
- Placing a spare mattress on the floor of the baby's room for late night cuddling and nursing away from other family members (McKenna, Mosho, & Richard, 1997)

This last option works best for those near-toddlers and larger babies who tend to "sing" when they eat, sometimes loudly enough to awaken nearby sleepers.

Maintaining an Adequate Milk Supply

As discussed throughout this book, insufficient milk supply is a common reason mothers give for premature weaning. Maintaining an adequate milk supply is a common problem for women after they return to work (Auerbach, 1984; Hills-Bonczyk, 1993), and it can contribute to weaning (Chezem, Montgomery, & Fortman, 1997). Women who return to employment and discontinue breastfeeding before they had planned may develop negative feelings, such as guilt, sadness, and depression (Chezem, Montgomery, & Fortman, 1997; Yimyam & Morrow, 1999). Pumping to express milk during the work hours is important to maintaining the milk supply. Women who maintain regular pumping breastfeed for longer durations than those who do not pump regularly (Auerbach & Guss, 1984). If mothers notice their supply dropping after returning to work, they should increase their pumping during the workday and increase feedings at the breast during the evening, night, and early morning. Child-care providers should be informed not to feed the infant in the hour preceding the mother's return from work so that she may feed the infant at the breast soon after arrival at the center or upon arrival at home.

The Day-Care Dilemma

Whether to use a day-care facility, where such care will be provided, when the baby will be enrolled and for how many hours and days, and the effects of day care on the child are issues that figure into the decision making of the early postpartum period. In some cases, the father may take on child care, particularly when the parents' work hours differ or when the father's work schedule is flexible. In other families, however, the mother may not have a partner who is available, or she may be a single parent. Other relatives may not be potential caregivers, because of geographical distance, disinclination to provide such assistance, physical or psychological incapacity, and many other reasons.

Parents must address the likelihood of childhood illness as a result of out-of-home care during the early years. It is now common knowledge that children cared for in child-care facilities have higher rates of upper respiratory tract infections as well as diarrheal illnesses. The frequency with which the young child will become ill has implications for where he can receive care. Generally, when an infant or young child becomes ill, the usual day-care arrangement is no longer available, thus forcing the family to use an alternative arrangement. Often that arrangement is the mother's loss of one or more days at work because she must stay home to care for the baby. However, continuing to breastfeed following return to work can actually help prevent infant illness and mater-

nal absenteeism due to such illness. Cohen, Mrtek, and Mrtek (1995) compared maternal absenteeism and infant illness rates among breastfeeding and formula-feeding women in two corporations that had a corporate lactation program. They found that in the first year of infants' lives 28 percent remained illness free; 86 percent of those infants were breastfed and 14 percent were formula fed. When illness occurred, 1-day absences occurred more often in mothers of formula-fed infants (75 percent) than in mothers of breastfed infants (25 percent).

Alternatives to infant day care need to be developed and supported by the government. One such alternative is a system that enables—perhaps even encourages—parents to remain with their infants during the first few months of life. This could be accomplished with paid infant-care leaves, not to be confused with maternity leaves, which are often viewed as a form of disability. In Sweden, a mother may receive up to 1 year of paid leave—and take another 6 months of unpaid leave—without fear of losing her job. In Denmark, women receive paid maternity leave for the first 6 months after birth. Most babies enter day care in their seventh month of life, when their mothers return to full-time employment.

Workplace Strategies

Women in paid employment can be helped to continue breastfeeding by being provided with minimum enabling conditions such as paid maternity leave, part-time work arrangements, on-site child care, facilities for expressing and storing breastmilk, and appropriate break time. Studies have shown that breastfeeding can be enhanced if women have support to help them sustain breastfeeding (Bar-Yam, 1998; Cohen, Mrtek, & Mrtek, 1995; Dodgson & Duckett, 1997; Hills-Bonczyk, 1993; Thompson & Bell, 1997). Four important elements related to breastfeeding and the workplace have been identified (Bar-Yam, 1998):

- *Time:* An important element that enables a mother to perform those activities related to breastfeeding activities including expressing breastmilk with breast pumps, traveling time between the workplace and the nursing mothers' room (NMR) or child care, cleaning the breast pump, and storing breastmilk. The amount of time it takes to pump depends on the types and quality of the pumps—for example, double versus single pump, electric versus manual pump.

- *Space:* A private area or facility where mothers can be comfortable expressing breastmilk for their babies. Women who do not have an office of their own may face some difficulties and become frustrated trying to find an area in which to pump routinely at work. Many large companies provide their employees with nursing mothers' rooms that are centrally located so that women can conveniently go there in a short amount of time. The nursing mothers' room is clean and has electrical outlets, a sink to wash hands, a comfortable chair, and a refrigerator to store breastmilk.

- *Gatekeeper:* The support person, office manager, human resource department, or employee health department that facilitates lactation management for the working mothers who desire to maintain breastfeeding while they are employed. Gatekeepers also extend to understanding colleagues, supervisors, and coworkers.

- *Support:* A supportive environment that enables working women to maintain lactation while separated from their infants. This support may include a work policy that allows mothers' access to their infants or to an NMR for expressing and storing milk, flexible hours, reasonable break time to pump breasts, and extended maternity leaves. Other sources of support may include the spouse, significant others, friends, coworkers, health-care providers, and employers. Table 17–2 presents an assessment checklist that health-care providers may use when discussing return to work with their breastfeeding patients.

Lactation Programs in Work Sites

Lactation support programs for childbearing female employees at hundreds of work sites in the United States have been instituted—from hospitals and health maintenance organizations to large companies and corporations. Examples include CIGNA Corporation, a giant national insurance and benefits company; Genentech, a California biotech company; Arthur Andersen, a national accounting firm; Johnson & Johnson, the famous health-care product company; and Gymboree, a large children's music and clothing company (Riccitiello, 2003). Hallmark Corporation of Kansas City, Missouri, has had a lactation support program since 1985 (Choplin, 2003). A group of three to four breastfeeding mothers started the program informally by co-renting a breast pump and garnered support from the employee health department. They started off using a medical exam room for pumping and, eventually, they were moved to a different space of their own. In 1990, private funding provided for the construction of a "mothers' room" that contains four small pumping rooms, each with a pump, bulletin board, chair, sink, and secure door (Figure 17–3). A larger sink, storage shelves, and a refrigerator adjoin the pumping rooms. The entire "mothers' room" is accessed through an unmarked door that requires users to enter a security code for entry. Breastfeeding employees state that they feel very supported by their employer as well as their coworkers. Hallmark also has four outlying production facilities, each with various levels of lactation support, but all include space for milk expression.

Published research on the effectiveness of such programs is still sparse. Cohen and Mrtek (1994) found that of women working in two settings where lactation programs were in place, 75 percent who returned to work still breastfeeding continued to do so for 6 months or longer. In addition, when formula-feeding and breastfeeding infants of employees were compared, 75 percent of illnesses occurred among the formula-feeding group. Of the 28 percent of infants who had no illnesses in their first year of life, 86 percent were breastfed (Cohen, Myrtek, & Myrtek, 1995). These findings translated into far fewer employee absences related to infant illness and thus less lost time to the company that employed them. Dodgson and Duckett (1997) described and evaluated a university-based lactation support program in Minneapolis, Minnesota. Eighteen months after the program was started, 46 of the 52 users responded to an evaluation survey. Over 90 percent of the respondents perceived that the nursing mothers' room had a positive impact on the amount of human milk they could provide for

Table 17–2

AN ASSESSMENT CHECKLIST FOR COMBINING WORK AND BREASTFEEDING

Type of work

What is your work setting? (office, factory, on the road)

Do you have your own office?

Do you keep your own schedule/control your own time?

Does your job involve travel?

Are most of your colleagues women?

Space

Is there a facility or private breastfeeding/pumping area in the workplace?

Can you use the same space every day?

Does the room have a sink, chair, electrical outlets?

Are breast pumps available there?

Is the nursing/pumping area near your work space?

Is there a refrigerator to store your milk?

If there is no designated space, where will you pump?

Time

How old will baby be upon your return to work?

Do you plan to express milk/breastfeed when you return to work?

Will you have time to pump?

Will you use an electric or manual pump? Is there a double pump?

Is the pump easy to clean with each use?

Can a break be taken reliably at the same time every day?

If there is on-site or near-site day care, can you go there to nurse the baby?

Support

Does your supervisor need to be informed or consulted?

Does your supervisor feel supportive about your breast-feeding plan?

Are there other colleagues breastfeeding or planning to breastfeed at work?

Are there mothers at work who have done so in the past?

Does your partner feel supportive of your plan to nurse and work?

Do day-care providers recognize the importance of breastfeeding?

Do they know how to handle breastmilk?

Will an on-site or near-site provider call the mother to nurse, if you request?

Work Allies

Who can help you find the time and space to pump or breastfeed?

Who is responsible for signing up spare offices/rooms?

Did you discuss the breastfeeding issue with your supervisor?

What is his/her response or concerns about breastfeeding at workplace?

Are there any policies in the workplace regarding nursing mothers?

Are there any policies regarding flexibility for new mothers returning to work?

Do you have any of the following programs at your workplace?
   Earned time
   Flex-time
   Compressed work week
   Telecommuting
   Part-time
   Job-sharing
   Phase back
   On-site or near-site day care

Do you plan to take advantage of one or more of them?

Who is the person you need to contact to arrange one or more of these programs?
   Supervisor(s)
   Human resources officer
   Benefits officer
   Employee relations officer

Source: Adapted from Bar-Yam (1998).

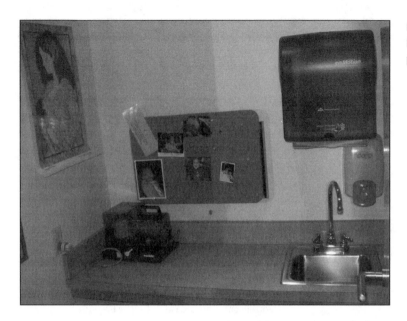

FIGURE 17–3.
Breastfeeding room at Hallmark Corporation, Kansas City, Missouri.

their infants instead of formula; 70 percent of the participants felt it contributed to an increased length of breastfeeding.

An important study, not yet published in the professional literature but described at the Breastfeeding.com Web site, involves the evaluation of the lactation support program (Working Well Moms) at CIGNA Corporation that started in 1995. This program includes lactation consultant contacts before and after birth, a private nursing room with hospital grade pumps and refrigeration, carrying case/cooler and other pumping supplies, educational seminars during pregnancy, and written breastfeeding information. The evaluation study conducted by University of California, Los Angeles, studied 363 women from multiple sites across the United States over 1 year. Results indicate that CIGNA saved $240,000 a year in health-care costs for breastfeeding mothers and infants and $60,000 in reduced absenteeism. Seventy percent of the women enrolled in the program were still nursing at 6 months postpartum and 36 percent of participants were still breastfeeding at 1 year, both rates higher than the published national rates of breastfeeding among employed women.

Although the increase in work-site programs and their effectiveness are impressive and promising, most are in higher skill level workplaces. Lit-

tle is known about the experiences of women who work in lower skilled and service jobs, a relatively large segment of working women in the United States. Barriers to continued breastfeeding after return to work are likely much higher for these women. Some preliminary findings (Rojjanasrirat, 2003) indicate that women in low-income WIC populations who attempt to combine breastfeeding and work face multiple challenges. Using focus group interviews, the 17 WIC women in this study perceived barriers to breastfeeding in terms of the difficult nature of their job (e.g., waitress, sales clerk, cashier, teacher); time issues such as no break time, too busy, no flexible time allowed; support issues such as lack of support from coworkers and feeling intimidated by male coworkers; lack of privacy; lack of space or facility to pump; and child-care issues such as high cost and low levels of trust.

The Employer's Perspective

Employers are pivotal in creating a work environment for women to succeed at combining breastfeeding and employment. Unfortunately, studies on employers' attitudes toward breastfeeding indicate that they lack knowledge about benefits of breastfeeding and see very little value to their business in supporting breastfeeding in the work environment (Bridges, Frank, & Curtin, 1997; Libbus & Bullock, 2002).

Brown, Poag, and Kasprzycki (2001) conducted a study of employers' knowledge, attitudes, and practices in providing breastfeeding support for lactating employees. They used focus groups of human resource personnel from a large-employer and a smaller-employer group, neither of which had a breastfeeding policy in place. Participants identified a major barrier to breastfeeding support in the workplace as an adverse effect on employee morale due to taking too much work or break time to breastfeed or express milk. Clearly employers need more information about creating breastfeeding support in their workplace and about the benefits of breastfeeding for employees, the company, and society.

Community Strategies

Health-Care Providers and Lactation Consultants

Throughout this chapter we have discussed how the health-care professional can assist the breast-feeding mother who works away from home. Physicians, nurses, midwives, and lactation consultants play an important role in promoting breastfeeding. Every health-care encounter should be utilized to inform and support the mother who plans to or is currently combining breastfeeding and employment. In the prenatal period, efforts to assist the pregnant woman to plan her return to work include information sharing and prenatal breastfeeding classes. Referral to a community or health plan-affiliated lactation consultant during the prenatal period can facilitate establishment of a therapeutic relationship that will promote successful breastfeeding and preparation for return to work. The lactation consultant can provide assistance to the mother once she has returned to work related to milk expression and pumping, maintaining her milk supply, and assisting with other issues that may arise related to continued breastfeeding. La Leche League International is another community resource for breastfeeding women who return to work.

Breastfeeding Support Groups

La Leche League International (LLLI) provides information on combining breastfeeding and employment through their pamphlets and books, as well as on their Web site. One feature that utilizes telecommunications technology is their "Balancing Act" online discussion site. This forum includes postings on balancing work, breastfeeding, and the home; pumping issues; family matters; and time demands. For those who prefer face-to-face contact, support can also be gained at LLLI local group meetings. Finally, LLLI has available to corporations a kit for implementing a workplace lactation support program (http://www.lalecheleague.org/corporate.html).

Other Internet resources for the health-care provider and breastfeeding mothers are listed at the end of this chapter. Breastfeeding.com provides a wealth of information to mothers on combining work and breastfeeding, including how to choose pumps, pumping and storage guidelines, relaxation tips to mothers from mothers, dealing with the employer regarding breastfeeding, choosing clothing, and many other issues of relevance. Rightonmom.com also has informative Web pages on working and breastfeeding.

National and International Strategies

Legislative Support and Public Advocacy

The United States lags behind several developed countries in legislative and federal policy regarding protection of families, mothers, and breastfeeding. The enactment of the Family Medical Leave Act in 1993 provided for the employee to take up to 12 weeks of unpaid leave during a 1-year period for various family and medical reasons. This legislation helps to provide mothers who can afford to take unpaid leave beyond the traditional 6-week maternity leave so that they can establish breastfeeding solidly before returning to work. Legislation in the United States related to breastfeeding, and specifically to breastfeeding and employment, is progressing, albeit slowly.

In 1999, US Representative Carolyn Maloney from New York made possible the enactment of the

Right to Breastfeeding Act, which ensures a woman's right to breastfeed her infant anywhere on federal property where she and her child are authorized to be (Baldwin & Friedman, 2003). Maloney also introduced the Breastfeeding Promotion Act in 1998. This bill and its components did not pass and different versions of it were reintroduced at later sessions, including the last one in 2001 (H.R. 285). This bill, if enacted, would help employed breastfeeding mothers by amending the Pregnancy Discrimination Act of 1978 (Civil Rights Act of 1964) to clarify that it extends to breastfeeding and thereby protect them from discrimination in the workplace when breastfeeding or expressing their milk during lunch or breaks. In addition, it would provide tax incentives to employers who make expenditures for breast pumps and other lactation equipment, and would regulate performance standards for breast pumps through the Food and Drug Administration. The last major action on the bill was on March 15, 2001, when it was referred to the Subcommittee on Employer-Employee Relations.

Senator Olympia Snowe of Maine also introduced the Pregnancy Discrimination Act Amendments of 2001 and again in 2003 in the 108th Congress. This bill would amend the Civil Rights Act of 1964 to protect breastfeeding by new mothers by inserting "breastfeeding" into the text after childbirth and defining "breastfeeding" as feeding of a child either directly from the breast or expression of milk from the breast. The bill, which does not contain the proposals for tax incentives and breast pump performance standards, as did Maloney's bill, was referred to the Committee on Health, Education, Labor, and Pensions on February 14, 2003. None of these federal initiatives have been enacted into law at this point.

Unlike the federal government, several states have enacted breastfeeding legislation and many have pending legislation (Baldwin & Friedman, 2003). In 1984, New York was the first state in the nation to enact a law that exempted breastfeeding from the criminal statutes on exposure. In 1993, Florida was the first state to enact comprehensive breastfeeding legislation related to breastfeeding in public and paved the way for other states to follow suit in protecting women from legal retribution and protecting their right to breastfeed their children in public places. The next year, Florida became the

first state to pass legislation regarding breastfeeding in the workplace by authorizing a demonstration project for public-sector employees to determine appropriate breastfeeding support policies for breastfeeding mothers who return to work. In 1995, Texas passed a comprehensive breastfeeding bill protecting breastfeeding mothers in public and providing for businesses' designation as "Mother-Friendly" by accommodating pumping breaks and facilities.

In 1998, Minnesota became the first state in the nation to require employers to accommodate breastfeeding mothers when they return to work by allowing mothers adequate time and an appropriate place to express breastmilk during their workday. Similar laws were enacted in Tennessee and Hawaii in 1999 and in Illinois, California, and Connecticut in 2001. States having laws that allow and/or encourage, but do not require, employers to accommodate breastfeeding mothers include Georgia and Washington, passing their laws in 1999 and 2001, respectively. At least two states, Wisconsin and New York, have pending breastfeeding-employment bills. For additional information, readers are encouraged to visit La Leche League's Web site to learn more about breastfeeding legislation (see the Internet Resources listed at the end of this chapter). In addition, readers may access state and federal legislative Web sites to follow legislation through the process of becoming law (e.g., Thomas Legislative Information can be found at http://thomas.loc.gov/).

The US Breastfeeding Committee is an overarching group formed in 1995 to coordinate breastfeeding advocacy activities in the United States. The committee is composed of representatives from health professional associations, breastfeeding support organizations, relevant government departments, and nongovernmental organizations. Their mission is to improve the nation's health by working collaboratively to protect, promote, and support breastfeeding. In 2001 they unveiled their strategic plan for breastfeeding in the United States. Goal four of this plan relates directly to breastfeeding and employment: Increase protection, promotion, and support for breastfeeding mothers in the work force. Therefore, strides are being made in the United States, but there is plenty yet to do in the whole area of protecting and promoting family and maternal interests. We turn next to the efforts of the

International Labour Organization to support breastfeeding women in the workplace.

International Labour Organization

One of the primary goals of the International Labour Organization (ILO) is to protect the maternity health needs of women workers and their babies and to promote the retention of women in the workforce throughout their child-bearing years. The ILO is composed of representatives of governments, workers, and employers, and it is a member of the United Nations. It sets international labor standards through Conventions and Recommendations. Upon ratification of an ILO Convention, its articles are binding on member states through a regulatory mechanism that influences national law and practice. To illustrate this, many African countries have at least 12 weeks of maternity leave, in spite of the fact that only three countries in the region actually ratified the 1952 Convention that stipulates 12 weeks as a minimum.

The ILO has issued three Conventions related to maternity protection for working women. In 1919, Convention 3 recognized the need to give women workers maternity leave and breastfeeding breaks. In 1952, maternity leave was increased to 12 weeks in Convention 103. The latest ILO Maternity Protection Convention 2000 (183) provides for at least 14 weeks of paid maternity leave and the right to one or more breastfeeding breaks daily. (For additional information, go to www.ilo.org/ilolex/english/convdisp1.htm.) The Convention also allows for a reduction of working hours, which gives added flexibility in settings where short breaks are not feasible.

The widened scope of Convention 183 affects all employed women. Provisions relating specifically to breastfeeding women are health protection at the workplace; paid maternity leave of not less than 14 weeks; 6 weeks of compulsory leave after childbirth; cash benefits at no less than two thirds of previous earnings; and nondiscrimination and employment protection in relation to pregnancy and breastfeeding.

The Convention also emphasizes that maternity protection is a social responsibility and that the burden of costs should thus be shared by all of society. Recommendation 191, which accompanies Convention 183, further encourages an extension of maternity leave to at least 18 weeks and the adaptation of the frequency and length of nursing breaks to the particular needs of mothers and babies, and it promotes the establishment of adequate hygienic facilities at or near the workplace for nursing mothers (see www.ilo.org/ilolex/english/recdisp1.htm).

Breastfeeding advocates can make use of several areas within ILO standards where the needs of breastfeeding women are addressed. When national or workplace policies are being created or updated, the ILO works to ensure that, for example, breastfeeding breaks are sufficient in number and frequency and that minimum requirements for a hygienic facility for breastfeeding or expression of milk are met. Flexibility is the key word. In light of the new World Health Organization recommendation of exclusive breastfeeding for 6 months, maternity leave should be long enough to enable working women meet this goal.

Improvements in maternity protection measures for working women can best be achieved by working together with the trade unions and other social partners. Two global trade union bodies—Public Services International (PSI) and the International Confederation of Free Trade Unions—have launched a campaign for ratification of Convention 183. Campaign materials can be downloaded from the PSI Web site. Affiliates of these international bodies can be found in most countries of the world and can be contacted to find out the most appropriate course of action related to ongoing efforts.

Clinical Implications

When providing information about breastfeeding and employment, the lactation consultant (LC) or other health-care provider is wise to sprinkle such information throughout several discussions of breastfeeding, maintaining a matter-of-fact attitude and establishing a positive expectation that this combination of roles is possible. The LC should discuss breastfeeding with the mother well in advance of her return to work (Bocar, 1997). The mother should be encouraged to identify her breastfeeding goals early in pregnancy and be aware of several breastfeeding options available based on the individual work circumstances (see Box 17–3). The combined breastfeeding and work assessment

Decisions the Employed Breastfeeding Mother Must Make

When to Return to Work

- *Work intensity:* Women must determine the status or intensity of their employment whether they choose to work part-time or full-time, or to not return to work after childbirth.
- *Breastfeeding goals:* Breastfeeding goals can be determined by considering factors such as length of maternity leave, breastfeeding intensity (exclusive or partial breastfeeding), work intensity, work circumstances, and amount of support available.

How Long to Breastfeed

- The decision regarding how long to breastfeed depends on a mother's breastfeeding goals and if weaning would occur due to mother-led reasons or baby-led reasons.

How Often to Pump

- The frequency of milk expression or pumping when a mother returns to work depends on the age of the baby and the duration of separation time between the mother and her child.
- The older the baby, the less frequent is the time needed to pump each day. Generally, mothers should express at least twice within 8 to 10 hours of work to maintain milk supply.

How Much Supplementation to Use

- How much supplementation or breast-milk substitute is used depends on breastfeeding intensity. For mothers who plan to breastfeed exclusively, they should avoid supplementation to prevent decreased milk production.
- Breastmilk substitutes are used for missed breastfeeding when mothers choose to breastfeed partially. The disadvantage of this option is that the mother's milk supply will decline as the baby receives more supplementation.

Child-Care Decisions

- Decisions on using child-care services depend on several factors, such as issues of trust, convenience, and finances.
- The options for child care include the following: in the baby's own home, in a neighbor's or friend's home, in the home of a someone who provides day-care services, or in a day-care center.

checklist presented earlier in Table 17–2 may be used to assess the important work-related elements so the appropriate planning can be done to fit with a mother's breastfeeding goal.

The role overload of the full-time employed mother necessitates that she learn how to organize her time for maximum efficiency. In breastfeeding, she has found an ideal combination for meeting the physical and psychological needs of her young child. In returning to work, she need not feel that she must shorten the period of lactation that she had planned. Some mothers may choose to breastfeed exclusively whereas some may elect to breast-feed partially and supplement with artificial milk. It is crucial that mothers understand clearly the consequences of each option. Mothers who choose to return to work early and desire to breastfeed exclusively may anticipate pumping frequently to maintain their milk supply.

Other mothers may choose not to express their milk at all. These women will need to know that expressing for comfort, at least during the first week or two, may be necessary if they are to avoid unpredictable, potentially embarrassing leak spots while their body is adjusting to the lack of breast stimulation during the workday. Additionally, these mothers should be encouraged to have someone introduce a bottle or cup of formula to the baby well in advance of her first day at work in case the baby develops an allergic reaction or does not tolerate formula well.

Some mothers will choose to return to work as soon as possible, often because they are financially unable to do otherwise; other women will make every effort to delay returning to work. The type of job that the woman has, the degree of involvement of coworkers and bosses, and her relationship with them, her seniority, and a wide array of other factors will influence these decisions. The health-care worker can provide information about maternal employment and breastfeeding, but only the mother can implement the final plan.

The lactation consultant can share with the mother how other women have coped with similar situations and should answer her questions based on research findings whenever possible. Babies do know when a mother is not available and adapt to her absence by altering sleep patterns. Changes in wakeful and sleepy periods are typical in families in which the mother works at times when the baby has previously been awake a great deal. Increased breastfeeding frequency when the mother is home (reverse-cycle nursing) is a common reaction, particularly in very young babies who breastfeed often. Such a pattern needs to be pointed out to the child-care provider; the mother should ask that the provider not wake the baby for feedings. Instead, the provider should let the baby indicate when to be fed during the day. These reverse-cycle nursing episodes do not always increase during the mother's nighttime sleeping hours; rather, they tend to be more frequent during the early daytime hours when she is preparing to leave for work and during the evening hours after she has returned home. Many mothers find that setting the alarm an hour earlier than they plan to be up reminds them to offer the baby the breast before heading for the shower or the kitchen to start the day. If she is encouraged to see this as the baby's touching and social time, the mother is more likely to view such behavior as a sign of the baby's attachment to her.

No "magic bullet" will resolve day-care issues. Unlike other countries, in which government subsidies enable many mothers to stay home for a substantial period following the birth of their babies, the United States has no federal policy supporting paid maternity leave. At the same time, increasing numbers of families make economic choices that mandate a two-worker household. In addition, day-care workers, often because they are so poorly paid, represent a workforce that has a high turnover, inadequate training, and lack of job commitment.

Summary

The role of the health-care worker is to inform the mother that she is not alone and other women have in most cases faced what she is likely to encounter. In some cases, the mothers found partial solutions; in other cases, their solutions enabled them, and will enable others, to proceed with breastfeeding with minimal interruption. Whatever the mother's individual situation, the person providing information needs to do so from a perspective of what has worked for others, recognizing that each mother's situation has unique strengths and pitfalls.

In settings in which institutionalized day care is well-organized and carefully supervised, many families' concerns can be set aside. In other day-care situations, the increased illness rates and other issues related to meeting the infant's and child's many needs warrant considerable concern. At-home care is both more expensive and more difficult to obtain; in addition, it provides no guarantee that some of the problems that have surfaced in group settings, including child neglect or abuse, will not also occur.

The length of time that a child breastfeeds (even if it is 2 years) represents a very small amount of the total time that the child will live in the par-ents' home. The length of the mother's employ-ment is likely to last far longer than her child's in-fancy. The longer the mother is home during the baby's early weeks and months, the shorter the time that breastfeeding is most likely to be negatively af-fected by that employment.

Key Concepts

- Currently 51 percent of married women return to the labor force while their children are under the age of 1.

- More women are choosing to breastfeed and many will continue to breastfeed after they re-turn to work.

- Research indicates that return to work does not impact breastfeeding initiation, but adversely effects duration of breastfeeding.

- Working full-time versus part-time impacts breastfeeding duration negatively.

- The sooner a mother returns to work, the shorter the duration of breastfeeding.

- The longer a mother stays at home before re-turning to work, the longer the breastfeeding duration.

- Level of job skill is associated with combining breastfeeding and employment: combined breastfeeding and employment increase as job skills increase.

- Prenatal planning is important to women who choose to combine breastfeeding and employ-ment. Key to planning is learning about breast-feeding and combining it with employment, decisions regarding work options and timing of return to work, assessing workplace support of breastfeeding, and child-care decisions.

- Four elements have been identified as en-hancers of breastfeeding in the workplace: time, space, gatekeeper, and support.

- Benefits of combined breastfeeding and em-ployment to employers include decreased ab-senteeism due to decreased infant illness—which translates into decreased health-care costs and increased worker productivity.

- There is evidence that lactation support pro-grams in the workplace reduce health-care costs, absenteeism, and infant illness while in-creasing breastfeeding duration.

- Breastfeeding problems may depend on the age of the infant and the timing of return to work.

- Common concerns and issues for women who breastfeed and work outside the home include loss of sleep, fatigue, maintaining an adequate milk supply, and day-care issues. Decisions re-garding exclusive or partial breastfeeding upon returning to work and the baby's age will de-termine the need and frequency of milk ex-pression.

- There are several factors to consider in breast pump choice including cleanliness, ease of use, comfort, efficiency, and cost.

- Human milk storage guidelines exist to pro-mote safety and are based on research.

- Community resources for the breastfeeding-employed woman include health-care pro-viders, lactation consultants, La Leche League, breastfeeding support groups, and online infor-mation and support.

- Legislative support and public advocacy is in-creasing to promote and protect women's rights to breastfeed after returning to work.

- The International Labour Organization has been instrumental in protecting maternal rights, including breastfeeding in the work-place, since 1919.

Internet Resources

Balancing Act Billboard, an online discussion forum for support and information for breastfeeding and working mothers: www.lalecheleague.org/cgi-bin/Ultimate.cgi? action=intro

The Balancing Act: Breastfeeding and Working, an 11-page pamphlet on employment and breastfeeding, available from online catalog (No 1165–17, $.95): www.lalecheleague.org/Web_store/web_store.cgi

Information on going back to work and breastfeeding. Extensive advertising: www.rightonmom.com

Public Services International (PSI) http://www.world-psi.org/psi.nsf

World Health Organization 55th World Assembly Provisional Agenda Item http://www.who.int/gb/EB_WHA/PDF/WHA55/ea5515.pdf

Other Resources

La Leche League International: *Working and Breastfeeding,* a 1-page double-sided tear-off sheet with information on planning for breastfeeding while employed.

La Leche League International: *The Womanly Art of Breastfeeding,* 6th ed. Schaumburg, IL: La Leche League International, 1997.

Pryor G. *Nursing Mother, Working Mother.* Boston, MA: Harvard Common Press, 1997.

References

Auerbach KG. Employed breastfeeding mothers: problems they encounter. *Birth* 11:17–20, 1984.

———. Assisting the employed breastfeeding mother. *J Nurse Midwifery* 35:26–34, 1990a.

———. Sequential and simultaneous breast pumping: a comparison. *Int J Nurs Stud* 27:257–65, 1990b.

Auerbach KG, Guss E. Maternal employment and breastfeeding: a study of 567 women's experiences. *Am J Dis Child* 138:958–60, 1984.

Baldwin E, Friedman KA. A current summary of breastfeeding legislation in the U.S. La Leche League International. Available at: www.lalecheleague.org/LawBills.html. Accessed February 28, 2003.

Bar-Yam NB. Workplace lactation support, Part I: a return to work breastfeeding assessment tool. *J Hum Lact* 14:249–54, 1998.

Begun AM, Blair C, Quiram JF. *Women's changing roles.* Wylie, TX: Information Plus, 1998.

Biancuzzo M. Selecting pumps for breastfeeding mothers. *JOGNN* 28:417–26, 1999.

Bocar D. Combining breastfeeding and employment: increasing success. *J Perinat Neonat Nurs* 11:23–43, 1997.

Breastfeeding.com. Supporting Moms is good business. CIGNA's corporate lactation program pays off. Available at: www.breastfeeding.com/workingmom/corp_lact.html Accessed February 27, 2003.

Bridges CB, Frank DI, Curtin J. Employer attitudes toward breastfeeding in the workplace. *J Hum Lact* 13:215–19, 1997.

Brown CA, Poag S, Kasprzycki C. Exploring large employers' and small employers' knowledge, attitudes, and practices on breastfeeding support in the workplace. *J Hum Lact* 17:39–46, 2001.

Buss IH et al. Vitamin C is reduced in human milk after storage. *Acta Paediatr* 90:813–15, 2001.

Carbonare SB et al. Effect of microwave radiation, pasteurization and lyophilization on the ability of human milk to inhibit *Escherichia coli* adherence to Hep-2 cells. *J Diarrhoeal Dis Res* 14:90–94, 1996.

Chezem J, Montgomery P, Fortman T. Maternal feelings after cessation of breastfeeding: influence of factors related to employment and duration. *J Perinat Neonat Nurs* 11:61–70, 1997.

Choplin M. Personal communication. Kansas City, Missouri, February 7, 2003.

Cohen R, Mrtek MB. The impact of two corporate lactation programs on the incidence and duration of breast-feeding by employed mothers. *Am J Health Prom* 8:436–41, 1994.

Cohen R, Mrtek MB, Mrtek RG. Comparison of maternal absenteeism and infant illness rates among breast-feeding and formula-feeding women in two corporations. *Am J Health Prom* 10:148–53, 1995.

Daly SEJ, Hartmann PE. Infant demand and milk supply: the short-term control of milk synthesis in lactating women. *J Hum Lact* 11:27–37, 1995.

Dodgson JE, Duckett L. Breastfeeding in the workplace: building a support program for nursing mothers. *AAOHN Journal,* 45:290–98, 1997.

Duckett L. Maternal employment and breastfeeding. *NAACOG's Clin Iss Perinat Women Health Nrsg* 3:701–12, 1992.

Fein SB, Roe B. The effect of work status on initiation and duration of breastfeeding. *Am J Pub Health* 88:1042–46, 1998.

Fetherston C. Risk factors for lactation mastitis. *J Hum Lact* 14:109, 1998.

Hager WD, Barton JR. Treatment of sporadic acute puerperal mastitis. *Infec Dis Obstet Gyn.* 4:97–101, 1996.

Hamosh M et al. Digestive enzymes in human milk: stability

at suboptimal storage temperatures. *J Pediatr Gasteoenterol Nutr* 24:38–43, 1997.

Hamosh M et al. Breastfeeding and the working mother: effect of time and temperature of short-term storage on proteolysis, lipolysis, and bacterial growth in milk. *Pediatrics* 97:492–98, 1996.

Hills-Bonczyk SG. Women's experiences with combining breastfeeding and employment. *J NurseMidwif* 38: 257–66, 1993.

———. Women's experiences with breastfeeding longer than 12 months. *Birth* 21:206–12, 1994.

International Labour Organization. *ABC of women workers' rights and gender equality.* Geneva, Switzerland: ILO Bureau of Publications, 2000.

———. C3 Maternity Protection Convention, 1919. Available at: www.ilo.org/ilolex/english/convdisp1.htm. Accessed February 27, 2003.

———. C103 Maternity Protection Convention (Revised), 1952. Available at: www.ilo.org/ilolex/english/convdisp1.htm. Accessed February 27, 2003.

———. C183 Maternity Protection Convention, 2000. Available at: www.ilo.org/ilolex/english/convdisp1.htm. Accessed February 27, 2003.

———. R191 Maternity Protection Recommendation, 2000. Available at: www.ilo.org/ilolex/english/recdisp1.htm. Accessed February 27, 2003.

Killien M. Returning to work after childbirth: considerations for health policy. *Nursing Outlook* 41:73–78, 1993.

Killien M, Habermann B, Jarrett M. Influence of employment characteristics on postpartum mothers' health. *Women's Work, Health, and Quality of Life* 33:63–81, 2001.

Libbus MK, Bullock FC. Breastfeeding and employment: an assessment of employer attitudes. *J Hum Lact* 18:247–51, 2002.

Lindberg LD. Women's decisions about breastfeeding and maternal employment. *J Marr Fam* 58:239–51, 1996.

Marshall R, Paulin B. Employment and earnings of women: historical perspective. In: Koziara KS, Moskow MH, Tanner LD, eds. *Working women: past, present, future.* Washington, DC: Bureau of National Affairs, 1987.

McKenna J, Mosho S, Richard C. Bedsharing promoted breastfeeding. *Pediatrics* 100:214–19, 1997.

Meek J. Breastfeeding in the workplace. *Ped Clin N A* 48:461–74, 2001.

Myrdal A, Klein V. *Women's two roles.* London: Routledge & Kegan Paul, 1956.

Neifert M. *Dr. mom's guide to breastfeeding.* New York: Penguin Putnam, 1998.

Ogundele MO. Techniques for the storage of human breastmilk: implications for antimicrobial functions and safety of stored milk. *Eur J Pediatr* 159:793–97, 2000.

Ovesen L et al. The effect of microwave heating on vitamins B_1 and E, and linoleic and linolenic acids, and immunoglobulins in human milk. *Int J Food Sci Nutr* 47:427–36, 1996.

Pardou et al. Human milk banking: influence of storage processes and of bacterial contamination on some milk constituents. *Biol Neonate* 65:302–9, 1994.

Piper S, Parks PL. Predicting the duration of lactation: evidence from a national survey. *Birth* 23:7–12, 1996.

Pugh L, Milligan R. A framework for the study of childbearing fatigue. *Adv Nurs Sci* 15:60–70, 1993.

Rea MF et al. Factors which facilitate and constrain breastfeeding among women working in factories in Sao Paulo, Brazil. *J Hum Lact* 13:233–39, 1999.

Riccitiello R. Corporate efforts: what some companies are doing to accommodate nursing moms. Available at: www.breastfeeding.com/workingmom/corp_lact.html. Accessed February 27, 2003.

Rojjanasrirat W. *The effects of a nursing intervention on breastfeeding duration among primiparous mothers planning to return to work* [dissertation]. University of Kansas, 2000.

Rojjansrirat W. Perceptions and attitudes toward breastfeeding and employment among low-income women. Unpublished manuscript, 2003.

Ryan AS, Wenjun Z, Acosta A. Breastfeeding continues to increase into the new millennium. *Pediatrics* 110:1103–9, 2002.

Thompsen AC, Espersen T, Maigaard S. Course and treatment of milk stasis, noninfectious inflammation of the breast, and infectious mastitis in nursing women. *Am J Obstet Gynecol* 149:492–95, 1984.

Thompson PE, Bell P. Breast-feeding in the workplace: how to succeed. *Iss Comp Pediatr Nurs* 20:1–9, 1997.

Tully MR. Recommendations for handling of mother's own milk. *J Hum Lact* 16:149–51, 2000.

US Bureau of Labor Statistics. *Families with their own children: employment status of parents by age of youngest child and family type, 2000–2001 annual averages.* Washington, DC: Division of Labor Force Statistics, 2001.

US Census Bureau. The official statistics. *Statistical abstract of the United States.* Washington, DC: 1998.

———. Profile of selected economic characteristics: 2000. Available at: www.factfinder.census.gov. Accessed February 2, 2003.

US Department of Labor. *Facts on working women* (No. 96–2). Washington, DC: US Department of Labor, Women's Bureau, September 1996.

Vanek EP, Vanek JA. Job sharing as an employment alternative in group medical practice. *Med Group Manage J* 48:40–24, 2001.

Visness CM, Kennedy KI. Maternal employment and breastfeeding: findings from the 1988 National Maternal and Infant Health Survey. *Am J Public Health* 87:945–50, 1997.

Wambach K. Maternal fatigue in breastfeeding primiparae during the first nine weeks postpartum. *J Hum Lact* 14:219–29, 1998.

World Health Organization. Infant and young child nutrition: global strategy on infant and young child feeding. Fifty-fifth World Health Assembly, Provisional Agenda Item 13.10, April 16, 2002.

Wyatt SN. Challenges of the working breastfeeding mother: workplace solutions. *AAOHN J* 50:61–66, 2002.

Yimyam S. Breastfeeding, work, and women's health among Thai women in Chiang Mai. *Breastfeed Rev* 6:17–22, 1998.

Yimyam S, Morrow M. Breastfeeding practices among employed Thai women in Chiangmai. *J Hum Lact* 15:225–32, 1999.

Youngblut J et al. Factors influencing single mothers employment status. *Health Care Women Int* 21:125–36, 2000.

18

CHILD HEALTH

Jan Riordan

This chapter reviews child health issues, beginning with the fundamentals of normal growth and development of infants and children and then a review of the prominent theories of child development. The discussion then focuses on the rich textures of mother-infant social interaction. Woven from the sophisticated sensory abilities of the newborn, they create a lifelong bond. Next, questions about such children's health issues as immunization and dental health are answered. The chapter concludes with the practical considerations of introducing solids and a discussion of weaning.

Developmental Outcomes and Infant Feeding

Before addressing specific elements of growth and development, it is useful to consider studies that compare developmental outcomes between breast-fed and bottle-fed babies. A number of studies suggest that breastfeeding has a long-term benefit on cognitive and intellectual development in childhood, which extends to young adulthood (Table 18–1).

These findings raise questions: What elements of breastfeeding play a role in promoting development and intelligence? Is it the nutritional or immunological aspects of breastmilk, or are there

environmental and emotional interactions connected with breastfeeding that cannot be controlled? Lucas et al. (1992) controlled for maternal interaction by studying preterm infants who received their mothers' milk via tube feedings, and compared them with children who got formula or children whose mothers intended to provide them with breastmilk but did not. Because all the infants were fed only by tube, the effects of breastmilk per se were separate from the normally intertwined effect of intimate maternal contact. The IQ scores of the children fed human milk were 8.5 points higher than those of the groups not fed human milk.

If human milk and breastfeeding are linked with higher intelligence, the mechanism of this effect on brain development is unknown at this time. It has been suggested that the presence of longer-chain polyunsaturated fatty acids, particularly arachidonic (AA) and docosahexanoic acid (DHA) in human milk are responsible. These fatty acids are essential nutrients for infants, because they are present in structural lipids in brain and nervous tissue (Farquharson et al., 1992). Differences in visual performance between breastfed and formula-fed full-term infants, for example, are thought to result from the provision of AA and DHA in breastmilk. Randomized trials have demonstrated improved vi-

Table 18–1

STUDIES ON BREASTFEEDING AND CHILDREN'S INTELLIGENCE

Source	Method	Findings
Richards, Hardy, & Wadsworth, 2002 (United Kingdom)	1946 birth cohort (n=1739) measured at age 53 years; cognitive test sores for reading ability, timed visual search, and verbal memory.	Breastfeeding is significantly and positively associated with educational attainment, an effect that was independent of early social background.
Jain, Concato, & Levanthal, 2002 (United States)	Meta-analysis of 40 published studies; 68% concluded that breastfeeding promotes intelligence.	Two of the studies on full-term infants met standards of high-quality feeding data. Of these two, one concluded that the effect of breastfeeding on intellect was significant and the other did not.
Mortensen et al., 2002 (Denmark)	Sample of 973 young adult men and 2280 women. Weschler Adult Intelligence Scale used to measure IQ. Controlled for marital and social status, education, mother's age, parity, and birth events.	IQ score 104 if breastfed for over 9 months compared with 99.4 for less than 1 month. No additional intellectual benefit from breastfeeding beyond 9 months.
Rao et al., 2002 (Norway, Sweden)	529 full-term small for gestational age (SGA) and normal weight Norwegian and Swedish infants followed up to 5 years. Norwegian version of Weschler Intelligence-Revised and Raven Progressive Matrices used to measure IQ.	Total IQ increased linearly with duration of exclusive breastfeeding for durations over 12 weeks giving an 11-point advantage in total IQ for SGA children exclusively breastfed for 24 weeks compared to those exclusively breastfed for 12 weeks.
Wigg et al., 1998 (Australia)	Cognitive assessments on 375 children at 2, 4, 7, and 11 to 13 years. Bayley Mental Development and Wechsler Full-Scale IQ.	Small, nonsignificant effect of breastfeeding on scores. Breastfed children had higher scores on Bayley Mental Development at ages 2 and 4, and higher IQ at ages 7 and 11.
Horwood & Fergusson, 1998 (New Zealand)	1000 children followed through age 18.	Small but consistent tendencies for increasing duration of breastfeeding to be associated with increased IQ, increased performance on standardized tests, higher teacher ratings, and high school achievement.
Johnson et al., 1996 (United States)	204 children measured at 3 years of age. Stanford-Binet, Hollingshead Index of Social Status used; controlled for socioeconomic status, mother's intelligence, smoking behavior, gender, and birth order of child.	Initiation of breastfeeding predicted scores on intelligence tests at age 3. Breastfeeding associated with 4.6 higher mean in intelligence.
Floury, Leech, & Blackhall, 1995 (United Kingdom)	592 first-born infants; Bayley Scales of Infant Development used.	Higher mental development (3.7–5.7 points) significantly related to breastfeeding at 2 weeks after discharge after control for social and demographic factors. No differences for psychomotor development or behavior.

Table 18–1 *(cont.)*

Temboury et al., 1994 (Spain)	364 healthy infants measured between 18 and 29 months of age. Bayley Scales of Infant Development used; controlled for maternal age, number of children, educational level, social class, job, psychosocial risk, and infant variables.	Low results on the Index of Mental Development associated with bottle-fed infants, lower-middle and lower social class, mother education, temper tantrums, and having siblings.
Rogan & Gladen, 1993 (United States)	855 newborns; Bayley Scales of Infant Development and McCarthy Scale used; prospective case control.	Statistically significant but small increases in scores among breastfed children on cognitive skills, not motor skills. Slightly higher English grades on report cards after adjusting for confounding variables.
Lucas et al., 1992 (United Kingdom)	926 low birth weight infants tube-fed with human milk or formula. Measured at 8.5 years of age; Weschler Intelligence Scale for Children used; randomized controlled trial of feeding mode; controlled for maternal contact, social class, education.	Dose-response relationship between proportion of breastmilk and IQ. Breastfed children scored 8.3 points higher.
Morley et al., 1988 (United Kingdom)	771 low birth weight infants; Bayley Mental Scale and Developmental Profile 11 used; measured at 18 months postterm; randomized controlled trial of feeding mode.	Breastfed children had a significant 8-point advantage on the Bayley Mental Developmental Index over the children who received only formula. After adjustment for social and demographic influences, the advantage was 4.3 points ($p < 0.005$).

sual and mental development in infants receiving a formula supplemented with DHA (Birch et al., 2000).

Another possible reason for enhanced cognitive function of breastfed children is the high concentration of sialic acid in breastmilk. Maturation of the brain is associated with total sialic concentration. Breastfed infants have higher brain sialic acid levels than do formula-fed infants because human milk is a rich source of sialic acid containing oligosaccharides, while formula contains very little (Wang et al., 1998).

Growth and Development

Physical Growth

Infant and child growth is affected by genetic makeup, general health, and nutrition. Infants and children vary in their tempo of growth and development, which tends to be marked by spurts of growth separated by plateaus. Still, there are universal patterns of growth for all children. These universal patterns include cephalocaudal growth (growth that proceeds from head to foot), proximodistal growth (growth that occurs from the center outward), and general-to-specific movements. The infant's head accounts for about one fourth of the infant's length at birth and illustrates cephalocaudal direction of growth. Maturation of motor skills also follows the cephalocaudal pattern: an infant masters control of his head before he masters arm and trunk control, which is followed by leg control (Figure 18–1).

Proximodistal and general-to-specific development is illustrated by the sequence of muscle control: infants control large muscles before they control small muscles. For example, the child is

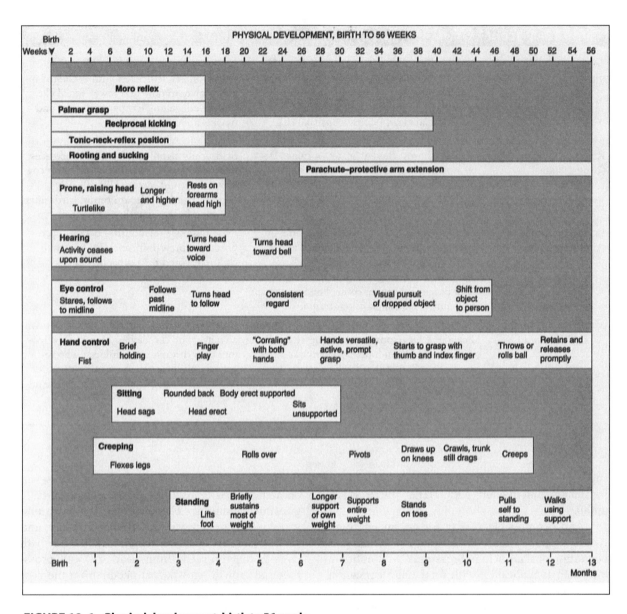

FIGURE 18–1. Physical development, birth to 56 weeks.

able to wave "bye-bye" before he is able to grasp with his whole hand and before he is able to hold a small object with his thumb and forefinger (pincer grasp). There is some evidence that breastfeeding has a beneficial effect on neurological development in children. Lanting et al. (1994) found a small advantageous effect of breastfeeding on the neurological status of children 9 years of age.

Weight and Length

Change, rather than stability, is the hallmark of infancy; weight increases faster in infancy than at any other time of life. The average neonate weighs about 3000 to 4000 gm (6.5–8.5 lb). Because full-term infants are born with excess fluid, they lose 5 to 10 percent of their birth weight following birth and then stabilize within a few days. Generally speaking, infants double their birth weight by about 5 months of age, triple it by 1 year of age, and quadruple it by 2 years of age.

As discussed earlier in this book, weight patterns of formula-fed infants differ from those of infants who are fed exclusively at the breast. Their weights are similar for the first few months, but at 3 to 4 months, formula-fed infants begin to weigh more than do their breastfed counterparts. This appears to hold crossculturally: formula-fed Japanese babies 6 to 8 months old weigh significantly more (135 gm) than do those breastfed (Yoneyama, Nagata, & Asano, 1994). As discussed in Chapter 4, North American breastfed babies gain an average of 35 gm (approximately 1 oz) per day at 1 month and 19 gm (0.6 oz) per day at 4 months, whereas formula-fed infants gain an average of 34.4 gm per day at 1 month and 23 gm per day at 4 months. Despite their slightly slower weight gain, breastfed infants at 4 months have more body fat (Butte et al., 1995).

Length at birth is about 50 to 53 cm (20–21 in.) and, on the average, male infants tend to be 5 oz heavier and 0.5 in. longer than females. A baby grows about 1 in. each month for the first 6 months and about 0.5 in. per month for the next 6 months. By the infant's first birthday, his length has increased by 50 percent. Length and head-circumference growth are similar for both breastfed and formula-fed infants (Butte et al., 1990). The weight of the baby's brain increases most rapidly during infancy as nerve cells enlarge, become longer and branched, and gain myelin sheathing. By 18 months of age, the infant's brain is 75 percent of its adult weight. If the infant becomes malnourished, the first growth factor to be affected is weight. Only when malnourishment is severe and longstanding are the infant's length or head circumference compromised.

Senses

Neonates and young infants have remarkably well-developed sensory capabilities. At birth, the infant's auditory nerve tracts have sufficient myelin sheathing to allow them to hear well; they can differentiate various tastes and smells. This ability to selectively respond through their senses enhances the infant's early attempts to locate and attach to the nipple and to distinguish between his own mother and other individuals.

Within several days after birth, breastfeeding infants respond preferentially to breast or axillary odors from their mother. In striking contrast, bottle-feeders display no evidence of recognizing axillary odors from their mothers. While feeding at the breast, the neonate's nostrils are in close proximity with the mother's bare skin, which provides the opportunity to become familiar with her characteristic odor (Makin & Porter, 1989).

As early as 2 months before birth, hearing develops in the womb. The fetus is already responding to both internal sounds from the mother and to noises outside the mother. Some young infants, for instance, appear to recognize their mother's favorite soap opera when it comes on television. Neonates discriminate between differences in pitch and can detect the direction of the source of sound.

Loud, low sounds are likely to disturb and alarm the infant, whereas soft, high-pitched sounds have a calming effect; therefore, the higher-range tones of the female voice tend to quiet and focus the baby's attention. When one baby starts crying in a nursery, others will do the same. Newborns respond to sound by differentiating the caregiver's voice from that of strangers. They also sense heat, cold, pressure, and pain.

The neonate's vision is less developed because retinal structures and the optic nerve are not yet complete. A neonate focuses mainly on large objects close to his face and sees best at a range of 8 to 12 in., with 9 in. as the optimum—just about the distance between the baby's face and the mother's face while the baby is being held at the breast level. Neonates are able to follow and track a moving object with their eyes and prefer moving objects to stationary ones.

Babies seem to have an innate visual preference. They prefer more complex stimuli, such as the human face, to a plain surface and will look at a face longer than at other visual patterns. All infants have dark, smoky eyes at birth. Their lids are puffy, and the tear ducts do not function. Eye muscles may occasionally drift to a crossed position.

Reflexes

The fragile appearance of neonates belies the sophistication of their reflexes, which are designed to enhance survival. Reflexes protect the infant and give the central nervous system and brain time to mature and to begin to govern coordinated behaviors (see Chapter 19).

Rooting, suckling, swallowing, and gag reflexes are directly applicable to breastfeeding. The rooting reflex initiates the act of suckling milk from the mother's breast and is considered vital to life. The suck-swallow reflex is presumably developed at 34 weeks of gestation. Synchronized coordination of suckling and swallowing with breathing appears to be achieved consistently by infants of more than 37 weeks postconception age (Bu'Loc, Woolridge, & Baum, 1990), but as discussed in Chapter 13 on prematures, many low birth weight infants can suckle at the breast. By 3 to 4 months after birth, the rooting reflex begins to diminish. In Chapter 3, we described the infant's oral/suckling capabilities as the cockpit of the nervous system. The presence of rooting, sucking, swallowing, and gag reflexes are barometers that indicate an intact, functioning central nervous system.

Levels of Arousal

Young infant behavior can be described by several levels of arousal states (Gill et al., 1988; Prechtl & Beintema, 1975). The Anderson Behavioral State Scale (Gill at al., 1988) lists 15 categories, with states ranging from very quiet sleep to hard crying (Box 18–1). The infant's most complex interaction with his environment is made in the quiet awake state; at this time, the neonate fixates on and follows objects and turns his head toward any sound. The neonate becomes more alert when he senses a new stimulus; if it is repeated, the infant responds less or habituates to the stimulus (Als & Brazelton, 1981). This decrement in response allows the neonate to control his behavioral state. Overactive infants are said to lack this ability to habituate (respond less to repeated stimuli).

Theories of Development

Nature Versus Nurture

Which is more important in a child's development, nature (genes, heredity) or nurture (environment)?

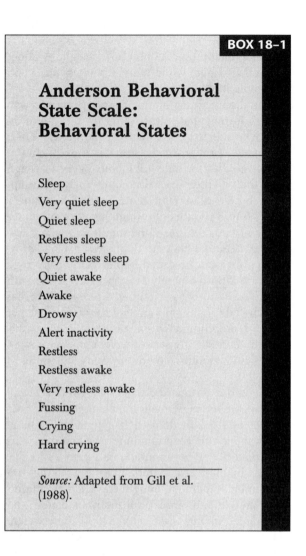

BOX 18–1

Anderson Behavioral State Scale: Behavioral States

Sleep
Very quiet sleep
Quiet sleep
Restless sleep
Very restless sleep
Quiet awake
Awake
Drowsy
Alert inactivity
Restless
Restless awake
Very restless awake
Fussing
Crying
Hard crying

Source: Adapted from Gill et al. (1988).

At one end of the spectrum, how a child develops is thought to be determined at conception; at the other end, development is seen as a product of the environment. Although we can demonstrate that breastfeeding appears to optimize development, the issue is still complex. For example, are the overall parenting patterns of a woman who chooses to breastfeed different from those of a woman who chooses to bottle-feed? We cannot say that any one aspect of child development is determined exclusively by either nature or nurture; clearly each plays a role. The extent of influences from nature versus nurture differ among developmental theorists. How these two issues interact are addressed in two classic theories about child development.

Erikson's Psychosocial Theory Eric Erikson (1963, 1968) identified stages of development that center around conflicts. These conflicts are central issues of crucial importance to the personality at each stage of life. Characteristics of the first two stages (infant and toddler) of Erikson's theory are shown in Table 18–2. Each stage requires resolution of its particular conflict, and each stage widens the social radius of the infant's influence. The first conflict is trust versus mistrust. According to Erikson, the first year is when confidence in having one's needs met and feeling physically safe results in the infant's either trusting or mistrusting his environment.

Once trust, as opposed to mistrust, is established, the toddler moves into the next stage, in which autonomy must be mastered over shame and doubt. By then (18 months to 3 years of age), he walks, runs, and expresses himself verbally, eagerly exploring his exciting new world but still needing reassurance and returning to his mother for "emotional refueling." If an infant is lovingly fed and his biological needs are cared for, he develops a sense of trust in the world. Being left hungry or crying for long periods results in a sense of mistrust of the world. Breastfeeding for nourishment becomes breastfeeding for reassurance and comfort in this stage. The process of individuation, a realization that he is a separate individual, unfolds gradually as the child begins to assert control over his life.

Table 18–2

THEORIES OF DEVELOPMENT

Theorist	Infant	Toddler
Erikson (psychosexual)	Trust versus mistrust (birth–1 year)	Autonomy versus shame and doubt (1–3 year)
	Requires basic needs (food, comfort, warmth) to be met	Increasing independence in eating, dressing, toileting, and bathing
	Learns to trust self (and environment)	Father becomes important
	Mutual giving and getting between self and caregivers	Limits (firm and consistent) lead to security
	Mistrust results if needs not met consistently or inadequately	Acquires "will"; feeling of self-control, bias for self-esteem
Piaget (cognitive)		Excessive criticism and expectation of perfection leads to shame and doubt about ability to control self and world
	Sensorimotor (birth–2 years); uses senses, motor skills, reflexes to explore	Proconceptual (2–7 years)
	Object permanence	Self-centered; other centeredness begins
	Trial and error	Perception from own point of view
	"Insight" problem solving	Use of symbols, especially language
	Able to think before acting (18–24 months)	Literal interpretation of works and action
		Judges thing for outcome, consequence to self
		Transductive reasoning

Source: Adapted from Erikson (1963); Piaget & Inhelder (1969).

Piaget's Cognitive Theory Jean Piaget (1952) identified the major periods through which humans pass in the course of intellectual maturation. The first is the sensorimotor stage, in which an infant's knowledge of the world comes primarily through his sensory experiences and motor activities. Its main features are presented in Table 18–3.

Table 18–3

CHARACTERISTICS OF INFANTS' THINKING: SENSORIMOTOR STATE

Major Task
Conquest of Object
Throughout this stage, infants are unable to think. Intelligence proceeds from directly acting, as a whole, on the environment to more goal-directed attending to and action on particular objects to make specific events occur. All the senses and motor skills are actively used to define and interpret objects and events.

Perception
- *Birth–3 months:* View of world and self undifferentiated; unconscious of self.
- *4–6 months:* View of world centered around body: self-centered.
- *After 6 months:* View of world as centered around objects.
- *6–12 months:* Self seen as separated from objects.
- *12–18 months:* Objects seen to have constancy and permanence.
- *18–24 months:* Represents spatial relationships between objects and between objects and self (e.g., knows smaller things fit inside larger things).

Thought
- *Birth–3 months:* Not present. Uses inborn reflexes and senses.
- *4–6 months:* Questions presence of thought. Uses combination of reflexes and senses purposively. Develops habits.
- *6–12 months:* Knows objects by how he or she uses them. Knows objects have constant size before knows objects have same form; serially acts out two previously separate behaviors in goal-directed sequences.
- *12–24 months:* Object permanence stimulates purposive, intentional use of behaviors to find hidden objects and to cause event via trial and error—problem solve via "insight": can now see effect when given the cause (e.g., knows where train will come out when it goes into tunnel). Symbolism and memory begin—uses deferred imitation to discover new ways of acting (e.g., when "pretends" sleep means "know" symbolic sleeping).

Reasoning
- *Birth–6 months:* Not present.
- *6–24 months:* Syncretism (1) perceives "whole"—impression without analysis of parts or synthesis of relations, (2) lacks systematic exploratory behavior until end of state, (3) begins to connect series of ideas into a confused whole.

Language
- *Birth–3 months:* Undifferentiated cry. Use of different intensities, patterns, and pitches of cry for different feelings (e.g., pain, hunger, fatigue).
- *6–8 weeks:* Cooing: contented and happy sounds.
- *3–6 months:* Babbling: repeated various sounds for sensation of pleasure. Laughing: when happy or excited.
- *6–12 months:* Spontaneous vocalization: imperfect imitation. Echolalia: conscious imitation of sounds.
- *12–18 months:* Expressive jargon: use of information, rhythms, and pauses to imitate sentence sounds. Holophrases: use of one word to convey meaning. Gestures: substitute for or add meaning to speech.
- *18–24 months:* Telegraphic speech: use of noun and verb to convey many meanings.

Play
- *Birth–6 months:* Exercise play—repetition of actions and sounds for pleasure (e.g., rolling over, babbling).
- *6–12 months:* Exploratory play: pleasure from causing effect and reconfirming skill (e.g., "peek-a-boo," "drop and retrieve, " "pat-a-cake").
- *12–24 months:* Deferred imitation—imitates previously observed actions (not reasons for or purposes of actions) from memory (e.g., pretends to be "Daddy" and goes through getting dressed, shaving, then walks outside, and gets in the "car").

Source: Adapted from Servonsky & Opas (1987, p. 22).

As infants experience sensory and motor activities, they construct schemas (concepts or models) for dealing with information and experiences. These schemas are put into play through complementary processes of assimilation and accommodation. Assimilation refers to the process of absorbing new information from the environment and using current structures to deal with the information. Accommodation refers to the process by which the infant alters his behavior and adjusts existing schemas to the requirements of objects or events to integrate new learning with old (and thus adapt to his ever-expanding environments). For example, if a child is breastfed, and a pacifier is given to him, the pacifier nipple may be sufficiently different so that the old sucking patterns do not work well. When this happens, disequilibrium occurs, and the child must restructure the existing view of suckling so that it fits with the new information or experience. This process is called *accommodation.* Through these processes, schemas are developed and refined.

The concept of object permanence is a feature of the sensorimotor period. Piaget (1952) suggested that the infant younger than 6 to 9 months of age lacks the ability for mental representation of the unseen. For instance, when an object such as a toy is out of sight, it ceases to exist, and the infant does not search for it. With the ability for mental representation, the infant realizes that an object or person continues to exist when out of sight, and he searches for a hidden object. It is now quite certain that person permanency precedes object permanency; an infant does recognize his mother, father, or caretaker long before 8 months and thus experiences loss or anxiety when an all-important person is not present. Later, as the child broadens the ability to recognize a separate existence from his mother, he begins to tolerate brief periods of separation from different caretakers. The ability roughly coincides with diminishing separation anxiety and with Erikson's establishment of trust progressing to the beginnings of autonomy.

Social Development

As infants grow, their periods of waking and socializing lengthen. By 2 to 8 weeks of age, a baby smiles spontaneously to pleasurable stimuli, particularly at human faces. Babies coo and babble to their parents and other fascinated adults who coo and bab-

ble back. By 3 months, the infant is interested in his environment and playfully reaches out to grasp objects, including breasts, nipples, noses, and hair. By 6 months of age, the infant reaches out to be picked up, squeals with pleasure at recognition of his mother, and enjoys games such as peek-a-boo.

Language and Communication

Because infants hear well from birth, they are able to discriminate between different intonations and between vowels and consonants. This ability to understand the spoken word is called *passive,* or *receptive, language.* The ability to produce meaningful utterances is called *expressive language.* The speech center in the brain borders on the areas of the motor cortex that control both mouth-tongue movement and hand movement. This proximity explains why we tend to express ourselves with both our hands and our mouths. Infants, as well, use many gestures in association with sounds and expressive language. Children consistently acquire language communication in a definable sequence:

- *Crying:* From birth; different rhythms signifying emotions and needs (hunger, anger, pain)
- *Cooing and gooing:* After 2 weeks; a wide variety of meaningless speech sounds (Figure 18–2)
- *Babbling:* 3 to 12 months ("mama-mama," "dada-dada")
- *Holophrasing:* 12 months; one-word sentences
- *Telegraphic speech:* 18 months; subject-verb-object
- *Complete sentences:* 2 years

The duration of a baby's crying during the early months of life typically increases until about 6 weeks of age, followed by a gradual decrease until 4 months of age. Infants cry more and are more wakeful during the late afternoon and evening. If the infant is carried during fussy periods, crying and fussing decrease, but the number of feedings and the duration of his sleep do not change (McKenna, Mosko, & Richard, 1997).

Although infants differ in the number of hours of sleep, each baby gets as much sleep as he needs. Newborns sleep an average of 16.5 hours per day; some sleep a total of about 10 hours, others sleep up to 23 hours. Generally, infants fuss and cry before

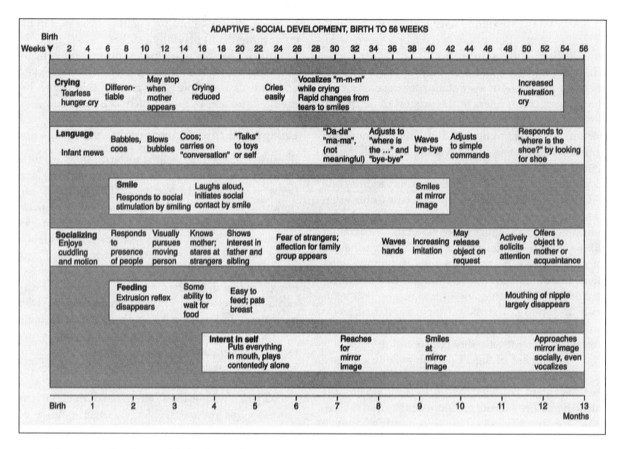

FIGURE 18–2. Adaptive-social development, birth to 56 weeks.

falling asleep. The sleeping pattern of breastfed infants differs from that of formula-fed infants. Breastfed infants wake more often during the night and have shortened sleep patterns (Elias et al., 1986; Mosko et al., 1996, 1997). The expression "He sleeps just like a baby" simply is not true during the first few months of life for any infant. The typical pattern is one of frequent, short periods of sleep interrupted by crying and fussing. This occurs night and day. The so-called infant sleep disorders being diagnosed today are not disorders at all but normal sleep patterns.

Mothers and babies interact with one another using a variety of communications that are visual, vocal, tactile, and postural. Babies coo, goo, and babble whenever they are alert and content. These sounds change from week to week and are elicited by the smiling faces of adults, by voices, or by touch. Any mother who has breastfed knows that feeding at the breast is a prime time for her baby to

communicate actively with coos, babbling, and speech sounds as he looks into the eyes of his mother (Figure 18–3). These exquisite sensory interchanges further bond the mother and baby. Epstein (1993) videotaped breastfeeding mothers and their babies during feedings to investigate maternal-infant interactions. These videos were later observed and analyzed.

The interactions between the mother and infants were elaborate and complex, with each breastfeeding dyad interacting with its own individual style. All of the mothers and babies looked at their partners' bodies, not just at their faces, during the breastfeeding session. All of the mothers had happy and affectionate expressions on their faces as they watched their babies, yet the amount of time they maintained the positive expression differed between mothers. Certain babies in the study even smiled and laughed with

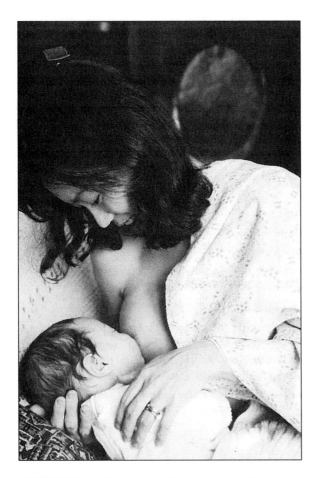

FIGURE 18–3. Mutual caregiving promotes the maternal role-taking process.

their mother's nipples in their mouths. Babies and mothers were observed vocalizing to one another. In some dyads, intricate vocal interactions occurred. Babies made sounds that their mothers initiated and this resulted in the babies continuing to make sounds and the mothers continuing to imitate them. In all of these cases, the sounds that the babies made seemed to be expressions of pleasure.

Mothers speak to their infants in a universal dialogue that instinctively uses exaggerated upbeat tones and facial gestures to talk to babies. Mothers use slowly rising crescendo and decrescendo allowing the baby time to process each short vocal package before the next communication arrives. How a mother talks to her baby is more important than what she says.

This sing-song quality of the mother's speech is tailored to the baby's listening abilities. Smiling, grasping, and talking all play important roles in the attachment process (i.e., the reciprocal development of an affectional tie between the mother or caregiver and the baby) (Pridham & Chang, 1992). During these interactions, the mother not only gives care to her infant but the newborn gives care back to his mother. For this reason, Anderson (1977) called the mother and infant "mutual caregivers" (p. 53):

As the mother holds her infant to her breast, assumes the en face position, and talks to her newborn, her eyes are the optimal distance away and her head, mouth and eyes move slowly and within a closely circumscribed range. Her newborn will also be sending stimuli, such as changes in facial expression, vocalizations, and eye-to-eye contact. The mother's response to such stimuli is immediate.

In a review of the theoretical framework for studying factors that affect the maternal role, Mercer (1981) emphasized the role of the infant in his mother's maternal role-taking process. The newborn's ability to see, hear, and track the human face shows socialization capabilities at birth that allow the infant to be an active partner with the mother in the attachment process. Each new infant presents a challenge to maternal adaptation and that previous experience with infants makes little difference to becoming the parent of a new child. Moreover, the transition process of being mother to a new infant is different in the second and third months from the process in the first month (Pridham & Chang, 1992). Breastfeeding plays an important role in a mother's feelings of competence. Tarkka (2003) reported that breastfeeding was a main predictor of a woman's competence as a mother. Competence was measured as the ability to make independent child-care decisions, to find pleasure in parenthood, and to meet the demands of being a parent.

The infant uses play as a part of the communication process. During the earliest (sensorimotor) stage of life, infants begin with exercise play, such as repeating newly learned actions for pleasure. Stick out your tongue at a young infant, and he will stick out his tongue at you. Next, infants play in order to explore their skills, crawling backward down the stairs, for example, or pushing a finger into the mother's mouth while breastfeeding and then squealing with glee when she pretends to bite the finger (Figure 18–4). The older baby's playful activities as he breastfeeds are a part of communication and attachment with his mother. Deferred imitation play begins at around 18 months of age, when toddlers begin to imitate the behavior and language they see and hear. For example, little girls, who are already adopting the gender role of their mothers, will very seriously and readily "nurse" their dolls at their breasts (Figure 18–5).

Attachment and Bonding

This exquisite dance of reciprocal reinforcement in the mother-infant dyad leads to the mother's "taking-in" her maternal role, cementing the mother-infant bond. Early theorists paved the way for understanding the processes of bonding and attachment. Konrad Lorenz (1935) noted the behavior and imitation of the mother animal by the young, which is necessary for survival, and labeled it *imprinting*. It is believed that attachment and bonding are the human equivalent of imprinting.

Bowlby's seminal paper (1958), which introduced the principles of attachment theory, empha-

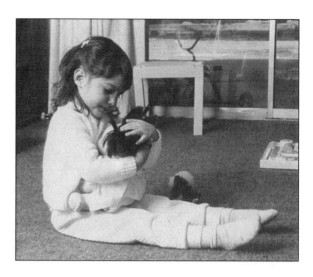

FIGURE 18–5. Child "nursing" doll.

sized the importance of an infant's developing a primary attachment to a caring, responsible adult. Later, Harlow and Harlow (1965) demonstrated the importance of contact comfort for the attachment and emotional well-being of the newborn rhesus monkey. When presented with "surrogate" mothers—one formed out of unpadded chicken wire and equipped with milk-filled bottles, the other made out of padded terry cloth but without bottles—the baby monkeys spent much more time with the warm, cloth-covered mothers, going only briefly to the bottles for food.

Mothers who room-in with their infants after birth touch their infants' face and head more often than do mothers who have minimal contact with their newborn (Prodromidis et al., 1995). Rubin (1967) showed a progressive attachment that results from touching: a mother first explores her newborn's extremities with her fingertips, rapidly moves to the baby's arms and legs, and finally caresses the trunk with the palm of her hand. A conceptual model for the maternal-infant bonding might well be like the weaving of a tapestry. Rubin described bonding as, " not a cord, nor a bond, nor a welding job, rather a large creative work, framed between the child and the mother's own significant social world, systematically and progressively developed for durability against time and stress to form the substance of her own personal identity and the fabric of her relationship with this particular child."

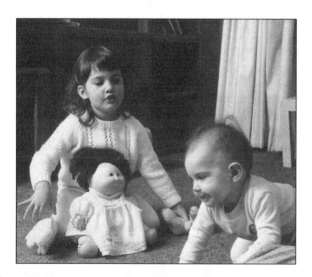

FIGURE 18–4. Developing motor skills by exploring the environment.

Ainsworth et al. (1978) studied brief infant separation from mothers in a laboratory situation to measure the degree of attachment. Mothers defined by the researchers as "securely attached" to their infants were most sensitive to their baby's needs, whereas mothers identified as "insecurely attached" to their infants were less emotionally expressive, felt more aversion to close body contact with the babies, and were more frequently irritated, resentful, and angry. A multitude of circumstances affect the mother-child relationship, which begins before the child is born; even though the baby is unseen, the mother imagines or fantasizes about her child.

The mother's perceptions of the "dream child" and, subsequently, her relationship with that child will not only be influenced by her self-concept but also by her total life experience. Her culture, social relationship, economic status, and state of health can all add to or detract from her relationship with her unborn child. If she experiences social isolation and economic deprivation during her pregnancy, her emotional reserves will be lowered. If she experiences physical discomfort and ill health, her physical stamina may be depleted. Thus the support she receives during pregnancy and from her total environment will affect her acceptance and readiness for mothering.

The infant's birth forces the mother to compare her real-life baby with her dreams, fantasies, and expectations. If reality and expectations are congruent, attachment begins soon after birth; if they are divergent, the mother must first work through the loss of the "dream child" and strive to fall in love with this stranger who bears little resemblance to the child of her fantasies.

Klaus and Kennell (1975) moved the concept of attachment one step further by popularizing the existence of a sensitive period for attachment shortly after birth. Barring excessive medication of the mother during delivery, a newborn will normally be in an alert state for at least 1 hour following birth. During this period, the mother will spend a significant amount of time gazing en face (face-to-face) into her infant's eyes, touching, and stroking. The neonate is born in a state of readiness for this human interaction. The infant's remarkable perceptual and sensory abilities (hearing, seeing, smelling, and tasting) at birth facilitate the attachment process. As attachment becomes established, the newborn is observed to move his arms and legs in rhythm to the cadences of the mother's voice, in a synchronous pattern that may be the foundation for later speech (Condon & Sander, 1974). Such interaction is known as *entrainment,* and its effects carry over into later life (Figure 18–6).

An active partner in the attachment process, the infant initiates about one half of parent-infant interaction. Through predictable and clear-cut transmission of cues or nonverbal signals, neonates are capable of producing the desired behavior in the parent and selectively reinforcing parent behavior. In many ways, the infant is as competent as the parents, perhaps even more so than young, inexperienced parents.

The baby's cry is an impossible-to-ignore cue for attention, and his mother responds by picking up, feeding, or carrying him. The perceptive mother is attuned to her baby's cues and reacts to them appropriately. If he coos and smiles, she reacts happily to his pleasure. The infant's contentment or irritability signal the mother to increase or decrease stimulation. If parents are aware of these cues as a method of communication for their infant, they respond by viewing their infants as individuals. Informing mothers about the behavioral characteristics of their babies is an effective means of enhancing the interaction between mothers and their infants (Anderson, 1981).

Breastfeeding, with its frequent touching, holding, and eye-to-eye contact, offers enhanced opportunities for attachment and responding to infant cues. Certainly, the frequency of subjective verbal responses by mothers who state that they "feel closer" to the breastfed child merits serious consideration. Through breastfeeding, the infant may exert more control: for example, the decision to end the feeding is a shared decision between the mother and baby when the mother "reads" and responds to her baby's behaviors. In bottle-feeding, on the other hand, the mother is chiefly responsible for ending the feeding. Maternal bonding consists of two global aspects: the first is related to preoccupations with infant safety, the second concerns developing a selective and unique bond with the baby. Even mothers of normal healthy babies ex-

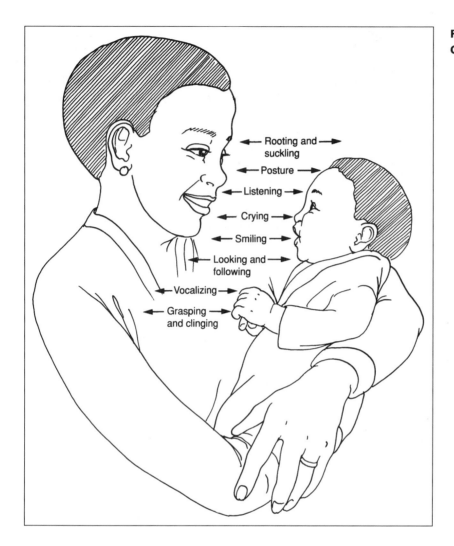

FIGURE 18–6.
Components of attachment.

Rooting and suckling

Posture

Listening

Crying

Smiling

Looking and following

Vocalizing

Grasping and clinging

perience thoughts and worries. Initial separation increases these preoccupations (Feldman et al., 1999).

The common practices today of rooming-in and mother-baby care in maternity care were the result of many studies of maternal-infant attachment and bonding in the 1970s that demonstrated that mother-baby contact was associated with stronger attachment. Now a flurry of research on skin-to-skin touching (Kangaroo Care) is similarly influencing this type of care for low birth weight infants (Anderson et al., 2003c). Numerous published reports relating to the safety, efficacy, and feasibility of Kangaroo Care have associated it with both immediate and long-term effects (Anderson et al., 2003a). In a survey of US neonatal intensive

care units, about 80 percent practice some form of Kangaroo Care in their units (Engler et al., 2002).

Kangaroo Care is now commonly practiced in neonatal care units in the United States and worldwide. Case Western Reserve University nurse researchers Gene Cranston Anderson (2001, 2003) and Susan Ludington-Hoe (1996, 2000) have led clinical research teams that study Kangaroo Care.

The intervention of skin-to-skin contact may be critical for mothers, especially those who have low birth weight babies or are otherwise unable to take their infants home. By promoting skin-to-skin touching, Kangaroo Care builds the components of bonding and even has been shown to increase the volume of breastmilk production (Hurst, Valentine,

& Renfro, 1997). The positive encounter of skin-to-skin provides a bonding experience that helps to offset the mother's experience of loss avoiding bonding failure (Anderson et al., 2003c). Kangaroo Care is also discussed in Chapter 13.

Although immediate postpartum mother-child contact is desirable, it is no longer considered critical. Almost all parents are attached to their babies, even if they experience marked disruption of the early parent-child contact, which most healthy mothers and babies now take for granted (see Chapter 9). For example, Hedberg-Nyqvist and Ewald (1997) found that Swedish infants who were separated from their mothers on the first day because they were ill or because of a complicated delivery breastfed for as many months as did those who had immediate contact with their mothers. Parents should be assured that not having the opportunity to interact and bond with their baby soon after birth will not cause irreparable damage to their child.

Temperament

During the past two decades, researchers have studied the temperament of the infant and how it influences parenting. The longitudinal work of Thomas and Chess (1977) suggested that every child exhibits a particular temperament from birth and that (1) infants have individual characteristics even as newborns, (2) these characteristics differentiate infants one from another, and (3) they remain constant over time. Categories of response that influence a child's temperament include activity level, regularity of body functions, adaptability, response to new situations, sensory threshold, intensity of reaction, quality of mood, distractibility, and attention span and persistence. These characteristics were rated for three temperaments: the easy child, the difficult child, and the slow-to-warm-up child. Characteristic temperament styles of each are seen in Table 18–4.

Sears (1987) reduced these three temperament characteristics into two categories in which he identified high-need and low-need babies and popularized the concept for parents to understand and use. High-need babies are fussy, seem to breastfeed "all the time," and cry if put down; low-need babies are content and cuddly and do not need constant carrying or attention. Two questionnaires or tools for assessing the temperament of an infant or child are the Infant Temperament Questionnaire (ITQ) for infants 4 to 12 months of age (Carey & McDevitt, 1978) and the Toddler Temperament Scale for children 1 to 3 years of age (Hegvik, McDevitt, & Carey, 1982). The ITQ scores identify a child's temperamental style; the results may be used as an opportunity for making parents aware of their child's temperament and for suggesting appropriate parenting skills.

Stranger Distress

As the infant grows older, the significance of his major caregiver is recognized and, during the second half of the first year of life, another developmental phenomenon appears: stranger distress. The infant who up to that time has been curious about everything in his environment, including strangers, suddenly frowns and cries and may even attempt physical escape when a stranger approaches. Stranger distress appears quite suddenly as early as 6 months but more commonly at 8 months. It is more pronounced when the mother or primary caretaker is not present. As a consequence, exposure to a variety of strangers is disruptive to an infant at this age. Although stranger distress occurs at about the same period of development as that of separation anxiety, it is a separate phenomenon.

Separation Anxiety

As mother or father leave the room, anxious eyes follow. Almost instantly, the child's face is contorted by rage; he cries loudly and may throw himself wildly about, kicking and screaming. No action brings solace at this point. This behavior is the first phase of separation anxiety, a phenomenon that emerges toward the middle of the first year of life, peaks from 13 to 20 months, and decreases after the second birthday. Separation anxiety, according to psychoanalytic theory, is the painful effect of anxiety engendered by the threat of actual separation from a loved one. Bowlby (1973) and Robertson (1958) delineated three phases of separation anxiety in young children: (1) protest, (2) despair, and (3) denial.

Protest. In an angry and yearning attempt to recover his mother or primary caregiver, the child violently cries and throws himself about, kicking and screaming. He is angry with the world and with

Table 18–4

CHARACTERISTICS OF TEMPERAMENT STYLES IN CHILDREN

Factor	Easy Child	Slow-to-Warm-Up Child	Difficult Child
Activity level—amount of physical activity during sleep, feeding, play, dressing	High	Medium	Low
Regularity—of body functions in sleep, hunger, bowel movements	Fairly regular	Variable	Fairly irregular
Adaptability to change in routine—ease or difficulty with which initial response can be modified in socially desirable way	Generally adaptable	Variable	Generally slow to adapt
Response to new situations—initial reaction to new stimuli, foods, people, places, toys, or procedures	Approach	Variable	Withdrawal
Level of sensory threshold—amount of external stimulation, such as sounds or changes in food or people, necessary to produce a response	High threshold (much stimulation needed)	Medium threshold	Low threshold (little stimulation needed)
Intensity of response—energy content of responses regardless of their quality	Generally intense	Variable	Generally mild
Positive or negative mood—energy content of responses regardless of their quality	Generally positive	Variable	Generally negative
Distractibility—effectiveness of external stimuli (sounds, toys, people) in interfering with ongoing behavior	Easily distractible	Variable	Nondistractible
Persistence and attention span—duration of maintaining specific activities with or without external obstacles	Persistent	Variable	Nonpersistent
Percentage of all children	40%	15%	10%

Source: From Carey (1978); Servonsky & Opas (1987, p. 180).

his mother for leaving him. He feels that she must be angry with him also, because she left him. The protest phase can last from a few hours to several days, depending on the energy of the child, his age, his relationship with his mother, and the quality of the new environment.

Despair.   Gradually, the child moves into quiet grieving and mourning as he begins to accept his fate. He shows little interest in his environment but suffers intensely; his expression is one of great sadness. Regressive behavior, such as thumb-sucking, occurs as the child turns inward for solace.

Detachment or Denial. The child develops a defense mechanism to deal with his loss by detaching himself from the importance of his mother's love. He gradually begins to interact with others, approaching anyone and even appearing cheerful. This stage is often misinterpreted as adapting or "settling in." Actually, he is coping with his loss by indiscriminately attaching to caretakers. When he is reunited with his mother at this point, he may appear uninterested and may not seem to recognize her.

Clinical Implications

Deviations from normal patterns of attachment signal that a problem may be present; hence assessing the infant's or child's growth and developmental level—and being able to apply a working knowledge of developmental patterns—is as important as knowing the specifics of a child's health problem. If a baby is being examined, for example, the close proximity of his mother helps to reduce stranger distress. Although clothing that appears "friendly" (nonwhite) helps to ameliorate the baby's distress, by no means does it prevent his crying and avoidance behavior as the examiner approaches him, especially for the first time.

How can health-care workers who are strangers to the child minimize this fear? First, take advantage of his attachment to his mother by relating to the mother first in the presence of the child. During this interaction with his mother, the child is carefully observing her response to and acceptance of the "stranger" and will take cues from her. Even body position is important; turning slightly sideways away from the child to avoid en face contact while talking with the mother is less threatening to the child. Spitz (1946) demonstrated in one of his films that when a stranger approaches with his back to the child, the child becomes curious and will even reach out after a bit and tug at the stranger. Using a soft, low voice rather than a loud or high-pitched tone is more pleasing to the child and facilitates his acceptance of this new person in his life.

Nursing and medicine have made great progress in recognizing and applying development theories in practice. Because a comprehensive listing and discussion of developmental assessment and screening tools is not within the scope of this book, we refer the reader to the many excellent references that discuss child development in detail. In addition, we remind the reader of the use of assessment tools, such as the Bayley Scales of Infant Development, the Denver Development Screening Test, and the Brazelton Neonatal Behavior Assessment Scale.

Immunizations

Immunizations have greatly reduced the incidence of childhood diseases worldwide. Many infections that contributed to high infant mortality in the past can now be prevented through a series of immunizations. Smallpox, for example, has been eliminated and poliomyelitis, rubella, and rubeola have decreased markedly since the rigorous enforcement of a series of immunizations.

Recommendations for immunizations are the same for breastfed children as for non-breastfeeding children. In the United States, the recommended age for beginning primary immunizations of infants is at birth. The usual schedule is for three immunizations for DTaP/Hib or DTP/Hib vaccine (diphtheria, tetanus, pertussis, and *Haemophilus influenzae* type b). DTaP is the preferred vaccine because it produces fewer side effects. A combination product containing measles, mumps, and rubella (MMR) vaccine is administered at 12 to 15 months of age, with a second dose recommended for school-age children. All children should receive four doses of inactivated polio vaccine at 2 months, 4 months, 6 to 18 months, and 4 to 6 years. Oral polio virus can be given only in special circumstances. This is to reduce the risk of vaccine-associated paralytic polio. The United States Recommended Childhood Immunizations Schedule (2003) is available on the Internet at www.cdc.gov/nip/recs/child-schedule.pdf.

The *H. influenzae* type b vaccine has been approved by the Food and Drug Administration for use at 2, 4, and 6 months of age, with a booster at 15 to 18 months of age. Children aged 6 to 12 months are at highest risk of *H. influenzae* type b infection. The exact timing of the immunizations is not nearly as important as the fact that the child eventually receives all of the immunization doses. A relatively new vaccine (Prevnar pneumococcal conjugate vaccine [PCV]) that protects infants and toddlers against pneumococcal disease was approved by the FDA in 2000. The recommendation is for all infants to be given the vaccine at 2, 4, and 6 months of age followed by a booster dose at 12 to 15 months. The rotavirus vaccine that was added to the schedule in 1999 was removed later. The action was in response to studies showing that the vaccine appears to be associated with intussusception. A new vaccine (Pediarix) combines three separate series of shots: one to protect again diphtheria, tetanus, and whooping cough; a second for polio, and a third for hepatitis B. Formerly, it took nine injections to get that much protection.

Infection with hepatitis B is becoming a major public health problem. In 1992, the American Academy of Pediatrics (AAP) recommended universal immunization of newborns in the United States against the HBV. The schedule calls for the initial vaccine to be given to all infants soon after birth; the first dose may also be given by age 2 months if the mother is HbsAg-negative. Only monovalent hepatitis B vaccine can be used for the birth dose. Either monovalent or combination vaccine can be used to complete the series. Infants born to HbsAg-positive mothers should receive the vaccine and hepatitis B immune globulin (HBIG) within 12 hours after birth at separate sites, a second dose of vaccine at 1 to 2 months of age, and a third dose at 6 months. Not everyone agrees with this recommendation, claiming that this decision marks the first time that a vaccine is recommended for children to prevent a disease that primarily occurs in adults. Hepatitis A vaccination is recommended only for selected states (AZ, AK, CA, ID, NV, NM, OK, OR, SD, UT, and WA) and for high-risk groups.

As a result of the vaccine supply shortage, deferral of some doses of tetanus and diphtheria toxoids, and pertussis vaccine and pneumococcal conjugate has been recommended (Centers for Disease Control and Prevention, 2002).

Generally, vaccines that contain attenuated "live" organisms are more effective than are inactivated or "killed" vaccines. Live vaccines induce long-lasting immunity, but they are also likely to cause adverse reactions. Although killed vaccines are noninfectious and can be prepared in a purified form, they usually induce a shorter period of protection; therefore, booster injections may be needed. Most vaccines are given parenterally; an

exception is the live oral polio vaccine (OPV) now given only in special circumstances.

When a measles-mumps-rubella vaccine is given during the immediate postpartum period in the rubella seronegative woman, the live attenuated virus will be found in her breastmilk. This poses no harm to the infant (Wolfe, 1990). Krogh et al. (1989) compared breastfed and formula-fed infants of a group of mothers who had been immunized with the rubella vaccine postpartum with a second group of naturally immune women who were seropositive for rubella and did not receive immunization after childbirth. Subsequent immunization with rubella vaccine of breastfed infants whose mothers had received postpartum immunization resulted in a serum antibody response that was similar to the response observed in formula-fed infants or the infants of naturally immune mothers who had not received immunization. Thus, early neonatal exposure to the rubella virus in breastmilk neither enhances nor suppresses subsequent responses to rubella vaccination in early childhood.

Breastfed infants are also successfully immunized if they are given OPV while receiving breastmilk. The same is true for the oral rotavirus vaccine (Rennels, 1996; World Health Organization, 1995). In fact, breastfeeding may enhance immunity in some cases. Pabst et al. (1989) found that infants who were breastfeeding had enhanced cell-mediated immune response to Bacillus Calmette-Guérin vaccine given at birth. In another study by the same group of investigators, breastfed infants immunized with *H. influenzae* type b vaccine had higher antibody levels at 7 months and at 12 months of age—strong evidence that breastfeeding enhances the active immune response in the first year of life.

Questions about risks of vaccination have been publicly raised by concerned citizens and advocacy groups. In response, Congress created the Vaccine Adverse Event Reporting System (VAERS), a national surveillance system administered by the Food and Drug Administration (FDA) and the Centers for Disease Control (CDC). VAERS maintains a database of reports of adverse events following vaccinations. More information on reporting adverse cases to VAERS can be found on the CDC Web site (www.cdc.gov/).

Vitamin D and Rickets

Vitamin D may constitute an exception to the general rule that breastfed infants do not need vitamin supplements. Recent national recommendations in the United States to prevent rickets and vitamin D deficiency are to give a daily vitamin D supplement to all breastfed infants unless they are weaned to at least 500 ml per day of vitamin D-fortified formula or milk (American Academy of Pediatrics [AAP], 2003). Vitamin D—which is actually a sterol, a compound that behaves like fats—is classified as a lipid. Vitamin D is essential to the development of healthy bones and when deficient can cause rickets (soft, malformed bones) in children. Although rickets is still uncommon, reports of rising numbers of rickets in breastfed children worldwide have triggered an international debate about the need for vitamin D supplementation (Welch et al., 2000).

Increased vitamin D intake results in higher levels in human milk. Women in the United States usually take multivitamins and eat vitamin D dairy foods so rickets and vitamin D deficiency is less a problem than in developing countries and in northern Europe. In studying Wisconsin infants, Greer and Marshall (1989) found that unsupplemented, exclusively breastfed white infants maintained normal vitamin D serum concentrations and had no evidence of vitamin D deficiency.

The risk of rickets is greatest for dark-skinned children living in inner city areas, children whose clothing lowers skin exposure to the sun, and breastfeeding children of women eating vegetarian diets that exclude meat, fish, and dairy products. The child who is adequately exposed to the sun (and thus to radiation-formed precursors of vitamin E) and whose mother consumes adequate nutrients does not need vitamin D supplements. Since the negative effect of sunlight exposure is well known, care providers recommend sunscreen and are reluctant to recommend placing infants in the sun. Giving daily vitamin D supplements in recommended dosages to infants is considered safe and without harmful side effects; however, there is a danger that accidental ingestion of concentrated liquid solutions of pure vitamin D available for pediatric use could cause toxicity. Most physicians in North Carolina already prescribe vitamin D supplements for African-American breastfed infants in their practice (Kreiter et al., 2000).

Dental Health and Orofacial Development

The first primary (deciduous) teeth to erupt are the lower central incisors, which appear at about 6 to 8 months of age. By two and a half years of age, children have a full set of primary teeth that will be replaced by permanent teeth. Although breastfeeding helps to protect the teeth, healthy dental practices should in no way be neglected because the child is breastfeeding.

Nursing-bottle caries is a term applied to progressive dental caries aggravated by sucking on a bottle while sleeping and is associated with a high count of lactobacilli in dental plaque, low socioeconomic status, and nutritional deficiencies (Smith & Moffatt, 1998). In developed countries, the prevalence is reported to vary between 1 and 12 percent (Milnes, 1996). Decay usually starts with the maxillary (upper) incisors and often spares the mandibular (lower) incisors. Several studies suggest that breastfed children have less dental decay than do those who are fed otherwise (Al-Dashti, Williams, & Curzon, 1994; Oulis et al., 1999; Weerheijm et al., 1998). The probable reasons for this include the mechanical differences between breastfeeding and bottle-feeding. Drawn deep into the child's mouth, the human nipple rests at the junction of the hard and soft palate during breastfeeding, posterior to the child's teeth. A suckle is automatically followed by a swallow, thus preventing the teeth from being bathed in pooled milk. In contrast, the milk from a bottle flows out spontaneously with only the slightest pressure into the anterior part of the mouth, permitting stagnation of the milk on and around the teeth.

A few studies have reported a condition similar to nursing-bottle caries that occurred in breastfed children, especially those who breastfed for 2 to 3 years and have spent long, uninterrupted periods at the breast. Although these cases represent a small percentage of young children who breastfeed, nursing caries is associated with the practice of breastfeeding at night "at will" after 6 months of age (Al-Dashti, Williams, & Curzon, 1994; Matee et al., 1994). As the numbers of breastfeeding toddlers increase, however, it is reasonable to expect that some of them will develop dental disease, especially after the introduction of solids that often contain sugar.

A lack of methodological consistency in studies on dental caries in breastfed children makes it difficult to draw conclusions. For example, none of the studies reported the dietary habits of the remainder of the children's diet. If a child ingests a sugar-rich food and then breastfeeds, the lips are pressed against the teeth, thus restricting flow of saliva and facilitating caries development (Bowen et al., 1997). As a result, when Valaitis et al. (2000) reviewed 151 articles on caries and breastfeeding, she was unable to come to a conclusion. Erickson (1999) conducted a unique in vitro study on caries development and human milk. She found that when children's teeth were exposed to human milk as the only carbohydrate source, caries did not occur. When breastmilk was supplemented with 10 percent sucrose, caries development was rapid.

Dental caries is also thought to be an inherited trait; therefore, these children probably represent a group who are more susceptible, and prolonged nocturnal exposure to human milk becomes a risk factor. It could be argued that some breastfed children develop caries not because they were breastfed but in spite of it. The susceptibility of the child's teeth to decay cannot be clinically predicted, and caries may be extensive before they become evident.

Orofacial development is a health issue in which breastfeeding has a measurable impact (Palmer, 1998). The orofacial development of a child is affected by feeding methods, swallowing patterns, and finger sucking (Sanger & Bystrom, 1982). The mechanisms by which bottle-feeding might contribute to the development of malocclusion include a forward thrusting of the tongue, which in turn leads to underdevelopment of the masseter and buccinator muscles (Stanley & Lundeen, 1980), abnormal swallowing patterns, and increased prevalence of nonnutritive sucking. In Czechoslovakia, Adamiak (1981) found that the longer the duration of breastfeeding, the lower the incidence of malocclusion anomalies. Among children breastfed fewer than 3 months or not at all, 36 percent had anomalies, whereas 24 percent of those breastfed for longer than 6 months had anomalies. This trend was constant for all variables tested and remained even when adjusted for age and

maternal educational level as a proxy of socioeconomic status.

Solid Foods

Every breastfed infant reaches a point when breastmilk alone no longer fulfills his nutritional needs. If breastfeeding is continued exclusively, the baby will eventually become malnourished. How long exclusive breastfeeding can satisfy the nutrient needs of babies is a crucial public health issue, especially in areas with an unsafe water supply and poor sanitation, where early supplements are likely to be associated with infections.

Introducing Solid Foods

Solid foods are not necessary, nor are they recommended, before a baby is 4 to 6 months of age (AAP, 1997). Developmental cues for introducing solid foods to the infant are the fading of his tongue-extrusion reflex, eruption of teeth, the ability to sit, and purposeful movement of the baby's hands and fingers, all of which normally occur during the middle months of the first year of life. Most infants will at first actively resist the advances of even the most enterprising parent in attempts to spoon-feed them during the early months of life. Before 6 months of age, a baby has a tongue-extrusion reflex and is unable to push food to the back of his mouth. In the full-term baby, the prenatal storage of iron acquired during the last trimester of pregnancy gradually begins to diminish by 4 to 5 months of age, and external sources of iron are needed (Pisacane et al., 1995).

Early introduction of solids is still a common practice in the United States, even though the American Academy of Pediatrics' Committee on Nutrition has consistently held that no nutritional advantage results from the introduction of supplemental foods prior to 4 to 6 months of age. A study of mothers in Kentucky found that by 1 month of age, 12 percent of mothers reported that their infant had received solid food and cereal added to the bottle. Fruit juices were given to one fifth of the study infants by 1 to 2 months of age (Barton, 2001).

In fact, mothers sometimes competitively seek to outdo one another in initiating solid food, as if how soon an infant eats adult food is a measure of his maturity. Despite official recommendations and a concerted effort to teach parents to delay solids, many infants still receive solid foods during their first few months of life. The first solid food is usually cereal, which is given in the evening because some parents wrongly believe or have been told that feeding solids to the baby will help him sleep through the night. However, feeding infants solids prior to bedtime is not related to evening sleep patterns; according to well-controlled studies, babies who receive solids before bedtime have the same sleep patterns as do babies who are not given solids (Keane et al., 1988; Macknin, Medendorp, & Maier, 1989).

Energy-intake patterns between breastfed and formula-fed infants discussed earlier in this book indicate that breastfed infants maintain energy-intake levels below those of formula-fed infants. These patterns persist even after solid foods are introduced. If breastfeeding infants are given solids at from 3 to 6 months, their milk intakes decline significantly; the energy from solids generally replaces that from breastmilk. Although the infant breastfeeds fewer times during the day, the frequency of night feedings remains the same (Heinig et al., 1993). This is not true for formula-fed infants, who continue to take about the same amount of formula when early solids are given. In industrialized countries, infants fed solids early appear to have about the same incidence of illness as do infants who are fed solids later. In developing countries, however, the risk of diarrhea is such that the risks of introducing solids before 6 months outweighs any potential benefits.

Choosing the Diet

If solids are started after 6 months of age, the sequence of foods is not critical. If solids are introduced earlier, the following order is suggested: cereals, yellow vegetables, fruits, meats, and (last) legumes. For cereal that requires mixing with a liquid, breastmilk (rather than cow's milk) avoids any potential allergic reaction. Egg yolk, if carefully separated from the white (which is highly allergenic), is high in protein and iron, is hypoallergenic, and is therefore safe.

Infants need additional water when solids are started because of their added osmolar load. His-

torically, fruit juice was recommended by pediatricians as a source of vitamin C and water. Because fruit juice tastes sweet, children readily accept it. Although fruit juice has some benefits such as the vitamins and in some cases calcium that it contains, it also has potential detrimental effects (AAP, 2001). Children can become addicted to consuming fruit juices at the expense of eating other foods, especially healthy, fresh foods.

A basic rule is to feed the infant foods in as close to a natural state as possible: pieces of raw, peeled apples, slices of banana, toasted whole wheat bread, orange sections, and a chicken leg with the skin removed are all good choices. They can be picked up and held and are tasty, nutritious, and satisfying to chew. Small amounts at first followed by gradually increased amounts (along with continued breastfeeding), avoids constipation. Mothers should be prepared for changes in consistency, odor, and frequency of stool when solids are begun. Generally, all foods eaten by the family can be given to the infant in a consistency that he can handle. The beginning eater enjoys foods of all kinds and relishes the tactile pleasures of squeezing, smearing, and crushing his food—an activity he should be allowed with impunity because it is also a learning experience. General guidelines for initiating solid foods are found in Table 18–5.

Breastfed babies are exposed to a variety of flavors of whatever is transmitted in their mothers' breastmilk (Mennella, 1995). As a result, it seems likely that they would be more accepting of novel flavors in solid foods than are formula-fed infants who are not so exposed. Likewise, flavors from the mother's diet during pregnancy are transmitted to amniotic fluids and swallowed by the fetus. Consequently, food flavors eaten by women during pregnancy are experienced by infants before their first exposure to solid foods (Mennella, Jagnow, & Beauchamp, 2001). To test this assumption, Sullivan and Birch (1994) compared acceptance of vegetables by 4- to 6-month-old infants. These infants were randomly assigned to be fed one vegetable on ten occasions for 10 days. They found that breastfeeding infants ate more vegetables than did formula-fed infants. Thus breastmilk may facilitate the acceptance of solid foods during the important transition from suckling to feeding solids. Babies who are given cereal were more accepting of it if it is

Table 18–5

INTRODUCING SOLID FOODS INTO A BREASTFED INFANT'S DIET

When to Introduce	Approximate Total Daily Intake of Solids*	Description of Food and Hints About Giving Them
6–7 months if infant is breastfed	*Dry cereal:* Start with 1/2 tsp (dry measurement); gradually increase to 2–3 tb. *Vegetables:* Start with 1 tsp; gradually increase to 2 tb. *Fruit:* Start with 1 tsp; gradually increase to 2 tb. Divide food among 4 feedings per day (if possible).	*Cereal:* Offer iron-enriched baby cereal. Begin with single grains. Mix cereal with an equal amount of breastmilk. *Vegetables:* Try a mild-tasting vegetable first (carrots, squash, peas, green beans). Stronger-flavored vegetables (spinach, sweet potatoes) may be tried after infant accepts some mild-tasting ones. *Fruits:* Mashed ripe banana and unsweetened, cooked, bland fruits (apples, peaches, pears) are usually well-liked. Apple juice and grape juice (unsweetened) may be introduced. Initially, dilute juice with an equal amount of water. Introduce one new food at a time and offer it several times before trying another new food. Give a new food once daily for a day or two; increase to twice daily as the infant begins to enjoy the food. Watch for signs of intolerance. Include some foods that are good sources of vitamin C (other than orange juice).
6–7 months if infant is breastfed	*Meat:* Start with 1 tsp and gradually increase to 2 tb. Divide food among 4 feedings per day (if possible). *Dry cereal:* Gradually increase up to 4 tb. *Fruits and vegetables:* Gradually increase up to 3 tb of each.	*Meat:* Offer pureed or milled poultry (chicken or turkey) followed by lean meat (veal, beef); lamb has a stronger flavor and may not be as well-liked initially. Liver is a good source of iron; it may be accepted at the beginning of a meal with a familiar vegetable. Continue introducing new cereals, fruits, and vegetables as the infant indicates he is ready to accept them, buy always one at a time; introduce legumes last.
7–9 months if infant is breastfed	*Dry cereal:* Up to 1/2 cup. *Fruits and vegetables:* Up to 1/4 to 1/2 cup of each. *Meats:* Up to 3 tb. Divide food among 4 feedings per day (if possible).	Soft table foods may be introduced—for example, mashed potatoes and squash and small pieces of soft, peeled fruits. Toasted whole grain or enriched bread may be added when the infant begins chewing. If introduction of solids is delayed until now, it is not necessary to use strained fruits and vegetables.
8–12 months if infant is breastfed	*Dry cereal:* Up to 1/2 cup. *Bread:* About 1 slice. *Fruits and vegetables:* Up to 1/2 cup of each. Divide food among 4 feedings per day (if possible).	Continue using *iron-fortified* baby cereals. Table foods cut into small pieces may be added gradually. Start with foods that do not require too much chewing (cooked, cut green beans and carrots, noodles, ground meats, tuna fish, soft cheese, plain yogurt). If fish is offered, check closely to be sure there are no bones in the serving. Mashed, cooked egg yolk and orange juice may be added at about 9 months of age. Sometimes offer peanut butter or thoroughly cooked dried peas and beans in place of meat.

Some infants do not need or want these amounts of food; some may need a little more food.

mixed with mother's milk rather than water (Mennella & Beauchamp, 1997). And, in situations in which families are unable to provide high-quality solids, continued breastfeeding beyond 1 year of age is recommended to enhance linear growth in toddlers (Marquis et al., 1997).

Foods prepared at home are not only more wholesome and nutritious but cost less than do commercially prepared baby foods. Carrots and applesauce, for example, cost about one half the store price when prepared at home, and blended beef or chicken provide more nutrients by weight than do their commercial counterparts, chiefly because they contain less water. With the aid of an electric blender, food mill, or grinder, preparing baby food is easily accomplished. The foods should be selected from high-quality fresh or frozen fruits, vegetables, or meats, with special attention to hygienic preparation and storage. For convenience, small individualized portions can be stored safely in the refrigerator or freezer for reasonable periods. A list of foods that can be quickly and easily prepared appears in Box 18–2. Fun finger foods are listed in Box 18–3.

Some parents prefer to buy commercial baby food rather than to make their own. In addition to being expensive, commercial baby foods are generally produced by pulverizing fruit, grain, vegetable, and meat ingredients with water and adding filler ingredients such as colorings, additives, and preservatives (Randle, 1999).

For families on vegan diets, their infants may need supplements of vitamin B_{12} when dairy products and eggs are excluded from the diet. Older infants may need zinc supplements and reliable sources of iron and vitamin D as well as vitamin B_{12}. Timing of solid-food introduction is similar to that recommended for nonvegetarians. Tofu, dried beans, and meat analogs are introduced as protein sources around the middle of the first year (Mangels & Messina, 2001).

Choosing Feeding Location

The best place to feed a baby is at the family table at mealtime, in a high chair or on someone's knee. Young children love to be considered one of the family and to sit at the same height as the rest of the family. Even before the infant is ready to take solids, he enjoys being nearby during meals and

---

> **BOX 18-2**
>
> ## Quick, Easy-to-Prepare Infant Foods
>
> - Yogurt (low-fat)
> - Fresh fruit: cut-up apples, pears, oranges, bananas, grapes, or any fruit in season
> - Cheese, cut into chewable pieces
> - Toast of whole grain bread, cut into strips
> - Chicken: leg, wing, or cut-up pieces
> - Egg: soft-boiled; hard-boiled as finger food
> - Vegetables: mashed; whole (e.g. peas); in strips or pieces as finger food
> - Crackers: whole grain; cheese spread
> - Custard
> - Cottage cheese
> - Dried fruit: apples, dates, figs, prunes (pitted)
> - Liver: sauteed and cut into strips
> - Tuna: drained; with grated cheese

---

can "join in" by chewing on such food as a bread crust or a carrot.

Delaying Solid Foods

Babies who are started on solid food early (before 5 to 6 months) and who have a family history of allergy are more likely to develop atopic disease (allergic asthma, allergic rhinitis, atopic dermatitis, food allergy). Delaying solids, especially wheat, egg whites, pork, and legumes, from the potentially allergic child until the immature immunity period has passed, minimizes or even prevents the symptoms

---

BOX 18–3

Fun Finger Foods

- Pieces of ripe avocado
- Pieces of steamed apple or pear
- Dried fruit soaked in water to make it softer
- Pieces of baked or boiled white or sweet potato
- Pieces of baked or steamed squash
- Well-cooked beans
- Soft tofu cubes

Source: From Lair (1998).

(Arshad, 2001). At age 6 months, the infant produces sufficient IgA antibody to prevent absorption of food antigens through the intestinal wall, thus reducing food allergy.

IgE, which is associated with allergy, rises in direct time sequence to the introduction of solid foods. IgE is also associated with allergy verified by a positive skin test later in life. Before the age of 6 months, the infant's intestine lacks the necessary digestive enzymes to completely digest complex proteins and starches down to amino acids and simple sugars. At the same time, the infant's intestinal mucosa is permeable to some intact proteins and starches. These incompletely digested peptides and starches can be absorbed and serve as sensitizing agents to the infant's immune system. IgE is then produced and allergy results in some (perhaps many) infants.

Obesity

Childhood obesity is a growing problem throughout the world. Thirteen percent of young children in the United States are obese. Children are driven to school, and when they come home they watch television many hours each day. Children of obese parents are more likely to be overweight themselves (Hediger et al., 2001; Maffeis, 1999). In addition to lack of exercise and genetic endowment, early diet plays a role in obesity. Breastfed infants regulate their food intake according to their caloric needs and, at the same time, control their mother's milk production. In contrast, the satiated bottle-fed baby is encouraged to empty the bottle and may not ever develop control over food intake. Are breastfeeding children then less likely to become obese? It depends on who is asked and the culture where a study takes place.

Dewey (2003) and Butte (2001) extensively reviewed breastfeeding and childhood obesity studies worldwide. Dewey concluded that breastfeeding reduces the risk of a child becoming overweight to a moderate extent. Butte found the association to be insignificant. Many large studies have shown that breastfed babies are less likely than bottle-fed infants to become obese (Armstrong & Reilly, 2002; Bergmann et al., 2003; Gillman et al., 2001; Kramer 1981; Toschke et al., 2002; von Kries et al., 1999). In the Bergmann et al. and Kramer studies, the findings were robust and could not be accounted for by confounding variables. Other research showed no such relationship between breastfeeding and later obesity (Baranowski et al., 1992; Li, Parsons, & Power, 2003), and one even found that breastfed children were more likely to become fat (Agras et al., 1990).

The literature is contradictory in part because many studies are based on small sample sizes, missing data, lack of adequate control for confounding factors (e.g., the mother's nutritional awareness, exercise patterns), and methodological problems (e.g., operational definitions of obesity, the distinction between a "breastfed" infant versus a "bottle-fed" infant, and the timing of feedings). Moreover, differences in exercise patterns of children were not included in studies as a confounding factor. Breastfeeding, along with genetic, racial, socioeconomic, and behavioral factors, affects later obesity. Policymakers and clinicians cannot ignore the growing body of evidence that breastfeeding lowers the risk of becoming overweight later in life (Gillman, 2002).

Co-Sleeping

Mothers who breastfeed are also likely to co-sleep with their babies. The closeness and convenience of having the baby nearby during the night facilitates both breastfeeding and the mother's sleep. Babies who sleep in their parent's bed breastfeed more frequently (Ball, 2003; Pollard et al., 1999). Yet, co-sleeping is an emotionally charged subject that is debated heatedly in the United States. It evokes strong feelings in supporters and opponents because it touches basic philosophies about parenting: mainly pitting the child-guided philosophy against parents who believe in strict discipline and scheduling from an early age.

Historically, parents have slept with their infants until recent times but concerns about suffocation and sudden infant death syndrome (SIDS) have led the US Consumer Product Safety Commission and the AAP (1999) to recommend against allowing children younger than 2 years of age to sleep in a bed with adults. Concerned parents reacted immediately to this widely publicized warning. Grossman (2000) reviewed the studies that the consumer commission used in making their recommendation. He pointed out several troubling errors, among them that of the 38 deaths investigated, the specific cause of death was misclassified in 18 cases.

Parents across the globe take co-sleeping for granted. In Japan, for example, most infants and toddlers co-sleep and have adult company and body contact as they fall asleep (Latz, Wolf, & Lozoff, 1999). Despite the warning by the AAP against co-sleeping, the practice is growing in the United States. The practice seems to be widespread as more parents let their infants sleep with them. The percentage of infants who sleep in a bed with parents or a caregiver more than doubled from 1993 to 2000 (Willinger et al., 2003).

James McKenna, an anthropology professor and expert on the subject of co-sleeping, believes that the practice can be a positive experience and not considered dangerous if the following precautions are taken (McKenna, Mosko, & Richard, 2000):

- Bedding should be tight fitting to the mattress. Use only light blankets—never a duvet, quilt, or comforter that could cover a baby's nose.

- The mattress should be firm. Never sleep with a baby on a sofa or a water bed.

- Remove all loose pillows or soft blankets near the baby's face.

- Make sure there is no space between the bed and headboard or adjoining wall because a baby's small head could slip between them. Cram any spaces and crevices with towels and check them nightly.

- Do not place the baby on his stomach.

- Do not allow an adult who smokes or has taken alcohol or drugs to bed-share with the baby.

Long-Term Breastfeeding

Long-term breastfeeding is considered "comfort nursing"—a form of nurturance and a special bonding rather than nourishment. Nutritional benefits are considered secondary. The conceptual difference is that breastfeeding is considered as a "process" rather than a "product" (Van Esterik, 1985). Do older breastfeeding children receive sufficient nutriment to grow? Nutrition in long-term breastfeeders in the United States appeared to be adequate in one study. When daily food intake of these children was measured, their nonbreast intake of complementary foods met RDA energy requirements (Buckley, 2001).

Weaning

In the United States, weaning usually takes place during the first year of life. Women who breastfeed longer than this have difficulty with acceptance by relatives, peers, and health professionals (Page-Goertz, 2002). If "baby-led weaning" is practiced, weaning usually takes place between the child's second and fourth birthdays (Sugarman & Kendall-Tackett, 1995). To counteract social pressures for early weaning, women with breastfeeding toddlers find peer support for each other, sometimes changing their circle of friends.

In a study by Wrigley and Hutchinson (1990) of 12 mothers who practiced long-term breastfeeding, one mother reported that her obstetrician told her anyone who breastfed an infant past 6 months of age was "perverted." Another said that her father thought she was "strange." Many health-care workers, who wholeheartedly support breastfeeding and would never advocate taking a security blanket away from a baby reel in horror when a mother breastfeeds a walking child. Page-Goertz (2002) advises "To avoid embarrassing moments at the mall due to the toddler's increasing language skills, parents may want to teach their child a code word for breastfeeding. Examples are "pillow" and "nums" This can prevent a child from yelling 'BOOBY mom—now!' "

Ideally, the time for weaning is a joint decision in which both the mother and the baby reach a state of readiness to begin weaning around the same time; however, this is not always the case. The child may be ready before his mother; more often, the mother is ready before her child. In a unique study of weaning times of 36 primates, anthropologist Dettwyler (1995) determined what would be a natural duration of breastfeeding in modern humans. Her evidence suggests that two and one half years is the minimum duration of time for breastfeeding. And that four or five years, or longer, is within the normal range for humans.

Sometimes, the decision is made to wean quickly. Although the literature offers considerable advice about gradual weaning, there is little information for the anxious mother in a situation in which weaning must be rapid and will necessarily be traumatic. The following nondrug therapies may make deliberate weaning easier and at the same time avert plugged ducts or mastitis:

- Shower and allow the warm water to run over the breasts, or soak the breasts by lying down in the tub.
- Use a breast pump or manual expression to relieve breast fullness.
- Wear a supportive, comfortable bra.
- Observe for signs of plugged ducts or a breast infection.
- Expect to feel very emotional during this time and seek support from people who will listen sympathetically.
- Give the baby extra cuddling and holding.

It may take several days before the mother finds it is no longer necessary to express breastmilk for comfort. As described earlier in this book, an Australian method for reducing engorged breasts is to wear cool raw cabbage leaves in the bra. Doing so has been reported to quickly relieve engorgement.

Implications for Practice

Care providers assume responsibility for educating families in optimal infant-feeding practices and for providing rationale and support when they are needed. The introduction of foods other than breastmilk is culturally influenced and common worldwide. Some mothers encourage their babies to eat as much as possible, believing that a plump baby represents the picture of health. Competition among mothers can also lead to the early introduction of baby foods. Mothers who feel pressure to give their babies solids may misinterpret the baby's cries as hunger, when the baby merely needs stimulation by holding and interacting. Education is a powerful tool for teaching healthy food practices. To counteract early solid food introduction, a videotape was incorporated into an adolescent mothers' home-visiting program. This simple intervention significantly reduced the practice of adolescent mothers giving early solids (Black et al., 2001). Several important points should be shared with new parents:

- Continue frequent breastfeedings with lots of cuddling and holding.
- Crying is not always a sign of hunger. It can mean that the infant has nonfood needs—for example, to be held, rocked, and soothed.
- Delay the introduction of solid foods until around the middle of the first year of life when the baby indicates that he is ready for them.
- Prepare foods for the infant in as close as possible to a natural state.
- Have easy-to-prepare foods available for quick meals for the infant.
- Bring the baby to the family meal table whenever possible.

It is not unusual for children, usually from about 2 years of age, to become very fussy about food and to refuse to eat certain items; they may especially dislike vegetables. Children will go through periods of eating very little for a period from as short as a week to as long as a few months; then they gradually start eating more again. The mother should be reassured that "this too shall pass" and that her child will start eating again. Meanwhile, she should make the food he does like easily available and neither force the child to eat nor mask his natural appetite by offering sugary foods.

Choices about weaning should be based on the mother's own wishes rather than on the expectations of others and should call for active listening to her feelings. If the mother enjoys breastfeeding but feels pressure to wean, pointing out the advantages of continued breastfeeding and the cultural differences in weaning practices may be all the reinforcement she needs. On the other hand, if she expresses resentment each time her baby breastfeeds and is impatient for each feeding to end, she is entitled to know options for safe and comfortable weaning techniques. Some women report that after weaning their baby, they experienced improvement in mood, and sexuality and felt less fatigue (Forster et al., 1994).

Summary

Imperative to assisting a breastfeeding family is recognition and knowledge of a wide array of areas of child health. Taking the holistic view, breastfeeding is but one aspect of the child's overall health and welfare. This chapter has offered readers basic information derived from research findings and clinical experiences. Teaching parents and incorporating research findings into the daily lives of families are the linchpins of effective practice.

Key Concepts

- Worldwide studies indicate that breastfed infants are more likely to have higher intellectual ability and cognitive development compared with those who were not breastfed.

- Universal child growth patterns include cephalocaudal and proximodistal growth.

- Generally, both breastfed and bottle-fed infants double their birth weight by the middle of the first year of life and triple it by 1 year. Breastfeeding infants weigh slightly more than their formula-fed counterparts for the first 3 to 4 months.

- The infant's brain grows rapidly during infancy.

- Neonates are born with well-developed sensory abilities of hearing, smell, and taste. Visual preference is for human faces and moving objects.

- Theories about early developmental stages include (1) trust versus mistrust and autonomy versus shame and doubt (Erickson), and (2) sensorimotor, assimilation, and accommodation (Piaget).

- Breastfed infants tend to be more wakeful, cry more often during the late afternoon, and evening and wake more frequently during the night.

- Attachment and bonding is a series of physical contact and sensory interactions between mother and baby as "mutual caregivers."

- Stranger distress and separation anxiety, which occur during the second year of life, is a normal phenomenon where the child fears strangers and being apart from his primary caretaker.

- Developmentally speaking, the ability to tolerate solids offers no evidence that their early introduction is advantageous. In fact, the practice may initiate a chain of disadvantages that include allergies and obesity.

- Recommendations for immunizations are usually the same for breastfed children as for non-breastfeeding children.

- The rise in cases of rickets in breastfed infants has led to a debate about the need for vitamin D supplementation of infants at risk.

- Breastfeeding infants generally have fewer dental caries. Reported cases of dental caries are usually associated with nighttime feedings, genetic predisposition, and dietary sugar.

- Solids foods are not necessary before 4 to 6 months of age. Developmental cues for introducing solid foods are fading of the child's tongue-extrusion reflex, the eruption of teeth, the ability to sit, and purposeful movement of the baby's hands and fingers, all of which normally occur during the middle months of the first year of life. Full-term babies have storage of iron that begins to diminish by 4 to 5 months of age.

- Total solid food elimination for the first 6 months of life, in addition to exclusive breast-milk feeding, appears to reduce atopic disease in children who are at hereditary risk. The protective effect against eczema afforded by solid-food postponement lasts up to 1 year of age.

- Breastfeeding appears to have a slight protective effect against later obesity, but it appears to be weaker than genetic, racial, socioeconomic, and behavioral factors.

- Co-sleeping facilitates breastfeeding. Safe co-sleeping includes bedding that fits tightly to the mattress, no soft pillows or space between the bed and the wall, and placing the baby on his back or side.

- Ideally weaning takes place when both the mother and baby reach a state of readiness around the same time. Crossculturally, weaning takes place around two and one half years of age.

Internet Resources

Brian Palmer's Web site, focusing on child health topics: sleep apnea, SIDS, dental caries: www.brianpalmerdds.com/

Centers for Disease Control: www.cdc.gov/

The decade's progress on exclusive breastfeeding in 44 developing countries, 1989–1999: www.childinfo.org/eddb/brfeed/probl3/htm

Information about co-sleeping and Jim McKenna's mother and baby behavioral sleep laboratory at the University of Notre Dame: www.nd.edu/~alfac/mckenna

Information and statistical data for professionals and researchers. Brochures and pamphlets for family and community members: www.unicef.org

UNICEF Breastfeeding and Complementary Feeding: www.childinfo.org/eddb/brfeed/test/database.htm

References

Adamiak E. Occlusion anomalies in preschool children in rural areas in relation to certain individual features. *Czas Stomat* 34:551–55, 1981.

Agras WS et al. Influence of early feeding style on adiposity at 6 years of age. *J Pediatr* 116:805–11, 1990.

Ainsworth MDS et al. *Patterns of attachment.* Hillsdale, NJ: Lawrence Erlbaum, 1978.

Al-Dashti AA, Williams SA, Curzon MEJ. Breast feeding, bottle feeding and dental caries in Kuwait, a country with low-fluoride levels in the water supply. *Commun Dental Health* 12:42–47, 1994.

Als H, Brazelton TB. A new model of assessing the behavioral organization in preterm and full-term infants. *J Am Acad Child Psychol* 20:239, 1981.

American Academy of Pediatrics (AAP). Work Group on Breastfeeding. Breastfeeding and the use of human milk. *Pediatrics* 100:1035–39, 1997.

———. The use and misuse of fruit juice in pediatrics. *Pediatrics* 107:1210–13, 2001.

———. Prevention of rickets and vitamin D deficiency: new guidelines for vitamin D intake. *Pediatrics* 111:908, 2003.

Anderson GC. The mother and her newborn: mutual caregivers. *JOGN Nurs* 6:50–55, 1977.

———. Enhancing reciprocity between mother and neonate. *Nurs Res* 30:89–93, 1981.

Anderson GC, Dombrowski MA, Swinth JY. Kangaroo Care: not just for stable preemies anymore. *Reflect Nurs Leadersh* 27:32–34, 2001.

Anderson GC et al. Early skin-to-skin contact for mothers and their healthy newborn infants. (Cochrane Review). In: *The Cochrane Library, Oxford: Update Software,* Issue 2, 2003a.

Anderson GC et al. Mother-newborn contact in a randomized trial of Kangaroo (skin-to-skin) Care. *JOGN Nurs* 32:604–11, 2003b.

Anderson GC et al. Skin-to-skin for breastfeeding difficulties postbirth. In: Field T, ed. *Advances in touch.* New Brunswick, NJ: Johnson & Johnson, 2003c.

Armstrong J, Reilly JJ. Breastfeeding and lowering the risk of childhood obesity. *Lancet* 359:2003–4, 2002.

Arshad SH. Food allergen avoidance in primary prevention of food allergy. *Allergy* 56(suppl 67):113–16, 2001.

Ball HL. Breastfeeding, bed-sharing, and infant sleep. *Birth* 30:181–88, 2003.

Baranowski T et al. Height, infant-feeding practices and cardiovascular functioning among 3 or 4 year old children in three ethnic groups. *J Clin Epidemiol* 45:513–18, 1992.

Barton SJ. Infant feeding practices of low-income rural mothers. *MCN* 26:93–98, 2001.

Bergmann KE et al. Early determinants of childhood overweight and adiposity in a birth cohort study: role of breastfeeding. *Int J Obesity* 27:162–72, 2003.

Birch EE et al. A randomized controlled trial of early dietary supply of long-chain polyunsaturated fatty acids and mental development in term infants. *Dev Med Child Neurol* 41:174–81, 2000.

Black MM et al. Home and videotape intervention delays early complementary feeding among adolescent mothers. *Pediatrics* 107:E678, 2001.

Bowen WH et al. Assessing the carcinogenic potential of some infant formulas, milk and sugar solution. *JADA* 128:865–71, 1997.

Bowlby J. The nature of the child's tie to his mother. *Int J Psychoanalysis* 39:350–72, 1958.

———. *Attachment and loss: separation.* Vol 2. New York: Basic Books, 1973.

Buckley KM. Long-term breastfeeding: nourishment or nurturance? *J Hum Lact* 17:304–12, 2001.

Bu'Loc F, Woolridge MW, Baum JD. Development of coordination of sucking, swallowing and breathing: ultrasound study of term and preterm infants. *Dev Med Child Neurol* 32:669–78, 1990.

Butte NF. The role of breastfeeding in obesity. In: Schanler R, ed. Breastfeeding 2000, Part 1. *Pediatr Clinics No Amer* 48:189–98, 2001.

Butte NF et al. Energy utilization of breast-fed and formula-fed infants. *Am J Clin Nutr* 51:350–58, 1990.

———. Influence of early feeding mode on body composition of infants. *Bio Neonate* 67:414–24, 1995.

Carey WB, McDevitt SC. Revision of the Infant Temperament Questionnaire. *Pediatrics* 61:735–39, 1978.

Centers for Disease Control and Prevention (CDC). Recommended childhood immunization schedule—United States, 2002. *MMWR* 287(6):70–78, 2002.

Condon WS, Sander LW. Neonate movement is synchronized with adult speech: interaction participation and language acquisition. *Science* 183:99, 1974.

Dettwyler KA. A time to wean. In: Stuart-Macadam P, Dettwyler KA, eds. *Breastfeeding: biocultural perspectives.* New York: Aldine de Gruyter, 1995:39–73.

Dewey KG. Is breastfeeding protective against child obesity? *J Hum Lact* 19:9–18, 2003.

Elias F et al. Sleep/wake patterns of breast-fed infants in the first 2 years of life. *Pediatrics* 77:322–29, 1986.

Engler AJ et al. Kangaroo Care: national survey of practice, knowledge, barriers and perceptions. *MCN* 27:146–52, 2002.

Epstein K. The interactions between breastfeeding mothers and their babies during the breastfeeding session. *Early Child Dev Care* 87:93–104, 1993.

Erikson EH. *Childhood and society.* 2nd ed. New York: Norton, 1963.

———. *Identity, youth and crisis.* New York: Norton, 1968.

Erickson PR. Investigation of the role of human breastmilk in caries development. *Pediatr Denistry* 21:86–90, 1999.

Farquharson J et al. Infant cerebral cortex phospholipid fatty-acid composition and diet. *Lancet* 340:810–13, 1992.

Feldman R et al. The nature of the mother's tie to her infant: maternal bonding under conditions of proximity, separation, and potential loss. *J Child Psychol Psychiat* 40:929–39, 1999.

Floury CV, Leech AM, Blackhall A. Infant feeding and mental and motor development at 18 months of age in first-born singletons. *Int J Epidemiol* 24(3)(suppl 1):S21–26, 1995.

Forster et al. Psychological and sexual changes after the cessation of breast-feeding. *Obstet Gynecol* 84:872–76, 1994.

Gill NE et al. Effect of nonnutritive sucking on behavioral state in preterm infants before feeding. *Nurs Res* 37:347–50, 1988.

Gillman MW. Breast-feeding and obesity [editorial]. *J Pediatr* 141:749–50, 2002.

Gillman MW et al. Risk of overweight among adolescents who were breastfed as infants. *JAMA* 285:2453–60, 2001.

Greer FR, Marshall S. Bone mineral content, serum vitamin D metabolite concentrations and ultraviolet-B exposure in human milk-fed infants with and without vitamin D_2 supplements. *J Pediatr* 114:204–12, 1989.

Grossman ER. Less than meets the eye: the consumer product safety commission's campaign against bed-sharing with babies. *Birth* 27:277–80, 2000.

Harlow HF, Harlow M. The affectional systems. In: Schrier A, Harlow H, Stollnitz F, eds. *Behavior of nonhuman primates.* Vol. 2. New York: Academic, 1965.

Hedberg-Nyqvist K, Ewald U. Successful breast feeding in spite of early mother-baby separation for neonatal care. *Midwifery* 13:24–31, 1997.

Hediger ML et al. Association between infant breastfeeding and overweight in young children. *JAMA* 285:2453–60, 2001.

Hegvik R, McDevitt SC, Carey W. The Middle Childhood Temperament Questionnaire. *J Dev Behav Pediatr* 3:197–200, 1982.

Heinig MJ et al. Intake and growth of breast-fed and formula-fed infants in relation to the timing of introduction of complementary foods: the DARLING study. *Acta Paediatr* 82:999–1006, 1993.

Horwood LJ, Fergusson DM. Breastfeeding and later cognitive and academic outcomes. *Pediatrics* 101:1621, 1998.

Hurst N, Valentine CK, Renfro L. Skin-to-skin holding in the neonatal intensive care unit influences maternal milk volume. *J Perinatol* 27:213–17, 1997.

Jain A, Concato J, Leventhal JM. How good is the evidence linking breastfeeding and intelligence? *Pediatrics* 109:1044–53, 2002.

Johnson DL et al. Breast feeding and children's intelligence. *Psychol Rep* 79:1179–85, 1996.

Keane V et al. Do solids help baby sleep through the night? *Am J Dis Child* 142:404–5, 1988.

Klaus MH, Kennell JH. *Maternal-infant bonding: the impact of early separation and loss on family development.* St Louis: Mosby, 1975.

Kramer MS. Do breast-feeding and delayed introduction of solid foods protect against subsequent obesity? *J Pediatr* 98:883–87, 1981.

Kreiter SR et al. Nutritional rickets in African American breast-fed infants. *J Pediatr* 137:153–57, 2000.

Krogh V et al. Postpartum immunization with rubella virus vaccine and antibody response in breast-feeding infants. *J Lab Clin Med* 113:695–99, 1989.

Lair C. *Feeding the whole family.* Schaumburg, IL: La Leche League International, 1998.

Lanting CI et al. Neurological differences between 9-year-old children fed breast-milk or formula-milk as babies. *Lancet* 344:1319–22, 1994.

Latz S, Wolf AW, Lozoff B. Cosleeping in context. *Arch Pediatr Adolesc Med* 153:339–46, 1999.

Li L, Parsons TJ, Power C. Breastfeeding and obesity in childhood: cross sectional study. *BMJ* 327:904–5, 2003.

Lorenz KZ. The companion in the environment of the bird. *J Ornithol* 83:137–215, 289–413, 1935.

Lucas A et al. Breastmilk and subsequent intelligence quotient in children born preterm. *Lancet* 339:261–64, 1992.

Ludington-Hoe S, Swinth JY. Developmental aspects of Kangaroo Care. *JOGN Nurs* 25:692–703, 1996.

Ludington-Hoe S et al. Kangaroo Care compared to incubators in maintaining body warmth in preterm infants. *Biol Res Nurs* 260–73, 2000.

Macknin ML, Medendorp SV, Maier MC. Infant sleep and bedtime cereal. *Am J Dis Child* 143:1066–68, 1989.

Maffeis C. Childhood obesity: the genetic—environmental interface. *Endocrinol Metab* 13:31, 1999.

Makin JW, Porter RH. Attractiveness of lactating females' breast odors to neonates. *Child Devel* 60:803–10, 1989.

Mangels AR, Messina BV. Considerations in planning vegan diets: infants. *J Am Diet Assoic* 101:670–77, 2001.

Marquis GS et al. Breastmilk or animal-products foods improve linear growth of Peruvian toddlers consuming marginal diets. *Am J Clin Nutr* 66:1102–9, 1997.

Matee MIN et al. Nursing caries, linear hypoplasia, and nursing and weaning habits in Tanzanian infants. *Commun Dent Oral Epidemiol* 22:289–93, 1994.

McKenna J, Mosko S, Richard C. Bedsharing promotes breastfeeding. *Pediatrics* 100:214–19, 1997.

Mennella JA. Mothers' milk: a medium for early flavor experiences. *J Hum Lact* 11:39–45, 1995.

Mennella JA, Beauchamp GK. Mothers' milk enhances the acceptance of cereal during weaning. *Pediatr Res* 41:188–92, 1997.

Mennella JA, Jagnow CP, Beauchamp GK. Prenatal and postnatal flavor learning by human infants. *Pediatrics* 107:E88, 2001.

Mercer R. A theoretical framework for studying factors that impact on the maternal role. *Nurs Res* 30:73–77, 1981.

Milnes AR. Description and epidemiology of nursing caries. *J Public Dent* 56:38–50, 1996.

Morley R et al. Mother's choice to provide breastmilk and developmental outcome. *Arch Dis Child* 63:1382–85, 1988.

Mortensen EL et al. The association between duration of breastfeeding and adult intelligence. *JAMA* 287:2365–71, 2002.

Mosko S et al. Infant sleep architecture during bedsharing and possible implications for SIDS. *Sleep* 19:677–84, 1996.

———. Infant arousals in the bedsharing environment: implications for infant sleep development and SIDS. *Pediatrics* 100:841–49, 1997.

Oulis CJ et al. Feeding practices of Greek children with and without nursing caries. *Pediatr Dent* 21:409–16, 1999.

Pabst HF et al. Effect of breast-feeding on immune response to BCG vaccination. *Lancet* 1(11):295–96, 1989.

Page-Goertz S. Breastfeeding beyond 6 months. *Advance Nurs Pract* (February):45–48, 2002.

Palmer B. The influence of breastfeeding on the development of the oral cavity: a commentary. *J Hum Lact* 14:93–98, 1998.

Piaget J. *The origins of intelligence in children.* Cook M, trans. New York: International Universities Press, 1952.

Piaget J, Inhelder B. *Psychology of the child.* New York: Basic Books, 1969.

Pisacane A et al. Iron status in breast-fed infants. *J Pediatr* 127:429–31, 1995.

Pollard K et al. Night-time non-nutritive sucking in infants aged 1 to 5 months: Relationship with infant stage, breastfeeding, and bed-sharing versus room-sharing. *Early Hum Dev* 56:185–204, 1999.

Prechtl J, Beintema D. *The neurological examination of the full term infant* (Child Development Medical Series, 12). Philadelphia: Lippincott, 1975.

Pridham KF, Chang AS. Transition to being the mother of a new infant in the first 3 months: maternal problem solving and self-appraisals. *J Adv Nurs* 17:204–16, 1992.

Prodromidis M et al. Mothers touching newborns: a comparison of rooming-in versus minimal contact. *Birth* 22:196–2000, 1995.

Randle J. Starting solids. *New Beginnings*, La Leche League International, May-June, 1999.

Rao MR et al. Effect of breastfeeding on cognitive development of infants born small for gestational age. *Acta Paediatr* 91:267–74, 2002.

Rennels MB. Influence of breast-feeding and oral poliovirus vaccine on the immunogenicity and efficacy of rotavirus vaccine. *J Infectious Dis* 174(suppl 1):S107–11, 1996.

Richards M, Hardy R, Wadsworth ME. Long-term effects of a breast-feeding in a national birth cohort: educational attainment and midlife cognitive function. *Public Health Nutr* 5:631–35, 2002.

Robertson J. *Young children in hospital.* New York: Basic Books, 1958.

Rogan WJ, Gladen BC. Breast-feeding and cognitive development. *Early Hum Dev* 31:181–93, 1993.

Rubin R. Attainment of the maternal role. *Nurs Res* 16:237, 342, 1967.

Sanger R, Bystrom E. Breastfeeding: does it affect oral facial growth? *Dent Hygiene* 56:44–47, 1982.

Sears W. *Growing together.* Franklin Park, IL: La Leche League International, 1987:30, 71.

Servonsky J, Opas SR. *Nursing management of children.* Boston: Jones and Bartlett, 1987.

Smith PJ, Moffat ME. Baby-bottle decay: Are we on the right track? *Int J Circumpolar Health* 57(suppl 1):155–62, 1998.

Spitz R. Anaclitic depression. *Psychoanal Study Child* 2:313–42, 1946.

Stanley E, Lundeen D. Tongue thrust in breast-fed and bottle-fed school children: a cross-cultural investigation. *Int J Oral Myol* 6:6–16, 1980.

Sugarman J, Kendall-Tackett KA. Weaning ages in a sample of American women who practice extended breastfeeding. *Clin Pediatr* 34:642–47, 1995.

Sullivan SA, Birch LL. Infant dietary experience and acceptance of solid foods. *Pediatrics* 93:271–77, 1994.

Tarkka MT. Predictors of maternal competence by first-time mothers when the child is 8 months old. *J Adv Nurs* 41:233–40, 2003.

Temboury MC et al. Influence of breast-feeding on the infant's intellectual development. *J Pediatr Gastroenterol Nutr* 18:32–36, 1994.

Thomas A, Chess S. *Temperament and development.* New York: Brunner/Mazel, 1977.

Toschke AM et al. Overweight and obesity in 6- to 14-year-old Czech children in 1991: protective effect of breast-feeding. *J Pediatr* 141:764–69, 2002.

Valaitis R et al. A systematic review of the relationships between breastfeeding and early childhood caries. *Canadian J Public Health* 91:411–17, 2000.

Van Esterick P. Commentary: an anthropological perspective on infant feeding in Oceania. In: Marshall LB, ed. *Infant care and feeding in the South Pacific.* New York: Gordon & Breach Science Publishers, 1985:331–43.

von Kries R et al. Breast feeding and obesity: cross sectional study. *BMJ* 319:147, 1999.

Wang B et al. Sialic acid concentration of brain gangliosides: Variation among eight mammalian species. *Comp Biochem Physio* 119:435–39, 1998.

Weerheijm KL et al. Prolonged demand breast-feeding and nursing caries. *Caries Res* 32:46–50, 1998.

Welch TR et al. Vitamin D-deficient rickets: the reemergence of a once-conquered disease [editorial]. *J Pediatr* 137:143–45, 2000.

Wigg NR et al. Does breastfeeding at six months predict cognitive development? *Aust N Z J Public Health* 22:232–36, 1998.

Willinger M et al. Trends in infant bed sharing in the United States, 1993–2000: The National Infant Sleep Study. *Arch Pediatr Adolesc Med* 157:43–48, 2003.

Wolfe MS. Vaccine for foreign travel. *Pediatr Clin North Am* 37:757–69, 1990.

World Health Organization. Collaborative Study Group on Oral Poliovirus Vaccine: factors affecting the immunogenicity of oral poliovirus vaccines: a prospective evaluation in Brazil and the Gambia. *J Infect Dis* 171:1097–1106, 1995.

Wrigley EA, Hutchinson SA. Long-term breastfeeding: the secret bond. *J Nurse Midwifery* 35:35–41, 1990.

Yoneyama K, Nagata H, Asano H. Growth of Japanese breast-fed and bottle-fed infants from birth to 20 months. *Ann Hum Biol* 21:597–608, 1994.

THE ILL CHILD: BREASTFEEDING IMPLICATIONS

Sallie Page–Goertz and Jan Riordan

When a child becomes ill, or when a baby is born with problems that cause breastfeeding to be very difficult, the treasured breastfeeding relationship is threatened. Nurses and other health-care providers who are aware of the effect of a child's illness or health condition on breastfeeding and lactation can help to prevent unnecessary weaning. For ill or hospitalized children who have already established breastfeeding, the breastfeeding relationship helps normalize the routine during unfamiliar circumstances, and it provides important comfort and security for the baby. Breastfeeding is much more than nutrition—it is comfort and love shared between a mother and her baby. When an illness or other health problem makes the breastfeeding relationship difficult or impossible, emotional support and encouragement are needed for the family. This chapter presents strategies for helping parents of breastfeeding children who need special health care.

Team Care for the Child with Feeding Difficulties

A variety of health-care specialists may be helpful in assessing and treating a child who has ongoing feeding difficulties. A team might include a physical

or occupational therapist, neurologist, developmental medicine specialist, lactation consultant, speech-language pathologist, dentist, social worker, psychologist, and dietitian. Box 19–1 describes the services that each has to offer the child and family. When several people are involved in the child's care, one of them should serve as the coordinator to facilitate communication with the family and the child's primary health-care provider, and among the health team members themselves. Families will need both verbal and written instructions, and they should be encouraged to perform return demonstrations of recommended feeding techniques. Videotaping the breastfeeding mother and child while teaching special techniques allows the family to take with them a customized teaching aid.

Feeding Behaviors of the Ill Infant/Child

A child who is not feeling well commonly has a diminished appetite. A nursing infant may feed less vigorously and less often or more frequently but in brief bouts; the magnitude of the change in feeding routine varies with the severity of the illness. The child's condition may impair ability to suckle

BOX 19–1

Members of the Health-Care Team for the Breastfeeding Child with Special Health-Care Problems

Nurse

Assesses the global needs of child and family

Assists in identification of referral needs

Provides initial assessment of breastfeeding status

Ensures that the health-care plan is implemented

Provides family education

Provides direct nursing care to the child as needed

Lactation Consultant

Assesses the breastfeeding dyad

Identifies strengths and weaknesses

Identifies referral needs for the child with complex oral-motor difficulties

Develops a breastfeeding plan of care

Physician/Subspecialist

Diagnoses underlying illness/condition

Develops medical plan of care

Refers to other professionals as needed

Refers to neurologist or developmental specialist to assist in evaluation

Physical Therapist

Assesses gross motor capabilities

Develops plan of care to optimize baby's skills

Geneticist/Genetic Counselor

Provides risk counseling related to inherited conditions

Occupational Therapist

Assesses oral-motor/feeding capability as well as fine and gross motor skills as needed

Works with the mother to identify optimal positioning for the baby at breast

If breastfeeding is not possible, helps identify a preferred alternative feeding method

Develops plan of care to optimize baby's skills

Speech-Language Pathologist

Assesses oral-motor/feeding capabilities

May provide similar services to the OT related to oral-motor issues

Develops plan of care to optimize baby's skills

Dietitian

Assesses nutritional status of child

Develops plan of nutrition care

Identifies preferred supplements if needed

Mental Health Therapist

Assists families with the adaptation to a child with acute or chronic health care problem

Social Worker

Assesses family's needs for practical and psychosocial support

May provide counseling services

vigorously or frequently enough to take in sufficient calories to meet requirements for growth. In the face of illness such as congential heart defect or harlequin ichthyosis (Ripmeester & Dunn, 2002), the metabolic needs of the child may increase beyond the normal recommended daily allowances for age and height.

Milk supply may diminish fairly quickly with waning demand. Mothers may have uncomfortable breast fullness due to the child breastfeeding less. Any time that a baby has diminished appetite or is unable to maintain normal weight gain with direct breastfeeding, the mother must augment breast stimulation by expressing breastmilk by hand or pump (see Chapter 12) to maintain her milk supply and to prevent engorgement. Milk obtained in excess of a baby's immediate need can be stored for use at a later date. Box 19–2 provides milk collection and storage guidelines for the hospitalized infant.

If the infant is unable to feed orally for prolonged periods of time (days or weeks), he should receive oral stimulation by other means—typically a pacifier, despite the concern that sucking on an artificial teat may create problems in getting the baby back to the breast. Suckling the empty breast is an alternative. The baby who experiences uncomfortable procedures in and around the mouth such as suctioning, intubation, or operative intervention may be reluctant to breastfeed and requires special attention.

Skilled feeding assessment of the child with special health-care needs is vital. Assessment includes observation of at least one complete breastfeeding and monitoring of the infant's weight in order to determine the adequacy of milk transfer and caloric intake. If the child is not gaining weight normally, the amount of milk ingested is inadequate, regardless of what that amount might be.

BOX 19–2

Milk Collection and Storage Guidelines for the Hospitalized Nursling

- Hands are washed before initiating milk expression, with careful attention to fingernails and nail beds.
- A hospital grade electric breast-pump is preferred.
- Each mother must use her own collection kit.
- All parts of the kit that are touched by milk must be cleaned after each use with soapy water, rinsed well, placed on a clean towel, covered with another clean towel, and air dried. Cleaning in a dishwasher is an acceptable alternative.
- In areas where water is contaminated, boiled or bottled water must be used for cleaning pump kits.

- Expressed milk is labeled with the date, baby's name, baby's hospital identification number, any illnesses in the family, and any medication the mother is taking.
- Milk is stored in single feeding portions; aliquots larger than 8 oz should not be used.
- Colostrum and early milk may be "layered." Mother may chill and then add these small amounts of milk to the same container in order to get a full feeding.
- Storage containers should be made of glass, polycarbonate (clear, hard plastic), or polypropylene (cloudy, hard plastic) with solid caps that provide an airtight seal.

Source: Adapted from Arnold (1999).

Even if before- and after-feed weights indicate good intake for age (e.g., 3 oz per feeding in a 7+ pound infant), this volume may not be adequate for a daily weight gain of to 1/2 to 1 oz (15–30 gm, or 1 percent of the child's weight). An ill infant may have well-developed, effective oral-motor skills but may lack the energy to maintain suckling long enough to obtain sufficient calories for normal weight gain, as in the case of complex congenital heart disease.

What to Do If Weight Gain Is Inadequate

If a child is not gaining sufficiently, several strategies can be tried. General strategies will be discussed in this section, and a condition-specific section will look at special strategies and techniques.

The first suggestion is to simply change the baby's position at the breast. The upright posture shown in Figure 19–1 increases the baby's alertness through stimulation of the vestibular system and may increase breastfeeding vigor. Providing extra support for the baby's cheeks and jaw using the "Dancer-hand" position (Figure 19–2) may also

help. "Burp and bother" and other techniques are described in Chapter 10. Strategies for helping the child with abnormal tone (see Box 19–5, discussed later in this chapter) are useful for a baby who is neurologically normal but has a weak suckle. Trying to feed a soundly sleeping baby usually results only in frustration for both baby and mother, and it is not recommended. Supplementation with mother's milk, particularly high calorie hindmilk, or calorie-enriched mother's milk may be needed to improve weight gain. For the child with greatly increased metabolic demands, such as the infant with congenital heart disease, continuous or intermittent feeding with higher calorie milk through a nasogastric tube is often necessary to meet the increased caloric requirements for growth (Figure 19–3).

What to Do When Direct Breastfeeding Is Not Sufficient

When a child is incapable of or does not thrive with direct breastfeeding, health-care providers are faced with two challenges: (1) they must develop a feeding plan that will lead to optimal weight gain, and (2) they must help a family come to a peaceful acceptance of at least a temporary change in their

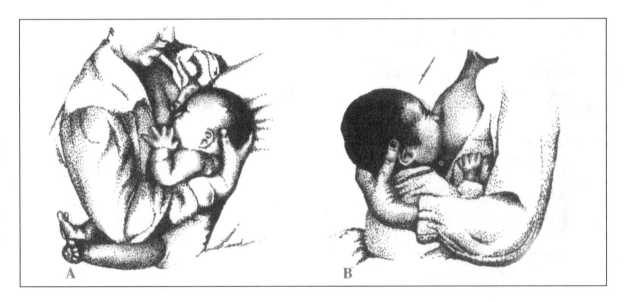

FIGURE 19–1. Upright Positioning. Either (A) side sitting, or (B) straddling the mother's thigh may serve to maximize the baby's breastfeeding efficiency. (Courtesy of the Cleft Palate Foundation, 1-800-24-CLEFT, http://www. cleftline.org.)

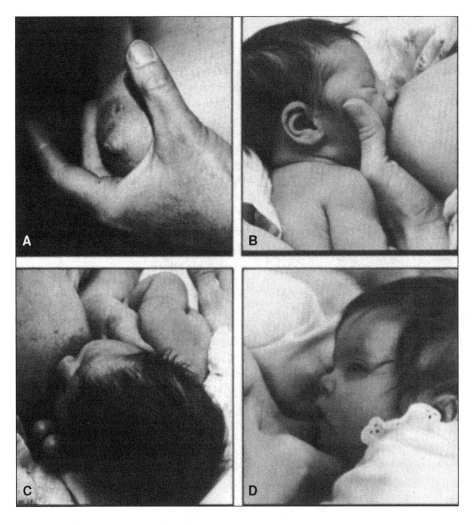

FIGURE 19–2.
Dancer-hand support. Dancer-hand positioning provides stability to the baby's jaw and support to weak masseter muscles. (A) The hand under the breast slides forward so that the breast is supported by three fingers rather than four. A "U" is formed with thumb and index finger. (B) The baby's head rests in the U where the jaw is supported, and cheeks are gently squeezed. (C) View from over the mother's shoulder shows how the hand supports both the mother's breast and the baby's head. (D) A modified dancer-hand position can provide just chin support, with the index finger applying pressure behind the mandible to support the tongue. (Source: From Danner & Cerutti, 1989.)

breastfeeding dreams. The health provider can make a difference in how a family comes to view these early experiences with their child. Some will remember brusque interactions and feelings that the provider had no understanding of the important nurturing aspect of breastfeeding. Other families may work with professionals who are so enthusiastic about breastfeeding that they lose sight of the importance of the infant's growth and development, even putting children at risk for severe dehydration or failure to thrive. The fortunate family interacts with professionals who are skilled in feeding assessment, understand the importance for optimal growth, and know when the child needs something different than exclusive or direct breastfeeding, and can communicate this with sensitivity.

According to Auerbach (1993), helping a mother to stop breastfeeding (or reframe breastfeeding) while supporting the infant-family relationship is one of the hardest things for lactation consultants to do.

When families of children with chronic conditions are interviewed about their experiences, they express appreciation for advice that is straightforward and, most importantly, accurate. Mothers of babies with cleft palate report how frustrating it was to realize that the enthusiasm of the pamphlets and the professionals they spoke to about the possibility of exclusive breastfeeding were in fact extraordinarily misleading (Miller, 1998). These mothers experienced feelings of failure, because their babies did not breastfeed "like the story in the pamphlet." Such pressure often leads to unrealistic, exhausting

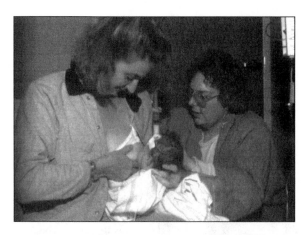

FIGURE 19–3. Baby is receiving calorie-enriched breastmilk via a supplementer made of a 5 Fr nasogastric tube and a 60 ml syringe. She is sitting upright—straddling her mother's lap to maximize suckling efficiency. (Courtesy of Sallie Page-Goertz.)

breastfeeding efforts that undermine the developing relationship between mother and baby.

When it is evident that direct or exclusive breastfeeding is not working, the skilled lactation consultant will focus on the positive aspects of the situation—for example, finding something complimentary to say about the child: "Look how the baby is watching you." "Isn't it wonderful how she follows your voice?" "He's trying hard—but when he's breathing so fast, it's just too much work for him." "What a wonderful snuggler you have." The goal is to reframe what's happening: Mothers and babies aren't breastfeeding failures—rather they're presented with a special challenge. It is also helpful to separate the two components of breastfeeding: the milk (nutrition) and the love (nurture) that happens with breastfeeding. The milk can continue to be offered, or saved until the baby can have oral feedings; the love continues on without interruption.

Alternative Feeding Methods

Breastfeeding specialists disagree about how to supplement children with special health-care needs. Unfortunately, there is insufficient data upon which to base the majority of recommendations, especially for infants and for children who are failing to thrive due to a myriad of other underlying health problems or conditions. Lacking such evidence, we base the recommendations presented here on understanding the child's condition, the anatomy and physiology of breastfeeding, the occasional case report, discussions with colleagues, and one's best clinical judgment. Consultation with an occupational therapist, physical therapist, and speech-language pathologist, as well as a dietitian, should be considered when working with a child who is not thriving with direct breastfeeding. These professionals provide valuable input into the assessment of how a particular child's strengths and weaknesses determine a plan of care that will optimize feeding and growth. If the child is not taking in sufficient volume of mother's milk to thrive, the dietitian provides input as to the preferred way to enrich the caloric content of the milk. Hindmilk or the addition of carbohydrate, fat, and/or protein supplement to breastmilk may be preferred, depending on the particular child's health condition.

Replacement feeding methods and supplementation devices such as cup, finger, and syringe feeding are discussed in detail in Chapters 7 and 10. Although a supplementation device is suitable for a prolonged period, the infant must be able to generate negative intraoral pressure to pull milk from the device. If the reservoir of the device is flexible, the mother can squeeze it so that a bolus of milk goes directly into the child's mouth and normal suckling skills may not be needed to accomplish sufficient intake. If the baby can latch onto the breast, supplementing at the breast is always the preferred way to provide extra calories. If the child is unable to gain adequate weight, other feeding methods need to be explored. Neither cup, or finger, or syringe feeding is conducive to long-term provision of large volumes of milk. Dowling et al. (2002) found that with cup-feeding, volumes of milk ingested were small and about one third of the amount taken from the cup was recovered on the bib.

For some children, bottle-feeding may be the best alternative feeding method. The feeding bottle can be used in ways that help develop or mimic breastfeeding skills (Kassing, 2002; Noble & Bovey, 1997). A squeezable bottle allows the caregiver to deliver a milk bolus into the baby's oral pharynx for swallowing, even when the baby is unable to generate negative intraoral pressure to accomplish milk flow. Higher volumes of milk or normal volumes of calorie-enriched milk can be provided to maximize weight gain for many children who are not thriving with direct breastfeeding.

Choice of feeding bottle and teat depends on a particular infant's need. Some children will be successful with a standard baby bottle—a firm reservoir with a variety of teats. Figure 19–4 illustrates one such bottle, which has a teat with a very wide base that encourages a wide-open latch. In general, it is best to select a wide-based teat that encourages latch with a wide-open mouth, that has a soft texture like the breast, and that has a nipple length that goes deep into the child's mouth but does not cause the child to gag. Longer teats may be helpful for the child with cleft lip/palate to avoid milk going directly into the cleft. Bottles that have been recommended for children who are not thriving with direct breastfeeding or use of a traditional feeding bottle include the Haberman feeder and the Mead-Johnson cleft palate feeder (Figure 19–5). Each of these bottles has a flexible reservoir allowing the caregiver to release a bolus of milk into the child's mouth. The Haberman has a specially designed

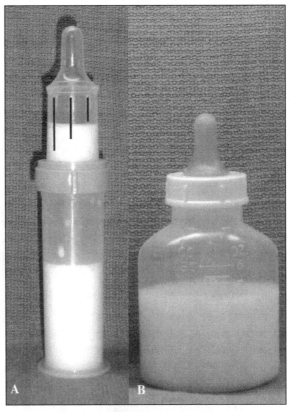

FIGURE 19–5. Bottles recommended for children who are not thriving with direct breastfeeding. (A) The Haberman feeder allows the caregiver to adjust the flow for the baby by aligning the marks with the baby's nose—the longer line provides greater flow. The one-way valve limits the negative pressure required to withdraw milk, and the flexible nipple reservoir allows the caregiver to squeeze a bolus of milk into the baby's mouth. (B) The Mead Johnson cleft palate feeder has a flexible reservoir allowing the caregiver to squeeze milk into the baby's mouth. The nipple is somewhat flattened and long so that milk can be released well into the baby's oral cavity. (Courtesy of Sallie Page-Goertz.)

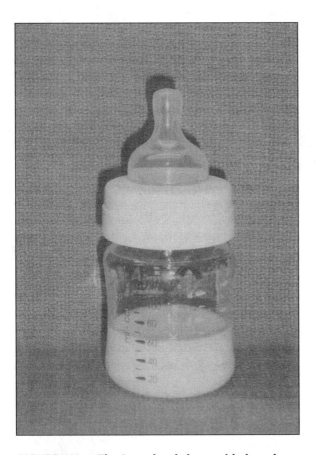

FIGURE 19–4. The Avent bottle has a wide-based teat to encourage a wide-open mouth. (Courtesy of Sallie Page-Goertz.)

valve and teat that allows the feeder to adjust milk flow to suit baby's needs. There is a slit in the nipple rather than a hole, which closes when the baby is not compressing/sucking the teat, preventing the flow of an unexpected bolus of milk into the mouth. The Pigeon nipple (Figure 19–6) has a flow valve that reduces the amount of negative intraoral pressure needed for milk transfer, similar to the Haberman feeder; the Pigeon nipple is softer and more flexible. It can be used on any standard infant feeding bottle. Fadavi et al. (1997) found that the Playtex nipple set flowed faster with less negative pressure and thus represented an increase in risk of choking and decreased oxygenation because of in-terrupted breathing patterns, particularly in hypotonic and preterm babies.

The baby can be fed with a bottle in ways to maximize closeness that naturally occurs with breastfeeding. Mothers and children need to be comfortable; babies can be skin-to-skin with their mothers or other caregivers during feeding. Eye contact, singing, and reading of stories is not precluded with bottle-feeding. Families should be taught to alternate the baby to left and right arms for holding, to provide equal visual stimulation, as normally happens with breastfeeding. When presenting the bottle to the baby, touch his lips to stimulate root/gape, and if possible, allow the baby to draw the teat deeply into his mouth. If the baby is unable to ingest the milk on his own, use a flexible bottle, or feeders using nurser bags to offer intermittent small boluses into the baby's pharynx for swallowing.

If bottle-feeding, even with calorie-enriched milk, is not sufficient for improving weight gain, more invasive feeding methods must be considered. Nasogastric feeding with a feeding tube, either by bolus or continuous drip for part or all of the day with regular or enriched milk, may need to be added to breast- or bottle-feedings. If oral feedings are not possible, enteral feedings can be given via gastrostomy or jejunostomy tube.

Care of the Hospitalized Breastfeeding Infant/Child

Hospitalization—whether it is planned or an emergency—disrupts family equilibrium. Unexpected admission to a pediatric intensive care unit of a previously healthy child causes parents to be near a panic level of anxiety (Huckaby & Tilem-Kessler, 1999). Parents find that the hospital setting presents uncertain boundaries regarding their roles and responsibilities for their own children. Tomlinson, Swiggum, and Harbaugh (1999) found that these uncertainties were lessened in an environment where the child was treated as a normal child and where the parent was free to continue to provide comfort care:

Seeing the nurse with her paralyzed/sedated infant, a mother said, "It is really nice to see the nurse touch

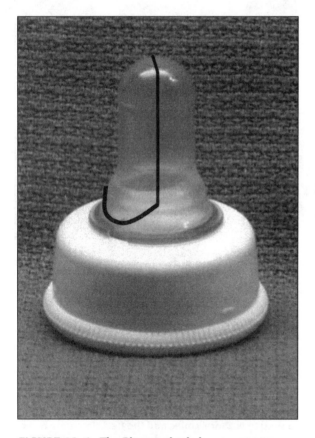

FIGURE 19–6. The Pigeon nipple has a one-way valve that decreases the amount of negative pressure required to withdraw milk. The outlined area of the nipple is slightly firmer and is positioned against the roof of the mouth. (Courtesy of Sallie Page-Goertz.)

her head to calm her. . . to see that the nursing staff doesn't only put stuff in the IVs and read the monitor." (p. 36)

It was also important that personnel recognized and respected family rights—keeping them informed, understanding the importance of family input, and providing appropriate explanations for medical problems and treatment decisions.

As with any crisis, hospitalization can be a time for learning and growth. Chances for a positive experience increase when the family stays with the child and all are supported by competent, caring staff. The goal for the hospitalized infant or child is to minimize disruption of normal routine. A secondary goal is to maintain and strengthen family unity. Families of breastfeeding children have a unique set of needs. Box 19–3 lists key characteristics of breastfeeding-friendly pediatric units. The stress of dealing with an ill child, perhaps hospitalization, and unexpected diagnoses makes intake of new information challenging for family members. Popper (1998) relates that families appreciate having a customized folder containing helpful information regarding the child's condition. Contents might include specific information about the child's illness and medications, breastfeeding tips, support group contacts, and the names of health-care team members. They can also include important family contact information, self-adhesive notes to use for communicating to staff when family members are away from the bedside, and blank paper to jot down questions or concerns for the health-care team. Family members may also place notes with their own observations about their baby into this folder (Popper, 1998).

BOX 19–3

Characteristics of a Breastfeeding-Friendly Pediatric Unit

- Has written breastfeeding policies in place.
- Employs or trains staff capable of skilled breastfeeding assessment and breastfeeding intervention when needed.
- Provides parents with written and verbal information about the benefits of breastfeeding and breastmilk.
- Facilitates unrestricted breastfeeding.
- Facilitates milk expression by mothers who wish to provide milk for infants who are unable to breastfeed. The following services should be available:

  Breast pump and privacy for pumping.
  Storage place for expressed milk.
  Referral to lactation services and pump rental sources if needed.

- Provides breastfed children only age-appropriate or medically indicated supplementation of food or drink.

- Uses alternative feeding methods most conducive to successful breastfeeding and appropriate weight gain.
- Provides 24-hour rooming-in of parents and their children.
- Provides meals and snacks for the breastfeeding mother.
- Plans medication schedule and procedures to avoid interfering with the breastfeeding relationship.
- Provides information about breastfeeding support available in the hospital and the community.
- Assesses compliance with policies through quality assurance activities and research.

Source: Adapted from Minchin et al. (1996) and Popper (1998).

For the child who is breastfed, feeding and nurturing patterns should approximate as closely as possible the normal home situation. Only by acquiring information can personalized and individualized care be given to families. Box 19–4 lists elements of the admission history that focus on breastfeeding issues. If the breastfeeding child is old enough to talk, the family may use a "code" word for breastfeeding, such as *nummies, yum-yum, nursie, snugglies, night-night,* or *side.* Acceptance of the normalcy of a walking and talking child who breastfeeds is discussed in Chapter 24.

If the infant is not feeding effectively, the hospital will ideally provide the mother with access to hospital grade electric pumps, and the maternal attachments that allow for dual collection, to maximize effectiveness of milk expression. Health-care workers should assist mothers in initiating milk expression as soon as it is noted that the infant's suckling abilities are not sufficient to maintain weight, or when oral feedings are not possible. Mothers may initially need assistance in negotiating any monitoring or therapeutic paraphernalia that is attached to

her baby as she puts the child to breast (Figures 19–7 and 19–8).

Home from the Hospital: The Rebound Effect

The child's reactions following hospitalization depend on the extent of trauma that has been experienced and the availability of coping mechanisms for self-protection. Almost all hospitals now encourage a parent to stay with the child during hospitalization. When parents room-in with the child, very few behavior changes occur on returning home. The young child who has experienced a painful separation may withdraw as a coping strategy, refusing to breastfeed and showing little interest in family members. The baby may cry a great deal and want to be held and breastfed exceptionally often, vigorously protesting having the mother out of sight for even a moment. For toddlers, emotional upheaval, including nightmares and insomnia, is common in the first few weeks following hospitalization. Short separations during hospital-

---

BOX 19–4

Admission History for the Breastfeeding Patient

- Usual feeding routine
  - Frequency of breastfeeding
  - Length of breastfeeding
  - Behavior of the baby during and after feeding
  - Special equipment needs
  - Preferred positioning for feedings
  - Special words for breastfeeding
  - If parent not present, preferred alternative feeding method
- Use of supplements
  - What is used for supplementation?
  - How much is given per feeding and during a 24-hour period?

  - How is it given?
  - When is it given?
- Use of herbal or other complementary therapies for mother or baby
- Solid foods
  - Preferred foods
  - Schedule for solid foods
- Recent changes in feeding routine
- Recent changes in weight gain
- Other approaches to feeding that have been utilized
- Solitary or co-sleeper

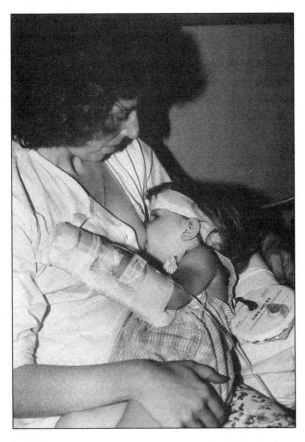

FIGURE 19–7. Breastfeeding with intravenous infusion. Mother may need some help negotiating the baby's equipment at first so baby can settle into the comfort of breastfeeding. (Courtesy of Debi Leslie Bocar.)

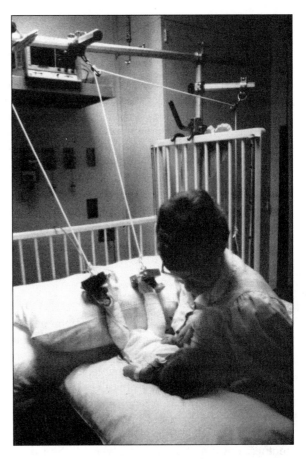

FIGURE 19–8. Breastfeeding while in traction. Mothers and babies can breastfeed under most any circumstances—even while the baby is in Bryant's traction for the treatment of congenital hip dysplasia.

izations are usually inevitable; however, when children feel safe and securely attached to their parent's love, trauma from the illness and temporary separations give way to restoration of trust after being reunited with their family. Helping parents to recognize this is vital to nursing care of the hospitalized child. Inherent in any crisis is the potential for bringing family members closer together with new awareness and appreciation of one another.

Perioperative Care of the Breastfeeding Infant/Child

Perioperative issues include the preoperative fasting period and postoperative recovery. The fasting period should be as short as physiologically appropriate for reducing anesthesia risk due to aspiration and also hypoglycemia. Separation of child and family should be minimized to reduce stress on all. The preoperative patient who is breastfeeding does *not* need to be NPO (nothing by oral route) for as long as the formula-fed infant because human milk is digested more quickly. For the infant who is receiving only breastmilk, fasting 3 hours prior to anesthesia induction should be sufficient to prevent vomiting (Feldman, Reich, & Foster, 1998). Another approach is for the mother to pump her breasts first and then let her baby suckle at the breast for comfort.

Littman, Wu, and Quinlivan (1994) found no differences in residual gastric volume and pH between children fed breastmilk and those fed clear liquids before surgery. He recommended that breastfeeding should be terminated 3 hours prior to induction, compared to 2 hours prior for clear liquids. In the case of breastfed babies, this distinction raises the question, "Why are 3 hours of fasting before surgery mandated rather than 2?" (Nicholson & Schreiner, 1995). Although some feel shorter fasting periods for breastfeeding infants are safe, this is not reflected in current guidelines for pediatric anesthesia (American Society of Anesthesiologists, 1999). Following surgery, breastfeeding should resume as soon as the physician indicates oral feeds can safely begin. There is no need for a first glucose water feeding. Mother may need to express milk until the infant is ready to resume breastfeeding.

Emergency Room

Nurses in the emergency room environment face the need to respond with split-second reactions and require a thorough background in a wide range of areas. It is very helpful for emergency room personnel to understand basic breastfeeding issues, so that inadvertent words or actions with the potential to undermine breastfeeding relationships are avoided. An example is a situation in which the mother, not the child, became very ill. She overheard the harried nurse say, "If she had given that baby a bottle, we wouldn't be in this mess," when the infant first refused and later vomited bottle-feedings. This example can serve as a lesson. The registered nurse reacted defensively to a life need. The parents may then have mistrusted that their medical needs would be handled well. How do health-care workers avoid insensitivity in care when they are faced with a situation beyond their experience or understanding? They should attempt to look at the family's needs through the eyes of each family member, actively seek to support their wishes when an emergency threatens the symbiosis of the breastfeeding relationship, and call upon colleagues in the maternal-child area for advice.

Often, emergency room medical providers do not have basic knowledge regarding breastfeeding. We are frequently told of situations where mothers were counseled to suspend or stop breastfeeding when there was in fact no medical indication to do so. For example, when the child presents with gastroenteritis, typical advice is to suspend all milk feedings and begin an oral electrolyte solution, as the physicians may be unaware that guidelines recommend continuation of breastfeeding during diarrheal illness. Or, a newborn with hematemesis (bloody vomitus) is given an invasive gastrointestinal work-up before someone thinks to ask if the mother's nipples are sore and bleeding. Or a breastfeeding mother is prescribed pain medication or antibiotic without consideration of its effect on the baby. Having a nurse in the emergency room who is aware of breastfeeding management concerns for the ill child may prevent inappropriate treatment.

Care of Children with Selected Conditions

Infection

Numerous research studies demonstrate that breastfeeding—even short-term, nonexclusive breastfeeding—reduces the risk of a variety of infections, both minor and major (Lopez-Alarcon, Villapando, & Fajardo, 1997; Scariati, Brummer-Strawn, & Fein, 1997). Protection from infection is afforded in a dose-response manner—the greater the dose, the greater the protection (Raisler, Alexander, & O'Campo, 1999; Scariati, Brummer-Strawn, & Fein 1997). The reduction in risk is most dramatic in resource-poor countries, but it is also significant in developed countries. Nonetheless, any child may experience infection at some point during the breastfeeding period. Breastfed children lose less weight during an infectious illness and are less likely to require hospitalization than if they are not breastfed. There is no reason to interrupt breastfeeding during infectious illnesses. However, the infant occasionally may be so severely ill that feeding capability is temporarily impaired. In these situations, the mother can express her breastmilk and save it until the baby resumes breastfeeding. Expressed milk can be provided to the child via nasogastric feeding when appropriate or stored for use at a later date.

Gastroenteritis

Gastroenteritis is caused by a number of viral and bacterial pathogens. Symptoms include vomiting, diarrhea, fever, anorexia, and fussiness presumably due to nausea and abdominal cramping. Sometimes new parents mistakenly believe that the normally loose breastmilk stools they observe in their newborn or the normal spitting up that babies do are signs of illness. (The emergency room physician might think so as well!) Viral gastroenteritis is responsible for more than 3 million deaths annually worldwide, primarily in resource-poor areas; in the United States it is estimated that there are about 200 deaths and 200,000 hospitalizations for treatment of dehydration (Iovino, 2003). The acute danger with gastroenteritis is the risk of dehydration when the infant takes in less fluid than is lost through vomitus and stools. With repeated gastrointestinal infections, the child also risks becoming chronically malnourished, increasing the probability of significant morbidity and mortality from a variety of causes. Infants are at greater risk for dehydration than older children or adults due to increased body surface area and therefore greater evaporative losses. Diarrhea and vomiting can also result in electrolyte imbalance caused by the losses of sodium and potassium. Electrolyte imbalance may be more severe if families have been supplementing with either high sodium fluids, such as broth, or very low sodium fluids such as water or soda pop, transforming a straightforward isotonic dehydration to a more complex hypotonic or hypertonic dehydration (Eliason & Lewan, 1998).

Babies with dehydration are listless, and they look and act sick. The degree of dehydration is most accurately determined by the extent of weight loss. Dehydration is classified as mild with 5 percent weight loss, moderate with 10 percent loss, and severe with 15 percent loss. However, the clinician rarely has access to a known pre-illness weight that is necessary to make this calculation and must depend on history and clinical findings. With just the clinical history of vomiting, the child is probably at least 3 percent dehydrated. Table 19–1 describes

Table 19-1

CLINICAL FINDINGS IN THE DEHYDRATED INFANT

Signs and Symptoms	Severity of Dehydration		
	None/Mild	**Moderate**	**Severe**
General Condition			
Infants	Thirsty, alert, restless	Lethargic/drowsy	Limp; cold, cyanotic extremities; may be comatose
Older children	Same	Alert; postural dizziness	Apprehensive; cold, cyanotic extremities; muscle cramps
Radial pulse	Normal	Thready/weak	Feeble/impalpable
Capillary refill	Immediate	Delayed	> 1.5–2 seconds delay
Respiration	Normal	Deep	Deep and rapid
Skin turgor	Pinch, immediate retraction	Pinch retracts slowly	Pinch retracts very slowly (> 2 seconds)
Eyes	Normal	Sunken	Very sunken
Tears	Present	Absent	Absent
Mucous membranes	Moist	Dry	Very dry
Urine output (parent report)	Normal	Reduced	None for many hours

Source: Adapted from Gorelick, Shaw, & Murphy (1997) and Armon et al. (2001).

the clinical signs of dehydration and the correlation with severity of dehydration. Gorelick, Shaw, and Murphy (1997) found that the diagnosis of clinically important dehydration could be based on the presence of at least three of these signs and symptoms. Capillary refill greater than 2 seconds, absent tears, dry mucous membranes, and ill general appearance predicted dehydration as well as a full set of 10 possible clinical signs (Gorelick, Shaw, & Murphy, 1997). Normally, six to eight cloth diapers wet with urine in a 24-hour period is an indication of adequate hydration; however, frequent stools can confuse estimates of urine output.

The child with mild illness needs no special intervention other than increased frequency of breastfeeding and close monitoring for signs of dehydration, especially number of wet diapers. If the infant has fewer than 4 wet diapers in 24 hours, refuses to nurse, or becomes either inconsolable or somnolent (sleepy), evaluation by the health-care provider is necessary. The child who is having more significant water losses or who is not interested in nursing may benefit from the addition of oral hydration solution (e.g., Pedialyte, Lytren, or the World Health Organization solution) in addition to breastfeeding (Armon et al., 2001). If the child is unable to keep fluids down, and has reduced voiding, intravenous fluid may be required.

Breastfeeding Implications. It is never necessary to interrupt breastfeeding during either the rehydration or recovery phase of illness (Armon et al., 2001). Human milk is a very well tolerated, easy to digest fluid. However, the nausea and abdominal cramping that accompany gastroenteritis may cause a period of anorexia and decreased interest in breastfeeding. If the youngster is reluctant to breastfeed for more than a couple of breastfeedings, the mother might want to express her milk both for comfort and to protect her milk supply.

Respiratory Infections

Respiratory infections, the most common cause of illness in infancy and childhood, are usually caused by viral pathogens. Infants with few outside contacts develop fewer respiratory infections than do children in day-care settings. Breastfeeding has a protective effect against respiratory illness, even when important confounding variables (birth weight, number of siblings, maternal age, smoking) are controlled (Beaudry, Dufour, & Marcoux, 1995; Wilson et al., 1998). In a retrospective review assessing morbidity based on maternal report in a cohort of infants, children were significantly less likely to be hospitalized for respiratory illness during breastfeeding weeks as compared to formula-feeding weeks (Beaudry, Dufour, & Marcoux, 1995). The protective effect of breastfeeding against lower-respiratory-tract infections is greatest for children exposed to environmental tobacco smoke (Nafstad et al., 1996, 1997; Horta et al., 1997).

Symptoms of an upper-respiratory-tract infection are fever, rhinorrhea, cough, sneezing, hoarseness, sore throat, and dysphagia. Symptoms of lower-respiratory-tract infection are somewhat different and include fever, tachypnea, wheezing, rhonchi, rales, and hyperresonance. Nasal flaring, expiratory grunting, and cyanosis are worrisome signs that require emergency referral for medical evaluation. The intervention needed depends on the severity of symptoms. Acetaminophen or ibuprofen will reduce the fever and make the child more comfortable. There are no data to suggest that a vaporizer adds therapeutic benefit. A warm air vaporizer is potentially dangerous (Colombo, Hopkins, & Waring, 1981), and both cool and warm air vaporizers may introduce mold into the environment if they are not meticulously cleaned.

Breastfeeding Implications. Breastfeeding difficulties commonly occur during both upper- and lower-respiratory-tract infections due to the baby's difficulty in coordinating suckle, swallow, and breath with nasal congestion, tachypnea (fast breathing), or pain of swallowing with pharyngitis. During coughing episodes, babies may gag and then vomit. Anorexia (loss of appetite) and vomiting is common. The child may be disinterested in breastfeeding, feed fretfully, or want frequent but short feedings. Pinnington et al. (2000) report that formula-fed infants with bronchiolitis had less effective coordination of breathing with swallowing, devoted less time to sucking, took in less volume per swallow, and had a total feeding volume that was about half that of well peers. It is not known if breastfeeding babies would have such dramatic differences in feeding. It is possible the differences might be less dramatic, in view of Mizuno, Veda, and Takeuchi's report (2002) that healthy children who were bottle-fed breastmilk had better coordination of suckle, swallow, and breathing than did infants fed formula or water.

Symptoms of respiratory distress may worsen while feeding at the breast if the child is moderately to severely ill. The nurse should observe the child's respiratory status during feeding; if the child becomes hypoxic, has cyanotic episodes, or has other signs of worsening distress, oral feedings may need to be suspended until the child's condition stabilizes. One should note respiratory and pulse rates before and during feedings, as well as oxygenation status. If the child is extremely tachypneic (respiratory rates of 60 to 80 or more for a young infant), they may not be able to tolerate oral feedings.

To make it easier for the infant to breathe, the mother can feed the baby held upright in a sitting position. Saline nose drops before feedings help thin the nasal secretions, which can then be aspirated. Saline drops can be purchased, or can be prepared at home if the parent is able to carefully measure the water and salt—1/4 tsp salt to 1 cup (8 oz) water. For infants older than 6 months who can tolerate vasoconstricting nose drops such as phenylephrine 0.16 percent, 1 to 2 drops twice daily for no more than 3 days can be administered. This reduces edema of the nasal mucosa. However, these nose drops must be used with caution as infants are at particular risk for rebound mucosal edema. It is critical that instructions for limited use of infant vasoconstricting nose drops be followed. Oral decongestants such as psuedoephedrine may be prescribed for the infant older than 3 to 4 months instead of vasoconstrictive drops.

If oxygen is required, the child may have a low-flow nasal cannula in place. This can remain in place without interfering with breastfeeding. For the infant who refuses to keep a canula or mask in place, a mist tent may be used. Although this imposes separation of the child from the parent, there is no reason for it to interfere with breastfeeding if the child is interested. The mother can join her baby under the tent if the child becomes hypoxic with feeding in room air environment—her presence may quickly quiet a crying, unhappy infant who has little energy to spare. Once the acute symptoms have passed, appetite will return, usually in a day or two. Until then, the mother should express her breastmilk to keep up her supply.

Pneumonia

Pneumonia is inflammation or infection of the lungs. More than 2 million children die of pneumonia worldwide each year, though mortality is rare in developed countries. Common pathogens tend to vary according to age:

- Neonates: Group B streptococci, gram negative enteric bacteria, cytomegalovirus, and listeria

- Age 3 weeks–3 months: *Chlamydia trachomatis,* Respiratory Syncytial Virus (RSV), parainfluenza, *Streptococcus pneumoniae*

- Age 4 months–4 years: RSV and other viruses, and *Streptococcus pneumoniae* (McIntosh, 2002).

Hospitalization may be necessary for closer monitoring, respiratory support, and intravenous fluids and antibiotics. Infants with pneumonia develop signs of acute illness often abruptly—high fever, productive cough (with emesis after coughing bout), and possibly, signs of systemic toxicity (tachypnea, lethargy, delayed capillary refill). Investigators have not been able to distinguish a constellation of symptoms that distinguish between bacterial and viral pneumonia (McIntosh, 2002). The infant may receive humidified oxygen as needed.

Bronchiolitis

Bronchiolitis is a viral illness distinguished by increased secretions and coughing that is sometimes severe. Infants will be tachypneic, have prolonged expiratory phase of respiration, and be in varying degrees of distress. Treatment is supportive care. Beta$_2$ agonists, such as albuterol, or corticosteroids are often prescribed but neither has been proved effective and both have significant side effects. Antibiotics are used only if a secondary bacterial infection develops. Most cases of bronchiolitis are self-limiting, and hospitalization is not necessary unless the child is in severe respiratory distress with hypoxia. Feeding may be somewhat disrupted for a day or two due to the cough and respiratory distress.

Respiratory Syncytial Virus

Respiratory syncytial virus (RSV) causes respiratory infection in people of all ages and is the most common cause of bronchiolitis and pneumonia in infants and young children. Breastfeeding has a protective effect against RSV (Holberg et al., 1991). The most striking symptom is the paroxysms of coughing with mild to severe respiratory distress. Children who are only a few weeks old, or who are premature may not have typical respiratory symptoms associated with RSV. Rather they may present with lethargy, irritability, poor feeding, and sometimes apnea. RSV occurs in epidemics in winter and early spring in temperate climates. Infants and toddlers younger than 2 years with chronic lung disease, and infants born before 32 weeks gestation are advised to receive palivizumab to prevent RSV infection. Medical treatment involves the provision of supportive care—ensuring hydration and providing supplemental oxygen, and mechanical ventilation if needed. The use of ribavirin treatment is controversial due to conflicting reports about effectiveness, the high costs, and concerns about potential toxic effects to exposed personnel. Corticosteroids are not effective and therefore not indicated.

Otitis Media

Otitis media (OM), inflammation of the middle ear, is the second most prevalent childhood disease after respiratory tract infections. It occurs most often in children between 6 months to 3 years of age. Common causative bacterial pathogens include *Streptococcus pneumoniae, Haemophilus influenzae,* and *Moraxella catarrhalis* in addition to viral pathogens. *S. pneumoniae* is the most common agent, and the least likely to resolve without treatment. There is growing concern about drug-resistant organisms (Dowell et al., 1999). It is well established that breastmilk feeding decreases the risk of otitis media (Aniansson et al., 1994; Aniansson et al., 2002; Duffy et al., 1997; Froom et al., 2001; Sassen, Brand, & Grote, 1994). The greater the dose of breastfeeding, the greater the benefit. Harabuchi et al. (1994) suggested that one mechanism for the protective effects of human milk against otitis media may be the inhibition of nasopharyngeal colonization with *H. influenzae* by a specific secretory IgA antibody. Exposure to smoke and day-care attendance are the most significant risk factors (Uhari, Mantysaari, & Niemela, 1996). Preventive strategies for otitis media include breastfeeding; avoidance of environmental smoke; avoidance of pacifier use (Niemela et al., 2000); avoidance of propped bottle-feeding of liquids other than breastmilk or water; and avoidance of day care.

Otitis media generally occurs following an upper respiratory infection. The child begins to feel worse rather than better. Many, though not all, develop fever. Pain behaviors include refusal to suckle, crying when put in a supine position, and general fussiness. Some children pull on their ears only with an ear infection. Recommendations for treatment might include expectant monitoring for the child who does not have a fever, antibiotics (amount and type dependent on the incidence of resistant *S. pneumoniae* in the community), and analgesia. Anesthetic pain drops placed into the ear canal will numb the tympanic membrane and afford immediate pain relief. These can be given on an as needed basis, particularly before feedings or bedtime, until the infection improves with time and/or antibiotic treatment. Oral analgesia such as acetaminophen or ibuprofen will help pain as well as fever. If the child continues to be symptomatic after 48 to 72 hours, the antibiotic treatment needs to be reassessed.

Breastfeeding Implications. An infant with a middle-ear infection may refuse to breastfeed, or feed very briefly due to the discomfort caused by changes in middle ear pressure with suckling. This leads to more frequent requests for brief nursings until the ear pain subsides. The child will be more comfortable nursing in an upright position to diminish middle-ear discomfort during suckling. Local anesthetic drops prior to feedings will help the child be more comfortable with feeds.

Meningitis

Meningitis is an acute inflammation of the meninges caused by viral or bacterial pathogens. The most common causative pathogens in infants and toddlers are pneumococci and meningococci. In areas with high rates of *Haemophilus influenza* vaccination the incidence of meningitis caused by *H. flu* has plummeted (Peltola, 2000). It is anticipated that the new pneumococcal vaccine will have similar effects on incidence of pneumococcal meningitis. Meningitis is also associated with other viral diseases, such as enteroviruses, measles, mumps, and herpes. The range of clinical symptoms and their severity varies widely and may be sudden or gradual in onset, depending on the age of the child and the causative pathogen. Signs of meningeal irritation include changes in level of consciousness, nausea and vomiting, and a tense anterior fontanel. Another neurological sign is pain with neck flexion. Infants may not exhibit positive Brudzinski or Kernig signs (see Chapter 20 on infant assessment).

One should suspect meningitis in the infant who prefers not to be held when ill (snuggling causes pain), and make urgent referral for medical evaluation. The child with meningitis requires emergent hospitalization. Lumbar puncture is done to culture cerebrospinal fluid, intravenous antibiotics are administered, and the child is isolated until the causative organism is ascertained. Length of isolation will depend on which pathogen is identified.

Breastfeeding Implications. Infants are sometimes uninterested in breastfeeding for a day or two during the acute phase but with effective treatment, and recovery, usually resume breastfeeding as eagerly as before. During the time the child is anorexic, mothers should be counseled to express their milk to keep their supply up. Children who have meningitis are at risk for a wide range of neurologic sequelae, and require ongoing assessment to identify any deficits, which could include difficulty with reestablishing effective breastfeeding.

Alterations in Neurological Functioning

The suck-swallow reflexes in a full-term, healthy infant are usually well developed at birth so the infant has little difficulty in establishing a pattern of effective suckling. This is not always true for children with neurologic impairment. Any deficit that affects neuromuscular function carries the risk that the child will have feeding difficulties. Suckling, swallowing, and breathing are integrated under medullary (brainstem) control. When this control is impaired, the normal muscle tension involved in these functions is affected. As a result, oral feeding can be difficult for both the baby and the caregiver. Children with neurologic impairment need careful assessment to determine the safety and the effectiveness of their feeding skills. The risks of oral feeds for the child with neurologic impairment include aspiration and failure to thrive. The overall muscle tone of the child will determine in part which interventions might be most helpful in facilitating oral feeding.

If breastfeeding is not going smoothly, it is important to seek expert intervention, calling on speech-language pathologists or occupational therapists to assist with the evaluation and treatment plan. Swallowing coordination and safety may need to be assessed using video-fluoroscopy or ultrasound. Experienced pediatric occupational therapists and speech-language pathologists understand the importance of looking at the whole child's development in the context of a feeding evaluation. Inappropriate oral exercises may not only be ineffective but may also exacerbate the child's difficulties (Bovey, Noble, & Noble, 1999).

When an infant is born with special healthcare needs, nothing should be assumed a priori about the child's capabilities before actually putting the baby to breast. One may be pleasantly surprised! A study of 59 breastfed infants with Down syndrome found that half had no difficulty in establishing suckling right after the birth. Four babies took less than 1 week to establish suckling; eight took 1 week, and 16 took longer than 1 week to do so (Aumonier & Cunningham, 1983).

Helpful techniques to improve suckling abilities in children with neurologic impairment are presented in Box 19–5. Signs of hypotonia related to breastfeeding include weak suck, lack of effective tongue movement, poor lip seal, inability to generate adequate suction, and inability to keep the breast inside the oral cavity. Positioning, head support, maternal breast support, and easy milk flow may assist these children. If latch-on and sustained suckling are not progressing, a nipple shield might help. The firmer texture provides a more dramatic stimulus for the baby compared with the nipple/areola. The use of a nipple shield to help infants achieve more effective milk transfer has been successful for premature infants and others (Bodley & Powers, 1996; Brigham, 1996; Meier, 2000).

BOX 19–5

Breastfeeding the Child with Altered Neuromuscular Tone

Action	Rationale
Getting started (both Hypo- and Hypertonia)	
• Arrange for a comfortable, quiet, low-light environment for feedings.	• A comfortable mother will be able to attend to teaching more readily.
• Encourage the mother to find a comfortable position for herself first.	
• Teach her the Dancer-hand position (see Figure 19–2).	• Enhances sucking efficiency with support of mandible (jaw) and masseter muscles (cheek) (Einarsson-Backes et al., 1994).
	• Shows the mother how to support her breast without interfering with latch-on.
• As with any special situation, ongoing assessment for breastfeeding effectiveness must be carried out.	• Feeding effectiveness may improve slowly for children with altered neuromuscular tone. Weight gain must be checked to assure the baby continues to thrive while working on improving direct breastfeeding.
• If strategies below are not successful in moving a baby to effective breastfeeding, consider referral to a therapist (occupational therapist, speech-language pathologist, or more experienced lactation consultant).	• Special diagnostic studies, such as a suck-swallow study, and special therapeutic measures may be needed to achieve improved breastfeeding.
• Provide the family with detailed written instructions, and observe return demonstration of prescribed techniques or devices.	• This assists the family's ability to replicate recommended strategies at home.
Baby with Hypotonia (low tone)	
• Help mother position the baby in an upright posture (Figure 19–1).	• Stimulates the arousal center.
• Teach mother how to tap gently and quickly around the baby's lips.	• Increases baby's ability to grasp the nipple.
	• Oral motor stimulation may enhance latch and suckling ability.
• Provide support with a finger under the chin, behind the mandible, to support the tongue.	• This support may enhance suckling effectiveness.

- Try an extensor position with arms and legs extended if the upright position is not helpful.
- Massage the breast so that milk is available for the baby to swallow or use a supplementer at the breast.
- Use a nipple shield to facilitate latch-on and sustained suckling.

- Some infants with low tone have more effective oral-motor function when positioned in extension.
- Milk flow into the oral pharynx stimulates swallow and subsequent suckling efforts.

- Massage or use of the device helps to provide a liquid bolus with minimal suckling effort on the part of the infant.
- The firmer texture of the nipple shield provides additional oral-motor stimulation, assists the mother to place the nipple over the baby's tongue, and in many cases stimulates more effective breastfeeding.

Baby with Hypertonia (high tone)

- Provide smooth gentle massage around the lips prior to feeding.
- Help mother position the baby in an upright posture.

- Support the trunk in a more forward position, rather than perpendicular to the hips (see stick drawing below).

- Pre-feeding massage may help relax the baby's oral tone.
- Upright posture stimulates the arousal center, facilitates hip flexion, and helps drop the tongue to the floor of the mouth.
- Positioning with the head coming downward onto the breast may prevent rapid flow of milk directly into the oralphyarnx, which may cause the hypersensitive baby to gag and choke.

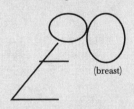

(breast)

- Avoid direct pressure on the back of the baby's head by placing a cloth between the back of the baby's head and the supporting hand, or moving the hand down to support the upper trunk and neck to avoid direct pressure on the head.
- Use a nipple shield to help get the baby's tongue down from the palate.

- Direct pressure on the occiput causes an infant to arch the head backwards, towards the pressure, rather than bringing the head forward to the breast.

- The firmer nipple may facilitate moving the tongue to the floor of the mouth in the baby with increased oral-motor tone.

Source: Compiled from Morbacher and Stock (2003), McBride and Danner (1987), Danner (1999), and the assistance of the feeding team, Developmental Disabilities Center, University of Kansas School of Medicine.

Babies with hypertonia have a hypersensitive, "tight" mouth and an easy gag reflex. When feeding at the breast, they tend to arch backward, hyperextend their head, thrust or retract their tongue. This baby will need help to come to a more flexed, relaxed posture in order to feed effectively. Swaddling or placing the baby in a sling to bring the shoulders forward and arms to midline helps accomplish this. If the mother cannot get the baby's tongue down to the floor of the mouth for latch-on, a nipple shield may be of assistance.

Down Syndrome or Trisomy 21

Down syndrome (DS) or Trisomy 21 is the duplication of the twenty-first chromosome, resulting in a constellation of abnormalities. Children with DS have characteristic physical features that include epicanthal folds, a flat nasal bridge, broad hands with shortened fingers, a simian crease (single crease across the upper palm), a flattened forehead, a small mouth, macroglossia (large tongue), and marked hypotonia. About half of DS children have congenital heart disease, and some have anomalies of the gastrointestinal tract as well. Most have mild to severe developmental delays.

Breastfeeding Implications. Difficulties with feeding may be encountered for some children with DS, but this is not universal. Hypotonia, tongue protrusion, and significant congenital heart disease are among the factors that may impact the child's effectiveness at breast. Mizuno and Ueda (2002) documented sucking behavior in 14 children with DS, using sucking pressure waveform and ultrasonography during bottle-feeding. They concluded that the babies' sucking difficulties may have been in part due to deficiencies in the peristaltic movement of the tongue as well as to the hypotonicity of perioral muscles, lips and masticatory muscles, and active tongue protrusion. The tongue was observed to fall to the back of the mouth, and touch the posterior palate. It is not known if these same sucking patterns are exhibited during breastfeeding. Interventions for the child with hypotonia as discussed will help maximize the child's feeding skills. Very close monitoring is necessary to evaluate the child's ability to maintain normal growth trajectory. As children with DS are shorter than the general population, a growth chart specifically for children with DS provides the most accurate tool to assess the adequacy of their growth.

Neural Tube Defects

Neural tube defects are anatomical abnormalities along the neural axis. These include encephalocele (protrusion of brain tissue), meningocele (protrusion of meninges), and myelomeningocele (protrusion of meninges and spinal cord) through bony defects of the skull or spine. The most common is myelomeningocele or spina bifida, which occurs most commonly in the lumbosacral region. The infant may have variable neurologic deficits below the level of the lesion. Alteration in sensory-motor function of the lower extremities and altered bladder and bowel control are common. Eighty to 90 percent of affected children have hydrocephalus requiring a shunt. The goal of early care is to prevent infection and further loss of neuromuscular function. Surgical correction to repair the myelomeningocele is performed as early as possible, preferably in the first 24 hours of life. If the defect is large, incisions lateral to the lesion will be made to allow the skin to cover the defect. Some centers are performing fetal surgery for closure of myelomeningocele at 24 to 30 weeks gestation. Bruner et al. (1999) have reported their outcomes with fetal surgery: significantly fewer babies developed hydrocephalus, and those that did develop it were 50 days old versus only 5 days old in a control group. Children having fetal repair were more likely to be premature. With successful surgical interventions, most infants affected by neural tube defects are able to breastfeed.

Nearly all children with myelomeningocele have a Chiari II malformation, a downward displacement of the brain into the neck. Anatomic differences in the whole brain accompany such a malformation. Infants are at risk for a Chiari crisis—brain stem malfunction causing potentially life-threatening apnea and bradycardia. Nurses and lactation consultants need to be alert for symptoms of a Chiari crisis: weak or absent cry, stridor, apnea and associated color changes, feeding and swallowing problems, arching of the neck, gastroesophageal reflux, and failure to thrive. About one in three children with myelomeningocele will have milder symptoms—typically related to feeding.

Breastfeeding Implications. Feeding difficulties frequently encountered by infants with myelomeningocele are due to oral hypersensitivity, poor oral-motor control, and a tendency to gag easily. These symptoms are probably due to the Chiari malformation which affects cranial nerves involved with sucking and swallowing (Sandler, 1997). When a baby is ready for oral feedings, the nurse can help with positioning to maximize breastfeeding effectiveness, while protecting the surgical site. A typical cradle hold can be used, taking care that the mother's arm does not put pressure over the defect/surgical site.

Postoperatively, a side-lying positioning of the mother and child may be the most comfortable. Until the surgical site is healed, the infant cannot be burped by patting the back. Gently rubbing between his shoulders or rocking on a firm surface may help to release any air bubbles. Sandler (1997) suggests feeding the baby in a semireclined position (as with cradle hold) and good head support, avoiding neck extension. If significant brainstem impairment is involved, the baby may not be able to feed effectively by mouth for a long time, if ever, in which case the mother can be supported to express breastmilk for her infant.

Hydrocephalus

Hydrocephalus is the accumulation of fluid in the cerebral ventricles caused by interference in the flow or in the absorption of cerebrospinal fluid. It may occur in isolation or along with myelomeningocele. As fluid accumulates within the ventricles, the infant's head enlarges to accommodate the increasing volume of fluid. With progressive hydrocephalus, sutures begin to separate and fontanels become distended. Children with marked hydrocephalus develop striking signs and symptoms, including the "setting sun" sign (the white of the eye showing above the iris and below the upper lid as a result of intracranial pressure), a high-pitched cry, muscle weakness, and severe neurological defects. Diagnosis of hydrocephalus is confirmed by a variety of imaging techniques, including ultrasound, CAT scan, or MRI. Surgery for placement of a ventricular shunt to decompress the ventricles is performed. The shunt drains the cerebrospinal fluid to another area, usually the peritoneum, where it is absorbed and finally excreted. Children are at increased risk for seizure disorder and meningitis.

Breastfeeding Implications. For the infant with advanced hydrocephalus, rarely seen in developed countries, care must be taken in positioning and supporting the infant's large, heavy head; side-lying positioning with the infant's head supported by a pillow is probably the most comfortable. For the child who has had shunt placement, care with the incision sites is needed during the immediate postoperative period. If the tender site is pressed during a feeding, the pain experience may lead to breast aversion (Merewood & Philipp, 2002). The neurosurgeon will prescribe specific limits to head elevation in the immediate postoperative period. Usually the child is required to stay completely flat, to avoid decompressing distended ventricles too rapidly. To prevent regurgitation due to increased intracranial pressure, feedings should be frequent and on demand. If there is severe brain damage associated with the hydrocephalus, effective breastfeeding may not be possible.

Congenital Heart Disease

Congenital heart disease (CHD) is the most common of structural birth defects (see Table 19–2). Symptoms range from none to severe depending on the particular defect, and effectiveness of medical/surgical management. Presence of CHD does not preclude breastfeeding; however, children with critical CHD, associated with cyanosis/hypoxia or congestive heart failure, are likely to face challenges with feeding and normal growth. Although most significant defects are identified shortly after birth, with 24-hour dismissal from the birthing facility, it is possible that a child may be discharged with undiagnosed critical heart disease. So, the nurse/lactation consultant who is assisting a newborn with breastfeeding difficulties should be very aware of the child who tires quickly, becomes tachypneic with feedings, or has color changes with feedings. Such a child may in fact have significant heart disease. The baby may begin with vigorous suckling, pulling away after a few minutes to rest, then again grasp the breast, and repeat the cycle. Feedings may become very lengthy, with limited intake due to the need for such frequent pauses to rest.

With a severe defect, the infant may exhibit signs of congestive heart failure: tachypnea, initially effortless and then progressing to more labored respiratory effort, tachycardia, progressively more difficult feedings, and sweating. Some children may exhibit hypoxic ("tet") spells during feeding—episodes of crying with intense cyanosis and deep and rapid breathing. While parents hold their infant, the heartbeat may be so prominent that they are aware of it. Any of the symptoms described, along with auscultation of abnormal heart sounds, palpation of a thrill or diminished femoral pulses, should lead the health-care worker to suspect a cardiac defect. The child should be immediately referred for medical evaluation.

Table 19–2

INCIDENCE OF CONGENITAL CONDITIONS

Birth Defects	Estimated Incidence
Heart and circulation	1 in 115 births
Muscles and skeleton	1 in 130 births
Club foot	1 in 735 births
Cleft lip/palate	1 in 930 births
Genital and urinary tract	1 in 135 births
Nervous system and eye	1 in 235 births
Anencephaly	1 in 8000 births
Spina bifida	1 in 2000 births
Chromosomal syndromes	1 in 600 births
Down syndrome	1 in 900 births
Respiratory tract	1 in 900 births
Metabolic disorders	1 in 3500 births
PKU	1 in 12,000 births

Note: All numbers are based on the best available estimates, which underestimate the incidence of many birth defects.

Source: March of Dimes Perinatal Data Center, 2000. Unpublished review of the literature and information from various state and regional birth defects surveillance systems (California, Iowa, Metropolitan Atlanta, New York, and Texas).

Breastfeeding Implications. Combs and Marino (1993) compared patterns of weight gain for 45 infants with CHD who had any breastfeeding to those who were exclusively formula-fed. The weight of the majority of infants in each group had dropped below their birth percentile at 5 months of age (66 percent of the breastfed, 75 percent of the bottle-fed infants). More formula-fed infants significantly fell off their individual growth curves than did the breastfed infants. One third of each group was below the fifth percentile for age at 5 months. Contrary to conventional wisdom, the severity of the cardiac defect was not a predictor of the infant's ability to breastfeed or of the duration of breastfeeding; rather it was the mother's commitment to continuing with breastfeeding that determined duration of any breastfeeding. Mothers in this study reported that they spent 1 of every 2 to 3 hours feeding their babies. The authors hypothesized that babies who were breastfeeding had improved growth due to the fact that breastfeeding was less physiologically taxing to infants, had less hypoxia, and spent less energy during feedings. A later study of seven children confirmed this hypothesis. While breastfeeding, none of the children with CHD dropped their SaO_2 below 90 percent, while four of the children dropped below 90 percent during bottle-feeding sessions (Marino, O'Brien, & LoRe, 1995). The volume of intake during breastfeeding or bottle-feeding was not reported.

Boctor, Pillo-Blocka, and McCrindle (2001) reported very different findings in their study of 24 infants who were also followed postoperatively. Exclusively breastfed infants lost a median of 49 gm/day. Partially breastfed babies gained a median of 5 gm/day, as compared to exclusively bottle-fed infants who gained a median of 20 gm/day. Babies in the partial and no breastfeeding groups were supplemented with calorie-enriched milks. Rate of weight gain was not related to the particular cardiac lesion or hospital length of stay. Possibly, the difference in conclusions between these two studies is that Boctor's group was able to look at exclusively, partially, and no breastfeeding as distinct groups, while the earlier study looked at "any breastfeeding." Both of these studies make it clear that achieving normal weight gain is a challenge, irrespective of feeding method.

Problems with weight gain stem from several issues. The child with congestive heart failure also has congestion of the gut, and may feel anorexic or nauseated because of the effects the congestion has on gut motility. Pressure on the gut from an enlarged liver or ascites may contribute to early satiety (Gervasio & Buxchanan, 1985). Gastroesophageal reflux disease is common in children with heart failure. Medications given to treat congestive heart failure also may cause nausea and anorexia. In addition, the energy needs of a child with significant CHD frequently exceed the normal RDA of 100 to 110 kcal/kg/day of the breastfed infant. Some children may require up to 140 to 160 kcal/kg/day to achieve positive weight gain (Gervasio & Buxchanan, 1985). This incredible increase in metabolic demand is related to the extra energy required to support the child's increased respiratory rate and effort, and to the increase of circulating catecholamines (stress hormones). The healthy newborn that is breastfeeding perfectly could not achieve this degree of caloric intake—and it is certainly impossible to expect in the face of symptomatic heart disease. Weight gain and sufficient protein calorie intake is important so that the child's operative risks are minimized. Thus, every effort must be made to help the child achieve as normal a growth rate as possible. The youngster with severe cyanotic heart disease or with congestive heart failure often requires very invasive methods to facilitate growth. When the baby has significant heart failure, a more comfortable breastfeeding position is a more stretched out posture, rather than a flexed one, as this avoids pressure on a distended and perhaps tender liver. Supplementation with hindmilk or calorie-enriched milk with a nursing supplementer during breastfeeding may be all that is required to push a baby into normal weight gain. However, others will require more intensive support with nasogastric feeding of calorie-enriched milk, with comfort time at the breast. Once the child's defect has undergone repair, the return to oral feeding should happen very quickly. Thankfully, advances in surgical care of the child with CHD allow for definitive repairs much earlier in infancy, minimizing disruption of normal feeding.

Oral/Facial Anomalies

The majority of infants with oral/facial anomalies—cleft lip/palate or Pierre Robin sequence—require continuous feeding evaluation and support. Most are unable to gain weight or maintain hydration with only direct breastfeeding. Mothers will need continued support to maintain their breastmilk supply. There are strategies to maximize the child's capabilities to breastfeed, with the understanding that health providers must frequently monitor growth, reevaluate feeding capability, and adjust feeding plans accordingly.

Cleft Lip and Palate

Cleft lip and palate are congenital malformations caused by incomplete fusion of the structures of the oral cavity and the palatine plates very early in gestation. This results in alteration in structure of the upper lip, maxilla, alveolar ridge, nose, and hard and soft palates. The clefting may involve only the lip, may extend into the hard and soft palate, and may be unilateral or bilateral. The general classifications include: lip only (CL); both the lip and the palate (CLP); and hard and/or soft palate only (CP). Cleft lip and cleft palate each account for 25 percent of the malformations; clefting of both structures is found in 50 percent of all cases; therefore, the nurse or lactation consultant will work most frequently with children with clefting of both the lip and the palate. Occasionally, small, isolated clefts of the soft palate are not identified until feeding difficulty becomes apparent. The lactation consultant may be the first to identify a problem during a feeding assessment.

One might think that children with CL would be at higher risk for parent-infant attachment disorders because of their unattractive appearance. However, Coy, Speltz, and Jones (2002) found that this was not the case. In a sample of families whose babies had CLP, CP, and no clefts, it was found that the CL affected babies demonstrated more secure attachment than those with CP or no cleft. The authors hypothesized that the perceived vulnerabilities of the children engendered extraordinary protectiveness and responsiveness in their mothers.

For the infant with CL, preoperative orthopedics may be used to help align the alveolar segments, decreasing the width of the cleft (Denk, 1998). These orthopedic interventions may be as low tech as the use of adhesive tape or steri-strips approximating the lip segments, or they may involve splints made of acrylic or soft dental material.

Surgical repair of cleft lip and palate is done in stages. First, the lip defect is corrected within the first 2 to 3 weeks of life (Denk, 1998). Early lip surgery appears to have no greater risks than does later surgery, and may serve to enhance the developing relationship between the family and their infant. Surgical closure of the palate is performed between 6 months and 2 years of age. Some surgeons are willing to contemplate repair of the palate prior to 6 months, which increases the possibility that the mother and child might then be able to enjoy direct breastfeeding. Denk (1998) reported on 21 infants who underwent palate repair within the first month of life. Babies returned to breastfeeding or bottle-feeding once they recovered from anesthesia. Limited follow-up indicates that the children have done well, but the authors feel longer follow-up is needed to assess long-term outcomes related to speech and facial development before a general recommendation to operate during the neonatal period is appropriate. Clearly, early palatal repair would facilitate the possibility of direct breastfeeding; more reports are awaited.

Multiple prospective studies find that return to direct breastfeeding or bottle-feeding, rather than cup- or dropper-feeding, immediately following cleft lip repair is best for the baby (Darzi, Chowdri, & Bhat, 1996; Cohen, 1997). Furthermore, it is more cost-effective as hospitalization time is shorter and the need for intravenous fluids is reduced (Darzi, Chowdri, & Bhat, 1996). Less is known about breastfeeding after repair of a cleft palate. No studies have discussed feeding method post palate repair. Typically, if a child is bottle-fed, weaning is recommended prior to surgery to avoid disruption of the palatal suture-line from the artificial nipple. However, for the breastfed infant/toddler, the mother's soft nipple would not be expected to traumatize this suture line. However, having the nipple inside the mouth may be initially painful to the youngster's tender postoperative site.

Breastmilk is particularly important for infants with CLP and Pierre Robin sequence as it reduces the risk of otitis media even beyond the time of weaning (Paradise et al., 1994; Aniansson, 2002). Trenouth and Campbell (1996) reported that half of the mothers of neonates with cleft lip or palate attempted to breastfeed. Almost all were dissatisfied with the information they had received while in the hospital and with the backup care when they went home. Young et al. (2001) queried parents of 40 children, and as one would predict, found that they wanted basic information in the immediate newborn period, especially about feeding. Only half of the families recalled having specific feeding instruction, while 97 percent felt it was critical not only to be informed but also to be shown how to feed their babies and what difficulties to expect. Feeding challenges are foremost on parents' minds and must be addressed very clearly.

Breastfeeding Implications. Children with clefts are very interested in breastfeeding, approach the breast eagerly, and in many instances appear to latch-on well. Their jaw movements appear effective, but usually swallows are very infrequent, particularly for the baby with cleft palate. All babies with CLP must have expert breastfeeding assistance, a written feeding plan, a support phone number, and a follow-up outpatient appointment within 24 to 48 hours of dismissal from the newborn nursery.

The ease with which the baby takes the breast is related to the severity and extent of the defect. The child who has an isolated CL can usually breastfeed effectively with minimal intervention. The baby may require some assistance from the mother in maintaining lip seal. Positioning the infant with the cleft as tightly to the breast as possible and placing the mother's thumb or index finger over the cleft can create sufficient closure for the infant to effectively milk the breast. According to Danner (1992a, p. 625), the baby may do best if the breast enters the mouth from the side on which the defect is located: "An infant with a right-sided defect should be held so that the right cheek touches the breast . . . the mother can go from cradle-hold on one side, to the football or 'clutch' hold on the other."

With a CP, it is very unlikely that the child will ever achieve normal growth with exclusive breastfeeding. The opening in the palate dramatically alters suckling mechanics. Because the baby is unable to generate negative intraoral pressure, it is hard to maintain breast tissue inside the oral cavity and impossible to generate the negative pressure that is a necessary part of milk transfer. As Wilson-Clay (1995) stated, "Try sucking on a straw with a hole in it." A recent review of pamphlets for parents and materials for health professionals noted that the information was unrealistically optimistic regarding the cleft-affected child's ability to thrive with exclusive breastfeeding (Miller, 1998). Miller interviewed several well-known clinicians and surveyed CLP centers in Canada and the United States. All respondents reported that their clinical experience revealed that it was in fact exceedingly rare for the child with CP to accomplish normal weight gain with exclusive breastfeeding. Pandya and Boorman (2001) found that 32 percent with unilateral CL, 38 percent with bilateral CL, and 49 percent with CLP had FTT in a retrospective review. Details of infant feeding method were not described for this cohort.

Oral feeding can be uncomfortable for the child due to regurgitation of the milk into the nostrils. Regurgitation is minimized with upright positioning during feeding and with quick milk flow into the back of the oral cavity where it can be swallowed rapidly. A baby with a bilateral cleft suckles best when straddled on the mother's lap or sitting on one side of her body with his legs under her arm (see again Figure 19–1). The soft breast fills the alveolar-ridge defect as well as the palate defect and can be moved to one side or the other as needed. It is important to note that cleft palate centers in the United States report that it is extremely rare to see a child that is able to breastfeed effectively, despite Danner's eloquent description of optimal positioning (Miller, 1998). One of the authors of this chapter has observed videos of babies at the breast who are drinking milk that the mother has hand expressed into the baby's mouth. The baby is not at all an active participant in the milk transfer, but rather a passive recipient of expressed milk.

The use of a palatal obturator is recommended by some cleft palate teams both to facilitate development of the oral cavity and to achieve suckling effectiveness. The dentist or plastic surgeon makes this appliance, which covers the cleft in the palate and may improve the infant's ability to suckle (Figure 19–9). It may take the baby weeks or months, if ever, to learn to effectively breastfeed using this device. Supplemental feedings are usually required to accomplish normal weight gain. Two groups report outcomes for infants who had obturators. Kogo et al. (1997) found that of ten babies in whom a Hotz-type palate was used, four were able to suckle the

breast directly and obtain milk. These four babies required supplemental feeding to sustain appropriate growth; however, the investigators viewed such assisted feeding at the breast as a first step in direct breastfeeding for these babies. Turner et al. (2001) report on eight infants who participated in a prospective feeding intervention study using a palatal obturator and Haberman feeders (see again Figure 19–5) for infants who were unable to achieve effective breastfeeding. None of the babies in their cohort were able to achieve sustained effective breastfeeding with any of the interventions. The use of the palatal obturator and Haberman feeder allowed the children to drink larger volumes in less time and to achieve normal growth. Feedings without the obturator in place were longer and significantly lower in volume. Lactation support for the

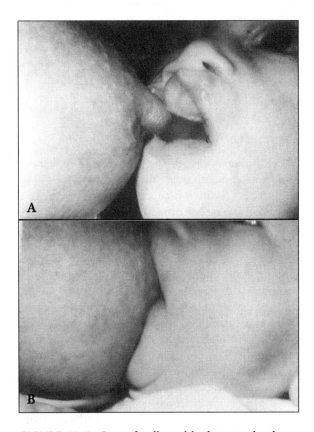

FIGURE 19–9. Breastfeeding with obturator in place. (A) Infant with cleft lip and palate with palatal obturator in place. (B) Same infant attempting breastfeeding. (Photos courtesy of David Barnes, DDS.)

mothers facilitated continued milk expression, among a highly motivated group.

While the parents and health-care team are working to maximize the infant's capacity for breastfeeding, milk expression is critical to maintaining the mother's milk supply. The infant can be fed breastmilk by alternative methods. Some parents find that a small spouted cup works well. Others favor an eyedropper, a rubber-tipped syringe (Brecht feeder), or a pipette. Feeding-tube devices have been used successfully for the occasional infant with cleft palates. Most children will do best with a flexible infant feeding bottle such as the Mead Johnson cleft palate or Haberman feeders (see again Figure 19–5). Shaw, Bannister, and Roberts (1999) found that a squeezable bottle was more effective and better accepted than a rigid feeding bottle for providing supplement. As with any child having suckling difficulty, bottle-feeding is no guarantee for appropriate weight gain for the same reasons that breastfeeding is so difficult. Thus such children continue to need frequent monitoring, and many benefit from calorie-enriched feedings. Box 19–6 discusses a typical case of a family whose 5-day-old baby with a CLP was extremely distressed.

Pierre Robin Sequence

Pierre Robin sequence is a complex of oral facial abnormalities including micrognathia (small jaw) and glossoptosis (tongue with retropharyngeal placement). Micrognathia is the hallmark feature of Pierre Robin sequence (Color Plate 34). Most children also have clefts of the palate. Up to 80 percent have other associated anomalies. Diagnosis is usually made very shortly after birth when the child's respiratory distress is noted. The position of the tongue causes interference with patency of the upper airway. Duskiness and apnea occur with feeding or supine positioning. The facial anatomy, particularly the placement of the tongue, leads to difficulties with airway obstruction and feeding, with or without presence of a cleft palate. The feeding problems, primarily due to difficulties in maintaining the airway (Marcellus, 2001), are complicated by difficulties in attaching to the breast and the presence of a cleft palate. A number of inter-

ventions may be required to prevent airway obstruction—from prone positioning to prolonged nasopharyngeal intubation to glossopexy (tongue is sutured so that it cannot occlude the airway), or tracheostomy for children who do not show clinical improvement with nasopharyngeal intubation (Marques et al., 2001). Nasopharyngeal intubation is preferred, as the child can then usually receive oral feedings.

Breastfeeding Implications. Effective breastfeeding is possible in mild cases, if the infant can maintain normal oxygenation. During initial feedings, oxygen saturation should be monitored. To facilitate airway maintenance, the child may do better with upright positioning, rather than the cradle or football position, in terms of more forward tongue placement. Unfortunately, it is rare for most babies with Pierre Robin sequence to be able to breastfeed or bottle-feed effectively in the first weeks of life, due to difficulties with airway, tongue placement, and receding mandible. In a prospective review of 35 children with Pierre Robin sequence, Baujat et al. (2001) found that 86 percent required nasogastric feedings to accomplish safe feeding and appropriate weight gain. None of the initially breastfed babies were able to feed effectively. In Baujat's series, 50 percent had abnormalities of esophageal motility that did not respond to standard gastroesophageal treatment. Baudon et al. (2002) used electromyography and esophageal manometry to evaluate motor function of the upper digestive tract (tongue, pharynx, and esophagus) in a group of 28 neonates during a bottle-feeding. Their findings demonstrate that most had sucking-swallowing disorders along with abnormal esophageal peristalsis and abnormal lower esophageal sphincter pressures and relaxation—many reasons for difficulties with feeding. If a trial of breastfeeding fails, oral feeding devices that are used for infants with clefts can be tried, though frequently nasogastric feeding is required initially for normal weight gain.

Parents will need continued support to maintain breastmilk production for their baby. Over time, the micrognathia resolves, so that the older infant has a completely normal facial appearance and no longer has problems with airway maintenance.

BOX 19–6

Case Study—An Unhappy Baby (and Family) with Cleft Lip and Palate

History

Baby Anna and her parents came to the breastfeeding clinic on the child's fifth day of life. Her primary care physician referred them for assistance with breastfeeding. Anna was the couple's first child. Pregnancy, labor, and delivery were uneventful and she was healthy except for the unilateral CLP, which was unexpected. Birth weight was 3650 grams, dismissal weight was not known.

The family reported that during the newborn stay, the baby was nursed every 3 hours. They thought that nurses in the nursery might be supplementing the baby, but were not specifically told this. Dismissal instructions were to breastfeed on demand.

At 5 days of age, they reported that she was inconsolable, at the breast continuously, and had orange stuff in her diaper. They had been to the doctor's office, where her bilirubin was 17 mg/dl.

Observation

The baby was jaundiced down to her shins, crying, and slim. Her mucous membranes were moist, and her skin turgor was good. She had a wide, unilateral cleft lip and palate. Her weight was 3190 grams—12 percent below birth weight.

Breastfeeding was observed. In cradle hold, the baby eagerly rooted, but never latched onto the breast. She was placed in the upright position (see Figure 19–1) and latched onto the breast. Rhythmic jaw movements were noted. She did not demonstrate swallowing until the mother had let down, and then she lapped a little milk off the surface of the breast. No sustained suck-swallows were noted during 10 to 15 minutes of attempted breastfeeding. A tube at breast was attempted without success.

Held in an upright position to avoid nasal regurgitation, Anna's mother fed her with a Mead Johnson cleft palate feeder (see Figure 19–5). Anna was able to take 3 oz in about 10 minutes and became relaxed, falling asleep in her mother's arms.

Assessment

Ineffective breastfeeding with resultant excessive weight loss, breastfeeding-associated jaundice, and mild dehydration based on history and weight loss.

Plan

Encourage breastmilk expression, feed Anna with cleft palate feeder on demand, follow-up with primary provider in 24 hours. Parents were given an intake and output sheet to monitor hydration. Parents expressed relief at being able to satisfy their infant and anger at the nursing care they had received in the hospital—noting that their child had been put at risk. The baby gained 2 oz within the next 24 hours.

Feeding difficulties improve with age, beginning after about 4 months (Baujat et al., 2001).

Choanal Atresia

Choanal atresia is the membranous or bony occlusion of the posterior nares, such that air cannot reach the pharynx via the nose. It may present as a component of the CHARGE syndrome (C, coloboma; H, heart disease; A, atresia choanae; R, retarded growth and development; G, genital hypoplasia; and E, ear anomalies and/or deafness). A rare congenital anomaly, complete bilateral atresia is a potentially life-threatening emergency in the neonate who will develop respiratory distress with hypoxia within a few hours of birth. An oral airway must be placed securely to allow for breathing. Surgery is usually attempted early in the newborn period, depending on the condition of the infant. Surgical repair of the blocked passageway is performed to create a nasopharyngeal airway. Depending on the characteristics of a particular child's anomaly, and the surgical repair required, nasal stents may be in place for 4 to 8 weeks postoperatively to maintain the integrity of the repair, and prevent restenosis of the tissue.

Breastfeeding Implications. The baby with choanal atresia may resist taking any type of oral feeding until the problem is corrected. Initially, oral feeding is not usually possible with bilateral choanal atresia, as the baby is unable to suck, swallow, and breathe. Feeding requires oral-gastric tube placement until surgery is accomplished. With stents in the nasopharynx postoperatively, the baby will be able to feed orally—the stent length may need to be adjusted to accommodate breastfeeding.

Gastrointestinal Anomalies and Disorders

Esophageal Atresia/ Tracheoesophageal Fistula

Esophageal atresia/tracheoesophageal fistula (EA/TEF) occurs in about 1 in 3000 live births. In the most common form of EA/TEF, the upper end of the esophagus ends in a blind pouch, with a fistula connecting the lower segment of the esophagus to the trachea (Spitz et al., 1994). This disorder may be suspected prenatally when polyhydramnios and the absence of identification of a fetal stomach bubble are observed during ultrasonography. Within a few hours after birth, classic symptoms of esophageal atresia with tracheoesophageal fistula include copious, white frothy bubbles of mucus from the mouth, which return after suctioning. The child may have noisy respirations, and experience coughing, choking, and cyanosis, which become worse with feeding. In the past, milk feedings were delayed for all infants until an initial water feed was well tolerated in the mistaken belief that water was less dangerous to aspirate if an infant had EA/TEF. This practice is no longer recommended.

If the infant is symptomatic, a catheter is passed into the esophagus to see whether gastric secretions can be aspirated. If gastric content cannot be determined and other symptoms are present, medical attention should be obtained at once. X-ray and sonography confirm the diagnosis. About 10 percent of children will have other malformations, primarily of the urinary tract or the musculoskeletal systems. VACTERL is an acronym describing the range of anomalies that might be found: V, vertebral defects; A, anorectal malformation; C, cardiac anomalies; T, tracheoesophageal fistula; R, radial and renal dysplasia; and L, limb anomalies.

Prior to surgery, care is provided to reduce the risk of aspiration. The child is maintained in an elevated position. The infant is not fed by mouth. Continuous suction to the blind pouch is required. Parenteral nutrition is provided until surgical correction is accomplished, usually in the first few days of life (Spitz, 1996). The premature or medically unstable baby will be provided parenteral nutrition; with gastrostomy and upper pouch to suction until stable enough for surgery. For children with more complex forms of EA/TEF, repair may be delayed by many months, necessitating placement of a gastrostomy tube for enteral feedings. Enteral feeding typically begins 5 to 7 days postoperatively. A common long-term problem for these children following surgery is gastroesophageal reflux (see below).

Breastfeeding Implications. Until the infant can take oral feedings, the mother can maintain lactation by expressing her milk. Until oral feeding is allowed, a plan for providing nonaversive oral stimulation is important.

Gastroesophageal Reflux

Gastroesophageal reflux is the effortless regurgitation of gastric contents into the oral cavity, or out of the mouth—i.e., "spitting up." Children who become symptomatic with chronic gastroesophageal reflux have gastroesophageal reflux disease (GERD). Although Heacock et al. (1992) noted that breastfed newborns have shorter episodes of reflux and lower gastric pH values than formula-fed babies (only during active sleep), it is not uncommon for breastfed infants to have GERD. There is a wide spectrum of GERD—from the happy, spitting up baby who is thriving to the miserable, fussy baby who may be either thriving or failing to thrive. Thankfully, the majority of infants are happy thriving spitters, and families simply require reassurance and support for what is mainly a problem of way too much laundry. Most children who have GERD improve as they mature. Eighty-five percent are symptom-free by 1 year of age; 10 to 15 percent have persistent problems off and on over the life span.

Children who have persistent symptoms affecting their weight gain, feeding behavior, or happiness require referral for evaluation. Symptoms of problematic GERD include anorexia, difficult or painful swallowing, arching of the back during feedings, irritability, failure to thrive, and very late signs of hematemesis due to esophagitis. GERD is also a common cause of life-threatening events and chronic respiratory disorders such as pneumonia, asthma, chronic cough, and stridor (GER Guidelines Committee, 2001). Parents may report that the child is happiest when prone (there is less reflux in this position). If the baby becomes increasingly fussy, has difficulty sleeping, refuses to feed, or wants to feed often, intervention is needed. Children with projectile vomiting or persistent vomiting may have other problems such as pyloric stenosis or malrotation of the bowel. Hirschsprung's disease or neurologic disorders also need to be considered in the medical evaluation.

Diagnosis of GERD is primarily based on the clinical history and observation of the child's behavior, particularly during and after feeding. An esophageal pH probe (a probe inserted in the baby's esophagus to monitor the pH) assesses frequency and duration of GER episodes, while an endoscopic examination establishes the presence of esophagitis, and allows for a biopsy of the esophagus if indicated. A barium swallow is not useful for establishing the diagnosis of GERD, but will identify the rare anatomic anomaly that may cause the reflux (GER Guidelines Committee, 2001). GERD is quite common in children with neurologic impairments such as cerebral palsy, in premature infants, and in infants with other congenital gastrointestinal tract anomalies such as gastroschisis and EA/TEF.

If the child's symptoms are interfering with normal weight gain, or causing pain behaviors, medications may be ordered that promote gastric motility and reduce acidity of gastric secretions. Medications that reduce acidity of gastric contents, such as ranitidine (Zantac), omeprazole (Prilosec), or lansoprazole (Prevacid), may be recommended. Metoclopramide (Reglan), a dopamine blocker, is the most easily available motility agent in the United States that is appropriate for infants (bethanacol is no longer recommended). Metoclopramide can cause extrapyramidal symptoms in infants, such as jitteriness and increased fussiness. Domperidone (Motilium), a motility agent that does not have the extrapyramidal side effects, is available through compounding pharmacies in the United States, or it can be purchased from other countries via the Internet.

Cisapride had been the preferred motility agent because it does not have limiting central nervous system side effects. However, as of this writing, it is only available under compassionate-use protocol in the United States due to case reports of cardiac arrythmias in infants and deaths related to cardiac side effects reported in adult patients. If medical management is not helping, surgical intervention may be required, particularly for children with underlying neurologic impairment. The Nissen fundoplication or modified Nissen are the most common procedures used. These procedures wrap the antrum of the stomach around the esophagus to limit reflux of gastric contents into the esophagus. However, it does not resolve underlying gastrointestinal motility disorders, and it has significant complications.

Breastfeeding Implications. Typical challenges for parents include the symptomatic child's difficulty with feeding and sleeping. Mathisen et al.

(1999) reported that infants with GERD aged 5 to 7 months in a case match control study had significantly more feeding problems affecting behavior, swallowing, food intake, and mother-child interaction. Children with GERD wake at night and sleep more during the day (Ghaem et al., 1998). When mothers are faced with a very fussy baby, more nursings are offered. Thus one may see a chubby baby who is nearly continuously breastfeeding—and a vicious cycle quickly develops of fussing, short feeding, and more fussing that occurs with high volume/high lactose/low fat foremilk feedings (Woolridge & Fisher, 1988). Encouraging several same-sided nursings in a row may break the cycle of fussing associated with relative lactose intolerance observed in these breastfeeding situations.

When the infant is unable to gain appropriate weight with direct breastfeeding, supplemental calories can be provided with fortified mother's milk via a supplementation device or other method. Bottlefeeding may facilitate increased caloric intake, as it is not entirely dependent on the child's cooperation. Rarely, a nasogastric (NG) feeding may be needed while fine-tuning medical management strategies to reduce discomfort with oral feedings. Box 19–7 presents interventions that may reduce the frequency and amount of gastroesophageal reflux.

Children with GERD need ongoing monitoring of growth. Breastfeeding does not need to be interrupted, but increased calories may be needed for normal growth. Some infants with GERD are found to have cow's milk protein allergy, thus the breastfeeding mother may be advised to try a dairy elimination diet to assess the effect on the child's symptoms. Occasionally, providers will suggest thickening feedings with cereal. When cereal is added to breastmilk, enzymes break it down very quickly, and it is an ineffective thickening agent. Furthermore, thickened feedings are not found to be effective. The frequency of reflux episodes may be reduced, but exposure of the esophagus to acidic gastric material is increased, probably because thickened gastric contents do not clear as quickly (Bailey et al., 1987). In addition, use of cereal thickened feedings is associated with coughing in infants with GERD (Orenstein, Shalaby, & Putnam, 1992). For the child who is the happy spitter and gaining well, no changes in routine are needed. Parents do need acknowledgement of their concerns, reassur-

---

BOX 19–7

Interventions for the Infant with Symptomatic Gastroesophageal Reflux

- Feed the baby in a more upright position, avoiding abdominal compression.
- Use one breast per feeding to reduce the volume of each feeding and increase access to higher calorie hindmilk.
- Feed more frequently.
- Elevate the bed to a 30 to 45 degree angle. (A baby who is sleeping on the parent's chest is in this position.)
- Avoid placing child in an infant seat or car seat after feedings. This compresses the stomach, increasing reflux episodes.

- Avoid using cereal to thicken feedings, a commonly advised treatment that does not help (Bailey et al., 1987).
- Avoid prone positioning for sleep. Due to the association with increased risk of SIDS, this is not recommended by pediatric gastroenterologists (GER Guidelines Committee, 2001).
- Left-lateral positioning significantly reduces reflux frequency and duration (Tobin et al., 1997; Ewer, James, & Tobin, 1999).

ance regarding how well their baby is doing, and sympathy for the increased laundry load.

Pyloric Stenosis

Pyloric stenosis (PS) is hypertrophy of the pyloric sphincter. It occurs more commonly in males. The relationship of feeding method to the incidence of pyloric stenosis is unclear. Habbick (1989) and Pisacane et al. (1996) found that formula-feeding was significantly more prevalent among infants with pyloric stenosis than among control subjects; however, others have found no relationship to feeding method and incidence of PS (Hitchcock et al., 1987; Lammer & Edmonds, 1987).

Symptoms of progressively more severe projectile vomiting develop at about 4 to 6 weeks of age. The typical clinical picture is of a hyperalert, emaciated baby who nurses, promptly vomits a large amount, and then requests immediate refeeding. Children may have dehydration and electrolyte imbalance if diagnosis and treatment are delayed. During and after a feeding, it is possible to see peristaltic waves that pass from left to right; the experienced examiner can palpate an olive-shaped tumor (the hypertrophic pylorus) in the right upper quadrant of the abdomen. Ultrasound studies confirm the presence of a pyloric mass, and barium studies show the elongated and narrow pyloric canal. Surgery is done after the infant is rehydrated and electrolyte balance is restored with intravenous fluids.

Breastfeeding Implications. Lactation consultants should have PS on their list of concerns for any baby that they see who is struggling with weight gain and is spitting up—remembering there are lots of causes for vomiting in infants in addition to GER. Ad libitum breastfeeding once the child has recovered from anesthesia is safe, decreases length of hospital stay, and saves an average of $400 per patient compared to a more lengthy fasting period with incremental feedings (Garza et al., 2002). Mothers will need to express their milk for the few feeds that are missed during the perioperative period.

Imperforate Anus

Imperforate anus ranges from no opening at all to a normal-appearing rectum that ends in a blind rectal pouch just above the opening. Presence of an imperforate anus is confirmed only by careful examination and by a diagnostic x-ray examination. As with EA/TEF, there is an association of a number of other VACTERL defects. Thus careful examination of the baby is critical to establish the presence of associated anomalies. Depending on the severity of the defect, anal reconstruction may be done in the immediate newborn period. More commonly, a three-step approach is required—colostomy, anal reconstruction, and colostomy reversal (Hendren, 1998). After colostomy placement surgery, feeding can begin as soon as bowel sounds are present—usually within 24 hours. When the colostomy is reversed, enteral feedings are suspended for 4 to 7 days—until nasogastric tube drainage is clear, and the child begins passing gastric secretions from the anus.

Breastfeeding Implications. The baby cannot have enteral feedings until there is either a reconstructed anus or a functioning colostomy. Parenteral nutrition is usually required for a period of time both pre- and postoperatively. Mothers will need to express their milk until the child can have oral feedings. The normally loose stools of the breastfed infant lessen the risk of constipation with subsequent breakdown of the surgical area and local infection.

Metabolic Dysfunction

More than 100 metabolic diseases can be detected in infancy. Diseases for which screening is performed vary from region to region, based in part on ethnic, financial, and political issues. Newborn screening for phenylketonuria and congenital hypothyroidism is done in all 50 US states and in most western countries (Clague & Thomas, 2002). Other metabolic disorders for which screening is commonly performed include galactosemia, amino-acidemias and organic acidemias, and cystic fibrosis. Private companies now make extensive newborn screening available directly to parents. A special filter paper is saturated with the infant's blood and mailed to the service for testing and interpretation. Other acquired metabolic conditions such as diabetes are not screened for in the newborn period and may not become symptomatic until much later in infancy or childhood.

Phenylketonuria

Phenylketonuria (PKU) is an autosomal recessive inherited metabolic disorder of phenylalanine (PHE) metabolism. A defect in the enzyme phenylalanine hydroxylase decreases conversion of phenylalanine to tyrosine. Abnormal metabolites accumulate in blood and tissues, including the brain, interfering with central nervous system development. In order to prevent brain damage, the amount of dietary PHE must be strictly limited, and PHE blood levels are monitored very closely. Current thinking is that it is best to be on a special PKU diet for life. Earlier, the PKU diet was liberalized in early school age, after the period of greatest brain development.

Breastfeeding Implications. Human milk has lower levels of PHE than does any commercial infant formula. Parents of children with PKU will be interested in knowing that infants with PKU who are breastfed have significantly higher intelligence quotient scores—a 12.9-point advantage even after adjusting for social and maternal education status (Riva et al., 1996). Breastfeeding along with supplemental use of PHE-free formula is prescribed. Breastfed infants who receive a daily amount of 362 ml (first month) to 464 ml (fourth month) of breastmilk each day, in addition to supplemental PHE-free formula, have a lower PHE intake than do infants who are fed exclusively on low-PHE formula during their first 6 months of life (McCabe et al., 1989). Thus fluctuations in the volume of breastmilk the baby takes are less worrisome than in formulas with higher PHE levels.

Recommendations for incorporating breastfeeding into a PKU diet include weighing of infants before and after breastfeeding to ensure correct dietary intake, a time-consuming task that may not be accurate. Greve et al. (1994) developed a less cumbersome method of calculating the low-PHE dietary prescription (see Box 19–8). The child's health-care provider uses this information to calculate the daily amount of PHE-free formula that is needed to keep PHE at the appropriate level. The child receives the prescribed amount of PHE-free formula, along with breastfeeding. The PHE-free formula can be provided either via supplementer at the breast or with some other alternative method prior to breastfeeding. A physician and dietician who specialize in metabolic disorders manage the dietary plan for the infant with PKU. In the United States, there is at least one medical center in each state designated to serve as a consultant and treatment facility for metabolic defects, including PKU (Duncan & Elder, 1997).

Women who have PKU should be on a diet prior to conception and throughout the pregnancy to reduce the chances of harming the developing fetus. PHE levels in milk of identical twins with PKU breastfeeding women, and the PHE status of their infants, were reported by Fox-Bacon et al. (1997). They found that high maternal PHE serum levels and high milk PHE levels did not result in abnormal PHE levels in their breastfeeding infants who did not have PKU.

Galactosemia

Galactosemia, a disorder of the metabolism of galactose-1-phosphate that is transmitted as an autosomal-recessive trait, occurs in only one in about every 60,000 to 80,000 births. The liver enzyme that changes galactose to glucose is absent and as a result, the infant is unable to metabolize lactose. Any intake of galactose results in liver dysfunction. These infants appear normal at birth but soon start having feeding difficulties. Other symptoms include vomiting, poor weight gain, jaundice, hepatosplenomegaly, and bleeding. Without treatment, liver failure and mental retardation follow. Untreated galactosemia leads to fatal liver disease. Treatment within the first 10 days of life is associated with the best neurodevelopmental outcomes.

Breastfeeding Implications. Abrupt weaning is necessary due to the galactose content of human milk. Avoidance of all galactose is required to prevent irreversible damage to the infant. Positive newborn screening tests are not always accurate, so results should be confirmed before recommending that women stop expressing milk while waiting confirmation. Nurses and lactation consultants working with babies that have jaundice and poor weight gain need to remember to check newborn screening results as galactosemia as well as congenital hypothyroidism can also cause these symptoms. If the diagnosis is confirmed, the mother will need instruction for relief of engorgement as

BOX 19 –8

Calculating Breastmilk and PHE-Free Formula Intake for the Infant with PKU

Given: Maximum phenylalanine (PHE) intake allowed is 25 to 45 mg/kg/day depending on the age of the infant. Mature breastmilk has .41 mg/ml PHE.

Calculate the amount of PHE-free formula supplementation for the breastfed baby:

1. Find the estimated volume of daily milk intake in ml (110 kcal/kg/day):

   (Infant weight in kg) times 110 = total calories/day

   (Total calories) divided by 20 = total number of oz/day

   (Total number of oz) times 30 = total volume in ml/day

2. Calculate the maximum allowable PHE/day (breastmilk has 0.41 mg PHE/ml):

   45 mg times infant weight in kg = total number of mg PHE allowed

   Total mg divided by .41 = total volume in ml of breastmilk allowed

3. Calculate amount of replacement PHE-free formula required:

   Total daily volume minus maximum volume allowed = amount of replacement feeding needed

Below are the calculations for a 4.0 kg infant:

1. Estimate volume of daily intake in ml:

   110 kcal times 4.0 = 440 calories

   440 divided by 20 = 22 oz

   22 oz times 30 = 660 ml

2. Calculate maximum allowable breastmilk/24 hours:

   45 mg times 4.0 kg = 180 mg PHE maximum per day

   180 times 0.41 = 439 ml of breastmilk

3. Calculate amount of PHE-free replacement feedings needed in order for infant to not drink more breastmilk than allowed:

   660 ml minus 439 ml = 221 ml replacement PHE-free formula required daily

The PHE-free formula can be given via a nursing supplementer during breastfeeds or with a bottle prior to breastfeeding. The total daily amount needed can be divided into several aliquots. For example, the baby above needs about 220 ml/day of PHE-free formula. This could be given in 30 ml aliquots with each breastfeeding for 8 feedings. The PHE-free formula should be offered prior to the breastfeeding, or along with the breastfeeding using a supplementer, rather than being offered after the breastfeeding.

well as emotional support for the loss of the breastfeeding relationship. (See Box 19–9 for A Mother's Guide to Saying Goodbye to Breastfeeding/Milk Expression.)

It is safe for women who have galactosemia to breastfeed. A case study reported that although the mother had galactosemia, her milk was normal in nearly all respects; her baby thrived on ex-

BOX 19–9

A Mother's Guide to Saying Goodbye to Breastfeeding/Milk Expression

- When the time comes to stop breastfeeding or milk expression, you may have very mixed emotions. The following are all normal responses when saying goodbye to breastfeeding.
  - If you are not ready to give up breastfeeding or the hope for a breastfeeding relationship, you may feel regret or sadness.
  - If you are so tired, you may feel a bit glad that the time committed to milk expression is available for other demands.
  - You may be glad to have your body back to yourself, but you may feel guilty that you have those feelings.
  - Your hormones will also be changing, and that may affect your mood.

- As you stop breastfeeding/milk expression, you can express a small amount of milk to make you comfortable. This will keep your breasts from being uncomfortably full, and reduce your risk of developing a breast infection.
- A firm, but not tight, bra may provide comfort.
- Cold compresses may be soothing, and pain medication such as acetaminophen or ibuprofen can provide pain relief if your breasts become uncomfortably engorged.
- If you find yourself feeling unbearably sad, please call on your health-care provider for advice.
- Know that you gave your baby a wonderful gift of love.

clusive breastfeeding for 5 months and continued to breastfeed while receiving solids thereafter (Forbes et al., 1988).

Congenital Hypothyroidism

Congenital hypothyroidism (CH) is caused by a lack of thyroid secretion, either because the thyroid gland is absent or because there is an inborn enzymatic deficiency in the synthesis of thyroxine. Routine screening results show that congenital hypothyroidism occurs in one of every 3500 births (VanVliet, 2001). A transient form of hypothyroidism can occur from transfer *in utero* or during breastfeeding of antithyroid drugs or topical application of povidone-iodine on the mother at the time of delivery (Bartalena et al., 2001; Casteels, Punt, & Bramswig, 2000). Prompt treatment is required to prevent irreversible developmental delay and growth problems. Hypothyroidism is rarely di-

agnosed based on clinical findings in the early weeks—yet this is when the child is most vulnerable to irreversible brain damage. In the early weeks, parents of an untreated infant may praise their "good baby" because he cries so little. Without treatment, the symptoms of hypothyroidism become noticeable in 3 to 6 months: coarse, brittle hair; anemia; a large, protruding tongue; a wide forehead; and lack of skeletal growth. Untreated cases result in severe mental retardation. Treatment for congenital hypothyroidism is daily thyroid replacement for life. Blood levels are monitored periodically to adjust the dose as the child grows. Synthetic levothyroxine sodium (Synthroid or Levothroid) is usually given.

Breastfeeding Implications. Lactation consultants involved with newborns who are jaundiced or not thriving need to make sure that neonatal thyroid screening results are normal—as nonspecific early symptoms of CH may include feeding difficulties and hyperbilirubinemia.

Type I Diabetes

The delayed exposure to cow's milk protein provided with exclusive breastfeeding may reduce incidence of type I diabetes in the at-risk individual (Kimpimaki et al., 2001). It is very unusual for the onset of type I diabetes to occur during infancy. Diabetes management for the infant and toddler is challenging as feeding schedules and activity level are not predictable, and the child is not able to communicate symptoms of low blood glucose to parents or caregivers. This increases the risk of severe hypoglycemia, which could result in coma, seizures, and subsequent learning and behavioral disorders. Target blood sugars are in the range of 100 to 200 mg/dL (5.56 to 11.11 mmol/L). Insulin administration is tailored to the child's feeding schedule—usually given 2 to 4 times per day. Insulin doses are quite low and can be difficult to measure precisely. Litton et al. (2002) reported the effective use of insulin pumps in the diabetic management of toddlers. The children had improved hemoglobin A_{1c} levels, and fewer episodes of hypoglycemia, and parents felt much more confident in their ability to manage their child's diabetes.

Breastfeeding Implications. No research has been found that discusses breastfeeding and management of the infant with diabetes; however, the most important considerations for insulin dosing would be estimating the quantity of breastmilk the baby is taking. Night-time breastfeedings and demand breastfeedings are difficult to measure. Newer rapid-acting insulin can be given after feedings (contrary to the usual method of giving insulin prior to feedings), which facilitates incorporating breastfeeding into the diabetes management plan. If the health-care team finds it critical to quantify the amount of breastmilk ingested per feeding in order to develop a treatment plan, the child could be weighed before and after feedings for a day or two using a rented scale. This would assist in estimating the contribution of breastmilk to the child's total caloric intake, as well as to quantify carbohydrate, fat, and protein points. Another way to make sure the milk is measured is to have the mother pump and give the breastmilk via a

bottle or other feeding device. Weaning is usually not advised because of the additional stress it imposes on the baby and the mother.

Celiac Disease

Celiac disease, often called malabsorption syndrome or gluten enteropathy, is characterized by changes in the intestinal mucosa or villi that prevent the absorption of foods, mainly fat. The mucosal damage appears to stem from a sensitivity to gliadin, the protein fraction of gluten found in wheat, rye, barley, and other grains. Celiac disease is thought to be a genetic disorder causing either an inborn error of metabolism or an immune system disorder. Formula-feeding and the early introduction of solids accelerate the appearance of symptoms of celiac disease (Greco et al., 1988; Kelly et al., 1989; Hernell, Ivaarsson, & Persson, 2001; Peters et al., 2001). This may explain why the incidence of celiac disease has declined in the United States as breastfeeding rates have risen and solids are introduced later. The infant with this disorder is asymptomatic until solids containing gluten are introduced into the diet. Clinical symptoms are insidious and chronic. Because fat is not absorbed, the child's stools become frothy appearing, foul smelling, and excessive. Deficiencies of the fat-soluble vitamins (A, D, K, and E) appear. If the disease progresses without treatment, abdominal distension and general wasting are evident. The affected child's diet must be modified and vigorously maintained to exclude gluten, thus improving food absorption and preventing malnutrition.

Breastfeeding Implications. Primary prevention is family teaching and encouraging women with a family history of this disease to breastfeed for a long period and to delay introduction of solid foods.

Cystic Fibrosis

Cystic fibrosis (CF) is a genetic disorder caused by a defect in a single gene on chromosome 7. This leads to abnormalities in the apical membrane of epithelial cells that line the airways, biliary tree, intestines, vas deferens, sweat ducts, and pancreatic ducts. Secretions of these sites become more viscid and obstruct ducts, leading to dysfunction at the organ level. The exocrine glands of the affected child produce abnormally thick and sticky secretions that block the flow of pancreatic digestive enzymes, clog hepatic ducts, and impede the movement of cilia in the lungs. The increased sodium chloride in the child's sweat provides an important diagnostic clue: the family reports that the child tastes salty when kissed. In the newborn, CF may present as a meconium ileus (intestinal obstruction caused by a plug of meconium). Signs of intestinal obstruction include abdominal distention, vomiting, and failure to pass stools. This is a surgical emergency. At birth, about half of the affected children are already pancreatic insufficient. Nutrient absorption—particularly of fat-soluble vitamins—is thus impaired from the beginning. Because of problems with fat absorption, the infant fails to gain weight, despite reports of a voracious appetite. When solid foods are introduced, the stools become bulky, more frequent, foul smelling, and frothy. Pulmonary complications are almost always present, and the child often suffers persistent, severe respiratory infections because of inability to clear thick secretions.

Prevention of respiratory complications and malnutrition are the mainstay of management for the child with CF. Protection from and aggressive treatment for respiratory infection is accomplished by airway clearance procedures (postural drainage and percussion, chest vest, and others), aerosol therapy, and medications, such as bronchodilators, inhaled corticosteroids, and antibiotics. The use of aerosolized recombinant human DNase to decrease the viscosity of secretions has been a breakthrough in CF treatment (Jackson & Vessey, 1996).

Breastfeeding Implications. Breastfeeding offers many special advantages to children with CF. The protection from infection as well as the easy digestibility of breastmilk are particularly important for this high-risk group. Children with CF who were exclusively breastfed were found to be taller and heavier than those who were exclusively formula-fed (Holliday et al., 1991). A survey of CF centers in the United States found that most of them recommended breastfeeding alone or combined with pancreatic enzyme supplement or hydrolyzed formula (Luder et al., 1990). Babies with CF produce normal levels of gastric lipase, which is a major digestive enzyme. This enzyme, together with milk lipase in breastmilk, may help the infant

with CF to absorb fat more efficiently. Human milk contains appreciably greater amounts of lipase than cow's milk. Rooney (1988) suggested that some breastfed infants with CF developed symptoms only after breastfeeding stopped.

Nutrition management includes promoting breastfeeding, providing fat-soluble vitamin supplements, and prescribing pancreatic enzyme replacement (Pancrease) (Koletzko & Reinhardt, 2001). The enzyme microspheres are mixed in a tiny amount of applesauce. The enzyme dose is based on estimated fat intake, not abdominal symptoms such as bloating or cramping, or on weight of the infant (Anthony et al., 1999). Because salt content in the infant diet is very low, salt supplementation may be recommended. For breastfed children, this is especially important during hot weather or periods of increased fluid losses (diarrheal illness, fever). If the child is not gaining weight well, or presents with failure to thrive at the time of late diagnosis, calorie supplementation may be needed. Extra calories may be added in a number of different ways—for example, with glucose polymers or fat added to breastmilk. The child's medical provider will ensure that enzyme replacement dose is sufficient. Other comorbid problems such as GERD, or cow's milk protein allergy, among others may also interfere with weight gain.

Allergies

The issue of the preventive nature of breastfeeding for allergic disease continues to be controversial. At present, there is no consensus about whether breastfeeding protects against the development of asthma and allergy. There are studies documenting that breastfeeding reduces risk, ameliorates severity, or delays onset of atopic conditions (Bloch et al., 2002; Chandra, 1997b; Saarinen & Kajosaari, 1995). However there are also those finding that breastfeeding either has no effect on risk, or even increases risk (Bergmann et al., 2002; Sears et al., 2002). As with many health-care issues, the data at this time are unclear.

Allergic disease is multifactorial, depending on family history, sensitization, and triggers. Family history has the best predictive value for identifying at-risk neonates who should be targeted for allergy prevention (Zeiger, 2000). The atopy prone infant is at increased risk to sensitization to allergens prior to birth, and early after birth. Antigen exposure is evident as early as the 22nd week of gestation (Jones et al., 1996).

Food allergy is generally defined as an adverse reaction to a foreign substance or antigen accompanied by immunological changes, notably a rise in IgE. It occurs in about 4 to 6 percent of children (Zieger, 2000). As shown in Table 19–3, the most common offending foods in the United States are cow's milk, peanuts, nuts, chicken eggs, soy, and fish (Zieger, 2000). The initial exposure is sensitization, which does not usually result in allergic symptoms. With a subsequent exposure, however, allergic symptoms may become evident. This distinction helps to make it clear why a baby given a routine cow's milk formula in the hospital may not experience a reaction until the next exposure several days or weeks later. If the mother is not informed that supplement was given in the nursery, she may not recognize that a sensitizing event occurred. This is one reason why parents must be asked for permission before any supplementation is given to their baby.

Breastfeeding Implications. When someone asks if an infant can be allergic to breastmilk, the answer is "Yes." Proteins of ingested foods pass into the breastmilk, where they may trigger an allergic response in the at-risk child who has been sensitized. Antigens in human milk have been detected for peanuts, beta-lactoalbumin, and ovoalbumin (Casas et al., 2000; Vadas et al., 2001). Furthermore, there can be cross-reactivity between cow's milk and human milk proteins (Bernard et al., 2000). The amount of allergen needed to sensitize or trigger symptoms is minute. For bovine b-lactoalbumin, only 1 ng (that's 1 nanogram, which is one billionth of a gram!) is required for sensitization. The amount of bovine b-lactoalbumin in mother's milk ranges from 0.5 to 32 ng/L. A 40 ml feeding of cow's milk formula contains bovine b-lactoalbumin in the equivalent to the amount found in 21 years of breastfeeding (Businco, Bruno, & Giampietro, 1999).

The list of symptoms caused by food allergy is long: vomiting, diarrhea, colic, colitis, bloody stools (hematochezia), eczema, urticaria, rhinitis, fussiness, and poor sleep patterns are among them. Some exclusively breastfed infants develop allergic

Table 19–3

SELECTED SOURCES OF ALLERGENIC FOODS THAT MAY AFFECT THE NURSLING

Food*	Sources
Cow's milk in any form	Butter, bread, pudding, yogurt, cheese, baked goods, sherbet, ice cream, creamed soups, powdered-milk drinks, gravies, casein or whey used as additives
Eggs	Baked goods, custard, French toast, root beer, mayonnaise, breaded foods, some cake icings, meatloaf, noodles
Wheat	Bread, baked goods with wheat flour, pasta, hot dogs, bologna, some canned soups, some puddings and gravies, textured vegetable protein
Peanuts, legumes	Peanut butter, beans, peas, lentils as well as foods containing soy protein, soy flour, or oil
Nuts, kola nut	Candy, granola, baked goods, chocolate, cocoa, cola beverages
Corn	Cereal, chips, Cracker Jacks, corn tortillas and other Mexican foods with corn masa, popcorn, cornstarch, cornmeal
Fish, shell fish	Fish sticks, appetizers
Citrus fruits	Orange, lemon, lime, grapefruit, fruit deserts, fruit punch, sorbet
Tomatoes	Ketchup, tomato juice, meatloaf, stew or other mixed dishes, spaghetti sauce, pizza sauce

This is not an exhaustive list of foods containing allergens. Patients need to be provided with detailed written information to allow them to avoid a particular allergen.

symptoms following exposure to cow's milk or other proteins because they have been sensitized to them transplacentally, through inadvertent exposure via supplementation, or through their own mother's milk (Fukushima et al., 1997). Individual infants may respond differently to allergenic foods. From the same food one infant may develop diarrhea, colic, or other GI complaints; another may have a central nervous system response, becoming irritable or hyperactive; while a third may have dermatological symptoms, such as urticaria or eczema.

Cow's milk protein allergy is the most common food allergy during infancy. Two studies have reported a series of children with proctocolitis during exclusive breastfeeding, which resolved within 48 to 72 hours with maternal dietary exclusion of cow's milk protein (Patenaude et al., 2000; Pumberger, Pomberger, & Geissler, 2001). When a child's symptoms are suspected to be due to allergies, maternal elimination diets may be prescribed. If the offending food has been eliminated, symptoms should improve within 48 to 72 hours, though some recommend a full 2-week elimination trial (Mohrbacher & Stock, 2003).

Clinicians approach this problem in a variety of ways. One is to have the mother begin an extreme diet, eliminating a list of common offenders. Food groups can then be reintroduced one at a time, from the least likely suspect to the most suspect food group. Others will have the mother begin with a more "simple" elimination diet (no elimination diet is really simple) of omitting all dairy products, as that is the most common offending food group. If the elimination diet is to be of any value, it has to be carefully followed and clearly spelled out: written instructions are the most helpful, and scrupulous reading of labels on packaged foods helps to avoid inadvertent consumption of foods that should be eliminated. Especially if several foods are contributing to the baby's adverse reaction, the mother may find food-elimination plans difficult to implement (de Boissieu et al., 1997). It is necessary in some cases to remove all dairy foods. The difficulty of following an elimination diet is described by a mother whose son developed eczema while she was exclusively breastfeeding (Sutin, 1988):

I stopped drinking milk and expected instant miracles, but nothing changed. I cut cheese and yogurt out of my diet and still saw no improvement. Eventually, I had to eliminate all dairy products as well as products containing even trace amounts of milk. Then I could see the improvement.

Repucci (1999) and Schach and Haight (2002) report success of a novel approach to helping the allergic breastfeeding dyad when the child's symptoms do not resolve with maternal elimination diets. Mothers of infants with severe bloody stools due to allergic colitis were prescribed Pancrease MT4, digestive enzymes normally used in the treatment of cystic fibrosis for improving breakdown of foods in the gastrointestinal tract. With more thorough food digestion, fewer intact proteins would be available to enter the mother's milk. In these two reports, colitis symptoms in the infants resolved in most of the treated dyads.

Occasionally, the health-care provider recommends that the child interrupt breastfeeding, substituting a hypoallergenic formula for a short or long period of time to relieve severe symptoms (severe colic, significant gastrointestinal bleeding, severe eczema) before reintroducing breastfeeding. Soy-based formulas are not appropriate breastmilk substitutes for the atopic child.

To prevent or reduce severity of atopic conditions for infants with family history of allergies and asthma, it is recommended that the mother do the following:

- Avoid the allergen beginning prior to the 22nd week of gestation.
- Continue to avoid maternal allergen during breastfeeding.
- Exclusively breastfeed until about 6 months.
- Continue breastfeeding with cautious introduction of complimentary foods thereafter (Fergusson & Horwood, 1994).

Common offenders (see again Table 19–3) should be avoided if possible during the first year of life. If the mother removes dairy products and other foods from her diet, she must take sufficient calcium from other foods or from calcium supplements, and monitor her nutritional status (Holmberg-Marttila et al., 2001).

Food Intolerance

Most children do not care at all what their mothers eat or drink. This is why it is not necessary to provide mothers with a list of foods to avoid. However the occasional child may have a consistent uncomfortable response to the food ingested by the mother. Children who do not tolerate specific foods, but do not have true allergic responses, may have similar gastrointestinal and dermatologic symptoms. Chandra (1997a) describes common causes of nonallergic adverse reactions to foods: (1) gastrointestinal symptoms due to reduced activity of lactase (lactose intolerance); (2) vasoactive responses to amines in foods causing urticaria, angioedema, difficulty in swallowing, wheezing, and migraine; (3) toxins and food additives causing urticaria and other symptoms; and (4) foods such as prunes or onions that may cause local gastrointestinal irritation when consumed in large amounts.

Typical offenders according to retrospective maternal reports include chocolate, onion, and cruciferous vegetables such as broccoli or cauliflower (Lust et al., 1996). Some babies are sensitive to caffeine and become irritable when their mothers drink too much. Mothers can be instructed to titrate their caffeine intake to their baby's behavior. If a mother notes that her baby is always excessively cranky after she has a huge serving of chocolate cake, then she can decide to reduce the size of the portion next time and see if the baby is happier.

Lactose Intolerance

Fortunately, primary lactase deficiency is a rare problem in infancy as lactose is the carbohydrate in human milk. Humans normally produce sufficient lactase for lactose digestion until childhood, when selected populations begin to have problems with insufficiency. However, infants may experience symptoms related to secondary lactase deficiency following gastrointestinal illness or antibiotic use, or as a result of feeding mismanagement. Symptoms of lactose intolerance include escalating fussiness, excessive gassiness, and bright green, irritating, slimy stools.

Woolridge and Fisher (1988) describe very clearly the problem of colicky symptoms and feeding mismanagement. When mothers rather than babies control the child's time at the breast, the child may receive high volume, low fat feedings that result in a higher than normal lactose load for the baby to digest. When a baby is allowed to nurse as long as desired on the first breast before being moved to the second, the feeding is more likely to have the appropriate balance of volume, fat, and lactose. Following gastrointestinal illness, or antibiotic administration, the brush border of the gastrointestinal tract where lactase is located may be damaged, leading to transient lactose intolerance.

Psychosocial Concerns

Anytime families face the unexpected with their children, the myriad of feelings and concerns that bombard them can be overwhelming. Nurses have an absolutely instrumental role in supporting a family's adaptation to whatever is facing them. Each family differs in their response to the birth of a child with a defect or who is diagnosed with a serious or chronic illness, and each will need support from their health-care team. It is important for professionals to have a working knowledge of crisis and grief theories to support their clinical work with families.

Family Stress

All parents of ill children are under stress, but consider the effects of stress on a parent who must deal with it over many months and perhaps years when a child has a chronic health problem, such as the family described here:

Driving to the hospital and back from their home 100 or more miles away, so as to alternate staying with their sick infant, a breastfeeding mother and her husband try to cope. With three other children at home, they can snatch only a few hours of sleep at a time. It is the third surgical procedure for their infant, who was born with a congenital defect. Although their physician encourages them with the news that the prognosis is good, the worry and strain seem endless. The mother expresses her milk with a pump when necessary, and her baby is able to breastfeed part of the time. Lately she has been able to express only a few drops at a time, and she wonders how long she will be able to continue lactating.

The first response of parents whose children are diagnosed with a chronic illness is shock. This initial disorganization and upheaval does not last long, however. At some point after the diagnosis, the family begins to pull together their resources and develop a support system. Although for many parents their child's diagnosis is the worst problem they have ever faced, they are able to make many adjustments in a short period of time. With support, most families are able to develop adaptive coping mechanisms.

Issues that challenge families include financial concerns, caretaking, fatigue, depression, altered family image, and goal diffusion. However, these stresses are not fixed or predictable (Burke et al., 1998). Reframing these burdens as tasks that need to be mastered can give families direction to take rather than seeing themselves as victims (Burke et al., 1999). The degree of stress may relate more to issues of social support rather than to the specific health problem that the child faces (Smith, Oliver, & Innocenti, 2001; Visconti et al., 2002). Pelchat et al. (1999) compared parents of children with congenital heart disease, Down syndrome, cleft lip and palate, and children without disabilities. They discovered that parents with Down syndrome and congenital heart disease reported higher levels of parenting and psychological stress and that parents of babies with cleft lip and palate and nondisabled children had lower stress levels.

Stress affects all of the child's caregivers and family—mother, father, sister, brother, and others. Each may react differently to unexpected changes in their lives. During the child's illness, attention is often focused primarily on the mother and the ill child. When the mother is breastfeeding a hospitalized child, she most likely will be the one spending most of the time at the bedside. While a child is in the hospital, the father must pick up the responsibility for caring for the household, perhaps while continuing to work full-time, as well as nurturing the ill child and mother; he is expected to be the Rock of Gibraltar, an anchor in a sea of distress.

These stresses may affect the partners' bond. The divorce rate in families with a child born with a neural-tube defect was nine times greater than the divorce rate for the normal population (Tew et al., 1977). When a sick child becomes the focus of a mother's attention, other relationships and responsibilities become secondary. Some men sensing this withdraw emotionally until the crisis is over. Yet, for other couples, their mutual concern causes them to grow closer and draw emotional support from each other. Some parents feel guilty about making love while their child lies ill. If it seems appropriate, point out that sexual enjoyment reinforces their relationship.

The family's response to a chronic illness involves not so much the event itself as it does a particular family's definition or perception of the event as well as the family's resources—social, financial, and emotional—to help them cope. A family with no health insurance and little or no savings may perceive their child's chronic illness as more stressful than would a family with health insurance, sufficient income, and savings on which to draw if necessary. Unreasonable as such feelings may be, both parents may harbor feelings of guilt for bringing on the illness or for not recognizing how sick the child was in early stages. Such questions as "What have I done?" or "What should I have done?" torment them. It may be easier for the breastfeeding mother, who continues to have close contact with her child to deal with these feelings than it is for the father. Picking up cues about the father's feelings and encouraging him to talk about them helps; it also provides the opportunity to reassure him that his feelings are normal. The therapeutic value of "talking it out" reduces stress (Foster, 1974). Hearing their own statements aloud releases the parents' tension and speeds resolution of their inner conflicts.

Hospitalization brings about a disruption of lifestyle and environment to the family and is tantamount to culture shock. A barrage of unfamiliar stimuli is thrust on them: infusion pumps that periodically sound an alarm, mist tents, and a constantly rotating staff of new faces all place tremendous stress on the family. Normally affable people can become demanding and even hostile as a by-product of their stress and guilt, and perceived or actual unmet needs. These defensive behaviors are part of the parents' coping strategies for managing their feelings and help to protect families from painful realities. They are not necessarily maladaptive. Although it can be difficult and even painful to deal with such parents, it is far preferable to work with these concerned parents than with those who are unconcerned or passive. Sympathetic listening and simple, understanding statements, such as "I can see you are upset," or "This is such a difficult time," can help parents through this trying time. If hospital nurses rationally assess parents' behaviors and use of defenses, their interactions with parents will be more therapeutic.

Parents who are many miles from home during their child's hospitalization must arrange for sleeping accommodations in the area if both are not allowed to stay overnight at the hospital. Fortunately, many cities now have Ronald McDonald Houses that shelter these families. Support groups of other parents experiencing a similar life crisis are effective, because each person in the group understands the day-to-day issues and problems of caring for an ill child or rearing one with a chronic disease. Nevertheless, support groups are not for all parents; some are so overwhelmed by their own problems that they are not able to reach out and support others.

Coping with Siblings

Siblings are often the forgotten members of the family when attention and concern is focused on the sick child. The concept of family-centered care extends to every person in the family, including the children at home, who frequently react to their brother's or sister's illness with anger, resentment, jealousy, and guilt. The situation is especially difficult when an older child is hospitalized and a younger breastfeeding baby or toddler is at home. The mother is emotionally torn between being with her sick child and attending her breastfeeding baby, who so obviously needs her. If the baby is one of breastfeeding twins or if the mother is breastfeeding both a walking child and a baby, the problem is further compounded. Most hospitals encourage siblings (who are not infectious) to visit their brother or sister in the hospital. Institutions that do not do so may add to the family's stress by enforcing isolation when contact would be most beneficial to all parties. When the ill child is at home, siblings may bear additional responsibilities of child care or helping with household tasks.

Chronic Grief and Loss

When the breastfeeding child is chronically ill or has a disabling defect, the disappointment, sorrow, and frustration of parents can be overwhelming. Instead of the perfect child expected during the pregnancy, there is an intense feeling of loss. If the child requires indefinite special care and attention, there is a persistent effect described in Olshansky's classic work, *Chronic Sorrow* (1962). Unlike acute grief, which is limited in time, chronic sorrow is prolonged and recurrent. Through grieving, coping processes evolve, and parents can find satisfaction and joy from their child: "The shock and numbness linger for days, even months. . . . It is only after you have gotten over that first crisis that you begin to realize a life and soul have been given into your care" (Good, 1980). The onset of chronic sorrow is variable among families and sometimes difficult to identify; however, this condition is a natural outgrowth of parenting and is an adaptive response.

Breastfeeding has an ameliorating effect for both the child and the parents when chronic illness is involved. The baby receives added protection from infection and also benefits from close contact and stimulation. The mother of a breastfed baby has the satisfaction of giving something special to her child, which helps her deal with her feelings of loss.

The Magic-Milk Syndrome

In the process of grieving over their child's special needs, parents move through several stages of adjustment. After the initial shock and emotional numbness, they reach a stage characterized by rationalization, denial, and sometimes a search for a magic cure. If the baby is not being breastfed, some desperate parents will search for donated breastmilk, hoping that it will help or cure their child. The unique properties of breastmilk are so well known that it is sometimes perceived by parents to contain magic properties. The health-care provider needs to validate the value of human milk while helping the parents to recognize that their baby may need more than breastmilk can offer. In some cases, breastmilk may in fact be therapeutic. For example, children with allergies and metabolic disorders may respond well to breastmilk feedings (see the discussion of donor milk in Chapter 14). In a situation in which the need is real and substantiated by medical opinion, the child can receive breastmilk from a human milk bank.

The Empty Cradle . . . When a Child Dies

Parents must face the tremendous task of coping and somehow continuing with life when their child dies. The first reactions of shock, disbelief, and denial are all the more intense when the death is unexpected. Parents need to be able to express their feelings by crying, yelling, or quietly talking about how they feel. Compassionate care assists closure after death. Giving the parents the opportunity to hold their child and to say goodbye helps this process. Afraid at first, the members of one family changed their minds and cradled their dead baby in their arms. "Holding him is what helped us most to accept the death of our baby; it made us feel he was really our own. He smelled sweet and felt soft, and we just stroked him and talked with him for a while."

Fathers and mothers grieve differently and have their own ways of coping with grief (Wallerstedt & Higgins, 1996). These differences are called incongruent grief and result from societal expectations based on gender; whereas the father may not grieve openly, the mother may be more emotional (Klaus & Kennell, 1982). Moreover, the focus of concern often falls on the mother. The father, who has had a significant, loving relationship with his child, is sometimes forgotten. The cultural stereotype of male stoicism belies his feelings of shock, grief, and pain. Fathers also need to grieve, but their response is affected by what is perceived as their responsibilities, such as informing family and friends of the child's death and making funeral arrangements. As the shock subsides, acute mourning and bereavement are followed by a developing awareness of the full impact of their loss. Parents may feel less than whole, that they have lost a part of themselves. Guilt, silent or expressed, is an almost universal emotion during this period. Questioning the health professional about the possible effects of heredity on the disease is likely as their grief turns inward in the form of self-blame. Explanations of hereditary factors must be honest and factual, tempered with an understanding of what the parents are able to accept.

Physical symptoms, such as sleeplessness or a lack of appetite, often accompany the parents' feelings of loss and pain. Some parents describe feeling "dead inside" or having a "hole inside that nothing can fill." The breastfeeding mother may have to cope with the physical discomfort of breast fullness and leaking for a while and needs advice for management of involution (see again Box 19–9). Occasionally, a mother will continue to pump her milk for several weeks, donating it to a milk bank so that other children may benefit from it. Doing so is her way of coping by maintaining visible evidence of the existence of the lost child. When she offers to do so, the best approach is to put her in touch with a milk bank whose staff members can assist her.

For many parents, the peer support system that previously helped them in parenting and breastfeeding changes its significance; seeing other breastfeeding mothers and their babies may be a painful ordeal. The mother may assiduously avoid them, choosing only one or two especially close peers with whom she can privately talk about her feelings and emotional pain.

Caring for Bereaved Families

When an infant dies, memories that tie the parents to the child must be relived before they can be put aside. Especially important to them is the acknowledgment that their child was special: they should never be denied the right to their sorrow. Remarks such as "It just wasn't meant to be," or "You can always have another baby," are hurtful. They provide no consolation whatsoever regarding the loss of this baby. Statements such as "I'm sorry about your baby," or "If you want to talk, call me," are consoling and show sensitivity. The following suggestions for health-care providers who are assisting parents and families through the grief process are based on the authors' experiences as well as those of other health-care professionals:

- Call the baby by name.
- If the mother was lactating, help her to remain comfortable. Mothers who lose a baby after 20 weeks of gestation may become engorged. This sometimes comes as a complete shock. Often, women are reluctant to relieve their discomfort by expressing milk for fear of stimulating more milk (see again Box 19–9).
- Help parents anticipate how to share the bad news with other children and family members.

- Refer the parents to bereavement support groups such as AMEND (Aiding Mothers and Fathers Experiencing Neonatal Death).

- Acknowledge the parents' loss by sending cards or calling. If you do not know the parents well, anything more may be too much.

- Attend the funeral if it seems like the right thing to do.

- Call the family several weeks after the death to check in on them. After the immediate flurry at the time of death, many people are now ready for a listening ear, and most will then have a list of questions about what happened to their baby. Encourage them to have a follow-up appointment with their baby's primary provider to clear up these questions or concerns when they feel ready.

- Allow the parents to verbalize feelings of anger, fear, guilt, and anxiety by validating them.

- Feel your way through the conversation, getting feedback from the parent; wait for him or her to lead the way. Most parents appreciate a chance to talk about their baby and their experience with someone who will understand. Ensure that they know you are available to talk whenever needed.

Families very much appreciate contact with their child's health-care team after the death. It affirms for them that people really cared about their family and their beloved child.

Summary

There are unique considerations for helping the breastfeeding family when their infant or young child has special health-care needs or illness. These special needs can be met by recognizing the developmental stage, assessing family lifestyle, reducing parental stress, involving parents in direct care of their child, and most of all, minimizing separation between family members. Discontinuing breastfeeding is rarely necessary for the child with a health problem. However, feeding patterns may need to be modified. Too often, weaning from the breast is assumed to be necessary. This is rarely the case.

Each family is unique. The experience of one situation can never be duplicated; therefore, care providers helping families must be versatile and have solid knowledge about the nature of the health problem so that the best possible care can be provided. Competent care, and then compassionate care, are the top priorities (compassion without competence is a disservice to the family).

If the child dies, understanding the impact of the parents' grief and their coping styles requires a special sensitivity, along with the crisis-intervention skills needed to help support a family. Informing the parents about every aspect of the health problem, including them in decision making, and developing a working relationship between the health-care team members and the family is what creates mutual respect and allows for effective problem management.

Key Concepts

- The health, nutrition, and growth of the infant with special health-care needs are of primary concern.

- Breastfeeding may be adversely affected when a child is ill or has special health-care needs.

- Infants with certain special health-care needs may not thrive on only direct breastfeeding.

- Babies and their mothers can often experience a better breastfeeding experience with the help of competent nurses and lactation consultants.

- Supplementation and alternative feeding methods may be needed to provide optimal nutrition in selected situations.

- The use of adaptive devices and positioning techniques can maximize breastfeeding effectiveness.

- The milk supply can be maintained/supported until the child is able to breastfeed directly, or for as long as is necessary.
- Direct breastfeeding rarely requires suspension or cessation.
- Galactosemia is the only condition requiring complete cessation of human milk feeding.
- With phenylketonuria, human milk can be part of the PKU diet.
- Families who have a child with special health-care needs face many stressful issues and may be chronically grieving for the loss of the healthy baby they dreamed of.
- The loss of a "normal" breastfeeding experience may add to family stress.
- The breastfeeding mother whose child has died requires sensitive support.
- Breastfeeding-friendly pediatric hospital units can ease the unique stresses of the breastfeeding family.

Internet Resources

Birth Defects Foundation (support for families affected by congenital conditions):
www.birthdefects.co.uk

Exceptional Parent (publishers of magazine and resource guide for children with special health care needs):
www.eparent.com

International Birth Defects Information System (information and support about congenital problems in multiple languages):
ibis-birthdefects.org

March of Dimes Birth Defects Foundation (information and support about birth defects):
www.modimes.org

MOBI (support and advice for women who are/were unable to breastfeed, feel unsuccessful in breastfeeding, are/were experiencing severe breastfeeding problems, or experienced untimely weaning):
www.internetbabies.com/mobi

Mothers United for Moral Support (information and support for parenting children with special needs):
www.netnet.net/mums

National Organization for Rare Disorders (information for families and professionals):
www.rarediseases.org

Allergies

Milks Soy Protein Intolerance Guide (information on maternal dietary restriction for babies with milk and soy protein allergies, ordering information for cookbook for MSP restricted diets):
www.mspiguide.org

Celiac Disease

Celiac Disease Foundation:
www.celiac.org

Celiac Sprue Association (family support and information):
www.csaceliacs.org

Congenital Heart Disease

American Heart Association:
www.americanheart.org

Diabetes Mellitus

American Diabetes Association (information and support):
www.diabetes.org

Down Syndrome

National Association for Down Syndrome (parent support and information):
www.nads.org

National Down Syndrome Congress (parent support):
www.ndsccenter.org

National Down Syndrome Society (parent support and information):
www.ndss.org

Gastroesophageal Reflux

Esophageal Atresia / Tracheoesophageal Fistula (child and family support connection):
www.eatef.org

International Association of Reflux Parents ("The GERD WORD"):
www.geocities.com/HotSprings/Villa/2193

International Foundation for Gastrointestinal Disorders (about kids' GI disorders):
www.aboutkidsgi.org

PAGER (Pediatric and Adolescent Gastroesophageal Reflux Association):
www.reflux.org

Metabolic Problems

Children Living with Inherited Metabolic Disease:
www.climb.org.uk

Parents of Galactosemic Children (parent information and support):
www.galactosemia.org

Neural-Tube Defects

National Hydrocephalus Foundation (information and support):
www.hydroassoc.org

Spina Bifida Association of America (information and support):
www.sbaa.org

Oral-Facial Anomalies

Cleft Palate Foundation (information for families and professionals):
www.cleftline.org

FACES (support group of the National Craniofacial Association):
www.faces-cranio.org

Pierre Robin Network (connects families of children with Pierre Robin sequence):
www.pierrerobin.org

Wide Smiles (parent-to-parent support):
www.widesmiles.org

REFERENCES

American Society of Anesthesiologists. Practice guidelines for preoperative fasting and the use of pharmacologic agents to reduce the risk of pulmonary aspiration: application to healthy patients undergoing elective procedure—a report by the American Society of Anesthesiologists. Task Force on Preoperative Fasting. *Anesthesiology* 90(3):896–905, 1999.

Aniansson B et al. Prospective cohort study on breast-feeding and otitis media in Swedish infants. *Pediatr Infect Dis J* 13:183–88, 1994.

Aniansson G et al. Otitis media with breast milk of children with cleft palate. *Scand J Plast Reconstr Surg Hand Surg* 36(1):9–15, 2002.

Anthony H et al. Pancreatic enzyme replacement therapy in cystic fibrosis: Australian guidelines. *J Paediatr Child Health* 35:125–29, 1999.

Armon K et al. An evidence- and consensus-based guideline for acute diarrhoea management. *Arch Dis Child* 85:132–42, 2001.

Arnold L. *Recommendations for collection, storage and handling of a mother's milk for her own infant in the hospital setting.* 3rd ed. Sandwich, MA: Human Milk Banking Association of North America, 1999.

Auerbach K. Last resort help-seeking and breastfeeding failure. *J Hum Lact* 9(2):73–74, 1993.

Aumonier ME, Cunningham CC. Breastfeeding in infants with Down's syndrome. *Child Care Health Dev* 9:247–55, 1983.

Bailey DJ et al. Lack of efficacy of thickened feeding as treatment for gastroesophageal reflux. *J Pediatr* 110:187–89, 1987.

Bartalena L et al. Effects of amiodarone administration during pregnancy on neonatal thyroid function and subsequent neurodevelopment. *J Endocrinol Invest* 24(2):116–30, 2001.

Baudon JJ et al. Motor dysfunction of the upper digestive tract in Pierre Robin sequence as assessed by sucking-swallowing electromyography and esophageal manometry. *J Pediatr* 140:719–23, 2002.

Baujat G et al. Oroesophageal motor disorders in Pierre Robin syndrome. *JPGN* 32:297–302, 2001.

Beaudry M, Dufour R, Marcoux S. Relation between infant feeding and infections during the first six months of life. *J Pediatr* 126:191–97, 1995.

Bergmann RL et al. Breastfeeding is a risk factor for atopic eczema. *Clin Exp All* 32:205–9, 2002.

Bernard H et al. Molecular basis of IgE cross-reactivity between human beta-casein and bovine beta-casein, a major allergy in milk. *Mol Immunol* 37:161–67, 2000.

Bloch AM et al. Does breastfeeding protect against allergic rhinitis during childhood? A meta-analysis of prospective studies. *Actae Paediatr* 91:275–79, 2002.

Boctor DL, Pillo-Blocka F, McCrindle BW. Nutrition after cardiac surgery for infants with congenital heart disease. *Nutr Clin Pract* 14:111–15, 1999.

Bodley V, Powers D. Long-term nipple shield use—a positive perspective. *J Hum Lact* 12(4):301–4, 1996.

Bovey A, Noble R, Noble M. Orofacial exercises for babies with breastfeeding problems? *Breastfeed Rev* 7(1):23–28, 1999.

Brigham M. Mothers' reports of the outcome of nipple shield use. *J Hum Lact* 12(4):291–97, 1996.

Bruner JP et al. Fetal surgery for myelomeningocele and the incidence of shunt dependent hydrocephalus. *JAMA* 282(19):1819–25, 1999.

Burke SO et al. Stressors in families with a child with a chronic condition: an analysis of qualitative studies and a framework. *Canad J Nursing Reseach* 30:71–95, 1998.

———. Assessment of stressors in families with a child who has a chronic condition. *MCH* 24:98–106, 1999.

Businco L, Bruno G, Giampietro PG. Prevention and management of food allergy. *Acta Paediatr Suppl* 88 (430):104–9, 1999.

Casas R et al. Detection of IgA antibodies to cat, beta-lactoalbumin and ovoalbumin antigens in human milk. *J Allergy Clin Immunol* 105:1236–40, 2000.

Casteels K, Punt S, Bramswig J. Transient neonatal hypothyroidism during breastfeeding after post-natal maternal topical iodine treatment. *Eur J Pediatrics* 159(9):716–17, 2000.

Chandra RK. Food hypersensitivity and allergic disease: a selective review. *Am J Clin Nutr* 66:526S–29S, 1997a.

———Five-year follow-up of high-risk infants with family history of allergy who were exclusively beast-fed or fed partial whey hydrolysate, soy, and conventional cow's milk formulas. *J Pediatr Gastroenterol Nutr* 24(4):380–88, 1997b.

Clague A, Thomas A. Neonatal biochemical screening for disease. *Clin Chim Acta* 315(1–2):99–110, 2002.

Cohen M. Immediate unrestricted feeding of infants following cleft lip and palate repair. *Br J Plastic Surgery* 50:143, 1997.

Colombo JL, Hopkins RL, Waring WW. Steam vaporizer injuries. *Pediatr* 67:661–63, 1981.

Combs VL, Marino BL. A comparison of growth patterns in breast and bottle-fed infants with congenital heart disease. *Pediatr Nurs* 19:175–79, 1993.

Coy K, Speltz ML, Jones K. Facial appearance and attachment in infants with orofacial clefts: a replication. *Cleft Palate Craniofacial J* 39(1):66–71, 2002.

Danner SC. Breastfeeding the infant with a cleft defect. *Clin Iss Perin Wom Health Nurs* 3:634–39, 1992a.

———Breastfeeding the neurologically impaired infant. *Clin Iss Perin Wom Health Nurs* 3:640–46, 1992b.

Danner SC, Cerutti ER. *Nursing your baby with Down's syndrome.* Rochester, NY: Childbirth Graphics, 1989.

Darzi MA, Chowdri NA, Bhat AN. Breast feeding or spoon feeding after cleft lip repair: a prospective, randomised study. *Br J Plastic Surg* 49:24–26, 1996.

de Boissieu D et al. Multiple food allergy: a possible diagnosis in breastfed infants. *Acta Paediatr* 86:1042–46, 1997.

Denk MJ. Advances in neonatal surgery. *Ped Clin No Amer* 45(6):1479–506, 1998.

Dowell SF et al. Acute otitis media: management and surveillance in an era of pneumococcal resistance—a report from the Drug-Resistant *Streptococcus pneumoniae* Therapeutic Working Group. *Pediatr Infect Dis J* 18(1):1–9, 1999.

Dowling D et al. Cup-feeding for preterm infants: mechanics and safety. *J Hum Lact* 18(1):12–20, 2002.

Duffy LC et al. Exclusive breastfeeding protects against bacterial colonization and day care exposure to otitis media. *Pediatr* 100(4):e7, 1997.

Duncan LL, Elder SB. Breastfeeding the infant with PKU. *J Hum Lact* 13:231–35, 1997.

Einersson-Backes et al. The effect of oral support on sucking efficiency in preterm infants. *Am J Occup Ther* 48(6):490–8, 1994.

Eliason BC, Lewan RB. Gastroenteritis in children: principles of diagnosis and treatment. *Am Fam Physician* 58:1769–76, 1998.

Ewer AK, James ME, Tobin JM. Prone and left lateral positioning reduce gastro-esophageal reflux in preterm infants. *Arch Dis Child Fetal Neonatal Ed* 81:F201–5, 1999.

Fadavi S et al. Mechanics and energetics of nutritive suckling: a functional comparison of commercially available nipples. *J Pediatr* 130:740–45, 1997.

Feldman D, Reich N, Foster JMT. Pediatric anesthesia and postoperative analgesia. *PCNA* 45(6):1525–37, 1998.

Fergusson DM, Horwood LJ. Early solid food diet and eczema in childhood: a 10-year longitudinal study. *Pediatr Allergy Immunol* 5(6):44–47, 1994.

Forbes GB et al. Composition of milk produced by a mother with galactosemia. *J Pediatr* 113:90–91, 1988.

Foster SB. An adrenal measure for evaluating nursing effectiveness. *Nurs Res* 23:118, 1974.

Fox-Bacon C et al. Maternal PKU and breastfeeding: case report of identical twin mothers. *Clin Pediatrics* 36(9):539–42, 1997.

Froom J et al. A cross-national study of acute otitis media: risk factors, severity, and treatment at initial visit. Report from the International Primary Care Network (PCN) and the ambulatory sentinel Practice Network (ASPN). *J Am Board Fam Pract* 14(6):406–17, 2001.

Fukushima Y et al. Consumption of cow milk and egg by lactating women and the presence of beta-lactoglobulin and ovalbumin in breast milk. *Am J Clin Nutr* 65:30–35, 1997.

Garza JJ et al. Ad libitum feeding dcreases hospital stay for neonates after pyloromyotomy. *J Pediatr Surg* 37(3):493–95, 2002.

GER Guidelines Committee, North American Society for Pediatric Gastroenterology and Nutrition. Pediatric GE reflux clinical practice guidelines. *J Pediatr Gastoenterol Nutr* 32 (suppl):2, 2001.

Gervasio MR, Buchanan CN. Malnutrition in the pediatric cardiology patient. *Crit Care Q* 8:49–56, 1985.

Ghaem M et al. The sleep patterns of infants and young children with gastrooesophageal reflux. *J Paediatr Child Health* 34(2):160–63, 1998.

Good J. *Breastfeeding the Down's syndrome baby.* Franklin Park, IL: La Leche League International, 1980.

Gorelick MH, Shaw KN, Murphy KO. Validity and reliability of clinical signs in the diagnosis of dehydration in children. *Pediatr* 99(5):E6, 1997.

Greco L et al. Case-control study on nutritional risk factors in celiac disease. *J Pediatr Gastroenterol Nutr* 7:395–99, 1988.

Greve L et al. Breast-feeding in the management of the newborn with phenlketonuria: a practical approach to dietary therapy. *J Am Diet Assoc* 94:305–9, 1994.

Habbick BF. Infantile hypertrophic pyloric stenosis: a study of feeding practices and other possible causes. *Clin Commun Stud* 140:401–4, 1989.

Harabuchi Y et al. Human milk secretory IgA antibody to nontypeable *Haemophilus influenzae*: possible protective effects against nasopharyngeal colonization. *J Pediatr* 124:193–98, 1994.

Heacock HJ et al. Influence of breast versus formula milk on physiological gastroesophageal reflux in healthy, newborn infants. *J Pediatr Gastroenterol Nutr* 14:41–46, 1992.

Hendren H. Pediatric rectal and perineal problems. *PCNA* 45(6):1353–72, 1998.

Hernell O, Ivaarsson A, Persson LA. Coeliac disease: effect of early feeding on the incidence of the disease. *Early Hum Develop* 65 (suppl):S153–60, 2001.

Hitchcock NE et al. Pyloric stenosis in western Australia 1971–1984. *Arch Dis Child* 62(5):512–13, 1987.

Holberg KJ et al. Risk factors for respiratory syncytial virus-associated lower respiratory illnesses in the first year of life. *Am J Epidemiol* 133:1135–51, 1991.

Holliday KE et al. Growth of human milk-fed and formula-fed infants with cystic fibrosis. *J Pediatr* 118:77–79, 1991.

Holmberg-Marttila D et al. Do combined elimination diet and prolonged breastfeeding of an atopic infant jeopardise maternal bone health? *Clin and Experimental Allergy* 31:88–94, 2001.

Horta BL et al. Environmental tobacco smoke and breast-feeding duration. *Am J Epidemiol* 146:128–33, 1997.

Huckabay LM, Tilem-Kessler D. Patterns of parental stress in PICU emergency admission. *Dimens Crit Care Nurs* 18(2):36–42, 1999.

Iovino LA. Astroviruses are now a significant source of gastroenteritis in children. *Infectious Dis Child* 16(2):35, 2003.

Jackson PL, Vessey KJ. *Child with a chronic condition.* 2nd ed. St Louis: Mosby, 1996.

Jones AC et al. Fetal peripheral blood mononuclear cell proliferative responses to mitogenic and allergenic stimuli during gestation. *Pediatric Allergy Immunology* 7:109–16, 1996.

Kassing D. Bottle-feeding as a tool to reinforce breastfeeding. *J Hum Lact* 18(1):56–60, 2002.

Kelly DW et al. Rise and fall of coeliac disease 1960–1985. *Arch Dis Child* 64:1157–60, 1989.

Kimpimake T et al. Short-term exclusive breastfeeding predisposes young children with increased genetic risk of Type I diabetes to progressive beta-cell autoimmunity. *Diabetologia* 44(1):63–9, 2001.

Klaus M, Kennell J. *Parent infant bonding.* St.Louis: Mosby, 1982.

Kogo J et al. Breast feeding for cleft lip and palate patients, using the Hotz-type plate. *Cleft-Palate Craniofac J* 34:351–53, 1997.

Koletzko S, Reinhardt D. Nutritional challenges of infants with cystic fibrosis. *Early Human Development* 65 (suppl): S53–S61, 2001.

Lammer EJ, Edmonds LD. Trends in pyloric stenosis incidence, Atlanta, 1968–1982. *J Med Genet* 24(8):482–87, 1987.

Littman RS, Wu CL, Quinlivan JK. Gastric volume and pH in infants fed clear liquids and breastmilk prior to surgery. *Anesth Analg* 79:482–85, 1994.

Litton J et al. Insulin pump therapy in toddlers and preschool children with type 1 diabetes mellitus. *Pediatr* 141(4):490–95, 2002.

Lopez-Alarcon J, Villapando S, Fajardo A. Breast-feeding lowers the frequency and duration of acute respiratory infection and diarrhea in infants under six months of age. *J Nutr* 127:436–43, 1997.

Luder E et al. Current recommendations for breast-feeding in cystic fibrosis centers. *Am J Dis Child* 144:1153–56, 1990.

Lust K et al. Maternal intake of cruciferous vegetables and other foods and colic symptoms in exclusively breast-fed infants. *Am Diet Assoc* 96(1):46–48, 1996.

Marcellus L. The infant with Pierre Robin sequence: review and implications for nursing practice. *J Ped Nurs* 15(1):23–33, 2001.

Marino Bl, O'Brien P, LoRe H. Oxygen saturations during breast and bottle feedings in infants with congenital heart disease. *J Pediatr Nurs* 10(6):360–64, 1995.

Marques IL et al. Clinical experience with infants with Robin Sequence: a prospective study. *Cleft Palate-Craniofacial Journal* 38(2):171–78, 2001.

Mathisen B et al. Feeding problems in infants with gastro-oesophageal reflux disease: A case controlled study. *J Paediatr Child Health* 35:163–69, 1999.

McBride MC, Danner SC. Sucking disorders in neurologically impaired infants. *Clin Perinatol* 14:109–30, 1987.

McCabe L et al. The management of breastfeeding among infants with phenylketonuria. *J Inherit Metal Dis* 12:467–74, 1989.

McIntosh K. Community-acquired pneumonia in children. *N Engl J Med* 346(6):429–37, 2002.

Meier P. Nipple shields for preterm infants: effect of milk transfer and duration of breastfeeding. *J Hum Lact* 16(2):106–14, 2000.

Merewood A, Philipp BL. *Breastfeeding: conditions and diseases.* Amarillo, TX: Pharmasoft Publishing, 2002.

Miller JH. *The controversial issue of breastfeeding cleft-affected i nfants.* Innisfail, AB, Canada: InfoMed Publications, 1998.

Minchin M et al. Expanding the WHO/UNICEF Baby Friendly Hospital Initiative (BFHI): eleven steps to optimal infant feeding in a pediatric unit. *Breastfeeding Review* 4:87–91, 1996.

Mizuno K, Ueda A. Development of sucking behavior in infants with Down's syndrome. *Acta Paediatr* 90:1384–88, 2002.

Mizuno K, Ueda A, Takeuchi T. Effects of different fluids on the relationship between swallowing and breathing during nutritive sucking in neonates. *Biol Neonate* 81(1):45–50, 2002.

Mohrbacher N, Stock J. *The Breastfeeding Answer Book*. 3rd ed. Schaumburg, IL: La Leche League International, 2003.

Nafstad P et al. Breastfeeding, maternal smoking and lower respiratory tract infection. *Eur Respir J* 12:2623–29, 1996.

———. Weight gain during the first year in relation to maternal smoking and breast feeding in Norway. *J Epidemiol Commun Health* 51:261–65, 1997.

Nicholson SC, Schreiner MS. Feed the babies. *Breastfeed Abstr* 15:3–4, 1995.

Niemela M et al. Pacifier as a risk factor for acute otitis media: a randomized, controlled trial of parent counseling. *Pediatrics* 106(3):483–8, 2000.

Noble R, Bovey A. Therapeutic teat use for babies who breastfeed poorly. *Breastfeed Rev* 5(2):37–42, 1997.

Olshansky S. Chronic sorrow: a response to having a mentally defective child. *Soc Casework* 43:190–93, 1962.

Orenstein SR, Shalaby TM, Putnam PE. Thickened feedings as a cause of increased coughing when used as therapy for gastroesophageal reflux in infants. *J Pediatr* 121:913–15, 1992.

Pandya AN, Boorman JG. Failure to thrive in babies with cleft lip and palate. *Br J Plast Surg* 54(6):471–75, 2001.

Paradise JL et al. Evidence in infants with cleft palate that breast milk protects against otitis media. *Pediatrics* 94:853–60, 1994.

Patenaude Y et al. Cow's-milk-induced allergic colitis in an exclusively breast-fed infant: diagnosed with ultrasound. *Pediatr Radiol* 30:379–82, 2000.

Pelchat D et al. Longitudinal effects of an early family intervention programme on the adaptation of parents of children with a disability. *Int J Nurs Stud* 36(6):465–77, 1999.

Peltola H. Worldwide *Haemophilus influenzae* type b disease at the beginning of the 21st century: global analysis of the disease burden 25 years after the use of the polysaccharide vaccine and a decade after the advent of conjugates. *Clin Microbiol Rev* 13(2):302–17, 2000.

Peters U et al. A case control study of the effect of infant feeding on celiac disease. *Ann Nutr Metab* 45:135–42, 2001.

Pinnington LL et al. Feeding efficiency and respiratory integration in infants with acute viral bronchiolitis. *J Pediatr* 137:523–26, 2000.

Pisacane A et al. Breast feeding and hypertrophic pyloric stenosis: population based case-control study. *BMJ* 312(7033):745–47, 1996.

Popper PK. *The hospitalized nursing baby. Unit I/Lactation Consultant Series Two*. Schaumburg, IL: La Leche League International, 1998.

Pumberger W, Pomberger G, Geissler G. Proctocolitis in breast-fed infants: a contribution to differential diagnosis of haematochezia in early childhood. *Posgrad Med* 77(906):252–54, 2001.

Raisler J, Alexander C, O'Campo P. Breastfeeding and infant illness: a dose–response relationship. *Am J Public Health* 89:25–30, 1999.

Repucci A. Resolution of stool blood in breast-fed infants with maternal ingestion of pancreatic enzymes. *J Ped Gastro Nutr* 84:353–60, 1999.

Ripmeester P, Dunn S. Against all odds: breastfeeding a baby with Harlequin Ichthyosis. *JOGN Nurs* 31:521–25, 2002.

Riva E et al. Early breastfeeding is linked to higher intelligence quotient scores in dietary treated phenylketonuric children. *Acta Paediatr* 85:56–58, 1996.

Rooney K. Breastfeeding a baby with cystic fibrosis. *New Beginnings* 4:43–44, 1988.

Saarinen UM, Kajosaari M. Breastfeeding as prophylaxis against atopic disease: prospective follow-up study until 17 years. *Lancet* 346(8982):1065–69, 1995.

Sandler A. *Living with spina bifida: a guide for families and professionals*. Chapel Hill, NC: University of North Carolina Press, 1997.

Sassen ML, Brand R, Grote JJ. Breast-feeding and acute otitis media. *Am J Otolaryngol* 15:351–57, 1994.

Scariati PD, Brummer-Strawn LM, Fein SB. A longitudinal analysis of infant morbidity and the extent of breastfeeding in the United States. *Pediatr* 99:E5, 1997.

Schach B, Haight M. Colic and food allergy in the breastfed infant: Is it possible for the exclusively breastfed infant to suffer from food allergy? *J Hum Lact* 18(1):50–52, 2002.

Sears MR et al. Long-term relation between breastfeeding and development of atopy and asthma in children and young adults: a longitudinal study. *Lancet* 360:901–7, 2002.

Shaw WC, Bannister RP, Roberts CT. Assisted feeding is more reliable for infants with clefts—a randomized trial. *Cleft Palate-Craniofacial J* 36:262–68, 1999.

Smith TB, Oliver MN, Innocenti MS. Parenting stress in families of children with disabilities. *Am J Orthopsychiatry* 71(2):257–61, 2001.

Spitz L. Esophageal atresia: past, present, and future. *J Pediatr Surg* 31:19–25, 1996.

Spitz L et al. Oesophageal atresia: at-risk groups for the 1990's. *J Pediatr Surg* 29:723–25, 1994.

Sutin R. Eliminating foods worked wonders. *New Beginnings* 4:145, 1988.

Tew BJ et al. Marital stability following the birth of a child with spina bifida. *Br J Psychiatry* 131:79–82, 1977.

Tobin JM, McCloud P, Cmaeron DJS. Posture and gastroesophageal reflux: a case for left lateral positioning. *Arch Dis Child* 7:254–258, 1997.

Tomlinson PS, Swiggum P, Harbaugh BL. Identification of nurse-family intervention sites to decrease health-related family boundary ambiguity in PICU. *Issues Comp Pediatr Nurs* 22(1):27–47, 1999.

Trenouth MJ, Campbell AN. Questionnaire evaluation of feeding methods for cleft lip and palate neonates. *Int J Paediatr Dent* 6:241–44, 1996.

Turner L et al. The effects of lactation education and a prosthetic obturator appliance on feeding efficiency in infants with cleft lip and palate. *Cleft Palate Craniofacial J* 38(5):S510–24, 2001.

Uhari M, Mantysaari K, Niemela M. A meta-analytic review of the risk factors for acute otitis media. *Clin Infect Dis* 22(6):1079–83, 1996.

Vadas P et al. Detection of peanut allergens in breast milk of lactating women. *JAMA* 285:1746–48, 2001.

VanVliet G. Treatment of congenital hypothyroidsm. *Lancet* 358(9276):86–87, 2001.

Visconti KJ et al. Influence of parental stress and social support on the behavioral adjustment of children with transposition of the great arteries. *J Dev Behav Pediatr* 23(5):314–21, 2002.

Wallerstedt C, Higgins P. Facilitating perinatal grieving between the mother and the father. *JOGNN* 25:389–94, 1996.

Wilson AC et al. Relation of infant diet to childhood health: seven-year follow-up of cohort of children in Dundee infant feeding study. *BMJ* 316:21–25, 1998.

Wilson-Clay B. *Clefts.* LACTNET Accessed December 12, 1995.

Woolridge M, Fisher C. Colic, "overfeeding" and symptoms of lactose malabsorption in the breast-fed baby: a possible effect of feed management? *Lancet* 2(8605):382–84, 1988.

Young Jl et al. What information do parents of newborns with cleft lip, palate, or both want to know? *Cleft Palate Craniofacial J* 38(1):55–58, 2001.

Zieger RS. Dietary aspects of food allegy prevention in infants and children. *J Pediatr Gastroenterol Nutr* 30:S77–S86, 2000.

INFANT ASSESSMENT

Mary Koehn, Kathy Gill-Hopple, and Jan Riordan

Breastfeeding is dependent not only upon the mother but also on the behaviors of the infant. In the normal, healthy, full-term infant, the reflexes needed for breastfeeding are strong and support the capability of the infant to obtain sufficient nutrition from the breast. Therefore, a complete infant assessment is critical to breastfeeding. The infant assessment includes evaluation of perinatal history, gestational age assessment, breastfeeding assessment, physical assessment, and behavioral assessment.

Perinatal History

Infant assessment is incomplete without the perinatal history. A perinatal history focuses on the preconception, prenatal, and intrapartum periods. This history provides the context for the physical and behavioral assessment of the infant and may identify existing infant problems. However, it is important to remember that the presence of maternal obstetrical and infant prenatal risk factors does not automatically indicate an infant problem. Table 20–1 summarizes the essential components of the perinatal history (Evans et al., 2002; London et al., 2003; Moore & Nichols, 1997).

Gestational Age Assessment

Gestational age assessment determines the degree of maturity of the infant at birth. Knowing the gestational age helps to identify potential infant mortality and morbidity risk. Because gestational age affects his ability to suckle/swallow/breathe, this classification of the infant is useful in determining the infant's vulnerability to feeding problems (Table 20–2).

Historically, gestational age was based on the mother's estimated date of delivery and/or the infant's birth weight. However, these methods are unreliable, as the infant's maturity is influenced by other factors, such as maternal nutritional status, maternal exposure to environmental hazards, maternal disease, and genetic disorders of the infant. The following classification terms are now used in gestational age assessment (Sansoucie & Cavaliere, 2003):

- *Preterm:* An infant born at less than 37 weeks' gestation, regardless of weight.
- *Term:* An infant born between 37 and 42 weeks' gestation.
- *Postterm:* An infant born at the onset of 42 weeks' gestation or anytime thereafter.

Table 20–1

ESSENTIAL COMPONENTS OF THE PERINATAL HISTORY

Component	Required Data
Family history	• Family history of genetic disorders such as cystic fibrosis, sickle cell anemia, trisomy, phenylketonuria
	• Family history of diseases such as diabetes, seizures, chronic disorders
Social history	• Marital status and support systems
	• Substance abuse
	• Tobacco use
	• Exposure to environmental hazards
Maternal medical history	• Maternal age
	• Surgical procedures
	• Hospitalizations
	• Endocrine disorders (diabetes, hyperthyroid, or hypothyroid)
	• Cardiovascular disorders (hypertension, heart disease)
	• Respiratory disorders (asthma, pneumonia)
	• Renal (frequent infections, chronic kidney disease)
	• Hematologic (sickle cell disorders, blood type and Rh factor, blood disorders, Rh isoimmunization)
	• Cancer
	• Infections
	• Medications taken prior to pregnancy
Maternal reproductive history	• Gravidity, parity
	• Previous perinatal loss
	• Infant with cogenital anomaly
	• Spontaneous/elective abortions
	• Malformations of cervix, uterus
Pregnancy history	• Last known menstrual period
	• EDC (estimated date of confinement)
	• Nutrition and general health
	• Prenatal care (when first obtained and frequency of visits)
	• Prenatal laboratory tests (VDRL or RPR, screening for hepatitis B, HIV, STDs, rubella)
	• Weight gain during pregnancy
	• Results of prenatal testing (ultrasonography, amniocentesis, chorionic villus testing, alpha-fetoprotein, triple screen)
	• Medications (prescription, over-the-counter, recreational)
Intrapartum history	• Length of labor
	• Type of birth (vaginal or cesarean)
	• Rupture of membrane (spontaneous or artificial, time from rupture until birth)
	• Appearance of amniotic fluid
	• Complications
	• Instrumentation
	• Analgesia and anesthesia
	• Apgar scores and resuscitation of infant

Source: From Moore & Nichols (1997).

Table 20–2

PHYSIOLOGIC CHARACTERISTICS ASSOCIATED WITH GESTATIONAL AGE THAT AFFECT FEEDING/NUTRITION

Gestational Age Classification	Characteristic	Risk
Prematurity	Coordination of sucking and swallowing not present until 28 weeks (with wide variability); full coordination after 36–37 weeks	Aspiration
	Tires easily	Slow feeding
	Immature gag reflex < 36 weeks	Aspiration
	Poor muscle tone in the area of the lower esophageal sphincter < 37 weeks	Regurgitation into the esophagus
	Limited stomach capacity	Overdistention; compromises respiration
	Carbohydrates and fat poorly tolerated Secretion of lactase low < 34 weeks	Absorption of nutrients
	Inefficient in digesting and absorbing lipids—low levels of pancreatic lipase and low bile acid	Absorption of nutrients
	Low reserve of calcium, iron, phosphorus, proteins, and vitamins A and C	Inadequate nutrition
	Decreased muscle mass; decreased deposits of brown fat	Hypoglycemia
Postmaturity	Decreased efficiency of the placenta, macrosomia, meconium aspiration, polycemia	Respiratory distress Hypoglycemia
Large for gestational age	Transient hyperinsulinism	Hypoglycemia
Small for gestational age	Intrauterine malnutrition	Hypoglycemia

Source: From Wilson (2003).

- *Small for gestational age (SGA):* An infant whose birth weight is below the 10th percentile for a given gestational age.
- *Large for gestational age (LGA):* An infant whose birth weight is above the 90th percentile for a given gestational age.
- *Appropriate for gestational age (AGA):* An infant whose birth weight falls between the 10th and 90th percentiles for a given gestational age.
- *Low birth weight: (LBW):* An infant whose birth weight is between 1500 and 2500 gm.
- *Very low birth weight (VLBW):* An infant whose birth weight is 1500 gm or less.

The New Ballard Score

The New Ballard Score (Ballard et al., 1991) is a commonly used objective tool that includes the assessment of six external physical characteristics and six neurological signs to estimate the gestational age of the infant. This scoring system has its highest reliability when performed within 48 hours of birth and is considered accurate within 2 weeks of actual gestation (Ballard et al., 1991). Although the New Ballard Score has been expanded to include extremely premature infants, the Donovan et al. study (1999) failed to demonstrate a close relationship between gestational age and fetal maturation, as measured by this scoring system, in infants less than 28 weeks gestation. Thus, possible inaccuracies in gestational age based on New Ballard Scores should be considered when implementing treatment for infants less than 28 weeks.

Each item on the New Ballard Score is scored from –1 to 4 (or 5 with two of the signs) by comparing the infant with the descriptor on the scoring sheet (Figure 20–1). The numbers of points assigned per item are added to obtain a total score. The total score is then used to determine an estimate of gestational age in weeks by comparing the infant's score with the maturity rating score on the New Ballard Score. The following neuromuscular and physical signs are used for scoring (Buschbach, 1999; Wilson, 2003):

Neuromuscular Signs of Maturity

- *Posture:* Observe the posture when the infant is quiet. A term newborn's arms and legs are flexed with good body muscle tone. A preterm infant's arms and legs are extended with the body flaccid (Figure 20–2).

- *Square window:* Flex the infant's wrist down toward the ventral forearm and estimate the angle between the hand and forearm. Do not rotate the wrist. Measure the degree of flexion against the New Ballard Score chart. There is no downward angle with the full-term infant (i.e., a score of 3 or 4). The angle decreases with decreasing gestational age.

- *Arm recoil:* Fully flex the infant's arms for 5 seconds. Release. Score the degree of immediate return of arm flexion against the score sheet. A vigorous, fully flexed response is a score of 4. A slow response receives a lower score.

- *Popliteal angle:* With the infant's hips flat on the examining table, place one of the infant's thighs on the abdomen. Slowly, attempt to straighten the leg toward the infant's head. Do not force. Stop when resistance is met. Score the angle of the flexed leg according to the chart. A full-term infant will usually score a 3 or 4.

- *Scarf sign:* Pull the infant's arm across the chest and around the neck. Observe the infant's elbow in relation to the midline of the body. Score according to the chart. A full-term infant will usually score a 2, 3, or 4.

- *Heel to ear:* With the infant's hips on the examining table, slowly pull the heel toward the ear until resistance is felt. Observe the distance between the foot and the head as well as the degree of knee extension. Score according to the chart. A full-term infant will usually score a 3 or 4.

Physical signs of maturity

- *Skin:* Observe the skin for color and texture. Observe the trunk area for opacity. With increasing gestational age, the skin becomes less transparent and develops more texture. Blood vessels are generally not visible on the trunk of a full-term infant. Some peeling of the hands and feet is common in full-term infants. A preterm infant's skin is thin and smooth with visible vessels. Score the infant according to the chart. A full-term infant will usually score a 3 or 4.

- *Lanugo:* Observe the skin for this fine, downy hair. Lanugo covers the body of the fetus from about 24 to 28 weeks. After 28 weeks, it begins to disappear. Score the infant according to the descriptors on the chart. Note that a very premature infant will have no lanugo or it is sparse, thus scoring a 0 or -1. A full-term infant will usually score a 3 or 4.

- *Plantar surface:* Observe the soles of the feet for creases. The creases on the anterior surface of the foot begin to appear between 28 and 30 weeks. As gestational age increases, so do the number and depth of creases. Score according to the descriptors on the chart. A full-term in-

MATURATIONAL ASSESSMENT OF GESTATIONAL AGE (New Ballard Score)

NAME_____ DATE/TIME OF BIRTH_____ SEX_____

HOSPITAL NO._____ DATE/TIME OF EXAM_____ BIRTH WEIGHT_____

RACE_____ AGE WHEN EXAMINED_____ LENGTH_____

APGAR SCORE: 1 MINUTE_____ 5 MINUTES_____ 10 MINUTES_____ HEAD CIRC._____

EXAMINER_____

NEUROMUSCULAR MATURITY

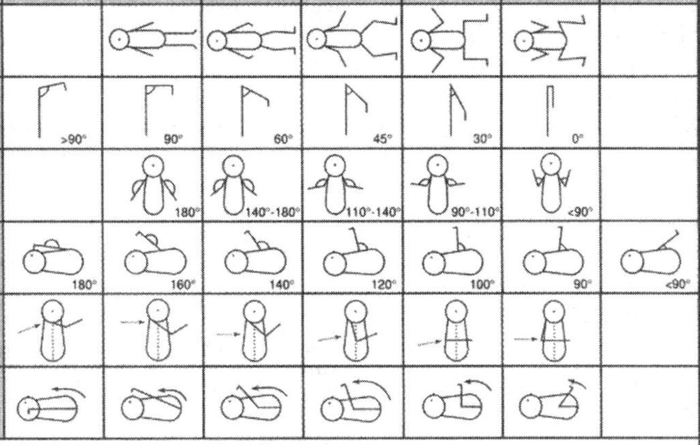

NEUROMUSCULAR MATURITY SIGN	SCORE							RECORD SCORE HERE
	-1	0	1	2	3	4	5	
POSTURE								
SQUARE WINDOW (Wrist)	>90°	90°	60°	45°	30°	0°		
ARM RECOIL		180°	140°-180°	110°-140°	90°-110°	<90°		
POPLITEAL ANGLE	180°	160°	140°	120°	100°	90°	<90°	
SCARF SIGN								
HEEL TO EAR								

TOTAL NEUROMUSCULAR MATURITY SCORE

PHYSICAL MATURITY

PHYSICAL MATURITY SIGN	SCORE							RECORD SCORE HERE
	-1	0	1	2	3	4	5	
SKIN	sticky friable transparent	gelatinous red translucent	smooth pink visible veins	superficial peeling &/or rash, few veins	cracking pale areas rare veins	parchment deep cracking no vessels	leathery cracked wrinkled	
LANUGO	none	sparse	abundant	thinning	bald areas	mostly bald		
PLANTAR SURFACE	heel-toe 40-50 mm:-1 <40 mm:-2	>50 mm no crease	faint red marks	anterior transverse crease only	creases ant. 2/3	creases over entire sole		
BREAST	imperceptible	barely perceptible	flat areola no bud	stippled areola 1-2 mm bud	raised areola 3-4 mm bud	full areola 5-10 mm bud		
EYE/EAR	lids fused loosely: -1 tightly: -2	lids open pinna flat stays folded	sl. curved pinna; soft; slow recoil	well-curved pinna; soft but ready recoil	formed & firm instant recoil	thick cartilage ear stiff		
GENITALS (Male)	scrotum flat, smooth	scrotum empty faint rugae	testes in upper canal rare rugae	testes descending few rugae	testes down good rugae	testes pendulous deep rugae		
GENITALS (Female)	clitoris prominent & labia flat	prominent clitoris & small labia minora	prominent clitoris & enlarging minora	majora & minora equally prominent	majora large minora small	majora cover clitoris & minora		

TOTAL PHYSICAL MATURITY SCORE

SCORE

Neuromuscular_____
Physical_____
Total_____

MATURITY RATING

score	weeks
-10	20
-5	22
0	24
5	26
10	28
15	30
20	32
25	34
30	36
35	38
40	40
45	42
50	44

GESTATIONAL AGE (weeks)

By dates_____
By ultrasound_____
By exam_____

FIGURE 20–1. New Ballard Score. (From Ballard (1991). Reprinted with permission.)

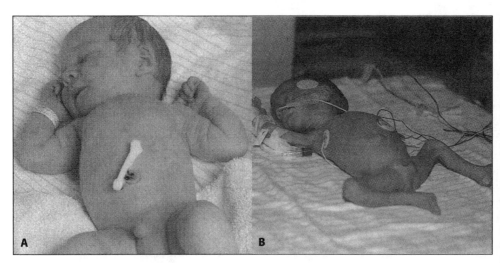

FIGURE 20–2. Neonate posture. (A) Full-term infant. (B) Premature infant. (Moore ML, Nichols FH: Neonatal assessment. In Nichols FH, Zwelling E eds. *Maternal-newborn nursing: theory and practice.* Philadelphia: WB Saunders, 1080–1131, 1997. Reprinted with permission of Elsevier Publications.)

fant will usually score a 3 or 4. Note that after 12 hours, the validity of plantar creases as an indicator of gestational age decreases because the skin begins to dry.

- *Breast:* Place two fingers of one hand on either side of the areola bud tissue. Measure (in millimeters) the diameter of the bud with a tape measure. Score according to the chart. A full-term infant will usually score a 3 or 4.

- *Eye/ear:* Prior to 26 to 30 weeks gestation, the eyelids are fused. After the eyes are open, there is no maturity scoring on the New Ballard Score. The ears are assessed for formation and amount of cartilage that is present in the pinna. Examine the pinna between the thumb and forefinger for amount of cartilage that is present. Fold the ear anteriorly. After approximately 36 weeks when some cartilage has developed, the pinna will spring back from being folded. Score according to the chart. A full-term infant will usually score a 3 or 4.

- *Genitalia (male):* Gently feel for the presence of the testes by examining the scrotum between the thumb and fingers of one hand. Observe the degree of descent into the scro-

tum and the development of rugae. The testes begin to descend at 28 weeks and descent is normally complete by 40 weeks. The scrotum of a full-term infant is also covered with deep rugae.

- *Genitalia (female):* Observe the genitalia of the female infant without spreading the labia majora. At full term, the infant's labia majora covers the labia minora. The premature infant will have a more prominent clitoris with small, widely separated labia.

After these assessments, complete the scoring by adding the total neuromuscular maturity score to the total physical maturity score. Compare that score, found on the left side of the maturity rating scale, with the corresponding gestational age on the right side of the rating scale. To complete the assessment of gestational age, plot the infant's weight, length, and head circumference in relation to maturity rating from the New Ballard Score on the Classification of Newborn by intrauterine growth and gestational age (Figure 20–3). The infant's maturity level can then be classified according to the previously defined classification terms.

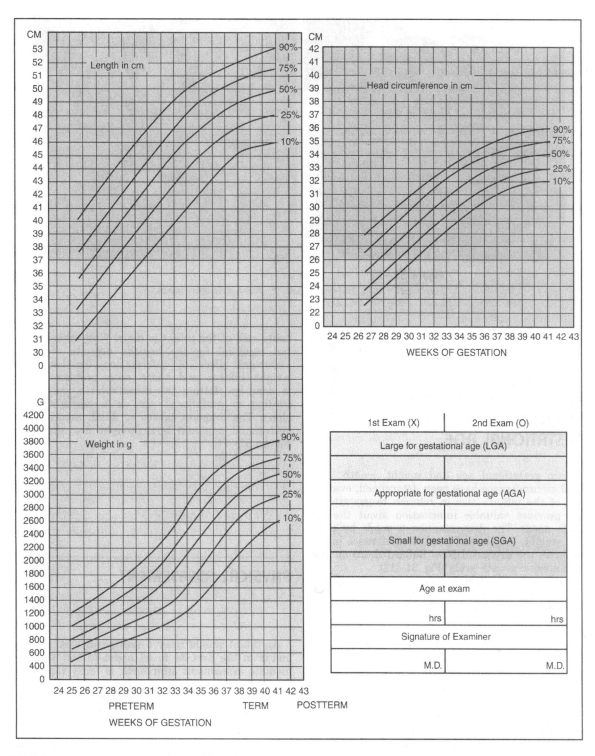

FIGURE 20–3. Intrauterine growth grids. Lubchenko LO, Hansman C, Boyd E. Intrauterine growth in length and head circumference as estimated from live births at gestational ages from 26 to 42 weeks. *Pediatrics* **37:403–8, 1996. Adapted with permission.**

Indicators of Effective Breastfeeding and Assessment Scales

This section defines behaviors that indicate whether breastfeeding is going well and reviews several breastfeeding assessment scales.

Breastfeeding Behaviors and Indicators

Breastfeeding is not a single behavior of suckling but a series of behaviors that can be described, assessed, and measured. Breastfeeding infants who are feeding effectively spontaneously turn their mouth to their mothers' nipples when put to breast, grasp the nipple firmly, suckle rhythmically, and pause to rest between bursts of suckling while continuing to hold the nipple in the mouth. Swallowing is observed during the first 3 days postpartum; swallowing is both observed and heard beginning 4 days postpartum or earlier for some mothers. In a recent study, audible swallowing was the only significant predictor of how much breastmilk the baby ingested at a feeding (Riordan & Gill-Hopple, 2002). Characteristics of frequently used breastfeeding indicators are defined below.

Rooting. Rooting is a reflexive behavior in which the infant turns his head in the direction of the stimulus and opens his mouth wide anticipating feeding. Rooting enables the infant to "catch" the mother's nipple and keeps the infant's tongue on the bottom of the mouth, important for compressing milk ducts (Figure 20–4). Licking movements typically precede and follow rooting in the early neonatal period.

Length of Time Before Latch-on. The time before latch-on is the amount of time in minutes before the infant latches on and remains on the breast.

Latch-on. Latch-on refers to the ability of the infant to grasp the nipple, flange the upper and lower lips outward against the breast areola, and remain firmly on the breast between bursts of suckling.

Suckling. Coordinated and rhythmic suckling, swallowing, and breathing characterized by a pattern of suckling burst, pause, suckling burst, pause: that is, alternating between nutritive (milk ingested) and nonnutritive (no milk ingested) suckling. The infant's lips should be visibly flanged outward dur-

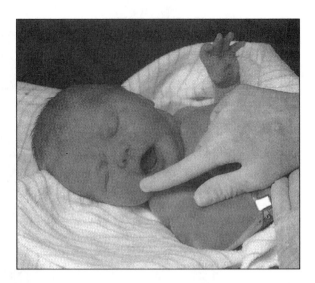

FIGURE 20–4. Rooting reflex. (Moore ML, Nichols FH: Neonatal assessment. In Nichols FH, Zwelling E eds. *Maternal-newborn nursing: theory and practice.* Philadelphia: WB Saunders, 1080-1131, 1997. Reprinted with permission of Elsevier Publications.)

ing suckling to prevent friction and abrasion of the mother's areolar tissue and to provide the seal that allows negative intraoral pressure.

Swallowing. In swallowing, the back of the tongue elevates and presses against the posterior pharyngeal wall. The soft palate rises and closes off the nasal passageways. The larynx then moves up and forward to close the trachea and propels the milk into the esophagus, thus initiating the baby's swallow reflex. Afterward, the larynx returns to its previous position. A sufficient volume of milk is needed to trigger swallowing. Swallowing can usually be observed during the first several days following birth and becomes audible following lactogenesis at approximately 4 days postpartum (or earlier). Swallowing produces observable movements of the infant's jaw (long, rhythmic jaw excursions) and throat muscles.

Breastfeeding Scales and Tools

Early feeding assessment scales were developed for and tested on infants who were bottle-fed. When breastfeeding became more common, hospital nurses documented breastfeedings with subjective phrases such as "breastfed well" or "breastfed poorly." Since then, breastfeeding assessment has evolved to use quantitative scales also known as "tools." Matthews (1988) separated and labeled indicators of infant feedings at the breast into the first scored assessment tool for breastfeeding. Around the same time, Shrago and Bocar (1990) published a list of breastfeeding behaviors for assessing feedings; however, they did not add a scoring system. Since then, several other scales have been developed; their description is below. The tools are shown in Appendix 20-A–20-D. In addition to assessing feedings at the breast, a breastfeeding scale can serve as an outcome measure for research, as a method of documentation and communication among health-care workers, and as a teaching tool for mothers to show them normal breastfeeding patterns of their babies (Riordan, 1998).

Infant Breastfeeding Assessment Tool (IBFAT).
A Canadian midwife developed the IBFAT, the first such scale, as her master's thesis (Matthews, 1988). The IBFAT has four indicators: (1) readiness to feed, (2) rooting, (3) fixing, and (4) sucking. A numerical score (0 to 3) is given for each indicator; the total score can range from 0 to 12. Breastfeeding is considered to be effective when scores range from 9 to 12. Reliability and validity of the IBFAT is supported. Matthews (1988) found that the observer and mother agreed on the breastfeeding score 91 percent of the time and that the higher the score, the more pleased the mother was with the feeding (Matthews, 1990). Riordan et al. (2001) found the same high agreement in another study. Low IBFAT scores have been associated with the use of labor analgesia (Crowell, Hill, & Humenick, 1994; Riordan et al., 2000). Mothers with low IBFAT scores breastfed for a significantly shorter period than those with medium or high scores (p < 0.001) (Riordan et al., 2000).

Mother-Baby Assessment Tool (MBA).
The MBA scoring system divides the process of breastfeeding into five steps: (1) signaling, (2) positioning, (3) fixing, (4) milk transfer, and (5) ending (Mulford, 1992). For each step, both a maternal and an infant behavior are scored. Ten is the highest possible feeding score: 5 for infant indicators and 5 for maternal indicators. Reliability and validity testing had mixed results. Percentage of agreement among the nurses rating videotapes of breastfeeds using the MBA ranged from 37 to 95 percent. The indicator receiving the greatest agreement was readiness of the baby and mother to feed (97 percent); the lowest was the milk transfer indicator (37 percent) (Riordan & Koehn, 1997). Morrison et al. (2002) reported a strong correlation between the MBA and the next tool described here—the LATCH Tool.

LATCH Assessment Tool.
The LATCH tool (Jensen, Wallace, & Kelsay, 1994) evaluates five indicators of breastfeeding. A numerical score (0, 1, or 2) is assigned to each measure for a possible total score of 10. Each letter of the acronym title denotes a category. "L" represents how well the infant latches onto the breast, "A" represents audible swallowing, "T" describes the mother's nipple type, "C" represents the mother's degree of breast or nipple comfort, and "H" evaluates the amount of help the mother needs to position her baby at breast. The LATCH scale appears to measure different aspects of breastfeeding behavior than the IBFAT, because another study found that the correlations between the two scales were not significant (Schlomer, Kemmerer, & Twiss, 1999).

When LATCH scores were compared with the overall duration of breastfeeding, women still breastfeeding at 6 weeks postpartum had significantly higher LATCH scores than those who had weaned (Riordan et al., 2001). Although this finding supports the scale's validity overall, it should be noted that this prediction was due to the item "comfort of nipples." Mothers who had very sore nipples stopped breastfeeding early. In other testing of the LATCH tool, scores of lactation consultants, scores determined by raters, and scores determined by mothers were positively correlated (r = .53 to .67) (Adams & Hewell, 1997), an indication of reliability.

Via Christi Breastfeeding Assessment Tool.
The Via Christi breastfeeding assessment tool is modified from the LATCH and IBFAT scales. It is a combination of indicators from other assessment scales that were selected because they demonstrated positive agreement with mother's evaluation and amount of breastmilk ingested during feedings—indicators of reliability and validity—in previous studies (Adams & Hewell, 1997; Riordan et al., 2001; Riordan & Koehn, 1997; Schlomer, Kemmerer, & Twiss, 1999). Mothers' evaluations of the

feedings were added to the scale because of a high positive correlation with other indicators. Mothers can gauge the effectiveness of the feed; only they can feel sensations of breastfeeding (baby's firm latch on the breast, "letting down," uterine contractions, etc.). Audible swallowing was included because it predicts the amount of breastmilk taken by the baby (Riordan & Gill-Hopple, 2002).

Preterm Infant Breastfeeding Assessment Scale.
The Preterm Infant Breastfeeding Behavior Scale (PIBBS) was developed as an observational tool to study preterm infant feeding behavior (Hedberg-Nyqvist & Ewald, 1999). Hedberg-Nyqvist, Rubertsson, and Ewald (1996) found acceptable agreement of scores between nurses and raters but not as satisfactory agreement between nurses and mothers. This tool appears in Chapter 13.

Neonatal Oral-Motor Assessment Scale.
The Neonatal Oral-Motor Assessment Scale (NOMAS) was originally developed to assess feedings in premature and medically compromised newborns (Palmer, Crawley, & Blanco, 1999). NOMAS is a nonnutritive sucking assessment done with the examiner's finger in the infant's mouth. The revised version has four parts that test normal and abnormal characteristics of the jaw and tongue. The examiner assesses and rates the newborn for these characteristics. The rating ranges from 0 to 16 (MacMullen & Dulski, 2000). NOMAS has some evidence of validity (Case-Smith, Cooper, & Scala, 1988).

Summary of Breastfeeding Assessment Scales

As more women choose to breastfeed and are discharged early with uncertain breastfeeding support, the need for tools that measure breastfeeding is obvious. Because the scoring must take place quickly in busy maternity units by overworked nurses, the scale should be short and easy to use. Which scales are best for full-term babies? At the time of this writing, three tools have support for their clinical use: (1) the IBFAT, (2) the LATCH, and (3) the Via Christi. In addition to having evidence of validity and reliability, all are brief and are being successfully used in clinical settings. Although further study of the PIBBs is needed, it is being successfully used in neonatal units to assess feeding readiness of low birth weight babies. NOMAS is seldom used

for routine breastfeeding assessment because of its complexity, intrusiveness, and required training. Finally, the journey to find the "best" breastfeeding assessment scale has only begun. Existing tools will be revised and new tools developed as new knowledge becomes available.

Physical Assessment

Transitional Assessment

During the first 24 hours of life, the newborn undergoes a typical pattern of adjustment indicating normal adaptation to extrauterine life. The first several hours after birth are considered the first period of reactivity. During the first 30 minutes of this time, the healthy, full-term newborn is alert (unless affected by maternal medication), cries spontaneously, and when put to the mother's breast will root, lick, and otherwise "nuzzle" the mother's breast. This is followed by hand-to-mouth movements and later latching-on to the nipple and suckling. This is an ideal time to begin breastfeeding, as the newborn is wide-eyed, alert, and responsive to environmental cues.

Physiologic changes during this time include rapid respiration and heart rate, and increased mucous secretions. There may be a transient episode of tachypnea and nasal flaring, but this should resolve spontaneously within the first 30 minutes. The next phase of this period begins when the infant falls into a deep sleep. Heart and respiratory rate decrease, temperature continues to be unstable, and mucous production decreases. Stimulation of the newborn to breastfeed at this time usually results in little response. This is normal neonatal behavior but can be upsetting to parents and nurses who are anxious for the baby to breastfeed sooner than the baby is ready for it. Some acrocyanosis may still be evident, although it usually shows a steady improvement. Bowel sounds may become audible at this time.

The second stage of reactivity occurs when the newborn awakens from a deep sleep state and becomes alert and responsive. The newborn's heart and respiratory rate increase; however, the baby can have periods of apnea associated with a decrease in heart rate. Tactile stimulation is used to improve the heart and respiratory rate. When apneic periods are associated with skin color changes further evaluation is necessary. It is not unusual for the newborn to gag, choke, and regurgitate as gastric and respiratory secretions increase. The gastrointestinal system is active, and most newborns will pass the first meconium stool within 8 to 24 hours of birth. Many newborns void immediately after birth. If the infant was not fed during the first period of reactivity this is an ideal time to initiate a feeding.

When performing a head to toe physical assessment (Table 20–3) a warm surface must be provided for the newborn. Exposing the newborn's body to uncontrolled temperatures increases the

Table 20–3

NEWBORN PHYSICAL ASSESSMENT

	Normal	Normal Variations	Abnormal
Vital Signs	• Temperature Axillary 36.5–37.4° C 97.9–98° F		• < 36.5 C • > 37.4 C
	• Pulse 120–140 beats/minute	• Increased with crying • Decreased when sleeping	• Tachycardia • Bradycardia < 80 to 100 • Associated with color changes
	• Respirations 30–60/minute	• Increased during first period of reactivity and with crying • Decreased when sleeping	
Measurement	• Head circumference 33–35 cm (13–14 in.) • Chest circumference 30.5–33 cm (12–13 in.) • Head to heel length 48–53 cm (19–21 in.) • Birth weight 2700–4000 gm (6–9 lb)	• Molding may decrease head circumference	• Head < 10th or > 90th percentile • Weight < 10th or > 90th percentile
Skin	• Bright red, smooth at birth • Vernix caseosa, lanugo	• Acrocyanosis • Cutis marmorata—mottling when exposed to low temperature, stress, or overstimulation • Milia • Erythema toxicum • Mongolian spots • Telangiectatic nevi • Harlequin color changes • Jaundice after first 24 hours	• Jaundice in the first 24 hours • Central or generalized cyanosis • Pallor • Mottling • Plethora • Persistent petechiae or hemorrhage or ecchymosis • Café au lait spots • Nevus flammeus
Head	• Anterior fontanelle 2.5–4.0 cm (1–1.75 in.), diamond-shaped • Posterior fontanelle 0.5–1 cm (0.2–0.4 in.), triangular-shaped • Soft, flat fontanelles	• Molding after vaginal birth • Fontanelle bulging when crying • Caput succedaneum • Cephalhematoma	• Fused sutures • Depressed or bulging fontanelles when quiet

Table 20–3 (cont.)

	Normal	Normal Variations	Abnormal
Eyes	• Edematous lids • Absence of tears • Slate gray, dark blue, or brown • Positive red, corneal, pupillary, and blink reflex • Fixes on objects, follows to midline	• Subconjunctival hemorrhages • Epicanthal folds in Asian newborns	• Purulent discharge • Upward slant of eyes • Iris pink color • Constricted or dilated pupil • Absence of red, corneal, papillary reflex • Inability to follow objects to the midline • Sclera yellow
Ears	• Pinna flexible, well formed, level with outer canthus of the eye	• Pinna flat against the head • Irregular shape, size • Skin tags	• Low placement of ears
Nose	• Patent • Thin, white nasal discharge	• Flattened, bruised, or slightly deviated	• Nonpatent • Thick, bloody discharge • Nasal flaring
Mouth/Throat	• Intact, arched palate • Midline uvula • Tongue centered in the mouth • Reflexes: sucking, rooting, gagging, extrusion • Vigorous cry	• Natal teeth • Epstein's pearls	• Cleft lip • Cleft palate • Large, protruding tongue • Drooling or copious salivation • Candidiasis—white, adherent, thick patches on tongue, palate, buccal surfaces • Weak, high-pitched cry
Neck	• Short, thick • Tonic neck reflex	• Torticollis	• Extra skinfolds or webbing • Resistant to flexion • Absence of tonic neck reflex
Chest	• Equal anteroposterior and lateral diameter • Smooth clavicles • Breast enlargement	• Supernumerary nipples • Thin breast secretions	• Crepitus or asymmetry over clavicle • Depressed sternum • Marked retractions • Asymmetrical expansion • Wide-spaced nipples
Lungs	• Bilateral bronchial breath sounds • Periodic breathing	• Crackles immediately after birth	• Inspiratory stridor • Expiratory grunting • Retractions • Unequal breath sounds • Apnea • Persistent fine crackles or wheezing • Peristaltic sounds
Abdomen	• Cylindrical shape • Soft to palpation • Umbilical cord bluish white at birth, with 2 arteries and 1 vein • Bowel sounds present • Femoral pulses equal bilaterally	• Firm to palpation when crying • Umbilical hernia • Diastasis recti	• Abdominal distention • Localized bulging • Absent bowel sounds • Drainage or blood at umbilical cord • Absent or unequal femoral pulses • Visible peristaltic waves

Table 20–3 (cont.)

	Normal	Normal Variations	Abnormal
Genitalia	*Female* • Labia majora and clitoris edematous • Urethral meatus behind clitoris • Vernix caseosa between labia • Urination within first 24 hours *Male* • Urethral opening at tip of penis • Palpable testes • Scrotum: rugae, edematous, pendulous, deeply pigmented in dark-skinned newborns • Smegma • Urination within first 24 hours	• Blood-tinged, mucous discharge • Hymenal tag • Nonretractable foreskin • Urethral opening covered by prepuce • Testes palpable in inguinal canal • Small scrotum	• Fused labia • Absence of vaginal opening • Masses in labia • Enlarged clitoris with urethral meatus at tip • Ambiguous genitalia • No urination within first 24 hours • Hypospadius • Epispadius • Chordee • Testes nonpalpable in scrotum or inguinal canal • Hypoplastic scrotum • Hydrocele • Masses in scrotum • Discoloration of testes • Ambiguous genitalia • No urination within first 24 hours
Back/Rectum	• Spine intact, no deviations, openings, or masses • Trunk incurvation reflex • Patent anal opening • Anal reflex • Meconium passed within first 24 hours		• Anal fissures or fistulas • Imperforate anus • Absent anal reflex • No meconium within 36–48 hours • Pilonidal cyst or sinus • Tuft of hair • Spina bifida
Extremities	• Ten fingers and toes • Full range of motion • Pink nail beds • Creases on anterior two thirds of sole • Symmetrical extremeties • Equal muscle tone bilaterally • Equal bilateral brachial pulses • Equal leg and gluteal folds	• Partial syndactyly between second and third toes • Second toe overlapping third toe • Wide gap between hallux and second toes • Asymmetric length of toes • Dorsiflexion and shortness of hallux	• Polydactyly • Syndactyly (webbing) • Persistent nail bed cyanosis • Nail beds yellowed • Transverse palmar crease • Fractures • Decreased or absent range of motion • Unequal leg or gluteal folds • Limited hip abduction • Audible click with abduction • Asymmetry

risk of hypothermia. Placing the baby in a radiant warmer for the initial examination after birth avoids this problem. For subsequent examinations, expose one area of the body at a time to minimize the amount of time the newborn is exposed to cold air. The Moro or startle reflex is elicited by loud noise or sudden movement of the surface the infant is lying on (Figure 20–5).

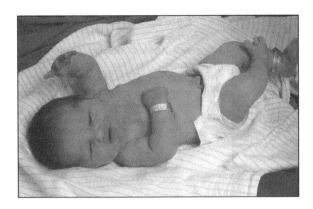

FIGURE 20–5. Moro reflex. (Reprinted with permission of Elsevier Publications.)

Skin

Observe the condition of the skin for color, opacity, thickness, and consistency. Dryness, cracking, and peeling are signs of full- or post-term maturity. A full-term newborn is likely to have flaking skin in the major creases at the ankles. Vernix caseosa—a combination of discarded epithelial cells, lanugo, and sebaceous gland secretions—is evident on term newborns and usually becomes less visible after 40 weeks gestation. Vessels will not be visible over the trunk of the body of the full-term newborn. Inspect the skin for color as well as bruises, lesions, rashes, or discolorations in natural light.

The skin should be warm, dry, and smooth. Skin color of the newborn will depend on the ethnicity of the parents. African-American newborns may appear pink or yellow-brown. Asian descent newborns may have a tan or rose color. Caucasian newborns are usually pink to red, and Hispanic newborns may have pink skin with an olive or yellow tint. Native American newborns may vary from pink to light brown or darker brown. Blanch the skin by gently pressing, then releasing a finger over the chest or forehead. The skin should show its own color when the finger is removed. The skin should not be jaundiced during the first 24 hours of life (see Chapter 11). Jaundice usually appears on the head first and progresses to the lower portion of the body and extremities as the bilirubin level rises. Jaundice noted in the first 24 hours is an abnormal finding and requires documentation and report to the physician. In Hispanic and African-American babies, the color of the mucous membranes is used to assess for jaundice.

The color of the skin changes with the activity state of the newborn. When the newborn is crying, the skin is likely to be darker in color. Within the first few hours of birth, the newborn may have brief periods of cyanosis not associated with heart rate changes or apnea. Generally, this resolves within the first few hours of life. Transient mottling may be apparent, especially when the newborn is exposed to cool temperatures. A common variation in the first 24 to 48 hours of life is acrocyanosis, a bluish discoloration of the hands and feet. As peripheral circulation improves, this will resolve and disappear within a few days after birth. Acrocyanosis lasting longer than the first 48 hours after birth needs to be investigated. Newborns with plethora, a ruddy color, have an excess of red blood cells contributing to the bright red skin color. This occurs more often in infants of mothers with diabetes. Hemoglobin and hematocrit need to be assessed in the newborn with plethora. Hematocrit results over 65 percent indicate polycythemia. These infants should be monitored closely for signs of hypoglycemia, cyanosis, respiratory distress, and jaundice (Vargo, 1996). Pallor is most often associated with anemia, hypoxia, or poor peripheral perfusion, and it needs to be evaluated. Harlequin color changes may occur as a result of the dependent half of the newborn's body reacting to a temporary autonomic imbalance of the cutaneous vessels. The skin on the dependent portion of the body becomes deep red, while the upper portion appears pale. When the newborn is turned to the opposite side the color variation reverses. This is a benign condition occurring more often in low birth weight infants (Lund & Kuller, 2003).

Observe and note the location of petechiae, pinpoint superficial hemorrhages that occur due to pressure during descent and rotation through the birth canal. Petechiae are more likely to be seen if there has been a nuchal cord, and they will usually fade within 24 to 48 hours after birth.

Skin turgor is the result of the outward pressure of interstitial fluid on the cells. Assess skin turgor by gently grasping and lifting the skin of the chest, abdomen, or thigh between the thumb and finger. Skin that readily springs back to its original shape indicates the newborn has adequate skin turgor, a sign of appropriate hydration. Dimpling, wrinkling, or folding of the skin indicates possible dehydration.

Milia are common variations that may occur on the skin of the newborn, commonly visible over the nose, cheeks, and brow. Milia are sebaceous glands that have swollen under the influence of maternal hormones. Treatment is not required for milia, as they resolve spontaneously within the first few weeks after birth. A common newborn rash, erythema toxicum, is a pink, papular rash with vesicles occurring first on the face, then spreading to the chest, abdomen, back, and buttocks that is often visible by the first or second day. This will disappear within 1 week. The rash may reappear and dissipate spontaneously without treatment.

Birthmarks

A bluish-black area of pigmentation over the buttocks and back of the newborn with dark skin may be apparent. This can easily be confused with bruising, however it is a common variation known as a Mongolian spot caused by a collection of melanocytes in the dermal layer (Figure 20–6). Mongolian spots are most often observed in African-American and Hispanic infants. The macular lesion or patch may also be seen on the legs or flank of the newborn, appearing gray or blue-green, and usually fades over time. Café au lait spots are light brown or tan macular areas with well-defined edges. As long as there are fewer than six spots and are less than 3 cm in length, they do not hold significance. Infants with larger or more numerous spots may have cutaneous neurofibromatosis (Landau & Krafchik, 1999; Margileth, 1994).

Telangiectatic nevi, "stork bites," are flat, deep pink areas over the eyelids or on the forehead or bridge of the nose that blanch with pressure. Most nevi fade with time, although they may become brighter in color when the newborn is crying. Nevus flammeus, "port wine nevus," is a reddish or flat pink lesion that does not blanch with pressure and is caused by dilated capillaries below the epidermal surface. This lesion usually remains constant in size and does not fade with time. It often appears over the face but may also be observed over the upper body.

Approximately 1 to 3 percent of newborns have hemangiomas present at birth, and another 10 percent will develop hemangiomas within the first 3 to 4 weeks (Lund & Kuller, 2003). Strawberry hemangiomas are soft, raised, lobed tumors with a bright red color, usually occurring on the head, neck, trunk, or extremities. The red color derives from the dilated mass of capillaries formed in the dermal and subdermal layers of the skin. Although spontaneous regression usually occurs, this may take several years. There will be no permanent

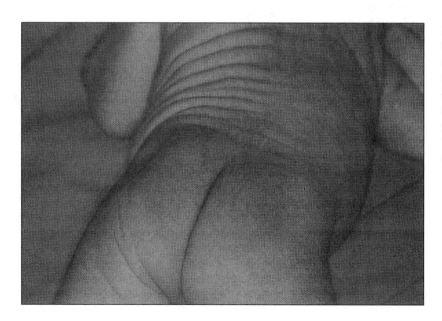

FIGURE 20–6.
Mongolian spot. (Moore ML, Nichols FH: Neonatal assessment. In Nichols FH, Zwelling E eds. *Maternal-newborn nursing: theory and practice.* Philadelphia: WB Saunders, 1080-1131, 1997. Reprinted with permission of Elsevier Publications.)

scars if these lesions are left alone. Tumors that interfere with feeding, respiration, and vision require treatment. Infection, bleeding, ulceration, and compression of the vital organs are rare complications of strawberry hemangiomas.

Head

Observe the head for shape, symmetry, bruises, and lesions. Palpation of the head may reveal swelling, masses, or bony defects. Move the head through its full range of motion to assess flexion, extension, bending, and rotation. The normal newborn's head is easily mobile in all directions, although the infant is not able to turn its head from side to side until two weeks of age. Common variations are molding, caput succedaneum, and cephalhematoma. The negative pressure created when the amniotic sac ruptures and draws a portion of the scalp into the cervical os causes a caput succedaneum. Dilated capillaries cause the edema and bruising that occurs over the occipitoparietal area of the head. Swelling usually resolves within 24 hours after birth. Overriding suture lines are common in the infant born vaginally in a vertex position. This irregular shape resolves within a few days in the full-term infant and may persist for several weeks in the premature infant. A soft area over the suture lines indicates that the sutures are separated.

The intersections of the cranial sutures are called fontanelles. The anterior fontanelle, diamond in shape, is the largest and most important for assessment (Figure 20–7). The anterior fontanelle is normally described as soft and flat but may appear to be bulging when the infant is crying vigorously, coughs, or vomits. Palpate the tension in the fontanelle with the infant in an upright and a recumbent position. A newborn with a soft sunken fontanelle in the prone position is dehydrated. The anterior fontanelle usually closes at 18 to 24 months. The posterior fontanelle—triangular-shaped, at the junction of the sagittal and lambdoidal suture—is small, 0.5 – 1 cm (0.25 – .5 in.) and closes at 2 to 3 months of age (Hoekelman, 1999).

Newborns have varying degrees of head control. When held in a supine position and pulled forward from the arms into a sitting position by the examiner, hyperextension and head lag are normal. While in a supported sitting position, the

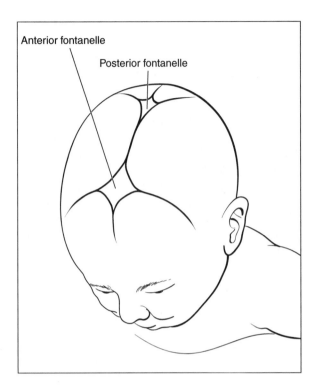

FIGURE 20–7. Fontanelles.

newborn may attempt to raise the head. The head will be in a straight line with the spine when the newborn is held in a ventral suspension position (Wilson, 2003).

Ears/Eyes

Inspect the infant's facial features for symmetry, shape, bruising, or dysmorphic features. Asymmetry may result from compression of the fetal head in the uterus or from nerve injury related to birth trauma. The sclera of the eyes should be white and without drainage. The eyelids are usually edematous immediately after birth, with no tears present. Scleral and small conjunctival hemorrhages may be present.

Able to fix on objects and follow objects to the midline, the newborn can focus on objects 7 to 12 in. (17.8 to 30.5 cm) away, the distance of the mother's face when the infant is at the breast. It is common in the newborn for the eyes to remain fixed when the head is moved through its full range of motion. Conjugate eye movements will develop rapidly after birth. The newborn is able to visually fix on objects at 2 to 4 weeks, and demonstrate coordinated eye movements at 5 to 6 weeks. By 3 months of age, the eyes converge and the infant is able to reach for objects (Hoekleman, 1999).

The ear should be horizontal with the outer canthus of the eye. The pinna is flexible and well formed in the full-term infant. There should be no drainage from the ears. Fold the ear forward to examine the undersurface of the ear for skin tags. Hearing assessment can begin early in the infant's life with simple observation of reaction to auditory stimuli. The newborn responds with a startle reflex, head turning, eye blinking, and a pause in body movements, particularly when a familiar voice is heard. The degree of the infant's alertness will affect response; however, it is wise to be observant for signs of normal behavior. Routine auditory screening of all newborns is common.

Nose

Inspect the nose for shape, symmetry, patency, and skin lesions. Observe each naris for a visual opening and gently occlude one side of the naris to observe breathing through the other side. Repeat the same process for the other naris. Newborns are nose breathers but should be able to tolerate occluding one naris during assessment. There should be no visible drainage from either naris. The nose may be misshapen at birth, due to uterine or vaginal compression, but this resolves within a few days. Obstructions or deformities, such as choanal atresia, may indicate congenital syndromes or anatomic malformations. Since clefting of the oral area may include the nose, close assessment is necessary.

Mouth

Inspect the mouth for size, shape, symmetry, color, and the presence of abnormal structures and masses when the newborn is both at rest and crying. Birth trauma may result in facial asymmetry owing to nerve damage. The midline region between the nose and the lips, the philtrum, should be well defined. The lips are fully formed and the maxilla rounded. Newborns with at least two dysmorphological characteristics of the face may have fetal alcohol syndrome or fetal alcohol effects: microcephaly (head circumference below the third percentile), short palpebral fissures, flattened upper lip, philtrum and midface (Kenner & D'Apolito, 1997).

The sucking reflex, so important for breastfeeding, can be elicited right after birth by stimulating the mucous membranes of the mouth with a gloved finger (see Figure 20–8). Assess the buccal pads on the sides of the mouth. A full-term newborn has adequate buccal pads that assist in the negative pressure created when suckling at the breast. Preterm or malnourished newborns may not have full buccal pads. The mucous membranes and tongue are pink and moist, and the tongue protrudes symmetrically over the alveolar ridge (gum line) when the mouth is open. The tongue fits easily within the mouth when closed. Macroglossia, an abnormally large tongue, may be seen in some congenital syndromes such as Beckwith-Wiedeman syndrome, and in hypothyroidism. Underdevelopment of the jaw, micrognathia, may be seen in certain malformation syndromes such as Pierre Robin syndrome.

The lingual frenulum has a consistency that may vary from thick and fibrous to very thin. The frenulum may be attached at the tip or midway along the undersurface of the tongue. Ankyloglossia, tongue-tie, occurs when the frenulum extends

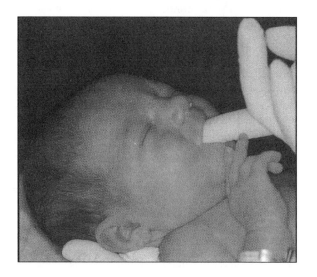

FIGURE 20–8. Suckling reflex. (Moore ML, Nichols FH: Neonatal assessment. In Nichols FH, Zwelling E eds. *Maternal-newborn nursing: theory and practice.* Philadelphia: WB Saunders, 1080–1131, 1997. Reprinted with permission of Elsevier Publications.)

in a fibrous cord to the tip of the tongue (see Chapter 10). The newborn should be able to move the tongue forward sufficiently to cup the mother's elongated nipple and areola while breastfeeding. If the tongue is able to extend to the anterior mandibular gum line, there should be little difficulty with breastfeeding. A V-shaped appearance at the tip of the tongue may indicate a frenulum that is unusually short or tight. If the tongue appears to have limited movement when the infant is crying, further assessment is warranted.

Along the gums—which are smooth and raised—or the palate, there may be retention cysts known as Epstein's pearls, which are yellow or white in color and occasionally mistaken for teeth. However, they resolve spontaneously within 1 to 2 months. (Hoekelman, 1999). Occasionally an infant will be born with supernumerary teeth. These teeth are soft with no enamel and are usually shed spontaneously. If not shed, they may need to be removed to minimize the risk of aspiration. Primary teeth will normally erupt in a wide range of ages. At age 10 months most Anglo infants have two upper and two lower central incisors. Approximately every 4 months 4 more teeth will erupt, so that there will be 8 teeth, by 14 months of age, 12 by 18 months, 16 by 22 months and 20 by 26 months.

Palpate the soft and the hard palate, which should be smooth, gently arched, and intact with the uvula in the midline. While a gloved finger is in the mouth, assess the suck reflex. It should be strong and coordinated in the full-term newborn. The newborn should be able to completely form a seal around the examiner's finger. Saliva will be either minimal or absent. Excessive drooling or oral secretions indicate an inability to swallow, or the presence of a pharyngeal or esophageal obstruction.

Neck

The newborn's neck is short and thick, which makes it difficult to observe swallowing, a cardinal sign of breastmilk intake. Palpate the clavicles for crepitus or shortening which may indicate fracture. The tonic neck reflex elicited by rotating the baby's head to one side (Figure 20–9) is seen as early as 35 weeks. Observe the neck for excess folds or webbing that may indicate congenital malformations.

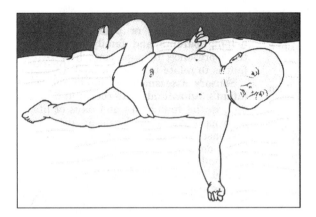

FIGURE 20–9. Tonic neck reflex. (Moore ML, Nichols FH: Neonatal assessment. In Nichols FH, Zwelling E eds. *Maternal-newborn nursing: theory and practice.* Philadelphia: WB Saunders, 1080–1131, 1997. Reprinted with permission of Elsevier Publications.)

Chest

Inspect the chest for size, symmetry, musculature, and bony structure. The chest is barrel shaped with equal anteroposterior and lateral dimensions. Chest circumference is approximately 2 cm smaller than the head. Newborn breast tissue is usually hypertrophied as a result of exposure to maternal hormones. Examination of the chest includes an assessment of respiratory stability of the newborn necessary to initiate feedings. The respiratory rate is 30 to 60 breaths per minute, with no retractions or signs of distress. The chest should rise equally on the right and left side during inspiration. Auscultate the lung sounds bilaterally and in all lung fields. It is not unusual for the lungs to sound coarse immediately after birth. Respirations will usually be shallow and slow, alternating with rapid and deep respirations. When the head is turned to one side, it is not unusual for lung sounds to be diminished on the side toward which the head is turned.

Auscultate the heart at the second intercostal space, to the right of the sternum for the aortic valve; auscultate at the second intercostal space, to the left of the sternum for the pulmonic valve; auscultate at the fourth intercostal space, to the left of the sternum for the tricuspid valve; auscultate at the fourth intercostal space, to the left of the midclavicular line for the mitral valve. Murmurs heard during the first 48 hours after birth are often due to the transition from fetal circulation to neonatal circulation. These murmurs will be audible during the systolic phase and usually disappear spontaneously.

Abdomen

The abdomen is rounded with no discoloration or visible bowel loops. Auscultate bowel sounds with the diaphragm of the stethoscope. Bowel sounds should be audible within the first hour after birth, and meconium is usually passed within the first 24 hours after birth. Observe the rise of the abdomen with the chest during respiration. Palpate the abdomen for consistency and masses. Using deep palpation, assess the abdominal organs. The liver is 1 to 3 cm below the right costal margin. The kidneys are 1 to 2 cm above and to both sides of the umbilicus. Observe the umbilical cord stump for drainage and bleeding. After the cord has been clamped for several hours, the vessels will no longer be visible. Prior to that time, observe for two umbilical arteries and one umbilical vein.

Genitalia

Male.   Observe the penis in the male newborn for the urinary meatus in the midline and at the tip of the glans penis. Since the foreskin is tightly adhered to the glans penis, the best way to assess the meatal opening is by observing the stream of urine. An opening on the dorsal side of the penis is epispadius, on the ventral side it is known as hypospadius. The scrotum is large and edematous in the full-term newborn. African-American and Hispanic newborns may have a deeply pigmented scrotum. Note the presence of rugae on the scrotal sac. Palpate the testes by placing one finger at the inguinal ring and pressing lightly. This prevents the testes from moving up into the inguinal canal while palpating the scrotal sac. The testes should feel firm, about the size of a pea. The cremasteric reflex may be observed by stroking the upper thigh or the scrotal sac. When stimulated, the testes appear to recoil in toward the inguinal canal.

Female.   The labia majora and the clitoris of the full-term female newborn are normally large and cover the labia minora, and may have a darker pig-

mentation. A small amount of white or blood-tinged discharge may be present at the vaginal opening. This is a response to the elevated estrogen levels the newborn has been exposed to during fetal development. Observe for the presence of hymenal tags. Tags usually disappear within the first few weeks and are of no great significance.

Back and Spine

Observe the back and spine for symmetry and closure. There should be no sign of openings, masses, curves, dimples, or hairy tufts. The anal opening should be visually patent and the gluteal folds even. A positive trunk incurvation reflex, the Galant reflex, is observed when suspending the newborn supine in the examiner's hand and stroking along the spine in a downward manner. The infant will curve his body inward to the side the examiner is stroking (Figure 20–10).

Extremities

The extremities of the full-term newborn are symmetrical, should remain flexed, and yet straighten out easily when moved by the examiner. Ortolani's and Barlow's maneuvers are used to assess the hips of the newborn for dislocation. To perform the Ortolani test, bend the knee and grasp the infant's

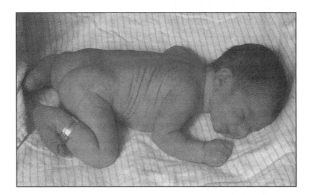

FIGURE 20–10. Trunk incurvation (Galant Reflex). (Moore ML, Nichols FH: Neonatal assessment. In Nichols FH, Zwelling E eds. *Maternal-newborn nursing: theory and practice*. Philadelphia: WB Saunders, 1080–1131, 1997. Reprinted with permission of Elsevier Publications.)

thigh and lower leg between the thumb and fingers. The examiner's middle finger is placed over the greater trochanter. Flex the hip approximately 90 degrees while bending the knee. This gently abducts the infant's leg. An audible click sound will be heard if the femoral head slides into the hip socket. Then adduct the hip. A second click will be heard as the femoral head is displaced out of the acetabulum. Barlow's test is used to determine hip instability and will help to identify the hip that can be easily displaced with manipulation. Placing the middle finger over the greater trochanter, as with Ortolani's test, and the thumb over the medial aspect of the thigh, apply gentle pressure downward and out to the side. A dislocated hip will again make a click sound and the hip will be reduced as the examiner releases the thumb pressure. Further evaluation is necessary when a hip dislocation is suspected, although many such cases are temporary and resolve without treatment.

The stepping reflex seen in Figure 20–11 is elicited by holding the infant upright so that the sole of a foot is in firm contact with a flat surface. This reflex appears at 34 weeks gestation and disappears at approximately 1 to 2 months of age. Parents may mistakenly interpret this reflex for the ability of the baby to take his first steps.

Palpate the clavicle for any signs of fracture, which may be detected by crepitus. Rotate the arm through a full range of motion in the shoulder. At this time observe under the arm for any skin tags. Palpate the humerus, radius, and ulna for symmetry. Compare the right and left brachial pulses bilaterally; they should be equal. Compare the brachial pulse with the femoral pulse again for equality.

Spread the fingers, count and observe for webbing, the presence of extra digits, (polydactyly), and observe the color of the fingernails. Infants who have been in meconium stained amniotic fluid may have yellow stained fingernails. Long fingernails are an indication that the newborn may be full-term or postmature.

Elimination

The urine of the newborn is pale yellow to clear in color and is odorless. The first urination usually occurs within the first 24 hours of life. The normal newborn will void two to six times per day for the

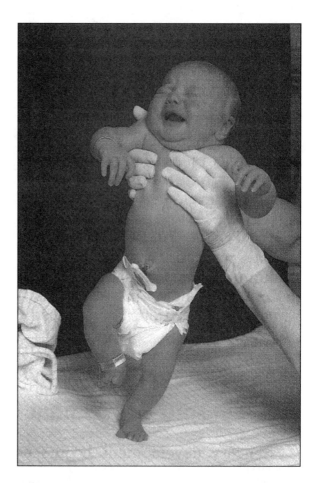

FIGURE 20–11. Stepping reflex. (Moore ML, Nichols FH: Neonatal assessment. In Nichols FH, Zwelling E eds. *Maternal-newborn nursing: theory and practice.* Philadelphia: WB Saunders, 1080–1131, 1997. Reprinted with permission of Elsevier Publications.)

first 2 days, up to 20 times per day after 2 days, owing to the kidneys' inability to concentrate urine, and later on five to eight times per day. By the end of the first week, the newborn's urine output is approximately 200 to 300 ml per 24 hours (Wilson, 2003). Superabsorbent disposable diapers make it difficult to determine the amount of urine. The presence of uric acid crystals, pink or red stains in the diaper, while usually insignificant during the first week of life, may indicate poor hydration.

Stool progression in the breastfed newborn follows a fairly predictable pattern relative to feedings.

The first stool, meconium, usually occurs within the first 24 hours. Composed of intestinal secretions, mucosal cells, and other fluids, the stool is black, thick, and tarry. Within 2 to 3 days, the stools will appear greenish black to greenish brown, then yellow or golden in color. These transitional stools may be watery or thick in texture, and they are odorless and less sticky than meconium.

Behavioral Assessment

The infant's behavior is a reflection of his capacity for self-organization (Brazelton, 1984). Self-organization refers to the infant's ability to control reactions, motor responses, responses to people and events associated with external stressors, and the ability to maintain an appropriate degree of alertness (Blackburn & Loper, 1992). An infant's reaction to stimuli affects how mothers, as well as other caregivers, react to him. This has important implications for breastfeeding as well as parent-child relationships.

Infant state is the foundation for interpreting an infant's behavior. Initially, newborns exhibit a period of alertness (2 to 4 hours) followed by a longer period of sleep. A newborn may sleep most of the next 2 to 3 postbirth days, most likely to recover from the birth experience. Subsequently, infants will demonstrate more organization of behavioral states. Infant behavior is state dependent. Infant behaviors while feeding at the breast follow a pattern as the baby develops. Table 20–4 shows infant behaviors at certain points of development.

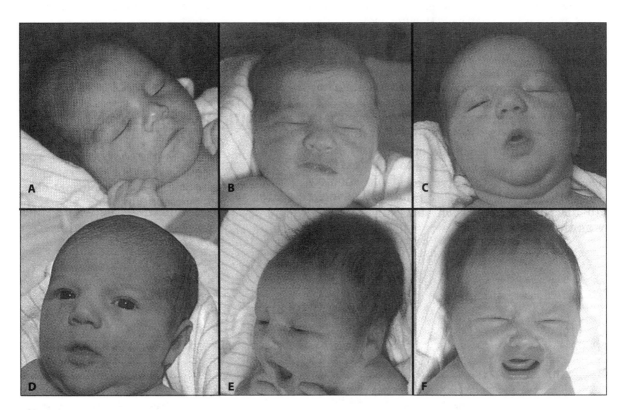

FIGURE 20–12. Infant states. (A) Deep sleep. (B) Light sleep. (C) Drowsy. (D) Quiet alert. (E) Active alert. (F) Crying. (Moore ML, Nichols FH: Neonatal assessment. In Nichols FH, Zwelling E eds. *Maternal-newborn nursing: theory and practice.* **Philadelphia: WB Saunders, 1080–1131, 1997. Reprinted with permission of Elsevier Publications.)**

Table 20–4

Infant Psychosocial and Breastfeeding Behaviors by Age

Age	Psychosocial Behavior	Breastfeeding Behavior
First day postpartum	• Quiet alert state after birth, followed by long sleep.	• May or may not feed following delivery; sleepy, learning how to suckle.
1 month	• Follows objects with eyes; reacts to noise by stopping behavior or crying.	• Becoming efficient at suckling; feedings last approximately 17 minutes. • Feedings now 8–16 times per day.
2 months	• Smiles; vocalizes in response to interactions.	• Easily pacified by frequent breastfeeding.
3 months	• Shows increased interest in surroundings; voluntarily grasps objects. • Vocalizes when spoken to. • Turns head as well as eyes in response to moving objects.	• Will interrupt feeding to turn to look at father or other familiar person coming into room and to smile at mother.
4–5 months	• Shows interest in strange settings. • Smiles at mirror image.	• Continues to enjoy frequent feedings at the breast.
6 months	• Laughs aloud. • Shows increased awareness of caregivers versus strangers. • May become distressed if mother or caregiver leaves.	• Solids offered; fewer feedings. • Feeds longer before sleep for the night. • May begin waking to nurse more often at night.
7–8 months	• Imitates actions and noises. • Responds to name. • Responds to "no." • Enjoys peek-a-boo games. • Reaches for toys that are out of reach.	• Will breastfeed anytime, anywhere. • Actively attempts to get to breast (i.e., will try to unbutton mother's blouse).
9–10 months	• Distressed by new situations or people. • Waves bye-bye. • Reaches for toys that are out of reach.	• Easily distracted by surroundings and interrupts feedings frequently. • May hold breast with one or both hands while feeding.
11–12 months	• Drops objects deliberately to be picked up by other people. • Rolls ball to another person. • Speaks a few words. • Appears interested in picture books. • Shakes head for "no."	• Tries "acrobatic" breastfeeding (i.e., assumes different positions while keeping nipple in mouth).
12–15 months	• Fears unfamiliar situations but will leave mother's side to explore familiar surroundings. • Shows emotions (e.g., love, anger, fear). • Speaks several words. • Understands meanings of many words.	• Uses top hand to play while feeding: forces finger into mother's mouth, plays with her hair, and pinches her other nipple. • Pats mother's chest when wants to breastfeed. • Hums or vocalizes while feeding. • Verbalizes need to breastfeed; may use "code" word.

Table 20–4 (cont.)

Age	Psychosocial Behavior	Breastfeeding Behavior
16–20 months	• Has frequent temper tantrums. • Increasingly imitates parents. • Enjoys solitary play or observing others. • Speaks 6 to 10 words.	• Verbalizes delight with breastfeeding. • Takes mother by the hand and leads her to favorite nursing chair.
20–24 months	• Helps with simple tasks. • Has fewer temper tantrums. • Engages in parallel play. • Combines 2 or 3 words. • Speaks 15 to 20 words.	• Stands up while nursing at times. • Nurses mostly for comfort. • Feeding before bedtime is usually last feeding before weaning. • When asked to do so by mother, willing to wait for feeding until later.

Table 20–5

INFANT SLEEP/WAKE STATES WITH IMPLICATIONS FOR BREASTFEEDING

Infant State	Description	Implications for Breastfeeding
Deep or quiet sleep	• Closed eyes with no eye movement; regular breathing • Relaxed • Absent body movements with occasional isolated startles	• Only intense stimuli will arouse • Do not attempt to feed
Light or active sleep	• Closed eyes with rapid eye movements • Irregular breathing • Sucking, smiling, grimacing, yawning • Some slight muscular twitching of the body • Most infant's sleep is in this state	• More easily aroused by stimuli • Not alert enough to feed
Drowsy	• May have eyes open • Irregular breathing • Variable body movements with mild startles • Relaxed	• Stimuli may arouse infant but may return to sleep • May enjoy nonnutritive sucking
Quiet alert	• Eyes bright and wide open • Responsive to stimuli • Minimal body activity	• Interacts with others • Excellent time to initiate breastfeeding before becomes fussy and agitated
Active alert	• Eyes open • Rapid and irregular breathing • More sensitive to stimuli and discomfort • Active	• Comfort (change diaper, hold, talk quietly) • Initiate breastfeeding before progression to crying
Crying	• Eyes open or tightly closed • Irregular breathing • Crying, very active • Uncoordinated, thrashing movements of extremities	• Comfort (hold, swaddle, talk quietly, rock) before attempting to breastfeed

Sleep-Wake States

The normal, healthy infant demonstrates six sleep-wake states (Table 20–5; Figure 20–12). The first two are sleep states. In the first, "deep sleep," the infant cannot be easily aroused even when stimulated. While in the second state, "quiet sleep," the infant exhibits some bodily movements and facial expressions. In this state, the infant is more easily aroused by stimuli, either internal or external. The newborn infant may spend as much as 18 hours per day in a combination of these sleep states. Consequently, the infant will not easily latch onto the breast when in one of these two sleep states.

The third state, "drowsy," is a transitional state. The infant is relaxed; he exhibits irregular breathing and his eyes may be open or closed. The infant is more reactive to stimuli and may either return to a "sleep" state or progress to one of the three "awake" states.

In the fourth state, "quiet alert," the infant is attentive to external stimuli but exhibits little bodily movement. Because the infant is calm in this state, this is an excellent time for breastfeeding. If a stimulus is presented at this point, such as the stroking of the cheek or the lips, the infant will become more alert and search for the stimulus. As the infant moves into the "active alert" state, he will become more sensitive to external stimuli—i.e., increased handling, diaper changing, or bathing, or internal stimuli such as hunger. The last state, "crying," is a state of much activity with crying and color change (pink to red). The infant is highly sensitive to external and internal stimuli and may need to be calmed and comforted before he will latch onto the breast. Comforting interventions such as swaddling, rocking, and softly singing or talking may help the infant return to the "quiet alert" or "active alert" state.

As part of the complete assessment, assess the infant's ability to move from one state to another. Observe for any self-quieting activi-ties, such as the infant sucking on his own hand. Also, observe the infant's response to a caregiver's voice or other calming interventions. Is the infant able to move from a crying state to one of the "alert" states? As the infant matures, he should show increasing ability to move from one state to another.

Neurobehavioral Cues and Reflexes

The cues that an infant gives about his self-organizational abilities assist the caregiver in recognizing the infant's readiness for interactions. Early and late cues that indicate the baby is hungry are seen in Table 20–6. For example, if the infant displays disengagement cues such as yawning, facial grimacing, arching, or rapid state change, he may be indicating a lack of self-organization and the need for a period of rest. That is, instead of playing with the infant or attempting to breastfeed, it may be better to swaddle, hold, rock, or otherwise provide comfort. On the other hand, engagement cues such as alertness, sucking, mouthing, smiling, or smooth movements indicate good self-organization and readiness for interaction or feeding (Blackburn & Loper, 1992) (Figure 20–13). Neonatal reflexes that have important implications for breastfeeding are seen in Table 20–7.

Table 20-6

EARLY AND LATE FEEDING CUES

Early Feeding Cues
- Body wriggling
- Hand and foot clasping
- Bringing hands to mouth or face
- Light sucking motions followed by more vigorous sucking
- Rooting behavior
- Tongue extension
- Light sounds or whimpering
- Blood flexion
- Turing head to the side

Late Feeding Cues
- Crying
- Exhaustion
- Falls asleep

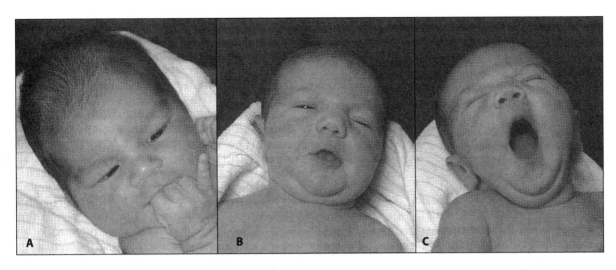

FIGURE 20–13. Infant behaviors. (A) Self-consoling. (B) Social. (C) Disengagement. (Moore ML, Nichols FH: Neonatal assessment. In Nichols FH, Zwelling E eds. *Maternal-newborn nursing: theory and practice*. Philadelphia: WB Saunders, 1080–1131, 1997. Reprinted with permission of Elsevier Publications.)

Table 20–7

DEVELOPMENTAL INFANT REFLEXES AND IMPLICATIONS FOR BREASTFEEDING

Reflex	Description	Implications for Breastfeeding
Moro (Startle)	• Elicited by any sudden noise or motion such as a handclap or jarring of the crib or cradle. • Extension of arm and opening of hands followed by flexion of arms on the chest and closing of hands. • Present by 34 weeks gestation. • Disappears at approximately 6 months of age.	• If the infant is exhibiting the Moro reflex, handle the infant more gently. • Avoid exposure to sudden, loud noises.
Sucking	• Elicited by stimulating the mouth/lips. • Infant will open the mouth and begin to suck. • Appears at 28 weeks gestation (weak and uncoordinated). • Mature at 34 weeks gestation. • Disappears at approximately 4 months of age.	• Cue for feeding (in quiet alert state). • Nutritive sucking: long, deep, suck-swallow-breathe pattern; audible. • Nonnutritive sucking: light, no audible sucking.
Rooting	• Elicited by lightly stroking the infant's cheek. • Infant will turn head in direction of stimulus. • Appears at 28 weeks gestation (immature). • Mature at 34 weeks gestation. • Disappears at approximately 4 months of age.	• May be difficult to elicit in a recently fed infant or one in a state of deep sleep. • Lightly stroking the mother's nipple on the center of the infant's lower lip will cause the infant to turn toward the breast. • Facilitates latch-on.

Summary

A complete infant assessment includes the perinatal history, gestational age assessment, breastfeeding assessment, physical assessment, and behavioral assessment. The purpose is to identify prenatal influences on the health status of the infant, create a baseline of the infant's health status, and provide early identification of actual or potential problems. Finally, a complete assessment is important when initiating breastfeeding, as well as educating and assisting the parents in understanding how to best meet the needs of their infant.

Key Concepts

- The perinatal history provides the context for the physical and behavioral assessment.

- The New Ballard scoring system has its highest reliability when performed within 48 hours of birth.

- Gestational age classification is useful for determining the infant's vulnerability to feeding/nutritional problems.

- The Infant Breastfeeding Assessment Tool, the LATCH, and the Via Christi Breastfeeding Assessment Tool are short and easy to use in the clinical setting, and they have evidence of validity and reliability.

- The quiet alert state is the most appropriate time to initiate breastfeeding.

- Behavioral assessment is useful for helping families understand how to meet their infant's needs as well as how to foster positive attachment.

- Providing a warm surface when performing physical assessment is necessary to maintain thermogreulation.

- Inspect the mouth for size, shape, symmetry, color, and the presence of abnormal structures and/or masses both when the newborn is at rest and when crying.

- The tongue is pink and moist and protrudes symmetrically over the alveolar ridge when the mouth is open.

- Bowel sounds should be audible within the first hour after birth.

- The first stool, meconium, usually occurs within the first 24 hours.

- Transitional stools may be watery or thick in texture, and are odorless and less sticky than meconium.

References

Adams D, Hewell SD. Maternal and professional assessment of breastfeeding. *J Hum Lact.* 113:279–83, 1997.

Ballard J et al. New Ballard Score, expanded to include extremely premature infants. *J Pediatr* 119:417–23, 1991.

Blackburn ST, Loper DL. The neuromuscular and sensory systems. In: Blackburn ST, Loper DL, eds. *Maternal, fetal, and neonatal physiology: a clinical perspective.* Philadelphia: W. B. Saunders, 1992:522–80.

Brazelton TB. *Neonatal assessment scale.* 2nd ed. Philadelphia: JB Lippincott, 1984.

Buschbach D. Physical assessment of the newborn infant. In: Deason J, O'Neill P, eds. *Core curriculum for neonatal intensive care nursing.* 2nd ed. Philadelphia: W. B. Saunders, 1999:74–100.

Case-Smith J, Cooper P, Scala V. Feeding efficiency of premature infants. *Am J Occup Therapy* 43:245–50, 1988.

Crowell MK, Hill PD, Humenick SS. Relationship between obstetric analgesia and time of effective breastfeeding. *J Nurse Midwifery* 39:150–156, 1994.

Donovan EF et al. Inaccuracy of Ballard scores before 28 weeks' gestation. *J Pediatr* 135:147–52, 1999.

Evans JC et al. Newborn assessment. In: Fox JA, ed. *Primary health care of infant, children, and adolescents.* St. Louis: Mosby, 2002:107–36.

Hedberg-Nyqvist K, Ewald U. Infant and maternal factors in the development of breastfeeding behaviour and breastfeeding outcome in preterm infants. *Acta Paediatr* 88: 1194–203, 1999.

Hedberg-Nyqvist K, Rubertsson C, Ewald U. Development of the preterm infant breastfeeding behavior scale (PIBBS): a study of nurse-mother agreement. *Jr Hum Lact* 12:207–19, 1996.

Hoekelman RA. Physical examination of infants and children. In: Bickley LS, Hoekelman RA, eds. *Bates guide to physical examination and history taking.* 7th ed. Philadephia: Lippincott, 1999:621–704.

Jensen D, Wallace S, Kelsay P. LATCH: a breastfeeding charting system and documentation tool. *JOGN Nurs* 23:27–32, 1994.

Kenner CD, D'Apolito K. Outcomes of children exposed to drugs in utero. *JOGN Nurs* 26:595–603, 1997.

Landau M, Krafchik B. The diagnostic values of café au lait macules. *J Am Acad Dermatol* 40:877–90, 1999.

London ML et al. Nursing assessment of the newborn. In: London ML et al., eds. *Maternal-newborn and child nursing: family-centered care.* Upper Saddle River, NJ: Peasron Education/Prentice Hall, 2003:526–65.

Lubchenko LO, Hansman C, Boyd E. Intrauterine growth in length and head circumference as estimated from live births at gestational ages from 26 to 42 weeks. *Pediatrics* 37:403–8, 1996.

Lund CH, Kuller JM. Assessment and management of the integumentary system. In: Kenner C, Lott JW, eds. *Comprehensive neonatal nursing.* Philadelphia: W. B. Saunders, 2003:700–24.

MacMullen NJ, Dulski LA. Factors related to sucking ability in health newborns. *JOGN Nurs* 29:390–96, 2000.

Margileth A. Dermatologic conditions. In: Avery GB, Fletcher MA, MacDonald MG, eds. *Neonatology: pathophysiology and management of the Newborn.* 4th ed. Philadelphia: Lippincott, 1994:1229–68.

Matthews MK. Developing an instrument to assess infant breastfeeding behaviour in the early neonatal period. *Midwifery* 4:154–65, 1988.

———Mothers' satisfaction with their neonates' breastfeeding behaviors. *JOGN Nurs* 20:49–55, 1990.

Moore ML, Nichols FH. Neonatal assessment. In: Nichols FH, Zwelling E, eds. *Maternal-newborn nursing: theory and practice.* Philadelphia: W. B Saunders, 1997:1080–131.

Morrison B et al. Psychometric validation of the Mother Baby Assessment Instrument. Presented at: State of the Nursing Science Congress, Washington DC, September 29, 2002.

Mulford C. The mother-baby assessment (MBA): an "Apgar Score" for breastfeeding. *J Hum Lact.* 1992:8:79–82.

Palmer MM, Crawley K, Blanco IA. Neonatal Oral-Motor Assessment Scale. *J Perinatol* 13:28–34, 1999.

Riordan J. Predicting breastfeeding problems. *AWHONN Lifelines, 2*(6):31–33, 1998.

———The effect of labor pain relief medication on neonatal suckling and breastfeeding duration. *J Hum Lact* 16:7–12, 2000.

Riordan J, Riordan S. The effect of labor epidurals on breastfeeding. Unit 4: Lactation consultant series 2. Schaumburg, IL: La Leche League, International, 1999, p. 8.

Riordan J, Gill-Hopple K. Testing relationships of breastmilk indicators with actual breastmilk intake. Presented at: NINR State of the Science Nursing Congress, Washington, DC, September 26, 2002.

Riordan J, Koehn M. Reliability and validity testing of three breastfeeding assessment tools. *JOGN Nurs* 26:181–87, 1997.

Riordan J et al. Predicting breastfeeding duration using the LATCH tool. *J Hum Lact* 17:20–23, 2001.

Sansoucie DA, Cavaliere TA. Newborn and infant assessment. In: Kenner C, Lott JW, eds. *Comprehensive neonatal nursing: a physiologic perspective.* 3rd ed. Philadelphia: W. B. Saunders, 2003:308–47.

Schlomer JA, Kemmerer J, Twiss, J. Evaluating the association of two breastfeeding assessment tools with breastfeeding problems and breastfeeding satisfaction. *J Hum Lact* 15:35–39, 1999.

Shrago LC, Bocar DL. The infant's contribution to breastfeeding. *JOGN Nurs* 19:211–17, 1990.

Vargo L. Cardiovascular assessment. In: Tappero EP, Honeyfield ME, eds. *Physical assessment of the newborn.* 2nd ed. Petaluma, CA: NICU Ink, 1996:77–92.

Wilson D. Health promotion of the newborn and family. In: Hockenberry MJ et al., eds. *Wong's nursing care of infants and children.* 7th ed. St. Louis: Mosby, 2003:240–94.

Appendix 20-A

INFANT BREASTFEEDING ASSESSMENT TOOL (IBFAT)*

Indicator	3	2	1	0
Readiness to feed	No effort needed	Needs mild stimulation	Need more stimulation to rouse	Cannot be roused
Rooting	Roots effectively at one	Needs coaxing prompting or encouragement	Roots poorly, even with coaxing	Did not root
Fixing/latch-on	Latches on immediately	Takes 3–10 minutes	Takes over 10 minutes	Did not latch-on
Suckling	Suckles well on one or both breasts	Suckles on and off but needs encouragement	Weak suckle, suckles on and off	Did not suckle

*Scored 0–12
Source: Matthews (1988).

Appendix 20-B

LATCH ASSESSMENT TOOL*

Indicator	0	1	2
Latch-on	Too sleepy, reluctant, no latch	Repeated attempts; holds nipple in mouth; needs stimulus to suck	Grasps breast; tongue down; lips flanged; rhythmic suckling
Audible swallowing	None	A few with stimulation	Spontaneous and intermittent, 24 hours old; spontaneous and frequent > 24 hours old
Type of nipple	Inverted	Flat	Everted after stimulation
Comfort (breast/nipple)	Engorged, cracked, bleeding, blisters, bruises	Filling; reddened; small blisters or bruises; moderate discomfort	Soft; tender
Hold (positioning)	Full assistance needed	Minimal assistance; teach one side, mother does other; staff holds, mother takes over	No assistance needed; mother able to position/hold infant

*Scored 0–10.
Source: Jensen, Wallace, & Kelsay (1994).

Appendix 20-C

MOTHER-BABY ASSESSMENT SCALE

Indicator	Mother Score = 1	Baby Score = 1	Score 0–10
Signaling	Watches and listens for baby's cues; holds, strokes, rocks, talks to baby; stimulates baby if he is asleep, calms if he is fussy.	Gives readiness cues: stirring, alertness, rooting, suckling, hand-to-mouth, cries.	
Positioning	Holds baby in good alignment within latch-on range of nipple; body is slightly flexed; entire ventral surface facing mother's body; head and shoulders are supported.	Roots well; opens mouth wide, tongue cupped and covering lower gum.	
Fixing	Holds her breast to assist baby; brings baby in close when his mouth is wide open; may express drops of milk.	Latches on, takes all of nipple and about 2 cm (1 in.) of areola into mouth, then suckles, has burst-pause suckling pattern.	
Milk transfer	Reports feeling any of the following: uterine cramps, increased lochia, breast ache or tingling, relaxation, sleepiness; milk leaks from opposite breast.	Swallow audibly; milk is observed in baby's mouth; may spit up milk when burping. Rapid "call-up suckling" rate (2 suckles/second); changes to nutritive suckling, about 1 suckle/second.	
Ending	Breasts are comfortable; lets baby suckle until he is finished. After nursing, breasts feel softer; has no lumps, engorgement, or nipple soreness.	Releases breast spontaneously; appears satiated. Does not root when stimulated. Face, arms, and hands relaxed; may fall asleep.	

Source: Mulford (1992).

Appendix 20–D

Via Christi Breastfeeding Assessment Tool

Indicator	0	1	2	Score
Latch-on	No latch-on achieved	Latch-on after repeated attempts	Eagerly grasped breast to latch-on	
Length of time before latch-on and suckle	Over 10 minutes	4-6 minutes	0-3 minutes	
Suckling	Did not suckle	Suckled but needs encouragement	Suckled rhythmically and lips flanged	
Audible swallowing	None	Only if stimulated	Under 48 hours, intermittent; Over 48 hours, frequent	
Mom's evaluation	Not pleased	Somewhat pleased	Pleased	
				TOTAL SCORE

The Via Christi Breastfeeding Assessment Tool assigns a score of 0, 1, or 2 to five factors. Scores range from 0 to 10.

Immediate high risk: All mothers who have had breast surgery. All babies who have lost >10 percent birth weight.

0 to 2 = High risk: Close, immediate post-discharge follow-up needed. Phone call and visit to provider within 3 days.

3 to 6 = Medium risk: Post-discharge phone call within 2 days. Follow-up as per protocol.

7 to 10 = Low risk: Information given to mother and routine phone call.

Source: Derived from Riordan & Riordan (1999); Jensen, Wallace, & Kelsey (1994); Matthews (1988).

FERTILITY, SEXUALITY, AND CONTRACEPTION DURING LACTATION

Kathy I. Kennedy

Fertility, sexuality, and contraception are interrelated aspects of reproduction. Breastfeeding affects each of these entities; thus the reproductive aspects of women's lives are more complex during lactation than during the nonlactating state (Figure 21–1). Although breastfeeding clearly has a fertility-reducing effect on the nursing mother, the nature of this effect is not fully understood. In general, the child's suckling initiates a cycle of neuroendocrinologic events that results in the inhibition of ovulation. One consequence of this inhibition is the creation of the hypoestrogenic state in the woman. Consequently, the dry, sometimes atrophic, vaginal mucosa may result in pain upon intercourse. Because of this and other circumstances, many breastfeeding women have sexual relationships infrequently and are thus at reduced risk of pregnancy for behavioral reasons. Emotions related to motherhood, such as intensive (albeit normal) involvement with the infant, and feelings of undesirability on the part of a woman who has not recovered her prepregnancy body, may affect her sexual behavior as well. Fear of subsequent pregnancy may also play a role in coital behavior and therefore risk of pregnancy. Since some contraceptives may relieve the vaginal symptoms of hypoestrogenicity as well as lessen the fear of pregnancy, coital frequency may also be related to family planning choice. These are but a few examples of the interrelationships among fertility, sexuality, contraception, and lactation. It is fitting that they should be explored together.

Reviewing current research on fertility and contraception, and critiquing the conventional wisdom and insights from research on sexuality during breastfeeding, this chapter explores lactation as it relates to fertility, sexuality, and contraception.

Fertility

The Demographic Impact of Breastfeeding

The natural birth-spacing effect of breastfeeding has been recognized for many years. In the past few decades, demographers have been able to quantify, in various ways, the degree of contraceptive protection that results from breastfeeding. In the early 1970s, it was determined that in the developing world nearly universal breastfeeding provided more woman-months of contraceptive protection than all other modern family planning methods combined (Rosa, 1975). It is not clear

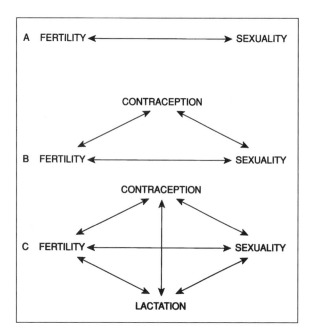

FIGURE 21–1. The interrelationships among fertility, sexuality, contraception, and lactation. (A) In the absence of a family planning intention, the phenomena of reproduction and sexual behavior (fertility and sexuality) are related in the most simple and direct manner. (B) When a family planning method is used for spacing or limiting pregnancies, it clearly affects fertility, and sometimes also sexual behavior (e.g., coitus-dependent methods). (C) Lactation can have independent effects on fertility, sexual behavior, and contraceptive decisions and patterns of use.

whether this situation still holds since the expansion of contraceptive choices to women in the developing world. In populations without access to modern methods of family planning, birth spacing is the major determinant of total fertility (the total number of children a woman will bear) and the birth interval is dependent for the most part on breastfeeding (Bongaarts & Menken, 1983; Bongaarts & Potter, 1983).

Demographers have described the fertility-suppressing effect of breastfeeding as the extent to which contraceptive prevalence would need to increase in order to offset a projected decline in breastfeeding—with its concomitant decrease in natural contraceptive protection (Bongaarts & Potter, 1983). For example, in countries where contraceptive prevalence is low and breastfeeding

prevalence is high, modest erosions in breastfeeding duration would require the tripling or better of contraceptive prevalence in order to prevent an increase in the existing, already high fertility in the country (Thapa, Short, & Potts, 1988).

In general, those more developed settings in which the erosion of breastfeeding practices has been profound are the very countries in which contraceptive prevalence is high. Thus, in the United States and the United Kingdom the contraceptive effects of breastfeeding are demographically insignificant.

Mechanisms of Action

During the normal menstrual cycle in the nonlactating woman, the hypothalamus secretes gonadotropin-releasing hormone (GnRH) in a pulsatile fashion, which in turn triggers a pulsatile release of luteinizing hormone (LH) from the anterior pituitary. LH pulses play a major role in follicular growth and estrogen secretion. In the first days of the cycle, the growing ovarian follicles produce increasing amounts of estrogen, which in turn appear to increase the frequency of LH pulses. When estrogens reach a critical level, there is a surge of LH followed by ovulation in about 17 hours. After ovulation, a corpus luteum is formed that produces estrogens and progesterone, and GnRH and LH secretion declines.

By about 4 weeks postpartum, plasma levels of LH return to a normal level in nonbreastfeeding women, and cyclicity begins anew, although the first few cycles are not always normal. In lactating women, LH levels are below normal and, more importantly, pulsation is not normal. In fully breastfeeding women, baseline levels of LH remain below normal even in the presence of follicular development. Presumably, suckling interferes with the normal secretion of GnRH by the hypothalamus, in turn disrupting normal pulsatile LH secretion (Figure 21–2). Thus, normal follicular development does not ensue. Small amounts of estrogen are secreted but they are insufficient to cause an LH surge and ovulation. An experiment to test this presumption involved the administration of pulsatile GnRH to breastfeeding women, after which follicular development, ovulation, and luteinization were observed (Glasier, McNeilly, & Baird, 1986; McNeilly, 2001a, 2001b).

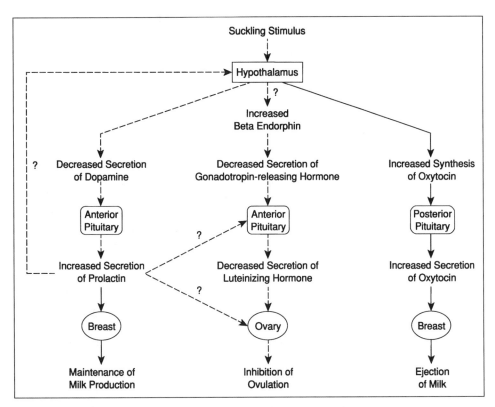

FIGURE 21–2. Physiological mechanisms involved in lactational infertility. (Adapted from Short, 1984. Reprinted with permission.)

Increased levels of prolactin are clearly associated with breastfeeding patterns (Gross & Eastman, 1985). Inhibitory effects of prolactin on gonadotropin secretion and/or ovarian function have been postulated. However, the role of prolactin is uncertain since some lactating women show normal ovulatory cycles despite high levels of prolactin (Diaz et al., 1995), and because pulsatile GnRH infusion can induce follicular development and ovulation in hyperprolactinemic breastfeeding women (Glasier, McNeilly, & Baird, 1986). Possibly, the decline in suckling causes both the decrease in prolactin and the improvement in LH pulsation, while the relationship between prolactin and hypothalamic inhibition is only coincidental (McNeilly, 2001a, 2001b).

The current understanding of the neuroendocrinologic mechanisms relative to lactational infertility is by no means complete. A summary of the existing neuroendocrinologic questions and suggestions for the next generation of studies is available (Diaz et al, 1995). The complexity of the process is appreciated, as is the irony that the baby is in charge of it all.

Lactational Amenorrhea

The period of lactational amenorrhea rather than the period of breastfeeding should be considered the phase of natural infertility (Short et al., 1991). Reviews of the international literature have shown that between 3 and 10 percent of women conceive during lactational amenorrhea if they are not otherwise practicing contraception (Van Ginnekin, 1974; Rolland, 1976; Badroui & Hefnawi, 1979; Simpson-Hebert & Huffman, 1981). These percentages are crude indices of the contraceptive efficacy of lactational amenorrhea and are not directly comparable to Pearl pregnancy rates or lifetable rates. Also, these percentages are uncontrolled for the time postpartum when the mothers conceived. (Some women may have become pregnant soon after delivery, but others may have remained amenorrheic for 2 or more years before they conceived.) They also do not control for the amount of breastfeeding that was going on before and around the time of conception.

Many studies suggest that the expected protection afforded by amenorrhea is significant—and competitive with reversible methods of fertility regulation such as pills or IUDs. In several retrospective studies, the researchers calculated rates of ovulation or pregnancy during lactational amenorrhea with reference to time postpartum. An analysis of 236 urban women in Chile found only a 0.9 percent probability of pregnancy at 6 months among amenorrheic women who did not feed their babies any breastmilk substitutes. In contrast, menstruating, breastfeeding mothers who gave milk supplements had cumulative probabilities of pregnancy of 35.6 and 54.7 at 6 and 12 months respectively (Diaz et al., 1991). In a study of 101 Australian women, an estimated cumulative probability of conception during lactational amenorrhea was calculated from the observed rate of the recovery of ovulation. The estimated probabilities of pregnancy were 1.7 percent at 6 months and 7.0 percent at 1 year postpartum (Short et al., 1991; Lewis et al., 1991). An analysis of data on 346 amenorrheic women who were not practicing contraception was pooled from nine studies in eight countries. It yielded a 12-month cumulative lifetable pregnancy rate of 5.9 percent (Kennedy & Visness, 1992). This study reflects the combined effects of many different breastfeeding patterns and styles or timings of weaning. These three analyses support the earlier, more crude estimates of 3 to 10 percent pregnancy rates during lactational amenorrhea, which did not control for time postpartum.

Obviously, a small proportion of women experience their first normal postpartum ovulation and conceive during the period of lactational amenorrhea. To the best of our knowledge, a woman will have no more than one ovulation during amenorrhea. If she does ovulate during amenorrhea, it will usually occur shortly (0 to 3 weeks) before the first postpartum menses.

Some women repeatedly experience "inadequate" menstrual cycles—i.e., cycles in which too little progesterone is produced to sustain a fertilized ovum after the end of lactational amenorrhea. Indeed some women who wish to conceive are unable to do so until after the breastfeeding child has been totally weaned, as even token breastfeeding may provide enough inhibitory stimulus to prevent ovulation or to allow adequate progesterone production.

Generally, the earlier in the postpartum period that a woman experiences her first menses, the less likely it is that this first bleeding episode will be pre-

ceded by ovulation (Howie et al., 1981, 1982b; Perez et al., 1972). The earlier in the postpartum period that the first ovulation occurs, the less likely it is to be characterized by a luteal phase of adequate duration and progesterone production (Howie et al., 1982a).

The Suckling Stimulus

The child's suckling is the stimulus that controls the negative feedback inhibition of the normal cycling of the hypothalamic-pituitary-ovarian axis, but accurate measurement or quantification of the suckling stimulus is difficult. In general, researchers have relied on measures such as the frequency of breastfeeding episodes, the duration of each episode, total minutes of suckling, and intervals between suckling episodes, as well as each of these measures classified by day and by night. All of these approaches result in indices of how often suckling occurred but not of other suckling characteristics, such as the strength of the stimulus or the volume of milk obtained. Various creative approaches to measuring suckling strength and milk volume have been attempted, such as breastmilk expression, test weighing mothers and babies before and after a breastfeed, isotope dilution, and moire topography. Unfortunately, the methodology required to measure, for example, pounds of pressure per square inch on the nipple, or tiny changes in the baby's weight before and after a feeding, have rendered measurement of these variables impossible on a large scale.

A different approach was taken in a study of the recovery of ovulation during lactation in the Philippines (Manila) and Baltimore. Researchers determined that breastfeeds as a proportion of all feeds (a reflection of the relative frequency of breastfeeds) was the best correlate of the risk of ovulation during breastfeeding. Women whose first ovulation occurred before 6 months had a significantly lower percentage of breastfeeds to total feeds in the first 6 months (84 percent) than did women whose first ovulation occurred later (88 percent) (Gray et al., 1990; Eslami et al., 1990). Even this simple measure, however, may be impractical for mothers to calculate each day (i.e., whether she is giving more or less than 85 percent of the baby's feedings as breastfeeds). Finally, although the difference in breastfeeds as a proportion of all feeds was statistically significant (84 percent versus 88 percent) this difference is clinically insignificant, so this factor could not be used practically as a sign of impending fertility.

The Manila study is one of a number that sought to develop simple guidelines for the optimum time for breastfeeding women to start using a modern contraceptive and/or to take full advantage of the natural protection from pregnancy that is provided by breastfeeding. Such guidelines usually involve some simple sign or behavior, such as a number of breastfeedings per day needed to prevent ovulation. The guideline must be based on phenomena easily observed or recorded by the woman in order to have widespread applicability.

Breastfeeding Frequency and Duration.
Studies in Scotland and Denmark showed that no woman ovulated if she breastfed her baby at least 6 times in 24 hours for a total of at least 65 minutes (McNeilly, Glasier, & Howie, 1985; McNeilly et al., 1983; Andersen & Schioler, 1982). A study in central Africa found that six suckling episodes per day were effective in maintaining levels of prolactin consistent with anovulation (Delvoye et al., 1977). However, subsequent prospective studies on the return of ovulation during lactation found no such minimum value of breastfeeding frequency that could be relied upon to suppress ovarian activity (Rivera et al., 1988; Israngkura et al., 1989; Shaaban et al., 1990; Elias et al., 1986). In these studies, some women ovulated despite up to 15 breastfeeding episodes per day (Israngkura et al., 1989), and a case of conception in the face of 12 breastfeeds per 24 hours has been reported (Khan et al., 1989).

The wide range of minimal feeding frequency required to prevent ovulation may be due to measurement differences across studies and between individual women. Additionally, the nature of a breastfeed changes from setting to setting and from woman to woman. For example, for some women, a breastfeed is a highly ritualized affair that takes some time to accomplish. It involves changing the baby's diaper, preparing a beverage for the mother to consume during the feed, taking the phone off the hook, settling into a particular rocking chair, suckling for 20 minutes or so, and putting the baby

(who may have slipped off to sleep) back into the crib. These breastfeeds occur, for example, five to six times a day and one to two times per night, perhaps with the baby nursing in the parents' bed. By contrast, another woman may identify her baby's cue to feed before the first whimper. She breastfeeds for 3 to 4 minutes until the baby regains serenity, as often as 15 to 20 times day and night. It is not surprising, then, that a "magic number" of breastfeeds has not been identified which will keep all women ovulation-free.

Having concluded that there is no universally reliable breastfeeding frequency associated with anovulation, it is important to note that when studying a large number of women, frequent breastfeeding remains an important correlate of lactational infertility (Jones, 1988, 1989). In fact, almost any valid measure of the amount of breastfeeding that occurs could be linked to the duration of infertility if the sample studied is large enough, depending on what other variables are measured and controlled.

The relationship between daily suckling frequency and duration (the total number of minutes of suckling) is difficult to generalize across mother-baby pairs. Many investigators assume that since frequent suckling produces higher milk yields than occasional suckling, mothers who feed frequently will also feed for a longer total duration. The more milk there is, the longer it will take for the baby to obtain it. Howie et al. (1981) found this relationship to be so strong that one characteristic could be substituted for the other.

Like every other aspect of breastfeeding (and fertility), this generalization needs to be tempered by recognition of normal individual variations. For example, the need of a given baby to suckle for comfort may affect both breastfeeding frequency and duration. Some babies are efficient sucklers and obtain milk quickly while others are more methodical and unhurried, just as children and adults vary in their speed of food consumption at the dinner table.

Although Howie et al. (1981) reported a very high positive association between suckling frequency and duration, this has not been reported in all studies. In an investigation of breastfeeding mothers in Manila (Benitez et al., 1992), the association between suckling frequency and duration at 1 month postpartum (r = 0.52) was not significant. This finding suggests that if such an association exists, it does not hold for all women. Figure 21–3 displays the breastfeeding frequency and minutes of suckling for four women in this study, including their individual correlation coefficients. Across the four panels, the gamut of possibilities can be seen: high-positive, low-positive, high-negative, and low-negative associations.

One of the most promising correlates of the duration of lactational infertility is actually a measure of not breastfeeding. The interval between breast-

feedings is an inverse expression of both frequency and duration because the number of intervals will be high if the frequency is high, and the length of the average interval will be low if the duration or the frequency of breastfeeds is high. Measuring average intervals between feedings yields no new information or advantage over measuring frequency and duration of feedings. However, the longest interval between feedings reflects a different characteristic from all others mentioned thus far.

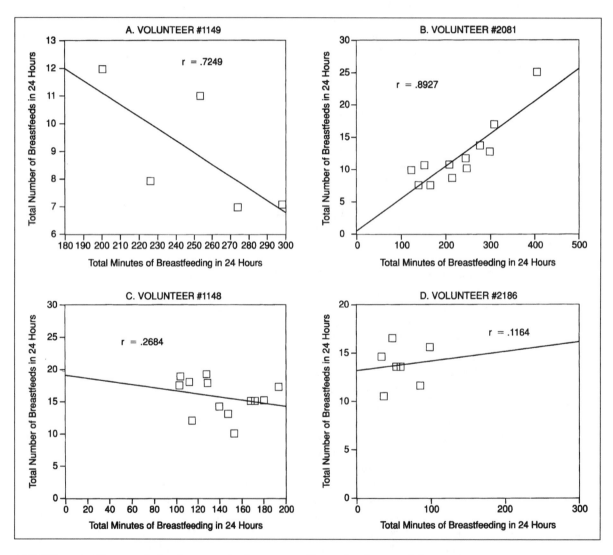

FIGURE 21–3. The association between the frequency of breastfeedings and the number of minutes of suckling within the same woman. This appears to be sometimes strong (A and B), sometimes weak (C and D), sometimes negative (A and C), and sometimes positive (B and D). (*Source:* Unpublished data derived from Benitez et al., 1992.)

Recognizing that the duration of lactational infertility is strongly influenced by infant feeding patterns, the World Health Organization (WHO) conducted a prospective study of more than 4000 breastfeeding women in seven countries to learn whether the duration of lactational infertility could be predicted (WHO, 1998a, 1998b). Eighty-three variables were available for analysis—32 were infant feeding variables and 51 were other characteristics of the mother and/or infant. Many measures of the suckling stimulus (such as breastfeeding frequency, duration, intervals between feeds, etc.) were tested. As should be expected, not all of the 32 breastfeeding (or infant feeding) factors were significant predictors of the duration of lactational amenorrhea because these factors are often interrelated, or simply slightly different ways of defining the same variable. After controlling for center-related differences across the five developing and two developed country settings, ten factors were found, in a multivariate analysis, to be significantly related to the duration of amenorrhea, and seven of the ten were infant feeding characteristics (Box 21–1). Whether the infant was breastfeeding versus totally weaned was, not surprisingly, a highly significant predictor of lactational amenorrhea. The total duration of breastfeeding per 24 hours and the interval between birth and the first breastfeed were also significant determinants of the duration of amenorrhea. Several significant factors were related to supplementation, such as the time until regular supplementation commenced and the percent of all feeds that were breastfeeds. This WHO Multinational Study of Breastfeeding and Lactational Amenorrhea clearly demonstrated a profound effect of suckling on the duration of amenorrhea. It also suggested that, among a large number of ways of defining the suckling stimulus, the simple presence of breastfeeding and the 24 hour duration of breastfeeding were the breastfeeding factors most closely associated with the duration of amenorrhea. Had the study not measured

---

BOX 21–1

Factors Related to Duration of Amenorrhea

Nonfeeding Variables

1. (High) number of live births = longer amenorrhea***

2. (High) maternal body mass index at 6 to 8 weeks postpartum = shorter amenorrhea***

3. (High) percent follow-up visits in which infant was ill = longer amenorrhea***

Feeding Variables

4. (Long) time from delivery to first breastfeed = shorter amenorrhea**

5. (Yes) regular supplementation with any food or drink = shorter amenorrhea**

6. (High) total 24-hour duration of breastfeeding = longer amenorrhea*

7. (High) percent of feeds constituted by breastmilk = longer amenorrhea***

8. (High) frequency of water/noncaloric supplements = longer amenorrhea***

9. (Yes) weaned = shorter amenorrhea***

10. (Yes) supplements comprise 50 percent of feeds = shorter amenorhea**

---

*$p < 0.05$
**$p < 0.01$
***$p < 0.001$

Source: World Health Organization (1998b).

the suckling stimulus in these particular ways, some other quantification of the suckling stimulus, such as the frequency of breastfeeding or the longest interval between suckling episodes, would have proven to be statistically significant.

Supplemental Feeding. The role supplementation plays in the return of fertility is anything but straightforward. A prevailing assumption is that anything that decreases the child's suckling behavior or the need to suckle will be a secondary cause of the recovery of fertility. Supplementation may have the effect of decreasing hunger, thirst, and possibly the emotional need for comfort, thereby reducing suckling at the breast.

The pioneering work of the Medical Research Council in Edinburgh found this to be the case (Howie et al., 1981). In a sample of Scottish women, the initiation of supplements to the infant occurred very shortly before the first ovulation. Supplementation was thought to be causally related to the recovery of ovulation because of the close temporal relationship between the two events. By contrast, in studies in developing countries, instances have been observed in which supplements are introduced to the baby without an impact on the underlying maternal ovarian hormone profile (see Figure 21–4). In such cases, the supplements are usually gradual additions to the baby's diet, and, like the maternal ovarian hormone levels, the breastfeeding behaviors remain essentially unchanged. A study of well-nourished Australian women who breastfed for an extended period of time also did not find supplementation to be associated with returning fertility (Lewis et al., 1991), presumably because the introduction of supplements was gradual and quantities were small. By contrast, in the Scottish studies, a supplement was generally a milk substitute that was given as a replacement for a breastfeed, and the suckling stimulus was thus decreased.

Supplementation has also been shown to have an effect on the duration of lactational amenorrhea independent of breastfeeding frequency and duration (Jones, 1989; Benitez et al., 1992). It is possible that supplementation changes some of the more elusive characteristics of breastfeeding, such as suckling strength, rather than just frequency and duration.

As seen in Box 21–1, five of the seven significant infant feeding variables that predicted the return of menses in the large WHO study were actually measures of supplementation (WHO, 1998a). The effect of supplementation on the return of fertility is likely to be a function of the degree to which weaning foods replace the suckling stimulus.

The strength and the nature of the relationship between infant feeding characteristics (such as breastfeeding frequency and time until supplementation) and the return of fertility changes with the duration of lactation. For example, if the duration of lactation is short, supplementation is probably more strongly associated with the return of fertility than if lactation extends over a long period.

The Repetitive Nature of the Recovery of Fertility

Unpublished studies in France, the Philippines, Australia, and Canada (reviewed in Kennedy, 1993) found that a significant association exists between the duration of lactational infertility after one pregnancy and the duration in the same woman after her next pregnancy. These and anecdotal observations prompted the secondary analyses of large, existing datasets about the relationship between the durations of lactational amenorrhea reported in consecutive pregnancies.

In a large prospective study of Bangladeshi women, 418 women were observed through the course of breastfeeding two consecutive babies. The length of amenorrhea while breastfeeding the first child had significant predictive value for the subsequent length of amenorrhea. The author concluded that information on previous experience with lactational amenorrhea should be incorporated into guidelines for the introduction of family planning during lactation (Ford, 1992).

In the WHO Multinational Study of Breastfeeding and Lactational Amenorrhea (WHO 1998b), the duration of lactational amenorrhea after the previous pregnancy was recorded at the time of admission. This single predictor was so highly significant and explained so much of the variance in the duration of lactational amenorrhea in the prospective study that no other factor in a multivariate analysis was significantly associated with the duration of lactational amenorrhea.

If a woman is to experience the same duration of infertility (or of amenorrhea) while breastfeeding two consecutive babies, the breastfeeding behavior

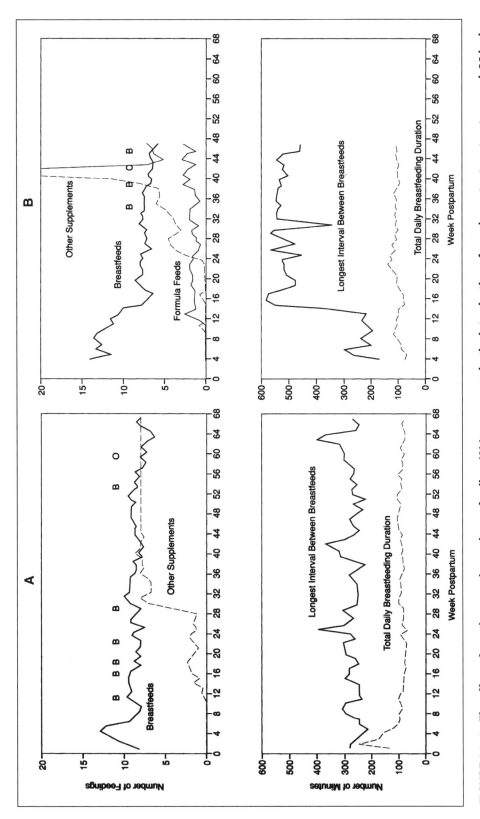

FIGURE 21-4. The effect of supplementation on breastfeeding. (A) In one example, the introduction of supplements at postpartum week 28 had no effect on breastfeeding frequency, duration, or the interval between feedings. (B) In another example, the introduction of supplements at about week 9 coincided with a decrease in breastfeeding frequency and an increase in the longest interval between breastfeeds. Ovulation was still postponed for about 10 months, probably because breastfeeding frequency and duration were high enough. (*Source:* From Rivera, 1988.)

is presumed to be roughly similar in both cases. Then the amount of neurosensory stimulation received by the mother through suckling would be roughly the same, eliciting roughly the same fertility repressing effect in the woman. We can suppose that this is likely to happen in many cases because two factors would be roughly the same in both breastfeeding couplets:

- The organism of the woman is the same; that is, her basic physiology is roughly the same. (If many years have passed between the pregnancies, then the woman's organismic responses to reproductive hormones may have changed somewhat with age.)

- The woman's orientation to infant feeding, and her ideas and habits about breastfeeding, probably remained constant across the two experiences. Differences also are likely to occur if her pattern of breastfeeding has also changed markedly. However, the research to date suggests that women generally can expect a similar pattern of recovery of fertility from one birth to the next, provided that the breastfeeding pattern does not change dramatically.

Of course, two infants with markedly different feeding needs and personalities could cause different effects on the mother's return to fertility.

In a later section, the timing of the introduction of postpartum contraception will be addressed. As suggested by Ford (1992), when the duration of the previous length of lactational amenorrhea is known, this may be a useful factor when making an individual decision about the commencement of postpartum contraception. In whole communities, information about the average duration of lactational amenorrhea may inform programs as to the most effective community approaches to postpartum contraception (Weiss, 1993).

The Bellagio Consensus

By the late 1980s, researchers on five continents had completed prospective studies of the changes in ovarian hormones in breastfeeding women. Many of these researchers assembled in Bellagio, Italy to determine whether their various findings about women with vastly different patterns of breastfeeding behavior could be synthesized into a statement about how breastfeeding women might predict their recovery of fertility (Box 21–2).

BOX 21–2

The Bellagio Consensus

Lactational amenorrhea should be regarded as a potential family planning method in all maternal and child health programs in developing and developed countries.

Postpartum women should be offered a choice of using breastfeeding as a means of family planning, either to help achieve optimal birth spacing of at least 2 years, or as a way of delaying the introduction of other contraceptives. They should be informed of how to maximize the antifertility effects of breastfeeding to prevent pregnancy.

Breastfeeding provides more than 98 percent protection from pregnancy during the first 6 months postpartum if the mother is "fully" or nearly fully breastfeeding and has not experienced vaginal bleeding after the 56th day postpartum.

Source: Family Health International (1988); Kennedy, Rivera, & McNeilly (1989).

The basis for the consensus in 1988 was a body of published and unpublished studies of the pregnancy rates (three studies in two countries), as well as data on the probability of a recognizable pregnancy from prospective studies of the recovery of ovulation during lactation (10 studies in seven countries). Among these studies, the highest pregnancy rate reported in fully breastfeeding amenorrheic women during the first 6 months postpartum was lower than 2 percent (Family Health International, 1988; Kennedy, Rivera, & McNeilly, 1989).

The Bellagio Consensus states that bleeding in the first 56 days postpartum can be ignored. This claim is supported by a prospective study of postpartum bleeding in 477 experienced breastfeeding women in the Philippines. A median duration of postpartum bleeding of 27 days was reported, which did not vary by age, parity, breastfeeding frquency, or level of supplementation. Furthermore, over a quarter of these women experienced a subsequent bleeding episode beginning not later than postpartum day 56. Only 10 women may have had their first cyclic menses before day 56. None became pregnant, although not all were yet sexually active. (Visness, Kennedy, & Ramos, 1997). A prospective study of 72 fully breastfeeding women in developed countries found that nearly half experienced some bleeding or spotting between the sixth and eighth weeks postpartum. Despite ovarian follicular development in seven of the 72 cases, there was no ovulation in any woman in the first 8 weeks postpartum. (Visness et al., 1997). Findings from the WHO Multinational Study of Breastfeeding and the return of menses are consistent with the advice to ignore bleeding prior to postpartum day 56 (WHO, 1999a).

The Bellagio Consensus is important because it reflects principles that are believed to be applicable cross-culturally. Yet this aspect of the consensus is also one of its weaknesses: by making generalizations that apply to a range of breastfeeding patterns and practices, some possible situations could not be accommodated. For example, in societies in which a child is breastfed for 2 years or more, or among La Leche League mothers in industrialized countries who choose to breastfeed for these longer periods, lactational amenorrhea alone may be a viable marker of returning fertility. Cognizant of this, Kennedy, Rivera, and McNeilly (1989, p. 485) cautioned as follows:

Guidelines specific to a particular country or population for using breastfeeding as a postpartum family planning method can be developed based on this consensus. Local infant feeding practices, the average duration of amenorrhea and the ongoing changes in women's status and health practices should be considered in adapting these general guidelines.

The consensus is also important because it represents the framework for the actual use of lactational amenorrhea as a method of contraception. Guidelines on how to integrate the Lactational Amenorrhea Method (LAM) into family planning and breastfeeding support programs have been developed based on the Bellagio Consensus (Labbok et al., 1994).

During the 8 years after the Bellagio Consensus, a new body of research was undertaken to test the consensus prospectively. Four clinical trials of the contraceptive efficacy of LAM were conducted in Chile (Perez, Labbok, & Queenan, 1992), Pakistan (Kazi et al., 1995), the Philippines (Ramos, Kennedy, & Visness, 1996), and in a multinational study (Labbok et al, 1997). These studies found cumulative 6-month lifetable rates of pregnancy during correct use of the method of 1.0, 0.5, 1.5, and 0.6 percent, respectively. These studies observed women who chose to use LAM as their postpartum contraceptive method and were taught and actually used the method. Other researchers conducted secondary data analyses on existing datasets (Short et al., 1991; Weiss, 1993; Rojnik, Kosmelj, & Andolsek-Jeras, 1995), and found that the protection from pregnancy under the LAM conditions can outlast the parameters set in the Bellagio Consensus. The largest secondary analysis is from the WHO Multinational Study of Breastfeeding and the Return of Menses in which the findings on pregnancy during lactation also uphold the Bellagio Consensus (WHO, 1999b).

On the basis of these studies, as well as unpublished research from a variety of sources, scientists who reconvened at Bellagio in 1995 were able to conclude that "the Bellagio Consensus has clearly been confirmed" (Kennedy, Labbok, & Van Look, 1996).

Having accumulated data and experience from prospective clinical trials, the group at "Bellagio II" was able to draw conclusions about the modification of LAM on a local level:

(1) It is not possible to eliminate the amenorrhea criterion.

Once menstruation has resumed, fertility is returning, or already has returned. Menses is an absolute indication of the need for another contraceptive method if continued protection is desired.

(2) It may be possible to relax the full or nearly full breastfeeding criterion.

If breastfeeding behaviors are sound and the introduction of weaning foods is not accompanied by a decline in any breastfeeding parameter, then theoretically the full/nearly full breastfeeding criterion may be relaxed. However, this possibility requires more research since the breastfeeding stimulus is what causes lactational amenorrhea, and supplementation can (but does not always) affect that stimulus.

(3) It may be possible to extend LAM beyond six months postpartum.

In the clinical trials and the secondary analyses, the protection provided by lactational amenorrhea beyond the sixth postpartum month—and hence during supplemented breastfeeding—was found to be relatively low in some settings—for example, 4–9 percent in the multinational study (Labbok et al., 1997) and 0–5 percent in the Philippine clinical trial (Ramos, Kennedy, & Visness, 1996). These rates are not surprising since decades of retrospective research reviewed above showed that 3–10 percent of women conceive during lactational amenorrhea. While these rates indicate significant protection among successfully breastfeeding women using LAM, many other modern contraceptives used correctly can provide better protection in the second 6 months postpartum. Although programmatic experience with the extension of LAM beyond 6 months has produced some useful observations (Wade, Sevilla, & Labbok, 1994; Cooney et al., 1996), no rigorous, prospective data on "extended LAM" from clinical trials are yet available.

A study of the efficacy of LAM among working women in Chile reported a 6-month cumulative pregnancy rate of 5.2 percent (Valdes et al., 2000). This elevated pregnancy rate was among fully breastfeeding women and suggests that despite adequate milk production, frequent suckling as well as full breastfeeding may be necessary to obtain the full protection from LAM.

Sexuality

Human sexuality in the 21st century is as complex as ever. Although the following discussion will presuppose a stable union between a breastfeeding woman and her male partner, this presupposition is simply for convenience. Nevertheless, the majority of lactating mothers are heterosexual, and there is little if any research about the sexuality of breastfeeding single and lesbian women. It is likely that much of the following discussion will apply to all women.

This discussion is also based on the assumption that libido or sexual desire is the main driving force or motivation for sexual expression (although the desire to please one's partner is also recognized as a motivation). Yet many women have intercourse against their will and/or without sexual desire. This chapter does not consider the role of breastfeeding in coercive or indifferent sexual relationships.

Libido

There are at least five categories of factors that may influence sexual drive or desire during lactation:

- Common situational factors unrelated to breastfeeding
- Libido-inhibiting influences related to parturition
- Libido-inhibiting influences of lactation
- Libido-enhancing factors related to pregnancy, birth, and lactation
- Lactation factors related to the breastfeeding woman's partner

Common Situational Factors Unrelated to Breastfeeding. Many preexisting factors that either facilitated or inhibited sexual arousal before pregnancy or birth will remain a part of a woman's living experience, family routine, or personal preference after the birth of the child. Preexisting factors that inhibit libido—such as the chronic illness of one of the partners, fear of pregnancy, or lack of privacy—persist and are unrelated to breastfeeding. If a couple has a dysfunctional or unsatisfying sexual rapport, this is no more likely to be spontaneously remedied by lactation than a faltering marriage is to be "saved" by adding a child to the family chemistry.

Conversely, there is no reason to assume that individualized stimuli per se, such as a preferred cologne, a special song, or candlelight, should lose their excitatory effects because a baby joins the family. Opportunity to attend to the old stimuli, however, is another matter. Some of the preexisting sexual stimuli or circumstances associated with sexual opportunity may be decreased due to having a young baby in the home. For example, the couple may find that they now lack time alone and that they endure constant interruptions—especially, it seems, at night. The quiet evening at home may seem gone forever.

Libido-Inhibiting Influences Related to Parturition. Much of the natural process of physical recovery from vaginal delivery takes about 6 weeks, although there is some variation across women. Postpartum abstinence is sensible until the woman decides that she has sufficient physical comfort to resume sexual intercourse.

The tenderness from episiotomy or vulvo-vaginal or perineal stress following vaginal delivery usually lasts for several months. Although the woman's stitches may have healed, she may still experience discomfort upon intercourse. A study in London found that 62 percent of 403 primiparas reported dyspareunia (pain upon intercourse) in the first 3 months after birth, dropping to half that percentage by 6 months (Barrett et al., 2000). In a study of 93 parturients in New South Wales, Australia, the median time required to achieve comfort during intercourse was 3 months, with a range of from 1 month to more than 12 months. Whether or not the women had episiotomies (58 yes, 35 no) did not affect the time until pain-free intercourse was experienced, but this may be because of the commonness of tearing (69 percent) of the vulval tissues, which required sutures in the women who did not have an episiotomy (Abraham et al., 1990). In a longitudinal study of 119 primiparous women attended at a London teaching hospital, 40 percent complained of soreness and occasionally painful intercourse at 3 months postpartum (Robson, Brant, & Kumar, 1981). Another study of British women reported dyspareunia during the first postpartum intercourse in 40 percent of mothers; of these, 64 percent refrained from further coitus after the initial distressing event (Grudzinskas & Atkinson, 1984). The anticipation of pain during intercourse may cause the woman to avoid sexual suggestion. A clear understanding of feelings and ongoing communication may help the couple to defer intercourse until some future time and to express their love and caring in other ways.

Soon after delivery, women experience a precipitous decline in ovarian steroid levels. This drastic hormonal change is sometimes associated with noticeable mood changes. The immediate effect is usually temporary and probably overlaps with the period of postpartum abstinence. In some women, postpartum depression can follow delivery immediately or occur after a few days or weeks. Although the etiology of postpartum depression is not well understood, this depression probably has both endogenous and exogenous sources. Some women experience emotional vulnerability when their progesterone levels are low, as happens during the postpartum period. (By way of analogy, the symptoms of premenstrual syndrome in the nonpregnant woman are often relieved by progesterone administration.) The overwhelming needs of the new baby plus other familial and extrafamilial responsibilities are more than enough to make a normal person weary (Figure 21–5). Thus exogenous sources of postpartum depression should not be underestimated. Depression is commonly characterized by a lack of sexual drive, and the "postpartum blues" is no exception.

Even if the mother does not experience postpartum depression, she will probably be spending most of her emotional energy caring for and bond-

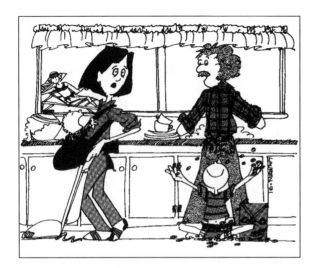

FIGURE 21–5. The postpartum domestic scene. The overwhelming needs of the new baby plus other familial and extrafamilial responsibilities are more than enough to make a normal person weary.

ing with her newborn. This process is sometimes likened to a love affair in which infatuation with one's beloved is like an obsession. It is difficult to refrain from thinking about and doing things for the object of one's affection. Between mother and child, this bonding serves exceedingly important functions by creating an enduring parental talent and commitment in the mother and a sense of trust and security in the infant. However, this process can preclude opportunity and emotional availability for the partner.

Psychological factors unrelated to hormones or to attachment can also be strong inhibitors of libido. Fear of pregnancy can be an important inhibitor of sexual drive. If the new baby was unplanned, especially if a contraceptive failure occurred, sexual inhibition could understandably be great. Parents of a firstborn sometimes have trouble synthesizing the roles of "lover" and "mother" or "father," because the parental role was previously understood subconsciously to be asexual. Colic or minor or major problems with the infant can decrease sexual interest in either partner, and if a difficult parenting challenge is faced by a mother who has no previous parenting experience, she may be even less emotionally available to her partner. Pre-existing marital difficulties may manifest them-

selves in an exclusive emphasis on the child and neglect of the adult love relationship. One mother suggested that the factors contributing to a decrease in the frequency of sexual relations were not very complex or deeply rooted and were probably unrelated to any particular psychological construct. She declared simply, "Our priorities changed! When you have kids, there are lots of other things to do, and your values change."

Libido-Inhibiting Influences of Lactation. Libido is thought to be elevated during the middle of the menstrual cycle in normal, nonlactating women. The midcycle is the period during which peaks in follicle stimulating hormone (FSH), LH, and estrogen are observed. Accordingly, libido in the breastfeeding woman may be linked to one or more of these substances, or to a drop in prolactin which, during breastfeeding, is elevated above the levels in normally cycling women. The study of parturients in New South Wales showed that breastfeeding duration longer than 5 months was associated with longer duration of discomfort during intercourse as well as longer periods of lactational amenorrhea (Abraham, 1990). This finding supports an association between the hormonal milieu during breastfeeding and sexual activity. Alder and Bancroft (1988) found that women who bottle-fed tended to resume coitus earlier and had intercourse more frequently than breastfeeders, which similarly supports a hormone-libido association. However, these same researchers had earlier found no relationship between basal prolactin levels, estrogen levels, or even the return of follicular development with measures of sexuality in breastfeeding women (Alder et al., 1986). Some design problems could account for these results—namely, the retrospective nature of the data collected, the small number of women under study, and the infrequent intervals of data collection. A possible explanation is that hormones may in fact exert some influence over sexual desire, but that there are other factors with greater influence over sexual behavior than the hormonal milieu.

Nonbreastfeeding, postpartum women produce low levels of estrogen until they begin to recover fertility at 1 to 2 months postpartum. Among breastfeeding women, the period of hypoestrogenemia can endure for the entire lactation course. As in menopause, lactation-related hypoestrogenemia can cause the vaginal epithelium to be very thin and to secrete little fluid during arousal. Dryness and pain are experienced during intercourse and vaginal tears are possible. The London study by Barrett et al. (2000) found that although dyspareunia declined greatly by the sixth postpartum month, breastfeeding is one of the few predictors of this extended period of discomfort or pain, probably due to vaginal dryness. Atrophy of the vaginal mucosa can be relieved quickly and easily by the use of inert, water-based lubricants. Estrogen cream is sometimes prescribed for vaginal application and yields satisfactory results in many cases (Wisniewski & Wilkinson, 1991). However, the vagina is so absorptive that users should be alert to the possible consequences of estrogen administration, such as the recovery of ovulation and a decrease in breast-milk production.

As if the emotional demands of parenthood are not enough, breastfeeding adds another dimension of complexity. Exhaustion may be the most pervasive inhibitor of sexual desire. The London study of primiparous women by Robson, Brant, and Kumar (1981) reported that 25 percent of mothers indicated that tiredness reduced their libido and/or enjoyment of sex. Of course, the non-breastfeeding woman with a new infant is also vulnerable to exhaustion, especially if she has other small children to care for. Yet breastfeeding women may be more vulnerable if frequent night feeding disturbs their sleep. If the breastfeeding child sleeps in the parents' bed, this may afford the mother a better night's sleep. Conversely, the presence of the child could inhibit sexual expression, in which case the couple could choose another site for lovemaking.

Emotional attachment between the mother and child is thought to be more intense if the dyad is breastfeeding rather than bottle-feeding (Bottorff, 1990; Virden, 1988; Wrigley & Hutchinson, 1990). Emotional availability of the mother for her sexual partner may be correspondingly reduced. One mother described these feelings during lactation:

When you are home and you touch, hold, hug, and nurse all day, you're not so interested in it when your husband walks through the door. But then his day has been all talk all day and no touch, and he's ready. It creates a problem. (Riordan, 1983)

Some men may feel that they are in competition with the baby, not only for the breastfeeding woman's attention but for her breasts. The woman's breasts are often an important aspect of eroticism for the couple. If either or both partners feel that the breasts are "off limits" for sexual play because the woman is producing milk, then the couple's sexual expression may be negatively affected. Even if the couple feels no taboo about the woman's breasts, there may be a dislike of milk leakage and a fear of eliciting it. The breasts may be tender, and the new mother may be tired of having her breasts "handled" (Figure 21–6). Conversely, there is little harm in breast stimulation and even suckling by the woman's partner, especially after the baby has had his fill. The partner may actually help to prevent or relieve engorgement by periodically stimulating milk secretion or ejection.

Libido-Enhancing Factors Related to Pregnancy, Birth, and Lactation. Especially in the context of a planned pregnancy, the birth can be a positive and fulfilling experience, and many couples express this mutual happiness in lovemaking. Childbirth is a major life event, and when this occurs under emotionally and physically healthy conditions, sexual expression can be particularly joyful and rewarding.

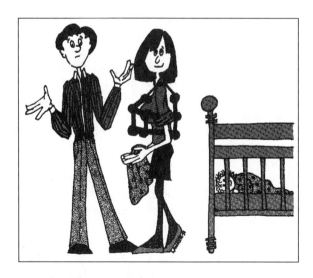

FIGURE 21–6. To touch or not to touch? If the breasts are "off limits," sexual expression may be negatively affected.

In contrast to the possible inhibitors mentioned earlier, pregnancy, childbirth, and breastfeeding can also have the effect of magnifying an appreciation of the womanliness of the mother by her partner. For example, to some men and women, the shape or fullness of the lactating breasts is particularly arousing.

The breastfeeding woman may feel more interested in sexual relations after a few months postpartum because of the interaction of some of the factors mentioned. Her perineum is less tender, she may be experiencing some ovarian activity, she no longer has the body shape of a pregnant woman, and she feels more normal. One mother described it this way:

To me, sex is best of all during the later breastfeeding period because (1) I feel physically better than at any other time, (2) no fear of pregnancy and no contraceptives needed because for me breastfeeding is a 100% effective contraceptive for at least one year after the birth of a baby, and (3) there is something about nursing a little baby that gives you an "all's right with the world" kind of feeling. I feel so happy and loving toward my whole family, husband, and other children as well as the baby. Sex just seems to be a nice, natural expression of this good feeling. (Kenny, 1973)

Human sexual expression can be a creative activity in addition to being procreative. It is also obviously a personal endeavor for the lovers as individuals and as a couple. For this reason, some potentially inhibiting factors may actually be arousing factors that add to the likelihood that the couple will have sexual intercourse. For example, one couple may make love more frequently in times of stress, while another couple may experience a paucity of emotional reserve for lovemaking under the same circumstances. The former pattern may be quite functional because orgasm helps to release tension and promotes relaxation and a feeling of well-being, thus providing one or both partners with more psychic energy with which to cope with the causes of stress. For some couples, pregnancy itself often stimulates erotic responses. Therefore to some people, having given birth and becoming nonpregnant again may be less sexually stimulating than being "great with child." Because each person and each couple is unique, any discussion of sexuality during lactation must be couched in generalities, recognizing that individual expression varies widely.

Barrett et al. (2000) reported that most women experience change in their sexual practices after delivery. The frequencies of intercourse and oral sex were reportedly lower after delivery, but 10 percent of women reported better quality in their sex lives. Very few women talk to their health-care professional about their sexual health. It seems possible that many couples could have better sexual satisfaction equipped with a few simple facts and some lubricant.

Factors Related to the Breastfeeding Woman's Partner. The possibility of role conflict has already been mentioned and is a reminder that men also experience psychological adjustments to accommodate the major life event of birth. No doubt the experience is most profound the first time that a man becomes a father. While the male partner is often assumed to be ever ready, willing, and wanting sex, this is an overgeneralization, possibly reflecting the relative lack of a cycle in the male capacity to fertilize. Men are subject to libidinal influences in everyday life, and, analogous to the female perspective discussed at the beginning of this section, these facilitators and inhibitors do not disappear with the birth of a child or during the lactation course of a partner.

When the man has witnessed his pregnant partner's metamorphosis into lactating mother, this may affect his perception of her as a sex partner, either because of her body's obvious changes or because of the meaning he ascribes to her maternity. Motherhood or lactation may make her more or less sexually appealing to him.

Fear of hurting a postpartum woman during vaginal intercourse may inhibit male sexual expression. A man may feel guilty for desiring his breastfeeding partner if he perceives that she has "more important" maternal matters. Identifying and talking about their sexual feelings, desires, and inhibitions, while earnestly caring for the welfare of each other, can help the couple through this sometimes awkward period.

Sexual Behavior During Lactation

In order to measure a level of sexual functioning or behavior in breastfeeding women, researchers have studied the resumption of postpartum intercourse and coital frequency. First, intercourse and coital frequency are relatively easy variables to quantify, although they certainly do not yield a complete understanding of sexual practices during lactation. Unfortunately, little qualitative information about sexual behavior during lactation is reported in the scientific literature. Few studies of sexual behavior during lactation contain large numbers of subjects, and the results of the studies are sometimes contradictory.

First Postpartum Intercourse. In one study in the postnatal hospital clinic of a city in England, 328 women were interviewed. By the time of the postnatal visit, 51 percent had already resumed intercourse, which was most frequently (the mode) during the fifth week postpartum (Grudzinskas & Atkinson, 1984). In the London study, 62 percent of women resumed sexual intercourse by the 7th or 8th week postpartum (Barrett et al., 2000). An intensive study of 25 breastfeeding women in Edinburgh, Scotland, found that 6 to 7 weeks was the mean time preceding initial postpartum intercourse. In a prospective study of 130 breastfeeding women in Santiago, Chile, the participants had "usually" resumed sexual relations by the beginning of the second month (Diaz et al., 1982).

A population-based survey of 3080 parturients was conducted in Cebu, the Philippines, where breastfeeding is the norm. The study included all identified pregnancies in 27 administrative districts in and around metropolitan Cebu. Sixty percent of women returned to coitus by 8 weeks postpartum (Udry & Deang, 1993). A study of 485 LAM users in Manila, the Philippines reported a median time to the resumption of coitus of 7 weeks (Ramos, Kennedy, & Visness, 1996). In a study involving 27 breastfeeding women in Bangkok, Thailand, the mean time until the first postpartum coitus was 7.8 weeks, although the range of time until the first coitus was from 3 weeks to more than 21 weeks postpartum (Israngkura et al., 1989). Although this is a small and nonrepresentative study, the women

recorded coitus data prospectively, unlike the methodology used in population-based surveys. In a study of 399 LAM users in Pakistan, three quarters of the volunteers were from the city of Karachi. By the end of the second month, 80 percent reported that they were sexually active, up from 14 percent in the first month (Kazi et al., 1995). The Cebu, Manila, Bangkok, and Karachi studies show that the postpartum resumption of sexual activity in urban areas of Asian developing countries typically occurs by 7 to 8 weeks.

Whether the average time to the resumption of sexual relations during breastfeeding is 4 weeks or 8 weeks, large numbers of women are sexually active before the traditional time of the postpartum check-up—i.e., 6 weeks postpartum. As will be discussed below, an argument can be made to schedule the postpartum visit on the basis of the time that the woman needs a provider to deliver her chosen contraceptive method. Of course, the new mother should always have access to care in the event of unexpected pain, vaginal discharge, or other physical concerns. Given that the majority of women have some sexual discomfort or concerns postpartum, health professionals should discuss sexual issues—actual or potential—when counseling on contraception.

Postpartum Coital Frequency. An analysis of retrospective and prospective data on coital frequency was performed using information provided by 91 nonpregnant, nonlactating women in North Carolina who were married or living with a male partner as if married. First, the women reported from memory their "usual" weekly frequency of sexual intercourse. Then they recorded each morning, for 1 to 3 months, whether they had intercourse during the previous 24 hours. The women reported a significantly higher frequency of coitus for the period prior to the first interview (2.5 times per week) compared with their later prospective recordings (1.7 times per week)—an average of 0.8 episodes per week. This overestimate occurred uniformly in subgroups of women and was thought to be caused by the women's tendency to report a frequency that would exist in the absence of travel, illness, menses, and other influencing factors. The prospective data showed trends toward decreased coital frequency with increasing age, education, income, and duration of relationship. Also, women currently using an intrauterine device (IUD) or who had had a tubal ligation had intercourse twice as often (2.0 times per week) as women with "no" contraceptive use (1.1 times per week) (Hornsby & Wilcox, 1989). Although the North Carolina analysis is a study of the methodology for obtaining information about coital frequency, it offers a clear example of the potential bias incurred with the use of retrospective data. Although it is a study of normally cycling women, it provides a good context in which to view studies of coital frequency during lactation.

In the aforementioned study in Santiago, Chile, the reported coital frequency ranged from one to six times per week in the first 6 months postpartum among breastfeeding women (Diaz et al., 1982). Conversely, the Cebu study found a remarkable lack of variance in coital frequency in the first 6 months postpartum. These women were asked every 2 months about the frequency of intercourse in the previous week. After controlling for a large number of potentially influential factors, coital frequency of 0.5 to 0.6 times per week did not vary meaningfully with any of the demographic or situational factors observed (Udry & Deang, 1993).

The variability in coital frequency in the Cebu study could not be well explained by factors such as age and education. Other factors, such as fear of pregnancy, may be stronger correlates of sexual behavior, as may psychological factors, such as perceived locus of control (the perception that one is in control of one's life and fate rather than the victim of forces outside oneself).

In the aforementioned study in Manila, coital frequency averaged three times per month among LAM users (Visness & Kennedy, 1997). In this study of breastfeeding women, the number of living children was unrelated to coital frequency, while maternal age was related in two ways: younger women reported an increase in frequency with time postpartum, and their overall frequency was greater than that reported by older women.

On an individual basis, coital frequency may only be important to know so that it may be compared with frequency before the pregnancy and/or the birth. An Edinburgh study prospectively measured coital frequency during weeks 12 to 24 postpartum and found a mean frequency of 1.2 times per

week. The recalled prepregnancy frequency was 2.6 times per week ($p < .01$) (Alder et al., 1986). In light of the findings of Hornsby and Wilcox (1989), it is possible that the retrospectively generated prepregnancy frequency was an overestimate. Also, it is not clear whether the prepregnancy period being recalled is a time in which pregnancy was actively sought, which could inflate sexual frequency above previous or later levels for the couple.

Does breastfeeding affect the resumption of sexual activity or coital frequency? Survey data from Bangladesh (Islam & Khan, 1993) and the Philippines (Udry, 1993) show lower coital frequencies among breastfeeding than nonbreastfeeding women. Alder and Bancroft (1988) reported that, when compared with bottle-feeders, breastfeeding women showed a lower preferred frequency of intercourse; delayed the resumption of coitus for a longer period; had a greater reduction in sexual interest and enjoyment compared with prepregnancy levels; experienced more pain during intercourse; and were slightly more depressed at 3 months postpartum. All of these differences disappeared by 6 months except for dyspareunia. The findings of Barrett et al. (2000) corroborate this conclusion.

By contrast, works by Masters and Johnson (1966) and by Kenny (1973) reported a more prompt return of sexual desire, plus a return to higher levels of sexual functioning, among breastfeeding women than among bottle-feeders. These earlier works were conducted during a time and at locations in which breastfeeding was not popular. It is unknown whether women who were less sexually inhibited were the ones who breastfed.

Robson, Brant, and Kumar (1981) reported that breastfeeding showed no influence over several indices of maternal sexuality in 119 primiparas in London. Grudzinskas and Atkinson (1984) reported that breastfeeding was not related to the resumption of coitus in their sample of 328 women. Nationally representative data from Thailand show that there is no overall difference in coital frequency between breastfeeders and nonbreastfeeders, except for a reduced frequency among women who breastfeed six or more times at night (Knodel & Chavoyan, 1991).

What do these conflicting results mean? Does breastfeeding stifle sexual experience, accelerate it, or neither? Conflicting results can be due to differences in research methodology or to cultural norms. Additional psychological, behavioral, and biological hypotheses are needed. Can breastfeeding have either an inhibiting or a stimulating effect? Perhaps breastfeeding is a swing factor, sometimes enhancing sexual feelings and sometimes acting as the obstacle to their expression.

Contraception

During lactation, the choice of whether to practice contraception, and if so which method, requires different considerations compared with the same choice during the nonlactating state (Figure 21–7). The array of available family planning methods has been put into a hierarchy according to their general advisability for use during breastfeeding (Labbok et al., 1994). The hierarchy of family planning options (Table 21–1) places nonhormonal methods as the first choice, progestin-only methods as the second choice, and methods containing estrogen as a distant third to be used only when other methods are unavailable. This hierarchy is consistent with guidelines published by the World Health Organization (2000, 2002), the International Planned Parenthood Federation (1996), and the Technical Guidance Working Group (1997).

The Contraceptive Methods

The following discussion describes the advantages and disadvantages of various contraceptive methods used during lactation. It is not intended to be an exhaustive exposition of the methods. Instead it emphasizes the implications of the use of the methods for the breastfeeding mother and baby. A fully detailed discussion of instructions for use, as well as the contraindications of each method unrelated to breastfeeding, can be found in the most recent edition of *Contraceptive Technology* (Hatcher et al., 1998).

Almost every method of family planning can be used during breastfeeding, but the timing of the introduction of the methods can vary profoundly. The question of when to start using a contraceptive will be revisited at the end of this section, and is also an integral aspect of LAM. It bears repeating that hormonal methods containing estrogen should be avoided during breastfeeding to the degree possible and reasonable.

Nonhormonal Methods. The permanent methods of family planning—now the most popular category of methods in the United States—all fall under the nonhormonal method category. They are highly appropriate methods provided that a couple wishes to prevent any future pregnancy, has been properly counseled, fully appreciates the irreversibility of the procedure, and is fully satisfied with the decision to use a permanent method.

When a permanent method is indicated, *vasectomy* is one of the most appropriate alternatives available, because it is safe and effective and should have no effect whatsoever on lactation. After the vasectomy, the male reproductive tract continues to clear itself of sperm during about 20 ejaculations. If the woman is not pregnant, the couple needs to use a second method of contraception for a period of time in order to be fully protected. The couple may feel that the vasectomy is ideally timed either during the pregnancy itself or in the first few months postpartum, especially if the current pregnancy was unplanned. In an era of only one or two children per family, however, the presumed final pregnancy often is highly planned. If so, couples may feel more comfortable postponing vasectomy until after the pregnancy, in case a miscarriage should occur, or even until after the infancy period of the child.

Female sterilization carries several advantages. It is safe, effective, and relatively convenient since it can be performed on the delivery table. Contrary to previous assumptions, a small risk of female sterilization failure can persist for at least a decade, but this risk is smallest after partial salpingectomy compared with other methods of tubal occlusion (Peterson et al., 1996).

There is a potential negative effect of the sterilization procedure on lactation, in that the general anesthesia used may synergistically interfere with the early breastfeeding pattern. The mother needs time to recover from the anesthesia, and during this period she is not breastfeeding. By the time she begins to breastfeed, the anesthetic agent has passed into her milk, contributing to the baby's drowsiness and making it difficult to feed effectively. In addition, any pain she feels may temporarily reduce her ability or desire to breastfeed, and it may limit her options for comfortably positioning herself or her infant for breastfeeding. If the mother is experienced and/or well counseled, and if hospital staff

Table 21–1

FAMILY-PLANNING OPTIONS AS THEY RELATE TO THE SPECIFIC CONCERNS OF BREASTFEEDING WOMEN

Method	Advantages	Disadvantages	Comments
First choice: nonhormonal methods			
Condoms	No effect on breastfeeding; very effective if used correctly.	May be irritating to vagina and require additional lubrication.	Offers some protection against sexually transmitted diseases. No risks to mother or child.
Diaphragms	No effect on breastfeeding; effective if used correctly.	Diaphragm must be refitted postpartum after uterus has returned to prepregnancy size.	Not widely available. Effectiveness depends on use with a spermicide.
Spermicides	No effect on breastfeeding; effective if used correctly.	May be irritating to genital area and to the male partner.	Small amount may be absorbed into maternal blood and some passage into milk: no known effect on infant.
Intrauterine devices (IUDs)	No effect from IUD itself on breastfeeding; effective.	Possible risk of expulsion and uterine perforation if not properly placed or if inserted prior to 6 weeks postpartum.	Delay insertion until after 6 weeks postpartum.
Natural family planning (periodic abstinence)	No effect on breastfeeding; effective if used correctly.	May require extended periods of abstinence. Requires ability to interpret fertility signs during breastfeeding.	Additional training may be necessary to interpret signs and symptoms of fertility during lactation. Calendar rhythm method alone has little value prior to first ovulation.
Vasectomy (voluntary male surgical sterilization)	No effect on breastfeeding; nearly 100% effective.	Minor surgery with chance of side effects; irreversible.	Recommended if no more children are desired. Counseling for couples. No risk to mother or child.
Tubal ligation (voluntary female sterilization)	No direct effect on breastfeeding; nearly 100% effective.	Minor surgery with chance of side effects; irreversible. Possible short-term mother–infant separation. Anesthesia can pass into milk in small amounts.	Recommended if no more children are desired. Counseling for couples.
Second choice: progestin-only methods			
Progestin-only methods (mini-pill, injectables, implants)	Effective; may increase milk volume. Effectiveness during breastfeeding approaches that of combined pill.	Some hormone passes into breastmilk.	No evidence of adverse effect on infant from small amount of hormone that passes into breastmilk.
Third choice: methods containing estrogen			
Combined oral contraceptives (estrogen and progestin)	Very effective.	Estrogens reduce milk supply. Some hormone passes into breastmilk.	No evidence of direct negative effect on infant; however, does suppress milk supply and leads to earlier cessation of breastfeeding. If these methods cannot be avoided, breastfeeding can and should continue.

Source: Labbok et al. (1994). Guidelines: breastfeeding, family planning, & the lactational amenorrhea method. Adapted with permission of the Institute for Reproductive Health, Georgetown University.

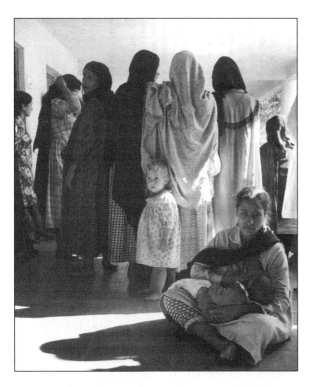

FIGURE 21–7. Family planning care at an Egyptian health center, where maternal and child health services are also included. According to the WHO perspective, family planning is concerned with the quality of life. It is a way of thinking and living that promotes the health and welfare of the family group and thus contributes to economic and social development.

does not interfere by bottle-feeding the baby, this interruption of early breastfeeding should not have serious consequences for lactation. Regional or local anesthesia is preferable to general anesthesia, and should be sought when reasonable. The mother should breastfeed just before the administration of the anesthetic and delay somewhat the breastfeed after the procedure to minimize the infant's exposure to the anesthetic agent (American Academy of Pediatrics, 2001).

Studies reviewed in the early 1980s have reported that up to 7 percent of women express regret about tubal sterilizations (Divers, 1984; Grubb et al., 1985). In general, regret over the procedure and/or desire for reversal has been associated with younger age (e.g., under 30) or low parity at the time of the procedure, as well as remarriage, the death of a child after the procedure, and having the procedure with a concurrent cesarean section or during the puerperal or postabortion period. Occasionally, lower socioeconomic class and lack of having a child of a specific gender have also been associated with regret over having the procedure. It is possible that regret is intensified when pre-, post-, and intraprocedural factors interact—for example, when a young woman with few children is sterilized immediately postpartum, and she later remarries.

Of more than 5000 women in the Collaborative Review of Sterilization, a multicenter prospective observational study conducted in the United States, 2.0 and 2.7 percent reported that they regretted their sterilization 1 and 2 years after the procedure, respectively. The preoperative risk factors for experiencing regret after 2 years were identified as an age of less than 30 and (for whites) concurrent cesarean section (Grubb et al., 1985). Chi et al. (1989c) also reported that women whose tubal ligations were combined with the cesarean procedure were more likely to have characteristics associated with later regret.

Counseling is crucially important when helping women or couples to select the best family planning approach for them. When a permanent method is a serious consideration, counseling must begin long before the procedure and be repetitive. This may be especially important when younger women of low parity express an interest in the procedure during the puerperium, as well as when young men under the same conditions consider vasectomy.

The *Lactational Amenorrhea Method (LAM)* is the proactive use of lactational infertility as a contraceptive method during the period of lactational amenorrhea, under very specific circumstances: (1) the woman is breastfeeding her child exclusively (or nearly exclusively)—i.e., no supplemental feedings; (2) the woman has experienced no vaginal bleeding or spotting after lochia ends (all bleeding, spotting, or bloody vaginal discharge before postpartum day 56 can be ignored); and (3) the child is less than 6 months of age. LAM is based on the Bellagio Consensus (Kennedy, Rivera, & McNeilly, 1989; Labbok et al., 1994). LAM is a temporary method of family planning. Another contraceptive method should be used immediately when LAM expires for continued pregnancy protection (Kennedy, Labbok, & Van Look, 1996; Van Look, 1996). Experience with LAM is growing, but it is still limited in the United States. LAM may prove to be a useful stopgap method for women who are delaying the use of a hormonal or a permanent method, but access to continuing protection should be ensured.

Nonhormonal *intrauterine devices (IUDs)* have been shown to have either no effect or a positive effect on lactation (Koetsawang, 1987). One study found Copper T-380A IUD insertion easier and less painful during lactation, with possibly higher continuation rates than in nonlactating women (Chi et al., 1989a, 1989b). IUDs inserted during the postpartum period tend to be expelled more frequently than IUDs inserted at other times. However, insertion immediately after delivery of the placenta (within 10 minutes) by an experienced person who places the device high in the fundus significantly reduces the chance of expulsion (Chi & Farr, 1989). IUDs inserted within 10 minutes of placental expulsion have not been associated with excessive bleeding or endometritis (Welkovic et al., 2001). Breastfeeding has not been found to increase the risk of expulsion when the device is inserted at this time or after the postpartum period (Chi et al., 1989a; Cole et al., 1983). Ideally, the IUD should be inserted immediately after placental delivery, or within 48 hours, or after 6 to 8 weeks, or with care and infection prophylaxis after 4 to 6 weeks, in this order (O'Hanley & Huber, 1992). An IUD can also be inserted following a cesarean delivery through the uterine incision.

Because of the advantages of immediate postplacental insertion, contraceptive counseling and informed consent to IUD insertion should occur long before labor and delivery. Counseling on postinsertion care is also important. Women should be encouraged to have early postpartum checkups and to return if the IUD thread is missing, because expulsion, if it occurs, often does so soon after insertion.

A study of US women found the risk of uterine perforation to be significantly elevated in women who were breastfeeding at the time of insertion (Heartwell & Schlesselman, 1983). A small, noncomparative study in Sweden drew the same conclusion (Andersson et al., 1998). However, large studies have been unable to confirm this (Chi, Feldblum, & Rogers, 1984; Farr & Rivera, 1992). Insertion by an experienced person is thought to minimize the risk of perforation.

Little research has been conducted on the effectiveness of *barrier methods* used during lactation.

Clinical trials of contraceptive efficacy have deliberately excluded breastfeeding women because their naturally subfertile state may influence pregnancy rates. The relative effectiveness of the various barrier methods vis-a-vis each other is probably maintained during lactation.

Barrier and/or spermicidal methods are widely used contraceptives among lactating US women. Several characteristics of these methods make them particularly attractive during the breastfeeding period. Condoms, diaphragms, and spermicides are all coitus-dependent methods. Even if couples prefer other methods, they may find these methods useful if they are having intercourse less frequently than before the pregnancy. The lubricative effect of the *spermicide* can be welcome if the woman experiences vaginal symptoms from estrogen suppression. The *contraceptive diaphragm* and the *cervical cap* should not be used in the first 6 weeks postpartum and may not be able to be fitted properly earlier. The *condom* is a good barrier method choice during the early postpartum period. Condoms can be purchased with or without a lubricant coating and/or a spermicide in the reservoir. A condom used with a spermicide, whether applied by the user or as part of the condom itself, should have better contraceptive efficacy than the condom alone.

The diaphragm that a woman used prior to her pregnancy is apt to be unsuitable in size after childbirth. A new diaphragm can usually be properly fitted at 6 weeks postpartum (and in some cases sooner), but some breastfeeding women may find the fitting process to be too uncomfortable for many weeks. In this case the couple may wish to abstain or to use lubricated condoms, a spermicide, or LAM until vaginal lubrication is more normal. If the woman will be sexually active before her diaphragm can be sized, she should use another method—such as condoms or LAM—in the interim. With the gain or loss of every 10 pounds, a new diaphragm may need to be sized in order to achieve effective protection, and a clinical gynecologic visit should be sought for this purpose. The diaphragm should always be used with a spermicidal cream or jelly.

Spermicidal cream, jelly, foam, or foaming tablets used alone are not as effective in preventing pregnancy as a spermicide used with a barrier, such as a sponge, diaphragm, or condom. However, spermicides used during breastfeeding, especially during the period of LAM protection, should result in a higher level of effectiveness due to double protection. They also represent a significant improvement over unprotected intercourse, and they have the advantage of being widely available and can be purchased over the counter.

The *Billings' Ovulation Method* and the *Symptothermal Method* are considered to be modern *natural family-planning (NFP) methods* because they are based on sound scientific research. The methods require abstinence from intercourse during the fertile period, which is identified by observing the woman's physical signs and symptoms—e.g., volume, color, stretchiness, sensation, and clarity of cervical mucus; basal body temperature; cervical position; and breast tenderness. The modern natural methods are highly effective when used correctly, but most studies observe a great deal of incorrect use. Incorrect use is usually the failure to abstain from intercourse during the fertile period rather than a misunderstanding of the method or how to use it. Knowledge of the fertile period is also useful for achieving pregnancy.

Modern NFP methods have been adapted for use during lactation. A Basic Infertile Pattern (BIP) of fertility symptoms (such as cervical mucus) is established during a two-week period of abstinence. Thereafter, every other night is available for intercourse unless there is a change in the BIP, which then requires additional abstinence according to method-specific rules (Parenteau-Carreau & Cooney, 1994).

The effectiveness of NFP methods during breastfeeding has seldom been systematically evaluated. As with the study of other contraceptives, most previous efficacy research has excluded all but ostensibly normally cycling women. One study of breastfeeding women observed a poor association between estrogen metabolite excretion and women's reports of the cervical mucus symptom that is regulated by estrogen (Brown, Harrison, & Smith, 1985). Basal body temperature is unknowable unless the woman has at least 6 hours of uninterrupted sleep; this requirement excludes many fully breastfeeding women, particularly in the early months of lactation. One prospective study of the symptothermal method used during breastfeeding found that the method is highly sensitive although not very specific in its ability to determine which days are fertile. That is, fertile days

are identified very well, but the method also requires abstinence on many days that probably are not fertile. Thus, correct use of the method during breastfeeding should result in a high degree of protection from pregnancy, but requires more abstinence than is necessary to prevent pregnancy (Kennedy et al., 1995). The requirement for somewhat more abstinence than is absolutely necessary is intentionally built into the method in order to err on the side of pregnancy avoidance. It is not at all clear whether the amount of abstinence required by NFP methods used during breastfeeding is a hardship on couples. If coital frequency is low at this time anyway, and if the BIP is clear and consistent, abstinence may not be a problem. Under opposite circumstances abstinence may be difficult. Thus, NFP leaders recommend that breastfeeding users first apply the rules of LAM in order to eliminate the need for abstinence for up to 6 months postpartum (Parenteau-Carreau & Cooney, 1994).

Although NFP methods can be taught and learned in simple terms (and illiterate women in many countries have learned to use the modern NFP methods), learning apparently is easier during normal cycles compared with the hypoestrogenic period of lactation. There may be an excess risk of unplanned pregnancy after the first postpartum menses in new users, since the changing fertility symptoms may be especially difficult to interpret (Labbok et al., 1991). Therefore, couples who wish to use natural methods to space or limit pregnancies during lactation are at an advantage if they have learned how to use their NFP method of choice prior to conception and subsequent lactation. However, one ovulation method study in Chile found a 12-month pregnancy rate of 11.1 percent during breastfeeding, but only 2 percent at 12 months were determined to be method failures (Perez et al., 1988).

Hormonal Methods. Hormonal contraceptive methods are not the category of first choice for breastfeeding women (International Planned Parenthood Federation [IPPF], 2002; WHO, 2000). The main reason is that steroid hormones, natural or synthetic, are transferred into the breastmilk to various degrees (Johansson & Odlind, 1987). The effect of the infant's exposure to exogenous hormones is presumed to be minor because very small amounts of hormone are excreted in the milk or absorbed by the infant. Since the fetus is exposed to very high levels of progesterone *in utero*, exposure to small quantities of progestins in breastmilk may be of no consequence. Nevertheless, the degree to which exogenous hormones can be cleared by the neonate is unknown. Plasma does not bind steroids well, the immature liver does not metabolize them well, and newborn kidneys are assumed to excrete inefficiently. Excess steroids or their metabolites may attach to receptor sites in the brain or reproductive organs (Harlap, 1987), which may be especially concerning in the first few months of life when extrauterine central nervous system growth is most rapid (Diaz, 2002). The long-term effects of consumption of exogenous steroid hormones on development are as yet unknown. Although the concern about infant exposure to exogenous hormones is theoretical, avoidance of exposure in the early weeks or months is urged because its effects are unknown, and other contraceptive methods are available.

Progestin-only Hormonal Methods. It is recommended that the use of progestin-only hormonal methods be delayed for at least 6 weeks postpartum (IPPF, 1996, 2002; WHO, 2000; TGWG, 1997) to avoid neonatal exposure to the steroid hormone. Since other temporary methods, such as barriers and LAM, should be available to the breastfeeding woman, and since coital frequency can be low during the first 6 weeks postpartum, the use of a stop-gap method in the early postpartum period is a reasonable approach.

Progestin transfer to the infant varies across formulations of progestin-only methods. The estimated dose consumed by the infant is much smaller with pills and implants than with injectables. An implant that delivers orally inactive progesterone (i.e., Nesterone or Elcometrine) is available in some countries and would be a better progestin-only alternative than Norplant or Implanon during breastfeeding (Diaz, 2002).

Progestin-only pills (McCann et al., 1989; Moggia et al., 1991; Sinchai et al., 1995), injections (Hannon et al., 1997), and subdermal implants (Coutinho et al., 1999; Reinprayoon et al., 2000; Massai et al., 2001; Schiappacasse et al., 2002) are not associated with reduced milk production,

breastfeeding frequency, or impaired infant growth or early development, even if initiated before 6 weeks postpartum. (WHO, 1994a, 1994b; Diaz, 2002; Curtis et al., 2002).

Although progestin-only methods should not interfere with breastfeeding (and may actually enhance lactation), anecdotal accounts of lactation failure associated with the very early use of progestin-only contraceptives are of concern. Despite the caution of experts to delay initiating progestin use for at least 6 weeks, some women receive progestin injections on the delivery table, or within 72 hours of delivery prior to hospital discharge. It seems likely that this early bolus of exogenous progestin could interfere with the establishment of lactation, since the physiological trigger for lactogenesis is the precipitous withdrawal of natural progesterone, which does not occur in humans until 2 to 3 days postpartum (Cowie, Forsyth, & Hart, 1980). Accordingly, progestin contraceptive initiation should be delayed for at least 3 full days (Kennedy, Short, & Tully, 1997), and preferably until after the mature milk has come in and lactation is rather well established. Two studies of the initiation of progestin-only pills during the first week postpartum found no deleterious effect on milk production (McCann et al., 1989; Moggia et al., 1991). However, the pill dose is relatively small compared with the injected amount, and pill consumption may have begun later than 3 days postpartum.

Progestin-only pills are marginally less effective than combined estrogen-progesterone formulations, but they are still highly effective when taken consistently and correctly. Progestin-only pills are somewhat unforgiving of incorrect use—e.g., missing a pill—although when used during breastfeeding their effectiveness is close to that of combined pills. Their lower effectiveness can be reasonably compensated by good counseling on method use (Chi, 1993).

Women who use the 3-month progestin-only injectable product Depo-Provera often experience amenorrhea after an interval of irregular bleeding/spotting. Studies in Bolivia and China have found that breastfeeding women tolerated this common side effect better than nonbreastfeeding women and were more likely to continue using the method (Hubacher et al., 2000; Danli, Qingxiang, & Guowei, 2000).

Combined Estrogen-Progestin Hormonal Methods. Hormone formulations containing estrogen have been observed to decrease the milk supply in several studies (Koetsawang, 1987; WHO, 1988). Therefore, combined estrogen-progesterone pills or injectables should not be used during breastfeeding unless there is no other acceptable alternative. If combined pills (including low-dose formulations) are the only choice, the World Health Organization (2000) and the International Planned Parenthood Federation (2002) recommend that they be avoided, or postponed for at least 6 months or until weaning, whichever comes first. Due to the elevated risk of thrombosis in the first few weeks postpartum, methods containing estrogen should be avoided for about 3 weeks regardless of breastfeeding status (WHO, 2000).

Clinical Implications

When a woman or couple makes a legitimate family planning decision and/or chooses a method for achieving their family planning ideal based on full and accurate information and reflection, that person or couple has maximized the likelihood of being satisfied with the decision or choice and of using the chosen method correctly and effectively.

Informed choice has been defined as "effective access to information on reproductive choices and to the necessary counseling, services, and supplies to help individuals choose and use an appropriate method of family planning, if desired" (Piotrow, 1989, p. 2). Informed choice should be viewed as a continuing process that parallels changing procreative desire and phase of life, as well as personal changes over time. Family planning intentions do not remain fixed throughout life, and one type of contraceptive is usually not appropriate for the same person throughout all the reproductive years. An appropriate range of available methods includes both male and female methods—and permanent methods as well as long- and short-acting temporary ones. If only a limited range of methods is available to the health-care provider, he or she should be prepared to offer referrals to help meet the patient's needs.

Information can be shared with patients in different ways, using the written word through pamphlets, books, and posters, or the spoken word through videos, audiovisual presentations, or "class-

style" (part lecture, part participatory) discussions. Providing information, however, is not sufficient. An interpersonal exchange is necessary to ensure that effective communication of information has been achieved and also to provide clarification and counseling. The desired result of counseling is a patient or couple who has made a choice based on full understanding of the alternatives—and who has made that choice freely, unaffected by the counselor. Information should flow freely between the provider/counselor and the woman/couple. This circumstance exists, ideally, between the lactation consultant and the breastfeeding woman. Accordingly, the lactation consultant needs to be well versed in available family planning services and alternatives in her community. Perhaps most important, the health-care provider should be aware of the possible interaction of various contraceptives with breastfeeding as discussed in this chapter. Both lactation consultants and family planning providers should be prepared to discuss common sexual issues as well.

A study in Scotland showed that postpartum counseling about family planning during the hospital stay after delivery is ineffective (Glasier, Logan, & McGlew, 1996). However, for the immediate postpartum insertion of an IUD or for postpartum sterilization, counseling is essential before delivery. A large multicenter study compared antenatal family planning counseling with standard postpartum counseling and found no difference in pregnancy and continuation rates at 1 year postpartum, except in Edinburgh where significantly more women counseled antenatally chose sterilization (Smith et al., 2002).

Ideally, a plan for postpartum contraception is decided before delivery, with postpartum follow-up timed to match the requirements of the chosen method. A postpartum checkup with an obstetrician/gynecologist is advised and can probably occur at any time from the third to the eighth week after delivery. The longer the consultation is delayed, the more comfortable a pelvic examination is likely to be for a breastfeeding woman. However, the woman should insist on seeing her clinician earlier than the traditional 6 weeks in the event of abnormal vaginal discharge or pain, or if she needs a contraceptive method before the sixth week or needs help with a postpartum sexual issue. All women who wish to avoid pregnancy should be ensured of a method for doing so before hospital discharge, but preferably before delivery. If a woman's method is not one that can be appropriately delivered in the hospital, then condoms or progestin-only pills—and clear instructions for their use—should be distributed generously at hospital discharge, and LAM should be taught prior to delivery with reinforcement at hospital discharge. Some kind of family planning follow-up (for example, by phone) should occur in the third to fourth week postpartum to revisit and support the chosen contraceptive strategy. Since the lactation consultant is one of the most likely health-care providers in the first month postpartum, the lactation consultant can check that a plan is in place, and facilitate or support the couple in procuring their contraceptive method.

Accurate information is an essential tool for lactation consultants, and posing the questions in Box 21–3 will help the LC ascertain some essential information. Additionally, such information will influence the ability of the woman or couple to make a decision without undue influence from the consultant. When the couple freely makes informed choices, the lactation consultant is better able to support the woman and her family in their choices.

BOX 21–3

Issues to Consider When Discussing Family Planning with the Breastfeeding Woman

Questions

1. Does the mother wish to limit or space any future pregnancies? If so, what method(s) of family planning does she prefer?

2. If she has breastfed a previous child, how long did she remain amenorrheic? What factors may have influenced the duration of her lactational amenorrhea?

3. If she has not breastfed before, how does she plan to do so? Is she familiar with the factors that can reduce the duration of lactational amenorrhea?

4. If she wishes to have no more children, how will her family be affected if a temporary method of contraception fails and she becomes pregnant before she had planned, or in the face of a desire to have no more children?

Information to Share

1. Discuss the effectiveness of the mother's preferred method(s) and offer additional information about other contraceptives as well. Include information about the effect of each method on lactation and on the suckling child.

2. This information may predict the degree of double protection she may experience by using both a contraceptive and breastfeeding to reduce the risk of an unplanned pregnancy.

3. Review the factors that reduce the duration of lactational amenorrhea and increase the early resumption of fertility. Pay particular attention to what is meant by exclusive or nearly exclusive breastfeeding, the impact of pacifier use, regular use of solid foods in the infant's diet, and supplementary bottle-feedings.

4. When the reproductive intention is to prevent any future pregnancies, it is especially important that a highly effective contraceptive method be chosen. Double protection is not an issue under this circumstance.

Summary

Fertility, sexuality, and contraception are normally related, but each of these aspects of reproduction also affects or is affected by lactation. A clear understanding of the interrelationships of these elements is essential if the health-care provider is to discuss issues and concerns of the lactating mother as she seeks to determine her fertility in concert with her sexual self. The health-care provider benefits from an understanding of the relationship between physiological responses to suckling stimulation and the resumption of fertility. Additionally, the breastfeeding woman needs to be prepared for the ways in which her own breastfeeding experience may alter her sexual experience as well as her fertility—in the early weeks after birth as well as when her breastfeeding child is weaning.

Nearly all modern contraceptive methods can be used during breastfeeding, but the timing of the introduction of the methods can vary profoundly. Permanent, long-term, short-term, nonhormonal, and hormonal methods are all viable options when introduced appropriately. Temporary, stopgap methods, such as condoms and LAM, may comprise a suitable bridge in the early weeks or months of breastfeeding—especially if coital frequency is low—until another method of the couple's choosing is appropriate. All breastfeeding women who wish to avoid pregnancy can be helped to do so, and should plan to do so from the first postpartum coitus. Lactation consultants are well-positioned to ensure that a family planning strategy is in place within the first few weeks postpartum.

In order to best serve the breastfeeding family, the health-care provider who is assisting the lactating mother should be thoroughly familiar with how lactation, fertility, sexuality, and contraception are intertwined threads in the cord of life experience.

Key Concepts

- The child's suckling initiates a cycle of neuroendocrinologic events that result in the inhibition of ovulation.

- Anything that decreases the child's suckling behavior or the need to suckle will be a secondary cause of the recovery of fertility. Supplementation may have the effect of decreasing hunger, thirst, and possibly the emotional need for comfort, thereby reducing suckling at the breast.

- A significant association exists between the duration of lactational infertility after one pregnancy and the duration in the same woman after her next pregnancy.

- Breastfeeding provides more than 98 percent protection from pregnancy during the first 6 months postpartum if the mother is "fully" or nearly fully breastfeeding and has not experienced vaginal bleeding after the 56th day postpartum.

- Once menstruation has resumed, fertility is returning or already has returned. Menses is an absolute indication of the need for another contraceptive method if continued protection is desired.

- The tenderness from episiotomy or vulvovaginal or perineal stress following vaginal delivery usually lasts for several months and can cause pain or discomfort during intercourse.

- Postpartum women produce low levels of estrogen until they begin to recover fertility. Among breastfeeding women, this period of hypoestrogenemia can endure for the entire lactation course, and it can cause the vaginal epithelium to be very thin and to secrete little fluid during arousal, which may be remedied by the use of inert, water-based lubricants.

- Most women experience change in their sexual practices after delivery. The frequency of sex is often lower, although some women report better quality in their sex lives.

- Very few women talk to their health-care professional about their sexual health.

- During breastfeeding, nonhormonal methods are the first-choice category of contraceptives and progestin-only methods comprise the second choice. Methods containing estrogen should be avoided during breastfeeding, especially in the first 6 months.

- Counseling is crucially important when helping women or couples to select the best family planning approach. When a permanent method is a serious consideration, counseling must begin long before the procedure and be repetitive.

- Nonhormonal intrauterine devices (IUDs) have been shown to have either no effect or a positive effect on lactation.

- Contraceptive steroid hormones, natural or synthetic, are transferred into the breastmilk to various degrees. Since the fetus is exposed to very high levels of progesterone *in utero*, exposure to small quantities of progestins in breastmilk may be of no consequence. Nevertheless, the degree to which exogenous hormones can be cleared by the neonate is unknown.

- It is recommended that the use of progestin-only hormonal methods be delayed for at least 6 weeks postpartum to avoid neonatal exposure. Other temporary methods, such as barriers and LAM, can be used, especially since

coital frequency can be low during the first 6 weeks postpartum.

- The physiological trigger for lactogenesis is the precipitous withdrawal of natural progesterone at about 2 to 3 days postpartum. Accordingly, progestin contraceptive initiation should be delayed for at least 3 full days and preferably until after the mature milk has come in and lactation is rather well established.

- Progestin-only pills, injections, and subdermal implants are not associated with reduced milk production, breastfeeding frequency, or impaired infant growth or early development.

- Hormone formulations containing estrogen have been observed to decrease the milk supply. Therefore, combined estrogen-progesterone pills or injectables should not be used during breastfeeding unless there is no other acceptable alternative.

- Serving as one of the most likely health-care providers in the first month postpartum, the lactation consultant can check that a plan for family planning is in place, and facilitate or support the couple in procuring their contraceptive method.

References

Abraham S. Recovery after childbirth. *Med J Aust* 152:387, 1990.

Abraham S et al. Recovery after childbirth: a preliminary prospective study. *Med J Aust* 152:9–12, 1990.

Alder E, Bancroft J. The relationship between breastfeeding persistence, sexuality, and mood in postpartum women. *Psychol Med* 18:389–96, 1988.

Alder EM et al. Hormones, mood and sexuality in lactating women. *Br J Psychiatry* 148:74–79, 1986.

American Academy of Pediatrics, Committee on Drugs. The transfer of drugs and other chemicals into human milk. *Pediatrics* 108(3):776–89, 2001.

Andersen AN, Schioler V. Influence of breastfeeding pattern on pituitary-ovarian axis of women in an industrialized community. *Am J Obstet Gynecol* 143:673–77, 1982.

Andersson K et al. Perforations with intrauterine devices—report from a Swedish study. *Contraception* 57:251–55, 1998.

Badroui MHH, Hefnawi F. Ovarian function during lactation. In: Hafez ESE, ed. *Human ovulation.* Amsterdam: Elsevier-North Holland Biomedical Press, 1979:233–41.

Barrett G et al. Women's sexual health after childbirth. *BJOG* 107(2):186–95, 2000.

Benitez I et al. Extending lactational amenorrhea in Manila: a successful breast-feeding education program. *J Biosoc Sci* 24:211–31, 1992.

Bongaarts J, Menken J. *Determinants of fertility in developing countries.* New York: Academic Press, 1983.

Bongaarts J, Potter RG. *Fertility, biology and behavior.* New York: Academic Press, 1983.

Bottorff JL. Persistence in breastfeeding: a phenomenologic investigation. *J Adv Nurs* 15:201–9, 1990.

Brown JB, Harrison P, Smith MA. A study of returning fertility after childbirth and during lactation by measurement of urinary estrogen and pregnanediol excretion and cervical mucus production. *J Biosoc Sci* 9(suppl.):5–23, 1985.

Chi IC. The safety and efficacy issues of progestin-only oral contraceptives—an epidemiologic perspective. *Contraception* 44:1–21, 1993.

Chi IC, Farr G. Postpartum IUD contraception—a review of

an international experience. *Adv Contraception* 5:127–46, 1989.

Chi IC, Feldblum PJ, Rogers SM. IUD-related uterine perforation: an epidemiologic analysis of a rare event using an international dataset. *Contracept Deliv Syst* 5:123–30, 1984.

Chi IC et al. Performance of the Copper T-380A intrauterine device in breastfeeding women. *Contraception* 39:603–18, 1989a.

———. Insertional pain and other IUD insertion-related rare events for breastfeeding and non-breastfeeding women—a decade's experience in developing countries. *Adv Contraception* 5:101–19, 1989b.

———. Tubal ligation at cesarean delivery in five Asian centers: a comparison with tubal ligation soon after vaginal delivery. *Int J Gynecol Obstet* 30:257–65, 1989c.

Cole LP et al. Effects of breastfeeding on IUD performance. *Am J Public Health* 73:384–88, 1983.

Cooney KA et al. An assessment of the nine month lactational amenorrhea method in Rwanda. *Stud Fam Plann* 27:162–71, 1996.

Coutinho EM et al. Use of a single implant of Elcometrine (ST-1435), a nonorally active progestin, as a long-acting contraceptive for postpartum nursing women. *Contraception* 59:115–22, 1999.

Cowie AT, Forsyth IA, Hart IC. *Hormonal control of lactation.* Berlin: Springer-Verlag, 1980.

Curtis KM et al. Contraception for women in selected circumstances. *Obstet Gynecol* 99:1100–12, 2002.

Danli S, Qingxiang S, Guowei S. A multicentered clinical trial of the long-acting injectable contraceptive Depo Provera in Chinese women. *Contraception* 62:15–18, 2000.

Delvoye P et al. The influence of the frequency of nursing and of previous lactation experience on serum prolactin in lactating mothers. *J Biosoc Sci* 9:447–51, 1977.

Diaz S. Contraceptive implants and lactation. *Contraception* 65:39–46, 2002.

Diaz S et al. Fertility regulation in nursing women: I. The probability of conception in full nursing women living in an urban setting. *J Biosoc Sci* 14:329–41, 1982.

———. Contraceptive efficacy of lactational amenorrhea in urban Chilean women. *Contraception* 43:335–52, 1991.

———. Neuroendocrine mechanisms of lactational infertility in women. *Biol Res* 28:155–63, 1995.

Divers WA. Characteristics of women requesting reversal of sterilization. *Fertil Steril* 41:233–36, 1984.

Elias MF et al. Nursing practices and lactational amenorrhea. *J Biosoc Sci* 18:1–10, 1986.

Eslami SS et al. The reliability of menses to indicate the return of ovulation in breastfeeding women in Manila, the Philippines. *Stud Fam Plann* 21:243–50, 1990.

Family Health International. Breastfeeding as a family planning method. *Lancet* 2:(8621):1204–5, 1988.

Farr G, Rivera, R. Interactions between IUD and breastfeeding status at time of IUD insertion: analysis of PCU 380A acceptors in developing countries. *Am J Obstet Gynecol* 167:2027–31, 1992.

Ford K. Correlation between subsequent lengths of postpartum amenorrhea in a prospective study of breastfeeding women in rural Bangladesh. *J Biosoc Sci* 24:89–95, 1992.

Glasier AF, Logan J, McGlew TJ. Who gives advice about postpartum family planning. *Contraception* 53:217–20, 1996.

Glasier A, McNeilly AS, Baird DT. Induction of ovarian activity by pulsatile infusion of LHRH in women with lactational amenorrhea. *Clin Endocrinol* 24:243–52, 1986.

Gray RH et al. Risk of ovulation during lactation. *Lancet* 335:25–29, 1990.

Gross BA, Eastman CJ. Prolactin and the return of ovulation in breastfeeding women. *J Biosoc Sci Suppl* 9:25–42, 1985.

Grubb GS et al. Regret after decision to have a tubal sterilization. *Fertil Steril* 44:248–53, 1985.

Grudzinskas JG, Atkinson L. Sexual function during the puerperium. *Arch Sex Behav* 13:85–91, 1984.

Hannon PR et al. The influence of medroxyprogesterone on the duration of breastfeeding in mothers in an urban community. *Arch Pediatr Adolesc Med* 151:490–96, 1997.

Harlap S. Exposure to contraceptive hormones through breast milk: Are there long-term health and behavioral consequences? *Int J Gynaecol Obstet* 25(suppl):47–55, 1987.

Hatcher RA et al. *Contraceptive Technology.* 17th ed. New York: Irvington Publishers, 1998.

Heartwell SF, Schlesselman S. Risk of uterine perforation among users of intrauterine devices. *Obstet Gynecol* 61:31–36, 1983.

Hornsby PP, Wilcox AJ. Validity of questionnaire information on frequency of coitus. *Am J Epidemiol* 130:94–99, 1989.

Howie PW et al. Effect of supplementary food on suckling patterns and ovarian activity during lactation. *Br Med J* 283:757–59, 1981.

———. Fertility after childbirth: adequacy of postpartum luteal phases. *Clin Endocrinol* 17:609–15, 1982a.

———. Fertility after childbirth: postpartum ovulation and menstruation in bottle- and breastfeeding mothers. *Clin Endocrinol* 17:323–32, 1982b.

Hubacher D et al. Factors affecting continuation rates of DMPA. *Contraception* 60:345–51, 2000.

International Planned Parenthood Federation (IPPF). IMAP statement on breastfeeding, fertility, and postpartum contraception. *IPPF Med Bull* 30:1–3, 1996.

———. IMAP statement on hormonal methods of contraception. *IPPF Med Bull* 36(5):1–8, 2002.

Islam MM, Khan HTA. Pattern of coital frequency in rural Bangladesh. *J Fam Wlfare* 39:38–43, 1993.

Israngkura B et al. Breastfeeding and return to ovulation in Bangkok. *Int J Gynaecol Obstet* 30:335–42, 1989.

Johansson E, Odlind V. The passage of exogenous hormones into breastmilk: possible effects. *Int J Gynaecol Obstet* 25(suppl):111–14, 1987.

Jones RE. A hazards model analysis of breastfeeding variables and maternal age on return to menses postpartum in rural Indonesian women. *Hum Biol* 60:853–71, 1988.

———. Breastfeeding and postpartum amenorrhea in Indonesia. *J Biosoc Sci* 21:83–100, 1989.

Kazi A et al. Effectiveness of the lactational amenorrhea method in Pakistan. *Fertil Steril* 64:717–23, 1995.

Kennedy KI. Fertility, sexuality and contraception during lactation. In: Riordan J, Auerbach K, eds. *Breastfeeding and human milk*. Sudbury, MA: Jones and Bartlett, 1993.

Kennedy KI, Labbok MH, Van Look PFA. Consensus statement—lactational amenonorrhea method for family planning. *Int J Gynecol Obstet* 54:55–57, 1996.

Kennedy KI, Rivera R, McNeilly AS. Consensus statement on the use of breastfeeding as a family planning method. *Contraception* 39:477–96, 1989.

Kennedy KI, Short RV, Tully MR. Premature introduction of progestin-only contraceptive methods during lactation. *Contraception* 55:347–50, 1997.

Kennedy KI, Visness CV. Contraceptive efficacy of lactational amenorrheoa. *Lancet* 339(8787):227–30, 1992.

Kennedy KI et al. Breastfeeding and the symptothermal method. *Stud Fam Plann* 26:107–115, 1995.

Kenny JA. Sexuality of pregnant and breastfeeding women. *Arch Sex Behav* 2:215–29, 1973.

Khan T et al. A study of breastfeeding and the return of menses and pregnancy in Karachi, Pakistan. *Contraception* 40:365–76, 1989.

Knodel J, Chaynovan N. Coital activity among married Thai women. In: *Demographic and health surveys world conference proceedings,* Vol. 2. Columbia, MD IRD/Macro International, 1991: 925–45.

Koetsawang S. The effects of contraceptive methods on the quality and quantity of breastmilk. *Int J Gynaecol Obstet* 25(suppl):115–28, 1987.

Labbok MH et al. Ovulation method use during breastfeeding: Is there increased risk of unplanned pregnancy? *Am J Obstet Gynecol* 165:2031–36, 1991.

———. *Guidelines: breastfeeding, family planning and the lactational amenorrhea method—LAM*. Washington, DC: Institute for Reproductive Health, 1994.

———. I. Multicenter study of the lactational amenorrhea method (LAM): duration and implications for clinical guidance. *Contraception* 55:327–36, 1997.

Lewis PR et al. The resumption of ovulation and menstruation in a well-nourished population of women breastfeeding for an extended period of time. *Fertil Steril* 55:529–36, 1991.

Massai MR et al. Contraceptive efficacy and clinical performance of Nesterone implants in postpartum women. *Contraception* 64:369–76, 2001.

Masters WH, Johnson VE. *Human sexual response*. Boston: Little, Brown, and Co., 1966.

McCann MF et al. The effects of a progestin-only oral contraceptive (levenorgestrel 0.03 mg) on breastfeeding. *Contraception* 40:635–48, 1989.

McNeilly AS. Lactational control of reproduction. *Reprod Fertil Dev* 13:583–90, 2001a.

———. Neuroendocrine changes and fertility in breastfeeding women. *Prog Brain Res* 113:207–14, 2001b.

McNeilly AS, Glasier A, Howie PW. Endocrine control of lactational infertility-I. In: Dobbing J, ed. *Maternal nutrition and lactational infertility*. New York: Raven Press, 1985.

McNeilly AS et al. Fertility after childbirth: pregnancy associated with breastfeeding. *Clin Endocrinol* 18:167–73, 1983.

Moggia AV et al. A comparative study of a progestin-only oral contraceptive versus nonhormonal methods in lactating women in Buenos Aires, Argentina. *Contraception* 44:31–43, 1991.

O'Hanley K, Huber DH. Postpartum IUDs: keys for success. *Contraception* 45:351–61, 1992.

Parenteau-Carreau S, Cooney KA. *Breastfeeding, lactational amenorrhea method and natural family planning interface: teaching guide.* Washington, DC: Institute for Reproductive Health, 1994.

Perez A, Labbok MH, Queenan JT. Clinical study of the lactational amenorrhoea method for family planning. *Lancet* 339:968–70, 1992.

Perez A et al. First ovulation after childbirth: the effect of breastfeeding. *Am J Obstet Gynecol* 114:1014–47, 1972.

———. Use-effectiveness of the ovulation method initiated during postpartum breastfeeding. *Contraception* 38:499–508, 1988.

Peterson HB et al. The risk of pregnancy after tubal sterilization. *Am J Obstet Gynecol* 174:1161–70, 1996.

Piotrow PT. *Informed choice: report of the Cooperating Agencies Task Force.* Baltimore: Johns Hopkins University, Center for Communication Programs, 1989.

Ramos R, Kennedy K, Visness C. Effectiveness of lactational amenorrhea in prevention of pregnancy in Manila, the Philippines: non-comparative prospective trial. *Br Med J* 313:909–12, 1996.

Reinprayoon D et al. Effects of the etonogestrel-releasing contraceptive implant (Implanon) on parameters of breastfeeding compared to those of an intrauterine device. *Contraception* 62:239–46, 2000.

Riordan J. *A practical guide to breastfeeding.* St. Louis: Mosby, 1983.

Rivera R et al. Breastfeeding and the return to ovulation in Durango, Mexico. *Fertil Steril* 49:780–87, 1988.

Robson KM, Brant HA, Kumar R. Maternal sexuality during first pregnancy and after childbirth. *Br J Obstet Gynaecol* 88:882–89, 1981.

Rojnik B, Kosmelj K, Andolsek-Jeras L. Initiation of contraception postpartum. *Contraception* 51:75–81, 1995.

Rolland R. Bibliography (with review) on contraceptive effects of breastfeeding. *Biblio Reprod* 28:1–4, 93, 1976.

Rosa FW. The role of breastfeeding in family planning. *WHO Protein Advisory Group Bull* 5:5–10, 1975.

Schiappacasse V et al. Health and growth of infants breastfed by Norplant contraceptive users: a six-year follow-up study. *Contraception* 66:57–65, 2002.

Shaaban MM et al. The recovery of fertility during breastfeeding in Assiut, Egypt. *J Biosoc Sci* 22:19–32, 1990.

Short RV. Breast Feeding. *Scient Am* 250(4):35–41, 1984.

Short RV et al. Contraceptive effects of extended lactational amenorrhea: beyond the Bellagio consensus. *Lancet* 337: 715–17, 1991.

Simpson-Hebert M, Huffman SL. The contraceptive effect of breastfeeding. *Stud Fam Plann* 12:125–33, 1981.

Sinchai W et al. Effects of a progestin-only pill (Exluton) and an intrauterine device (Multiload Cu250) on breastfeeding. *Adv Contracep* 11:143–55, 1995.

Smith KB et al. Is postpartum contraceptive advice given antenatally of value? *Contraception* 65:237–43, 2002.

Technical Guidance Working Group (TGWG). *Recommendations for updating selected practices in contraceptive use: results of a technical meeting,* Vol. 2. Chapel Hill, NC: Program for International Training in Health (INTRAH), School of Medicine, University of North Carolina at Chapel Hill, 1997.

Thapa S, Short RV, Potts M. Breastfeeding, birthspacing and their effects on child survival. *Nature* 335(6192):679–82, 1988.

Trussell J et al. Contraceptive failure in the U.S.: an update. *Stud Fam Plann* 21:51–54, 1990.

Udry JR. Coitus as demographic behaviour. In: Gray R, ed. *Biomedical and demographic determinants of reproduction.* Oxford, England: Clarendon Press, 1993.

Udry JR, Deang L. Determinants of coitus after childbirth. *J Biosoc Sci* 25:117–125, 1993.

Valdes V et al. The efficacy of the lactational Amernorrhea Method (LAM) among working women. *Contraception* 62:217–19, 2000.

Van Ginnekin JK. Prolonged breastfeeding as a birth spacing method. *Stud Fam Plann* 5:201–6, 1974.

Van Look PFA. Lactational amenorrhea method for family planning. *Br Med J* 313:893–94, 1996.

Virden SF. The relationship between infant feeding method and maternal role adjustment. *J Nurs-Midwif* 33:31–35, 1988.

Visness CM, Kennedy KI. The frequency of coitus during breastfeeding. *Birth* 24(4):253–57, 1997.

Visness CM, Kennedy KI, Ramos R. The duration and character of postpartum bleeding among breast-feeding women. *Obstet Gynecol* 89:159–63, 1997.

Visness CM et al. Fertility of fully breast-feeding women in the early postpartum period. *Obstet Gynecol* 89:164–67, 1997.

Wade KB, Sevilla F, Labbok MH. Integrating the lactational amenorrhea method into a family planning program in Ecuador. *Stud Fam Plann* 25:162–74, 1994.

Weiss P. The contraceptive potential of breastfeeding in Bangladesh. *Stud Fam Plann* 22:294–307, 1993.

Welkovic S et al. Postpartum bleeding and infection after post-placental IUD insertion. *Contraception* 63:155–58, 2001.

Wisniewski PM, Wilkinson EJ. Postpartum vaginal atrophy. *Am J Obstet Gynecol* 165:1249–54, 1991.

World Health Organization. Effects of hormonal contraceptives on breast milk composition and infant growth. *Stud Fam Plann* 19:36–69, 1988.

————. Progestin-only contraceptives during lactation: I. Infant growth. *Contraception* 50:35–53, 1994a.

————. Progestin-only contraceptives during lactation: II. Infant development. *Contraception* 50:55–68, 1994b.

————. The WHO multinational study of breastfeeding and lactational amenorrhea: I. Description of infant feeding patterns and the return of menses. *Fertil Steril* 70:448–60, 1998a.

————. The WHO multinational study of breastfeeding and lactational amenorrhoea: II. Factors associated with the length of amenorrhoea. *Fertil Steril* 70:461–471, 1998b.

————. The WHO multinational study of breastfeeding and lactational amenorrhea: IV. Postpartum bleeding and lochia in breastfeeding women. *Fertil Steril* 72(3):441–47, 1999a.

————. The WHO multinational study of breastfeeding and lactational amenorrhea: III. Pregnancy during breastfeeding. *Fertil Steril* 72(3):431–40, 1999b.

————. *Improving access to quality care in family planning: medical eligibility criteria for contraceptive use.* Geneva: WHO Reproductive Health and Research Division, 2000.

————. *Selected practice recommendations for contraceptive use.* Geneva: WHO Reproductive Health and Research Division, 2002.

Wrigley EA, Hutchinson SA. Long-term breastfeeding: the secret bond. *J Nurs-Midwif* 35:35–41, 1990.

SECTION

5

SOCIOCULTURAL AND RESEARCH ISSUES

Breastfeeding exists within the constraints of each culture. Theoretical constructs that allow us to examine the family—its members and their roles—also enable us to identify issues around breastfeeding and to understand breastfeeding women of all cultures. Breastfeeding education, interwoven within the threads of a culture, leads to better care and a more satisfying experience.

As the trend continues toward evidence-based health care, caring for breastfeeding mothers and infants also means measuring clinical outcomes. Thus, lactation consultants need to know about research methods. In addition, they need more research to expand the knowledge of lactation and the variations in breastfeeding behavior. Only with such research will myths about breastfeeding be put to rest.

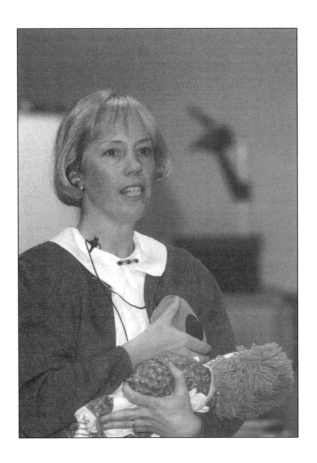

22

Research, Theory, and Lactation

Roberta J. Hewat

What is the base of lactation practice and education? Is it intuition, gut reaction, and use of traditional procedures? Or, is practice and education founded on knowledge generated or validated from data gathered and interpreted by systematic methods that practitioners continually question, study, and expand? Research is a process for developing a knowledge base for accountable and responsible practice. Theories provide the structure for systematically organizing and synthesizing knowledge derived from many sources in order to facilitate its use in research and to guide clinical practice. A body of knowledge founded on research and practice based on the best available evidence legitimizes professional care.

The intent of this chapter is to assist lactation practitioners to develop an interest in—and understanding of—lactation research and theories that support them in their role as research consumers. This entails a complex process: reading articles to learn about current practices; understanding research methods to evaluate and determine whether study findings are relevant; incorporating appropriate findings into their practice; and consistently questioning practices to develop questions for further research.

Theories Related to Lactation Practice

Lactation consultant practice is developing an abundance of rich and diverse literature in medicine, nursing, immunology, and psychosocial sciences, among other areas. This specialized and in-depth body of knowledge, increasingly based on scientific findings, is the foundation of lactation practice. Theories are conceptual constructions of concepts and their relationships that can be tested through research as well as a guide to practice. Theories provide structure for systematically organizing and synthesizing knowledge that may be from many sources, to facilitate its use in research, and to guide clinical practice. As the specialty advances, assumptions about breastfeeding and lactation are tested using theoretical frameworks and theories to guide the studies.

A *theoretical framework* is a representation of the concepts and relationships inherent in a theory that is the underpinning of a study. Other terms used—often interchangeably, which can be confusing—are *conceptual frameworks* and *models*. All are conceptual structures made up of concepts relevant to a phenomenon. Conceptual frameworks

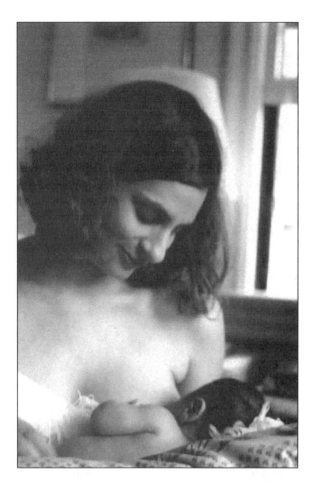

FIGURE 22–1. Theories provide structure for research that ultimately guides clinical practice.

and models, however, do not include a "deductive system of propositions that assert a relationship between the concepts" (Polit & Hungler, 1999, p. 107) that is part of a theoretical framework. All are useful in organizing studies and applying their findings to clinical practice (Figure 22–1).

Theories range from those that are exceptionally broad in scope such as grand theories to those known as micro theories. The grand theories are complex, often comprising several smaller theories; micro theories are a limited set of propositions about a well-defined phenomenon (Tomey & Alligood, 1998). Theories in the middle-range are considered to be most useful to both practice and research, and for highlighting the theory-practice research links (Lenz et al., 1995). The majority of the theories presented in this chapter are middle-

range theories. Their selection is based on the interest they have generated among researchers and their historical relationship to lactation and the care of childbearing families.

Maternal Role Attainment Theory

Rubin (1967a, 1967b) attempted to explain the process of taking on the maternal role as a learned rather than an intuitive experience. Based on role theory described by Sarbin (1954) and Mead (1934) and observations of and interviews with women throughout pregnancy and the postpartum period, Rubin proposed two fundamental processes of maternal role attainment: (1) acquisition of the maternal role and (2) identification of the partner, the infant.

Attainment of the maternal role is through psychological processes such as mimicry, role-play, fantasy, introjection-projection-rejection, and the grief work of letting go of a former role. The role attainment process ends when a new identity or sense of self in the maternal role is recognized. In 1984 Rubin updated her perspectives, replacing the term *maternal role attainment* with *maternal identity* and *maternal experience* and postulating that a new maternal identity was part of each birth.

Rubin's work provided a foundation for Mercer (1981, 1985), who developed a theoretical framework for studying maternal role attainment during the first year after delivery. Mercer postulates that "maternal role attainment is a process by which mothers achieve competence in the mothering role, integrating their mothering behaviors into their established roles so that they achieve confidence and harmony with their new identities" (Mercer & Ferketich, 1994). Mercer and associates have conducted numerous studies since 1985 to determine factors that influence maternal role attainment and predictors of role competence in a variety of childbearing populations. Associations between a mother's breastfeeding experience and maternal role attainment are highly relevant. For many, successful breastfeeding is viewed as part of the mothering role and when feeding problems occur many mothers question their competence and mothering abilities.

Parent-Child Interaction Model

Based on empirical research showing that mother-infant interactions influence the mother-child relationship and the psychosocial development of the child, and that characteristics of each of the interactive partners affect the interaction, the Barnard model was constructed to represent the caregiver-infant interaction system (Barnard & Eyres, 1978; Sumner & Spietz, 1994). The interaction is influenced by characteristics of the caregiver and the infant.

Caregiver/parent/mother characteristics important for positive interactions are showing sensitivity to the infant's cues, acting to alleviate the infant's distress, and using strategies that provide growth fostering experiences for the infant. The infant/child characteristics are clarity of cues and responsiveness to the caregiver or parent. Feeding is considered an excellent context for viewing mother-infant interactions. Practitioners throughout the world use the Nursing Child Assessment Feeding Scale (NCAFS) (1978) for assessing parent-child interactions during feeding. Certification is required to ensure that assessments and interpretations are correctly made.

The Child Health Assessment Interaction Model (Barnard & Eyres, 1978; Sumner & Spietz, 1994) is an overall framework that is exceptionally useful for practitioner assessments and as a guide for research. In this model, three concentric, overlapping circles represent the environment, the caregiver, and the infant/child. For use in breastfeeding assessments, the largest circle represents the environment, which can include breastfeeding support from family, friends, and health professionals as well as cultural influences, physical surroundings, and all other extrinsic factors influencing the breastfeeding dyad. The second largest circle, representing the mother, can include factors influencing breastfeeding such as maternal age, education, intent to breastfeed, physical attributes for breastfeeding, and postpartum depressive state. The smallest circle represents the infant and it includes what the infant brings to the interaction such as physical attributes and abilities for breastfeeding and interactional behaviors. A small area where all circles overlap represents the interaction of the infant, mother, and environment and the potential influence each has on the other.

Although numerous infant feeding studies using these conceptualizations have been done, those specific to breastfeeding are few. Furr and

Kiregis (1982) examined the quality of mother-infant interactions in an intervention study in which breastfeeding mothers received education on neonatal behaviors, and Hewat (1998) examined and compared mother-infant interactions during breastfeeding for dyads whose infants were perceived as problem breastfeeders and dyads whose infants were perceived to feed well.

Bonding and Attachment Theory

The concept of maternal attachment in health-care literature is generally founded in bonding theory proposed by Klaus and Kennel (1976). This theory attempts to explain maternal attachment to the infant as well as disruption in that attachment. Based on a study that compared women who had extended contact with their infant at birth and for the first 3 postpartum days with women whose contact with their infant was limited during this time, the findings showed the mothers with greater access responded differently to their infants, having more eye contact and positive interactions with their infant. Klaus and Kennel postulated that close parent-infant contact soon after birth was critical for optimal child development. In 1982 these claims were modified to include the premise that attachment can occur at a later period because of the adaptability of humans. In spite of critical reviews, this theory was the basis for recognizing the importance of parent-infant ties at delivery and in the early postpartum period. This led to changes in hospital practices that support breastfeeding women (Klaus & Kennel, 1982).

Theory of Darwinian and Evolutionary Medicine

The tenets of Darwinian medicine are founded in the theory of natural selection postulated by Charles Darwin in his 1859 publication, *On the Origin of Species by Means of Natural Selection.* The process of natural selection occurs whenever genetically influenced variation among individuals affects their survival and reproduction. Darwinian medicine is the application of Darwin's theory of natural selection to the understanding of human diseases. Emerging in the early 1980s, this biomedical research approach aims at finding evolutionary explanations of vulnerabilities of disease such as infection, injuries and toxins, genetic factors, and abnormal environments (Williams & Nesse, 1991). Evolutionary medicine has the same underpinnings and beliefs, although greater breadth in scope is evident in the publications. This view suggests that "many contemporary social, psychological, and physical ills are related to incompatibilities between the lifestyles and environments in which humans currently live and the conditions under which human biology evolved" (Trevathan, Smith, & McKenna, 1999, p. 1).

Studies based on this theory that are of interest to lactation practitioners are those related to the positive effects of kangaroo care, a practice that involves skin-to-skin contact for premature infants. Based on these findings, many neonatal intensive care units have adopted or are currently initiating this type of care.

Evolutionary theory was the basis for a study conducted by McKenna, Mosko, and Richard (1999) on the association of sudden infant death syndrome (SIDS) and breastfeeding and mother-infant cosleeping. Findings suggest that the interactive responses between mother and infant throughout the night are a protective mechanism for decreasing the occurrence of SIDS. It was also concluded that the notion of infants sleeping alone meets the beliefs and values of Western culture rather than the biological needs of the infant.

Two other evolutionary explorations and interpretations of interest to the field of lactation are the questioning of whether neonatal jaundice is a disease or an adaptive process (Brett & Niermeyer, 1999) and infant crying behavior and colic (Barr, 1999). The conclusions of these explorations question conventional knowledge and treatments for both conditions.

Self-Care Theory

Self-care can generally be described as the activities that individuals initiate and perform on their own behalf in maintaining life, health, and well-being. In the self-care approach to breastfeeding, the lactation consultant assists, encourages, and nurtures the mother and her family toward effective use of their own resources for achieving an optimal breastfeeding experience. Professional assistance is needed only when a problem prevents or hinders normal breastfeeding. This orientation is congruent with

health-care consumer participation. Self-care theory provides a framework that is especially appropriate for lactation practice where the clients are usually in a healthy state.

Self-Efficacy Theory

The basic proposition of self-efficacy theory, derived from social learning theory (Bandura, 1977, 1982), is described as an ongoing cognitive process in which individuals determine their confidence or their perceived ability for performing a specific behavior. The factors influencing this ability are their motivation, emotional state, and social environment. For measuring self-efficacy, a behavior-specific, task-related approach is suggested.

Dennis and Faux (1999; Dennis 1999) used this theory for developing a breastfeeding self-efficacy scale that reflects maternal confidence in breastfeeding. In keeping with the theory, researchers postulate that self-efficacy expectancies are based on the mother's previous breastfeeding experience, observations of successful breastfeeding, encouragement received from others, and her state of wellness. The developed 40-item scale is internally consistent and has construct validity. For mothers completing the scale before hospital discharge, the scores on the scale predicted breastfeeding patterns, which were defined as exclusive breastfeeding, breastfeeding and bottle-feeding, and exclusive bottle-feeding at 6 weeks postpartum. The scores from the exclusive breastfeeding and bottle-feeding groups were significantly different. The construction of a scale based on the self-efficacy of social learning theory exemplifies use of this theory in research for developing a tool appropriate to use in future research and for practitioners who may want to predict which mothers may terminate breastfeeding early because of lack of confidence in their ability to breastfeed.

Theory of Planned Behavior and Theory of Reasoned Action

The origins of the theory of planned behavior (TPB) is an expansion of the theory of reasoned action (TRA) (Ajzen & Fishbein, 1980). TRA and TPB are a function of intention to perform a behavior, and the intention is the main factor in predicting behavior. The original theory constructs are attitudes and social norms, and control was added to the revised theory, TPB. Intention, as the antecedent to behavior, includes an individual's determination as to whether a behavior is worthwhile performing (attitude), the perception about what others think one should do with respect to a certain behavior (social norm), and assessment as to whether or not a behavior is considered to be easy to perform (control). Both theories have been used to predict behavioral intentions.

TRA was used in a study that examined nurses' support of breastfeeding mothers (Bernaix, 2000). Findings showed that the nurses' knowledge and attitudes were the best predictors of the support they provided to mothers, but that a relationship between intentions and behavior were not found, which did not support the premise of this theory.

TPB is the theoretical foundation for the BAPT tool developed by Janke (1992). Dick et al. (2002) undertook a study for testing and revising the tool. Results of the study showed that the revised BAPT effectively predicted 78 percent of mothers who had stopped breastfeeding at 8 weeks and 68 percent of those that continued to breastfeed, concluding that the BAPT is a useful tool for clinicians to use in determining women at risk for premature termination of breastfeeding.

Theories that provide a base for lactation research and practice have been described. Incorporating theory into practice demonstrates cognitive awareness as to the meaning of the "what" and the "why" of practices used, which is a contributing factor to legitimizing a profession.

Types of Research Methods

Research methods are founded in the philosophical perspectives. Quantitative methods emanate from positivism and postpositivism, and qualitative methods from the narrative, humanistic, and interpretive perspective. The methods of each perspective and combinations of these methods can be used in studies based on critical or emancipatory perspectives. These methods, as well as observational, historical, and feminist research that are suitable for breastfeeding research, are described.

Qualitative Methods

The origins of qualitative methods are inherent in philosophy and the social sciences. Phenomenology, ethnography, and grounded theory are three methods commonly used, but studies using other methods, such as discourse analysis, and narrative and interpretive descriptions, are starting to appear in journals.

Phenomenology and grounded theory methods emanate from philosophy and sociology; ethnographic methods originate from anthropology and discourse analysis from sociolinguistics and cognitive psychology. Depending on the origin, there are variations of each method as well as specific practices and procedures for conducting the research.

Phenomenology. Phenomenology is a philosophy, research method, and humanistic scientific approach. The objective is to understand the meaning or nature of everyday life experiences or events from the perspective of those living the experiences. As the science developed, variations in phenomenological methods emerged. Two approaches are illustrated by the following studies.

Studies using the phenomenological approach advocated by van Manen (1990) are: *Woman to Mother: A Transformation* (Bergum, 1989); *Persistence in Breastfeeding: A Phenomenological Investigation* (Bottorff, 1990); and *The Experience of Living with an Incessantly Crying Infant* (Hewat, 1992). In all studies the meaning of lived experiences are captured through articulation of content, form, and language specific to phenomenological writing. Rich descriptions attempt to show how these experiences are lived in the everyday world. The deeper understanding that practitioners gain from reading these studies should contribute to more humanistic care when working with individuals who are living these experiences.

A more structured process for conducting phenomenological research is proposed by Giorgi (1985). A study using this structured method addresses women's perceptions of the breastfeeding experience (Hewat & Ellis, 1984). The findings describe similarities and differences of women who breastfeed for short and long durations and discuss a conceptualization of the mother-infant breastfeeding relationship. The complexity of the breastfeeding experience is explained and direction is provided for breastfeeding practitioners.

Ethnography.   Ethnography is a method used to explain the beliefs, practices, and patterns of behavior from the perspective of the individuals of a culture or subculture within the context of their environment. A "traditional" ethnography describes the many facets of an entire culture or subculture, whereas a "focused" ethnography portrays one aspect of a culture (Morse, 1991a). The purpose is to understand, from the study participants, the cultural meanings and perceptions they use to organize and interpret their experiences (Spradley, 1979).

Neander and Morse (1989) conducted a focused ethnography. The authors describe infant feeding practices of the Northern Alberta Woodlands Cree when infants were born at home and compared them with feeding practices after childbirth was relocated to the hospital. The decline in breastfeeding that occurred is associated with the mothers' loss of social support from native women and the lack of understanding by health professionals about Cree cultural beliefs and practices.

Grounded Theory.   Grounded theory is a research method for "generating explanatory theory that furthers the understanding of social and psychological phenomena" (Chenitz & Swanson, 1986). Using a rigorous and structured process, data based on individuals' realities are simultaneously collected and analyzed to develop theoretical constructs (Glaser, 1978; Strauss & Corbin, 1990). The emerging theory represents reality because it is "grounded" in the data. From this new understanding, relevant interventions for clinical practice can evolve.

Using grounded theory Leff, Jefferis, and Gagne (1994a) interviewed 26 mothers concerning successful and unsuccessful breastfeeding. The categories of successful breastfeeding were infant health, infant satisfaction, maternal enjoyment, desired maternal role attainment, and lifestyle compatibility. The overall theme or core concept was "working in harmony." The mothers described successful breastfeeding as a "complex interactive process resulting in mutual satisfaction of maternal and infant needs" (p. 99).

Wrigley and Hutchinson (1990) also used this method in a study examining the mother-infant breastfeeding relationship for dyads breastfeeding for more than 1 year. Two key processes were identified: (1) synchronization, defined as the mother proceeding in step with her infant and (2) reorientation, defined as the mother rearranging her life to meet the needs of her infant. For women breastfeeding more than 1 year, the authors suggest that a "secret bond" develops between mother and child, which limits intrusion and protects the breastfeeding relationship from a society that disapproves of long-term breastfeeding.

Discourse Analysis.   Discourse analysis examines language and how it is communicated in order to interpret and construct underlying meanings of participants' experiences, events, or practices (Potter & Wetherall, 1987). Accounts are critically analyzed in order to understand the social and cultural influences on the participants' perspectives and behaviors. Rich descriptions constructed to represent the meaning of the participants' dominant discourses lead to a deeper understanding of their experience.

This method was used by Schmied (1999) to examine the experiences of 25 women breastfeeding for 6 months following their infant's birth. The overall theme was that breastfeeding is an embodied experience, and for 35 percent of the study participants' experience was "connected, harmonious, and intimate embodiment" (p. 328). Mixed feelings were revealed by 40 percent of the women, and the remaining 25 percent found breastfeeding as "disrupted, distorted and a disconnected experience" (p. 329). It was concluded that recognition of the variance of women's personal experiences is important for practitioners working with breastfeeding women.

Quantitative Methods

The major types of quantitative research are nonexperimental, which includes descriptive and correlational studies, and experimental and quasi-experimental studies (Polit & Hungler, 1999). The type of inquiry chosen depends on the current state of knowledge of the study topic and the purpose of the research.

Descriptive Studies.   Descriptive studies are appropriate when there is little knowledge about a topic of interest and specific information is desired. For example, the research questions may address characteristics, influencing factors, or knowledge deficits related to a topic. Findings describe the studied phenomenon and may identify relationships among variables.

A study by Zimmerman and Guttman (2001) examined beliefs about breastfeeding and formula-feeding among 94 breastfeeding and 60 formula-feeding women. Major findings revealed that women in both groups rated breastfeeding higher than formula-feeding for health benefits, enhancement of the infant's development, and creation of a special bond between mother and infant, but breastfeeding was also viewed as restricting a mother's activity. Those who chose formula-feeding did so for lifestyle reasons in spite of their belief that breastfeeding is beneficial to an infant's health. The authors conclude that lifestyle issues should be part of breastfeeding promotion. The findings of some descriptive studies may identify relationships between variables that form the basis for further study.

Correlational Studies.

Correlational studies examine relationships between two or more variables and the type (negative or positive) and strength of the relationship(s). These studies require greater type of control than descriptive studies. The data collected is structured in order to allow for numerical representation for correlational analysis to determine if the relationships between variables are statistically significant.

A study by Oddy et al. (2003) that illustrates this method was conducted prospectively to examine the association between the duration of full breastfeeding and cognitive abilities measured by verbal IQ at 6 years of age and performance abilities at 8 years of age. Full breastfeeding was defined as breastfeeding "up to the introduction of milk other than breast milk and did not preclude the intake of solid foods" (p. 82). Data were categorized as never breastfed, full breastfeeding for less than 4 months, full breastfeeding from 4 to 6 months, and full breastfeeding for more than 6 months. Of the 2024 participants, longer periods of full breastfeeding were significantly associated with higher verbal IQ for children tested at 6 years and intellectual performance of children tested at 8 years. An interactive effect of longer breastfeeding and higher maternal education was a finding for the verbal IQ score but not for the performance score. These study findings add to the growing evidence that breastfeeding is positively associated with children's intelligence in the early school years.

Experimental Studies.

Experimental studies examine hypothesized relationships between variables to determine cause (often an intervention or treatment) and effect (the outcome). Rigorous control of variables is integral to conducting these studies. Several criteria are essential for a true experimental study:

- *Manipulation* of an experimental intervention or treatment (the independent variable) by the investigator.
- *Control* of the experimental situation to eliminate interference or confounding effect of extraneous variables (additional influencing factors) on the outcome (dependent variable).
- *Randomization* so that subjects are systematically allocated with all having an equal chance of participating in the experimental or control study groups (Burns & Grove, 1997).

Morrow et al. (1999) conducted an experimental study that was a randomized control trial to determine the effect of peer counselor visits on the duration of breastfeeding. The 130 participants were randomly assigned to either a control group, or one of two intervention groups. The high-intervention group received peer counsellor home visits in mid- and late pregnancy and in postpartum weeks 1, 2, 4, and 8. The low-intervention group received peer counselor home visits in late pregnancy and postpartum weeks 1 and 2. The control group mothers received standard care for the area, which consisted of visits to their physician if breastfeeding problems occurred. Findings revealed that at 3 months postpartum exclusive breastfeeding was significantly greater among both intervention groups than the control group and significantly higher for the high-intervention over the low-intervention group, inferring that the home visits by peer counselors were effective in assisting increased numbers of mothers to maintain exclusive breastfeeding during the first 3 postpartum months.

The results of this study are encouraging for the support of home visits by peer counselors to increase exclusive breastfeeding rates for longer durations. Additional studies that are similar and have comparable outcomes, however, are needed. Research is an ongoing process and many experimental studies about a topic are often necessary before conclusions are accepted as definitive.

The involvement of human subjects does not always permit the rigor necessary for a true experiment. In many situations it is not always practical, efficient, ethical, or feasible to randomly select subjects or to expose them to a specific treatment or experience. When an experimental method is used to study an intervention but only one of the two additional criteria for conducting a true experiment can be met, the research design is quasi-experimental. A study by Martens (2000) to determine the effectiveness of a 1-hour breastfeeding education intervention provided to nursing staff in a small rural hospital illustrates this method. Another hospital in a community of similar size was selected as a control because of similarities to the intervention site but randomization of sites was unfeasible. Hypothesized outcomes for the intervention site were to *increase*: exclusive breastfeeding rates for infants at hospital discharge, positive beliefs and attitudes among nursing staff, and compliance with the ten steps of the Baby-Friendly Hospital Initiative. In a 7-month period, the intervention hospital showed significant increases over the control site in all outcome measures except breastfeeding attitudes, demonstrating that a short and relatively inexpensive education session for nurses contributed to improved breastfeeding care and outcomes for mothers and infants.

Additional Methods and Approaches for Breastfeeding Research

Other research approaches suitable for breastfeeding studies that do not fit precisely into the qualitative or quantitative classification are observational, historical, participatory action, and feminist research. Either quantitative or qualitative methods or a combination of them may be used for these studies.

Observational Research. Observational research is important for studying human behavior or events that cannot be captured through interviews or self-report questionnaires. Originating in the discipline of biology, ethology is an observational method that explores and examines animal behaviors within natural settings. Behavioristic psychology also contributed structured methods for conducting observational research. Study outcomes can include frequencies of behavioral occurrences, timing of specific behaviors, and/or sequences of behaviors. Types and timing of behaviors during experiences, practices, and events can add a new perspective and greater understanding of a phenomenon.

Ethology was used in an observational study conducted by Hewat (1998). Videotapes examined and compared mother-infant interactions during breastfeeding between two sets of dyads: those whose infants were perceived by their mothers as problematic breastfeeders and those whose mothers perceived their infants as nonproblematic breastfeeders. From the initial assessment of the interactions, ethograms—detailed descriptions of behaviors and patterns—were created, hypotheses were generated, and a guide was developed for coding behaviors to further examine and compare the mother-infant interactions of the two groups. Differences in tempo and rhythm of the mother-infant interaction patterns were delineated as harmonic attunement, disharmonic attunement, and disattunement. The proportions of interactions that were disharmonically attuned and disattuned were significantly higher among the dyads whose infants were problematic breastfeeders. These findings provide insights for observing mother-infant interactions during breastfeeding and assisting mothers whose breastfeeding sessions are often active and disruptive rather than calm and restful.

Historical Research. Historical research methods are valuable for exploring past practices, examining patterns and trends during specific periods, discovering relationships, and drawing inferences. Past revelations can increase understanding of traditions and practices and guide decision making. Historical inquiry entails identifying, collecting, categorizing, and determining validity of evidence, critical analysis, synthesis, and writing to present meaningful discussion of the subject (Shafer, 1980).

Millard's work (1990) illustrates the value of historical research. Pediatric literature between 1897 and 1987 shows that although breastfeeding was advocated, advice centered on regimes and schedules. Even as flexibility in feeding times became more acceptable, advice including time limitations continued. Study findings suggest that emphasis on time in regard to breastfeeding and the allocation of control in breastfeeding to medical experts undermined breastfeeding during this 90-year period.

Participatory Action. Participatory action is a type of research method for conducting studies aimed at social action and change. It is based on a partnership between individuals and groups most closely affected by and involved with the phenomenon under study. All participants contribute and work together through all stages of the research process. Recognition, increased knowledge, and empowerment for those most affected by an unacceptable or substandard situation contribute to eventual change. This method is often used for community development to establish programs with those who desire and will attend a service. An example is development of a healthy lifestyle program that includes breastfeeding support for women living in difficult circumstances. Establishing working relationships and "equal" partnerships with participants and community representatives is complex and challenging.

Feminist Research. Feminist research is an approach that is congruent with but not overtly evident in current breastfeeding research. Whether there is a "feminist method" or whether any research method can be conducted from a feminist perspective is an unresolved issue (Kelly, Burton, & Regan, 1994). Feminist research is guided by the following principles: it is about women, for women, and done with, not to, women; it should be empowering for participants; it is directed toward positive social change; and it generally uses qualitative methods. A feminist perspective encourages the researcher to focus on women in a societal and political context and to consider cultural influences and attitudes within society as central to the experience of the women involved (Harding, 1987). Feminist researchers recognize the negotiated social act between the researcher and the participants. The researcher defines the study and interprets the findings and the participants decide what information they will share with the researcher (Maynard & Purvis, 1994).

Multimethod studies that use both qualitative and quantitative approaches simultaneously are an emerging trend, although they are not accepted by all researchers. Those who support this approach argue that using several methods can enhance theoretical insights, facilitate incremental growth of knowledge, augment validity of studies, and force investigators to reflect and find new views when, for example, findings from one method are incongruent with another method used (Polit & Hungler, 1999). Challenges include the ability of the investigator(s) to reconcile differences in philosophical underpinnings of differing approaches; expense; investigator knowledge about and skills for working with two approaches; analytic challenges; and acceptance of manuscripts by journals that publish studies (Polit & Hungler, 1999). Studies using multimethods are complex and should be conducted by an experienced researcher.

Elements of Research

The elements of research are essential to writing proposals and reports, conducting research, and evaluating studies. The major elements include the research problem and purpose; the review of literature; the protection of human subjects; the method; the analysis; and the results and discussion. Although the elements are similar for both qualitative and quantitative research approaches, the content and processes vary. The following section describes the elements and discusses the differences between qualitative and quantitative methods.

Research Problem and Purpose

The research problem is a critical component of a study. It identifies "what" is studied and with "whom." The purpose delineates "why" the study is conducted. There are many sources for generating research problems. Questioning clinical practice, observing clinical and societal patterns and trends, building on findings from previous studies, and examining theoretical propositions are ways of developing research questions.

A problem that is suitable for study should be important to the topic of breastfeeding and amenable to investigation by scientific inquiry. It should be meaningful to many individuals or have a distinct influence on a few. A study examining the effect of labor pain relief medication on neonatal suckling and breastfeeding duration conducted by Riordan et al. (2001) illustrates the importance to all childbearing women and their infants. In contrast, a study about the effect of sequential and simultaneous breast pumping on milk volume and prolactin levels among women who express milk for a prolonged period of time (Hill, Aldag, & Chatterton, 1996) has important implications for a few. Criteria that render a problem appropriate for scientific inquiry include the following:

- *Suitability* of the research design for the research question
- *Accessibility* of study participants
- *Feasibility* of the study with regard to time, funding, and equipment
- *Potentiality* of adhering to ethical requirements throughout all study phases

Reviewing the literature about a study topic provides direction for asking a relevant question and selecting an appropriate method. A qualitative method is indicated when literature is limited about a phenomenon or when more in-depth knowledge is desired. When many studies about a topic have been undertaken, however, the findings often provide a base and focus for further study, and a quantitative method may be most appropriate.

Research problems can be written as questions or declarative statements. Clearly identifying the topic, population, and variables for study is essential for quantitative methods. In qualitative studies, less is known about the topic of interest; therefore, the research question is broader. The purpose is to describe and interpret meanings of a phenomenon, to gain an in-depth understanding of an experience or situation, or to discover variables relevant to a topic rather than to examine variables previously identified. Examples of research questions that can be applied to specific methods are shown in Table 22–1. All questions pertain to breastfeeding pre-

---

TABLE 22–1

EXAMPLE OF RESEARCH QUESTIONS AND METHODS

Questions for Qualitative Methods	Research Method	Variables for Study
Topic of Interest: Breastfeeding preterm infants		
What are mothers' experiences of breastfeeding a preterm infant?	Phenomenology	
What are the cultural factors influencing feeding patterns of preterm infants among Chinese women?	Ethnography	
What is the experience of learning how to breastfeed a preterm infant?	Grounded theory	
Questions for Quantitative Methods		
Topic of Interest: Social support and breastfeeding*		
Population: Mothers of preterm infants		
What kinds of social support are most useful to breastfeeding mothers of preterm infants?	Descriptive	Social Support
Is there a relationship between social network and choice of feeding method and duration of breastfeeding for mothers of preterm infants? (Kaufman & Hall, 1989)	Correlational	Social network Feeding method choice Breastfeeding duration
What is the effect on breastfeeding duration of scheduled visits by a lactation consultant to breastfeeding mothers of preterm infants?	Experimental	Breastfeeding duration Scheduled visits by a lactation consultant (independent variable)

The topic and variables for study are usually more specifically identified in quantitative studies.

term infants. For quantitative methods this has been further delineated to social network and breastfeeding preterm infants, a topic and population studied by Kaufman and Hall (1989).

Variables, Hypotheses, and Operational Definitions

Variables. Variables are defined as "qualities, properties, or characteristics of persons, things, or situations that change or vary and are manipulated or measured in research" (Burns & Grove, 1997). Qualitative studies may aim to discover indicators that influence the study phenomenon, whereas quantitative studies identify specific variables for investigation. Experimental studies have at least one dependent and one independent variable. The *dependent variable*, also called the *outcome variable*, is what the investigator is most interested in understanding, explaining, or predicting. In the example of an experimental study cited in Table 22–1, the dependent variable is breastfeeding duration. The *independent variable* is thought to affect or change the dependent variable. It is the treatment or intervention that affects the outcome; in this example it is the scheduled visits by a lactation consultant. Uncontrolled, confounding, or extraneous variables are those elements in quantitative studies that may affect the dependent or outcome variable. Sometimes such variables come between the occurrence of the treatment (independent variable) and the measurement of the outcome variable. For example, if mothers with preterm infants view a television documentary on the advantages of breastmilk for preterm infants, the television program—rather than the scheduled visits by the lactation consultant—may be the motivating factor for prolonging breastfeeding. To "control" the effect of these variables on experimental study outcomes, subjects are randomly assigned to an experimental group receiving visits by a lactation consultant or to a control group receiving existing care that does not include such visits. The random placement of subjects in each group is expected to ensure that each group is similar in regard to background characteristics, practices, and opportunities. Therefore, if the experimental group breastfeeds longer than the control group (as determined by statistical procedures), the increased breastfeeding duration is attributed to the visits by the lactation consultant.

Hypotheses. "A hypothesis is the formal statement of the expected relationship(s) between two or more variables in a specified population" (Burns & Grove, 1997). Qualitative studies may generate hypotheses, whereas correlational and experimental studies examine and test relationships between identified variables.

Hypotheses for correlational studies focus on the association of variables. For the study by Kaufman and Hall (1989), a hypothesis may be written as the following: For mothers of preterm infants, there is a positive relationship between the mothers' perceptions of their social network and breastfeeding duration.

In experimental studies, a hypothesis represents a prediction of how an intervention specifically influences an identified outcome. The written hypothesis includes these components as well as naming the study groups. For the experimental study in Table 22–1, a research hypothesis is written as follows: Mothers of preterm infants who have scheduled visits by a lactation consultant will breastfeed longer than mothers of preterm infants who do not have scheduled visits by a lactation consultant. The experimental and control groups, the dependent and independent variables, and the predictor (longer breastfeeding duration) are identified.

For statistical purposes, some investigators prefer to write hypotheses in the null form. For example: There will be *no* difference in the duration of breastfeeding between mothers of preterm infants who receive scheduled visits by a lactation consultant and mothers of preterm infants who do not receive scheduled visits by a lactation consultant. In using the null hypothesis, outcomes for the groups are considered the same until it is established that they are statistically different. When this occurs, the null hypothesis is rejected, and an inference is made that the visits by a lactation consultant are the reason for the different group outcomes. The visits are then considered an effective intervention.

Operational Definitions. Operational definitions are explicit descriptions of how the major variables are observed and measured—and how they are integral to correlational and experimental studies. In the Kaufman and Hall (1989) study, both major variables are defined so that numerical comparisons can be made. Breastfeeding duration is specified as the number of postnatal days of any breastfeeding or expression, and social network is defined as a mother's perception of influence from social referents as measured by the Influence of Specific Referents (ISR) Scale.

In experimental studies, the independent variable must be clearly defined. In the fictitious experimental study shown in Table 22–1, a definition of the intervention regime—the scheduled visits by a lactation consultant—could be operationally defined in many ways. One example is a lactation consultant will visit a mother once a week from birth until 4 weeks after hospital discharge.

Operational definitions used in a study influence sample size, data collection, analyses, outcomes, interpretation, and the credibility of the study. In experimental studies and those examining breastfeeding relationships, the definitions of the major variables must be clearly and precisely described in order for findings to be considered accurate. Clear definitions are also necessary for comparing the results of studies that address similar topics, and they are essential for replication of a study. The numbers of categories included in a definition must be considered, however, as increasing categories require larger samples.

In a quasi-experimental study evaluating the efficacy of a breastfeeding clinic in prolonging breastfeeding duration, Ellis, Hewat, and Livingstone (1991) used precisely defined exclusive categories to measure breastfeeding outcomes over time. The following categories were used: *Exclusive:* total breastfeeding; *Primarily:* breastfeeding or expressed breastmilk (EBM) plus a maximum of 1 alternative milk feeding per week; *Mainly:* more than 1 breastfeeding or EBM per day plus more than 1 other milk feeding per week to a maximum of 1 per day; *Partial:* more than 1 breastfeeding or EBM per day plus more than 1 alternative milk feeding per day; *Minimal:* 1 or less than 1 breastfeeding or EBM per day to 1 breastfeeding or EBM feeding per week; and *Weaned:* breastfeeding or EBM has stopped for 1 week or more. For analysis, research assistants entered the type of feeding based on the mothers' responses and for some statistical procedures categories were collapsed. This precision in definitions was required by reviewers of the agency funding the study.

Another much less complex way of defining breastfeeding that has been found useful by researchers when duration of breastfeeding is a study outcome is to ask mothers if they are breastfeeding or not breastfeeding. Mothers not breastfeeding are then asked the number of days they breastfed before weaning and weaning is defined as not breastfeeding in the last 48 hours and not intending to breastfeed this child again (Cronenwett et al., 1992).

An intensity ratio was used in descriptive studies to determine breastfeeding exclusivity in a large national sample ($n = 1863$) over time (Piper & Parkes, 2001) and the intensity of breastmilk exposure for premature infants after hospital discharge (Piper, 2002). For the first study, the intensity ratio was the "number of reported breastfeeds per day for a specific month(s)" divided by "summed total of the number of reported breastfeeds, formula feeds, and cow's milk feeds for a specific month(s)" (Piper & Parks, 2001, p. 229). The range is 0 to 1.0 with 1 representing exclusive breastfeeding and numbers close to 1 indicating higher intensity of breastfeeding. The ratio was similar in the second study ($n = 40$) in that the number of breastmilk feeds to total liquid feeds of the premature infants was calculated (Piper, 2002). These studies show that this is a measure that can be used for studies with large and small samples, but that mothers again are asked specific questions and researchers use mothers' responses for calculating the ratio.

Lack of consistency in "how" breastfeeding is defined and at "what times" data are collected is a problem for comparing individual studies and collecting data and comparing breastfeeding rates in different regions and countries. In 1988, the Interagency Group for Action on Breastfeeding (IGAB), an international organization, started developing standard definitions for breastfeeding patterns that are recommended for international use (Armstrong, 1991; Labbok & Coffin, 1997). The definitions include full breastfeeding, which is further delineated into exclusive and almost exclusive breastfeeding; partial breastfeeding, with groupings of high, medium, and low; and token breastfeeding, which is described as minimal, occasional, and irregular breastfeeds (Labbok & Krasovec, 1990), although all categories were not precisely described and would not support rigorous investigations. Added to the dilemma, the World Health Organization/United Nations Children's Fund (WHO/UNICEF) published breastfeeding definitions that are used for the global databank on breastfeeding (Labbok, 2000). These include exclusive, predominant, and full breastfeeding as well as complementary feeding and bottle-feeding. As suggested by Labbock, it is the responsibility of all to be aware of the many breastfeeding definitions used by writers and researchers and to "be diligent to ensure that our decisions are evidence-based and our understanding reflects the definitions of breastfeeding used in the research" (p. 21). Consistent definitions for databases that could be used for comparing breastfeeding rates between regions and countries, however, are still an issue.

Review of Literature

Reviewing literature on a study topic provides knowledge and understanding about the phenomenon. Findings from studies help to formulate the research problem and provide direction for research methods. The purpose of a literature review can be different for qualitative and quantitative approaches. In qualitative studies, an initial review of literature is done for investigator awareness and knowledge of the studies conducted. Since the goal of qualitative methods is discovery or a new view of a phenomenon, literature should not influence the mindset of the investigator during initial data collection. In the analysis stage, study findings reported in the literature are used to compare, contrast, and verify findings of the current study. Findings from a new study may also be combined with those of a previous study to identify new insights and expand current knowledge about a phenomenon.

In quantitative studies, the existing literature will help to clarify the research problem and identify theories or concepts on which the study is based. Identification of key concepts and their relationships provides a conceptual framework or structure for the study. Literature is also useful in assisting with selection of a research design, providing strategies for data collection and analysis, and interpreting findings.

Protection of the Rights of Human Subjects

Most breastfeeding research involves human subjects. To protect the rights of study participants throughout the research process, investigators must adhere to ethical guidelines. The first international ethical standards are the Nuremberg Code, developed in 1949. This code is the basis of ethical standards developed by medicine and the behavioral science disciplines. The Declaration of Helsinki, adopted in 1964 and revised in 1975 by the World Medical Assembly provides further guidelines for investigators conducting clinical research. Governments and institutions stipulate ethical requirements for funded research, and individual codes of ethics have been developed by professional associations for researchers within the discipline to adhere to when conducting human research.

Four basic rights of human subjects are recognized (Wilson, 1989): (1) freedom from risk or injury from physical, emotional, financial, or social harm; (2) full knowledge of the study purpose, procedures to be used, time commitments asked of the participants, and any other factors that may affect the subjects; (3) the assurance of the right to self-determination, which means that subjects may refuse to participate or withdraw from a study *at any time* without any effect on the care they are receiving or will receive; (4) the affirmation of their privacy, anonymity, or confidentiality throughout all phases of the research.

Mechanisms developed to ensure that research is ethically conducted include the investigator's use of an informed consent document and review of the proposed study by ethical review boards. An informed consent document describes the study, addresses how the rights of subjects will be maintained, explains that the subject can withdraw from the study at any time without compromising health care, and provides a contact number for the investigator. It is presented to subjects when they are recruited. A subject's signature on the informed consent document indicates an understanding of the study and willingness to participate. Ethical review boards—established by universities and many health-care agencies, school boards, or organizations that are resources for human subjects—review study proposals to ensure that the research process protects the rights of study participants. The investigators are bound by the recommendations of these review boards during the research process.

Method

Each study method addresses setting, sample, data collection, and data analysis.

Setting.   Setting is the location of the study and/or source of participating subjects or sample. In all studies, the setting must be clearly described.

Population.   Population, which is often referred to as the target population, is the group of individuals in which the researcher is interested. For example, it could be all breastfeeding mothers, primiparas who breastfeed, mothers who work and breastfeed, or mothers of preterm infants. Or, in some cases, an object, such as breastmilk, may be the phenomenon of interest rather than individuals. Because it is difficult to study an entire population, researchers generally study a *sample* of the larger population.

Sampling.   Sampling is a process for selecting the sample from the population. The two basic types are probability and nonprobability sampling.

Probability sampling is specific to quantitative studies and is used when investigators want to generalize findings from the sample studied to larger populations. For these studies it is important that the sample be representative of the target population. This is accomplished by the *random selection* of subjects from the population, a process that requires that every individual in the population of interest has an equal and independent chance of being chosen. There are several methods of probability sampling.

Simple random sampling is achieved by numbering all members of the population and then selecting subjects by using a table of random numbers available in many quantitative research books. Other procedures include drawing subjects' names from a hat or flipping a coin.

Systematic sampling follows the procedure of choosing every "nth" (e.g., every eighth, 10th, or 100th) subject from a list of individuals in the target population. To ensure that all possible subjects have an equal chance, the names on the list must

not be grouped in any special way, such as alphabetical order or age of subjects. For example, in a study of the effect of hospital practices on early breastfeeding experience, selecting every nth case from the list of mothers admitted to a particular postpartum unit would be an appropriate sampling technique.

Stratified random sampling is a process of identifying subgroups of a population and selecting numbers of subjects that represent the distribution of the subgroups in the population. For example, if a researcher wishes to study a population of all mothers giving birth in a specific geographic location and learns that the population distribution is 40 percent primiparas and 60 percent multiparas, then the investigator will randomly select the numbers for each subgroup or "stratum" that reflects the population distribution.

In studies that involve human subjects, probability sampling is frequently not possible because all subjects in a population—for example, all breastfeeding mothers—cannot be identified. Or, depending on the purpose of the study, random assignment of women to feeding groups may be unethical. As a result, many breastfeeding studies utilize nonprobability sampling.

Nonprobability sampling is the nonrandom selection of subjects or participants for a study. Methods for selecting the study participants depends on the type of study that is being conducted.

Convenience sampling is a common method used for both qualitative and quantitative studies. The sample consists of consenting subjects from a readily available source—for example, all mothers giving birth at a hospital or attending a particular clinic.

Network, nominated, or *snowball sampling* is a strategy that bases recruitment on asking current study participants to identify other individuals, similar to themselves, who may also consent to be study subjects. This method is useful in the study of an ethnic group or individuals with a specific condition for which a support group has been established, such as parents who are experiencing a perinatal loss.

Solicited or *volunteer sampling* is used when the investigator wishes to broaden the sample. Advertisements in newspapers and notices on bulletin boards regarding the research often entreat interested participants (Morse, 1991b).

Purposive sampling occurs when the investigator selects participants "according to the needs of the study" (Morse, 1991b). Participants are selected either because they are thought to be knowledgeable about the study topic or because as much variation as possible is wanted for the sample.

Theoretical sampling is used with qualitative methods, and it is similar to purposive sampling. Sampling is generally initiated using one of the nonprobability methods, but as the study progresses the investigator determines that more information or greater diversity in views are needed to examine categories and their relationships for expanding the developing theory.

Methods of Data Collection. Data are collected by asking questions, observing, and/or measuring key variables identified in the research question. The data collection method must be appropriate to the research method and the study population.

Self-report questionnaires are an effective and common way of obtaining specific information from a large sample. However, the construction of questionnaires, which can be understood by all participants and are sufficiently broad in scope to reflect "true" meanings, can be time-consuming and expensive to develop. If they are too long or repeated frequently throughout a study, participants may not complete all questionnaires. This results in study attrition and if the sample size is sufficiently lowered, determination of statistically significant outcomes may be compromised.

Interviews elicit more in-depth information; however, they are more time-consuming and expensive to administer. A skilled interviewer is required to ensure explicit and valid collection of data. When more than one interviewer is used, varying degrees of bias on the part of the interviewer must be considered as a potential limitation of the data.

Observations are useful for collecting data about events, patterns of behavior, activities, or interactions. Observations can be unstructured and recorded as field notes, or they can be structured for specific recording on checklists. Developing a coding scheme that is congruent with the research question and specific to the level of behaviors that are of interest is essential. However, the process must be precise, and it is time-consuming. Methods of recording data include paper and pencil, a digital data acquisition system that is a hand-held keyboard for entering coded behaviors as they occur, or videotaping (Morse & Bottorff, 1990). The latter is a means for recording observations that can be coded more precisely and in greater detail at a later time.

Biophysiological measurements—for example, infant weight, length, head circumference, respirations, oxygen consumption, and heart rate, as well as the mother's temperature, prolactin levels, and milk composition—have been used in breastfeeding research. Measurements are only as accurate as the equipment used and the investigator responsible for measuring and recording.

Data Analysis

Data analysis is the process of examining, summarizing, and synthesizing the data collected to determine if study findings answer the research question. Strategies for data analysis are dependent on the research question, sample selection and size, and method and type of data collection.

Application of Methods to Qualitative Approaches

Specific methodological procedures, based on the philosophical foundations of each qualitative method, have been developed, but as qualitative research has become more recognized, the use of different kinds of methods have expanded and the blending of others has occurred. There is debate among qualitative researchers as to whether these changes enhance qualitative research or if mixing methods transgresses assumptions of data collection procedures and analysis, compromising the science (Morse, 1991a). It is inevitable that variation in method use will continue.

Sampling

All nonprobability sampling methods are suitable for recruiting study participants. As the study progresses, *theoretical sampling* may be used and this will also help to determine the number of participants. As data are simultaneously collected and analyzed from initial participants and as descriptions of experiences are revealed, additional informants are recruited on the basis of expanding the developing knowledge base. Participants are recruited until no new information is disclosed and data are fully explored (Chenitz & Swanson, 1986; Glaser, 1978). Sample size depends on the scope of the topic, the method used, and the type of data collection, but most qualitative studies have relatively few participants. Numbers may range from 10 to 50.

Data Collection

Methods of data collection include interviews, field observations, and review of documents. In-depth, unstructured interviews, which explore participants' perceptions and in many studies validate the investigator's subjective interpretation of the data, remain the most common method for the qualitative approaches. The interviews are usually taped on audiocassette and then transcribed for detailed analysis. Participant observation, another common method, is particularly suitable for ethnographic research. For the circumstance under study, the investigator observes the activities, people, and physical aspects of the situation while engaging, either passively or actively, in the activities (Spradley, 1980). Field notes of the observations are recorded for later analysis. In phenomenological studies, data resources may be expanded to include movies, pictures, poetry, stories, or any medium that portrays the nature of the meaning of the study topic. Focus groups are also used to augment data collection in some studies.

Data Analysis

Data analysis is ongoing throughout the period of data collection. Each piece of data, whether from transcriptions of interviews, detailed field notes, documents, or photographs, is compared and contrasted with each other. As the study progresses the investigator makes interpretations. Study participants validate investigator's interpretations to ensure that they are congruent with the participants' experiences.

In phenomenological studies, several processes of analysis have evolved. For example, Giorgi (1985) outlines specific steps for data analysis. They include: compiling and examining descriptions about the meaning of a phenomenon; identifying common elements or units of meaning; delineating

themes; naming abstract meanings; and generating what are called structural descriptions that embrace the meaning of the lived experience from the participants' perspectives. In contrast, van Manen (1990) describes methodological underpinnings of analysis as "the dynamic interplay of six research activities" (p. 30). These include selecting a phenomenon of great interest for study; investigating a lived rather than a conceptualized experience; reflecting on the themes representing the phenomenon; describing it through the art of writing and rewriting; maintaining a strong pedagogical orientation; and balancing the research context by considering parts and the whole (pp. 30–31). The lived experience is represented through language, which is achieved by writing and rewriting until the written word portrays a deep understanding of the meaning of a lived experience.

In ethnographic studies, participant observation in the field is often an important component of data collection. To understand the behaviors, activities, and experiences of individuals and how they interact with their environment the investigator becomes an interactive group observer. The environment or culture of interest may be that of an ethnic group, a neonatal intensive care unit, or a breastfeeding support group. In-depth interviews with participants and field note observations are qualitatively analyzed. Ethnographies may be descriptive or analytical. Descriptive ethnographies generally identify and describe social patterns or actions within a specific culture whereas analytic ethnographies examine social meanings and cultural biases or norms that guide the actions of individuals within the identified culture (Morse & Field, 1995).

Grounded theory research follows an exceptionally systematic analytic process. Data from transcribed interviews are coded and categorized, and connections between categories are made; a tentative conceptualization or theory is formulated, and the examination continues until a core variable emerges that is the focus of the theory. Concept modification and integration continue through two processes called *memoing* and *theoretical coding*. The process of analysis is not linear. Throughout the data analysis, codes, categories, conceptualizations, and theory are constantly compared, and the researcher moves between inductive and deductive reasoning. Conceptualizations of relationships are deductively proposed and these are inductively examined for verification. The analytic process is ongoing until a theory, substantiated by the data, is generated (Glaser, 1978; Strauss & Corbin, 1990).

Trustworthiness of Qualitative Research

Ensuring that study findings are trustworthy and reflect the truth is an essential component of qualitative research. This requires ongoing examination by the investigator throughout the research process. Sources of error can occur in sampling, data collection, and analysis. Factors to evaluate throughout the process include the integrity of key informants in providing accurate data; the interviewer's skill in obtaining the participants' true perspectives; the accuracy of field observations; the generation of codes or units of analysis that represent data accurately within a social context; and the interpretations of the data to determine whether they represent true meanings.

Criteria for assessing trustworthiness are outlined by Lincoln and Guba (1985) as credibility, dependability, confirmability, and transferability. *Credibility* is achieved by implementing and demonstrating that the processes in conducting the research are plausible. There are several practices that demonstrate study credibility: engaging in data collection and analyses for a sufficient length of time to ensure the aspects of participants' experiences are understood; using multiple data sources; engaging others to read and interpret transcripts; involving participants to review data, interpretations, and emerging theories for correctness; and illustrating the experience of the research conducting the study. *Dependability* reflects the reality that is that individual's views and situations. It is shown through an inquiry audit, which entails having another researcher review the data, process, and rigor undertaken during analysis. *Confirmability* is achieved by developing an audit trail of the data and recording interpretations and their meanings for review by another person. *Transferability* is the extent that findings can be transferred to another group or setting. Rich descriptions of the participants, settings, and experiences allow others to judge if study findings can be transferred to similar settings or populations (Polit & Hungler, 1999).

Application of Methods to Quantitative Approaches

Sampling and Sample Size

Probability sampling methods, particularly for correlational and experimental studies, are preferred, so that the study findings can be generalized to a larger population. However, as previously discussed, many studies involving human subjects must employ nonprobability sampling methods. The most common method is convenience sampling.

Deciding on the sample size can be a critical issue in quantitative studies. Factors to consider include the study purpose, level of inquiry, design, and type of analysis, as well as the availability of subjects, research funds, and the time frame of the study. For descriptive studies that identify and describe characteristics of a population, sample size will generally not affect study outcomes to the same degree as it will for other quantitative methods. Recommendations are to recruit as large a sample as possible after considering the previously described factors.

Sample size is critical in experimental and quasi-experimental studies that statistically test hypotheses. If the sample size is too small, group differences may not be detected when they actually exist and a null hypothesis (no difference between groups) is not rejected. The result is that an intervention or treatment that is effective is not recognized as making a difference.

For these kinds of studies, a sample size that is adequate to show true differences between groups can be estimated using a *power analysis* (Cohen, 1988; Kramer & Thiemann, 1987). Computer software programs are available for computing this statistical procedure. When a research proposal is being developed, researchers frequently consult with a statistician for advice about sample size, study design, and analyses procedures.

In experimental or quasi-experimental studies, *random assignment* of subjects to experimental and control groups is advised. This has two purposes: all subjects have an equal and independent chance of receiving the treatment, and it increases the probability that each group is similar in regard to background characteristics. The latter serves as a control of extraneous variables that may influence the effect of treatment. Random assignment should not be confused with random selection (previously discussed), which allows findings to be generalized to the population from which the sample was selected.

Correlational studies and those using survey questionnaires generally require large samples. The size is reflected in the number of variables to be examined and/or subgroups to be compared. As each of these factors increase, so must the sample size. If numbers are insufficient, statistical analyses and study findings can be compromised.

Two types of epidemiological studies examine associations between variables such as exposure (risk factors) and a disease or health condition: (1) case-control and (2) cohort studies. In case-control studies, subjects with a specific condition are compared, generally retrospectively, with a control group that does not have the condition. Differences between the two groups in the subjects' past experiences or life events are examined to identify factors that may lead to the onset of the condition. During the past decade, there has been increasing interest in the relationship of breastfeeding exclusivity and duration and diseases such as childhood leukemia, diabetes, and upper respiratory infections. Case-control studies are a method for providing this information.

Cohort studies are similar except that they are generally follow-up studies of subjects who are exposed or not exposed to a risk factor that is assumed to be associated with the onset of an identified health problem. An example is provided in a study by Wright et al. (1989) regarding breastfeeding and lower-respiratory-tract illness during the first year of life. Infants in a pediatric practice were followed from birth throughout their first year and comparisons were made between infants who were and were not breastfed as well the length of time they were breastfed. Comparisons were also made in regard to the incidence of lower-respiratory-tract illnesses. The findings showed that breastfeeding for any duration was associated with a decreased incidence of wheezing illnesses during an infant's first 4 months of life.

Data Collection

All methods of data collection previously described

are applicable to quantitative studies if they are applied consistently and objectively. Descriptive studies gather data that are broader in scope or more subjective than correlational or experimental studies. However, questionnaires, interview schedules, and observation criteria must be structured so that the same data are collected in the same manner from all subjects. Measurement studies, such as correlational, quasi-experimental, and experimental studies, require data that can be reduced to numbers in order to apply statistical procedures. Reliable and valid questionnaires and observation checklists used for measuring variable relationships often take years to develop. Once established, they may be used in numerous studies.

Reliability and validity estimates of existing breastfeeding questionnaires and tools are limited. Table 22–2 presents an overview of these tools and what is known about their reliability and validity. Some of the tools can be found in Chapter 20. For correlational and experimental studies, it is recommended that the questionnaires or measures used for data collection are reliable and valid.

Reliability and Validity

Reliability and validity are central issues concerned with error in research. Occurrence of error at any stage of the research process can affect study outcomes and limits the usefulness of the data. Reliability refers to the accuracy, consistency, precision, and stability of measurement or data collection. Validity reflects truth, accuracy, and reality. To be valid, measures and methods of data collection must also be reliable.

Reliability.   Accuracy and consistency in the way data are collected, as well as the tools or instruments used, are essential in quantitative studies. Several types of reliability should be addressed.

Interrater reliability refers to accuracy and consistency in data collection. When more than one individual or instrument (such as a thermometer) is used for data collection, the probability of error between the individuals or instruments used increases. To control this aspect, checks are made. Similar instruments should be calibrated until measurement is consistent. For individuals making similar obser-

TABLE 22–2

Breastfeeding Questionnaires and Assessment Tools

Title	Purpose	Reliability	Validity
Breastfeeding Attrition Prediction Tool (BAPT) (Janke, 1992, 1994; Riordan & Koehn, 1997). Modified BAPT Tool (Dick et al., 2002).	To identify women at risk for early, unintended weaning. Four factors measure negative and positive breastfeeding attitude, perceived maternal control, and social and professional support.	Cronbach alphas for all scales, .79–.85 (Janke, 1992, 1994); .80–.93 (Riordan & Koehn, 1997); and .81–.86 (Dick et al., 2002).	Prediction validity: 3 of 4 scales related to 8-week feeding outcome (Janke, 1992) and negative sentiment scale predicted early unintended weaning (Janke, 1994). Modified BAPT: 2 scales predicted 78% of women who discontinued breastfeeding at 8 weeks and 68% of those still breastfeeding (Dick et al., 2002).
Maternal Breastfeeding Evaluation Scale (MBFES) (Leff, Jefferis, & Gagne, 1994b; Riordan, Woodley, & Heaton, 1994).	To measure a mother's overall evaluation of the breastfeeding experience using a 30 item Likert scale. Subscales include: maternal enjoyment/ role attainment, infant satisfaction/growth, and lifestyle/maternal body image.	Test-retest correlations: .82–.93. Cronbach alphas for subscales: .80–.93 (Leff, Jefferis, & Gagne, 1994b) and .73–.83 (Riordan, Woodley, & Heaton, 1994).	Items developed from qualitative study (Leff, Jefferis, & Gagne, 1994a). Predictive validity: Significant positive correlation of total scale and subscales with maternal satisfaction and breastfeeding intent and duration (Leff, Jefferis, & Gagne, 1994b; Riordan, Woodley, & Heaton, 1994).
Breastfeeding Self-Efficacy Scale (BSES) (Dennis & Faux, 1999).	To assess and measure confidence in breastfeeding mothers. Factors include techniques/maternal skills and attitudes and beliefs.	Cronbach alpha: .96.	Content validity. Predictive validity: Feeding method (breast or bottle) at 6 weeks postpartum (Dennis & Faux, 1999).
LATCH breastfeeding assessment tool (Jensen, Wallace, & Kelsay, 1994).	To assess effective breastfeeding in first week after birth for latch-on, audible swallowing, nipple type, comfort of breast/nipple, and help needed to position baby.	Interrater reliability: Mothers' and nurses' total scores positively correlated (Riordan et al., 2001).	Requires further testing but mothers' total scores positively correlated with breastfeeding at 6 weeks postpartum (Riordan et al., 2001).
Infant Breastfeeding Assessment Tool (IBFAT). (Matthews, 1988).	To assess and measure infant breastfeeding competence. Four subscales measure readiness to feed, rooting, fixing, and sucking. Score range 0–12.	Interrater reliability: 91% agreement in co-assessed feeds (Matthews, 1988) Pairwise correlations of raters .58 (Riordan & Keohn, 1997).	Content validity and observation in clinical practice (Matthews, 1988).

vations, the degree of their accuracy can be statistically determined. Acceptable levels of reliability are dependent on the statistical method used—for example, for interobserver reliability an agreement of 90 percent is adequate. When using a Cohen's kappa statistic, a procedure that corrects for level of chance agreement, an acceptable level is .70 (Bakeman & Gottman, 1986). For the Infant Breastfeeding Assessment Tool (IBFAT) described in Table 22–2, interrater reliability was determined by comparing agreement of the mother's and the investigator's breastfeeding assessments. Overall, agreement was 91 percent accurate, although it was noted that infants who fed well or poorly were easier to assess than those who rated in the middle range and were classified as moderate feeders (Matthews, 1988, 1991).

Intrarater reliability refers to accuracy and consistency over time. When data are collected for more than 6 months, investigators may want to check the accuracy of the individual who is making the observations—and/or the instrument(s) used—every few months. Calculations and acceptability are similar to interrater reliability.

Test-retest reliability indicates the stability of a measure, such as a questionnaire, over time. Results of two questionnaire administrations to the same subjects, occurring approximately 3 weeks apart, are statistically compared. A coefficient reported as .80 or above is generally acceptable for measurement questionnaires that reflect attitudes or feelings. For some events, however, such as postpartum adjustment, a low correlation coefficient (such as .40 or .50) may be desired since differences in individual scores over a period of time reflect inconsistency and are then a possible indication that the individual is changing or adjusting to a different lifestyle. The Maternal Breastfeeding Evaluation Scale (MBFES) presented in Table 22–2 shows that this tool is highly reliable over time.

Internal consistency refers to the statistical agreement of several items on a questionnaire that reflect the meaning of a concept—for example, satisfaction with breastfeeding. Similarity in meaning or internal consistency of the items can be statistically determined. Cronbach's alpha is a reliability coefficient frequently computed to determine internal consistency. A coefficient of .70 to .80 is generally acceptable for a questionnaire measur-

ing a construct (Nunnally, 1978). Therefore, the Breastfeeding Attrition Prediction Tool (BAPT), the MBFES, and the Breastfeeding Self-Efficacy Scale (BSES) described in Table 22–2 are all internally consistent questionnaires for data collection.

Validity. Validity addresses the extent to which a questionnaire or measurement instrument reflects the meaning of the concept that is being measured. Types of validity referred to in quantitative studies are content, concurrent, and construct validity. Questionnaires and interview schedules used for descriptive studies should have *content validity,* which means that the questions reflect the study concepts. In developing questionnaires, investigators review the literature to include dimensions of the concept being studied and then submit the questionnaire to individuals who are considered experts on the research topic for review. This validation of content with literature and experts is known as content validity.

All other types of validity require psychometric testing and statistical validation, but this is important for assessment/measurement tools and questionnaires. *Concurrent validity* determines similarities or differences in the construct that two similar tools measure. *Predictive validity* ascertains whether a measure at one time can predict future outcomes. In Table 22–2 the BAPT, MBFES, and BFES all show some predictive validity for breastfeeding outcomes. *Construct validity* indicates that a tool measures what it is intended to measure. The use of questionnaires and tools with these types of validity enhances the credibility of study findings.

Data Analysis

Data analysis is the process of organizing, summarizing, examining, and synthesizing the data collected in order to reach conclusions about the research question. Numerical analysis of data is central to quantitative studies. The data collected is converted to numerical values in a variety of ways. Table 22–3 defines levels of measurement and provides examples. The level of measurement has implications for the statistical procedures applied.

Statistical procedures used for correlational, experimental, or quasi-experimental studies can be classified as parametric or nonparametric. Para-

TABLE 22–3

LEVELS OF MEASUREMENT

	Nominal	Ordinal	Interval/Ratio
Definitions	Discreet categories of data that do not have any implied order.	Assigned categories of data that can be ranked in order; intervals between categories are not equal.	Categories of data that are ordered and are equal distances apart. Ratio also has a known zero point.
Examples	Gender: male/female Breastfed/not breastfed Marital status	Most Likert-type scales BAPT, MBFES, BSES, and IBFAT scales (see Table 22–2)	Body temperature Blood pressure Weight or length Duration of breastfeeding measured in specified days, weeks, months, or years.

metric tests are more powerful and preferred because they permit inferences to be made from findings of the study sample to the larger population. The use of parametric procedures requires that three assumptions be met: (1) random selection of the sample; (2) variables are normally distributed among the study groups; and (3) measurement of the dependent variable(s) at an interval level. Nonparametric statistics are used in situations when the following characteristics are evident: (1) the sample size is small; (2) normal distribution of variables in the sample cannot be assumed; (3) parameters of the population are unknown; and (4) the level of measurement of variables is at a nominal or ordinal level.

The selection of an appropriate statistical procedure is dependent on the type of study, sample size, sampling procedure, and type of data to be analyzed. Table 22–4 indicates commonly used procedures for study type and level of data. In experimental or quasi-experimental studies, the level of data of the dependent variable dictates the type of statistical testing that can be done. The purpose of this table is to assist research novices to recognize the appropriate use of statistics for reviewing studies. Extensive knowledge about statistical procedures is beyond the scope of this chapter.

The choice of interval versus ordinal data is controversial. Human feelings and perceptions do not fit the interval scale and most psychosocial variables can only be superimposed on an ordinal scale. Therefore, statistical procedures that traditionally require interval data are often used in human research with ordinal data.

Descriptive Studies. Data collected to describe variables and their relationships are generally subjected to content analysis and descriptive statistics. Content analysis consists of examining the data, identifying similar content or meanings, and classifying those that are identified into mutually exclusive categories. These nominal data can then be used with the descriptive statistics identified in Table 22–4. Findings may be reported as frequencies, percentages, or modes; they may be displayed in graphs, histograms, or contingency tables.

Correlational Studies. Correlation coefficients are the outcomes of statistical procedures for determining the relationship between two variables. The type of relationship is reported as positive (as one variable increases so does the other), negative (variables both decrease), or inverse (as one variable increases the other decreases). The strength of the relationship is reported as a number between 1 and −1; stronger relationships are near 1 (positive) or −1 (negative), and 0 indicates no relationship.

Associations in epidemiological studies are estimated using relative risk or risk ratio (RR) and odds

TABLE 22–4

APPROPRIATE STATISTICS FOR TYPE OF STUDY AND LEVEL OF DATA

Type of Study	Nonparametric Tests and Level of Data	Parametric Tests and Level of Data
Descriptive		
• One variable	Frequency—*nominal*	
	Percentage—*ordinal*	
	Mode—*nominal*	
	Median—*ordinal*	
	Mean—*interval*	
	Standard deviation—*interval*	
• Two or more variables	Contingency table—*nominal*	
	Cross tabulation—*nominal*	
	Chi-square—*nominal*	
Correlational	Spearman's Rho—*ordinal*	Pearson-*r*—*ordinal*
	Kendall's Tau—*ordinal*	
Experimental/Quasi-experimental		
• Two independent groups	Median test—*ordinal*	*t*-test (pooled)—*interval***
	Mann-Whitney U—*ordinal*	
• Two dependent or paired groups	Wilcoxon signed-rank—*ordinal*	*t*-test (paired)—*interval***
	McNemar chi-square—*nominal*	
• Two or more groups	Chi-square—*nominal*	ANOVA (F test)—*interval***
	Kruskal-Wallis—*ordinal*	
	Friedman test—*ordinal*	

*Level of data of dependent variable.

ratio (OR). Cohort studies use relative risk, which indicates the probability of a group exposed to an identified factor developing a specific disease or condition in relation to a group not exposed to the factor. The risk ratio is expressed as the incidence rate of the disease in the exposed group to the incidence rate in the unexposed group (Harkness, 1995). It is calculated using the formula:

$$RR = \frac{\dfrac{a}{a+b}}{\dfrac{c}{c+d}}$$

See representations in Table 22–5. In case-control studies, subjects have developed the disease or condition of interest, and the relative risk is then estimated by calculating the ratio of the odds of exposure among the cases to that among the controls (Hennekens, Buring, & Mayrent, 1987). In a hypothetical case, the odds ratio for estimating the association of disease X and exposure to a factor such as being fed only milk substitutes in the first 6 months of life can be calculated using the formula OR = *ad/bc* as *a*, *d*, *b*, and *c* as represented in a 2 by 2 table, shown in Table 22–5.

A relative risk or odds ratio of 1.0 suggests that the incidence rate of disease is the same for both

TABLE 22–5

CALCULATION OF RISK RATIO AND ODDS RATIO

Factor	Disease X	
	Cases	Controls
Milk substitutes		
Yes	*a*	*b*
No	*c*	*d*

the exposed and nonexposed groups. However, a value above 1—for example, 1.5—indicates an increased risk of 1.5 times or 50 percent higher among those exposed to the factor. Ratios less than 1 indicate decreased risk among those exposed. Odds ratios are often reported with confidence intervals, which "represent the range within which the true magnitude of effect lies with a certain degree of assurance" (Hennekens, Buring & Mayrent, 1987).

Experimental/Quasi-Experimental Studies.

The statistical procedure used to determine differences between groups depends on the number of groups and the level of measurement of the dependent variable, as shown in Table 22–4. Statistical differences are calculated using probability theory. Before analysis, the investigator decides on a level of significance—or a "*p*-value"—that will be used to accept that a statistically significant result indicates true differences between groups. The *p*-value reflects the probability that the statistical result can occur by chance, and it establishes the risk of the investigator making a Type I error. This means that a null hypothesis is rejected when in reality the hypothesis is true, leading to an incorrect interpretation that an intervention was successful. Conversely, a Type II error is the acceptance of a null hypothesis when in fact it is false, and in this situation an intervention that is successful is not recognized as such. In research, *p*-values of .01 or .05 are most commonly used (meaning there is 1 or 5 chances out of 100, respectively) of making a Type I error. Reducing the chance of a Type I error, however, increases the

probability of a Type II error. For this reason, most investigators conducting breastfeeding research elect to use a *p*-value of .05.

Multivariate Analysis. Multivariate analysis is the concurrent analysis of three or more variables to determine patterns of relationships between variables. These advanced statistical procedures are suitable for analyzing complex correlational and experimental studies that have several independent and/or several dependent variables (Tabachnick & Fidell, 1989). Generally, large sample sizes are required to accommodate analysis of increasing numbers of variables. The procedures commonly used include multiple regression; path analysis; analysis of covariance (ANCOVA); factor analysis; discriminate analysis; canonical correlation; and multivariate analysis of variance (MANOVA). As research becomes more sophisticated, the use of multivariate statistics in studies increases. This is a dilemma for beginning researchers and research consumers because studies using complex analytic procedures may be more difficult to evaluate.

Results, Discussion, Conclusions, and Dissemination

Study results or findings should be clear, concise, and congruent with the research question(s) asked and the methods used. The presentation of results varies for the type of study conducted. Qualitative studies are descriptive narratives, which include participants' verbatim accounts that provide evidence of the researcher's data interpretations. The results may be rich descriptions or new constructions of the study phenomenon, hypothetical propositions generated from the data, or a proposed theory.

Quantitative studies frequently use tables and graphs to display results. Variables examined in descriptive studies should be precisely described, and responses should be numerically reported. Relationships of variables investigated in correlational studies and the procedures used to determine relationships must be clear. In studies that test hypotheses, the statistical procedures used, the results, and the decision for supporting or not supporting the hypothesized relationships must be evident for each hypothesis stated. Significant, nonsignificant, and unexpected results must be reported. Findings in studies that are not what the investigator anticipates also contribute knowledge about the study topic; they can be an impetus for asking more relevant or more detailed research questions for future studies.

Interpreting study results is an intellectual process that gives meaning to the study and addresses the implications of the study outcomes. The investigator considers the study results with regard to the study process as well as findings from other studies that support or contradict results of the current study. These can be addressed with the presentation of the results or separately in a section discussing the findings.

Limitations of a study acknowledge factors that may affect study outcomes. Compromises are often necessary in the study process for pragmatic and ethical reasons. These can create weaknesses in design, sampling process, sample size, methods of data collection, or data analysis techniques, and should be reported. The extent to which study findings can be generalized to populations beyond the study sample should also be discussed. Stating limitations assists readers to evaluate the scientific merits of the study and enhances the credibility of the investigator.

Conclusions are concise statements that synthesize the findings; they provide an overall account of the importance of the study and an understanding of the phenomenon in question. The conclusions must be pertinent to the findings and not expanded beyond the study parameters. Following the conclusions, implications of the findings for clinical practice are generally described, and suggestions for further research are identified.

Communicating the results of the study is the final step of conducting research. This is done through research reports, journal articles, and presentations at conferences, workshops, and educational rounds in institutions. Dissemination of research solicits review by peers and facilitates the likelihood of study findings contributing to improved clinical practice.

Evaluating Research for Use in Practice

Evaluation is an analytical appraisal that makes judgments about the scientific merits of a study. The analysis objectively addresses the study's strengths and weaknesses, poses questions about the research, and makes constructive recommendations. Purposes for evaluating studies include determining if study findings are useful to clinical decision-making, contributing to knowledge that could change clinical practice, or concluding whether further study of a topic is indicated.

Evaluation begins with reading the research report or journal article several times to become familiar with the study. Analysis of the research elements can then proceed. This chapter can serve as a base for understanding the research process as well as expectations for research approaches and specific methods. A key issue in reviewing a study is congruency. All elements—the research question, purpose, design, sampling procedures, methods of data collection, analysis, interpretation of the findings, and discussion—should be consistent with one another. Table 22–6 lists questions to ask when evaluating qualitative and quantitative studies. Although not exhaustive, the guidelines will assist in the systematic review of studies.

Following examination of the research elements, the reviewer identifies the strengths and weaknesses of the study. All studies have limitations; therefore, weaknesses are considered in relation to how they affect outcomes and the overall meaning of the study. Judgments are made regarding the relevancy of knowledge generated and the usefulness of findings to clinical practice. Legitimate criticisms of a study should be presented with rational and constructive recommendations. Evaluating studies is a skill that develops with practice, increased knowledge and understanding of the research process, and an awareness of the studies related to a specific topic.

Research articles published in professional journals are the most common source of research reports. The limitations, particularly the length of the report, must be considered in the appraisal. Journal articles lack the detail in accounts of full research reports. Studies in refereed journals are subject to review before publication. Members of journal review boards, generally regarded as experts in the field, critique articles to judge them for their scientific merit and make recommendations regarding whether they should be published. The beliefs that members of review boards have regarding the scientific value of qualitative research can influence their decision about publication.

Breastfeeding encompasses many disciplines in the natural, social, and health sciences; therefore, breastfeeding practitioners must consult numerous

TABLE 22– 6

GUIDELINES FOR EVALUATING QUANTITATIVE AND QUALITATIVE STUDIES

General Guidelines	Quantitative Studies	Qualitative Studies
1. Problem and purpose		
• Clearly stated?	• Provides direction for study?	• Broadly stated?
• Amenable to scientific investigation?		• Exploratory
• Significant to breastfeeding knowledge?		
2. Review of literature		
• Pertinent?	• Includes recent and classic references?	• Acknowledges the existence of (or lack of) literature on the topic?
• Well organized?	• Theoretical base or conceptual framework evident?	
3. Protection of human rights		
• Subject's protection from harm ensured?		
• Subject suitably informed by a written informed-consent?		
• Reviewed by an ethics board?		
• Means for ensuring privacy, confidentiality, or anonymity are explained?		
4. Method		
• Design congruent with research question?	• Deductive approach?	• Inductive approach used?
• Sampling procedure appropriate for research method?	• Variables identified and defined?	• Key informanats and theoretical sampling addressed?
• Method of data collection relevant for design?	• Sample representative of population and adequate size?	• Data collection and analysis concurrent?
	• Measuring tools suitable, reliable, and valid?	• Process for data collection and analysis described?
	• Control of extraneous variables is evident?	• Data saturated?
		• Credibility, dependability, confirmability, and transferability are evident?
5. Results and discussion		
• Analysis suitable for method and design?	• Statistical procedures used suitable for data and sample size?	• Examples of informants' accounts displayed?
• Results clearly presented?	• Tables clear and represent the data?	• Rich descriptions or theory presented?
• Interpretations clear and based on data?	• Successful and unanticipated results reported?	• Findings compared with literature?
• Research question answered?		• Theory logical and complete?
• Limitations of study identified?		
• Conclusions based on results?		
• Implications for practice and research described?		

and varied journals to remain current with new knowledge. Although a challenging task, remaining current is essential for professional practice.

Using Research in Clinical Practice

Bridging the gap between generating and utilizing knowledge is an ongoing process that takes motivation, commitment, persistence, and patience. Implementing research findings into clinical practice is a challenge for researchers and practitioners. The process is facilitated when researchers and practitioners work together to achieve the goal of implementing evidence-based practice. Researchers have the following responsibilities in assisting this process:

- Disseminating study findings directly to practitioners as soon as a study is completed through informal discussions; local, regional, and national presentations; and publications.

- Replicating studies that may improve clinical practice; changes are seldom made following the outcomes of one small study.

- Encouraging and assisting practitioners to participate in research to develop their interest and awareness.

- Listening to concerns about practice in order to generate problems for study that are relevant to a particular practice area.

- Collaborating with practitioners in research projects.

- Assisting practitioners with evaluation of research articles so they may increase their knowledge and competence in judging research findings.

Practitioners have the following responsibilities in translating research findings to the practice field:

- Developing a questioning attitude and openness to change.

- Sharing concerns about practice with researchers to develop pertinent clinical studies.

- Collaborating with researchers and participating in research projects.

- Critically reading and evaluating research articles and using relevant findings in practice.

- Attending professional conferences where research is presented and discussed.

- Telling other clinicians about study findings that reflect, assist, or may alter practice.

Evidence-based practice has increasingly been endorsed by health professionals as the gold standard for care. Initiated by medicine, evidence-based medicine (EBM) is based on systematic reviews and appraisals by experts of studies that address interventions for a specific clinical problem. For this purpose the studies most valued are randomized clinical trials. If findings from sufficient studies show that a specific practice or intervention is clinically significant, then the next step is to incorporate the intervention into clinical practice. The Cochrane Collaboration (http://www.cochrane.org) of systematic reviews of the effects of health-care interventions is internationally recognized and increasingly used by health-care professionals.

A broader perspective of evidence-based practice is taken by the discipline of nursing for evidence-based nursing (EBN). It is argued that EBM is narrow in scope, medicalizes health-care, discounts scientific evidence that is not based on experimental methods, and overlooks the knowledge of the expert practitioner and the context in which the intervention is being used (French, 1999). Although complex, a broader base of scientific evidence linked with the expertise of the practitioner is an approach that is appropriate for lactation practitioners and other health-care professionals who provide care to breastfeeding women. Findings from studies using different approaches and methods are relevant and can expand scientific knowledge related to breastfeeding to optimum practice that benefits mothers, infants, families, and society.

Perspectives of Research Methodologies

Research can be conducted in many ways and the basis of these diversities is often referred to as research paradigms (Polit & Hungler, 1999). Paradigms are worldviews that represent belief systems that are based on philosophical foundations and assumptions (Crotty, 1998). The type of research conducted by an individual is often closely linked to their beliefs in that they frame research questions congruent with how they view the world. The associated assumptions guide investigators in the research methods used and establish the parameters for conducting the study and interpreting the findings. Perspectives used for developing knowledge in health-care disciplines are the positivist/postpositivist perspective, the naturalistic/humanistic/interpretive perspective, and the critical/emancipatory perspective (Gillis & Jackson, 2002; Jacox et al., 1999). Extending the kinds of research perspectives contributes to developing a broader knowledge base for providing relevant health care.

Positivist and Postpositive Perspective

Positivism is the foundation of traditional science methods that are based on objectivity, precision, and a search for accurate, valid, and absolute truth. Often referred to as quantitative research, the ascribed methods are characterized by objectivity, measurement, and control that are context-free and void of investigator bias. Investigators use these methods to examine specific variables, control intervening variables, and determine associations or cause and effect relationships among variables using statistical procedures. The goal is to explain, predict, and generalize. Scientists with this worldview claim that new knowledge is attained only through traditional methods. As philosophers and social scientists challenged these claims during the twentieth century, the postpositivist perspective emerged. Based on the same worldview and scientific principles, this perspective is tempered in that certainties have changed to probabilities and truth seeking is approximate rather than a totality. Greater flexibility in use of methods and adherence to philosophical assumptions is evident, although the debate continues between scientists who hold on to the conservative view and those who accept multimethods to understand a phenomenon under study. This perspective has dominated health science inquiry throughout the twentieth century.

Naturalistic, Humanistic, or Interpretive Perspective

The naturalistic, humanistic, or interpretive perspective constructs understanding of the "meaning" that human values, beliefs, practices, or life experiences and events have for individuals. Through interactions between the investigator and participants, new information or a new perspective of a phenomenon, and its meaning, is created. Generally conducted in naturalistic settings, all possible variables that influence individuals' perspectives are considered data and these data are broad and frequently complex. Often referred to as qualitative research, this humanistic approach is congruent with a holistic philosophy of providing health care.

The outcomes of qualitative studies are mainly twofold, theory generation and/or rich descriptions that provide a deeper understanding of the meaning of experiences, events, or practices of individuals. Theory is generated primarily by the process of inductive reasoning, which means that specific ideas progress to more generalized statements. Thus, from the study of an everyday life phenomenon, variables and how they relate are identified. Further interpretation of the data can lead to a conceptualization of an experience from which theories are developed (Morse & Field, 1995). Or in some studies a rich, linguistic construction of the essence of a human experience showing meaning in a deeper manner can provide greater understanding of a phenomenon (van Manen, 1984).

Critical or Emancipatory Perspective

The critical or emancipatory perspective is based on both postpositivist and humanistic perspectives, as well as sociopolitical and cultural factors that influence experience (Jacox et al., 1999). It includes critical theory, action research, feminist research, and ethnocentric approaches of minority groups. The aim of emancipatory methods is to engender social change through or as a result of the research process for individuals or groups that are often unrecognized or considered oppressed. This perspective accentuates growth, change, and empowerment of individuals or groups as well as barriers that limit social change. Participant involvement and equity in every phase of the research process is critical. Research designs and methods may be combined and variable. The methods thought to have the greatest potential to generate the greatest amount of change for a particular group and situation are generally chosen.

It is important to understand and recognize these different perspectives as the underpinnings to research, but the perspectives themselves are not necessarily method specific. Recently, there is greater use of multimethods, particularly in large studies, to answer the research questions and study goals. In addition, increasing numbers of studies are undertaken by "teams" with representatives from different disciplines, academics to maintain the rigor of the research, and practitioners and at times patients to enhance clinical relevance. This trend of research teams conducting studies and use of multimethods not only broadens the purpose and outcomes of studies but also contributes to greater research complexity.

Summary

Research is a process and theory is a base for developing knowledge that serves as a foundation for accountable and responsible practice. The approaches and methods involved in conducting research originate from various philosophical systems: the positivist/postpositivist perspective; the natural science, human science, and interpretation perspective; and the critical and emancipatory perspective. These perspectives give rise to research approaches and methods used in qualitative, quantitative, observational, historical, and feminist research. The research question asked—and whether knowledge is generated inductively or deductively—directs the approach used.

The qualitative approach generates an understanding of the "meaning" that reflects human values, beliefs, practices, and life experiences or events. The three qualitative methods commonly used are phenomenology, ethnography, and grounded theory. The quantitative approach is characterized by objectivity, measurement, and control. The quantitative methods commonly used are descriptive, correlational, experimental, and quasi-experimental studies. The simultaneous use of qualitative and quantitative methods in one study is an increasing trend.

The major elements of research are the problem and purpose, review of literature, protection of human subjects, method, and results and discussion. The research problem identifies "what" is studied and with "whom," and the purpose delineates "why" the study is conducted. Research questions for quantitative methods are more specific than those of qualitative studies. In quantitative studies, variables are delineated and operationally defined. How breastfeeding and the duration of breastfeeding are defined is of particular importance when conducting or evaluating studies.

Reviewing literature about a study topic assists in formulating the research problem and directs the research method. Qualitative methods are frequently used when little is known about a topic.

Research that involves human subjects must ensure the study participants of basic rights. Ethical review boards or committees help protect subjects by reviewing the informed consent document and evaluating the study before it is conducted.

Study methods address setting, sample, data collection, and data analysis. The setting indicates the location of the study or the source of the participants. The sample is a subset of a larger population or group of individuals in whom the investigator is interested. Sampling is a process for selecting the sample from the population; the two types of sampling are probability and nonprobability. Nonprobability sampling is used in qualitative studies. Probability sampling is preferred in quantitative studies because findings can then be generalized from the study sample to the target population. This method requires random selection of subjects, which is not always possible; therefore, many quantitative studies involving human subjects use nonprobability sampling.

Data are collected when the researcher asks questions, makes observations, and/or measures key variables identified in the research question. In-depth interviews and observations are the most common methods used for qualitative studies, and data collection and analysis occur simultaneously. Systematic and rigorous methods for collecting and analyzing data are developed for all qualitative methods. Methods for data collection in quantitative studies are highly structured and must be the same for every subject.

Reliability and validity issues must be addressed for all research. Reliability refers to accuracy, consistency, precision, and stability of data collected; validity reflects the true meaning of data. In qualitative studies this aspect is referred to as trustworthiness. This includes building in checks in the data collection and analysis process. In quantitative studies, reliability of measurement tools and investigators collecting data can be statistically estimated, as can the validity of the measurements used.

Data analysis is the process of organizing, summarizing, examining, and synthesizing the data collected to identify study findings. Qualitative studies generate rich descriptions and posit hypotheses and/or theory. Descriptive narratives of participants' verbatim accounts support the investigator's interpretations. In quantitative studies, data are translated to numerical terms for statistical analysis. Depending on the type of study and the level of measurement of the data collected, a variety of statistical procedures can be employed. Results are displayed in tables and graphs.

Study results should be clear, concise, and congruent with the method used and they should answer the research question(s). Significant, nonsignificant, and unexpected results are reported. Limitations of the study and the extent to which findings can be generalized to additional populations must also be addressed. Study conclusions should reflect only the study findings.

Research reports or articles are evaluated to make judgments about their scientific merit and the usefulness of findings for clinical practice. A key issue in evaluation is study congruency.

Implementing research findings into clinical practice is a challenge for researchers and practitioners. This process can be expedited when both work together. Although findings from current studies are not generally definitive and further study is frequently recommended, using relevant findings in practice often serves to question effects and generate new studies. Breastfeeding research is an ongoing process that expands knowledge and facilitates evidence-based practice. The benefactors of health professionals who draw from a scientific body of knowledge and establish practices based on best evidence are mothers, children, families, and society.

Key Concepts

- Research is the systematic, logical inquiry of a phenomenon to discover new knowledge or to validate existing knowledge.

- Theory is a conceptual construction of a view of reality that describes, explains, or predicts something. It includes concepts and their relationships.

- Middle-range theories include well-defined concepts and relationships, but the propositions are more easily tested than those of grand theories. They are amenable to theories used in clinical practice.

- Inductive reasoning is the process of reasoning from specific observations or abstractions to a general premise.

- Deductive reasoning is the process of reasoning from a general premise to the concrete and specific.

- A conceptual framework is a basic structure representing concepts and relationships but not a specific theory that explains the relationships.

- A theoretical framework is a basic structure representing theories, concepts, and propositions that are the underpinnings of a study and in which the propositions can be tested.

- A core concept is the overall theme of a grounded theory study. It is central to and interelates the themes and categories identified in the study.

- A key informant is an individual who is most knowledgeable and who best articulates the meaning of the phenomenon under study.

- Bias is any factor, action, or influence that distorts the results of a study.

- Control is specific to quantitative research. It is the process of eliminating the influence of confounding variables that could compromise the research findings.

- Operational definitions are explicit descriptions of a concept or variable of interest. For quantitative studies, they are expressed in measurable terms.

- A dependent or outcome variable is the variable the investigator measures in response to the independent or treatment variable; the outcome variable is affected by the independent variable.

- An independent variable is the treatment or invention that is manipulated by the investigator to influence the dependent variable.

- Power is the probability that a statistical test will reject a null hypothesis when it should be rejected, or in other words, detect a significant difference that does exist.

- Reliability is the degree to which collected data are accurate, consistent, precise, and stable over time.

- Validity is the degree to which collected data are true and represent reality, and a measuring instrument reflects what it is intended to measure.

- Trustworthiness is the process of establishing the credibility of qualitative research.

Internet Resources

AWHONN Evidence-based clinical practice guidelines series (International):
www.guideline.gov/summary/summaryaspx?doc=2928&2154

Canadian Medical Association Infobase (Canada):
http://mdm.ca/cpgsnew/cpgs/index.asp

The Cochrane Collaboration: Cochrane database of systematic research reviews:
www.library.mun.ca/nsl/guides/cochrone.php

Cumulative Index to Nursing & Allied Health Literature (CINAHL):
www.library.ucsf.edu/db/cinahl.htm

Federal US health databases and research articles: MEDLINE:
www.nlm.nih/medlineplus/databases.html

Medscape:
www.medscape.com/

PubMed:
www.ncbi.nih.gov/entrez/query.fcgi?db=PubMed

References

Armstrong HC. International recommendations for consistent breastfeeding definitions. *J Hum Lact* 7:51–54, 1991.

Ajzen I, Fishbein M. *Understanding attitudes and predicting behavior.* Englewood Cliffs, NJ: Prentice Hall, 1980.

Bakeman R, Gottman JM. *Observing interaction: an introduction to sequential analysis.* Cambridge, England: Cambridge University Press, 1986.

Bandura A. Self-efficacy: toward a unifying theory of behavioural change. *Psych Review* 84:191–215, 1977.

———. Self-efficacy mechanism in human agency. *American Psychologist* 37:122–47, 1982.

Barnard K, Eyres S. Overview of the nursing child assessment project. In: Barnard K, ed. *Nursing child assessment training learning resource manual.* Seattle, WA: University of Washington School of Nursing, 1978:16–21.

Barr RG. Infant crying behavior and colic: an interpretation in evolutionary perspective. In: Trevathan WO, Smith EO, McKenna JJ, eds. *Evolutionary medicine.* Oxford, England: Oxford University Press, 1999:27–51.

Bergum V. *Woman to mother: a transformation.* Granby, MA: Bergin & Garvey, 1989.

Bernaix LW. Nurses' attitudes, subjective norms, and behavioural intentions toward support of breastfeeding mothers. *J Hum Lact* 16:201–9, 2000.

Bottorff J. Persistence in breastfeeding: a phenomenological investigation. *J Adv Nurs* 15:201–9, 1990.

Brett J, Niermeyer S. Is neonatal jaundice a disease or an adaptive process? In: Trevathan WR, Smith EO, McKenna JJ, eds. *Evolutionary medicine.* Oxford, England: Oxford University Press, 1999:7–25.

Burns N, Grove SK. *The practice of nursing research: conduct, critique and utilization.* 3rd ed. Philadelphia: W. B. Saunders, 1997.

Chenitz WC, Swanson JM. *From practice to grounded theory.* Menlo Park, CA: Addison-Wesley, 1986:96–98.

Cohen J. *Statistical power analysis for the behavioural sciences.* 2nd ed. New York: Academic Press, 1988.

Cronewett L et al. Single daily bottle use in the early weeks postpartum and breastfeeding outcomes. *Pediatrics* 90:760–6, 1992.

Crotty M. *The foundations of social research.* Thousand Oaks, CA: Sage Publications, 1998.

Dennis CL. Theoretical underpinnings of breastfeeding confidence: a self-efficacy framework. *J of Hum Lact* 15:195–201, 1999.

Dennis CL, Faux S. Development and psychometric testing of the breastfeeding self-efficacy scale. *Res Nurs Health* 22:399–409, 1999.

Dick MJ et al. Predicting early breastfeeding attrition. *J of Hum Lact* 18:21–28, 2002.

Ellis DJ, Hewat RJ, Livingstone V. *Report of an evaluation of the efficacy of a breastfeeding clinic in prolonging the duration of breastfeeding.* Vancouver, BC: University of British Columbia, School of Nursing and Department of Family Practice, 1991.

French P. The development of evidence-based nursing. *J Adv Nurs* 29:72–78, 1999.

Furr PA, Kiregis CA. A nurse-midwifery approach to early mother-infant acquaintance. *J of Nurse-Midwifery* 27:10–14, 1982.

Gillis A, Jackson W. *Research for nurses: methods and interpretation.* Philadelphia: FA Davis Company, 2002.

Giorgi A. Sketch of a psychological phenomenological method. In: Giorgi A, ed. *Phenomenology and psychological research.* Pittsburgh: Duquesne University Press, 1985: 8–22.

Glaser BG. *Theoretical sensitivity.* Mill Valley, CA: Sociology Press, 1978.

Harding S, ed. *Feminism and methodology.* Bloomington: Indiana University Press, 1987.

Harkness GA. *Epidemiology in nursing practice.* St Louis: Mosby, 1995:86–95.

Hennekens CH, Buring JE, Mayrent S. *Epidemiology in medicine.* Boston: Little, Brown, and Co., 1987.

Hewat RJ. Living with an incessantly crying infant. *Phenomenology Pedagogy* 10:160–71, 1992.

———. *Mother-interaction during breastfeeding: a comparison between problematic and nonproblematic breastfeeders* [doctoral dissertation]. Edmonton, AB: University of Alberta, 1998.

Hewat RJ, Ellis DJ. Breastfeeding as a maternal-child team effort: women's perceptions. *Health Care Wom Int* 5:437–52, 1984.

Hill PD, Aldag JC, Chatterton RT. The effect of sequential and simultaneous breast pumping milk volume and prolactin levels: a pilot study. *J Hum Lact* 12:193–99, 1996.

Jacox A et al. Diversity in philosophical approaches. In: Hinshaw AS, SL Feetham, JIF Shaver, eds. *Handbook of clinical nursing research.* Thousand Oaks: Sage Publication, 1999, 3 –17.

Janke J. Prediction of breast-feeding attrition: instrument development. *Applied Nurs Rese* 5:48–63, 1992.

———. Development of the breast-feeding attrition prediction tool. *Nurs Res* 34:100–4, 1994.

Jensen D, Wallace S, Kelsay P. LATCH: a breastfeeding charting system and documentation tool. *JOGNN* 26:181–87, 1994.

Kaufman KJ, Hall LA. Influences of the social network on choice and duration of breastfeeding in mothers of preterm infants. *Res Nurs Health* 12:149–59, 1989.

Kelly L, Burton S, Regan L. Researching women's lives or studying women's oppression? Reflections on what constitutes feminist research. In: Maynard M, Purvis J, eds. *Researching women's lives from a feminist perspective.* London: Taylor & Francis, 1994:27–48.

Klaus MH, Kennell JH. *Maternal-infant bonding.* St Louis: Mosby, 1976.

———. *Maternal-infant bonding.* 2nd ed. St Louis: Mosby, 1982.

Kramer HC, Thiemann S. *How many subjects? Statistical power analysis in research.* Newbury Park, CA: Sage Publications, 1987.

Labbok M. What is the definition of breastfeeding? *Breastfeeding abstracts* 19:19–21, 2000.

Labbok MH, Coffin CJ. A call for consistency in definition of breastfeeding behaviors. *Soc Sci Med* 44:1931–32, 1997.

Labbok M, Krasovec K. Toward consistency in breastfeeding definitions. *Stud Fam Plann* 21:226–30, 1990.

Leff EW, Jefferis SC, Gagne MP. Maternal perceptions of successful breastfeeding. *J Hum Lact* 10:99–104, 1994a.

———. The development of the maternal breastfeeding evaluation scale. *J Hum Lact* 10:105–11, 1994b.

Lenz ER et al. Collaborative development of middle-range nursing theories: Toward a theory of unpleasant symptoms. *Adv Nurs Sci* 17:1–13, 1995.

Lincoln YS, Guba EG. *Naturalistic inquiry.* Newbury Park, CA: Sage Publications, 1985.

Martens PJ. Does breastfeeding education affect nursing staff beliefs, exclusive breastfeeding rates, and Baby-Friendly Hospital Initiative compliance? The experience of a small, rural Canadian hospital. *J Hum Lact* 16:309–18, 2000.

Matthews MK. Developing an instrument to assess infant breastfeeding behavior in the early neonatal period. *Midwifery* 4:154–65, 1988.

———. Mothers' satisfaction with their neonates' breastfeeding behaviors. *JOGNN* 20:49–55, 1991.

Maynard M, Purvis J. *Researching women's lives from a feminist perspective.* London: Taylor & Francis, 1994.

McKenna J, Mosko S, Richard C. Breast-feeding and mother-infant cosleeping in relation to SIDS prevention. In: Trevathan WR, Smith EO, McKenna JJ, eds. *Evolutionary medicine.* Oxford, England: Oxford University Press, 1999:53–74.

Mead GH. In: Morris, CW ed. *Mind, self and society.* Chicago, IL: University of Chicago Press, 1934.

Mercer RT. A theoretical framework for studying factors that impact on the maternal role. *Nurs Res* 30:73–77, 1981.

———. The process of maternal role attainment over the first year. *Nurs Res* 34:198–204, 1985.

Mercer RT, Ferketich SL. Predictors of maternal role competence by risk status. *Nurs Res* 43:38–43, 1994.

Millard AV. The place of the clock in pediatric advice: rationales, cultural themes, and impediments to breastfeeding. *Soc Sci Med* 31:211–21, 1990.

Morrow AL et al. Efficacy of home-based peer counselling to promote exclusive breastfeeding: a randomised controlled trial. *Lancet* 353:1226–31, 1999.

Morse JM. Qualitative nursing research: a free-for-all? In: Morse JM, ed. *Qualitative nursing research: a contemporary dialogue.* London: Sage Publications, 1991a:14–22.

———. Strategies for sampling. In: Morse JM, ed. *Qualitative nursing research: a contemporary dialogue.* London: Sage Publications, 1991b:127–44.

Morse JM, Bottorff JL. The use of ethology in clinical nursing research. *Adv Nurs Sci* 12:53–64, 1990.

Morse JM, Field PA. *Qualitative research methods for health professionals.* 2nd ed. London: Sage Publications, 1995.

Neander WL, Morse JM. Tradition and change in the northern Alberta Woodlands Cree: implications for infant feeding practices. *Can J Public Health* 80:190–94, 1989.

Nunnally JC. *Introduction to psychological measurement.* Toronto: McGraw-Hill, 1978:245.

Oddy WH et al. Breast feeding and cognitive development in childhood: a prospective birth cohort study. *Birth* 17:1–90, 2003.

Piper S. Feeding patterns of preterm infants post NICU discharge. In: Auerbach KG, ed. *Current Issues in Clinical Lactation.* Boston: Jones and Barlett, 2002:11–21.

Piper S, Parks PL. Use of an intensity ratio to describe breastfeeding exclusivity in a national sample. *J Hum Lact* 17:227–32, 2001.

Polit DF, Hungler BP. *Nursing research: principles and methods.* 6th ed. Philadelphia: Lippincott, 1999.

Potter J, Wetherall M. *Discourse and social psychology: beyond attitudes and behavior.* London: Sage Publications, 1987.

Riordan J et al. Predicting breastfeeding duration using the LATCH breastfeeding assessment tool. *J Hum Lact* 17:20–23, 2001.

Riordan J, Gross A, Angeron J, Krumwiede B, Melin J. The effect of labor pain relief medication on neonatal sucking and breastfeeding duration. *J Hum Lact* 16:7–12, 2001.

Riordan JM, Koehn M. Reliability and validity testing of three breastfeeding assessment tools. *JOGN Nurs* 26:181–87, 1997.

Riordan JM, Woodley G, Heaton K. Testing validity and reliability of an instrument which measures maternal evaluation of breastfeeding. *J Hum Lact* 10:231–35, 1994.

Rubin R. Attainment of the maternal role: part I. *Nusr Res* 16:237–45, 1967a.

———. Attainment of the maternal role: part II. *Nurs Res* 16:342–46, 1967b.

———. *Maternal identity and the maternal experience.* New York: Springer, 1984.

Sarbin TR. Role theory. In: Lindzey G, ed. *Handbook of social psychology.* Reading, MA: Addison-Wesley Publishing Co., 1954:223–58.

Shafer RJ. *A guide to historical method.* 3rd ed. Belmont, CA: Wadsworth Publishing, 1980.

Schmied V. Connection and pleasure, disruption and distress: women's experience of breastfeeding. *J of Hum Lac* 14:325–34, 1999.

Spradley JP. *The ethnographic interview.* New York: Holt, Rinehart, & Winston, 1979:3–5.

———. *Participant observation.* New York: Holt, Rinehart, & Winston, 1980.

Strauss A, Corbin J. Basics of qualitative research: grounded theory procedures and techniques. Newbury Park, CA: Sage Publications, 1990:24–32.

Sumner G, Spietz A. *NCAST Caregiver/Parent-child interaction feeding manual.* Seattle: NCAST Publications, 1994.

Tabachnick BG, Fidell LS. *Using multivariate statistics.* 2nd ed. New York: HarperCollins, 1989:1–10.

Tomey AM, Alligood MR. *Nursing theorists and their work.* 4th ed. St. Louis: Mosby, 1998.

Trevathan WR, Smith EO, McKenna, JJ. *Evolutionary medicine.* Oxford, England: Oxford University Press, 1999:27–51.

van Manen M. Practicing phenomenological writing. *Phenomenology Pedagogy* 2:37–69, 1984.

———. *Researching lived experience: human science for an action sensitive pedagogy.* Ann Arbor, MI: Althouse Press, 1990.

Williams GC, Nesse RM. The dawn of Darwinian medicine. *Q Rev Biol* 66:1–22, 1991.

Wilson HS. *Research in nursing.* 2nd ed. Redwood City, CA: Addison-Wesley, 1989.

World Medical Association. *Declaration of Helsinki: recommendations guiding doctors in clinical research.* New York: World Medical Association, 1964.

Wright AL et al. Breastfeeding and lower respiratory tract illness in the first year of life. *Br Med J* 299:946–49, 1989.

Wrigley EA, Hutchinson SA. Long-term breastfeeding. *J of Nurse-Midwifery* 35:35–41, 1990.

Zimmerman DR, Guttman N. "Breast is best": knowledge among low-income mother is not enough. *J Hum Lact* 17:14–23, 2001.

Appendix 22–A

RESEARCH TERMS

Applied research: Research that focuses on solving or finding an answer to a clinical or practical problem.

Basic research: Research that generates knowledge for the sake of knowledge.

Bivariate: Statistics derived from the analysis of the relationship between two variables.

Chi-square: A statistical procedure that uses nominal level data and determines significant differences between observed frequencies in relation to the data and expected frequencies.

Concept: A word, idea, or phenomenon that generally has abstract meaning.

Construct: A cluster of several concepts that has abstract meaning.

Correlation coefficient: A statistic that indicates the degree of relationship between two variables. The range in value is +1.00 to −1.00; 0.0 indicates no relationship, +1.00 is a perfect positive relationship, and −1.00 is a perfect inverse relationship.

Design: The blueprint or plan for conducting a study.

Epidemiology: The study of the distribution and determinants of health-related states or events in specified populations, and the application of this study to control of health problems.

External validity: The extent to which study findings can be generalized to samples different from those studied.

Extraneous variable: Variables that can affect the relationship of the independent and dependent variables—i.e., that can interfere with the effect of treatment. In experimental studies, strategies for controlling these variables are built into the research design.

Incidence: The number of instances of illness commencing, or of persons falling ill, during a given period in a specified population. More generally, the number of new events—e.g., new cases of disease in a defined population—within a specified period of time.

Inductive reasoning: The process of reasoning from specific observations or abstractions to a general premise.

Internal validity: The extent to which manipulation of the independent variable really makes a significant difference on the dependent variable rather than on extraneous variables.

Likert scale: A scale that primarily measures attitudes by asking respondents their degree of agreement or disagreement for a number of statements.

Nonparametric statistics: Statistical procedures used when required assumptions for using parametric procedures are not met.

Parametric statistics: Statistical procedures used when a sample is randomly selected, represents a normal distribution of the target population, and is considered sufficiently large in size and interval level data are collected.

Prevalence: The number of instances of a given disease or other condition in a given population at a designated time; sometimes used to mean prevalence rate. When used without qualification the term usually refers to the situation at a specified point in time.

Population: The total set of individuals that meet the study criteria from which the sample is drawn and about whom findings can be generalized.

Sample: A subset of the population selected for study.

Sampling: The procedure of selecting the sample from the population of interest.

Target population: The population that is of interest to the investigator and about which generalizations of study results are intended.

Univariate: Statistics derived from analysis of a single variable—e.g., frequencies.

Variable: Attributes, properties, and/or characteristics of persons, events, or objects that are examined in a study.

BREASTFEEDING EDUCATION

Jan Riordan and Debi Leslie Bocar

Education is the cornerstone supporting the framework of lactation and breastfeeding. This chapter provides the health-care provider with tools to fashion meaningful educational experiences for breastfeeding families and colleagues. Two types of programs are addressed: those aimed at assisting families in having a positive breastfeeding experience and those designed to increase the knowledge base of the health-care providers so that they can effectively assist with breastfeeding. Because education permeates all activities in the field of breastfeeding, isolating the educational component is an enormous challenge. This chapter addresses a broad range of educational issues, from theory to practical application. An overview of research related to breastfeeding education is provided, along with strategies for teaching adult learners.

In traditional societies, an inexperienced woman turns to her mother, older sisters, cousins, aunts, or grandmothers for emotional support during childbearing and breastfeeding. Breastfeeding "education" involves lifelong immersion in a culture in which seeing a baby at breast is a normal, welcome sight. Even though formal breastfeeding and parental education is common in many parts of the world, it is still only a replacement for a time-honored family function that involves aunts and grandmothers (Bender & McCann, 2000).

The dramatic decrease in breastfeeding in industrialized societies during the first half of the twentieth century reduced the number of mothers who could share their breastfeeding experiences. Over time, expectant mothers were less likely to see an infant breastfeed or to know someone who could provide practical assistance. Geographical mobility further isolated young families from traditional support networks. Into the vacuum came alternative support systems for the few women who chose to breastfeed. Self-help groups such as La Leche League International, Australian Breastfeeding Association, and childbirth education groups began to organize. They flourished worldwide, providing accurate information, practical assistance, and emotional support for breastfeeding families using a mother-to-mother approach.

Educational Programs

As breastfeeding rates increased and health-care providers recognized the lifelong benefits of breastfeeding, health-care systems began to offer formal breastfeeding classes and educational opportunities.

689

Hospitals, clinics, health maintenance organizations, and medical practice groups increasingly offer classes of all types to parents, siblings, and grandparents. Although the primary purpose of these programs is educational, they are also effective public relations techniques for attracting families to those institutions. In an era in which health-care agencies are increasingly competitive, patient/client education can be an effective marketing strategy. Shifts in the US health-care industry affect breastfeeding education of parents. Third-party reimbursement rewards birth settings from which patients are discharged quickly. When families leave the hospital or birthing center within hours or days after birth, teaching opportunities shift to prenatal education or postdischarge follow-up.

Educational programs for health professionals and lactation consultants have proliferated along with parent education. Privately owned continuing education companies, medical centers, and academic institutions regularly offer systematic training in lactation management to health professionals. Some programs offer completion certificates or titles, such as breastfeeding educator. These programs, as well as many high-quality seminars offered throughout the world, are useful preparation for individuals seeking to improve their knowledge of breastfeeding. Many individuals attend educational offerings not only for professional development but also to qualify as continuing education for sitting the certification examination by the International Board of Lactation Consultant Examiners (IBLCE).

Distance Learning and Web Courses

Lactation education through distance learning and the World Wide Web is a rapidly growing area. Distance learning spans a rich heritage that began when the printing press met the pony express and continues today through the Internet. Distance learning offers a way for people worldwide to "attend" a course without leaving their home area. Breastfeeding Support Consultants of Philadelphia has offered long-distance education for lactation and breastfeeding since the mid-1980s. The first Internet course on breastfeeding came online in 1997 from Wichita State University School of Nursing (Riordan, 2000). It is taught entirely through the Internet. With the rapid changes in education toward teach-

ing on the Internet, other Web breastfeeding courses are becoming available. A current listing of lactation courses can be found on the Web site of the International Lactation Consultant Association (www.ilca.org/index.html). Lactation consultants take part in an Internet discussion group called LACTNET. In daily posts, LACTNET participants seek and receive help with difficult clinical cases and discuss current issues that relate to breastfeeding.

Learning Principles

Learning principles are most effective when individuals are ready to learn (i.e., when they feel a need to know something) (Redman, 1988). "Teachable moments" refer to those periods when learners perceive the need for information and skills. Motivation is further enhanced when the material to be learned is organized in a manner that makes it meaningful to the learner. Activities that are novel and interesting to learners encourage learning. Active rather than passive participation is associated with more meaningful and permanent learning (Brillinger, 1990). Learning is divided into three domains, and breastfeeding education incorporates all three (Bloom, 1956):

- Cognitive skills (gathering information, linking concepts, problem solving)
- Psychomotor skills (listening to instructions, observing skills, repetitive practice, mastery of skill performance)
- Affective learning (modifying attitudes, values, and preferences)

Individual learning styles need to be considered when planning teaching strategies (Lauwers & Shinskie, 2000). Some participants learn primarily through auditory perceptions; they listen intently and remember what they hear. Others learn best visually and retain information about what they see. These learners benefit from visual aids and printed materials (Figure 23–1). A third style is kinesthetic or psychomotor learning. Kinesthetic learners benefit from touching and handling equipment and models. Most learners use all three modalities. Therefore, in teaching about breast pumps, learning is strengthened by discussion coupled with the

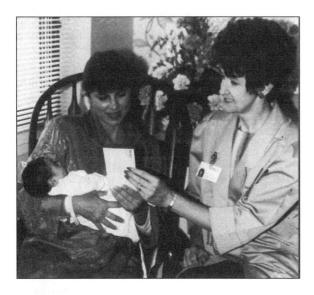

FIGURE 23–1. Visual learning. Pamphlets and other written materials reinforce one-to-one teaching. (Courtesy of Shira L. Bocar.)

Adult learners have a rich variety of backgrounds and motivations for participating in educational programs. They appreciate and expect respect as unique individuals. If the instructor identifies what these personal learning needs are and fulfills them, learning occurs quickly and easily. Adult learning should be self-directed and provide feedback about the learner's progress toward achieving these goals (Figure 23–2). Parents should be considered "co-learners" in that they teach each other as well as the instructor, who will invariably learn at least one new piece of information at every class. Principles of adult education are easily applied to breastfeeding education using the following approaches:

- Ensure that content and timing of teaching coincides with parents' "readiness" to learn (prior to conception, during pregnancy, immediately postbirth, later postpartum).

showing of slides that demonstrate how pumps work and by having the learners manipulate the equipment themselves.

Because success is predictably more motivating than is failure, dividing tasks and information into easily mastered segments keeps the adult learners motivated to continue the program. Learners respond to specific descriptions of their positive performance. Praise enhances feelings of self-confidence and conveys respect for the learner.

Adult Education

Adult learners differ widely from children in their learning styles. Unlike children, who are required to attend school, adults are self-directed when they choose to attend educational activities (Knowles, 1980). Adults perceive time as one of their most valued and scarce assets, and they are not willing to spend it in meaningless activity. Educational programs must therefore demonstrate a clear applicability to the adult's everyday life. For example, discussion of the anatomy of the breast and the physiology of breastfeeding is more meaningful when related directly to practical skills, such as latch-on techniques and how often to feed the baby.

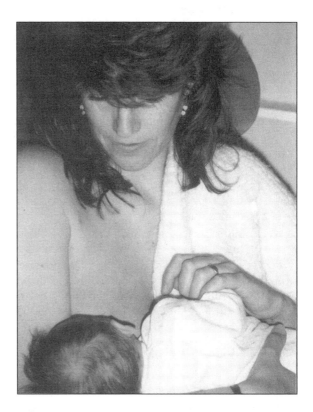

FIGURE 23–2. Adult learning. Adults are self-directed and have individual learning needs.

- Prioritize and present information in easily understood and easily mastered segments.

- Organize activities in increments to increase the likelihood of success.

- Give explicit instructions so that participants clearly understand what they are being asked to do.

- Provide specific, immediate feedback following each activity.

- Recognize the importance of body language and nonverbal communication.

- Use handouts and other media to reinforce and augment rather than to replace individualized assessment and teaching.

- Identify breastfeeding support resources, including telephone numbers of local resources.

There are several factors that enhance a positive learning climate for adult learners. Lighting, temperature, seating, the availability of writing surfaces furnished with paper and pencils, and the ability to view learning materials comfortably have a tremendous impact on learning. Adults appreciate physical comfort and knowing where drinks, food, and restroom facilities are located.

Adult education programs tend to be a social as well as a learning activity, because they afford opportunities to become acquainted with other adults. Greet each person warmly; demonstrate genuine concern for each one as an individual. It is a good idea to structure break periods with refreshments to encourage socializing. Adults enjoy sharing informal learning activities with others, and successful programs encourage adults to have fun as they learn. Adults also expect teachers to value student opinions about the usefulness of learning activities. One way to find out what areas of the program were helpful is to request informal verbal feedback or formal written evaluations. Evaluations are important data to modify and improve programs.

Curriculum Development

Assessing learning needs is mandatory when working with adult learners. There must be a "match" between what the learner needs to know and what

the teacher presents. If the teacher erroneously assumes that learners already possess a high level of knowledge, learners can be frustrated because the information is too complex. Conversely, learners may be offended if the instructor assumes they have minimal knowledge.

To assess levels of knowledge when working with small groups, the facilitator can ask nonthreatening questions—such as, "What are some of the myths about breastfeeding you have heard?" In larger class settings, the content cannot be customized to each participant. Asking participants at the beginning of class what specific topics they would like to discuss helps assess their learning needs and involves them in establishing the curriculum. The importance of a topic should be reflected in the time given to it, taking into consideration how frequently the information will be used. For example, positioning and latch-on are fundamental to breastfeeding and so deserve a more thorough discussion than adoptive nursing, which is relevant to a much smaller group of learners.

Too much information at one time is overwhelming and prioritizing teaching is critical. Basic physiologic requirements (e.g., adequacy of the infant's nutrient intake) help guide prioritization. Health-care providers must also be aware of additional family resources and defer some teaching for later health visits. Thus, when a family is in the birth setting, the health-care provider may share with the mother that breastfeeding can continue when she is employed outside the home. However, specific techniques for doing so will be taught after breastfeeding is established.

Parent Education

Facilitating the learning experience for parents requires an understanding of the tasks of adulthood. People seeking breastfeeding assistance are couples involved in a major life change: acquisition of the parental role. There are four stages of transition into parenthood: (1) anticipatory, (2) formal, (3) informal, and (4) personal. During the *anticipatory stage,* before the birth of the infant, expectant parents benefit from realistic information about infant care. It is important for parents to understand that, in the first weeks after the baby is born, they will experience loss of sleep, fatigue, and episodes of crying (by baby, mom, and possibly dad). In this phase, parents should be encouraged to perform in certain ways:

- Form realistic expectations of infant care.
- Identify responsibilities that they can relinquish to devote time and energy to infant care.
- Learn practical aspects of infant care (including psychomotor experiences with dolls or infants).
- Begin to identify philosophical approaches to infant care (such as how they will respond to a crying child).
- Learn about typical emotional responses to new parenthood so that their experiences can be placed in perspective.
- Review previous personal successful experiences to support self-confidence.
- Socialize with other new families to increase opportunities for incidental learning and for developing a support network.
- Identify community resources that can facilitate the transition into parenthood.

The *formal stage* begins with the birth of the infant. Parents are often surprised at their intense feelings about the responsibilities of parenthood. Although forming attachment bonds with their infant, they are simultaneously achieving parental roles. Attachment is enhanced if parents have rooming-in, which allows them more opportunities to get acquainted with their baby (Anderson, 1989). Health-care providers can also use the infant's given name frequently to establish the identity of the infant.

Parental caretaking behavior is often characterized by rigidity as parents seek to perform psychomotor tasks "the one best way." They are often overwhelmed if given too many equally attractive alternatives in child care. They may become noticeably frustrated if they receive conflicting information during this phase of role acquisition. New parents often feel awkward and inadequate because they lack experience and confidence in caretaking skills. They often equate their performance of infant care with their ability to parent effectively. During

this stage, new parents are extremely vulnerable to implied judgment of their caretaking abilities. They are quite sensitive to nonverbal communication regarding their performance. Health-care providers and experienced parents are particularly powerful role models as the self-image of the new parents emerges. The most persistent feelings during such role transition are those of inadequacy and lack of self-confidence.

During this time, mothers are fatigued and feel overwhelmed. In the days immediately after giving birth, women have impaired cognitive function, particularly in memory function (Eidelman, Hoffman, & Kaitz, 1993). Therefore, new parents benefit from simple, concrete instructions divided into easily mastered segments. Specific, positive feedback about their performance, coupled with encouragement by someone whose opinion is important to them, can greatly enhance their self-confidence. They need frequent assistance in placing their experiences in perspective.

The *informal stage* begins when parents feel that they have mastered child-care tasks. Self-confidence increases as a person accrues successful experiences (Coopersmith, 1967). Several weeks or months are required by most parents to amass adequate positive experiences so that they can proceed to the informal stage of role acquisition. Health-care providers are in a unique position to enhance parental self-confidence by providing enthusiastic praise of performance and reviewing positive experiences. The relatively restrictive behavior of the formal stage is replaced by a willingness to consider options. Behavior becomes more spontaneous, and there is less fear of imperfection. A reassuring environment that supports experimentation and provides stimulation through a variety of role models enables parents to progress to the final stage of parental role acquisition.

During the *personal stage*, behaviors are further modified, so that a parental role style evolves that is consistent with the parents' personalities. Relinquishing the fantasy of being the "perfect parent" frees parents to develop a unique set of behaviors with which they are comfortable. Support groups and classes provide ideal social settings in which parents can share their personal child-care techniques and approaches with other parents, thus integrating their new parental role into their personalities (Figure 23–3).

Prenatal Education

Most mothers make decisions about how they will feed their baby before they become pregnant and during pregnancy. Pregnancy is an appropriate time to support a mother's decision to breastfeed, to correct inaccurate information, to add to the information she already has about breastfeeding, and to encourage undecided expectant mothers to consider breastfeeding. Infant feeding should be discussed before mothers start feeling the baby's movements. (Quickening usually occurs around the fifth month of pregnancy.) When mothers begin to perceive their babies as separate beings, they start making concrete plans for care, including how they will feed their babies. Mothers need information about infant feeding before being asked, "How are you going to feed your baby?" Because of the influence of the baby's father or the mother's partner and other family members, breastfeeding education programs should include support persons by encouraging their attendance at classes and group meetings and by providing educational materials specifically directed to them (Freed, Fraley, & Schanler, 1993; Giugliani et al., 1994; Littman et al., 1994; Matich & Sims, 1992; Sciacca et al., 1995).

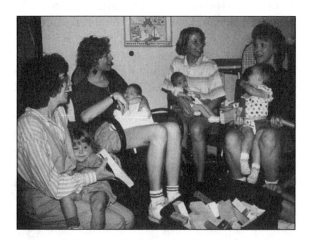

FIGURE 23–3. La Leche League meeting. Adult learning in action. (Courtesy of Debi Leslie Bocar.)

Breastfeeding education programs during early pregnancy must describe the benefits of breastfeeding both to mother and infant so that expectant parents can make an informed choice regarding infant feeding (Libbus, 1992). If an educational program is to influence the decision to breastfeed, it must address maternal concerns, including those related to convenience, modesty, participation of the father in infant care, and to incorporating breastfeeding into the mother's lifestyle, her return to employment, any previous negative experiences with breastfeeding by the mother or her peers, and contraceptive considerations (Jones, 1987; Young & Kaufman, 1988). An awareness of the values in a particular culture is essential.

Early Breastfeeding Education

Toward the end of pregnancy, breastfeeding education appropriately focuses on the basics of breastfeeding initiation and management during the early days and weeks following the baby's birth. Classes should be accessible (with parking) and offered at times convenient to families. Patients can read pamphlets and view videos while they are waiting for appointments. Health-care providers can also assess and add to the patients' knowledge during appointments. It is generally better to have frequent, short discussions about breastfeeding throughout the course of prenatal care rather than to attempt to say everything a mother may need to know in one discussion about breastfeeding. Freestanding classes can be provided by institutions and health-care professionals in the community—through hospitals, clinics, libraries, childbirth education programs, breastfeeding support groups, and lactation consultants.

The content of breastfeeding classes offered during pregnancy should include information necessary to initiate breastfeeding (e.g., timing of the first breastfeeding, positioning and assisting the infant to latch onto the breast, prevention of nipple trauma, management of engorgement, assessment of adequate milk intake, and establishing, maintaining, and increasing milk supply) (Box 23–1).

A variety of techniques can be used, including formal or informal classes, videos, and printed materials. Educational programs, however well developed, augment rather than replace the responsi-

BOX 23–1

Recommended Topics for Prenatal Breastfeeding Classes

Early Pregnancy

- Ask questions: "How do you plan to feed your baby?"

    Importance of decision about feeding choice

- Assess knowledge and perceptions regarding breastfeeding

    Reasons mothers choose (breastfeeding, bottle-feeding, combined feeding)

- Explore and identify concerns

    Personal feelings
    Families' feelings (including partner, significant other)
    Dealing with disapproval

- Acknowledge and validate feelings

- Educate using carefully targeted messages to address individual concerns

    Benefits of breastfeeding (infant, mother, community)
    Risks of formula-feeding
    Doctors' recommendations

    Ease of breastfeeding
    Breastfeeding with modesty
    Family involvement
    Lack of dietary restrictions and lifestyle changes
    Feasibility with employment or school
    Availability of people to assist

- Identify breastfeeding resource network

    Family and friends
    Health-care providers
    Mother-to-mother support group

Later Pregnancy

- Explain that nipple and breast preparation is *not* necessary (breastfeeding is easy)

- Assess nipple eversion; treat if necessary (after 37 weeks gestation only)

- Discuss nursing bras, clothes for discrete nursing

- Explain that there is no need for nipple creams, ointments during pregnancy

---

bility of the health-care professional for individualized assessment and one-to-one teaching specific to each breastfeeding family.

Although mothers can have a positive breastfeeding experience at the birth setting, breastfeeding continuance is influenced by situations she encounters after she returns home. Given the mother's limited stamina and inability to retain large quantities of new information, care should be taken not to overwhelm families with the sheer volume of material. Prioritize the content of classes in the birth setting, from most important to least important. For example, information that relates to continuing breastfeeding and ensuring infant well-

being is most important, whereas information that pertains to returning to employment and weaning can be covered later.

Individualize the content based on the mother's concerns (Box 23–2). For example, if a pregnant mother wants to select a pump to prepare for going back to work, the lactation consultant provides this information. Families do not attend to information that health-care providers *think* they should have until their own concerns have been addressed.

When special circumstances, such as prematurity, multiple births, congenital anomalies, or infant neurological impairment, affect the initiation of

BOX 23-2

Sample Content for "How-To" Breastfeeding Class (Based on Common Concerns of Mothers)

How Do I Get off to a Good Start?

- Best time for breastfeeding: within first hour after birth (importance of colostrum)
- Rooming-in
- What if separation is medically necessary?
- How often to breastfeed
    - Baby-led feedings
    - Identify early hunger cues
    - Feed at least every 3 hours during day (8–12 feedings each 24 hours)
    - Feed at least 5–10 minutes each side
    - Listen for swallowing
    - Watch infant for satiety cues
    - Avoid intense clock watching
- Will I have enough milk? What causes decreased milk production?
    - Long intervals between feedings
    - Formula or water supplements
    - Smoking
- Do I have to change my lifestyle?
- Nutrition, fluids, rest
    - Listen to your body: eat when hungry, drink when thirsty, rest when tired
- Medications, drugs, alcohol, nicotine
- What should I do if I get a cold?

Will Breastfeeding Hurt?

- Do I have to prepare my nipples?
    - Check for nipple protrusion
- Do I need special supplies or equipment?
- Positioning and latch-on
    - Alerting infants: techniques

Avoid overuse of swaddling
Mother's position and breast support
Infant's position (cradle hold, football hold, side-lying)
Demonstrate with visual aids, doll

- What is a good latch?
    Wide-open mouth
    Lips flanged
    Nose and chin to breast
    No sharp pain
- Can I prevent sore nipples?
    Break latch if it hurts, breastfeed frequently, start on less sore side
    Creams and ointments (not always helpful)
- What is engorgement? How do I manage engorgement?
    Breastfeed frequently
    Place cold packs on breasts
    Use breast pump if necessary
    Softer, smaller breasts (after engorgement) do not mean lost milk supply

Where Can I Get Help?

- Special role of father (or primary support person)
- Types of help: Practical help, emotional help, skilled assistance
- Dealing with advice and opinions
- Sources for expert help with breastfeeding
- How do I know if baby is getting enough?
    Can hear baby swallowing regularly
    Bowel movements (at least 4 per 24 hours)

Satisfied between feedings
    At least 8 feedings per 24 hours
- Family life with baby: Enjoying baby, consoling baby, and fear of "spoiling"
- When to call for help

    Baby feeding every hour
    Feedings lasting more than 1 hour
    Baby sleeping for more than 4–5 hours more than once each 24 hours
    Baby feeds fewer than 7 times in 24 hours

    Baby has fewer than 4 bowel movements in 24 hours
    Severe nipple pain
    Tender, swollen area in breast
- Learn and respond to baby's cues
- Use expert resources
- No supplements unless health-care provider recommends
- Realistic expectations

    What to expect during first weeks; commit to breastfeeding for 2 weeks

breastfeeding, the learning needs of the parents are complicated by the emotional ramifications of the experience. Families with special needs benefit from individualized teaching and assistance and from specific educational materials and ongoing group support. It's hard for parents to retain information when they are under stress. Prioritize content so that only important information is given first and is later repeated.

Continuing Support for Breastfeeding Families

The sharp decline in breastfeeding in the early weeks postpartum demonstrates the need that mothers have for assistance and follow-up. A systematic program to ensure contact with the new breastfeeding mother can be a powerful influence on breastfeeding duration. Where feasible, telephone contact, home care, or early return visits to a clinic are ideal. Each mother should be able to identify at least one resource person for information, support, and assistance.

Studies have compared mothers' expectations versus nurses' expectations regarding breastfeeding support and education. Berger and Cook (1998) studied postpartum teaching priorities of nurses and mothers. They found that nurses and mothers agreed that immediate physical health needs of both mothers and newborns were most important, but they differed on specifics. Nearly three fourths

of the nurses considered breast care to be a very important learning need, whereas only half of the mothers agreed. In a qualitative study, hospital nurses felt the provision of interpersonal and informational support was adequate for successful breastfeeding. The mothers at this facility, on the other hand, wanted encouragement as well as interpersonal and informational support (Gill, 2001).

In addition to needing information and assistance with solving breastfeeding challenges, mothers need support and encouragement to continue breastfeeding (Box 23–3). Family, peers, and community resources are often their primary sources of support. However, health-care professionals have a role to play in assessing, augmenting, or creating support systems.

How Effective Is Breastfeeding Education?

With short hospital stays and tight hospital budgets, we need to know what strategies work most effectively. Because education can change only those elements that are modifiable, we first need to identify what *can* be changed. When Janke (1993) extensively reviewed the research literature a few years ago, she found only six modifiable variables that predict breastfeeding outcomes:

- Mother intends to breastfeed for a long time.

BOX 23–3

Recommended Topics for an Ongoing Breastfeeding Support Class

Newborn Adjustment

- Parental fatigue, time management
- Physical changes during postpartum
- Maternal mood changes
- Management of fussiness, crying

    Concerns about "spoiling" infants
    Consoling techniques

- Infant sleeping issues, nighttime parenting
- Transition from being two to being three (when a husband feels left out)

    Being a person and partner as well as a parent
    Sexuality and contraception

- Dealing with unsolicited advice
- Blended families, sibling or pet adjustments

Breastfeeding Concerns

- Concerns about milk supply
- Assessing adequacy of infant intake

- Strategies to increase milk supply
- Appetite and growth spurts
- Frequency of breastfeeding as baby gets older
- Involving family members
- Obstructed ducts and mastitis
- Weaning

Returning to an Employment Setting

- Feasibility of combining breastfeeding and employment outside the home
- Feeding options
- Child-care considerations
- Time management
- Selecting a breastmilk expression technique (hand expression and breast pump options)
- Expressing and storing breastmilk
- Maintaining a milk supply; maintaining baby's interest in breastfeeding
- Keeping breastfeeding in perspective

- Mother is strongly committed to breastfeeding.
- Mother and family have a strong support system.
- Mother expresses a positive attitude toward breastfeeding.
- Baby has an early first feeding.
- Mother avoids supplemental feedings of water or formula.

Focusing on these modifiable factors and the timing of their contact with expectant parents can maximize the influence of health-care professionals. How the mother will feed her baby is a decision that often is made prior to conception. Therefore, educational efforts may have to target future parents prior to conception through the elementary and secondary school systems, the mass media, churches, community organizations, and other influential institutions.

Studies summarized in Table 23–1, and in Chapter 2, Table 2–1, which listed randomized trials in the discussion of work strategies, show that education and professional interventions make a positive difference in the birth setting and postpartum by extending the length of breastfeeding

Teaching Strategies

Good teaching involves organizing learning experiences that keep the participant's interest and use the

Table 23–1

OUTCOMES OF BREASTFEEDING EDUCATION

Source	Description and Results
Adams et al., 2001 Ontario, Canada	Hospital-based lactation services offered to all mothers in community. Open hours for outpatient visits. Mothers highly rated service. Positive association between number of visits and breastfeeding duration.
Akram, Agboativalla, & Shamshad, 1997 N =140 Pakistan	Group discussions and home visits until 6 months. Significantly higher percentage full breastfeeding at 4 months in intervention group (94 vs. 7%).
Alvarado et al., 1996 N = 138 Chile	Prenatal home visits, hospital visits, group sessions, individual consultation until 6 months, posters, and pamphlets. Significantly higher percentage full breastfeeding at 5 months in intervention group (53 vs. 3%).
Davies-Adetubgo, 1996 N = 256 Nigeria	One-to-one counseling, posters, monthly home visits until 4 months. Significantly higher percentage full breastfeeding at 4 months in intervention group (40 vs. 14%).
Greiner & Mitra, 1999 N = 10,128 Bangladesh	Home visits, radio jingles, printed matter, advertisements. No significant results of any breastfeeding 12–23 months (93 vs. 92%).
Houston et al., 1981 N = 80 Scotland	Hospital and home visits in 1st week and every 2 weeks until 24 weeks. Significantly higher percentage breastfeeding at 20 weeks in intervention group (89 vs. 65%).
Martens, 2000 Canada	Education program for nursing staff (1.5 hours). Increase in breastfeeding beliefs ($p < .01$), exclusive breastfeeding rates ($p < .05$), but no change in breastfeeding attitudes.
Palti et al., 1988 N = 310 Israel	Individual session from 7th month of pregnancy until 6 months postpartum. Mean duration of full breastfeeding was 9 weeks for intervention group compared with 7 weeks for control group.
Pugin et al., 1996 N = 422 Chile	Group session 3 to 5 times during last trimester. Significantly higher percentage full breastfeeding at 6 months in intervention group (80 vs. 65%).
Vega-Franco, Gordillo, & Meijerink, 1985 N = 50 Mexico	Group session 4 times: 30 minutes + pamphlet (after 6th month). Significantly higher percentage any breastfeeding at 4 weeks in intervention group (72 vs. 16%).
Valdes et al., 1993 N = 735 Chili	Individual consultation at d 7–10 and monthly until 6 months. Significantly higher percentage full breastfeeding at 6 months in intervention group (67 vs. 32%).
Westphal et al., 1995 Brazil	Improved knowledge of health-care provider and improved institutional scores related to WHO/UNICEF Ten Steps to Successful Breastfeeding after training course.
Zimmerman, 1999 United States	Prenatal education, support groups, discharge packets. Breastfeeding at 2 weeks increased from 35% to 57%.

facilitator's time efficiently. The lecture format yields an efficient use of the instructor's time; however, it requires that participants remain passive, and it is associated with decreased retention. An ef-fective strategy is to vary the teaching format. Team presentations, small group discussions, demonstrations, role playing, question-and-answer sessions with teacher-led or student-led questioning, observations and comments by participants, group projects, and individualized instruction modules are effective ways to break the monotony of lecture presentations.

Each teaching session should include an introduction, learning experience, and conclusion or summary. A fundamental axiom is to "explain what you're going to teach, teach, and then describe what you have taught." When using the lecture format, remember certain essential guidelines:

- Use a conversational tone (avoid reading notes word for word).
- Vary speech (inflection, speed, and tone).
- Wear bright, interesting clothing.
- Move around while lecturing and use gestures for emphasis.
- Use visual aids liberally (slides, charts, models, portions of videotapes and films).
- Use humor.
- Demonstrate psychomotor tasks.
- Encourage the audience to participate by practicing psychomotor skills and with questions, comments, and small group discussion.
- Schedule breaks every 50 minutes for maximum retention.

Charts, slides, line drawings, and role playing are useful in dividing a psychomotor skill, such as positioning and latch-on, into understandable steps. Follow this with a videotape presentation of the skill. The facilitator must always preview audiovisual materials and be knowledgeable about equipment operation so that each learner's time is used efficiently.

Small Group Dynamics

Formal classes and educational media might provide information to large numbers of people, but small-group teaching is a much more powerful method for behavior change. Group discussions enhance peer support and decision making, and they decrease dependence on health-care professionals. A group is two or more people who interact and influence each other, accomplish common goals, and derive satisfaction from maintaining membership in the group. The ideal group size ranges from 8 to 12 people. More than 10 people in a subgroup decreases productivity (Tubbs, 1984).

Small-group interaction has the advantage of stimulating a free flow of information and encouragement among participants as different questions are asked and new topics are raised. Small groups meet human needs for companionship, knowledge, and identity. Discussion in a small group is more likely to answer participants' information needs, because they usually feel more comfortable asking questions and changing the topic than when they are in a large group.

An informal, relaxed setting encourages participation. The group leader needs to be an expert in the subject content area and skilled in group dynamics. Familiarity with the different roles played by group members (initiator, elaborator, evaluator, coordinator, encourager, harmonizer, compromiser, aggressor, recognition-seeker, confessor, dominator) enhances the group leader's effectiveness in moving the group in a fruitful direction (Sampson & Marthas, 1981).

Although the group leader may have to actively guide the discussion initially, the goal is to act as a resource for information, encouraging participants to develop their own creative and problem-solving abilities (Nichols & Edwards, 1988). When participants share their personal experiences, it enhances learning and increases self-worth as individuals' efforts are reinforced and supported by the group.

Multimedia Presentations

Educational programs must compete with television, videotapes, compact discs (CDs), and the Internet. Audio or visual enhancements are almost mandatory for educational programs. In an age of television and computers, people expect visual and auditory stimulation. Speakers feel compelled to produce multimedia extravaganzas to compete. Some say our current expectations harken back to humankind's original visual communication style, before language and the printing press. The following items offer ways to present breastfeeding information visually:

- Use computer technology, such as PowerPoint software and LCDs (computerized slides that reside on a "floppy" computer diskette or on a CD). PowerPoint presentations are becoming the norm for presentations. It is easy to print professional-looking outlines of your talk for handouts and to make speaker's notes for each slide.

- Arrange for all necessary equipment (projectors, screens, video equipment, tape recorder, pointer, podium light, chart stands) well in advance of the presentation. If you need Internet access, ensure that the facility can provide it. It's probably best to bring overheads of your talk "just in case."

- Identify light switches and sound control panels; make certain that a responsible person is available to operate them.

- Adjust the volume of the microphone so that persons in the back of the room can hear easily. Make adjustments before beginning the presentation.

- Tape extension cords and cables to the floor to reduce the likelihood of an accident.

- Adjust the location of the slide projector so that images fill the entire screen and can be seen clearly by all participants.

- Adjust the position of the monitor(s) so that all participants can see.

- Adjust the lighting in the room to enhance the visual presentation and still allow for taking notes.

- Arrange equipment so that it does not block the view of the screen(s).

- When showing part of a videotape, preset the tape to the place where it is to begin.

- Meet with the equipment operator, review the audiovisual component of the presentation, and explain what the operator will need to do during the presentation (e.g., change slide trays, press "play" on the videotape player).

- Screen visual aids before the presentation (are PowerPoint slides in order?).

- Avoid facing the audiovisual aids when speaking or standing between them and the audience.

Audiovisual aids that are presented effectively greatly enhance teaching. Learners are frustrated when such aids are poorly presented or the instructor talks about a wonderful component that is not available. Adequate planning and preparation are the best insurance for an effective presentation.

Slides

Slides are easily stored and transported and are flexible; there is a wide variety of ways that they can be sequenced. Slides might be "worth a thousand words," but they can be expensive to make. Some lactation consultants working in hospitals and health-care agencies have access to audiovisual staff whose sole job is to produce audiovisual aids. Computer-generated slides are the standard for presentations. Presentation software such as PowerPoint create electronic slides that can be easily modified, so there is little or no expense in revising and updating them.

Transparencies

Transparencies or overhead projections are easy to make and the least expensive of all the media options. Almost every classroom has an overhead projector. However, transparencies are easily damaged, are difficult to combine with slide presentations, and may require a second person at the overhead projector. Transparencies are generally limited to charts and words (photographs do not reproduce well) and appear to be less "professional" than other formats.

Television, Videotapes, and DVDs

Parents today are children of the television age. Television, videotapes, or DVDs are excellent for demonstrating live-action psychomotor skills (e.g., positioning mother and baby for breastfeeding) and are easily transported and stored. Maternity facilities that provide a television set in mothers' rooms often have a closed "Newborn Channel" that airs teaching programs on early newborn care including breastfeeding. Almost all households in the United States have videotape players but DVD players are rapidly replacing them. As of this writing, many excellent videotapes on breastfeeding exist, but very few DVDs are available.

Compact Discs

Compact discs (CDs) are one of the newest technologies in education. They are individually paced and everyone receives consistent information.

When developing a presentation using a visual format, apply these principles:

- Identify key concepts to be emphasized. Before developing slides or transparencies, write them out an a storyboard—a sequence of the presentation's main points. Draw boxes on a paper pad and fill them in with the secondary points.

- Keep the content simple: one idea per slide; six points related to that idea.

- Ensure that all lettering is large enough to be read in the back of the room.

- Insist that all lettering, artwork, and photography are of professional quality.

- Use multiple colors to maintain interest.

- Avoid overuse of clip art. It can distract learners.

- Use simple, clearly labeled graphs and drawings.

- Avoid complicated, detailed artwork that is more suitable for print publications.

- Choose photographs that convey single key points. They should be sharp, clear, visually appealing, and uncluttered. Well-selected photographs help viewers to see how information can be used in their lives. A presentation on breastfeeding that uses attractive photos of breastfeeding mothers and infants is rated higher by participants than is one in which no such photos are used.

- Include photographs that are several feet away from the subject, within a few feet of the subject, and very close to the subject.

- Avoid photos with distracting, outdated hair or clothing styles.

Educational Materials

People retain new information in a shorter period of time when they are under stress. After the physical and emotional stress of childbirth, families benefit from written materials that reinforce verbal teaching throughout pregnancy and after childbirth in addition to one-on-one individualized teaching.

Adults retain only about 30 percent of the information they hear, but a multimodal approach (seeing and hearing) increases their retention to 50 percent (Becton & Dickenson, 1981). For example, if a mother practices positioning at the breast or assembles a breast pump in addition to reading printed matter, her retention is improved.

Materials must be scrutinized closely for their accuracy to determine that no outdated information is included. Information must be consistent. New parents are frustrated by conflicting recommendations. Because nonverbal messages have a more profound impact on behavior than do verbal instructions, materials must be carefully reviewed before using them. Mothers need to make informed decisions about how they will feed their babies, but they do not need to know how to manage every potential breastfeeding difficulty. Materials that dwell on the management of complications (i.e., breast abscess) may be frightening to mothers still considering how they will feed their baby. Materials should indicate when a mother should seek assistance and should always include a local resource telephone number.

Printed matter should be attractively packaged. Families from a variety of socioeconomic backgrounds have access to sophisticated printed materials and commercial television programs; they expect similar quality in materials about breastfeeding. Pamphlets must be inviting, easy to read, and organized (with bold headings and generous amounts of white space). Too many words on a page can overwhelm a reader. Pictorial learning is superior to verbal learning for recognition and recall (Redman, 1988). Pictures and drawings make materials more interesting. Assess the mother's interest in reading before making recommendations about written materials. Although some mothers welcome books on breastfeeding, women who have not read a book since they completed their formal education may think that if they have to read a book, breastfeeding may be too difficult for them.

More is not necessarily better when presenting printed materials. If families are bombarded with thick stacks of pamphlets and materials, the likelihood of their use is decreased. A few carefully selected pamphlets can convey the idea that breastfeeding is uncomplicated and enjoyable. Pamphlets and short audiovisual programs are preferable to lengthy materials that attempt to cover the gamut of breastfeeding experiences. Brief, focused materials should address the issues that the family perceives as meaningful and that they are motivated to learn. This concept applies especially to mothers and families in special circumstances (such as prematurity, birth anomalies, and relactation). Books that are divided into small segments and have detailed indexes help families to locate needed information. Visual materials are more effective if they depict parents with ethnic, socioeconomic, and cultural backgrounds that are similar to the target audience. For example, teenage mothers respond most favorably to visual representations of adolescent mothers. A lending library of books and videotapes conveys a commitment to empowering families.

The source of materials must be considered in evaluating educational materials. Organizations whose purpose is to promote and sell formula cannot be expected to genuinely promote breastfeeding (Valaitis & Shea, 1993). Underlying messages may communicate that bottle-feeding is the cultural norm and that breastfeeding is difficult, complicated, uncomfortable, immodest, and inconvenient. There is often an explicit message that when families begin using formula, the product of that company is optimal.

The target audience should be considered in evaluating educational information. Materials must be written at a reading level that the reader can understand. Most word-processing programs can calculate the reading level of material by a simple push of a button. Box 23–4 lists the criteria for evaluating education materials.

Education for At-Risk Populations

In the United States, women who have low incomes, who are minimally educated, or who are members of particular ethnic groups initiate and sustain breastfeeding at rates lower than those of the national average. Although mothers with limited formal education are likely to be economically disadvantaged, their breastfeeding concerns are similar to those of more affluent mothers: modesty, partner participation, lifestyle changes, contraception, and fear of difficulty or pain.

In addition, they are influenced by the relative absence of peer models and social support. Women with minimal formal education may be more influenced by advertisements and media portrayal of artificial feeding as the cultural norm. They may also lack self-confidence, control over their lives, and assertiveness skills that are likely to enhance their experience with breastfeeding. Thus, mothers with limited formal education should receive informational support and follow-up to enhance their breastfeeding experiences. Because partners, family members, and social-support people exert considerable influence on mothers with limited formal education, they should be included in breastfeeding education (Buckner & Matsubara, 1993; Gielen et al., 1992; Libbus, 1992; McClurg-Hitt & Olsen, 1994; McNatt & Freston, 1992).

US families who do not speak English create challenges regarding health education. Ideally, an interpreter will be available to assist in providing critical information. If a facility serves a large population that speaks English as a second language, the agency should consider translating educational materials and use pictures to teach the basics of breastfeeding. Also, they can purchase translated breastfeeding materials. La Leche League International sells pamphlets in many languages.

If the teacher or leader of a breastfeeding class comes from a different socioeconomic or ethnic group than do the mothers she is teaching, she may have a difficult time being accepted as a peer in whom the mothers can confide and trust. An example is a white, highly educated, articulate, and well-dressed woman leading an inner-city group of African-American or Hispanic mothers in a WIC program. On the other hand, peers who are especially trained to help other women in their community with breastfeeding (peer counselors) have a profoundly positive effect on initiation and continuation of breastfeeding among low-income urban women. Locklin (1993, p. 181) described peer counselors trained by members of the Chicago Breastfeeding Task Force, a grass-roots organization consisting of committed professionals whose mission is to train peer counselors. A compilation of study outcomes of peer counselor programs appears earlier in this chapter.

BOX 23–4

Criteria for Evaluating Educational Material

Content

- Specific to family's needs?
- Accurate, reliable information based on valid research reports?
- Accepted principles of anatomy and physiology?
- Up-to-date recommendations?
- Consistency between narrative and visual aids?
- Simple, uncomplicated approach?
- Avoids dwelling on difficulties or potential complications?

Presentation

- Attractive, inviting?
- Organized for easy scanning: bold headings, short paragraphs, ample white space?
- Appropriate reading level?

   Less than high school education: Need more visuals, less narrative.
   High school graduate: Newspapers are written at this level
   College graduate: Professional journals are written at this level.

- Generous use of appropriate pictures, drawings, and graphs that are consistent with the narrative?
- Visual aids depict families from similar backgrounds of audience?
- Appropriate length to maintain interest?

Promotional Materials

- Enthusiastically discusses benefits of breastfeeding?
- Includes risks of bottle-feeding?
- Models culturally appropriate breastfeeding?
- Includes practical tips for successful breastfeeding?
- Provides information for additional resources?

Source of Materials

- No underlying or hidden messages about the use of formula?
- Breastfeeding presented as complicated, uncomfortable, immodest, inconvenient?
- Complies with WHO Code, which precludes health-care providers from distributing materials provided by formula companies?

Adolescents

Adolescents' concerns regarding breastfeeding reflect their developmental stage (Flanagan et al., 1995). The primary focus of the adolescent is the development of a sense of personal identity. Self-consciousness and modesty may be so pronounced that the young mother may be reluctant to consider breastfeeding. Typical concerns of North American adolescent mothers include issues of modesty, sex-uality, mobility, lifestyle, peer approval, the wish to return to school, and the attitude of the baby's father (Alexy & Martin, 1994; Marchand & Morrow, 1994; Peterson & DeVanzo, 1992; Purtell, 1994; Robinson et al., 1993). A focus group of US teens identified fears related to breastfeeding, which included lack of confidence, dietary concerns, loss of freedom, pain and discomfort, and disfigurement (Bryant, 1992).

Peer role models exert a strong influence in favor of breastfeeding (Radius & Joffe, 1988). Teen mothers who have enjoyed breastfeeding should be encouraged to discuss their experiences among pregnant peers. Adolescents are typically interested in having new experiences; some teenage mothers show interest in breastfeeding because they do not want to miss the "novel" experience of breast-feeding. Some teens find that breastfeeding is a source of pride; they gain positive attention from health-care providers, family members, and peers. Choosing to breastfeed can demonstrate their maturity and show that they are individualists. Because adolescents want to be loved and to give love, it can be effective to emphasize that breast-fed babies and mothers feel a special closeness and love for each other.

"Whose baby is this?" is sometimes an issue between the adolescent mother and her baby's grandmother. Breastfeeding can be attractive, because only the mother can breastfeed. It is important to emphasize flexibility in feeding plans with teen mothers. Although there are numerous advantages to exclusive breastfeeding, an all-or-none approach will usually result in teens declining to breastfeed. It is more appealing for teens to discuss feeding plans in which the teen mother decides what the baby will be fed and by whom. Health-care providers can place their recommendations in perspective by remembering that partial breastfeeding provides more advantages to mothers and babies than no breastfeeding. Teens are especially sensitive to the opinions of others. Conveying confidence in the adolescent mother's ability to care for her baby validates her role as a mother.

When working with adolescent mothers, avoid rigid rules about positioning, dietary intake, and exclusive breastfeeding. As they complete their developmental tasks of adolescence, teenagers tend to distance themselves from (and sometimes actively rebel against) rules and regulations. It is more effective to suggest ideas that have worked for other young mothers. It is also important to emphasize the ease of breastfeeding (after the first weeks), because teens may lack self-confidence (Benson, 1996). Teenagers tend to think more concretely than abstractly and thus benefit from hands-on activities, such as positioning dolls and games (see Box 23–5). Learning activities should be fun,

geared to what the mothers believe is important, and quickly paced. It is helpful to remember that adolescents are used to being entertained with television and videotapes. Enthusiastic praise for any interest in breastfeeding, practical assistance in the birth setting, supportive social networks, and close follow-up during the week after birth are critical factors in facilitating successful breastfeeding among teenage mothers (Benson, 1996; Maehr et al., 1993).

Older Parents

Parents who have delayed childbearing, whether by choice or as a result of infertility, have unique concerns. Incorporating an infant and breastfeeding

---

BOX 23–5

Teaching Teenagers About Breastfeeding

Fill a "lunch box" with items that represent the benefits of breast-feeding. Ask the participants to create other items for the box.

- Clock (saves time)
- Diaper (stool doesn't smell bad)
- Doctor's Kit (fewer trips to MD)
- Diploma (smarter baby and child)
- Kotex or tampax (delays menses)
- Money (breastfeeding costs less)
- Syringe (antibodies "immunize" baby)
- Tape measure (return to prepregnant shape faster)
- Thermometer (milk always at the right temperature)
- Toothbrush (fewer cavities)

into their established lifestyle is not easy, and they may require frequent reassurance. On the positive side, older parents have more education, read more, have the advantages of varied life experiences, and perhaps have wisdom and patience that enhance parenting skills. They may need assistance to locate peers with whom they can relate. The older mother may need reassurance that the ability to breastfeed does not decrease with increasing maternal age.

Educational Needs and Early Discharge

As families are discharged from the birth setting more quickly, educational opportunities are abbreviated. There are fewer hours to discuss educational needs, there are more visitors, and the mother's retention of information is affected by sleep deprivation, discomfort, and analgesics.

In the birth setting, it is critical that health-care providers prioritize discharge teaching so that parents have information that is critical. *Infant hydration and nourishment is top priority.* Teaching latch-on and assessment of milk intake is far more important than is teaching bathing, which can be reviewed by other resource persons (family members, friends, or health-care providers) following discharge. Special concerns identified by the family and when and from whom to get help are other areas that should be covered before the family leaves the birth setting.

When teaching for discharge, be optimistic yet realistic. The maxim "Expect the best and prepare for the worst" is appropriate. Using a chronological approach, discussing what parents should expect in the first few days is helpful. Subsequent visits with a physician or nurse practitioner (ideally within a few days after discharge) provide opportunities to discuss ensuing concerns. Concrete time frames (i.e., "You will probably begin to notice that your breasts are fuller on Tuesday.") is easier for a new mother to comprehend than is professional "jargon" (i.e., "You'll probably notice that your breasts will become engorged four to five days postpartum."). Giving the parents written information on engorgement, nipple tenderness, and the like (ideally in separate pamphlets or fliers) can reinforce earlier teaching if the mother is experiencing these situations.

Continuing Education

Almost all large medical centers now offer at least some staff or continuing education related to breastfeeding. Some of these programs are highly successful and bring in welcome revenue (Box 23–6). Others that are less financially successful are considered "loss leaders." The strategy is to attract young families to a particular health-care system that employs nurses and other providers who are knowledgeable in and supportive of breastfeeding. As birth settings that support breastfeeding are recognized and rewarded by the community, families will in turn become lifelong paying "customers" of the health-care system offering them. Core components of developing and presenting continuing education programs follow these sequential steps:

- Assess the learning needs of the participants.
- Assess participants' motivation and readiness to learn.
- Plan and develop learning objectives, curriculum content, and teaching methods.
- Implement teaching strategies and assist participants in focusing attention on learning tasks.
- Evaluate the outcome of teaching activities.

Managers become aware of learning needs and deficits in the clinical staff through feedback from families and from other health-care providers. In addition to gaining administrative input regarding learning needs, potential participants of the educational program should be involved in assessing their own learning needs. Their involvement in the planning stage will enhance their belief that the program will benefit them in their clinical practice. Staff may attend educational programs either because their employer requires attendance or because they need to attend a certain number of continuing-education offerings to maintain their professional registration or certification (extrinsic motivation). However, if participants are there because they want to be (intrinsic motivation), they are self-directed learners who have identified their learning goals and are enthusiastic about learning. Relating the curriculum content directly to a clinician's practice is a key strategy for arousing and

BOX 23–6

Sample Continuing-Education Program

Program title: Insufficient Lactation and Infant Weight Gain

Description: This 2-hour course reviews the characteristics and interventions of a situation where the infant is gaining weight at below acceptable levels owing to apparent maternal lactation insufficiency.

Objectives

1. Correlate normal growth with expected nutritional intake.

2. Assess the mother and infant to determine probable causes of insufficient milk supply.

3. Identify variation in the lactating breast that may potentially impact a mother's milk supply.

4. Distinguish between primary and secondary lactation insufficiency.

5. Describe effective interventions supplementation of the infant while maintaining lactation and feedings at the breast.

(Three objectives can usually be adequately covered in 1 hour.)

Teaching Methodology: Lecture, slides, videotape, case study for discussion

Instructor: Jane Smith, RN, BSN, IBCLC

References

Hillervik-Lindquist C. Studies on perceived breast-milk insufficiency: a prospective study in a group of Swedish women. *Acta Paediatr Scand Suppl* 376:1–27, 1991.

Livingstone V. Problem-solving formula for failure-to-thrive infants. *Can Physician* 36:1541–45, 1990.

Powers N. How to assess slow growth in the breast-fed infant. In: Schanler RJ, ed. *Breastfeeding 2001*, Part 2. *Pediatr Clin No Amer* 48(2):345–63.

Evaluation: Program will be evaluated by participants using the standardized form, *The Comprehensive Evaluation Tool for Continuing Health Education Programs.* The faculty/presenter will receive evaluation results and participant comments.

---

maintaining interest in the program. Teaching strategies for staff or continuing professional education are similar to those used with breastfeeding families.

Evaluating professional educational programs includes the staff's own assessment of the usefulness of the program to their clinical practices and an appraisal of the speaker and the content. This information is invaluable in modifying future programs; it also helps to convey the goal of clinical applicability and communicates respect for participants as valuable individuals.

Objectives and Outcomes

In developing education programs for health-care professionals, it is useful to clearly identify what the learner is expected to master. Writing behavioral objectives is one concrete way of identifying learning goals. A behavioral objective states what the student will be able to do at the end of the session. Table 23–2 presents examples of the correct and incorrect ways to write behavioral objectives.

Program outcomes are different from objectives. Objectives have to do with what a learner is

Table 23–2

EXAMPLES OF BEHAVIORAL OBJECTIVES

Incorrect	Correct
The learner will understand the relationship between breastfeeding and jaundice. (*Note:* the student's "understanding" is not observable.)	The learner will list the types of neonatal jaundice and will describe the relationship of each type to breastfeeding.

Behaviors that are Not Observable	Behaviors that are Observable
Understand, know, appreciate, learn, perceive, recognize, be aware of, comprehend, grasp the significance of, gain a working knowledge of	State, list, define, identify, describe, compare, critique, rate, demonstrate, plan, design, choose, discuss, match, relate, categorize, distinguish between, select, locate

able to do as a result of an education program whereas outcomes are the *results* of clinical practice that may be an indirect result of educational programs. For example, staff nurses who become more knowledgeable about breastfeeding after attending a series of continuing-education programs will obtain new knowledge that ultimately results in an outcome—that fewer mothers will be weaning early. Outcomes must be relevant and measurable and a logical result of clinical practices or of institutional effort. The examples of breastfeeding outcomes of breastfeeding education are many:

- Number and percentage of mothers who initiate breastfeeding
- Length of time the mothers breastfed
- Rate of ER visits for breastfeeding infants with dehydration
- Cost savings to managed care organizations due to the better health of infants because they were breastfed

All of these outcomes are relevant and measurable, and they reflect staff and institutional knowledge and effort. Most managed care organizations now require reports of clinical-outcomes data periodically. An Excel spreadsheet is available to all health agencies that have desktop computers. Setting up a database of breastfeeding outcomes that reflect the impact of educational programs are one more way to document the importance and effectiveness of education.

The Team Approach

A team approach to breastfeeding education enhances the learning experiences of childbearing families by providing a comprehensive approach. The fragmented care that often typifies women's health care today is not conducive to effective breastfeeding education. Consistent information shared by a variety of providers on multiple occasions strengthens the impact of each breastfeeding education encounter. The breastfeeding team's exposure to current information (workshops, articles, etc.) strengthens consistency of education. To avoid unintentional contradiction, documenting what has been discussed with teaching checklists and care maps allows the educator to build on that foundation and to reinforce key points. Each health-care provider develops a unique relationship with a breastfeeding family and can make unique contributions to the family's education (Bocar, 1992).

Childbirth Educators

Childbirth educators develop rapport with breastfeeding families during their multisession classes. They provide invaluable anticipatory guidance by including breastfeeding information in general childbirth education programs. Following childbirth, families frequently seek breastfeeding assistance from childbirth instructors.

Nurses

Most certified lactation consultants are also nurses. Staff nurses not certified as specialists refer more complex cases to lactation consultants. Breastfeeding educator and lactation counselor are titles that indicate completion of a study of breastfeeding basics (Figure 23–4).

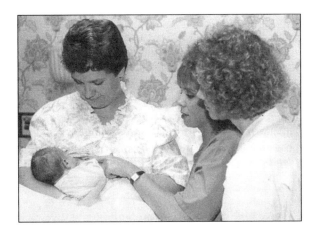

FIGURE 23–4. A perinatal nurse observes a new mother breastfeeding her infant. Learning new skills from a lactation consultant. (Courtesy of Debi Leslie Bocar.)

Lactation Consultants

Lactation consultants are health-care providers whose primary focus is providing breastfeeding assistance. They provide a variety of specialized services, including individual consultations for unusual breastfeeding situations, care plans developed in collaboration with other health-care providers, breastfeeding class sessions, and instruction in the use of specific breastfeeding products. They also serve as a resource for information and data, develop special programs or projects related to breastfeeding, provide continuing education programs for health-care providers, and conduct research. Lactation consultants have received certification from the International Board of Lactation Consultants (IBLCE), the internationally recognized certification body for this specialty area.

Physicians

Physicians can serve as powerful breastfeeding promoters. Their support of breastfeeding can be a potent force in a family's decision to begin and continue breastfeeding. About half of new physicians are young women, many of whom will become mothers who are likely to choose to breastfeed because of the health benefits and will later become strong advocates for breastfeeding. Physicians often refer families to lactation consultants for time-intensive treatment of breastfeeding difficulties or follow-up. A few physicians are themselves certified as lactation consultants and may have practices that are limited to breastfeeding families.

Dietitians

The responsibilities of dietitians include nutritional counseling for childbearing families. They can describe the influence of breastfeeding on maternal and infant nutrition needs. Many dietitians working with breastfeeding families are employed by WIC programs and in other community health settings.

Community Support Groups

Mother-to-mother support groups create an invaluable social support network for breastfeeding families. Practical tips and much incidental learning about parenting are derived from these important support groups. The largest and most effective self-care group for breastfeeding support is La Leche League International (LLLI). Founded in 1956, the organization's core service is mother-to-mother support and information provided through small neighborhood-based groups. Four monthly topics are provided throughout the year on a rotating basis.

Leaders are available between meetings for individual assistance and problem solving. The relaxed, friendly interchange between women with common interests in breastfeeding, childbearing, and childrearing is a basic strength of this highly successful organization. LLLI is effective in meeting the educational and support needs of breastfeeding women worldwide. More than 9000 volunteer leaders are estimated to serve more than 100,000 families in the United States each year.

Summary

Breastfeeding families are empowered for self-sufficiency when health-care providers furnish information in an accurate, well-organized manner. When good information is coupled with identification of the family's goals and assistance with problem solving, parents have greater self-confidence and self-reliance.

Underestimating a family's desire to breastfeed may be an unrecognized barrier to its continuance. This is particularly true with such groups as adolescent mothers, single mothers, immigrant women, mothers from ethnic minority populations, or mothers who are employed outside the home.

Developing and presenting educational programs for health-care providers who assist breast-feeding families requires significant time and energy. One needs to remember the ripple effect related to education; enormous numbers of breast-feeding families benefit from the enhanced knowledge of health-care providers. A successful education program—regardless of its subject matter—entails positive experiences for learners and educators. Identifying the components of effective breastfeeding education programs can assist health-care providers who are involved in planning, implementing, and evaluating breastfeeding services.

Key Concepts

- Learning is most effective when individuals are ready to learn (the teachable moment) and the material to be learned is organized in a manner that makes it meaningful to the learner.

- Learning is divided into three domains: (1) cognitive skills, (2) psychomotor skills, and (3) affective learning. Breastfeeding education incorporates all of them.

- Adults are self-directed and perceive time as one of their most valued and scarce assets, and they are not willing to spend it in meaningless activity. Educational programs must therefore demonstrate a clear applicability to the adult's everyday life.

- Assessing the learning needs of adults is mandatory. There must be a "match" between what the learner needs to know, what the teacher presents, and the time taken for important topics.

- Facilitating the learning experience for parents requires an understanding of the acquisition of the parental role as one of the tasks of adulthood.

- Frequent, short discussions about breastfeeding throughout the course of prenatal care is better than covering everything a mother needs to know in one information session on breastfeeding.

- The content of prenatal breastfeeding classes should include information necessary to initiate breastfeeding (e.g., timing of the first breastfeeding, positioning and assisting the infant to latch onto the breast, prevention of nipple trauma, management of engorgement).

- Families with special needs benefit from individualized teaching, assistance, and ongoing group support. Individualize the content based on family concerns and not what health-care providers *think* they should have.

- When special circumstances such as prematurity, multiple births, congenital anomalies, or neurological impairment affect the initiation of breastfeeding, the learning needs of the parents are complicated by the emotional ramifications of the experience. It is hard for parents to retain information when they are under stress. Prioritize content so that only important information is given and repeated.

- Numerous studies show that education and professional interventions can be provided throughout the breastfeeding period.

- A fundamental axiom is to "explain what you're going to teach, teach, and then describe what you have taught."

- Small-group teaching is a powerful method for changing behavior. The ideal small group size is 8 to 12 participants.

- To develop slides, identify key concepts and write them out on a storyboard—a sequence showing the presentation's main points and secondary points. It is best to present one idea and six points per slide.

- Adults retain only about 30 percent of the information they hear in a lecture but 50 percent of what is presented in a multimodal approach (both seeing and hearing).

- Peer role models exert a strong influence on teenage mothers. Adolescents are typically interested in having new experiences, and some will breastfeed because they do not want to miss the "novel" experience.

Internet Resources

Parent and staff breastfeeding education, including videos, print materials, links to books, articles, support groups, chat rooms:
www.lalecheleague.org

www.babycenter.com

www.breastfeeding.co.uk

www.wrsgroup.com

www.injoyvideos.com

www.noodlesoup.com

Courses on breastfeeding:
www.ilca.org

www.breastfeedingbasic.org

www.health-e-learning.com

References

Adams C et al. Breastfeeding trends at a community breastfeeding center: an evaluative survey. *JOGN Nurs* 30: 392–400, 2001.

Akram DS, Agboatwalla M, Shamshad S. Effect of intervention on promotion of exclusive breast feeding. *J Pak Med Assoc* 47:46–48, 1997.

Alexy B, Martin CA. Breastfeeding: perceived barriers and benefits/enhancers in a rural and urban setting. *Public Health Nurs* 11:214–18, 1994.

Alvarado R et al. Evaluation of a breastfeeding support programme with health promoters' participation. *Food Nutr Bull* 17:49–53, 1996.

Anderson GC. Risk in mother-infant separation postbirth. *Image* 21:196–99, 1989.

Becton LG, Dickenson CC. Patient comprehension profiles: recent findings and strategies. *Patient Couns Health Educ* 2:101–6, 1981.

Bender DE, McCann MF. The influence of maternal intergenerational education on health behaviors of women in peri-urban Bolivia. *Soc Sci Med* 50:1189–96, 2000.

Benson S. Adolescent mothers experience of parenting and breastfeeding—a descriptive study. *Breastfeed Rev* 5:19–26, 1996.

Berger D, Cook CA. Postpartum teaching priorities: The viewpoints of nurses and mothers. *JOGNN* 27:161–68, 1998.

Bloom BS. *Taxonomy of educational objectives.* New York: David McKay, 1956.

Bocar DL. The lactation consultant: part of the health care team. *NAACOG Clin Iss Perin Wom Health Nurs* 3(4): 731–37, 1992.

Brillinger MF. Helping adults learn. *J Hum Lact* 6:171–75, 1990.

Bryant CA. Promoting breastfeeding among economically disadvantaged women and adolescents. *NAACOG Clin Iss Perin and Wom Health Nurs* 3(4):723–30, 1992.

Buckner E, Matsubara M. Support network by breastfeeding mothers. *J Hum Lact* 9:231–35, 1993.

Coopersmith S. *The antecedents of self-esteem.* San Francisco: W. H. Freeman, 1967.

Davies-Adetugbo AA. Promotion of breast feeding in the community: impact of health education programme in rural communities in Nigeria. *J Diarrhoeal Dis Res* 14:5–11, 1996.

Eidelman A, Hoffmann AI, Kaitz M. Cognitive deficits in women after childbirth. *Obstet Gynecol* 81:764–67, 1993.

Flanagan PJ et al. Adolescent development and transitions to motherhood. *Pediatrics* 96:273–77, 1995.

Freed GL, Fraley JK, Schanler RJ. Accuracy of expectant mothers predictions of fathers attitudes regarding breastfeeding. *J Fam Pract* 37:148–52, 1993.

Gielen AC et al. Determinates of breastfeeding in a rural WIC population. *J Hum Lact* 8:11–15, 1992.

Gill SL. The little things: perception of breastfeeding support. *JOGNN* 30:401–9, 2001.

Giugliani ERJ et al. Effect of breastfeeding support from different sources on mothers decisions to breastfeed. *J Hum Lact* 10:157–61, 1994.

Greiner T, Mitra SN. Evaluation of the effect of a breastfeeding message integrated into a larger communication project. *J Trop Pediatr* 45:351–57, 1999.

Houston MJ et al. Do breast feeding mothers get the home support they need? *Health Bull* 39:166–72, 1981.

Janke JR. The incidence, benefits, and variables associated with breastfeeding: implications for practice. *Nurse Pract* 18(6):22–32, 1993.

Jones DA. The choice to breastfeed or bottle-feed and influences upon that choice: a survey of 1525 mothers. *Child Care Health Dev* 13:75–85, 1987.

Knowles M. *The modern practice of adult education.* New York: Cambridge University Press, 1980.

Lauwers J, Shinskie D. *Counseling the nursing mother.* 3rd ed. Sudbury, MA: Jones & Bartlett, 2000.

Libbus MK. Perspectives of common breastfeeding situations: a known group comparison. *J Hum Lact* 8:199–203, 1992.

Littman H et al. The decision to breastfeed: the importance of fathers approval. *Clin Pediatr* 33:214–19, 1994.

Locklin MP. Passionate advocacy: a look back, a look forward. *J Hum Lact* 9(3):12, 1993.

Maehr JC et al. A comparative study of adolescent and adult mothers who intend to breastfeed. *J Adolesc Health* 14:453–57, 1993.

Marchand L, Morrow MH. Infant feeding practices: understanding the decision-making process. *Fam Med* 26: 319–24, 1994.

Martens PJ. Does breastfeeding education affect nursing staff beliefs, exclusive breastfeeding rates, and Baby-Friendly Hospital Initiative compliance? *J Hum Lact* 16:309–18, 2000.

Matich J, Sims LS. A comparison of social support variables between women who intend to breast or bottle feed. *Soc Sci Med* 34:919–27, 1992.

McClurg–Hitt D, Olsen J. Infant feeding decisions in the Missouri WIC program. *J Hum Lact* 10:253–56, 1994.

McNatt MH, Freston MS. Social support and lactation outcomes in postpartum women. *J Hum Lact* 8:73–77, 1992.

Nichols FH, Edwards MR. Are your group process skills up to par? *Nurs Health Care* 9:205–8, 1988.

Palti H et al. Evaluation of the effectiveness of a structured breast-feeding promotion program integrated into a maternal and child health service in Jerusalem. *Isr J Med Sci* 24:342–48, 1988.

Peterson CE, DaVanzo J. Why are teenagers in the United States less likely to breast-feed than older women? *Demography* 29:431–50, 1992.

Pugin E et al. Does prenatal breastfeeding skills group education increase the effectiveness of a comprehensive breastfeeding promotion program? *J Hum Lact* 12:15–19, 1996.

Purtell M. Teenage girls attitudes to breastfeeding. *Health Visitor* 67:156–57, 1994.

Radius SM, Joffe A. Understanding adolescent mothers' feelings about breastfeeding: a study of perceived benefits and barriers. *J Adoles Health Care* 9:156–60, 1988.

Redman BK. *The process of patient education.* 6th ed. St Louis: Mosby, 1988.

Riordan J. Teaching breastfeeding on the Web. *J Hum Lact* 16:231–34, 2000.

Robinson JB et al. Attitudes toward infant feeding among adolescent mothers from a WIC population in northern Louisiana. *J Am Diet Assoc* 93:1311–13, 1993.

Sampson EE, Marthas M. *Group process for the health professions.* New York: Wiley, 1981.

Sciacca JP et al. A breast feeding education and promotion program: effects on knowledge, attitudes and support for breast feeding. *Commun Health* 20:473–82, 1995.

Tubbs SL. *A systems approach to small group interaction.* Reading, MA: Addison-Wesley, 1984.

Valaitis RK, Shea E. An evaluation of breastfeeding promotion literature: does it really promote breastfeeding? *Can J Public Health* 84:24–7, 1993.

Valdes V et al. The impact of a hospital and clinic-based breastfeeding promotion programme in a middle class urban environment. *J Trop Pediatr* 38: 142–51, 1993.

Vega-Franco L, Gordillo LC, Meijerink J. Prenatal education or breast-feeding (Spanish). *Boletin Medico del Hospital Infantil de Mexico* 42:470–75, 1985.

Westphal MF et al. Breast-feeding training for health professionals and resultant institutional changes. *Bull WHO* 73:461–68, 1995.

Young SA, Kaufman M. Promoting breastfeeding at a migrant health center. *Am J Public Health* 78:523–25, 1988.

Zimmerman DR. You can make a difference: increasing breastfeeding rates in an inner-city clinic. *J Hum Lact* 15:217–19, 1999.

24

The Cultural Context of Breastfeeding

Jan Riordan

Culture exerts a major influence on a mother's attitude toward breastfeeding that crosses the boundary between private and public. Attitudes and patterns of infant feeding cannot be understood without placing them in their specific cultural context. This chapter looks at breastfeeding as a human behavior that is sensitive to cultural influence and social change.

The fastest growing segments of the US population are minorities. Non-European ethnic minorities are fast becoming an aggregate majority. For example, Hispanics compose the fastest growing minority population in the United States. The Hispanic/Latino population is expected to quadruple its 1990 size by the middle of this century (Riordan & Gill-Hopple, 2001).

Culture is defined as the values, beliefs, norms, and practices of a particular group, which are learned and shared and guide thinking, decisions, and actions in a patterned way (Leininger, 1985). Culture provides implicit and explicit codes of behavior:

- It is *learned* both through language and socialization.

- It is *shared*, often unconsciously, by all members of a cultural group who are then bound together under one identity.

- It is an *adaptation* to specific conditions related to environmental and technical factors and to the availability of natural resources.

- It is a *dynamic,* ongoing process.

From a practical standpoint, a society's culture consists of whatever one has to know or believe to operate in a manner acceptable to its members. Culture is a blueprint for human behavior, a guide that helps us to gain a clearer understanding of individual behaviors. The new mother is the product of all of her history: what she has learned about infants and infant feeding, and what she has seen. If she grows up in a breastfeeding culture, she has many opportunities to observe how infants are fed and knows that her female relatives and neighbors with breastfeeding experience will support her when she becomes a mother (Mulford, 1995). Women and their families have a right to expect that their cultural needs will be met as they are helped with breastfeeding and lactation. Without an understanding of a mother's cultural practices, the care and intervention of health-care professionals can do more harm than good (Figure 24–1).

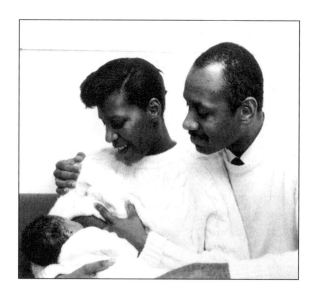

FIGURE 24–1. Expectations about breastfeeding. Each family has its own ideas, which are based in part on culture.

The Dominant Culture

Every society has a dominant culture, the values of which are shared by the majority of its members as a result of early common experiences. Although there are approximately 100 ethnic groups in the United States, the dominant cultural group is that of white, middle-class Protestants, descendants of northern Europeans who immigrated to the United States several generations ago. Norms characteristic of this group are a conservative value system, family orientation, commitment to higher education for one's children, a work ethic, materialism, a personal faith in God, the quest for physical beauty, cleanliness, high technology, punctuality, independence, and free enterprise. Given these prevailing values, it may be relevant to consider women's roles, their contribution to the economy, and the extent to which breastfeeding is perceived to hinder this.

The dominant health culture in the United States views birth as dangerous for the mother and neonate. Breastfeeding is seen as the optimal method of infant feeding but as difficult to accomplish and as a private act not to be practiced in public. These norms are slowly changing as waves of immigrating Asians and Hispanics become the

"new" Americans. In the United States, Western allopathic medicine is viewed as "professional" health care; any medical tradition outside this system is considered traditional folk medicine with its accompanying connotations of primitive, "useless," "lay," and "outdated." The dominant US health system marketplace is composed of the hospital, the health worker's office, and the community health department. The folk belief–system marketplace centers on the home of the clients or of their extended kin.

The role of women in a culture may also define the experience of breastfeeding. In some societies, male control (male physicians, for example) over breastfeeding serves to weaken the woman's role as mother and to emphasize her role as wife. Rather than viewing insufficient milk supply and early weaning as problems in themselves, these factors could be interpreted as reflecting insecurity about the abilities of women's bodies and the precariousness of their lives and as a symptom of broader self-questioning (Obermeyer & Castle, 1997).

Ethnocentrism Versus Relativism

Ethnocentrism may be defined as being centered in one's ethnic or cultural system (i.e., judging the world by one's standards or in the vernacular believing that "my group is best"). When caring for culturally diverse groups, nurses and health-care workers at first tend to ethnocentricity, believing that their professional, scientifically based practices are superior. Many of the health-care workers reading this book have been socialized into their profession within the framework of a Western health-care system that emphasizes the biomedical model and is based on the white, working- and middle-class value system. If this system is the only model used to evaluate and implement care, the nurse or lactation consultant is ethnocentric. When health-care workers are exposed to other cultures, they may begin to appreciate why certain behaviors and values are effective in that culture and may move beyond ethnocentric behaviors.

The opposite of ethnocentrism is *cultural relativism*, in which the health-care provider recognizes and appreciates cultural differences and treats individual clients with deference to their cultural backgrounds—building on and using cultural variations rather than seeing them as obstacles. To provide optimal assistance, caregivers must first understand their personal reactions to cultural differences and then appreciate how these cultural values affect the lives of their clients. By discovering areas of commonality between themselves and their patients, nurses or care providers will be better able to recognize and deal with cultural similarities and variations between the clients and themselves. This process is illustrated in Figure 24–2.

Cultural relativism likewise recognizes variation within cultures, such as the diverse ethnic groups in the United States. At one time, people expected and hoped that these ethnic and cultural groups would blend into one common whole: the melting-pot approach. It has not worked out that way; many third- and fourth-generation Americans proudly claim and identify with their original ethnic heritage. The tendency to label subpopulations to explain behaviors is responsible for many myths about new Americans.

Assessing Cultural Practices

A cultural assessment elicits shared beliefs and customs that affect how nursing care is given (Mattson, 2000). When a nurse examines cultural traditions, it is helpful to ask questions that indicate respect for cultural practices. A practice that seemingly does not provide any immediately visible benefit may be important to the mothers, and its value should be

acknowledged. Nurses who show that they respect the mothers' practices will gain respect in turn and better adherence to teaching.

Are They Helpful? All cultures have beliefs, myths, and rituals that may help breastfeeding. For example, the Lusi people in Papua New Guinea prohibit the lactating mother from having intercourse because it is believed that semen poisons her breastmilk (Maher, 1992). One result of this practice is eliminating the likelihood of a superimposed pregnancy. Such beliefs ensure that infants continue to be breastfed and are well nourished and nurtured. Cultural practices such as carrying a baby close, breastfeeding on demand, and spacing children by long-term breastfeeding are likewise considered beneficial.

Are They Harmless? Placing an amulet or charm of garlic around the baby's neck to protect him from harm or pinning a bellyband around his abdomen to prevent an umbilical hernia are harmless practices, assuming that such items are kept clean. If the mother eats garlic to prevent illness, the practice is harmless to her baby even though her milk will be garlic-flavored (Mennella & Beauchamp, 1991).

Are They Harmful? Unlike most of the rest of the world's people, white Europeans put mother and baby in separate sleeping rooms, sometimes even in the hospital, which hinders the establishment of breastfeeding. In rural southern Senegal the mother expresses and discards her colostrum and the infant is fed only water with sugar or honey until the "true" milk comes in, thereby depriving the baby of the concentrated immune properties of colostrum (Whittemore & Beverly, 1996).

Language Barriers

When working with families who speak a different language, the health-care provider ideally can understand and speak that language. If she cannot, she should study the language spoken by the breastfeeding families that she frequently serves. Rapport is difficult when language differences form a barrier.

Health-care workers who can speak Spanish are desperately needed in the southwestern United States and in large cities where Hispanics/Latinos

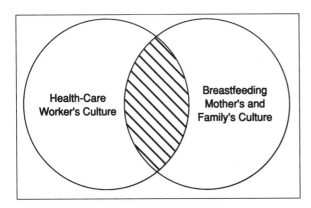

FIGURE 24–2. Shared values and beliefs. (From Orque MS, Block B, & Monrroy LS, 1983.)

are fast becoming ethnic majorities (Mattson, 2000). In towns with a high population of Hmong women, Hmong nurses are needed. In the northeast Canadian-border area, French is appropriate. Health agencies with large Hispanic/Latino populations should provide courses in Spanish for their employees (Berry, 1999).

When it is necessary to find someone fluent in a language, a trained interpreter is best able to rephrase words so that they are understandable and more acceptable to the member of the culture. When a translator is available, care providers should speak slowly in a normal voice and should avoid using slang and subjectives (e.g., *would* and *if*). It may also be wise to tape-record the discussion with the mother, so that the taped discussion may be referred to again. Even with a translator, there may be problems, because there are different dialects within some countries. Vietnamese, for example, is a language with many regional dialects. Also, a word may have different shades of meaning in different regions of the country. In preparing a flipchart and audiocassette for encouraging breastfeeding among mothers in the Dominican Republic, I used the word *amamantar* to mean *breastfeeding,* as it is used in many Spanish-speaking countries. This provided much amusement to the Dominican mothers, to whom it meant, "milk the cow."

Most people who are new to a culture are shy. Out of respect for the people with whom they are dealing, they may nod their head and say yes even though they may disagree or not understand what is being said. Whenever possible, printed materials regarding breastfeeding should be written in the family's language. Information sheets on breastfeeding in many different languages may be ordered from La Leche League International. Phrases that are frequently used when helping mothers breastfeed are presented in Spanish in Table 24–1.

The Effects of Culture on Breastfeeding

Immigrants tend to adopt the cultural practices of their new country; for newcomers to the United States, adaptation means bottle-feeding instead of breastfeeding. These mothers were breastfed themselves as infants and breastfed those children born in their native land; however in their eagerness to fit in with American cultural norms, these women turn away from their heritage of breastfeeding—hardly a surprise in a country where toy baby dolls are sold with formula bottles and women pump milk for their babies in the room reserved for evacuating bodily wastes (Morse, 1989). The longer a newly immigrated woman lives in the United States, the more likely she will choose to bottle-feed, even though she may come from a country where the breastfeeding rate is high. Mexican women in the United States are an example—the least acculturated are more likely to breastfeed than the more acculturated (Libbus, 2000). Breastfeeding becomes a choice for them, neither a cultural norm nor an economic necessity. The women may be wrongly told that it is the custom in the United States to bottle-feed babies.

Perception of breastfeeding support can be different for immigrants compared with women of the dominant culture. For example, immigrant mothers in Canada experienced more hospital practices detrimental to breastfeeding than did Canadian-born mothers. But they also received better professional support in the community (Loiselle et al., 2001).

US and Australian care providers' work increasingly with Asian families who have immigrated in search of a new life and opportunities. Few of these women choose to breastfeed (Rasbridge & Kulig, 1995; Rossiter, 1994). These mothers were breastfed as infants, and they breastfed those children born in their native land. However, in their eagerness to acculturate, these women turn away from their cultural heritage of breastfeeding. A local community health nurse asked a Vietnamese mother, "But didn't your mother breastfeed you?" The woman replied, "Yes, but that's the old way. We're in a new land now."

Hmong women living in Wisconsin stated that they bottle-fed rather than breastfed for the following reasons: "not enough milk in breasts;" "can go someplace without taking a baby;" "going back to school;" "stale milk in breasts" (Jambunathan & Stewart, 1995). The father of the baby is likely to agree with his wife, especially if their baby is a boy, in the belief that their son will grow to be physically larger (and more like American men) and to have "harder bones" if he is fed formula.

Consider the influences of a new culture when a mother receives a formula discharge pack from

Table 24–1

COMMONLY USED PHRASES WHEN SPEAKING WITH SPANISH-SPEAKING WOMEN ABOUT BREASTFEEDING

Spanish	English
Leche materna	Breastmilk
Calostro	Colostrum
Madre	Mother
Bebé	Baby
Consultor de lactancia	Lactation consultant
Consejera	Nurse
Masaje del pecho	Breast massage
Expresión manual	Hand expression
No usar chupetes	Do not use pacifiers
No usar biberones	Do not use bottles
Succionar los pechos	Pump breasts
Alimentación suplementaria	Supplemental feeding
Alimentación de pecho	Breastfeeding
Amamantar a su bebé	Breastfeeding
Pecho	Breast
Pezón	Nipple
Ya puede amammantar a su niño(a)	You can breastfeed your baby now.
¿Le va bien cuando da pecho?	How is breastfeeding going?
¿Cada cáundo el niño come cada ves que le da pecho?	How often does the baby breastfeed each day?
¿Esta recibiendo suficiente? Cinco a seis pañales mojados al día.	Getting enough? Five or six wet diapers each day?
¿Esta recibiendo suficiente? Cuatro o más deposiciónes al día?	Getting enough? Four or more bowel movements a day?
¿Cuantas veces hace pupu el niño al día?	How many dirty diapers does the baby have each day?
Le da pecho las veces que el niño quiere, usualmente ocho a doce veces al día.	Breastfeed as often as the baby wants, usually eight to twelve times a day.
Usted puede comer lo que quiera al menos que el niño se ponga malo después de que come algo en particular.	You can eat what you want unless you notice the baby is fussy after you eat certain foods.
Sus pezónes van a estar un paquito enflamados. Pero en unos cuantos dias se le va a quitar.	Your nipples may be sore for a few days. But the soreness will go away.

the hospital and free formula through the WIC program in the land "where babies don't die." The WIC office in a Dallas Cambodian community was universally referred to as the *kinlaeng baek tuk dah ko,* "the place to get formula" (Rasbridge, & Kulig, 1995). Consider, too, the messages the mother re-ceives when she sees the stacks of formula in the supermarket and the magazine pictures of attractive mothers bottle-feeding their babies. Rossiter (1994) noted that when breastfeeding classes for Vietnamese women living in Australia are geared to their language and their culture, these women have more positive attitudes toward breastfeeding and are more likely to breastfeed.

Why do African-American women choose to breastfeed less often? In a qualitative study using interviews (Corbett, 2000), an African-American woman described the curiosity of friends who wanted to watch her because they had never seen a woman breastfeed. Breastfeeding seemed to be an unfamiliar and uncertain activity, as is reflected in the lower rate of breastfeeding than among other groups.

When African-American women were asked why they chose bottle-feeding, they acknowledged that breastfeeding is more healthful than formula feeding (Riordan & Gill-Hopple, 2001), but they offered many reasons for not doing so: "if you've got a job you've got to pump"; "it ties women down"; "you've got formula given to you from WIC"; "it hurt too much and I couldn't take the pain"; and "I thought it was just a turn-off." Others said they chose not to breastfeed because they believed that the baby would be "spoiled" and also that the baby would not receive enough milk. Are there other, deeper, unstated reasons why African-American women turn away from breastfeeding? Blum (1999) thinks so and attributes their history of slavery and the common practice of Southern black women wet-nursing white infants as

a legacy of embodied exploitation where their sexuality and reproduction were appropriated by white men. Breastfeeding, in which the black baby was denied its mother's milk as she nursed the white infant, is a particularly charged symbol (p. 147).

In Baltimore, the baby's grandmother plays a key role in an African-American woman's decision to breastfeed and in when to introduce complementary foods and replacement feedings. Younger mothers in this population are often single and living at home with their own mother. The grandmother, the decision-maker in the family, wields the authority and experience (Bentley, Dee, & Jensen, 2003). In order for any breastfeeding promotion in this group to be successful, it must first educate and convince the grandmothers.

The US view of the breast as erotic and society's notion that motherhood is incompatible with sexuality also have negative ramifications for breastfeeding among Asian immigrants, who initially feel comfortable with breastfeeding but cannot reconcile this behavior with what they see in their new environment. They worry about how others will perceive them if they do breastfeed (Rodriguez-Garcia & Frazier, 1995). Native Ojibwe women in Canada express this same contradiction: they believe breastfeeding is the "right way to feed the baby" yet they are uncomfortable about breastfeeding being related to their view of the breast as sexual (Dodgson et al., 2002).

Breastfeeding in a public place or in the presence of friends is an activity that is extremely sensitive to cultural norms (Figure 24–3). For instance, in

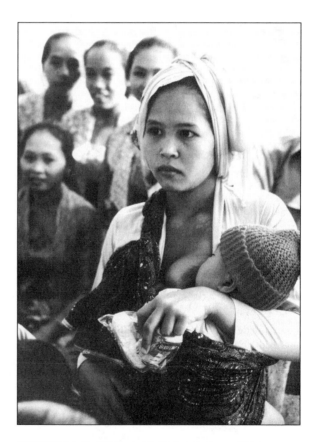

FIGURE 24–3. Well-nourished woman and breastfeeding infant in Searo. Breastfeeding is a basic part of the life process in this part of the world. (Courtesy of World Health Organization.)

Saudi Arabia it is not uncommon to see a totally veiled woman baring her breast to feed her infant in public with no one taking notice—except, perhaps, a foreigner. In France, women in topless swimsuits are perfectly acceptable on certain beaches. However, a French woman would hesitate, or at least cover herself carefully, while breastfeeding in public, even in a restaurant near the "topless" beach. Modesty is important for the Mexican-American mother and may be viewed as inconsistent with breastfeeding in public. Breastfeeding in public is becoming a more accepted practice in North America. When Canadian women tested public reaction by breastfeeding in a restaurant and a shopping mall, they received very little notice from passersby (Sheeshka et al., 2001).

Rituals and Meaning

Rituals and cultural meanings associated with infant feeding are critical elements in assessing the culture's infant-feeding practices. Unfortunately, the word *ritual* has come to connote a meaningless ceremonial act. Actually, rituals can have a significant effect if the individual believes in them. Eating a special food or praying to a patron saint to increase the milk supply are cultural rituals that work for some people, just as taking a pill on the advice of a Western-trained doctor may have a positive effect, even if the medicine is a sugar pill. Researchers call this the *placebo effect*, which is based on the observation that if one believes that a particular action will have a desired effect, it will.

In the Philippines, the ritual of *lihi* ensures a good flow of rich milk. The ceremony involves stroking the mother's breasts with broken papaya leaves and stalks of sugar cane. The white sap of the papaya ensures that the mother's milk will be copious, thick, and white, whereas the cane guarantees that it will be sweet. In certain rural areas of Japan, figurines and paintings depicting a woman with a bounteous milk supply are displayed in the belief that they increase the mother's milk (Figure 24–4). A picture of a breastfeeding mother seated in front of a waterfall has been used in the United States for similar effect. The use of nipple creams, popular in some Western countries, could be considered a ritual that is a comfort measure, even if it is not necessary from a physiological point of view.

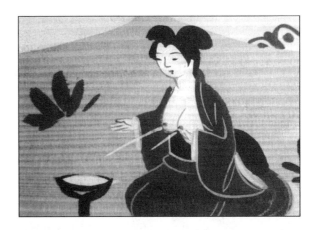

FIGURE 24–4. Votive picture (*ema* in Japanese). This wooden plaque is given to the breastfeeding mother by the temple. She in turn prays to the plaque for sufficient milk. If her wish is fulfilled, she writes her name and age on the plaque and dedicates it to the temple. (Courtesy of K. Sawada.)

Colostrum

In many cultures throughout the world, colostrum is accepted and encouraged as the first food for infants. In some cultures, however, colostrum is considered to be "old" milk that has been in the breasts for months and is unfit for the newborn and thus should be expressed and thrown away until the "true" milk appears on the second or third day (Conton, 1985; Fishman, Evans, & Jenks, 1988). In many developing countries, mothers do not give their babies this first milk because they fear it to be "pus" or "poison." This belief exists among people in countries thousands of miles apart, including the native peoples of Guatemala and Korea, and Africans in Sierra Leone and Lesotho. Lactation consultants have the opportunity and responsibility to encourage women to breastfeed their baby early by explaining that colostrum is "special" early milk made just for their baby and will help keep their baby healthy.

Sexual Relations

We are sexual beings and the breastfeeding woman is no exception. Although breastfeeding is usually a rich meaningful experience, its impact on a woman's sexuality is generally ignored. Historically, sex during the lactation period has been fraught with myths and prescribed behaviors. For example, the notion that semen contaminates breastmilk, a vestige of medieval European thought, is still widespread in many developing countries. It assumes that there is a physiological connection between the uterus and the breast and that the mother's milk may become contaminated by sexual contact. One negative result of a taboo against having sexual intercourse while lactating is that men pressure women to shorten breastfeeding so they can resume sexual relations and that women, concerned that their milk may be "contaminated" by sperm, are more likely to wean early (Maher, 1992). On the positive side, the taboo is an effective means of birth spacing.

When Avery, Duckett, and Frantzich (2000) surveyed 576 breastfeeding women in Minnesota about their sex life, overall they reported that breastfeeding had a slightly negative impact of some aspects of sexuality but did not greatly affect the woman's sexual relationship with her partner. The striking thing was their wide range of experiences. When asked if the sensations of suckling elicited arousal, most of the women (60 percent) reported negatively. Based on the information from this study, caregivers can help mothers deal with sexuality during the breastfeeding by doing the following:

- Teaching normal (and wide) variations of experiences of sexuality

- Discussing resumption of intercourse when she feels ready

- Providing good information about safe and efficacious contraceptives

- Describing methods of reducing perineal pain, such as vaginal lubricants

- Emphasizing that a priority should be placed on time for sleep

- Reminding couples that the window of time devoted to breastfeeding is relatively short compared to their total life together.

Wet-Nursing

Wet-nursing, a historic practice worldwide, may provide for a child whose mother has died or who is otherwise unable to breastfeed. Among Japanese, Chinese, and Thai mothers, breastmilk can be shared between infants of the same sex but not those of the opposite sex. Infants who had the same wet-nurse cannot marry in Arabic Moslem countries. In cultures that view breastmilk as a conduit for ancestral power, it is not unusual for wet-nurses to be restricted to women from the mother's or father's clan or lineage (van Esterik & Elliott, 1986). Americans practiced wet-nursing up until recent times; for example, Southern women sometimes used black slaves to wet-nurse their babies. Wet-nursing is now discouraged because of concerns about AIDS transmission. However, a few women still practice wet-nursing; for example, mothers in Northwest Indian tribes, especially sisters, regularly practice wet-nursing secretly.

Other Practices

A seclusion period of about 40 days after giving birth is common in many cultures. This time of support from female kin and seclusion for the mother and baby varies according to the culture. Generally, it permits a mother to become acquainted with her baby, to establish her milk supply, and to reduce both her and her infant's exposure to infectious disease. In Bedouin Arab Society, female relatives visit the new mother and baby and bring small gifts of money to mark the birth of the baby (Forman et al., 1990).

In Korea, the mother's mother-in-law traditionally takes care of her after the child's birth and serves as her "doula." During pregnancy, Korean women undergo *Thae Kyo* or education-teaching of the fetus. In this ancient tradition a mother-in-law trains her daughter-in-law to be a mother. *Thae Kyo* instructs the expectant mother that to avoid bad luck in having her baby, she should not see fires or fights, she must think pure thoughts and eat "pretty" foods, and she must always walk in a straight line. During the postpartum period, which lasts about 3 to 4 weeks, the woman is also cared for by her own mother and her husband. This perception that the mother is "sick" and requires care runs counter to the expectations of US-trained nurses and to early discharge from the hospital.

Contraception

Methods of contraception used by breastfeeding mothers of any culture should not interfere with lactation. Nurses who advise ethnic minority women in community family planning services play a key role in monitoring the type of oral contraceptive dispensed. Combination pills that contain both progestin and estrogen (Lo/Ovral, Ortho-Novum, Triphasil, Nordette) seriously diminish breast-milk production, and they almost invariably lead to giving formula supplements and weaning (American College of Obstetricians and Gynecolgists [ACOG], 2000). If mother does not speak English or if she is an illegal immigrant, she may hesitate to ask questions as to why her milk supply suddenly dried up after she started taking a combined oral contraceptive pill.

On the other hand, progestin-only oral contraceptives (Micronor, Nor-QD, Ovrette) and long-acting progestin-only injectables (Depo-Provera, Norplant) do not affect the quality of breastmilk and may increase the volume of milk (ACOG, 2000), especially if they are not started until 6 weeks postpartum when lactation is well established (Diaz & Croxatto, 1993). For nonhormonal contraception during the first 6 months after delivery, ACOG (2000) recommends exclusive breast-feeding meeting lactational amenorrhea method criteria and, if desired, using additional protection such as condoms and other barrier methods. (See Chapter 21 for a detailed discussion.)

Infant Care

Swaddling or bundling is an ancient practice still used today to soothe the infant and maintain his body temperature. Swaddling and carrying the baby on the mother's side or back also frees her hands for other tasks. In many parts of rural Nigeria, an infant is wrapped on the mother's back all day and sleeps with her at night. During the first 40 days, the baby is snugly wrapped, a practice that ensures that the infant stays warm and reduces his energy requirements (Omuloulu, 1982).

In parts of the world that do not have intensive care nurseries, premature infants who are clinically stable go directly to the mother as early as 2 to 3 hours after birth. By being held in an upright position, skin-to-skin between their mother's breasts, they are kept warm (Anderson, Marks, & Wahlberg, 1986; Anderson, 1992). This practice has spread to intensive care units worldwide in many countries and is now known as Kangaroo Care (Figure 24–5).

In any culture, swaddling and carrying the baby close typifies mothers who practice unrestricted breastfeeding. As early as 24 hours after delivery, the Zambian infant is secured to his mother's body with a *dashica,* or long piece of cloth. The baby rides on the mother's hip in the *dashica,* and his head is not supported. As a result, the Zambian infant maintains a strong shoulder girdle to keep his head steady and thereby develops early head control. The *aquawo*—a specially woven, strong cotton cloth folded in a special way—is the infant carrier in Bolivia. The *aquawo* can be turned around to several positions to facilitate breastfeeding. In Mexico, a woman uses a long, wide shawl called a *rebozo* for carrying her infant while she goes about her daily activities.

Many different types of baby carriers are used worldwide. Mothers and fathers, regardless of their cultural backgrounds, recognize and enjoy the convenience these carriers afford. Carrying the infant swaddled to his mother's body develops the child's muscle tone and seems to encourage alertness. Being carried about during daily activities offers many opportunities for tactile, visual, and social stimulation.

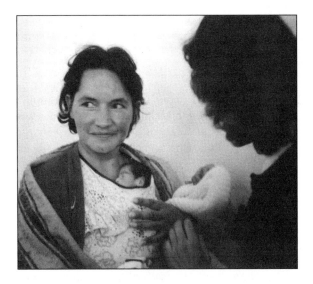

FIGURE 24–5. A premature infant in Bogota goes home. Twelve hours after birth, the baby cradled skin-to-skin with his mother. (Courtesy of G. C. Anderson.)

Babies in the Dominican Republic are not secured to their mother in any fashion but are carried in their arms in a horizontal position until they are old enough to sit up by themselves. Because it is believed that a baby can break his or her neck easily if the head is not held, a mother will become visibly anxious when the nurse assesses her baby's head control.

Diseases recognized only in a particular culture may affect an infant. In Spanish-speaking cultures, the most common is *mollera caida* (fallen fontanel). The health professional interprets a depressed fontanel in the baby as a symptom of dehydration, whereas a Hispanic mother may see it as curable illness caused by removing her nipple while the baby is still suckling, or by the baby falling.

Another Hispanic and Puerto Rican folk disease is *mal de ojo,* or evil eye, which is presumably caused by someone casting very strong glances at the baby or by someone who admired the baby but did not touch him. Symptoms of *mal de ojo* are sometimes vague, but the baby is usually very unhappy, cries continuously, cannot sleep, and may even die (Lacay, 1981). The cure is to find the person who is thought to have given the infant the evil eye and have her or him touch the baby. Lactation consultants working with such clients should take care to touch the baby when admiring him or her to avoid being thought of as the cause of a later case of *mal de ojo.*

Babies often are outfitted with special ornaments or bands that have a specific purpose. Hispanic grandmothers often worry a great deal about the infant's umbilicus and may insist that the baby wear a bellyband (*fajita*) to prevent an umbilical hernia. A traditional necklace protects the Laotian newborn. Babies in Papua New Guinea are protected from disease by special rituals, such as blackening the top of the baby's head with burnt coconut husk (Lepowsky, 1985).

Maternal Foods

Whether she lives on a mountaintop in remote Tibet, in a dusty Mexican village, or in an American suburb or urban high-rise apartment, the lactating woman produces milk that is amazingly homogeneous in composition, despite the wide diversity of foods she consumes. Only the milk of a woman who is severely malnourished will be measurably diminished in its nutrient content and volume because body nutrients are depleted before the milk suffers.

Part of understanding a culture involves becoming acquainted with its foodways—the way in which a distinct group selects, prepares, consumes, and otherwise uses portions of the available food supply. For more than half the inhabitants of this planet, including lactating women, beans, rice, and grains are daily fare. Fruits and vegetables appear seasonally, and meat is found in the family cooking pot only on special occasions. When it does appear, it is usually poultry, goat, horse, or dog, rather than beef. In most cultures, meat plays a minor part in flavoring rice, beans, and vegetables, not the major role it has served in affluent Western industrialized countries.

The daily food pattern of a breastfeeding Mexican mother who eats very little meat might concern us if we did not have a basic knowledge of amino acids and complementary proteins. Beans, a staple item in Mexican foodways, provide an incomplete protein when served alone, because they are low in methionine, an essential amino acid. This deficiency, however, is completely corrected when beans are served with a food high in methionine, such as whole grain breads or cereals. Complementary proteins can be obtained by numerous combinations. For example, eggs or a milk product will balance the protein and amino acids of a meal consisting primarily of plant proteins. However, two protein foods cannot complement each other if they have similar amino acids in their composition. For this reason, nuts and black-eyed peas are not complementary proteins, because both legumes lack the same amino acids.

"Hot" and "Cold" Foods

For many cultural groups, foods involve a balance that must be maintained to sustain health or be restored when illness occurs. Balance between opposing energy forces is based on the Greek theory of body humors. After centuries of dissemination throughout the world, this theory now appears as the hot (*caliente*) and cold (*frio* or *fresco*) system in Hispanic cultures. Other people, such as the Vietnamese, Chinese, East Indians, and Arabs, also use a hot–cold designation to some extent. Classifying foods as "hot" or "cold" in a given culture has little to do with their form, color, texture, or temperature, although hot foods are believed to be more easily digested than are cold foods. Instead, the classification is based on the food's effect on an illness or condition, which is itself categorized as hot or cold. During the last trimester of pregnancy, the unborn child is believed to be hot; therefore the mother is in a hot state. Once the child is born, accompanied by a loss of blood, a cold condition exists for both. To correct this imbalance, women believe that they need hot drinks and foods and to keep warm to replace heat and energy (Davis, 2001). Baths are taboo as exposure to water cools the body. Birthing in a hospital where postpartum showers are expected poses serious concerns for these mothers.

Traditional Chinese consider chicken, squash, and broccoli to be hot. Cold foods include melon, fruits, soybean sprouts, and bamboo shoots. In India, milk may be hot or cold, depending on where a person lives. In Hispanic cultures, cold foods include most fresh vegetables, tropical fruits, dairy products, beans, squash, and some meats. Hot foods—cereal grains, chili peppers, temperate-zone fruits, goat's milk, oils, and beef—serve to balance the cold foods. Because the potential listing of hot and cold foods in any particular culture is almost endless, health providers must do their ethnographic homework regarding the belief system of the cultures with whose members they are working. Among Southeast Asian women who delivered infants in the United States in the late 1990s, foods restricted after childbirth included all fruit. Postpartum foods are mainly rice and some boiled chicken. Garlic, black pepper, and ginger create warmth in the body and are encouraged (Davis, 2001).

Another belief system concerning food balance is the Chinese *yin-yang* theory. In America, people who use macrobiotics practice this system. Like the hot-cold theory, the basis of the *yin-yang* belief rests on a proper balance between opposing energy forces. On one side, yin represents "female," a negative force (cold, emptiness, darkness); on the other side, yang represents "male," a positive force (warmth, fullness, light). Too much of either yin or yang food is considered threatening to health. Whether a food is considered yin or yang depends on the effect it is thought to have on the body; the designation is not associated with color, texture, or other obvious characteristics. Without an extensive orientation for things Chinese, it is difficult to understand the "yin-ness" or "yang-ness" of food.

Herbs and Galactogogues

Almost all cultures abound with an array of certain foods for lactating women. In the past, beer and brewer's yeast have been touted as galactogogues—foods that are thought to increase milk secretion and improve let-down. Rice, gruel, soup, vegetables, and medicinal herbs may be used extensively by many cultures during the immediate postpartum period to promote the secretion of milk. Fenugreek tea is a popular galactogogue in the United States but is also used in many other parts of the world. Northern Mexicans make special teas from "hot" plants such as sesame and absinthe, and in some parts of Latin America herbal teas are drunk in the evening to stimulate milk for the morning (Baumslag, 1987). Herbs taken by the breastfeeding mother may have pharmacological effects on her baby, including irritation of the mucosal lining of the intestine and an increase in the release of flatus. Unless these symptoms become troublesome, it is more important for the mother to continue enjoying her favorite herbs in moderation than to stop using them because of her baby's minor stool changes. If the mothers within a particular ethnic group believe that certain foods can promote lactation, encourage these women to eat those foods. This practice gives a clear signal that the health-care system supports breastfeeding and respects these cultural beliefs.

Weaning

Weaning is a time when childhood illness and death are more likely in developing countries; thus it is a key issue in studies of crosscultural child-care practices. Cultural assessment includes the timing of feeding, types of foods given to infants, and weaning practices. When a substantial proportion of dietary intake comes from food other than breastmilk, growth rates falter, and the effects of morbidity come into play. Woolridge (1991) suggests, as a rule of thumb, that when 25 to 50 percent of a baby's kilocalories come from breastmilk, the milk will protect the baby from environmental pathogens. At the same time, every breastfed infant reaches a point at which breastmilk alone can no longer meet its nutritional needs and solid foods are necessary.

Early solid and semisolid infant foods given by mothers vary widely across cultures, as does the timing of their introduction. Worldwide, there is a high rate of both the initiation of breastfeeding and early supplementation with other foods, even in maternity units certified as "Baby Friendly" (Alikasifoglu et al., 2001). Although infants in Papua New Guinea are not introduced to supplemental foods until 6 months (Lepowsky, 1985) (an optimal age), this is not a usual pattern. In a comparison study of how mothers feed their infants in four diverse countries, Winikoff, Castle, and Laukaran (1988) noted that early introduction of other foods is common. The majority of Kenyan babies are given foods other than breastmilk before they are 4 months old (Dimond & Ashworth, 1987; van Esterik & Elliott, 1986); in East Java, force-feeding by hand is a common practice from as early as few days after birth (van Steenbergen et al., 1991). Clearly, much has to be done before reaching the goal of exclusive breastfeeding.

Types of Weaning

Weaning from the breast is a process during which mothers gradually introduce their babies to culturally assigned foods as they continue to breastfeed. Weaning begins with the introduction of sources of food other than breastmilk and ends with the last breastfeeding. Three types of weaning have been described:

- *Gradual weaning* that takes place over several weeks or months.

- *Deliberate weaning,* a conscious effort initiated by the mother to end breastfeeding at a particular point.

- *Abrupt weaning,* an immediate cessation of breastfeeding, which may be forced on the baby by the mother or on mother and baby by others.

Examples of gradual, deliberate, or abrupt weaning may be found in any culture. Gradual weaning, however, is the least traumatic, to both the infant and the mother.

Weaning practice can affect infant health, particularly in developing countries or in inner-city areas in which weaning diarrhea is prevalent. In cultures in which food is available sporadically or is meager, kwashiorkor, a severe form of protein deficiency, appears during the transition from breastmilk to other foods. In Ga, the language of Ghana, the term *kwashiorkor* means "the disease of the deposed baby." Identifying the reasons for women weaning early sheds considerable light on the beliefs and attitudes that influence the continuation of breastfeeding.

Various stages in infant development are sometimes used as cues to begin deliberate weaning. A common belief among African cultures is that the child should be walking before weaning is attempted. Some kind of independence is implicit in the concept of weaning, so it seems reasonable that the child be self-sufficient in locomotion before leaving the dependency of his/her mother's breast. In many Western cultures, teething is a developmental reference point thought to signal readiness to wean. In others, subsequent pregnancy signals the time to wean (Bohler & Ingstad, 1996). Usually a toddler or child will spontaneously wean with a new pregnancy. The reasons include a diminished milk supply, changes in the milk composition, and a less desirable taste.

For mammals, the length of lactation is positively correlated with adult female mass. Generally, larger mammals have long lactation periods (Hayssen, 1993). What is the "natural" age for weaning in humans? Dettwyler (1995) suggests four criteria associated with age at weaning in primates that range from 27 months to 7 years:

- *Weaning according to tripling or quadrupling of birth weight:* Using US data, male infants quadruple their birth weight by about 27 months and female infants by around 30 months.

- *Weaning according to attainment of one-third adult weight:* Weaning for the human would be predicted at between 4 and 7 years of age.

- *Weaning according to adult body size:* Using this comparison predicts the age for weaning in humans at between 2.8 and 3.7 years, with larger-bodied populations breastfeeding for the longest time.

- *Weaning according to time of dental eruption of permanent molars.* Modern humans' first molar eruption occurs around 5.5 to 6.0 years of age (the same time as that for adult immune competence).

Some rather harsh techniques have been used to bring about abrupt weaning. One time-honored method calls for pepper, garlic, ginger, or onion to be applied to the mother's breasts to discourage the baby from breastfeeding. In the Fiji Islands, weaning of kali ("to separate") is a four-day period during which the breast is denied to the infant and the baby's food is specially cooked in a separate pot. The infant is not allowed to sleep with the mother until after weaning and is sometimes cared for by one of the mother's female relatives in another household for this period.

In cultures in which early weaning is a common practice, a minority of people accept long-term breastfeeding. The sight of a walking child calmly sliding onto the mother's lap for milk and deftly opening her buttons to gain access to her breasts is considered shocking and subject to ridicule in some cultures. The term *closet nursing* describes a practice that has evolved in the United States in response to criticism of breastfeeding that extends beyond the culture's expectations. In closet nursing, breastfeeding continues by mutual consent of mother and child, but only in secret. The mother and baby usually have a code word for breastfeeding that can be used in public (Wrigley & Hutchinson, 1990). In many Western cultures, teething is a developmental reference point thought to signal readiness to wean. In others, subsequent pregnancy signals the time to wean. Many toddlers will spontaneously wean with a new pregnancy because of a diminished milk supply and a less desirable taste (Bohler & Ingstad, 1996). Regardless of the culture,

weaning is ideally a collaborative effort in which both the mother and baby reach a state of readiness to begin weaning.

Implications for Practice

Every culture has its visible elements (housing, clothing, food) and its invisible elements (attitudes, tradition, values); an understanding of both contributes significantly to communication between the breastfeeding client and the health-care provider. Some Spanish-speaking folkways and how to handle them are seen in Box 24–1. Immigrant mothers may be served foods that traditionally are forbidden to postpartum women, such as raw vegetables and fruit for Vietnamese mothers. Lactation consultants working in these birthing areas can make sure that alternate foods are provided to these women.

Many Indochinese women living in the United States formula-feed their infant, at least while in the hospital, and then both breastfeed and bottle-feed after leaving the hospital; therefore, formula discharge packs are not appropriate. It is advisable to have women health workers care for these mothers, because they regard it improper for men to touch a woman's body (especially the breasts). If mothers in any culture believe that certain foods can promote lactation, these women should be encouraged to bring these foods to the postpartum unit. This practice will enhance breastfeeding and provide a clear signal that the health-care system supports breastfeeding and is respectful of these cultural beliefs.

Regardless of the culture, weaning is ideally a collaborative effort in which both the mother and baby reach a state of readiness to begin weaning. In a culture in which unrestricted breastfeeding is practiced and in which the child breastfeeds for a prolonged period, the mother has very little ambivalence when she decides to wean and says, "You, child, have had enough milk!" (Mead & Newton, 1967).

Though weaning practices vary from culture to culture, weaning is thought to be the least traumatic when it is slow, gradual, and related to the needs of the child. It is essential to identify factors

BOX 24–1

Specific Folkways and Ways to Handle Them

- Touching the baby of a Spanish-speaking family while admiring him helps avoid giving the baby *mal de ojo*—the evil eye.
- An anemic breastfeeding mother who is not vegetarian believes that anemia is a yin condition. Suggest that she consume more meat, a yang food, to improve her iron status.
- A Korean mother refuses a cold pack for engorged breasts or for pain resulting from an episiotomy. Offer her cool water from a washcloth or from a peri bottle.
- A mother expects a 40-day period of special care postpartum. Respect the tradition and help her through early discharge with one or more home visits.

- A baby burps during feedings. According to some Hispanic mothers, this air goes to the breast and stops the flow of milk, causing her milk duct to become plugged. Ask her to switch to the other breast and then back to the first breast to release the "air."
- A mother believes that colostrum is "bad." Suggest that she express the first few drops of "impure" milk and discard it before putting the baby to breast, then say, "the sooner you breastfeed, the better the milk."
- Avoid serving ice water or cold drinks to a new mother from Southeast Asia.

that influence continuation or early termination of breastfeeding so as to develop appropriate programs to assist the mother who wishes to maintain breastfeeding. Women involved in long-term breastfeeding develop a special bond with their baby. The mother's choice of how long she wishes to breastfeed is an individual right that may not mesh with others' expectations. All breastfeeding families deserve to be treated in a nonjudgmental manner that accepts the cultural diversity that they represent.

Summary

The study of child-rearing patterns of a given culture is crucial to all health-care professionals who work with new and growing families. The seeds of a culture are planted, grow, and thrive in child-rearing patterns. Cultural awareness provides liberation from egocentric views in which one looks at the universe and sees only one's beliefs in the center. The study of any culture begins with critical self-reflection and awareness of the differences between one's cultural values and those of other people. By becoming aware of these differences, we begin a process of partnership in which all groups have something to contribute and something to learn. Although acculturation to the United States generally has a negative effect on breastfeeding, it can be offset if the mother receives support from health-care providers and from friends and family (Thiel de Bocanegra, 1998).

Analysis of infant feeding within its cultural context is critically linked to social action and policy decisions regarding breastfeeding promotion and teaching. For those who examine cultural issues carefully, so-called cultural obstacles to solving problems usually include the solutions, too. Within the cultural context of underlying infant-feeding problems, solutions must ultimately emerge. If changes are to last, they must originate from within a culture, rather than being imposed from without.

Key Concepts

- Culture is a blueprint for human behavior, one that helps us to gain a clearer understanding of individual behaviors. The new mother is the product of all of her history: what she has learned about infants and infant feeding, and what she has seen.

- *Culture* is defined as the values, beliefs, norms, and practices of a particular group, which are learned and shared and guide thinking, decisions, and actions in a patterned way.

- *Ethnocentrism*—being centered in one's ethnic or cultural system (i.e., believing that "my group is best") is the opposite of *cultural relativism*—the recognition and appreciation of cultural differences and backgrounds.

- A nonjudgmental way to assess a cultural practice is to ask certain questions: Is it helpful? Is it harmless? Is it harmful?

- Ideally, the care provider can understand and speak the language of the mother and her family. When it is necessary to translate a conversation, a trained interpreter should be used.

- Breastfeeding in public, time of weaning, and giving the neonate colostrum are all practices that are extremely sensitive to cultural norms.

- If a cultural ritual is important for a new mother and causes no harm to herself or her baby, the lactation consultant should respect the mother's wishes regardless of whether the ritual has been scientifically tested.

Internet Resources

Collection of papers in different languages (also artworks, stamps, and paintings):
www.geocities.com/HotSprings/Spa/3156

EthnoMed (cultural beliefs, medical issues, and other related topics pertinent to the health care of recent immigrants to Seattle, specifically, or to the United States):
http://ethnomed.org

La Leche League International (breastfeeding printed information and visuals in many languages):
www.lalecheleague.org

Mother discussions, photo gallery:
www.promom.org

Office of Minority Health:
www.omhrc.gov

Online guide to breastfeeding and baby care from India (including links, discussion forum, photo album):
www.breastfeedingindia.org

San Diego County Breastfeeding Coalition (breastfeeding information in Spanish and English):
www.breastfeeding.org

References

Alikasifoglu M et al. Factors influencing the duration of exclusive breastfeeding in a group of Turkish women. *J Hum Lact* 17:220–25, 2001.

American College of Obstetricians and Gynecologists (ACOG). *ACOG educational bulletin on breastfeeding.* No. 258, July 2000. The author.

Anderson GC. Current knowledge about skin-to-skin (kangaroo) care for preterm infants. *J Perinatol* 11:216–26, 1992.

Anderson GC, Marks EA, Wahlberg V. Kangaroo care for premature infants. *Am J Nurs* 86:807–9, 1986.

Avery M, Duckett L, Frantzich CR. The experience of sexuality during breastfeeding among primiparous women. *J Midwifery Womens Health* 45:227–37, 2000.

Baumslag N. Breastfeeding: cultural practices and variations. *Adv Int Matern Child Health* 7:36–50, 1987.

Bentley ME, Dee DL, Jensen JL. Breastfeeding among low income African-American women: power, beliefs and decision making. *J Nutr* 133:S305–9, 2003.

Berry AB. Mexican American women's expressions of the meaning of culturally congruent prenatal care. *J Transcultural Nurs* 10:203–12, 1999.

Blum L. *At the breast: ideologies of breastfeeding and motherhood in the contemporary United States.* Boston: Beacon Press, 1999.

Bohler E, Ingstad B. The struggle of weaning: factors determining breastfeeding duration in East Bhutan. *Soc Sci Med* 43:1805–15, 1996.

Conton L. Social, economic and ecological parameters of infant feeding in Usino, Papua New Guinea. *Ecol Food Nutr* 16:39–54, 1985.

Corbett KS. Explaining infant feeding style of low-income Black women. *J Pediatr Nurs* 15:73–81, 2000.

Davis RE. The postpartum experience for Southeast Asian women in the United States. *Maternal Child Nurs* 26(4):208–13, 2001.

Dettwyler KA. A time to wean: the homonid blueprint for the natural age of weaning in modern human populations. In: Stuart-Macadam P, Dettwyler KA, eds. *Breastfeeding: biocultural perspectives.* New York: Aldine De Gruyter, 1995:39–72.

Diaz S, Croxatto B. Contraception in lactating women. *Curr Opinions Obstet Gynecol* 5:815–22, 1993.

Dimond HJ, Ashworth A. Infant feeding practices in Kenya, Mexico, and Malaysia: the rarity of the exclusively breastfed infant. *Hum Nutr Appl Nutr* 41A:51–64, 1987.

Dodgson JE et al. An ecological perspective of breastfeeding in an indigenous community. *J Nurs Scholarship* 34:235–41, 2002.

Fishman C, Evans R, Jenks E. Warm bodies, cool milk: conflicts in postpartum food choice for Indochinese women in California. *Soc Sci Med* 26:1125–32, 1988.

Forman MR et al. The forty-day rest period and infant feeding practices among Negev Bedouin Arab women in Israel. *Med Anthropol* 12:207–16, 1990.

Hayssen V. Empircal and theoretical constraints on the evolution of lactation. *J Dairy Sci* 76:3213–33, 1993.

Jambunathan J, Stewart S. Hmong women in Wisconsin: what are their concerns in pregnancy and childbirth? *Birth* 22:204–10, 1995.

Lacay GI. The Puerto Rican in mainland America. In: Clark A, ed. *Culture and childrearing.* Philadelphia: Davis, 1981:211–27.

Leininger M. *Qualitative research methods in nursing.* Orlando, FL: Grune & Stratton, 1985.

Lepowsky MA. Food taboos, malaria and dietary change: infant feeding and cultural adaptation of a Papua New Guinea Island. *Ecol Food Nutr* 16:105–26, 1985.

Libbus MK. Breastfeeding attitudes in a sample of Spanish-speaking Hispanic American women. *J Hum Lact* 16:216–20, 2000.

Loiselle CG et al. Impressions of breastfeeding information and support among first-time mothers within a multiethnic community. *Canadian J Nurs Res* 33(3):31–46, 2001.

Maher V. Breastfeeding in cross-cultural perspectives, pardoxes and proposals. In: Maher V, ed. *The anthropology of breastfeeding.* Oxford, England: Berg, 1992.

Mattson S. Striving for cultural competence. *AWHONN Lifelines* 4(3):48–52, 2000.

Mead M, Newton N. Cultural patterning of perinatal behavior. In: Richardson SA, Buttmacher AF, eds. *Childbearing: its social and psychological aspects.* Baltimore: Williams & Wilkins, 1967:142–43.

Mennella JS, Beauchamp GK. Maternal diet alters the sensory qualities of human milk and the nursling's behavior. *Pediatrics* 88:737–44, 1991.

Morse JM. "Euch, those are for your husband!" Examination of cultural values and assumptions associated with breastfeeding. *Health Care Women Int* 11:223–32, 1989.

Mulford C. Swimming upstream: breastfeeding care in a nonbreastfeeding culture. *JOGNN* 24:464–73, 1995.

Obermeyer CM, Castle S. Back to nature? Historical and cross-cultural perspectives on barriers to optimal breastfeeding. *Med Anthropol* 17:39–63, 1997.

Omuloulu A. Breastfeeding practice and breastmilk intake in rural Nigeria. *Hum Nutr Appl Nutr* 36A:445–51, 1982.

Orque MS, Block B, Monrroy LS. *Ethnic nursing care: a multicultural approach.* St. Louis: Mosby, 1983:19.

Rasbridge LA, Kulig JC. Infant feeding among Cambodian refugees. *MCN Am J Matern Child Nurs* 20:213–18, 1995.

Riordan J, Gill-Hopple K. Breastfeeding care in multicultural populations. *JOGN* 30:216–23, 2001.

Rodriguez-Garcia R, Frazier L. Cultural paradoxes relating to sexuality and breastfeeding. *J Hum Lact* 11:111–15, 1995.

Rossiter JC. The effect of a culture-specific education program to promote breastfeeding among Vietnamese women in Sydney. *Int J Nurs Stud* 31:369–79, 1994.

Sheeshka J et al. Women's experiences breastfeeding in public places. *J Hum Lact* 17:31–38, 2001.

Thiel de Bocanegra H. Breast-feeding in immigrant women: the role of social support and acculturation. *Hispani J Behav Sci* 20(4):448–67, 1998.

van Esterik P, Elliott T. Infant feeding style in urban Kenya. *Ecol Food Nutr* 18:183–95, 1986.

van Steenbergen WM et al. Nutritional transition during pregnancy in East Java, Indonesia: I. A longitudinal study of feeding pattern, breastmilk intake and the consumption of additional foods. *Eur J Clin Nurs* 45:67–75, 1991.

Whittemore RD, Beverly EA. Mandinka mothers and nurslings: power and reproduction. *Med Anthropol Q* 10:45–62, 1996.

Winikoff B, Castle MA, Laukaran VH, eds. *Feeding infants in four societies: causes and consequences of mothers' choices.* New York: Greenwood Press, 1988:187–201.

Woolridge M. *Breastfeeding in the US and Thailand* [presentation]. Miami: International Lactation Consultant Association, 1991.

Wrigley EA, Hutchinson S. Long-term breastfeeding: the secret bond. *J Nurse Midwifery* 35:35–41, 1990.

FAMILIES

Jan Riordan and Kathleen G. Auerbach

When health-care professionals help a breastfeeding mother and baby, they help a family. The breastfeeding family exists in a social context; therefore, care providers must recognize "family" as a group that is variously defined and experienced. They need to know about the family from which the mother comes and into which her child will be born and reared. Although every family is expected to perform similar functions, the ways in which those functions are recognized and accomplished will vary.

This chapter examines the family from a developmental perspective. The birth of a baby has rightly been described as a crisis because it forces new ways of behavior on all family members. This chapter discusses issues pertaining to the development of spousal and parent-child attachment, paying particular attention to the father's role as a helpmate and supporter of his partner's role as mother and as breastfeeder. It also addresses the special needs of the adolescent mother and of women living in poverty and considers certain negative family experiences, including violence against women and children.

Family Forms and Functions

Every individual experiences many family forms during a lifetime. Each form meets different needs

and serves different functions. A *traditional family* is one in which the mother is a full-time homemaker and primarily responsible for rearing the children, while her husband is a full-time worker outside the home. He is committed to seeing that the children are raised to adulthood, but his role in child rearing is seen as secondary to that of his wife. Although this form has often been viewed as ideal, it is experienced by only a small percentage of families. A *nuclear family* includes one or both parents and their children, either born to or adopted by them. An *extended family* usually contains lateral kin (such as aunts, uncles, or cousins) who occupy the same generational status as the parents and children in a nuclear family; or vertical kin (such as grandparents or grandchildren), who represent generations different from the parents and children in the nuclear family. In some cases, an extended family may include "fictive" kin, individuals who cannot trace lineage through blood or marriage ties to the nuclear family members but who act, and are treated, as if they were related.

Examining how different family forms are likely to be experienced throughout an individual's lifetime can provide insight into the stresses that an individual is likely to encounter. It also reveals the people on whom an individual will lean as he or she attempts to cope with those stresses.

Today's families increasingly recognize that child rearing will occupy only a portion of the entire life experience of a couple (regardless of the number of relationships experienced). Though a baby may be the outcome and reflection of the love its parents feel for one another, the presence of a baby nearly always adds stress to the new family unit.

One way to identify how babies represent potential and ongoing stress for the young couple is to recognize how family interaction patterns are affected by the addition of a new member. The couple relationship is easy to understand. Each member of the couple relates to the other in a spousal relationship. Add one child and two new relationships are added: one linking mother to child and one linking father to child. In addition, the couple is now husband and wife and mother and father. In assuming these roles, each partner may view the other in new ways that are not always supportive of a continued spousal role. When another child is added, the relationships become even more complex. The mother and the father each have a new relationship with the new baby. And a sibling relationship is added. Thus, in a two-person household, two relationships exist. In a three-person household, three relationships exist; in a four-person household, six relationships exist (Figure 25–1). With each new person added to the family, more than one new relationship is also added, because each person interacts with all other family members.

How families interact with health-care workers in a hospital or clinic setting is often related to the structure of the family in its own environment. If the husband/father makes all decisions relating to the family's role with the outside world, it may not be surprising that when the woman is asked when she will register at the hospital, her husband answers! This may not reflect the woman's dependency on her partner so much as the couple's established way of organizing their life. Likewise, if one were to ask the husband something that is the responsibility of the wife/mother, he would expect her to answer, for that is part of her role in their family.

Family Theory

Numerous theories have been applied to understanding how families work, what influences them to work effectively, and how best to offer assistance when they do not. One approach that seems particularly appropriate to health-care providers assisting young families is to recognize that they expand and contract at different times. Thus, over time, a given family is likely to experience a couple stage, an expansion stage, a stable stage, and a contracting stage.

Most families begin as *couples* and then move to the *expansion stage,* which begins with the first pregnancy and continues until the birth of the last child. In some families, this stage may be very brief, the duration of one pregnancy only; in other families, it might last more than two decades as new infants are added to the family. The *stable stage* occurs when members are neither added nor taken away. This stage is followed by the *contracting stage,* which begins when the oldest child leaves home, and it continues until the only individuals remaining in the home are the original couple or their replacements in the family (if one or both of the original couple has remarried). However one views the family from a developmental perspective, the number of stages identified is not nearly as important as are the tasks expected of the family at different times in the life cycle.

The health-care worker assisting breastfeeding mothers is most likely to interact with members of families during the expansion phase of the family's

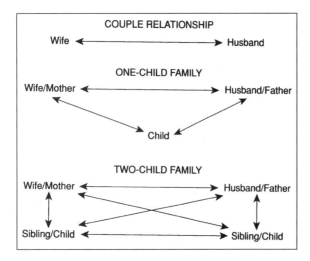

FIGURE 25–1. How relationships change with the addition of a new family member.

life cycle. It is important to recognize that varying tasks characterize this phase of the family, in order to identify how those tasks will influence decision making and behavior related to infant feeding and other aspects of the early mother-child relationship.

Social Factors that Influence Breastfeeding

The role of supportive significant others in the breastfeeding mother's life cannot be overemphasized. Social support is the mobilization and access to interpersonal resources when an individual attempts to deal with stress and the strains of life. Social support includes emotional support, esteem support, financial or skill support, and information or network support (McVeigh, 2000). Freedom of choice regarding infant-feeding decisions is always couched within the social context in which it occurs. Thus, in a family in which extended breast-

feeding is viewed as aberrant behavior, it is unlikely that the mother will choose to continue breastfeeding unless she receives a preponderance of positive, or at least neutral, reactions from her significant others. In another family in which breastfeeding is viewed as just another activity of two- or three-year-olds, extended breastfeeding is far more likely to occur. The interaction of mother and baby with significant others and their acceptance of such breastfeeding behavior must be taken into account when determining how best to assist her.

Table 25–1 summarizes some of the variables that impact breastfeeding and can be influenced by the health-care provider. The results of numerous studies have consistently revealed that the mother's *intention* to breastfeed is the single most important factor in deciding whether she will start breastfeeding and how long she will continue. Research findings have also shown us that intention is linked to social support, the mother's attitude, and her confi-

Table 25–1

HOW HEALTH-CARE PROVIDERS CAN INFLUENCE FACTORS THAT AFFECT BREASTFEEDING

Factor	Influence	Studies
Social support	Women with greater access to support choose to breastfeed more frequently and breastfeed longer. Support is manifested differently across ethnic and social groups.	Bar-Yam & Darby, 1997; Kessler et al., 1995; Balcazar, Trier, & Cobas, 1995
Intention to breastfeed	The majority of pregnant women decide how they will feed their baby before or early in pregnancy. A consistent positive association exists between intended and actual duration of breastfeeding.	Chapman & Perez-Escamilla, 2000; Grossman et al., 1990; Losh, Dungy, & Russell, 1995; Wambach, 1997
Attitude toward breastfeeding	There is increased breastfeeding initiation and duration by women with a positive attitude.	Avery et al., 1998; Janke, 1994; Tarkka, Paunonen, & Laippala, 1999
Mother's confidence	Women with high confidence breastfeed longer than women with low confidence.	Boettcher et al., 1999; Chezem, Friesen, & Boettcher, 2003; Dennis & Faux, 1999; O'Campo et al., 1992
Staff knowledge and attitudes toward breastfeeding	Lack of appropriate breastfeeding knowledge in hospital staff is a barrier to assistance from nurses and breastfeeding support.	Balcazar, Trier, & Cobas, 1995; Bernaix, 2000; Coriel et al., 1995; Freed et al., 1996; Lazzaro, Anderson, & Auld, 1995

dence in herself regarding breastfeeding. Age, education, employment, and previous breastfeeding experience are also factors that affect breastfeeding, but the health provider cannot change them. For example, most lactation consultants can report that they have worked with women whose firm intention to breastfeed resulted in their overcoming all types of adversity in order continue nursing; conversely, LCs can also describe cases where a mother has plenty of breastmilk and the baby is gaining weight well, yet for no obvious reason she weans the baby. We can assume that her intention was not to breastfeed (at least not for very long). Intention is invisible, but it can be measured with research tools (see Chapter 22).

Coupled with intention to breastfeed and maternal attitude toward breastfeeding, support systems influence choices (Kessler et al., 1995). In their study, Kaufman and Hall (1989) found that women who gave birth to preterm babies and who identified no source of support were six times more likely to stop breastfeeding than were women with a support system. Those most likely to continue breastfeeding could identify several persons who supported their feeding decision. As with mothers of preterm infants, teenage mothers also tend to breastfeed longer when they have a support system whose members affirm, aid, and affect in specific practical ways their mothering behavior, including breastfeeding.

Social support also influences the timing of weaning the baby from the breast. Usually pressure to wean from family members and others is more likely as the baby approaches or exceeds the age of 12 months. The support of others moves gradually from actively supporting breastfeeding in the first few months of the baby's life, to tolerating breastfeeding, to ignoring breastfeeding, to actively encouraging weaning. This last stage usually is manifested sometime after the baby's sixth month and may grow markedly stronger after the baby's twelfth month in the developed world, when others view the baby as too old to breastfeed.

Social support is especially important in the period immediately following any life stress. One such stress, insofar as it necessitates changes in relationships and life patterns, is childbirth. Another is breastfeeding, particularly if the mother has not breastfed an older child, or if she is the first in her family or group of friends to do so. Very often,

mothers and others assume that the mode of feeding is the cause of other infant behaviors. Working-class, first-time mothers are more likely to breastfeed, and to remain feeding the baby mother's milk when the mothers received support and information before, during, and after the baby's birth. Disadvantaged American mothers tend to follow the advice of grandmothers, especially if they live in the same house with the new mother. Health-care workers should recognize the grandmother as a key informant and network person and involve her in health care and advice giving.

Mothers who choose to combine breastfeeding and bottle-feeding have not been studied well but may make this choice to reap the infant health benefits of breastfeeding and to avoid embarrassment if they are not able to provide sufficiently for their infants (Boettcher et al., 1999). Lactation consultants may have the greatest influence on the mother who is undecided about infant feeding. Early studies indicated that health-care workers are not viewed as consistent support resources for breastfeeding. However, newer research and secondary analysis of these older data found that prenatal education was a strong predictor of intentions to breastfeed (Dennis, 2001).

The racial or ethnic group with which the mother identifies influences whose advice she seeks and follows relating to childbearing and breastfeeding. For example, among low-income Anglo-American women, the male partner, the mother's own mother, the grandmother, and the best friend tend to support breastfeeding. This pattern, with the exception of the best friend, is seen among Mexican-Americans as well.

Black women, by contrast, choose breastfeeding because of the information and encouragement they received from their physician during prenatal care (Bentley et al., 1999), and they reported minimal support from family members. In a qualitative study based on interviews (Corbett, 2000), an African-American woman told of the curiosity of friends who wanted to watch her because they had never seen a woman breastfeed. Breastfeeding seemed to them to be an unfamiliar and uncertain activity. This was reflected in a lower rate of breastfeeding than other groups.

For many Southeast Asian women, the mother-in-law is traditionally the person who makes decisions and gives advice about childbearing and child raising, including breastfeeding (Schneiderman, 1996). Most of the Vietnamese women who chose to breastfeed were encouraged by the experiences of significant others: "My mum breastfed all her nine children in Vietnam. She said breastmilk is good for a baby"; "My mother-in-law and my husband both wanted me to breastfeed, particularly because this is our first child" (Rossiter & Yam, 2000).

Generally, the more support a mother has for breastfeeding, the more likely she is to continue. Health-care workers should make clear their support of breastfeeding and encourage other family members to support this choice as well. After early discharge from the hospital, the degree of support that new mothers have at home is critical. It is imperative that the health-care provider learns whether the new mother will have someone to whom she can turn once she is at home. If she does not, steps need to be taken to provide follow-up support or to arrange for home visitation by one of the many social-service organizations that provide such assistance. In addition, much of the teaching that is viewed as appropriate during the postpartum period may have to be shifted to a prenatal setting in order to free what little time is available at discharge for key planning issues. Studies tell us that certain characteristics are associated with breast-

feeding over which health providers have no control, but it is helpful to be knowledgeable about their effects (Table 25–2).

When attempting to provide ongoing information and help, particularly when that help is provided outside an institutional setting, the LC needs to be aware of the social support system that the mother can tap.

Fathers

Fathers are often the most influential support persons in the early breastfeeding period (Bar-Yam & Darby, 1997; Gorman, Byrd, & VanDerslice, 1995; Pavill, 2002). In a study of culturally diverse fathers, 81 percent wanted their babies to be breastfed; more African-American men indicated they preferred their infants to be breastfed than had been reported in any previous study (Pollock, Bustamante-Forest, & Giaratano, 2002).

Fathers benefit from suggestions of specific ways by which they can support their partners. They can help the mother to achieve a comfortable breastfeeding position, provide nutritional support and household assistance, burp and console the infant, monitor the mother's fatigue level, limit visitors, and show delight in the decision to breastfeed.

Table 25–2

FACTORS THAT AFFECT BREASTFEEDING OVER WHICH HEALTH-CARE PROVIDERS HAVE NO INFLUENCE

Factor	Influence	Studies
Maternal age	Older women are more likely to choose to breastfeed and to breastfeed for a longer period.	Chapman & Perez-Escamilla, 2000; Nolan & Goel, 1995
Socioeconomic status	Varies by culture; women in higher SES levels in United States are more likely to breastfeed.	Raisler, 2000
Maternal education	Women with more education are more likely to breastfeed; varies according to culture.	Nolan & Goel, 1995
Maternal employment	Although not associated with breastfeeding initiation, employment is likely to shorten breastfeeding duration.	Chapman & Perez-Escamilla, 2000; Fein & Roe, 1998; Novotny et al., 2000; Visness & Kennedy, 1997
Previous breastfeeding experience	Experienced breastfeeders are more likely to breastfeed longer than those without previous experience.	Boettcher et al., 1999

Some investigators have emphasized the degree of similarity between mother-infant and father-infant behaviors in the attachment process in parents (Lamb, 1977). Classic among them is the observation of Greenberg and Morris (1974) that fathers present at the birth of their baby were more comfortable handling the baby sooner than those who were not present. Additionally, these investigators described a sequence of touching remarkably similar to that engaged in by mothers. The fingertips are used first to make tentative contact with the extremities of the newborn; a gradual movement of the hand follows this until the entire palm is in contact with the baby's chest, face, or head, progressing from gazing to touching in the first 15 minutes after birth (see Figure 25–2). Enthusiastic reactions to the neonate are more likely when the father is not anxious about the mother's postpartum condition (Tomlinson, Rothenberg & Carver, 1991).

When helping to care for a family breastfeeding a new baby, the lactation consultant can gather information by paying attention to the father. The fathers' reactions to their breastfeeding baby vary a great deal. Some will enthusiastically participate in putting the baby to breast, making suggestions, and generally helping. Others, often first-time fathers, will hang back and observe but not interact. A few

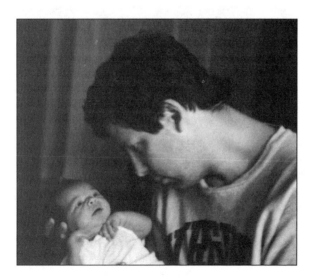

FIGURE 25–2. A father attaches to his baby in much the same way as the mother.

of these first-time dads look shell-shocked with the first few breastfeedings—perhaps partly due to the unfamiliarity of having their wife's breasts exposed.

When fathers enter into caregiving roles from the first with their infants, they are more likely to feel that they are an important part of the baby's life (Pavill, 2002). When teaching the mother how to put the baby to breast, involve the father by asking him to help with the breastfeeding—i.e., placing the baby, helping to control the baby's hands and arms, burping, etc. Likewise, when giving discharge instructions, address the father as well as the mother. The mother, already overloaded with stress, may not remember what you are saying, but fathers often pay close attention to what is said, sometimes adding questions of their own to the mother's questions.

Examinations of the ways in which men evolve into fathers suggests that the role remains relatively invisible to others; it is a relatively passive reflection of what is happening to the pregnant wife until after the baby's birth. When the baby begins to interact with the father directly, the father's role becomes more explicit—in his own mind as well as in the awareness of others (Jordan & Wall, 1993). Nurturing is a fundamental human quality that need not be gender-specific. That it is viewed as feminine by many must be seen as a cultural artifact rather than a reflection of inherent differences between males and females.

When a baby is born prematurely, Levy-Shiff et al. (1990) report that the frequency of the father's visiting the hospital predicted later positive fathering behavior after the baby's discharge. When the father visited frequently, the baby's weight gain was more rapid, and the father's involvement with the baby at 8 and 18 months after birth was more intensive, regardless of the mother's visiting patterns during the period when the baby was in the premature care unit.

Fathers play a vital role as a supporter of breastfeeding, particularly when they have a positive mind-set relating to breastfeeding (Earle, 2000; Pavill, 2002). Discussions of infant feeding in childbirth classes are effective in allaying concerns and dispelling myths. Humor is a perfect way to reach and help allay the father's anxieties about the coming baby. The use of Neil Matterson's cartoons in prenatal classes gets fathers to open up to discuss issues related to breastfeeding (see Internet Resources at the end of this chapter). Prenatal classes are also ideal for teaching fathers the benefits of breastfeeding and for informing a father of how he can help his breastfeeding wife without having to feed the baby.

The early days of fathering can be as stressful and disruptive to the father as mothering is to the mother; it is not at all unusual for a father to become disenchanted with his marriage after the first baby's birth. Jealousy of the physical and emotional closeness of mother and infant, feelings of uselessness during breastfeeding, sexual frustration, and repulsion from the sight of full, dripping breasts are all reported by some fathers. Some fathers feel ashamed of these emotions and tend not to talk about them; or they may joke about being jealous of the new baby (Gamble & Morse, 1993).

The most comfortable place for fathers to express these socially unacceptable but very real feelings is with other new fathers, many of whom may harbor the same feelings. Childbirth education classes and La Leche League groups often offer fathers-only classes, in which new fathers can openly share their feelings, tears, and perceptions about the realities of parenthood in an atmosphere of unconditional acceptance. Experienced fathers can help one another realize that they are not alone in having ambivalent feelings about the closeness between their breastfeeding wives and babies and about giving up certain pleasures in exchange for new responsibilities. One such father offered this report:

If I'd been more prepared that they would be this complete unit unto themselves, it would have been easier. For a while I felt left out, like I was around only to bring home the money and wasn't a part of it. I felt bad, then guilty about feeling bad. Before the baby came, my wife really spoiled me, you know, really adored and lavished attention on me. Then, whammo, she was pregnant three months after we were married and I wasn't getting that kind of treatment anymore. I resented it. Things really broke loose and we had a showdown; I finally had to open up and let her know how I really felt. After that, when it was all in the open, things got better. With the next baby, I don't think I'll go through those feelings again.

Support groups for new fathers validate a commitment to recognize the needs of new fathers—to help them develop coping strategies for optimal parenting of their breastfed baby. These father groups tend to attract men who are having more difficulty or who are more open in admitting to feeling stressed by making adjustments. These actions can potentially strengthen family relationships in the years ahead.

Implicit in the notion that breastfeeding prevents father-child closeness is acceptance of the assumption that the most (perhaps the only) significant way in which a father can interact with his child is by feeding her or him. Encourage the father to consider the many ways in which he can interact with the baby, particularly during the very early period when artificial feeding may increase the risk of breastfeeding failure (Figure 25–3). Several options are available:

- *Burping the baby after a feeding:* The necessity of burping is less an issue than is the opportunity to frequently hold the baby when the infant is likely to be relaxed and somnolent; if a burp is obtained, the father also gains a sense of having accomplished something tangible that can be translated to mean "I am a good father."

- *Changing the baby's wet diapers:* This activity occurs frequently.

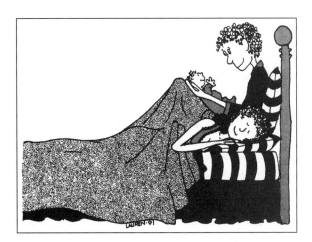

FIGURE 25–3. One of the many ways a dad helps with the care of a new baby.

- *Changing the baby's soiled diapers:* This, too, occurs frequently and, in breastfed infants, is far less unpleasant because the odor is less noxious than are the feces of an artificially-fed baby.

- *Giving the baby a massage:* Fathers who massage their babies often find that they can put a baby to sleep with little effort; such activity can assist an overstimulated or colicky baby to relax sufficiently to fall asleep.

- *Bathing the baby:* Assisting with the baby's bath is usually most happily accomplished after the baby begins to enjoy the bath.

- *Rocking the baby:* The father's involvement with the baby frees the mother to engage in other activities.

- *Singing or reading to the baby:* This activity can begin as soon after birth as the father wishes. Often, repeating the same songs that were played during the pregnancy will result in clear signals of recognition by the baby.

- *Playing with the baby:* Although the last item in this list, playing is usually the first thing that mothers will say fathers do best. Often, babies quickly identify fathers as "playthings" and mothers as "caregivers" because fathers spend far more time tickling or playing with an infant and less time in caregiving activities, such as changing, feeding, and cleaning. Such patterns are most likely to emerge in families in which clearly different gender roles are exhibited by mothers and fathers.

The Adolescent Mother

Few situations are fraught with more difficulties than that in which a child has a child. The younger the mother when her first baby is born, the more likely she is to encounter problems that will impede her ability to care for herself and her baby. Wherever young women are expected to complete a high school education before they embark on adult roles, such as marriage and raising children, the adolescent mother is a visible reminder that society has failed to protect her from too early parenthood and that she has failed her society, which expects that parenthood comes after marriage and at least minimal schooling. For such young women, school-

ing may not be resumed or may be delayed for several years, and marriage—if it occurs—comes after, rather than before, the birth of her child.

Although fewer adolescents in the United States are becoming pregnant, US rates are higher than many other industrialized countries. Generally, breastfeeding rates of adolescents are lower than adult women and they breastfeed for a much shorter period of time. Older adolescents are more likely to breastfeed than younger ones (Wambach & Cole, 2000).

Many caregivers assume that the young mother is neither interested in giving nor ready to give to another person by breastfeeding. On the contrary, a significant percentage of adolescents consider breastfeeding an option even if they ultimately bottle-feed (Leffler, 2000). Those who breastfeed make their decision before pregnancy or in the early stages of pregnancy, which suggests that adolescent mothers may be responsive to prenatal intervention to promote breastfeeding. The volume and properties in breastmilk of adolescents and adults are almost the same. Study data that report that adolescents produce less milk than women beyond the teen years are drawn from adolescent subjects who typically breastfeed less frequently and introduce formula earlier than do adult mothers (Motil, Kertz, & Thotathuchery, 1997).

Role modeling and peer influence are powerful tools for altering adolescent behavior. Not surprisingly, Wieman, DuBois, and Berenson (1998) found that using a breastfeeding video geared to teens was a key intervention to help adolescents overcome perceived barriers to breastfeeding. Likewise when Volpe and Bear (2000) started a Breastfeeding Educated and Support Teen (BEST) Club, more teenagers subsequently breastfed than those not in the club. Martens (2001) randomized breastfeeding education sessions that included a video to Canadian Ojibwa adolescents whose beliefs about breastfeeding subsequently improved. In another study, almost all (82 percent) participants in an Australian program for pregnant teenagers decided to breastfeed after attending prenatal classes (Greenwood & Littlejohn, 2002).

Concern about keeping their figure and not gaining weight concerns new mothers of all ages, but it is of particular concern to adolescents (Wambach & Cole, 2000). A study of Korean adolescents tested an intervention using a video that explained misconceptions about breastfeeding including body changes. Following the video Korean adolescents remained skeptical that breastfeeding might make them gain weight and "lose" their figure (Kim, 1998). These adolescents reported that "embarrassment" was a major barrier to breastfeeding. Even in a society in which most infants are breastfed, privacy and modesty are concerns of teenage girls and boys.

Teen mothers, when asked to identify their needs after the birth of their baby, identified the infant's health and medical needs first, followed by daily physical care of the infant, psychosocial needs of mothers and babies, and, finally, the mother's physical care. Mothers rated information about how to breastfeed and care for the breasts as important or very important. This high level of interest in meeting their baby's needs suggests that teen mothers are likely to be motivated to follow advice when it is offered. However, because many teenage mothers often share social characteristics that are linked with the choice not to breastfeed—such as lower educational attainment, low income, and unmarried status—fewer of these young women will choose to breastfeed (Peterson & Da Vanzo, 1992).

Usually, questions of new adolescent mothers are no different from those of older, more experienced women except for concerns about embarrassment with public exposure (Hannon et al., 2000). Most new mothers are concerned about how to help a baby grasp the breast, how to avoid sore nipples, and how to provide sufficient milk. In contrast, the kind of assistance offered to teens depends on their life situation. The teen mother living alone may need more frequent assistance and referral to a breastfeeding support group. The teen mother living with her own mother—who may be caring for the baby while the teen is in school—may need to know about resources on which she can draw for additional information and support about breastfeeding. The teen mother living with the baby's father or another male adult needs to know how to balance her baby's needs and other people's plans for her. For example, if her friends want her to go to a school dance, she needs help in recognizing that the baby cannot be abandoned until she returns. A happy breastfeeding experience, of whatever duration, helps the young mother to progress toward adulthood with a stronger and more positive sense of self and of what she wants for her children in the future.

The Low-Income Family

In the United States and other developed countries, fewer low-income mothers than their more affluent countrywomen choose to breastfeed. Poor women, whose babies most need the benefits of human milk, including its far lower production cost and its marked safety as compared to artificial baby milk, are least likely to breastfeed. As more women in the developing world seek to emulate women in the developed world, the cost to these women and the countries in which they live will be even higher.

Background variables can predict whether a low-income woman will breastfeed. Grossman et al. (1989) found that if a poor woman was married, if she had at least a high school education, if she began prenatal care in the first trimester, and if she was white or Hispanic, she was more likely to breastfeed. Libbus and Kolostov (1994) report that if the maternal grandmother breastfed and if the male partner endorsed breastfeeding, the low-income women in their study were more likely to intend to breastfeed and to view it as a positive experience.

Lack of Information

Sometimes the reasons for not breastfeeding are related to lack of information. Kistin, Abramson, and Dublin (1994) studied low-income black women in the United States and found that prenatal education sessions that included in-depth discussions about breastfeeding not only increased the likelihood that the women would choose to breastfeed but also the likelihood that they would act on their choice when the baby was born. These sessions also positively influenced the duration of breastfeeding. The investigators concluded that "greater educational efforts in institutions and offices serving black, low-income, urban women might yield significant changes in breastfeeding rates."

According to Hill (1988), attendance at classes designed to inform low-income mothers about breastfeeding significantly increased the likelihood that these women would choose breastfeeding, assuming that they attended two or more classes. Recognizing the benefits of breastfeeding and acknowledging a desire to breastfeed may come only after being informed of the differences between artificial feeding and human milk feeding. Therefore, simply adding a session on infant feeding to childbirth-preparation classes, or offering a one-time-only class on breastfeeding may be insufficient to break down the barriers protecting the passive bottle-feeding choice so that breastfeeding can be considered and then implemented.

Brent, Redd, and Dworetz (1995) found that prenatal and postpartum instruction from a lactation consultant resulted in more low-income women choosing breastfeeding. One-on-one intervention by a lactation consultant has positive impact on breastfeeding for mothers of all income levels (see Chapter 2).

Hospital Practices

Sometimes the reasons for choosing not to breastfeed are related to hospital factors. Perez-Escamilla et al. (1992) found that rooming-in positively affected breastfeeding duration among primiparas (but not multiparas) in their sample of low-income urban Mexican women. Additionally, those women who were rooming-in *and* who received breastfeeding guidance during the hospital stay also breastfed longer than those women who did not room-in and/or who did not receive additional assistance before they went home.

Overall, hospital practices concerning breastfeeding have improved in the last decade. Much of this improvement comes from two sources: consumer demand and the Baby-Friendly Hospital Initiative (BFHI), an international program created by the World Health Organization and UNICEF. BFHI has successfully incorporated practices that support breastfeeding into hundreds of hospitals across the world (Turner-Maffei, 2002). As noted in Chapter 1, the Baby-Friendly Hospital Initiative highlights ten steps by which any institution caring for new postpartum mothers and their neonates can assist the initiation of breastfeeding. As of this writing, certifying records of Baby-Friendly USA, the certifying body for BFHI in the United States, showed that only 34 US hospitals had achieved Baby-Friendly designation, less than 1 percent of

the approximately 5000 hospital in the United States. Administrators' concerns about the added cost of buying formula (a hospital cannot receive free formula and qualify for Baby-Friendly designation) and lack of professional support from community physicians and nursing staff present barriers to pursuing Baby-Friendly certification.

When the "ten steps" recommended by the BFHI are part of the caregiving offered in a given institution, the mothers who give birth and begin breastfeeding there are more likely to have an optimal experience. Three studies in particular have identified the ways in which implementation (or the failure of implementation) of these ten steps has influenced the breastfeeding experiences of the mothers who gave birth and subsequently received care in the hospitals whose care patterns were examined.

A leading example is the PROBIT study, a large randomized trial carried out in Belarus. Hospitals and clinics were randomized into two groups: an intervention group where the Baby-Friendly ten steps were implemented and a control group where no practice changes were made. Infants ($n = 17,000$) born at the intervention sites were breastfed significantly more often and had fewer gastrointestinal infections and atopic eczema than infants at the control sites (Kramer et al., 2001).

Merewood and Philipp (2001) overcame numerous obstacles in an inner-city teaching hospital in Boston to become the first Baby-Friendly hospital in Massachusetts. Receiving free formula was a major roadblock. After two years of work, nine of the ten steps were in place except for dealing with the estimated cost ($72,000) for buying formula instead of receiving it free. Further investigation showed that the quantity of formula listed by the formula company was far in excess of the amount actually used by the hospital. Using a standard figure of 20 cents per bottle of formula, the estimated annual cost of formula came to only $20,000, a far cry from the original $72,000 figure and a proportionately small amount of money for a large hospital with 1800 births per year.

Which of the ten steps have the greatest impact on breastfeeding? Wright, Rice, and Wells (1996) compared the effects of these steps on the likelihood that the women were fully breastfeeding at 4 months postpartum. The duration of breastfeeding was longer for women who did not receive formula in the hospital, who were not given discharge packs and/or coupons, and who roomed-in more than 60 percent of the time.

The Importance of Peer Counselors

The availability of an outside source of support in the first 6 weeks postpartum nearly always lengthens breastfeeding duration in a group of low-income women. Generally, the more breastfeeding friends the mother has, the longer she is likely to breastfeed.

Peer counseling programs, where breastfeeding support is given by trained lay female advisors knowledgeable about breastfeeding, is an effective intervention (Bronner, Barber, & Vogelhut, 2001; Dennis, 2001). Women who receive support from trained peer counselors in WIC Peer Counselor Programs are more likely to initiate breastfeeding and to breastfeed longer than those who do not. Peer counselors know current information, establish supportive personal relationships with women enrolled in the WIC program, refer women to breastfeeding specialists for problems, show enthusiasm, and facilitate breastfeeding (Raisler, 2000).

In one example of a successful program, Sciacca et al. (1995) included incentives as well as contact with a peer role model and found that the rate of exclusive breastfeeding at hospital discharge (88.5 percent versus 55.2 percent), 2 weeks (80.8 percent versus 34.5 percent), 6 weeks (50 percent versus 24.1 percent), and 3 months postpartum (42.3 percent versus 17.2 percent) were significantly higher when the mothers had peer role modeling and received a variety of incentives to choose to breastfeed.

The message that "Breast Is Best" has reached most low-income mothers. Regardless of how they choose to feed their baby, low-income women acknowledge the health benefits from breastfeeding. The choice not to breastfeed is often accompanied by a nagging feeling of guilt (Guttman & Zimmerman, 2000). Although younger low-income women in this same study believed that their community viewed breastfeeding as the optimal feeding method, they reported that friends and peers thought it "nasty." In addition, some of the low-income mothers associated breastfeeding with socioeconomic privilege. When poor women do breastfeed, the empowerment these women gain from the breastfeeding experience is an overlooked secondary effect that has potentially long-term impacts on other aspects of these women's lives (Locklin & Naber, 1993). These programs should be supported and expanded. Studies of the effectiveness of peer counseling are listed in Table 25–3.

The Downside of Family Experience

Not all families meander into the sunset "happily ever after." When a marriage dies, the death of that relationship affects not only the spouses but also any children they may have, as well as other relatives and friends. When the mother is breastfeeding, issues surrounding custody may be colored by the fact that she feels (rightly or wrongly) that the court should take her feeding method into consideration in deciding on custody arrangements and contacts of her children with her soon-to-be former husband.

The role of the lactation consultant in such a situation must necessarily be limited to advocacy for breastfeeding. Unless the LC is an attorney, points of law are not her concern. Instead, she can perform a valuable service by educating the judge and the mother's (and perhaps the father's) attorney about the importance of breastfeeding for the child's continued physical and psychological health (Suhler, Bornmann, & Scott, 1991). Questions may surface pertaining to how the father's attachment to the child is enhanced when breastfeeding is protected. Questions relating to the frequency of breastfeeding may not arise. In most cases, if the child is older than a few months, short periods of time with the father (away from the mother) are unlikely to place the breastfeeding relationship at risk. In addition, maintaining the child's attachment with both parents requires that child and parent are together as often (as much as possible) as they would have been if the marriage and joint parenting experience had remained intact.

When the mother is seeking to maintain breastfeeding beyond the time when most people in her society—including the judge and the attorneys—are likely to find it acceptable, the lactation consultant can provide information that again focuses on the health-preserving aspects of breastfeeding (Wilson-Clay, 1990). Such longer-term breastfeeding

Table 25–3

STUDIES OF PEER COUNSELORS

Arlotti et al. (1998) (N =36)	Women in Florida WIC program contacted by telephone, letter, or in person 5 times postpartum. Significant difference between groups in breastfeeding exclusivity but not in overall duration.
Caulfield, Gross, & Betley (1998) (N = 548)	Low-income pregnant women in Baltimore WIC program. Prenatal and postnatal weekly contact. Peer support associated with breastfeeding initiation but no duration at 7 to 10 days postpartum.
Dennis et al. (2002) (N = 256)	Randomized trial of primiparous postpartum women near Toronto. Telephone contact occurred within 48 hours post discharge and as needed. Significant statistical difference between groups in breastfeeding duration and exclusivity at 12 weeks.
Gross et al. (1998)	Interventions: video and/or peer-counseling vs. control group. Higher proportion of breastfeeding in intervention groups vs. control.
Haider et al. (2000) (N = 720)	Prenatal and postnatal home visits for pregnant women in Bangladesh. Significant differences between initiation and duration of exclusive breastfeeding (70% vs. 6%).
Kistin, Abramson, & Dublin (1994)	Low-income US women who received support from peer counselors had significantly greater breastfeeding initiation, exclusivity, and duration than those who did not.
Long et al. (1995) (N = 141)	Pregnant Native American women in Utah WIC program. Prenatal and postpartum contact by home and clinic visits and by telephone. Significantly higher breastfeeding initiation (84% vs. 70%) in intervention group but not duration at 12 weeks (49% vs. 36%).
Mongeon & Allard (1995) (N = 194)	Prenatal and postnatal telephone contact with 194 pregnant women in Montreal. No significant difference between control and intervention groups in breastfeeding duration.
Morrow et al. (1999)	Prenatal and postnatal home visits. One control and two intervention groups (Group I: 6 home visits; Group II: 3 home visits). Significant difference between groups in breastfeeding exclusivity (6 visits = 67%; 3 visits = 50%; control = 12%) and duration at 12 weeks.
Schafer et al. (1998) (N = 134)	Prenatal and postnatal face-to-face and telephone contact for rural, low-income women in Iowa. Significant differences between intervention and control groups in breastfeeding initiation (82% vs. 32%) and duration.
Shaw & Kaczorowski (1999) (N = 192)	Prenatal clinic visit and postnatal phone contact for low-income women in Tennessee WIC program. Significant higher breastfeeding initiation and duration for the intervention group.

does not necessarily limit reasonable visitation periods with the noncustodial parent, nor does it prevent periods of separation of the child from the mother. It does place the issue squarely where it must remain: preserving the best interests of the child.

Violence

The lactation consultant may become involved if a woman wishes to breastfeed or is breastfeeding and living in a situation in which she or her children are being threatened or assaulted. Whenever the lacta-

tion consultant believes that such violence is occurring, she has a responsibility to report this to relevant authorities who are in a position to intervene and to provide a safe haven for the mother and her children if she chooses to use it. Assisting with breastfeeding in abusive households need not be any different from assisting any other woman, although sensitivity to the abuse situation is necessary.

The number of breastfeeding women who are in homes in which they are being abused is not known. Acheson (1995) reported that lack of breastfeeding was associated with physical and sexual abuse of the woman or her children or both. In her retrospective review of 800 pregnancies and births in one family practice, Acheson noted that postpartum depression occurred more frequently in the absence of breastfeeding, as did marital problems and domestic violence. The author suggested that the striking 38-fold decrease in frequency of violence against women or their children (or both) when breastfeeding is practiced warrants careful scrutiny. One must ask the question: what is it about the decision to breastfeed, or its practice, that is related to nonviolent households? In other words, is the social dynamic in families in which violence occurs such that breastfeeding is also unlikely and, if so, what factors compose that social dynamic?

Childhood Sexual Abuse

A history of abuse during childhood, including sexual abuse, is likely to result in a variety of reactions to the breastfeeding experience. For example, if a mother wishes to breastfeed but cannot bring herself to allow the baby to latch onto the breast, and if issues such as breast tenderness are not immediately evident, the consultant must consider the possibility that the breast area was involved in the sexual abuse that the mother may have suffered years earlier.

Depending on one's definition of sexual abuse, as many as 20 percent of US women were sexually abused as children (Prentice et al., 2002). Given such a high incidence of abuse, beliefs surrounding the breasts' function and emotions pertaining to these beliefs are very likely to include fears that stem from experiences outside the realm of most lactation consultants' field of expertise.

Sexual abuse can have both short-term and long-term effects on the victim. Those effects may be expressed in various ways, including symptoms of posttraumatic stress disorder, cognitive distortions, emotional distress, impaired sense of self, interpersonal difficulties, health problems, and numerous kinds of avoidance behavior (including amnesia for the abuse-related events, dissociation, and self-destructive behaviors such as drug abuse). Sometimes, pregnancy (Grant, 1992) or childbirth (Courtois & Riley, 1992; Kitzinger, 1992; Rose, 1992) or breastfeeding can trigger recall that has previously been suppressed. One woman first regained memories of her abuse when she tried to breastfeed her infant. Because she was so unprepared for the sensations and the accompanying memories, she was unable to tolerate putting the baby to breast (Heritage, 1998). Coping mechanisms will vary from one woman to the next and may or may not be manifested during pregnancy, childbirth, or breastfeeding (Kendall-Tuckett, 1998).

When she has established rapport with the lactation consultant and feels safe, the mother may admit that she has been a victim of childhood abuse. In many cases, however, she may be unaware of the reason for her extreme discomfort, owing to brain changes that occur as a result of abuse and the coping mechanisms, including amnesia relating to the abusive events, that she may have practiced for years in order to maintain a facade of normalcy (Mukerjee, 1995). Additionally, if the mother recalls the abuse, she may or may not view it as being connected in any way with her current situation, including difficulties she may be having with breastfeeding.

Survivors of past sexual abuse may have symptoms of posttraumatic stress disorder These survivors frequently re-experience the traumatic event through nightmares or intrusive thoughts, such as sudden flashbacks of the abuse experience. If breastfeeding triggers sudden recall, nurturing her baby in this manner may be frightening to the mother. See Box 25–1 for suggestions on how to deal with a new mother who may have been sexually abused.

One mother had no recall of being abused until she put her baby to her breast for the first time. This action triggered a flashback so frightening to her that she screamed and immediately dropped the baby onto her bed. By the time hospital staff reached her, she was weeping and begged them to take the baby to the nursery. She subsequently cried uncontrollably each time she attempted to put her baby to her breast. The staff began helping her by giving her permission to pump her breasts to give her baby her milk. This action was something she could completely control. Being able to determine the degree of suction the pump exerted was important to her. After a week of pumping, during which time she gradually increased the pump pressure, she was willing to "try the baby again." She gradually was able to tolerate feedings without fearing that she would harm her baby.

BOX 25–1

Interventions for Helping Sexual Abuse Survivors

- Be gentle and respectful when asking questions about sexual abuse. Whether the LC should ask directly depends on the rapport established with the mother.
- Teach the normal course of lactation, including the normalcy of pleasurable aspects of breastfeeding. Offer suggestions to make breastfeeding more comfortable.
- Suggest that the mother express her milk if she is unable or unwilling to feed at breast. This may be the most comfort-

able way for the mother to provide her milk to her baby while protecting herself from what she perceives emotionally (consciously or unconsciously) as an assault on her person.
- Make a referral to a mental health-care provider. Be cautious about becoming the main source of emotional support.

Source: Derived from Kendall-Tuckett (1998).

Despite incidences like these, the evidence is actually contrary to what may be expected. At least one research group (Prentice et al., 2002) found that mothers who self-identify sexual abuse as a child are *more* likely, not less, to initiate breastfeeding than women who report no such abuse. Could it be possible that women who were sexually abused as children are more concerned about parenting? If this is true, then these women may

be more likely to breastfeed because it is a healthier way to feed a baby.

Acceptance of each woman's decision to breastfeed—however that is defined at a given time—may enable her to move closer to a full breastfeeding relationship with her baby and to further cement a healthy ongoing relationship with all of her children, something she may not have enjoyed in her family of origin.

Summary

Different family forms reflect different members' needs. Family developmental theories enable the health-care worker to identify specific family functions throughout the life cycle. The goal of the health-care provider should be to help the family to meet its own needs without her or his assistance. Key issues related to family functioning are the family's place within the support system and larger

community. The early parenting period is characterized by patterns of attachment behavior and ways that these reflect the growing competence of the parents as parents. In some cases, the father may be the mother's single and most constant supporter; in other situations, he may be less involved in the family and unlikely to support breastfeeding.

Key Concepts

- Examining how different family forms and relationships are likely to be experienced throughout a lifetime can provide insight into the

stresses that a family with a new baby is likely to encounter.

- How families interact with health-care workers in a hospital or clinic setting often is related to the family structure, stage, and tasks related to childbearing.

- A mother's *intention* to breastfeed is the single most important factor in deciding whether she will start breastfeeding and how long she will continue. In turn, her intention in regard to breastfeeding is influenced by her attitude and her confidence in herself and the social support she receives. The more support she has for breastfeeding, the more likely she is to continue.

- The racial or ethnic group with which the mother identifies also has a major influence on her infant-feeding choices.

- Fathers are often the most influential support persons in the early breastfeeding period.

- When fathers are involved with taking care of their new baby, they are more likely to have positive feelings that they are an important part of the baby's life.

- Experienced fathers can help one another realize that they are not alone in having ambivalent feelings about the closeness between their breastfeeding wives and babies and about giving up pleasures in exchange for new responsibilities.

- Role modeling and peer influence are powerful

tools in teaching breastfeeding to pregnant adolescents especially when their concerns about keeping their figure and embarrassment are addressed.

- Breastmilk of adolescents is the same as that of adult mothers except that adults breastfeed more often and for a longer time.

- Imparting information of the benefits and importance of breastfeeding through classes and other educational means increases the likelihood that women with a low income will choose to breastfeed.

- The peer counseling program of WIC has a proven powerful effect to promote and maintain breastfeeding through one-on-one contact and support.

- Several international studies have demonstrated the positive impact of changes in hospital practices on breastfeeding initiation and duration because of the influence of the Baby-Friendly Hospital Initiative.

- The number of hospitals designated as Baby-Friendly in the United States has grown very slowly. The major obstacle US hospitals encounter when in compliance with the Baby-Friendly Ten Steps is paying for formula used in the hospital and not receiving it free from formula companies.

Internet Resources

Academy of Pediatrics, information on breast-feeding:
www.AAP.org/family/brstguid.htm

Baby-Friendly USA:
http://home.onemain.com/~ct1008688/bfusa.htm

Cartoons by Neil Matterson:
www.mako.com.au/babymall/itsababy.htm

La Leche League stories by fathers:
www.lalecheleague.org

References

Acheson L. Family violence and breastfeeding. *Arch Fam Med* 4:650–52, 1995.

Arlotti J et al. Breastfeeding among low-income women with and without peer support. *J Comm Health Nurs* 15:163–78, 1998.

Avery M et al. Factors associated with very early weaning among primiparas intending to breastfeed. *MCN* 2(3):167–79, 1998.

Balcazar H, Trier CM, Cobas, JA. What predicts breastfeeding intention in Mexican-American and non-Hispanic white women? Evidence from a national survey. *Birth* 22:74–80, 1995.

Bar-Yam NB, Darby L. Fathers and breastfeeding: a review of the literature. *J Hum Lact* 13:45–50, 1997.

Bentley ME et al. Source of influence on intention to breastfeed among African-American women at entry to WIC. *J Hum Lact* 15:27–33, 1999.

Bernaix LW. Nurses' attitudes, subjective norms, and behavioral intentions toward support of breastfeeding mothers. *J Hum Lact* 16:201–19, 2000.

Boettcher JP et al. Interaction of factors related to lactation duration. *J Perin Educ* 8:11–19, 1999.

Brent NB, Redd B, Dworetz A. Breast-feeding in a low-income population: program to increase incidence and duration. *Arch Pediatr Adolesc Med* 149:798–803, 1995.

Bronner Y, Barber R, Vogelhut J. Breastfeeding peer counseling: results from the National WIC Survey. *J Hum Lact* 17:135–39, 2001.

Caulfied LE, Gross SM, Bentley ME. WIC-based interventions to promote breastfeeding among African-American women in Baltimore: effects on breastfeeding initiation and continuation. *J Hum Lact* 14:15–22, 1998.

Chapman DJ, Perez-Escamilla R. Maternal perception of the onset of lactation is a valid, public health indicator of lactogenesis stage II. *J Nutr* 130:2972–80, 2000.

Chezem J, Friesen C, Boettcher J. Breastfeeding knowledge, breastfeeding confidence and infant feeding plans: effects on actual feeding practices. *JOGNN* 32:40–47, 2003.

Corbett KS. Explaining infant feeding style of low-income Black women. *Ped Nurs* 15:73–81, 2000.

Coreil J et al. Health professionals and breastfeeding counseling: client and provider views. *J Hum Lact* 11:265–71, 1995.

Courtois CA, Riley CC. Pregnancy and childbirth as triggers for abuse memories: implications for care. *Birth* 19:222–23, 1992.

Dennis C. Breastfeeding initiation and duration: a 1999–2000 literature review. *JOGN Nurs* 31:12–32, 2001.

Dennis CL, Faux S. Development and psychometric testing of the Breastfeeding Self-Efficacy Scale. *Res Nurs Health* 22:399–409, 1999.

Dennis CL et al. A randomized controlled trial evaluating the effect of peer support on breastfeeding duration among primiparous women. *Can Med Assoc J* 166:21–28, 2002.

Earle S. Why some women do not breastfeed: bottle-feeding and father's role. *Midwifery* 16:323–30, 2000.

Fein S, Roe B. The effect of work status on initiation and duration of breast-feeding. *Am J Pub Health* 88:1042–46, 1998.

Freed GL et al. Methods and outcomes of breastfeeding instruction for nursing students. *J Hum Lact* 12:105–10, 1996.

Gamble D, Morse J. Fathers of breast-fed infant: postponing and types of involvement. *JOGNN* 22:358–65, 1993.

Gorman T, Byrd TL, VanDerslice J. Breast-feeding practices, attitudes, and beliefs among Hispanic women and men in a border community. *Fam Commun Health* 18:17–27, 1995.

Grant LJ. Effects of childhood sexual abuse: issues for obstetric caregivers. *Birth* 19:220–21, 1992.

Greenberg M, Morris N. Engrossment: the newborn's impact upon the father. *Am J Orthopsychiatry* 44:520–31, 1974.

Greenwood K, Littlejohn P. Breastfeeding intentions and outcomes of adolescent mothers in the Starting Out program. *Breastfeed Rev* 10(3):19–23, 2002.

Gross SM et al. Counseling and motivational videotapes increase duration of breast-feeding in African-American WIC participants who initiate breast-feeding. *J Am Diet Assoc* 98:143–48, 1998.

Grossman LK et al. Breastfeeding among low-income, high-risk women. *Clin Pediatr* 28:38–42, 1989.

———. The infant feeding decision in low and upper income women. *Clin Pediatr* 29:30–37, 1990.

Guttman N, Zimmerman DR. Low income mothers' views on breastfeeding. *Soc Sci Med* 50:1457–73, 2000.

Haider R et al. Effect of a community-based peer counselors on exclusive breastfeeding practices in Dhaka, Bangladesh: a randomized controlled trial. *Lancet* 356:1643–47, 2000.

Hannon PR et al. African-American and Latina adolescent mothers' infant feeding decisions and breastfeeding practices: a qualitative study. *J Adolesc Health* 26:399–407, 2000.

Heritage C. Working with childhood sexual abuse survivors during pregnancy, labor, and birth. *JOGN Nurs* 27:671–77, 1998.

Hill PD. Maternal attitudes and infant feeding among low-income mothers. *J Hum Lact* 4:7–11, 1988.

Janke JR. Development of the breastfeeding attrition prediction tool. *Nurs Res* 43:100–04, 1994.

Jordan PL, Wall Vr. Supporting the father when an infant is breastfed. *J Hum Lact* 9:31–4, 1993.

Kaufman KJ, Hall LA. Influences of the social network on choice and duration of breast-feeding in mothers of preterm infants. *Res Nurs Health* 12:149–59, 1989.

Kendall-Tuckett K. Breastfeeding and the sexual abuse survivor. *J Hum Lact* 14:125–30, 1998.

Kessler LA et al. The effect of a woman's significant other on her breastfeeding decision. *J Hum Lact* 11:103–9, 1995.

Kim Y. The effects of a breastfeeding campaign on adolescent Korean women. *Ped Nurs* 24:235, 1998.

Kistin N, Abramson, R, Dublin P. Effect of peer counselors on breastfeeding initiation, exclusivity, and duration among low-income urban women. *J Hum Lact* 10:11–15, 1994.

Kitzinger JV. Counteracting, not reenacting, the violation of women's bodies: the challenge for perinatal caregivers. *Birth* 19:219–20, 1992.

Kramer MS et al. Promotion of breastfeeding intervention trial (PROBIT): a randomized trial in the Republic of Belarus. *JAMA* 285:413, 2001.

Lamb ME. Father-infant and mother-infant interaction in the first year of life. *Child Dev* 48:167–81, 1977.

———, ed. *The role of the father in child development.* New York: Wiley, 1976.

Lazzaro DE, Anderson J, Auld G. Medical professionals' attitudes toward breastfeeding. *J Hum Lact* 11:97–101, 1995.

Leffler D. U.S. high school age girls may be receptive to breastfeeding promotion. *J Hum Lact* 16:36–40, 2000.

Levy-Shiff R et al. Fathers' hospital visits to their preterm infants as a predictor of father-infant relationship and infant development. *Pediatrics* 86:289–93, 1990.

Libbus MK, Kolostov LS. Perceptions of breastfeeding and infant feeding choice in a group of low-income mid-Missouri women. *J Hum Lact* 10:17–23, 1994.

Locklin MP, Naber SJ. Does breastfeeding empower women? Insights from a select group of educated, low-income minority women. *Birth* 20:30–35, 1993.

Long DG et al. Peer counselor program increases breastfeeding rates in Utah Native American WIC population. *J Hum Lact* 11:279–84, 1995.

Losch M, Dungy CI, Russell D. Impact of attitudes on maternal decision regarding infant feeding. *J Pediatr* 126:507–14, 1995.

Martens PJ. The effect of breastfeeding education on adolescent beliefs and attitudes: a randomized school intervention in the Canadian Ojibwa Community of Sagkeeng. *J Hum Lact* 17:245–55, 2001.

Merewood A, Philipp BL. Implementing change: becoming Baby-Friendly in an inner city hospital. *Birth* 28:36–40, 2001.

McVeigh CA. Satisfaction with social support and functional status after childbirth. *Mat Child Nurs* 25:25–30, 2000.

Mongeon M, Allard R. Controlled study of a regular telephone support program given by volunteers on the establishment of breastfeeding in [French]. *Can J Public Health* 86:124–27, 1995.

Morrow A et al. Efficacy of home-based peer counseling to promote exclusive breastfeeding: a randomized controlled trial. *Lancet* 353:1226–31, 1999.

Motil KJ, Kertz B, Thotathuchery M. Lactation performance of adolescent mothers shows preliminary differences from that of adult women. *J Adolescent Health* 20:442–49, 1997.

Mukerjee M. Hidden scars: sexual and other abuse may alter a brain region. *Scientific American* October 1995:14–15.

Nolan L, Goel V. Sociodemographic factors related to breastfeeding in Ontario: results from the Ontario health survey. *Can J Public Health* 86:309–12, 1995.

Novotny R et al. Breastfeeding duration in a multiethnic population in Hawaii. *Birth* 27:91–96, 2000.

O'Campo P et al. Prenatal factors associated with breastfeeding duration: recommendations for prenatal interventions. *Birth* 19:195–201, 1992.

Pavill BC. Fathers and breastfeeding. *Lifelines* 6:324–31, 2002.

Perez-Escamilla R et al. Effect of the maternity ward system on the lactation success of low-income urban Mexican women. *Early Hum Dev* 31:254–40, 1992.

Peterson CE, Da Vanzo J. Why are teenagers in the United States less likely to breastfeed than older women? *Demography* 29:431–50, 1992.

Pollock CA, Bustamante-Forest R, Giaratano G. Men of diverse cultures: knowledge and attitudes about breastfeeding. *JOGNN* 31:673–79, 2002.

Prentice JC et al. The association between reported childhood sexual abuse and breastfeeding initiation. *J Hum Lact* 18:219–26, 2002.

Raisler J. Against the odds: breastfeeding experiences of low income families. *Midwif Womens Health* 45:253–63, 2000.

Rose A. Effects of childhood sexual abuse on childbirth: one woman's story. *Birth* 19:214–18, 1992.

Rossiter JC, Yam BMC. The perceptions of Vietnamese women in Australia. Midwif Womens Health 45:271–6, 2000.

Schafer E et al. Volunteer peer counselors increase breastfeeding duration among rural low-income women. *J Hum Lact* 25:101–6, 1998.

Schneiderman JU. Postpartum nursing for Korean mothers. *Am J Mat Child Nurs* 21:155–58, 1996.

Sciacca JP et al. Influences on breast-feeding by lower-income women: an incentive-based, partner-supported educational program. *J Am Diet Assoc* 995:323–28, 1995.

Shaw E, Kaczorowski J. The effect of a peer counseling program on breastfeeding initiation and longevity in a low-income rural population. *J Hum Lact* 15:19–25, 1999.

Suhler AM, Bornmann PG, Scott JW. The lactation consultant as expert witness. *J Hum Lact* 7:129–40, 1991.

Tarkka M, Paunonen M, Laippala P. Factors related to successful breast feeding by first-time mothers when the child is 3 months old. *J Adv Nurs* 29:113–18, 1999.

Tomlinson PS, Rothenberg MA, Carver LD. Behavioral interaction of fathers with infants and mothers in the immediate postpartum period. *J Nurs Midwif* 36:232–39, 1991.

Turner-Maffei C. Using the baby-friendly Hospital Initiative to drive positive change. In: Cadwell K, ed. *Reclaiming breastfeeding in the United States.* Sudbury, MA: Jones and Bartlett, 2002:23–73.

Visness C, Kennedy K. Maternal employment and breastfeeding. *Am J Public Health* 87:945–50, 1997.

Volpe EM, Bear M. Enhancing breastfeeding initiation in adolescent mothers through the Breastfeeding Educated and Supported Teen (BEST) Club. *J Hum Lact* 16:196–200, 2000.

Wambach KA. Breastfeeding intention and outcome: a test of the theory of planned behavior. *Res Nurs Health* 20:51–59, 1997.

Wambach KA, Cole C. Breastfeeding and adolescents. *JOGNN* 29:282–94, 2000.

Wiemann C, DuBois J, Berenson A. Strategies to promote breast-feeding among adolescent mothers. *Arch Pediatr Adolesc Med* 152:862–69, 1998.

Wilson-Clay B. Extended breastfeeding as a legal issue: an annotated bibliography. *J Hum Lact* 6:68–71, 1990.

Wright A, Rice S, Wells S. Changing hospital practices to increase the duration of breastfeeding. *Pediatrics* 97:669–75, 1996.

APPENDIXES

A–H

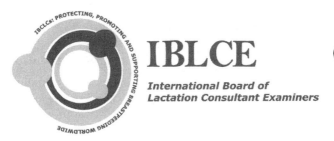

APPENDIX A

IBLCE
*International Board of
Lactation Consultant Examiners*

CLINICAL COMPETENCIES
FOR IBCLC PRACTICE

Much of the clinical practice of the International Board Certified Lactation Consultant (IBCLC) consists of systematic problem solving in collaboration with breastfeeding mothers and other members of the health care team. This checklist includes most of the clinical/practical skills that an entry level IBCLC needs in order to be satisfactorily proficient to provide safe and effective care for breastfeeding mothers and babies. The list is designed to encompass common breastfeeding situations and the challenges which are encountered most frequently by lactation consultants. Clinical instructors will be able to use this checklist as an appropriate guide in providing individualized education. A list of possible sites for obtaining clinical/practical experience appears at the end of the list of competencies.

Students are encouraged to become familiar with other documents that address the role of the IBCLC. The knowledge, skills and attitude inherent in the role of an IBCLC are summarized in a list of sixteen "Competency Statements" contained in the *International Board of Lactation Consultant Examiners Candidate Information Guide.* A more detailed description of the role is provided in the *Standards of Practice for IBCLC Lactation Consultants* published by the International Lactation Consultant Association (ILCA). Optimal breastfeeding care is clearly presented in twenty-four management strategies with rationales and references in *Evidenced-Based Guidelines for Breastfeeding Management during the First Fourteen Days,* also published by ILCA.

Communication and Counseling Skills

In all interactions with mothers, families, health care professionals and peers, the student will demonstrate effective communication skills to maintain collaborative and supportive relationships.

The student will:

- Identify factors that might affect communication (i.e., age, cultural/language differences, deafness, blindness, mental ability, etc.)

- Demonstrate appropriate body language (i.e., position in relation to the other person, comfortable eye contact, appropriate tone of voice for the setting, etc.)

- Demonstrate knowledge of and sensitivity to cultural differences

- Elicit information using effective counseling techniques (i.e., asking open-ended questions, summarizing the discussion, and providing emotional support)

- Make appropriate referrals to other health care professionals and community resources

The student will provide individualized breastfeeding care with an emphasis on the mother's ability to make informed decisions.

The student will:

- Assess mother's psychological state and provide information appropriate to her situation

- Include those family members or friends the mother identifies as significant to her

APPENDIX A (cont.)

- Obtain the mother's permission for providing care to her or her baby
- Ascertain mother's knowledge about and goals for breastfeeding
- Use adult education principles to provide instruction to the mother that will meet her needs
- Select appropriate written information and other teaching aides

History Taking and Assessment Skills

The student will be able to:

- Obtain a pertinent history
- Perform a breast evaluation related to lactation
- Develop a breastfeeding risk assessment
- Assess and evaluate the infant relative to his ability to breastfeed
- Assess effective milk transfer

Documentation and Communication Skills with Health Professionals

The student will:

- Communicate effectively with other members of the health care team, using written documents appropriate to the geopolitical region, facility and culture in which the student is being trained, such as: consent forms, care plans, charting forms/clinical notes, pathways/care maps, and feeding assessment forms
- Use appropriate resources for research to provide information to the health care team on conditions, modalities, and medications that affect breastfeeding and lactation
- Write referrals and follow-up documentation/letters to referring and/or primary health care providers that illustrate the student's ability to identify:
  - The mother's concerns or problems, planned interventions, evaluation of outcomes and follow-up

- Situations in which immediate verbal communication with the health care provider is necessary, such as serious illness in the infant, child, or mother
- Report instances of child abuse or neglect to specific agencies as mandated or appropriate

Skills for First Two Hours after Birth

The student will:

- Identify events that occurred during the labor and birth process that may negatively impact breastfeeding
- Identify and discourage practices that may interfere with breastfeeding
- Promote continuous skin-to-skin contact of the term newborn and mother through the first feeding
- Assist the mother and family to identify newborn feeding cues
- Help the mother and infant to find a comfortable position for latching-on/attachment during the initial feeding after birth
- Identify correct latch-on (attachment)
- Reinforce to mother and family the importance of:
  - Keeping the mother and baby together
  - Feeding the baby on cue—but at least 8 times in each 24 hour period

Postpartum Skills

Prior to discharge from care, the student will observe a feeding and effectively instruct the mother about:

- Assessment of adequate milk intake by the baby
- Normal infant sucking patterns
- How milk is produced and supply maintained, including discussion of growth/appetite spurts
- Normal newborn behavior, including why, when and how to wake a sleepy newborn

- Avoidance of early use of a pacifier and bottle nipple
- Importance of exclusive breast milk feeds and possible consequences of mixed feedings with cow milk or soy
- Prevention and treatment of sore nipples
- Prevention and treatment of engorgement
- SIDS prevention behaviors
- Family planning methods and their relationship to breastfeeding
- Education regarding drugs (such as nicotine, alcohol, caffeine and illicit drugs) and folk remedies (such as herbal teas)
- Plans for follow-up care for breastfeeding questions, infant's medical and mother's postpartum examinations
- Community resources for assistance with breastfeeding

Problem-Solving Skills

The student will be able to:

- Identify problems
- Assess contributing factors and etiology
- Develop an appropriate breastfeeding plan of care in concert with the mother
- Assist the mother to implement the plan
- Evaluate effectiveness of the plan

Skills for Maternal Breastfeeding Challenges

The student will be able to assist mothers with the following challenges:

- Cesarean birth
- Flat/inverted nipples
- Yeast infections of breast, nipple, areola, and milk ducts

- Continuation of breastfeeding when mother is separated from her baby
  - Milk expression techniques
  - Maintaining milk production
  - Collection, storage and transportation of milk
- Cultural beliefs that are not evidence-based and may interfere with breastfeeding (i.e., discarding colostrum, rigidly scheduled feedings, necessity of formula after every breastfeeding, etc.)
- Medical conditions that impact breastfeeding
- Adolescent mother
  - Strategies for returning to school
  - Maintaining milk production
- Nipple pain and damage
- Engorgement
- Plugged duct or blocked nipple pore
- Mastitis
- Breast surgery/trauma
- Overproduction of milk
- Postpartum psychological issues including transient sadness ("baby blues") and postpartum depression
  - Appropriate referrals
  - Medications compatible with breastfeeding
- Insufficient milk supply, differentiating between perceived and real
- Weaning issues
  - Safe formula preparation and feeding techniques
  - Care of breasts

Skills for Infant Breastfeeding Challenges

The student will be able to assist mothers who have infants with the following challenges:

- Traumatic birth

APPENDIX A (cont.)

- 35–38 weeks gestation
- Small for gestational age (SGA) or large for gestational age (LGA)
- Multiples/plural births
- Preterm birth, including the benefits of kangaroo care
- High risk for hypoglycemia
- Sleepy infant
- Excessive weight loss, slow/poor weight gain
- Hyperbilirubinemia (jaundice)
- Ankyloglossia (short frenulum)
- Yeast infection
- Colic/fussiness
- Gastric reflux
- Lactose overload
- Food intolerances
- Neurodevelopmental problems
- Teething and biting
- Nursing strike/early baby led weaning
- Toddler nursing
- Nursing through pregnancy
- Tandem nursing

Management Skills

The student will demonstrate the ability to:

- Perform a comprehensive breastfeeding assessment
- Assess milk transfer with:
  - AC/PC weights, using an electronic digital scale
  - Use of balance scale for daily weights
- Calculate an infant's caloric and volume requirements
- Increase milk production

Skills for Use of Technology Devices

The student will have up-to-date knowledge about breastfeeding-related equipment and demonstrate appropriate use and understanding of potential disadvantages or risks of the following:

- A device to evert nipples
- Nipple creams/ointments
- Breast shells
- Breast pumps
- Alternative feeding techniques
  - Tube feeding at the breast
  - Cup feeding
  - Spoon feeding
  - Eyedropper feeding
  - Finger feeding
  - Bottles and artificial nipples
- Nipple shields
- Pacifiers
- Infant scales
- Use of herbal supplements for mother and/or infant

Skills for Breastfeeding Challenges Which Are Encountered Infrequently

The following issues are encountered relatively infrequently, and may not be seen during the student's training. The entry-level lactation would not be expected to be proficient in these situations. The student will need to use basic skills to assist the mother and infant while seeking guidance from a more experienced IBCLC.

Infant:
- Infant with tonic bite/ineffective/dysfunctional suck
- Cranial-facial abnormalities, such as micronathia (receding lower jaw) and cleft lip and/or palate
- Down Syndrome

- Cardiac problems
- Chronic medical conditions, such as cystic fibrosis, PKU, etc.

Mother:
- Induced lactation and relactation
- Coping with the death of an infant
- Chronic medical conditions, such as MS, lupus, seizures, etc.
- Disabilities which may limit mother's ability to handle the baby easily, such as, rheumatoid arthritis, carpal tunnel syndrome, cerebral palsy, etc.
- HIV/AIDS: understanding of current recommendations based on the mother's access to safe replacement feeding

Skills for Meeting Professional Responsibilities

The student will demonstrate the following professional responsibilities:

- Conduct herself or himself in a professional manner, by complying with the *IBLCE Code of Ethics for International Board Certified Lactation Consultants* and the *ILCA Standards of Practice;* and by adhering to the *International Code of Marketing of Breastmilk Substitutes* and its subsequent World Health Assembly resolutions.
- Practice within the laws of the setting in which s/he works, showing respect for confidentiality and privacy.
- Utilize current research findings to provide a strong evidence base for clinical practice, and obtain continuing education to enhance skills and obtain/maintain IBLCE certification.
- Advocate for breastfeeding families, mothers, infants and children in the workplace, community and within the health care system.
- Use breastfeeding equipment appropriately and provide information about risks as well as benefits of products, maintaining an awareness

of conflict interest if profiting from the rental or sale of breastfeeding equipment.

Sites for Acquisition of Skills

The student may acquire clinical/practical skills in the following settings:

- Private practice IBCLC office
- Private practice OB, pediatric, family practice or midwifery office
- Public health department; Women, Infants and Children (WIC) Program (in the US)
- Hospital
  - Lactation services
  - Birthing center
  - Postpartum unit
  - Mother-Baby unit
  - Level II and Level III nurseries: Special Care Nursery, Neonatal Intensive Care Nursery
  - Pediatric unit
- Home health services
- Out-patient follow-up breastfeeding clinics
- Breastfeeding hotlines and warmlines
- Prenatal and postpartum breastfeeding classes
- Home births (if legally permitted)
- Volunteer community support group meetings

International Lactation Consultant Association (ILCA)
1500 Sunday Drive, Suite 102
Raleigh, NC 27607 USA
Phone: (919) 787-5181   Fax: (919) 787-4916
Email: info@ilca.org   Web: www.ilca.org

International Board of Lactation Consultant Examiners (IBLCE)
7309 Arlington BLVD, Suite 300
Falls Church, VA 22042 USA
Phone: (703) 560-7330   Fax: (703) 560-7332
Email: info@iblce.org   Web: www.iblce.org

APPENDIX B

CODE OF ETHICS

International Board of Lactation Consultant Examiners

Preamble

It is in the best interests of the profession of lactation consultants and the public it serves that there be a Code of Ethics to provide guidance to lactation consultants in their professional practice and conduct. These ethical principles guide the profession and outline commitments and obligations of the lactation consultant to self, client, colleague, society, and the profession.

The purpose of the International Board of Lactation Consultant Examiners (IBLCE) is to assist in the protection of the health, safety, and welfare of the public by establishing and enforcing qualifications of certification and for issuing voluntary credentials to individuals who have attained those qualifications. The IBLCE has adopted this Code to apply to all individuals who hold the credential of International Board Certified Lactation Consultant (IBCLC).

Principles of Ethical Practice

The International Board Certified Lactation Consultant shall act in a manner that safeguards the interests of individual clients, justifies public trust in her/his competence, and enhances the reputation of the profession.

The International Board Certified Lactation Consultant is personally accountable for her/his practice and, in the exercise of professional accountability, must:

1. Provide professional services with objectivity and with respect for the unique needs and values of individuals.

2. Avoid discrimination against other individuals on the basis of race, creed, religion, gender, sexual orientation, age, and national origin.

3. Fulfill professional commitments in good faith.

4. Conduct herself/himself with honesty, integrity, and fairness.

5. Remain free of conflict of interest while fulfilling the objectives and maintaining the integrity of the lactation consultant profession.

6. Maintain confidentiality.

7. Base her/his practice on scientific principles, current research, and information.

8. Take responsibility and accept accountability for personal competence in practice.

9. Recognize and exercise professional judgment within the limits of her/his qualifications. This principle includes seeking counsel and making referrals to appropriate providers.

10. Inform the public and colleagues of her/his services by using factual information. An International Board Certified Lactation Consultant will not advertise in a false or misleading manner.

11. Provide sufficient information to enable clients to make informed decisions.

12. Provide information about appropriate products in a manner that is neither false nor misleading.

13. Permit use of her/his name for the purpose of certifying that lactation consultant services have been rendered only if she/he provided those services.

14. Present professional qualifications and credentials accurately, using IBCLC only when certification is current and authorized by the IBLCE, and complying with all requirements when seeking initial or continued certification from the IBLCE. The lactation consultant is subject to disciplinary action for aiding another person in violating any IBLCE requirements

or aiding another person in representing herself/himself as an IBCLC when she/he is not.

15. Report to an appropriate person or authority when it appears that the health or safety of colleagues is at risk, as such circumstances may compromise standards of practice and care.

16. Refuse any gift, favor, or hospitality from patients or clients currently in her/his care which might be interpreted as seeking to exert influence to obtain preferential consideration.

17. Disclose any financial or other conflicts of interest in relevant organizations providing goods or services. Ensure that professional judgment is not influenced by any commercial considerations.

18. Present substantiated information and interpret controversial information without personal bias, recognizing that legitimate differences of opinion exist.

19. Withdraw voluntarily from professional practice if the lactation consultant has engaged in any substance abuse that could affect her/his practice; has been adjudged by a court to be mentally incompetent; or has an emotional or mental disability that affects her/his practice in a manner that could harm the client.

20. Obtain maternal consent to photograph, audiotape, or videotape a mother and/or her infant(s) for educational or professional purposes.

21. Submit to disciplinary action under the following circumstance: If convicted of a crime under the laws of the practitioner's country which is a felony or a misdemeanor, an essential element of which is dishonesty, and which is related to the practice of lactation consulting; if disciplined by a state, province, or other local government and at least one of the grounds for the discipline is the same or substantially equivalent to these principles; if committed an act of misfeasance or malfeasance which is directly related to the practice of the profession as determined by a court of competent jurisdiction, a licensing board, or an agency of a governmental body; or if violated a Principle set forth in the Code of Ethics for International Board Certified Lactation Consultants which was in force at the time of the violation.

22. Accept the obligation to protect society and the profession by upholding the Code of Ethics for International Board Certified Lactation Consultants and by reporting alleged violations of the Code through the defined review process of the IBLCE.

23. Require and obtain consent to share clinical concerns and information with the physician or other primary health care provider before initiating a consultation.

24. IBCLCs must adhere to those provisions of the International Code of Marketing of Breast-milk Substitutes which pertain to health workers.

To Lodge a Complaint

IBCLCs shall act in a manner that justifies public trust in their competence, enhances the reputation of the profession, and safeguards the interests of individual clients. To protect the credential and to assure responsible practice by its certificants, the IBLCE depends on IBCLCs, members of the coordinating and supervising health professions, employers, and the public to report incidents which may require action by the IBLCE Discipline Committee.

Only signed, written complaints will be considered. Anonymous complaints will be discarded. The IBLCE will become involved only in matters that can be factually determined, and will provide the accused party with every opportunity to respond in a professional and legally defensible manner.

Complaints which appear to fit the scope of the Discipline Committee's responsibilities should be sent to the:

Chair of the Discipline Committee
IBLCE
7309 Arlington Blvd., Suite 300
Falls Church, VA 22042-3215 USA

APPENDIX C

SUMMARY OF ELIGIBILITY PATHWAY REQUIREMENTS TO BECOME CERTIFIED BY IBLCE

An applicant for the IBLCE exam must document background or completion of courses in anatomy and physiology, sociology, psychology or counseling, child development, nutrition, and medical terminology. A degree (including diploma RN) in one of the licensed health care professions is sufficient documentation. Applicants with other academic backgrounds will need to provide specific documentation. Additionally, all applicants will need to provide evidence of a minimum of 45 documented clock hours of education in lactation, reflecting the Exam Content Outline, in the three years immediately proceeding the exam. The 45 documented clock hours are in place of the 30 hours of education previously required. You will still be required to accumulate the Breastfeeding Consultancy Practice hours for whichever standard pathway you qualify for.

Exam candidates are required to have extensive practical experience as breastfeeding consultants before taking the exam. Candidates must meet ALL of the requirements of ONE of these pathways:

Standard Pathways

Pathway A.*

- Four full years of post-secondary education, or a bachelor's, master's, or doctoral degree;
- Plus a minimum of 2500 hours of practice as a breastfeeding consultant;
- Plus a minimum of 30 hours of education specific to breastfeeding within three (3) years immediately prior to taking the exam.

Pathway B.*

- An associate degree, including a diploma RN, or at least two (2) full years of post-secondary academic credit;
- Plus a minimum of 4000 hours of practice as a breastfeeding consultant;
- Plus a minimum of 30 hours of education specific to breastfeeding within three (3) years immediately prior to taking the exam.

Pathway C.

- A bachelor's, or higher, degree with a concentration in human lactation from an accredited institution, including 900 precepted clinical hours in human lactation.

Recertification Pathways

Pathway T. Recertification by examination. Recertificants may recertify by 75 CERPs or by exam five (5) years after first passing the exam for certification. Ten (10) years after last passing the exam, recertificants must recertify again by exam.

Alternate Pathways

A candidate eligible to take the exam via an Alternate Pathway must have a minimum of 30 hours of education specific to breastfeeding within three (3) years immediately prior to taking the exam.

Pathway D.

- Doctor of Medicine;
- Plus a minimum of 900 hours of practice as a breastfeeding consultant;
- Plus a minimum of 30 hours of education specific to breastfeeding within three (3) years immediately prior to taking the exam.

Pathway E.* Exceptions based on individual cases for potential candidates who do not meet the educational background required by Pathway A or Pathway B.

- The total number of breastfeeding consultancy (BC) hours required is related to your post-secondary educational background.
- Usually 6000 to 8000 BC practice hours are required;
- Plus a minimum of 30 hours of education specific to breastfeeding within three (3) years immediately prior to taking the exam.
- Pathway E exceptions must be requested in a letter accompanying your completed exam application form.

Additionally, an exam candidate may also supplement Standard Pathway A or B or Alternate Pathway E with one or both of the following: Supplementary Pathways G and/or H.

Supplementary Pathways*

When applying to take the exam via Standard Pathway A or B or via Alternate Pathway E, a candidate may decrease (reduce) her/his total number of required breastfeeding consultancy practice hours by:

- 500 hours if they complete one of the following: Supplementary Pathways G or H.

- 1000 hours by participating in programs satisfying the requirements for both Supplementary Pathways G and H.

When you submit your application with one or both Supplementary Pathways, please be sure to circle your additional Pathway(s) on your Application Form.

Pathway G. An exam candidate who accumulates 150 Category L CERPs within three (3) years immediately prior to taking the exam will be credited with 500 practice hours toward her/his total number of required breastfeeding consultancy practice hours.

Pathway H. An exam candidate who completes 10–100 hours of planned, directly supervised clinical practice with an IBCLC who has been certified for at least five (5) years may reduce the required number of breastfeeding consultancy practice hours by a ratio of 5 to 1, up to 500 hours. That is, if the candidate interns for 10 hours:

- She/he will be credited with 50 BC hours;
- 20 hours of internship will be credited with 100 BC hours;
- 100 hours of internship will be credited with the maximum 500 BC hours.

This pathway does not include general supervised experience. Please consult the IBLCE office for further information.

Denotes pathways by which a candidate applying to take the exam via Standard Pathway A or B, or via Alternate Pathway E, can decrease her/his total number of breastfeeding consultancy practice hours by completion of one or both of the Supplementary Pathways (G and/or H).

Prototype Lactation Consultant Job Description

NOTE TO READER: This prototype job description is more inclusive than would be necessary in most settings.

QUALIFICATIONS NEEDED

1.0 Certification by the International Board of Lactation Consultant Examiners (IBLCE)

2.0 Minimum five years experience working with childbearing families or maternal health nursing.

OBJECTIVES

1.0 Document the need for a lactation consultant.

1.1 Establish baseline data on the numbers and percentages within the institution's patient base of mothers who initiate breastfeeding and the length of time they continue to breastfeed after hospital discharge.

1.2 Collect and analyze data to determine when and what kind of support the breastfeeding mother would like to receive prior to her baby's birth, while she is in the hospital, and after she returns home.

1.3 Survey other health-care providers who staff the institution and/or who work in the community which the hospital serves regarding their perceived need for the assistance and resources that a lactation consultant could provide.

2.0 Promote breastfeeding beyond the first few weeks of life and assist the mother to reach her goals for breastfeeding.

2.1 Develop and implement guidelines and standards of care for assisting breastfeeding mothers in all areas of the institution where they might be served (emergency room, obstetrics/gynecology, family medicine, the midwifery service, employee health, women's health service, pediatrics, and internal medicine).

2.2 Clarify roles of and perceptions about breastfeeding support among all health providers in the hospital, paying particular attention to those care providers who are most likely to serve lactating women and their breastfeeding infants.

2.3 Develop a reference library of breastfeeding materials appropriate for both health-care providers and mothers. Maintain and update a file of journal articles and references on the latest information on lactation.

2.4 Provide regular in-service education for all relevant medical, nursing, and ancillary staff.

2.5 Offer case conferences that highlight the particular needs of lactating mothers and/or their breastfeeding infants. Such case conferences may serve as a springboard for reexamining care routines and/or other aspects of the hospital experience of the mother–baby couple in question.

2.6. Set up a telephone warmline/hotline to provide continuing contact between the lactation consultant and the clients she has assisted in the hospital and others who may be referred to her for outpatient assistance.

2.7 Establish a regular follow-up system of continuing care for mothers first seen in the hospital. Such a system may be part of the warmline/hotline service, or it may consist of communication by postcard or letter, the incorporation of home visits by the hospital-based LC, or referral to a community-based breastfeeding counselor who makes home visits and reports back to the hospital LC.

2.8 Provide an outpatient service or clinic for persons who were not initially seen in the hospital and/or who are not in the immediate postpartum period.

2.9 Offer regularly scheduled prenatal breastfeeding classes to inform prospective mothers of the services available in the institution that support the breastfeeding course and to provide them with sufficient information to make an informed choice about infant feeding.

2.10 Offer regularly scheduled postpartum breastfeeding classes to mothers who give birth in the institution prior to their return home.

2.11 Provide breastfeeding equipment and devices when their use is appropriate to the lactating mother and her breastfeeding infant. Such equipment may include breast pumps, breast shells, breast shields, tube feeding devices, and the like. This equipment may be available for purchase or be rented. In situations where the lactation consultant is unable to provide rental or purchase options, she needs to develop an ongoing relationship with businesses in the community that offer such a service.

3.0 Coordinate the services of the professional staff to the benefit of the lactating mother and her breastfeeding baby.

3.1 Document care, teaching, and progress of the mother and baby on patient charts. In some cases, this may necessitate completing separate charts for the mother and the baby. Separate forms for documenting lactation can be appended to each patient's chart.

3.2 Confer regularly with the obstetrician, pediatrician, and nursing staff member on each patient's progress, special needs, and continuity of care.

3.3 Develop and/or review all literature relating to infant feeding that is distributed to patients in the hospital and those who return to the clinic.

3.5 Participate in a committee charged with evaluating relevant hospital policies that may influence the breastfeeding course of mothers and babies receiving care in the institution.

4.0 Participate in scholarly activities: research, publications, grants.

4.1 Maintain statistics on breastfeeding initiation and duration of all clients seen in the hospital or assisted in the outpatient clinic in order to periodically assess the contributions of lactation consultant services.

4.2 Implement "best practices" of patient care based on evidence from refereed, published articles.

4.3 Write and submit articles for publication in the health–profession journals and maternal–child literature.

4.4 Apply for grants to support new clinical care procedures, research protocols evaluating some aspect of the maternal lactation course, and/or infant breastfeeding patterns.

5.0 Serve as a speaker/participant in public and professional forums providing programs relating to lactation and breastfeeding.

RESOURCES NEEDED

1. Office space and supplies, including lockable file cabinets in which to store client information forms and other records relating to the performance of the LC's duties.

2. Electronic scale.

3. Supplies: washcloths, towels, diapers, drapes, comfortable couch and chairs, examination table and examining light, stethoscope, and blood pressure machine, in addition to breastfeeding pumps and devices.

4. Secretarial assistance in keeping with the needs of the LC or the LC practice.

5. Telephone with at least two lines. An answering machine and mobile phone are desirable in order that the LC may be reached when she is not at her desk.

APPENDIX D (cont.)

6. Small reference library.

7. Financial support for the LC to participate in regular continuing education at annual conferences, and the purchase of books and other resource materials relevant to the practice of lactation consulting.

8. Computer with Internet access, email, word processing, and spreadsheet software.

TABLES OF EQUIVALENCIES AND METHODS OF CONVERSION

METRIC

1 liter (L) = 10 deciliters (dl) = 1000 milliliters (ml) or 1000 cc
1 dl = 100 ml
1 ml = 0.001 L = 10^{-3} L = 1 cc = 1 gm (water)
1 kilogram (kg) = 1000 grams (gm)
1 gm = 100 milligrams (mg) = 0.001 kg
1 mg = 1000 micrograms (μg or mcg) = 0.001 gm = 10^{-3} gm
1 μg = 0.001 mg = 10^{-6} gm
1 nanogram (ng) = 0.001 μg = 10^{-9} gm
1 picogram (pg) = 0.001 ng = 10^{-12} gm

VOLUME

Household Measure	Fluid Ounces (Fl oz)	Metric Equivalent* (ml)	
1 cup (c)	8	240	1 c = 16 Tbsp
2 Tablespoons (Tbsp)	1	30	1 Tbsp = 3 tsp
1 Tbsp	not used	15	
1 teaspoon (tsp)	not used	5	
1 quart (qt)	32	960 ($\cong$ 1 L)	1 qt = 4 c = 2 pt
1 pint (pt)	16	480 ($\cong$ 500 ml)	1 pt = 2 c

WEIGHT

1 pound (1 lb or #) = 0.45 kg   1 oz = 28 gm $\cong$ 30 gm
1 kg = 2.2 lb
To convert lb to kg, divide lb by 2.2 *or* multiply lb by 0.45
To convert kg to lb, multiply kg by 2.2

LINEAR MEASURE

1 inch (in. or ″) = 2.54 centimeters (cm) ($\cong$ 2.5)
1 cm = 0.4 in.
To convert in. to cm, multiply in. by 2.5.
To convert cm to in., multiply cm by 0.4 *or* divide cm by 2.5.

TEMPERATURE

To convert Celsius (C) to Farenheit (F), °C = $\frac{5}{9}$ (°F − 32)
(Subtract 32, then multiply by $\frac{5}{9}$)
To convert Fahrenheit to Celsius, °F = $\frac{5}{9}$ °C + 32
(Multiply by $\frac{5}{9}$, then add 32)

Equivalent is given to nearest multiple of five. Number given in parentheses may sometimes be used to simplify calculations.
$\cong$ *means approximately equals.*

APPENDIX F

INFANT WEIGHT CONVERSION TABLE

The nurse or lactation consultant can use the table below to convert an infant's weight from pounds/ounces to grams (metric). Example: An infant weighing 5 pounds and 4 ounces (find 5 pounds in left column and then 4 ounces in top row) weighs 2381(intersecting number) grams. To convert grams to kilograms (kg), 1000 grams equal 1 kg, so the infant weighing 5 pound 4 ounces would weigh 2.38 kg. To convert from grams to pounds/ounces, find the gram number and read across the left (pounds) column and then read upward to the top (ounces) row to determine the infant's weight.

Ounces

	0	**1**	**2**	**3**	**4**	**5**	**6**	**7**	**8**	**9**	**10**	**11**	**12**	**13**	**14**	**15**
Pounds	**Grams**	28	57	85	113	142	170	198	227	255	283	312	340	369	397	425
1	454	482	510	539	567	595	624	652	680	709	737	765	794	822	850	879
2	907	936	964	992	1021	1049	1077	1106	1134	1164	1191	1219	1247	1276	1304	1332
3	1361	1389	1417	1446	1474	1502	1531	1559	1588	1616	1644	1673	1701	1729	1758	1786
4	1814	1843	1871	1899	1928	1956	1984	2013	2041	2070	2098	2126	2155	2183	2211	2240
5	2268	2296	2325	2353	2381	2410	2438	2466	2495	2523	2551	2580	2608	2637	2665	2693
6	2722	2750	2778	2807	2853	2863	2892	2920	2948	2977	3005	3033	3062	3090	3118	3147
7	3175	3203	3232	3260	3289	3317	3345	3374	3402	3430	3459	3487	3515	3544	3572	3600
8	3629	3657	3685	3714	3742	3770	3799	3827	3856	3884	3912	3941	3969	3997	4026	4054
9	4082	4111	4139	4167	4196	4224	4552	4281	4309	4337	4366	4394	4423	4451	4479	4508
10	4536	4564	4593	4621	4649	4678	4706	4734	4763	4791	4819	4848	4876	4904	4933	4961
11	4990	5018	5046	5075	5103	5131	5160	5188	5216	5245	5273	5301	5330	5358	5386	5415
12	5443	5471	5500	5528	5557	5585	5613	5642	5670	5698	5727	5755	5783	5812	5840	5868
13	5897	5925	5953	5982	6010	6038	6095	6095	6123	6152	6180	6209	6237	6265	6294	6322
14	6350	6379	6407	6435	6464	6492	6520	6549	6577	6605	6634	6662	6690	6719	6747	6776
15	6804	6832	6860	6889	6917	6945	6873	7002	7030	7059	7087	7115	7144	7172	7201	7228

BREASTFEEDING WEIGHT LOSS TABLE

Weight (grams)	5% Loss	10% Loss	Weight (grams)	5% Loss	10% Loss
2250	2138	2025	3250	3088	2925
2275	2161	2048	3275	3111	2948
2300	2185	2070	3300	3135	2970
2325	2209	2093	3325	3159	2993
2350	2233	2115	3350	3183	3015
2375	2256	2138	3375	3206	3038
2400	2280	2160	3400	3230	3060
2425	2304	2183	3425	3254	3083
2450	2328	2205	3450	3278	3105
2475	2351	2228	3475	3301	3128
2500	2375	2250	3500	3325	3150
2525	2399	2273	3525	3349	3173
2550	2423	2295	3550	3373	3195
2575	2446	2318	3575	3396	3218
2600	2470	2340	3600	3420	3240
2625	2494	2363	3625	3444	3263
2650	2518	2385	3650	3468	3285
2675	2541	2408	3675	3491	3308
2700	2565	2430	3700	3515	3330
2725	2589	2453	3725	3539	3353
2750	2613	2475	3750	3563	3375
2775	2636	2498	3775	3586	3398
2800	2660	2520	3800	3610	3420
2825	2684	2543	3825	3634	3443
2850	2708	2565	3850	3658	3465
2875	2731	2588	3875	3681	3488
2900	2755	2610	3900	3705	3510
2925	2779	2633	3925	3729	3533
2950	2803	2655	3950	3753	3555
2975	2826	2678	3975	3776	3578
3000	2850	2700	4000	3800	3600
3025	2874	2723	4025	3824	3623
3050	2898	2745	4050	3848	3645
3075	2921	2768	4075	3871	3668
3100	2945	2790	4100	3895	3690
3125	2969	2813	4125	3919	3713
3150	2993	2835	4150	3943	3735
3175	3016	2858	4175	3966	3758
3200	3040	2880	4200	3990	3780
3225	3064	2903	4225	4014	3803

APPENDIX H

Patient History

WELLSTART INTERNATIONAL℠

Patient History

Name:	☐ Boy Birthday: _____	Date of Visit: _____
Baby: _____	☐ Girl Age of Baby: _____	Birthplace (Hosp.): _____
Mother: _____	Age: _____	Home Phone: _____
Father: _____	Age: _____	
Obstetrician: _____		Phone: _____
Pediatrician: _____		Phone: _____
Mother's race/ethnicity (optional) _____		Mother's marital status _____

Reason for visit:	**For office use only**

MATERNAL HISTORY

1. Are you allergic to any medication?   ☐ Yes   ☐ No   If yes, please list: _____

2. Have you ever had any of the following? Please check (✔) all that apply.
   - ☐ Abnormal pap smear
   - ☐ Allergy/asthma
   - ☐ Anemia
   - ☐ Cancer
   - ☐ Constipation/hemorrhoids
   - ☐ Depression/blues
   - ☐ Diabetes
   - ☐ Diarrhea (chronic)
   - ☐ Heart disease
   - ☐ High blood pressure
   - ☐ Infertility
   - ☐ Kidney disease/bladder infection
   - ☐ Liver disease/hepatitis
   - ☐ Thyroid disorders
   - ☐ Tuberculosis
   - ☐ Venereal disease
   - ☐ None known
   - ☐ Other: _____

3. Have you ever had any of the following problems or procedures related to your breasts? Please check (✔) all that apply.
   - ☐ Biopsy
   - ☐ Lumps
   - ☐ Nipple problems: _____
   - ☐ Surgery: _____
   - ☐ None

4. Are you taking the following medications? Please check (✔) all that apply.
   - ☐ Prenatal vitamin-mineral
   - ☐ Other vitamins
   - ☐ Iron
   - ☐ Other minerals
   - ☐ Diet pills
   - ☐ Antihistamines/cold remedies
   - ☐ Laxatives/antacids
   - ☐ Diuretics/water pills
   - ☐ Aspirin/pain pills
   - ☐ Birth control pills
   - ☐ Antibiotics
   - ☐ None of the above
   - ☐ Other drugs _____
   - _____

PERINATAL HISTORY   List all pregnancies:

5.

Date Preg. Ended	Weeks Gesta- tion	Sex	Birth Weight	Complications of Pregnancy	Complications of Labor and Delivery	*Type of Anes- thesia	Type of Delivery		Breast- feeding Duration
							Vag.	C/S	

*Anesthesia: ① None   ② Local   ③ Epidural   ④ Spinal   ⑤ General (asleep)
              ⑥ Other _____

6. Did you have any of the following during this pregnancy? Please check (✔) all that apply.
   - ☐ Anemia (low iron level)
   - ☐ Fever
   - ☐ Gestational diabetes
   - ☐ High blood pressure
   - ☐ Nausea/vomiting (severe)
   - ☐ Premature labor
   - ☐ Urinary tract infection
   - ☐ Medication
   - ☐ None of the above
   - ☐ Other: _____

___/___/___/___

	For office use only
7. Did you have any of the following during this labor and delivery? Please check (✔) all that apply.	

7. Did you have any of the following during this labor and delivery? Please check (✔) all that apply.
☐ Drugs to induce or speed labor: If yes, for how long during labor was this drug administered? _____ hours
☐ Premature rupture of membranes
☐ Drugs to control high blood pressure
☐ Drugs to control pain
☐ Fever
☐ Antibiotics
☐ Hemorrhage
☐ None of the above
☐ Other:_____
_____

8. With this labor and delivery, did you have any of the following? Please check (✔) all that apply.
☐ Total labor longer than 30 hours
☐ Pushing stage longer than 2 hours
☐ Episiotomy or vaginal tear
☐ Tear that involved the rectum (a "third or fourth degree" laceration)
☐ Breech presentation
☐ Forceps delivery
☐ Vacuum extraction
☐ None of the above

9. How would you rate your labor and delivery experience? Please check (✔) all that apply.
☐ Easy
☐ Difficult
☐ Painful
☐ Long
☐ Short
☐ Average length
☐ Just what I'd expected
☐ Not what I'd expected
☐ Other_____

10. Postpartum complications? Please check (✔) all that apply.
☐ Urinary/other infection
☐ Excessive bleeding (hemorrhage)
☐ High blood pressure
☐ Low blood pressure (shock)
☐ None of the above
☐ Other_____

11. Did the baby have any of the following shortly after birth? Please check (✔) all that apply.
☐ Breathing problems
☐ Fever
☐ High hematocrit
☐ Jaundice
☐ Low blood sugar
☐ Meconium aspiration
☐ None of the above

☐ Medications:_____
☐ Other:_____

12. How soon after delivery did you first put your baby to your breast? _____

13. Were you and your baby separated for more than 2 hours while in the hospital?   ☐ Yes   ☐ No

14. While in the hospital, how many times in 24 hours did you breastfeed your baby?
☐ Less than 8 times   ☐ 8-12 times (every 2-3 hours)   ☐ More than 12 times

15. While in the hospital, what was the longest time between breastfeeding?   Day:_____   Night:_____

16. Did you have any of the following problems with your breasts or with breastfeeding your baby while in the hospital? Please check (✔) all that apply.
☐ Attachment difficulties
☐ Engorgement
☐ None
☐ Sleepy baby
☐ Sore nipples
☐ Other:_____
☐ Preference for one breast
☐ Not enough milk

17. While in the hospital, was your baby given any supplements?   ☐ Yes   ☐ No
If yes, please check (✔) all that apply.
☐ Formula
☐ Water (plain)
☐ Sugar water
How were supplements given?   ☐ Bottle   ☐ Syringe   ☐ Dropper   ☐ Other:_____

18. While in the hospital, was your baby given a pacifier?   ☐ Yes   ☐ No

19. Did you and your baby go home at the same time?   ☐ Yes   ☐ No

20. How old was the baby at discharge? _____

21. Are you currently having vaginal bleeding?   ☐ Yes   ☐ No
Have your menstrual periods returned?   ☐ Yes   ☐ No   Date of last menstrual period:_____

22. Which of the following family planning methods are you using or do you plan to use?   ☐ None
☐ Birth control pills   ☐ Other:_____

FEEDING HISTORY

23. How many times in 24 hours are you currently breastfeeding your baby?
☐ Less than 8 times   ☐ 8-12 times (every 2-3 hours)   ☐ More than 12 times

APPENDIX H (cont.)

24. What is the longest time between breastfeedings? Day:_____ Night:_____

25. How long does your baby nurse on each breast? _____

26. While nursing, do you sense any of the following in your breasts?
    ☐ Filling ☐ Burning ☐ Milk dripping from other breast
    ☐ Tingling ☐ Emptying ☐ None of the above
    ☐ Other_____

27. Who decides when the feeding is over? ☐ Mother ☐ Baby

28. At home, has your baby received:
    ☐ Water ☐ Formula ☐ Liquids, other than formula ☐ Any solids

29. How many times in 24 hours has your baby had: Wet diapers:_____ Bowel movements:_____

30. Does your baby spit up? ☐ Never ☐ Occasionally ☐ Often

31. Is the baby content or sleeping between feedings? ☐ Never ☐ Occasionally ☐ Often

32. Has your baby had any prolonged crying spells? ☐ Never ☐ Occasionally ☐ Often

33. Is your baby given a pacifier? ☐ Never ☐ Occasionally ☐ Often

34. Have you had any of the following problems with your breasts or with breastfeeding since coming home?
    ☐ Baby always hungry ☐ Cracked/bleeding nipples ☐ Painfully full breast(s)
    ☐ Baby prefers one breast ☐ Nipple pain ☐ Not enough milk
    ☐ Baby not interested ☐ Breast pain ☐ None of the above
    ☐ Other:_____

35. Have you used any of the following? Please check (✔) all that apply.
    ☐ Hand expression ☐ Nursing bra (no underwire) ☐ Breast or nipple shield
    ☐ Breast pump ☐ Nursing bra (with underwire) ☐ None of the above
    ☐ Breast cream
    ☐ Other:_____

36. Your bra size: before pregnancy_____ now_____

FAMILY HISTORY

37. Does anyone on either side of the baby's family have any of the following?
    ☐ Allergy (food) ☐ Allergy (hay fever) ☐ Genetic disease
    ☐ Allergy (asthma) ☐ Cancer (breast) ☐ Thyroid disease
    ☐ Allergy (eczema) ☐ Diabetes ☐ None of the above
    ☐ Other:_____

38. How are members of your family adjusting to the new baby?
    ☐ Very well ☐ Reasonably well ☐ Poorly ☐ Very poorly

39. Was your baby planned? ☐ Yes ☐ No

40. When did you decide to breastfeed this baby?
    ☐ Before pregnancy ☐ During pregnancy ☐ After delivery

41. How did you prepare for breastfeeding?
    ☐ Classes ☐ Reading ☐ Other:_____

42. Were you breastfed? ☐ Yes ☐ No ☐ Not known

43. Was your baby's father breastfed? ☐ Yes ☐ No ☐ Not known

44. How many previous babies have you breastfed?_____
    How long? _____ Why did you stop? _____

45. Why do you wish to breastfeed your baby? _____

46. Is there anyone in your household/family who feels you should **not** breastfeed this baby? ☐ Yes ☐ No

47. For how long do you plan to breastfeed this baby?_____

48. Why do you think you will discontinue breastfeeding at that time?_____

For office use only

49. What was the highest grade or year of regular school you have completed?
   - ☐ Less than 6 years
   - ☐ Elementary school (6 years)
   - ☐ Junior high school (9 years)
   - ☐ High school (12 years)
   - ☐ 2-year college (14 years)
   - ☐ 4-year college (16 years)
   - ☐ Graduate school (17+ years)

50. Usual occupation? Mother:_____ Father: _____
   When does mother plan to return to work? _____

NUTRITION

51. Did you see a nutritionist during your pregnancy? ☐ Yes ☐ No

52. Are there any foods that you avoid eating? ☐ Yes ☐ No If yes, what: _____
   Why? _____

53. Are you now on any of these special diets?
   - ☐ High protein
   - ☐ Low fat
   - ☐ Low salt
   - ☐ Weight loss
   - ☐ Diabetic
   - ☐ No special diet
   - ☐ Other:_____
   If yes, who suggested the diet?_____

54. Are you trying to lose weight at this time? ☐ Yes ☐ No If yes, how much?_____
   How? ☐ Less food/more exercise ☐ Program:_____ ☐ Other:_____

55. Are you a vegetarian? ☐ Yes ☐ No
   If yes, do you consume: ☐ Milk products (milk, cheese, yogurt) ☐ Eggs?

56. How would you rate your appetite presently? ☐ Good ☐ Fair ☐ Poor

57. How would you describe the type and amount of food in your household?
   - ☐ Enough of the kind you want
   - ☐ Sometimes not enough
   - ☐ Enough, but not always the kind you want
   - ☐ Often not enough

58. Are you receiving any of the following?
   - ☐ Food stamps
   - ☐ WIC
   - ☐ Other:_____
   - ☐ Medi-Cal
   - ☐ AFDC/welfare
   - ☐ Donated food/meals
   - ☐ None of the above

59. Do you have someone to help you shop and prepare meals? ☐ Yes ☐ No

60. How many times a day do you eat meals:_____ and snacks:_____

61. How many cups (8 oz.) of the following liquids do you usually drink per day?
   - _____ Water
   - _____ Juice
   - _____ Milk
   - _____ Sodas with sugar
   - _____ Diet soda, diet punch
   - _____ Punch, Kool-Aid, Tang
   - _____ Coffee
   - _____ Tea
   - _____ Other:_____

LIFESTYLE

62. How often are you now drinking beer, wine, hard liquor, or mixed drinks?
   - ☐ Daily ☐ Weekly ☐ Monthly ☐ Never
   When you drink, how many drinks do you have? ☐ One ☐ Two ☐ Three ☐ More

63. How many cigarettes do you smoke each day?
   - ☐ Do not smoke ☐ Fewer than 10 cigarettes ☐ 11-20 cigarettes ☐ More than 20 cigarettes

64. How often are you currently exercising (besides housework, child care)? _____
   What types of exercise do you do? _____

65. Do you feel you are getting adequate rest? ☐ Never ☐ Occasionally ☐ Often

66. Having a new baby can be a stressful time for the family. What other stresses are present in your home?
   - ☐ Relationship difficulties
   - ☐ Lack of help with home/child care
   - ☐ Moving
   - ☐ Financial concerns
   - ☐ Drug or alcohol use
   - ☐ Illness/death in the family
   - ☐ Other: _____
   - ☐ None of the above

67. Who lives with you in your home? _____

68. Do you have any other concerns about yourself, your baby, or your family's health that you would like to discuss during your appointment? ☐ Yes ☐ No
   If yes, what?_____

For office use only

APPENDIX H (cont.)

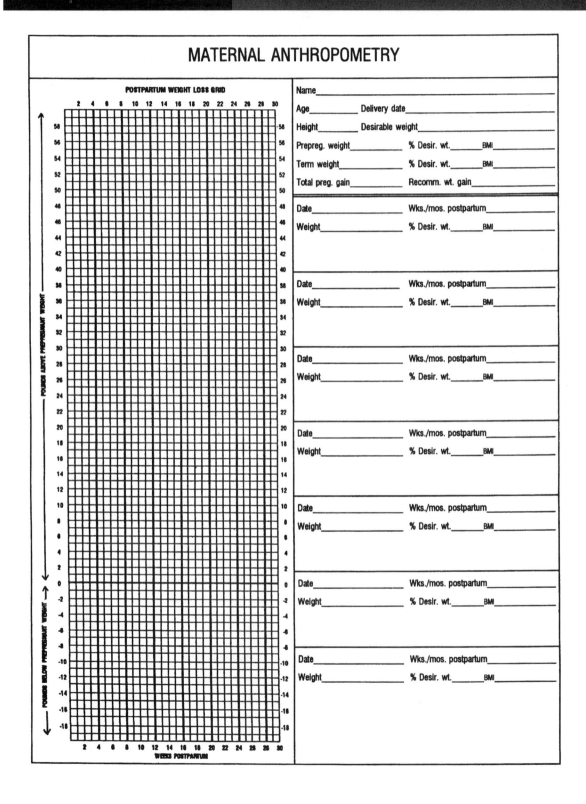

MATERNAL ANTHROPOMETRY

POSTPARTUM WEIGHT LOSS GRID

Name_____

Age_____ Delivery date_____

Height_____ Desirable weight_____

Prepreg. weight_____   % Desir. wt._____ BMI_____

Term weight_____   % Desir. wt._____ BMI_____

Total preg. gain_____   Recomm. wt. gain_____

Date_____   Wks./mos. postpartum_____

Weight_____   % Desir. wt._____ BMI_____

Date_____   Wks./mos. postpartum_____

Weight_____   % Desir. wt._____ BMI_____

Date_____   Wks./mos. postpartum_____

Weight_____   % Desir. wt._____ BMI_____

Date_____   Wks./mos. postpartum_____

Weight_____   % Desir. wt._____ BMI_____

Date_____   Wks./mos. postpartum_____

Weight_____   % Desir. wt._____ BMI_____

Date_____   Wks./mos. postpartum_____

Weight_____   % Desir. wt._____ BMI_____

Date_____   Wks./mos. postpartum_____

Weight_____   % Desir. wt._____ BMI_____

MOTHER'S PHYSICAL EXAM

Postpartum days/weeks	Height	Prepreg. wt.	Term wt.	Current wt.	Temperature	Blood Pressure

General Appearance	Thyroid

BREASTS RIGHT	LEFT

AREOLA	

NIPPLES	

SECRETION	

OTHER	

INFANT'S PHYSICAL EXAM

DATE	AGE	WEIGHT (pounds)	(kg.)	HEIGHT (inches)	(cm.)	H.C. (inches)	(cm.)
	Birth						
Discharge:							
Today:							

GENERAL/BEHAVIOR	Temp.

Head		Heart	
Eyes		Pulses	
Ears		Abdomen	
Nose		Genitalia	
Mouth		Extremities	
Thorax		Neuro	
Lungs		Skin	

APPENDIX H (cont.)

ORAL-MOTOR EXAMINATION/FUNCTION

MOUTH ☐ Normal	☐ Small	☐ Large		
JAW ☐ Normal	☐ Receding	☐ Asymmetrical	☐ Thrusting	☐ Tight/poor opening
LIPS ☐ Normal	☐ Cleft	☐ Passively pulled in	☐ Pursed/tight	
GUMS ☐ Normal	☐ Asymmetrical	☐ Excessive clenching/bite		
TONGUE ☐ Normal resting position	☐ Flat	☐ Clicking	☐ Elevated	☐ Up in back
☐ Behind gum line	☐ Thrust/protruding	☐ Sucking		
FRENULUM ☐ Normal	☐ Tight			
PALATE ☐ Normal	☐ High arch	☐ Cleft		

BREASTFEEDING OBSERVATION

Position used: ☐ Cradle   ☐ Side-sitting   ☐ Other:_____

Infant interest:
☐ Hungry, eager; goes easily to breast   ☐ Willing, falls asleep quickly   ☐ Awake, will not attach
☐ Willing but not insistent   ☐ Sleepy, totally disinterested   ☐ Awake, hungry, vigorously refuses
☐ Willing but distractable

Rooting:
☐ Normal   ☐ Depressed/absent   ☐ Tongue back/flat
☐ Frantic, disorganized

Attachment:
☐ Adequate   ☐ Lips retracted   ☐ Refuses
☐ Drops back   ☐ Arches   ☐ Other:_____
☐ Tongue malposition   ☐ Cries

Milk ejection reflex:
☐ Prior to attachment   ☐ After attachment, _____ sec / min   ☐ Not apparent after _____ sec / min
☐ Hyperactive

Effectiveness:
☐ Good suck/rhythm   ☐ Starts/stops repeatedly   ☐ Excessive vertical movement
suck:swallow _____:_____   ☐ Persistent flutter sucking only   ☐ Clenching/biting
☐ Becomes ineffective   ☐ Disorganized   ☐ Other:_____
☐ Weak suction   ☐ Cheeks dimple during suckling   _____
☐ Attached, not suckling   ☐ Tongue clicking   _____

Swallow: ☐ Normal   ☐ Uncoordinated

Comments:_____

Condition of nipple after nursing:
(Right)   Color_____ Shape_____   Color_____ Shape_____ (Left)

Infant stress
Mellow, relaxed — Disturbed slightly, not screaming — Screaming, resists positioning

Maternal stress: At ease, relaxed — Anxious — Extremely tense

Maternal interaction with infant:
☐ Hovering   ☐ Attentive   ☐ Harsh
☐ Over-stimulating   ☐ Affectionate   ☐ Detached

COMMENTS:

ASSESSMENT	PLAN
MOTHER	
INFANT	
BREASTFEEDING	

COUNSELING	☐ Attachment ☐ Bras ☐ Burping ☐ Expression/storage ☐ Family adjustment ☐ Feeding frequency, duration	☐ Hand expression ☐ How to tell if baby is getting enough ☐ Hydration ☐ Maternal nutrition ☐ Nipple care	☐ Positioning ☐ Rapid growth period ☐ Waking ☐ Other_____
HANDOUTS	☐ Blocked Duct ☐ Breastfeeding Record ☐ Calcium Rich Foods ☐ Candidiasis ☐ Daily Food Guide	☐ Engorgement ☐ Hand Expression ☐ How Much is Enough ☐ Is Baby Getting Enough ☐ Mastitis	☐ Mechanical Expression ☐ Increasing Milk Supply ☐ Milk Storage ☐ Nipple Trauma ☐ Other_____

Date	**Clinician**

Letter sent:_____

GLOSSARY

Achlorhydria Absence of hydrochloric acid in the gastric juice.

Acinus Acini (pl). Smallest division of a gland; a group of secretory cells arrayed around a central cavity. In the breast, an acinus secretes milk. *See also* Alveolus.

Acrocyanosis Bluish discoloration of the hands and feet in the newborn; also known as peripheral cyanosis. Normal after birth but should not persist beyond 24 hours.

Aerobic Requiring air for metabolic processes (e.g., aerobic bacteria). Normal skin, including the breast, is colonized with aerobic bacteria.

Allergen Any substance causing an allergic response. Foods, drugs, or inhalants may be allergens. Cow's milk protein is a common allergen of infants.

Allopathic medicine A form of medical care characterized by a focus on the cure of disease presenting in a given organ or organ system; also called *Western medicine;* nonallopathic medicine is sometimes called *traditional* or *folk medicine* to distinguish it from the allopathic form.

Alphalactalbumin The principal protein found in the whey portion of human milk; it assists the synthesis of lactose. The dominant whey protein in cow's milk and most artificial infant milks, betalactoglobulin, is not found in human milk. *See also* Noncasein protein.

Alveolar ridge The ridge on the hard palate immediately behind the upper gums. Movement of the infant's jaw during nursing compresses the areola between his tongue and alveolar ridge.

Alveolus Alveoli (pl). In the mammary gland, a small sac at the terminus of a lobule in which milk is secreted and stored. Groups of alveoli, organized in lobes, give the mammary gland the appearance of a "bunch of grapes." *See also* Acinus.

Anorectic abnormalities Anomalies of the rectum, the lower few inches of the large intestine, and the anus, the opening in the skin at the distal end of the rectum. An example is imperforate anus, in which the rectum ends in a blind pouch.

Antibody An immunoglobulin formed in response to an antigen, including bacteria and viruses. Antibodies then recognize and attack those bacteria or viruses, thus helping the body resist infection. Breastmilk contains antibodies to antigens to which either the mother or the infant has been exposed.

Antigen A substance that stimulates antibody production. It may be introduced into the body (as dust, food, or bacteria) or produced within it (as a by-product toxin).

Apoptosis Gk, *apo,* away, *ptosis,* falling. The sloughing off of a scab or other skin crust.

Applied research Research that focuses on solving or finding an answer to a clinical or practical problem.

Areola Pigmented skin surrounding the nipple. In order to suckle effectively, an infant should have his gums placed well back on the areola.

Artificial infant milk Any milk preparation, other than human milk, intended to be the sole nourishment of human infants.

Atopic eczema An inherited allergic tendency to rashes or inflammation of the skin. Exclusively breastfed infants are less likely to manifest this condition, as cow's milk protein is a common allergen.

Atresia, intestinal Congenital blockage or closure of any part of the intestinal tract.

Axilla The underarm area; in it lies the uppermost extent of the mammary ridge or milk line. Deep breast tissue (the axillary tail or tail of Spence) extends toward and sometimes into the axilla. This tissue may engorge the axilla along with the rest of the breast in the early postpartum period.

B cell A lymphocyte produced in bone marrow and peripheral lymphoid tissue; found in breastmilk. It attacks antigens and is one type of cell that confers cell-mediated immunity.

Bactericidal Capable of destroying bacteria. Breastmilk contains so many bactericidal cells that the bacteria count of expressed milk actually declines during the first 36 hours following milk expression.

Bacteriostatic Capable of inhibiting the proliferation of bacterial colonies.

BALT/GALT/MALT Bronchus/gut/mammary-associated immunocompetent lymphoid tissue. A lymphocyte pathway that causes IgA antibodies to be produced in the mammary gland after a lactating woman is exposed to an antigen on her intestinal or respiratory mucosa. These antibodies are then transferred through breastmilk to the breastfeeding infant, who thus may possess antibodies to antigens to which he has not been directly exposed.

Banked human milk *See* Donor milk.

Basic research Research that generates knowledge for the sake of knowledge.

Bioavailable That portion of an ingested nutrient actually absorbed and used by the body. Because the nutrients in breastmilk are highly bioavailable, low concentrations may actually result in more nutrients absorbed by the infant than do the higher, less bioavailable concentrations in cow's milk or artificial infant milks.

Bivariate Statistics derived from the analysis of the relationship between two variables.

Buccal pads Fat pads sheathed by the masseter muscles in young infants' cheeks. The buccal pads touch and provide stability for the tongue, which enhances the tongue's ability to compress breast tissue during suckling. Breastfed infants typically have a plump-cheeked appearance because of well-developed buccal pads.

Candidiasis A fungal infection caused by *Candida albicans;* also called "thrush." Common in the maternal vagina, it may inoculate the infant during delivery and be transferred from the infant's mouth to the mother's nipple. Candidiasis of the nipple and breast may produce intense nipple and breast pain. In the infant it may produce white spots on the oral mucosa and a bright red, painful rash ringing the anus. Formerly termed *moniliasis.*

Casein The principal protein in milks of all mammals. (The whey-to-casein ratio changes as lactation progresses).

Centers for Disease Control (CDC) An agency of the US Public Health Service established in 1973 to protect the public health of the nation by providing leadership and direction in the prevention and control of diseases and other preventable health conditions, and to respond to public health emergencies.

Certification The process by which a nongovernmental professional association attests that an individual has met certain standards specified by the association for the practice of that profession.

Chi-square A statistical procedure that uses nominal level data and determines significant differences between observed frequencies in relation to data and expected frequencies.

Colostrum The fluid in the breast at the end of pregnancy and in the early postpartum period. It is thicker and yellower than mature milk, reflecting a higher content of proteins, many of which are immunoglobulins. It is also higher in fat-soluble vitamins (including A, E, and K) and some minerals (including sodium and zinc).

Concept A word, idea, or phenomenon that generally has abstract meaning.

Conceptual framework A structure of interrelated concepts that may be generated inductively by qualitative research to provide a base for quantitative study.

Congenital infection An infection existing at birth that was acquired transplacentally. Infections that may be so acquired include HIV and TORCH organisms. *See also* Human immunodeficiency virus; TORCH.

Conjunctivitis Inflammation of the mucous membrane that lines the eyelid. In many traditional and some modern societies, fresh breastmilk is instilled into the eyes to alleviate this condition.

Construct A cluster of several concepts that has abstract meaning.

Contraception The prevention of conception. Breastfeeding provides significant contraceptive protection during the first few months postpartum—as long as the infant is fully breastfed and feeds during the night, and maternal menses have not resumed.

Cooper's ligaments Triangular, vertical ligaments in the breast that attach deeper layers of subcutaneous tissue to the skin.

Cord blood Blood remaining in the umbilical cord after birth.

Correlation coefficient A statistic that indicates the degree of relationship between two variables. The range in value is +1.00 to −1.00; 0.0 indicates no relationship, +1.00 is a perfect positive relationship, and −1.00 is a perfect inverse relationship.

Creamatocrit The proportion of cream in a milk sample, determined by measuring the depth of the cream layer in a centrifuged sample. An indicator of caloric content of milk, which must be used with care; the fat (and thus caloric) content of human milk varies between breasts, within a feeding, diurnally, and over the entire course of lactation.

Cross-nursing Occasional wet-nursing on an informal, short-term basis, usually in the context of child care.

Cultural relativism Recognition of the wide variation in beliefs and actions that pertain to given behaviors of humans living in different cultures.

Culture The values, beliefs, norms, and related practices of a given group that are learned and shared by the group members and that guide both the thoughts and behaviors of that group.

Cytoprotective Any condition or factor that protects cells from inflammation or death.

Deductive reasoning The process of reasoning from a general premise to the concrete and specific.

Dependent variable The variable the investigator measures in response to the independent or treatment variable; the outcome variable that is affected by the independent variable.

Design The blueprint or plan for conducting a study.

Diagnostic-related grouping (DRG) A group of diagnoses for health conditions that result in similar intensity of hospital care and similar length of hospital stay for patients hospitalized with those conditions.

Diffusion The process by which the molecules of one substance (e.g., a drug) are spread uniformly throughout a given substance (e.g., blood or plasma). *Passive diffusion* refers to movement from a higher to a lower concentration; *active diffusion* refers to movement from a lower to a higher concentration.

Disaccharide A carbohydrate composed of two monosaccharides. The principal sugar in human milk is lactose, a disaccharide; its constituent monosaccharides are glucose and galactose.

Donor milk Human milk voluntarily contributed to a human milk bank by women unrelated to the recipient.

Donor milk, pooled A batch of milk containing milk from more than one donor.

Dopamine The prolactin-inhibiting factor (PIF), or a mediator of the PIF, secreted in the hypothalamus. It blocks the release of prolactin into the bloodstream.

Drip milk Milk that leaks from a breast that is not being directly stimulated. Because its fat content is low, this milk should not be used regularly for infant feedings.

Ductules Small ducts in the mammary gland that drain milk from the alveoli into larger lactiferous ducts that terminate in the nipple.

Dyad A pair (e.g., the breastfeeding mother and her infant).

Eczema Skin inflammation or rash. *See also* Atopic eczema.

Eminences of the pars villosa Tiny swellings on the inner surfaces of the infant's lips that help the infant to retain a grasp on the breast during suckling.

Energy density The number of calories per unit volume; caloric density. Mature human milk averages 65 calories/dl, controlled largely by the fat content of the milk.

Envelope virus A virus that cannot infect other cells without its coat (envelope). If the envelope is destroyed (e.g., by heat or soap and water) the ability of the virus to produce infection is destroyed. Cytomegalovirus and the human immunodeficiency virus are two envelope viruses.

Epidemiology The study of the frequency and distribution of disease and the factors causing that frequency and distribution.

Epiglottis Cartilaginous structure of the larynx. An infant's epiglottis lies just below the soft palate. It closes the larynx when the infant swallows, ensuring passage of milk to the esophagus.

Estrogen A hormone that causes growth of mammary tissue during part of each menstrual cycle and assists in the secretion of prolactin during pregnancy; one of the hormones whose concentration falls sharply at parturition/birth.

Ethnocentrism A view that one's own culture and how it defines appropriate behavior is used as the basis for assessing all other cultures and behaviors.

Ethnography One research method that attempts to support an understanding of the beliefs, practices, and behavioral patterns within a (sub)culture from the perspective of the people living in that culture.

Exogenous Derived from outside the body—e.g., iron supplements that provide the infant with exogenous iron.

External validity The extent to which study findings can be generalized to samples different from those studied.

Extraneous variable Variables that can affect the relationship of the independent and dependent variables—i.e., interfere with the effect of treatment. In experimental studies, strategies for controlling these variables are built into the research design.

Foremilk The milk obtained at the beginning of a breastfeeding. Its higher water content keeps the infant hydrated and supplies water-soluble vitamins and proteins. Its fat content (1-2 gm/dl) is lower than that of hindmilk.

Frenulum Fold of mucous membrane, midline on the underside of the tongue, that helps to anchor the tongue to the floor of the mouth. A short or inelastic frenulum, or one attached close to the tip of the tongue, may restrict tongue extension enough to inhibit effective breastfeeding. Also called the *frenum.*

Galactagogue Any food or group of foods thought to possess qualities that increase the volume or quality of milk produced by the lactating woman who eats such foods.

Galactopoiesis Maintenance of established milk synthesis that is controlled by the autocrine system of supply and demand.

Galactorrhea Abnormal production of milk. It may occur under psychological influences or be a sign of pituitary tumor.

Galactose A monosaccharide present in small quantities in human milk. It is derived from lactose and, in turn, helps to produce elements essential for the development of the human central nervous system.

Gastroenteritis Inflammation of the stomach and intestines resulting from bacterial or viral invasion. Breastfed infants are at lower risk for this illness, as compared to nonbreastfed infants.

Gastroschisis An opening in the wall of the abdomen; a congenital malformation.

Gestational age An infant's age since conception, usually specified in weeks. Counted from the first day of the last normal menstrual period.

Half-life The length of time for half of a drug dosage to be eliminated; generally, it takes four to five half-lives for a drug to be considered completely or nearly completely eliminated. *Example:* Half-life of drug A is 12 hours; so 50 percent of the original drug dosage is eliminated in 12 hours; 25 percent of the drug remains after 24 hours; 12.5

percent remains after 36 hours; 6.25 percent remains after 48 hours; and only 3.12 percent remains after 60 hours (five half-lives from time of original dosage).

Harlequin sign Color change in which one side of the body is a deep color while the other side is light and pink; caused by vasomotor disturbances, which are usually transient.

Hematemesis Vomiting of blood. The bleeding is usually from the upper gastrointestinal (GI) tract. This means the bleeding may be from the upper small intestine (duodenum), the stomach, or the esophagus (the tube that connects the mouth and stomach).

Hindmilk Milk released near the end of a breastfeeding, after active let-down of milk. Fat content of hindmilk may rise to 6 percent or more, two or three times the concentration in foremilk.

Horizontal transmission Transmission of pathogens through direct contact. *See also* Vertical transmission.

Human immunodeficiency virus (HIV) A retrovirus that disarms the body's immune system, causing death from an opportunistic infection. The virus may be transmitted to unborn infants, and it is carried in the breastmilk, although not all breastfed infants born to HIV-positive mothers become ill themselves. The greatest risk to the infant is posed when a woman experiences her initial HIV-related illness while pregnant or breastfeeding.

Human milk Milk secreted in the human breast.

Human milk bank A service that collects, screens, processes, stores, and distributes donated human milk to meet the needs of infants, and sometimes adult recipients, for whom human milk has been prescribed by a physician.

Human milk fortifiers Nutrients added to expressed human milk to enhance the growth and nutrient balances of very low birth weight infants. Added protein may be derived from protein components of donor human milk or from cow's milk-based products. *See also* Lactoengineering.

Hydration The water balance within a body. Adequate hydration is necessary to maintain normal body temperature and for most other metabolic functions. Breastmilk is 90 percent water. Therefore, even in hot or dry climates, fully breastfed infants obtain all the water they require through breastmilk.

Hyperalimentation The intravenous feeding of an infant, commonly a very premature infant, with a solution of amino acids, glucose, electrolytes, and vitamins.

Hyperprolactinemia Higher-than-normal prolactin levels, which may result in spontaneous breastmilk production and amenorrhea. Causes include pituitary tumors and some pharmaceuticals. *See also* Prolactin.

Hypothalamus A gland that controls postpartum serum prolactin levels through release of dopamine. Inhibition of dopamine permits the release of prolactin, which controls the secretion of milk.

Hypoxia Inadequate oxygen at the cellular level, characterized by tachycardia, hypertension, peripheral vasoconstriction, dizziness, and mental confusion.

Immunity, active Immunity conferred by the production of antibodies by one's own immune system.

Immunity, passive Immunity conferred on an infant by antibodies manufactured by the mother and passed to the infant transplacentally or in breastmilk. Passive immunity is temporary but very important to the young infant.

Immunoassay Any method for the quantitative determination of chemical substances that uses the highly specific binding between antigen or hapten and homologous antibodies (e.g., radioimmunoassay, enzyme immunoassay, and fluoroimmunoassay).

Immunogen A substance that stimulates the body to form antibodies. *See also* Antigen.

Immunoglobulin Proteins produced by plasma cells in response to an immunogen. The five types are IgG, IgA, IgM, IgE, and IgD. IgG is transferred *in utero* and provides passive immunity to infections to which the mother is immune; IgA is the principal immunoglobulin in colostrum and mature milk; IgM is produced by the neonate soon after birth and is also contained in breastmilk. *See also* Noncasein protein.

Immunomodulator An agent in human milk that changes the function of another defense agent and thus enhances the quality or magnitude of the immune response.

Incidence How much a particular behavior is practiced at a given time. *Example*: How many women are initiating breastfeeding from time A to time B?

Incubation period The period between exposure to infectious pathogens and the first signs of illness.

Independent variable The experimental or treatment variable that is manipulated by the investigator to influence the dependent variable.

Inductive reasoning The process of reasoning from specific observations or abstractions to a general premise.

Infection control Practices—in hospitals formalized by protocols—that reduce the chance that infection will be spread between patients or between patients and staff. Hand washing and wearing of rubber gloves are two such practices.

Internal validity The extent to which manipulation of the independent variable really makes a significant difference on the dependent variable rather than on extraneous variables.

International Code of Marketing of Breast-Milk Substitutes A set of resolutions that regulate the marketing and distribution of any fluid intended to replace breastmilk, certain devices used to feed such fluids, and the role of health-care workers who advise on infant feeding. Intended as a voluntary model that could be incorporated into the legal code of individual nations in order to enhance national efforts to promote breastfeeding. Also referred to as the *WHO Code* or the *WHO/UNICEF Code*.

Intracellular Occurring within cells. Viruses live within other cells during part of their reproductive lives. Although viruses within cells may be passed to the infant in breastmilk, other cells in breastmilk enhance the destruction of these infected cells.

Intrauterine Within the uterus; *in utero*.

Intrauterine growth rate The normal rate of weight gain of a fetus. It is considered by many, but not all, physicians to be the ideal growth rate for premature infants.

Involution Refers to the return of the mammary gland to a nonproductive state of milk secretion.

Lactase Enzyme needed to convert lactose to simple sugars usable by the infant. Present from birth in the intestinal mucosa, its activity diminishes after weaning.

Lactase deficiency *See* Lactose intolerance.

Lactiferous ducts Milk ducts; the 15 to 24 tubes that collect milk from the smaller ductules and carry it to the nipple. They appear similar to stems on a bunch of grapes, the alveoli being the "grapes." The ducts open into nipple pores.

Lactobacillus bifidus Principal bacillus in the intestinal flora of breastfed infants. Low intestinal pH (5-6) of fully breastfed infants discourages the colonization of bacteria, which are common in feces of infants fed cow's milk-based infant milks.

Lactoengineering The process of fortifying human milk with nutrients (especially protein, calcium, and phosphorus) derived from other batches of human milk, in order to meet the special nutritional needs of very low birth weight infants. *See also* Human milk fortifiers.

Lactoferrin A protein that is an important immunological component of human milk. It binds iron in the intestinal tract, thus denying it to bacteria that require iron to survive. Exogenous iron may upset this balance. *See also* Noncasein protein.

Lactogenesis The initiation of milk secretion. The initial synthesis of milk components that begins late in pregnancy is termed *lactogenesis I;* the onset of copious milk production two or three days postpartum is termed *lactogenesis II*.

Lactose The principal carbohydrate in human milk, forming about 4 percent of colostrum and 7 percent of mature milk. A disaccharide, it metabolizes readily to glucose, which is used for energy, and galactose, which assists lipids that are laid down in the brain. Lactose also enhances calcium absorption, thus helping prevent rickets in the breastfed infant, and it inhibits the growth of pathogens in the breastfed infant's intestine.

Lactose intolerance The manifestation of lactase deficiency; the inability of the intestines to digest lactose, the principal carbohydrate in human milk. More common beyond early childhood because of diminished activity of intestinal lactase, especially in cultures that do not use milk or milk products as foods after early childhood.

Laryngomalacia Unusual flaccidity of laryngeal structures, a benign congenital condition that accounts for 70 percent of persistent stridor in infants.

Larynx The region at the upper end of the trachea (windpipe) through which the voice is produced. In the infant, the larynx lies close to the base of the tongue; during swallowing, it rises and is closed off by the epiglottis.

Lesion Circumscribed area of injured or diseased skin.

Let-down The milk-ejection reflex. Caused by contraction of myoepithelial cells surrounding the alveoli in which milk is secreted. It is under the control of oxytocin released during nipple stimulation and sometimes of psychological influences.

Leukocytes Living cells, including macrophages and lymphocytes, that inhabit breastmilk and combat infection.

Licensure The process by which an agency of state government grants permission to an individual, who is accountable for the practice of a profession, to engage in that profession. The corollary of licensure is that unlicensed individuals are prohibited from legally practicing licensed professions. The purpose of licensure is to protect the public by ensuring professional competence.

Ligand A small molecule that binds specifically to a larger molecule (e.g., the binding of an antigen to an antibody, or of a hormone to a receptor).

Likert scale A scale that primarily measures attitudes by asking respondents their degree of agreement or disagreement for a number of statements.

Lipase An enzyme that aids in the digestion of milk fats by reducing them to a fine emulsion.

Low birth weight The classification applied to infants weighing less than 2500 gm at birth.

Lymphadenopathy Abnormal swelling of the lymph nodes.

Lymphocyte A mature leukocyte; a lymph cell that is bactericidal.

Lyophilization A process of rapid freeze-drying of a fluid under a high vacuum. This process is used on human milk to obtain nutrient fractions used to fortify expressed human milk.

Lysozyme An enzyme in breastmilk that is active against *Escherichia coli* and *Salmonella*. *See also* Noncasein protein.

Mammary bud A clump of embryonic epithelial cells formed along the mammary ridge that extend into the underlying mesenchyme. It develops about 49 days postconception. From this bud sprout the precursors of the milk ducts.

Mammary ridge Also known as the milk line; the linear thickening of epithelial cells to each side of the midline of the embryo. Develops during weeks 5 through 8. Later this ridge differentiates into breast and nipple tissue.

Mammary secretory cells Cells capable of secreting breastmilk components. Also known as *lactocytes*.

Mammogenesis The development of the mammary gland and related structures within the breast.

Mandible The lower jaw. Strong, rhythmic closing of the mandible during breastfeeding drives the compression of the lacteriferous sinuses, one component of the infant's milking process.

Mature milk Breastmilk commonly produced after about 2 weeks postpartum and containing no admixture of colostrum. It is higher in lactose, fat, and water-soluble vitamins. Its exact composition varies in response to infant needs.

Median The middle number in a series of numbers; the number on either side of which exist an equal amount of numbers.

Mesenchyme The embryonic mesoderm.

Micrognathia Underdevelopment of the jaw, especially the mandible.

Milk/plasma ratio Quantity of a given drug or its metabolite in human milk in relation to its quantity in the maternal plasma or blood. Generally, if the M/P ratio exceeds 1.00, the drug is found in lesser quantities in milk than in plasma. If the M/P ratio is less than 1.00, the drug is found in lower quantities in milk than in plasma.

Mitosis A form of cell division in which each daughter cell contains the same DNA as the parent cell.

Morbidity The number of ill persons or instances of a disease in a specific population.

Mortality The number of deaths in a specific population.

Mucocutaneous Involving both mucous membranes and skin. Herpes blisters, for example, can form on both sites.

Multiparous Having carried two or more pregnancies to viability.

Myelination The process by which conducting nerve fibers develop a protective fatty sheath. The long-chain polyunsaturated fats that are important to myelination are abundant in human milk; they are much less abundant in cow's milk or cow's milk-based infant milks. Loss of myelin is a characteristic of the disease multiple sclerosis.

Myoepithelial cells Contractile cells. In the breast these cells surround the milk-secreting alveoli; their contraction forces milk into the milk ducts. When many of these cells contract at the same time, a let-down occurs. *See also* Let-down.

Necrotizing enterocolitis Inflammation of the intestinal tract that may cause tissue to die. Premature infants not receiving human milk are at markedly greater risk for this serious complication of premature birth.

Neurotransmitter A chemical that is selectively released from a nerve terminal by an action potential and then interacts with a specific receptor on an adjacent structure to produce a specific physiologic response.

Nipple A cylindrical pigmented protuberance on the breast into which the lactiferous ducts open. The human nipple contains 15 to 20 nipple pores through which milk flows.

Nipple, inverted A nipple that is retracted into the breast both when at rest and when stimulated.

Noncasein protein The protein in the whey portion of milk. Noncasein proteins in human milk include alphalactalbumin, serum albumin, lactoferrin, immunoglobulins, and lysozyme.

Nongovernmental organization (NGO) The title conferred by UNICEF on private organizations that command expertise valuable to UNICEF; such organizations are permitted to comment on and attempt to influence UNICEF activities. La Leche League International and the International Lactation Consultant Association are NGOs.

Nonparametric statistics Statistical procedures used when required assumptions for using parametric procedures are not met.

Nonprotein nitrogen (NPN) About one fourth of the total nitrogen in human milk is derived from sources, such as urea, other than protein. NPN contains several free amino acids, including leucine, valine, and threonine, which are essential in the young infant's diet because he cannot yet manufacture them.

Nutriment Any nourishing substance.

Oligosaccharide Carbohydrate, comprised of a few monosaccharides, present in human milk. Some oligosaccharides promote the growth of *Lactobacillus bifidus*, thus increasing intestinal acidity, which discourages the growth of intestinal pathogens.

Operational definition The explicit description of a concept or variable of interest in measurable terms.

Oxytocin A lactogenic hormone produced in the posterior pituitary gland. It is released during suckling (or other nipple stimulation) and causes ejection of milk as well as uterine contractions.

Palate, hard The hard, anterior roof of the mouth. A suckling infant uses his tongue to compress breast tissue against the hard palate.

Palate, soft The soft, posterior roof of the mouth, which lies between the hard palate and the throat. It rises during swallowing to close off nasal passages. Also called the *velum*.

Parametric statistics Statistical procedures used when a sample is randomly selected, represents a normal distribution of the target population, and is considered sufficiently large in size and interval level data are collected.

Parenchyma The functional parts of an organ. In the breast, the parenchyma include the mammary ducts, lobes, and alveoli.

Parenteral The introduction of fluids, nutrients, or drugs into the body by an avenue other than the digestive tract (intravenous, intramuscular).

Pasteurization The heating of milk to destroy pathogens. Milk banks commonly heat donor milk to 56° C for 30 minutes.

Pathogen A substance or organism capable of producing illness.

Peristalsis An involuntary, rhythmic, wavelike action. Commonly thought of in relation to food and waste products moving along the gastrointestinal tract. In order to strip milk from the breast, an infant's tongue uses a peristaltic motion that begins at the tip of the tongue and progresses toward the back of the mouth.

Pharynx The muscular tube at the rear of the mouth, through which nasal air travels to the larynx and food from the mouth travels to the esophagus. During infant feeding, contraction of pharyngeal muscles moves a bolus of fluid into the esophagus.

Pituitary An endocrine gland at the base of the brain that secretes several hormones. Prolactin, which is essential for production of milk, is secreted by the anterior lobe; oxytocin, which is essential for milk let-down, is secreted by the posterior lobe.

Placenta The intrauterine organ that transfers nutrients from the mother to the fetus. The expulsion of the placenta at birth causes an abrupt drop in estrogen and progesterone, which in turn permits the secretion of milk.

Polymastia The presence of more than two breasts. These additional structures, which usually contain only a small amount of glandular tissue, may occur anywhere along the milk line from the axilla to the groin.

Population The total set of individuals that meet the study criteria from which the sample is drawn and about whom findings can be generalized.

Power The probability that a statistical test will reject a null hypothesis when it should be rejected, or, in other words, detect a significant difference that does exist.

Premature infant One born before 37 weeks' gestational age, regardless of birth weight.

Primary infection The first incidence of illness after exposure to a pathogen.

Primiparous Having carried one pregnancy to viability.

Progesterone The hormone produced by the corpus luteum and placenta that maintains a pregnancy and helps develop the mammary alveoli.

Prolactin The hormone produced in the anterior pituitary gland that stimulates development of the breast and controls milk synthesis. Normal concentrations are 10-25 ng/ml in a nonpregnant woman; 200-400 ng/ml at birth.

Prone Lying on one's stomach.

Reliability The degree to which collected data are accurate, consistent, precise, and stable over time.

Respiratory syncytial virus (RSV) Organism causing a respiratory illness; breastfed infants are at less risk for this illness than are nonbreastfed infants.

Rickets Abnormal calcification of the bones and changes in growth plates that lead to soft or weak bones. Rarely seen in breastfed children; exceptions include those not exposed to the sun.

Rotavirus A class of viruses that are a major cause of diarrheal illness leading to hospitalization of infants. Breastfed infants are at less risk for illness caused by this organism, as compared to non-breastfed infants.

Rugae Corrugations on the hard palate behind the gum ridge that help the infant to retain a grasp on the breast during suckling.

Sample A subset of the population selected for study.

Sampling The procedure of selecting the sample from the population of interest.

Secretory IgA An immunoglobulin abundant in human milk that is of immense value to the neonate. It is synthesized and stored in the breast; after ingestion by the infant, it blocks adhesion of pathogens to the intestinal mucosa.

Secretory immune system The system that produces specific antibodies or thymus-influenced lymphocytes in response to specific antigens.

Sepsis The presence of bacteria in fluid or tissue.

Seroconvert A process by which serum comes to show the presence of a factor that previously has been absent, or vice versa. When antibodies to an infecting agent, such as cytomegalovirus, become present the person is said to have seroconverted.

Serological tests Tests performed on blood samples to ascertain the presence or absence of pathogens.

Seronegative Serum that does not demonstrate the presence of a factor for which tests were conducted; "tests negative."

Seropositive Serum that demonstrates the presence of a factor test for which tests were conducted; "test positive."

Serum Clear fluid portion of blood that remains after coagulation.

Serum albumin A protein in serum. *See also* Noncasein protein.

Smooth muscle The type of muscle that provides the erectile tissue in the nipple and areola.

Somatic Pertaining to the body, especially nonreproductive tissue.

Spontaneous lactation Secretion and release of milk unrelated to a pregnancy or to nipple stimulation intended to stimulate milk production.

Suck, suckle Used in this textbook interchangeably to mean the baby's milking action at the breast. In traditional usage, a baby at the breast "sucked," whereas a mother "suckled."

Sucking, nonnutritive Sucking not at the breast (e.g., as on a pacifier or on baby's own tongue); or, sucking at the breast characterized by alternating brief sucks and long rest periods during minimal milk flow. However, insofar as any milk is transferred, even this latter pattern of sucking may in fact be nutritive. *See also* Sucking, nutritive.

Sucking, nutritive Steady rhythmic sucking during full, continuous milk flow. Insofar as any milk is transferred, other sucking patterns also may be nutritive. *See also* Sucking, nonnutritive.

Supine Lying on one's back.

Symbiosis The intimate association of two different kinds of organisms. The breastfeeding dyad is considered by many to exemplify a mutually beneficial symbiosis.

Systemic immune system The nonspecific immune responses of the body.

Tachypnea An abnormally rapid rate of breathing.

Target population The population that is of interest to the investigator and about which generalizations of study results are intended.

T cells Any of several kinds of thymic lymphoid cells or lymphocytes that help to regulate cellular immune response. A subset of these cells (T4 cells) are preferentially attacked by the human immunodeficiency virus.

Teleological Describing the belief that all events are directed toward some ultimate purpose.

Thrombocytopenia Low levels of platelets in blood.

TORCH An acronym for organisms that can damage the fetus: toxoplasmosis, rubella, cytomegalovirus, herpes simplex.

Transcutaneous bilimeter A device that estimates bilirubin concentrations in the blood by measuring intensity of yellowish skin coloration.

Transitional milk Breast fluid of continuously varying composition produced in the first 2 to 3 weeks postpartum as colostrum decreases and milk production increases.

Transplacental Transferred from mother to fetus through the placenta. Nutrients and certain immunoglobulins are transferred to the fetus transplacentally; some infections also may be transferred.

Univariate The statistics derived from the analysis of a single variable—e.g., frequencies.

Universal precautions Guidelines for infection control, based on the assumption that every person receiving health care carries an infection that can be transmitted by blood, body fluids, or genital secretions.

Vaccine An infectious agent, or derivatives of one, given to a person so that his or her immune system will produce antibodies to that infection without a preceding illness.

Validity The degree to which collected data are true and represent reality; the extent to which a measuring instrument reflects what it is intended to measure.

Variable Attributes, properties, and/or characteristics of persons, events, or objects that are examined in a study.

Vertical transmission Transmission of infection from mother to child transplacentally or through breastmilk.

Very low birth weight Term applied to infants weighing less than 1500 gm at birth.

Virus Very small organisms that rely on material in invaded cells to reproduce. Viruses identified in breastmilk include cytomegalovirus, *herpes zoster, herpes simplex,* hepatitis, and rubella.

Water-soluble vitamins The B vitamins and vitamin C, pantothenic acid, biotin, and folate. These vitamins are present in serum; concentrations in breastmilk approximate those in serum. Concentrations reflect current maternal diet more directly than do fat-soluble vitamins (A, D, E, K).

Wet nurses Women who breastfeed infants who are not their own.

Whey The liquid left after curds are separated from milk. Alphalactalbumin and lactoferrin are the principal whey proteins. Whey forms soft, easily digested curds in the infant stomach. *See also* Casein; Noncasein protein.

Witch's milk Colostrum, formed under the influence of maternal hormones, which may be expressed from temporarily enlarged mammary tissue in the neonate's breasts.

World Health Organization (WHO) An agency of the United Nations charged with planning and coordinating global health care and assisting member nations to combat disease and train health-care workers.

Xerophthalmia Disease of the eyes caused by vitamin A deficiency; endemic in parts of Africa. Human milk is preventive.

INDEX

Note: *b* with page number indicates boxes, *f* indicates figures, *t* indicates tables.

FIGURE, TABLE, AND BOX CREDITS

p.1, Sergei Vasilev; p. 2, VH Brackett; p. 8, Courtesy of Children's Hospital, Islamabad, Pakistan; p. 10, Ladies Home Journal, 1895; p. 11, With permission from M.M. Coates; p. 13, Reproduced with permission from Pediatrics, Vol. 110, Pages 1103-1109, Figure 1, © 2002; p. 14, Reproduced with permission from Pediatrics, Vol. 110, Pages 1103-1109, Figure 1, © 2002; p. 19, Ross Laboratories, 2000; p. 22, From WHO/UNICEF, 1989; p. 24, Derived from Humenick & Gwai-Chore, 2001; p. 33, Adapted from de Oliveira, 2001; p. 35, IBLCE; p. 36, Derived from Steltzer, 2002; p. 37, Hafner-Eaton, 2000; p. 38, Derived from L. Smith, 2002; p. 41, With permission, Pardee Hinson; p. 48, Courtesy, St. Joseph Hospital; p. 52, With permission from Parris et al. Integrating nursing diagnoses, interventions, and outcomes in public health nursing practice, Nursing Diagnosis 10:49-56, 1999; p. 54, © Pat Lindsey; p. 65, Used with permission from WHO/PAHO, 1983; p. 69, Thomas Jefferson University Medical College Department of Radiology and Department of Pathology; p. 70, From DB Kopans, Breast Imaging, Philadelphia, 1989, JB Lippincott, p. 20/From DB Kopans, Breast Imaging, Philadelphia, 1989, JB Lippincott, p. 20; p. 71, Clement CD. Anatomy: a regional atlas of the human body. Philadelphia: Lea & Febiger, 1978; p. 73, Reproduced with permission, Victor B. Eichler, PhD; p. 74, With permission, Hale T. Medications and mother's milk, 9th ed. 2000:6; p. 87, From Woolridge, MW: The 'anatomy' of infant sucking. Midwifery 2:164-7, 1986; p. 89, Reproduced with permission from Hornell A et al. Breastfeeding patterns in exclusively breastfed infants: a longitudinal prospective study in Uppsala, Sweden. *Acta Pediatr* 88:203-11, 1999; p. 99, Humenick, 1987; p. 100, From Neville MC et al. *Am J Clin Nutr* 48:1375-86, 1988; p. 102, From Daly SE, Owens RA, and Hartmann PE, 1993; p. 107, Adapted from Anderson, 1985; p. 118, From Fan H, Conner R, Villarreal L. *The biology of AIDS*. Boston: Jones and Bartlett, 1989: 28; p. 121, Modified from Goldman AS et al. *J Pediatr* 100:663, 1982; p. 139, Reproduced with permission from Ross M, Gordon K, Paulina W. *Histology: a text and atlas*, 4th ed. Philadelphia: Lip-

pincott, Williams & Wilkins, 2002; p. 159, Adapted from Nuclear Regulatory Commission Guideline 8.39; p. 183, Sergei Vasilev; p. 191, From Anderson, 1989; p. 195, Adapted from Memorial Hospital, Colorado Springs, 2003; p. 199, Courtesy of Kay Hoover/Courtesy of Pat Bull; p. 201, Courtesy of Kay Hoover; p. 203, Adapted from Academy of Breastfeeding Medicine, 2002; p. 206, Snowden, Renfrew & Woolridge, 2002; p. 209, From Hall et al., 2002; p. 258, Reproduced with permission from Christina M. Smillie, MD, FAAP, IBCLC; p. 278, From Powers NG. *Clin Perinatol* 26(2)399-430, 1999, with permission from Elsevier; p. 279, From Powers NG. *Clin Perinatol* 26(2)399-430, 1999, with permission from Elsevier; p. 280, From Powers NG. *Clin Perinatol* 26(2)399-430, 1999, with permission from Elsevier; p. 284, From Dewey KG. *Pediatr Clin North Am* 48(1):87-104, 2001, with permission from Elsevier/From Dewey KG. *Pediatr Clin North Am* 48(1):87-104, 2001, with permission from Elsevier/From Dewey KG. *Pediatr Clin North Am* 48(1):87-104, 2001, with permission from Elsevier/From Dewey KG. *Pediatr Clin North Am* 48(1):87-104, 2001, with permission from Elsevier; p. 286, From Powers NG. *Clin Perinatol* 26(2)399-430, 1999, with permission from Elsevier; p. 287, From Nancy G. Powers, MD. Used with permission of the Academy of Breastfeeding Medicine, 2003; p. 288, Adapted from Powers NG. *Clin Perinatol* 26(2)399-430, 1999, with permission from Elsevier; p. 289, Adapted from Powers NG. *Clin Perinatol* 26(2)399-430, 1999, with permission from Elsevier; p. 290, With permission of Kathleen Auerbach/With permission of Kathleen Auerbach; p. 292, Courtesy of Gregory Notestine, with permission of Kathleen Auerbach; p. 298, Reproduced with permission of Pediatrics in Review. From Powers N, Slusser W. *Pediatr Rev* 18(5):147-161, 1997/Reproduced with permission of Pediatrics in Review. From Powers N, Slusser W. *Pediatr Rev* 18(5):147-161, 1997; p. 299, From Nancy G. Powers, MD. Used with permission of the Academy of Breastfeeding Medicine; p. 303, From Woolridge et al., 1984; Whitfield, Kay, & Stevens, 1981; p. 313, With permission from Bhutani, Johnson, & Silvier: *Pedi-*

atrics, 1999; p. 317, From Bhutani VK, Herschel M, Stevenson DK. *J Perinatol* 21:S01, 2001. Reproduced with permission.; p. 318, Academy of Pediatrics, 1994; p. 326, Courtesy of Neil Matteson, 1984; p. 332, Courtesy of Whittlestone, Benica, California; p. 333, Courtesy of WhisperWear, Marietta, Georgia; p. 324, Courtesy of Canon Babysafe Ltd., Suffolk, England/Courtesy of Hollister/Ameda-Egnell; p. 336, Courtesy of Medela Inc., McHenry, Illinois/Courtesy of Bailey Medical Engineering, Los Osos, California; p. 337, Courtesy of Medela Inc., McHenry, Illinois; p. 344, Derived from Hamosh et al., 1996; Williams-Arnold, 2000; Eteng et al., 2001; p. 347, Adapted from Curtis C. Frequently asked questions about used breastpumps. Available at: http://www.breastfeedingonline.com/; p. 350, (silicon nipple shields) Courtesy of Medela Inc., McHenry, Illinois; p. 379, With permission, The Lactation Support Program and Mothers' Own Milk Bank, Texas Children's Hospital, Houston, Texas/With permission, The Lactation Support Program and Mothers' Own Milk Bank, Texas Children's Hospital, Houston, Texas; p. 383, From Lucas et al., 1978; p. 385, With permission, The Lactation Support Program and Mothers' Own Milk Bank, Texas Children's Hospital, Houston, Texas/With permission, The Lactation Support Program and Mothers' Own Milk Bank, Texas Children's Hospital, Houston, Texas; p. 386, With permission, Rush Mothers' Milk Club, Rush-Presbyterian St. Luke's Medical Center; p. 389, Reproduced by permission of Royal Society of Medicine Press, London/Reproduced by permission of Royal Society of Medicine Press, London; p. 390, With permission, The Lactation Support Program and Mothers' Own Milk Bank, Texas Children's Hospital, Houston, Texas; p. 395, With permission, Rush Mothers' Milk Club, Rush-Presbyterian St. Luke's Medical Center; p. 407, Nyqvist KH et al. *J Hum Lact* 12:207-19, 1996; p. 411, Human Milk Banking Association of North America, Inc.; p. 415, Adapted from HMBANA, 2003, and Tully, 2002; p. 416, Human Milk Banking Association of North America, Inc.; p. 418, Arnold LDW. *J Hum Lact* 15:55-59, 1999. Reprinted by permission of Sage Publications, Inc.; p. 421, Human Milk Banking Association of North America, Inc., 2003; p. 422, With permission of the Mothers' Milk Bank, Denver, Colorado; p. 423, With permission of the Mothers' Milk Bank, Denver, Colorado; p. 424,

Arnold LDW. Donor milk banking in Scandinavia. *J Hum Lact* 15:55-59, 1999. Reprinted by permission of Sage Publications, Inc./Eitenmiller, 1990; p. 435, Sergei Vasilve; p. 444, Adapted from the American Dietetic Association, 1996; p. 445, Adapted from the Institute of Medicine, 1992; p. 447, Adapted from the Institute of Medicine, 1989; p. 469, Goldfarb L, Newman J. The protocols for induced lactation. Unpublished, 2002; p. 479, Adapted from Hale, 2002; p. 481, Adapted from Coakley & Mountford, 1985; p. 488, US Census Bureau, 1998, 2000; p. 490, From Hallmark Corporation, Kansas City, Missouri; p. 494, Adapted in part from Auerbach K, *J Nurs Midwifery* 35:26, 1990; Biancuzzo, 1999; Bocar, 1997; p. 499, Adapted from Bar-Yam, 1998; p. 500, From Hallmark Corporation, Kansas City, Missouri; p. 514, Adapted from Gill et al., 1988; p. 515, From Erikson, 1963; Piaget & Inhelder, 1969; p. 516, From Servonsky & Opas, 1987, p. 180; p. 522, From Mott S: Nursing care of children and families. Addison-Wesley Publication, 1993, p. 206; p. 543, Adapted from Arnold, 1999, p. 544, Provided courtesy of the Cleft Palate Foundation, 1-800-24-CLEFT, http://www.cleftline.org; p. 545, Childbirth Graphics Ltd., Rochester, New York; p. 546, With permission from Sallie Page-Goertz; p. 547, With permission from Sallie Page-Goertz/ With permission from Sallie Page-Goertz; p. 548, With permission from Sallie Page-Goertz; p. 549, Adapted from Minchin et al., 1996, and Popper, 1998; p. 551, (intravenous infusion), Courtesy of Debi Bocar; p. 553, Adapted from Gorelick, Shaw, and Murphy, 1997, and Armon et al., 2001; p. 562, March of Dimes Perinatal Data Center, 2000; p. 565, Courtesy of David Barnes, DDS; p. 592, Adapted from Moore & Nichols, 1997; p. 593, Adapted from Wilson, 2003; p. 595, Reprinted from the *Journal of Pediatrics*, Vol. 119, No. 3, Ballard et al., Maturational Assessment of Gestational Age (New Ballard Score), pp. 417-423, copyright 19991, with permission from Elsevier.; p. 596, With permission from Elsevier. From Nichols FH, Zwelling E. *Maternal-newborn nursing*. Philadelphia: W.B. Saunders, 1997; p. 597, With permission from Bataglia & Lubchenco, *J Pediatrics*, 1967; p. 598, With permission from Elsevier. From Nichols FH, Zwelling E. *Maternal-newborn nursing*. Philadelphia: W.B. Saunders, 1997.; p. 604, With permission from Elsevier. From Nichols FH, Zwelling E. *Maternal-newborn nursing*. Philadelphia: W.B. Saunders, 1997; p. 605, With permission from Elsevier. From Nichols FH, Zwelling E. *Maternal-newborn nursing*. Philadelphia: W.B. Saunders, 1997; p. 607, With permission from Elsevier. From Nichols FH, Zwelling E. *Maternal-newborn nursing*. Philadelphia: W.B. Saunders, 1997; p. 608, With permission from Elsevier. From Nichols FH, Zwelling E. *Maternal-newborn nursing*. Philadelphia: W.B. Saunders, 1997; p. 609, With permission from Elsevier. From Nichols FH, Zwelling E. *Maternal-newborn nursing*. Philadelphia: W.B. Saunders, 1997; p. 610, With permission from Elsevier. From Nichols FH, Zwelling E. *Maternal-newborn nursing*. Philadelphia: W.B. Saunders, 1997; p. 611, With permission from Elsevier. From Nichols FH, Zwelling E. *Maternal-newborn nursing*.

Philadelphia: W.B. Saunders, 1997; p. 615, (infant behaviors), With permission from Elsevier. From Nichols FH, Zwelling E. *Maternal-newborn nursing*. Philadelphia: W.B. Saunders, 1997; p. 623, Adapted from Short, 1984; p. 626, Derived from Benitez et al., 1992; p. 627, From WHO, 1998; p. 629, From Rivera, 1991; p. 630, From Family Health International, 1988; Kennedy, Rivera, & McNeilly, 1989; p. 641, From WHO; p. 653, Courtesy of Via Christi Health Systems; p. 691, (Visual learning), Courtesy of Shira Bocar; p. 694, Courtesy of Debi Bocar; p. 709, Courtesy of Debi Bocar; p. 715, From Orque, Block, & Monrroy. Ethnic nursing care: a multicultural approach. Mosby, 1983; p. 718, Courtesy of WHO; p. 719, Courtesy of K Sawada; p. 742, From Kendall-Tackett, 1998